Oral and Maxillofacial Surgery

Volume Two

by **W. HARRY ARCHER, B.S., M.A., D.D.S.**

FIFTH EDITION

1975

W. B. SAUNDERS COMPANY

Philadelphia London Toronto

W. B. Saunders Company: West Washington Square
Philadelphia, Pa. 19105

12 Dyott Street
London, WC1A 1DB

833 Oxford Street
Toronto, Ontario M8Z 5T9, Canada

Listed here is the latest translated edition of this
book together with the language of the translation
and the publisher.

Spanish (*4th Edition*), (2 Vols.) — Editorial Mundi S.R.L.,
                                Buenos Aires, Argentina.

German (*3rd Edition*) — Medica Verlag,
                Stuttgart, West Germany.

Japanese (*4th Edition*), (Vol. I, II, & III.) — Kenshin Imada,
                                Tokyo, Japan.

Italian (*4th Edition*), (Vol. I & II.) — Piccin Editore,
                            Padova, Italy.

Chinese — Shanghai, China.

Library of Congress Cataloging in Publication Data

Archer, William Harry.

Oral and maxillofacial surgery.

First and 2d editions published in 1952 and 1956 under title:
A manual of oral surgery. Third and 4th editions published in
1961 and 1966 under title: Oral surgery.

1. Mouth — Surgery.   I. Title. [DNLM: 1. Face — Surgery.
   2. Maxilla — Surgery.   3. Surgery, Oral. WU600 A672m]

RK529.A7 1975   617'.522   73–89931

ISBN 0–7216–1362–4 (v. I)

ISBN 0–7216–1363–2 (v. II)

	Volume I:	ISBN 0-7216-1362-4
Oral and Maxillofacial Surgery	Volume II:	ISBN 0-7216-1363-2

Last digit is the print number: 9   8   7   6   5   4   3   2   1

CHAPTER AUTHORS

RAMIRO ALFARO A., D.D.S., Professor of Oral Surgery, University of San Carlos, Facultad de Odontologia, Guatemala.

Rotation-Advancement Principle for Use in Wide Unilateral Cleft Lips

OSCAR ASENSIO DEL VALLE, D.D.S., Oral Surgeon and Director of Centro Infantil of Estomatologia, Antigua, Guatemala.

Rotation-Advancement Principle for Use in Wide Unilateral Cleft Lips

WILLIAM H. BELL, D.D.S., Associate Professor of Oral Surgery, Department of Surgery, University of Texas Health Science Center—Dallas. Staff, Parkland Memorial Hospital, Children's Medical Center, and Presbyterian Hospital, Dallas. Diplomate, American Board of Oral Surgery.

Orthognathic Surgery

HERBERT J. BLOOM, D.D.S., M.S., PhD., F.A.C.D., Adjunct Professor, Department of Speech and Hearing, and Adjunct Associate Professor, School of Medicine, Wayne State University, Detroit. Formerly Chief and now Consultant, Department of Oral and Maxillofacial Surgery, Sinai Hospital of Detroit. Chairman Emeritus, Department of Oral Surgery, Mount Carmel Mercy Hospital. Staff, United Hospitals of Detroit, Providence Hospital, and St. Joseph Mercy Hospital. Diplomate, American Board of Oral Surgery.

Surgical Repair of Cleft Lip and Palate

PHILIP J. BOYNE, D.M.D., M.S., F.A.C.D., Dean, Dental School, University of Texas Health Science Center—San Antonio. Staff, Department of Surgery, Bexar County Hospital, Santa Rosa Hospital, and Audie Murphy Veterans Administration Hospital. Diplomate, American Board of Oral Surgery.

Transplantation and Grafting Procedures

DONALD DAVIDSON, B.S., D.D.S., M.S., Consultant and Visiting Lecturer, West Virginia University Dental School and Medical Center, Morgantown. Chief of Oral Surgery, Uniontown Hospital, Uniontown, Pa. and Brownsville General Hospital, Brownsville, Pa. Staff, Connellsville State Hospital, Connellsville, Pa. and Mon Valley Hospitals, Charleroi and Monongahela Divisions, Charleroi and Monongahela, Pa. Diplomate, American Board of Oral Surgery.

Diagnosis and Treatment of Pain

CHARLOTTE P. DONLAN, M.D., F.A.C.R., Assistant Clinical Professor of Radiology, George Washington University Medical School, and Radiation Therapist and Consultant, St. Elizabeth's Hospital, Washington, D.C. Consultant in Radiation Therapy for Fairfax Hospital, Northern Virginia Doctors Hospital, and Arlington Hospital, Arlington, Va.

Radiation Therapy

J. CLIFTON ESELMAN, D.D.S., F.A.C.D., Formerly Associate Dean and Professor of Oral Roentgenology, University of Pittsburgh School of Medicine. Consultant in Oral Roentgenology, Veterans Administration Hospital, Pittsburgh, Pa.

Radiographs and Localization

LEWIS E. ETTER, M.D., F.A.C.R., Professor of Radiology, University of Pittsburgh School of Medicine, Falk Clinic, Presbyterian-University Hospital, University of Pittsburgh Medical Center. Consultant in Radiology, Western Psychiatric Institute and Clinic and C. Howard Marcy State Hospital, Pittsburgh, Pa.

Anatomy of Facial Bones and Jaws

JOHN COLLYER GAISFORD, M.D., F.A.C.S., Chief, Division of Surgery and Director, Burn Center, The Western Pennsylvania Hospital, Pittsburgh, Pa.

Oral Malignant Disease

T. CRADOCK HENRY, F.D.S., L.R.C.P., M.R.C.S., Consultant Oral Surgeon, The Hospital for Sick Children, Great Ormond Street, London, and Consultant Oral and Maxillo Facial Surgeon, Royal Surrey County Hospital, Guildford, Surrey, England.

Segmental Surgery

WILLIAM B. IRBY, D.D.S., M.S., F.A.C.D., Professor and Chairman, Department of Oral Surgery, and Assistant Dean for Postdoctoral Affairs, Medical University of South Carolina, College of Dental Medicine, Charleston. Consultant, U.S. Navy Hospital, Charleston, Fort Jackson, Fort Bragg, and Veterans Administration Hospital, Columbia. Staff, Medical University of South Carolina, Charleston County Hospital, and Veterans Administration Hospital, Charleston. Diplomate, American Board of Oral Surgery.

History of Oral Surgery and *Cast or Acrylic Splints*

A. D. MACALISTER, E.D., D.D.S.(N.Z.), F.D.S.R.C.S.(Eng.), F.R.A.C.D.S., Professor and Chairman, Department of Oral Medicine and Oral Surgery, University of Otago Dental School, Dunedin, New Zealand.

The Child Patient

ANDREW E. MICHANOWICZ, B.S., D.D.S., F.I.C.D., Associate Professor and Chairman of Graduate Endodontics, University of Pittsburgh School of Dental Medicine. Consultant in Endodontics, Children's Hospital, Pittsburgh. Staff, Montefiore Hospital, Pittsburgh, Pa.

Surgical Endodontics

MARVIN E. PIZER, D.D.S., M.S., F.I.C.D., Chief of Oral Surgery, Alexandria Hospital, Alexandria, Va. Consultant, National Orthopedic and

Rehabilitation Hospital, Arlington, Va. Courtesy Staff, Circle Terrace Hospital and Northern Virginia Doctors Hospital, Arlington, Va. Diplomate, American Board of Oral Surgery.

Diagnosis and Management of Oral Malignant Disease

H. B. G. ROBINSON, D.D.S., M.S., D.Sc.(Hon.), Dean Emeritus and Professor Emeritus of Oral Pathology and Diagnosis, School of Dentistry, University of Missouri – Kansas City.

Cysts of the Oral Cavity

MARSH ROBINSON, D.D.S., M.D., F.A.C.D., F.A.C.S., Professor and Chairman of Oral Surgery, School of Dentistry, University of Southern California, Santa Monica. Diplomate, American Board of Oral Surgery.

Orthognathic Surgery

VIKEN SASSOUNI, D.D.S., D.Sc., Professor of Orthodontics, University of Pittsburgh School of Dentistry. Chief Orthodontist, Children's Hospital and Western Pennsylvania Hospital, Pittsburgh, Pa.

Dentofacial Orthopedics

SIDNEY S. SPATZ, D.D.S., F.A.C.D., F.I.C.D., Professor and Chairman, Department of Oral Surgery, University of Pittsburgh School of Dental Medicine. Chief of Dentistry and Oral Surgery, Montefiore Hospital, Pittsburgh. Chief of Oral Surgery, Eye and Ear Hospital, Magee-Women's Hospital, Children's Hospital, and Central Medical Pavilion, Pittsburgh. Consultant, Veterans Administration Hospitals of Pittsburgh, Pa. Diplomate, American Board of Oral Surgery.

Antibiotic Therapy

CONRAD J. SPILKA, D.D.S., F.I.A.O.S., F.A.C.D., F.I.C.D., Clinical Professor of Oral Surgery and Anesthesia, Case Western Reserve University, Cleveland, Ohio. Chief, Department of Oral Surgery, Fairview General Hospital and Lutheran Medical Center, Cleveland, Ohio. Diplomate, American Board of Oral Surgery.

Orthognathic Surgery

IRVIN V. UHLER, D.D.S., F.A.C.D., F.I.C.D., Chief of Oral Surgery, Lancaster General Hospital, and Oral Surgeon, Lancaster Cleft Palate Clinic, Lancaster, Pa. Diplomate, American Board of Oral Surgery.

The Geriatric Patient

W. J. UPDEGRAVE, D.D.S., Professor Emeritus and Former Chairman, Department of Dental Radiology, Temple University School of Dentistry, Philadelphia, Pa.

Radiographs and Localization

YOSHIO WATANABE, D.D.S., M.D., D.Med.Sc., F.A.C.D., M.I.A.C., Director of Clinics and Professor and Chairman, Department of Oral Surgery, Tsurumi University School of Dentistry, Yokohama City, Japan.

Surgical Correction of Ankylosis of the Temporomandibular Joint

G. WREAKES, B.Ch.D., F.D.S., DIP.Orth., Consultant Orthodontist to the

Westminster Group of Hospitals and South West Thames Health Authority, Guildford, Surrey, England.

Segmental Surgery

HAROLD J. ZUBROW, A.B., D.D.S., F.A.C.D., Associate Professor of Oral Surgery, University of Pittsburgh School of Dental Medicine. Staff, Department of Oral Surgery, Montefiore Hospital, Eye and Ear Hospital, Magee-Women's Hospital, and Central Medical Pavilion, Pittsburgh, Pa.

Antibiotic Therapy

CONTRIBUTORS

JOSEPH ANDREWS, D.D.S., Departments of Oral Diagnosis and Oral Surgery, University of Pittsburgh School of Dental Medicine.

ABDEL K. EL-ATTAR, D.M.D., Assistant Professor, Department of Oral Surgery, University of Pittsburgh School of Dental Medicine.

STANLEY J. BEHRMAN, D.M.D., Clinical Assistant Professor of Surgery, Cornell University Medical College. Attending Oral Surgeon, The New York Hospital.

CARL J. BENDER, D.D.S., Formerly Senior Staff Dentist, Veterans Administration Hospital, Pittsburgh, Pa.

C. RICHARD BENNETT, D.D.S., Ph.D., Associate Professor and Chairman, Department of Anesthesia, University of Pittsburgh School of Dental Medicine.

JOSEPH L. BERNIER, D.D.S., M.S., Professor and Chairman, Department of Oral Pathology, Georgetown University School of Dentistry, Washington, D.C.

THOMAS C. BITHELL, M.D., Associate Professor of Internal Medicine, University of Virginia School of Medicine, Charlottesville.

HARRY BLECHMAN, D.D.S., Dean, College of Dentistry, New York University, New York, N.Y.

GERALD H. BONNETTE, D.D.S., School of Dentistry, University of Michigan, Ann Arbor.

JAMES L. BRADLEY, D.D.S., M.S.D., M.Sc., Oral Surgeon, St. John's Hospital, Memorial Hospital, and Passavant Hospital, Springfield, Ill.

PAUL M. BURBANK, D.M.D., M.S., Attending Oral Surgeon, Genesee Hospital and Highland Hospital, Rochester, N.Y.

D. LAMAR BYRD, D.D.S., M.S.D., Professor and Chairman, Department of Oral Surgery, Baylor College of Dentistry, Baylor University Medical Center, Dallas, Texas.

LESTER R. CAHN, D.D.S., President, New York Institute of Clinical Oral Pathology, New York, N.Y.

NOAH R. CALHOUN, D.D.S., M.S.D., Professor, Oral Surgery, Howard University. Professorial Lecturer, Georgetown University. Director of Oral Surgery Training, Veterans Administration Hospital, Washington, D.C.

RALPH J. CAPAROSA, M.D., Formerly Clinical Assistant Professor of Otolaryngology, University of Pittsburgh School of Medicine.

RICARDO CUESTAS CARNERO, M.D., Assistant Professor, Department of Oral Surgery, Part 2, Cordoba National University, Cordoba, Argentina.

A. P. CHAUDHRY, B.D.S., Ph.D., Professor of Oral Pathology, State University of New York at Buffalo School of Medicine.

LLOYD E. CHURCH, D.D.S., M.S., Ph.D., Assistant Professor of Anatomy, George Washington University School of Medicine, Washington, D.C.

LEON J. COLLINS, JR., M.D., Associate in Medicine, School of Medicine; Assistant Professor of Medicine, School of Dental Medicine, University of Pennsylvania, Philadelphia.

MARTIN P. CRANE, M.D., Quondam Chief Physician, The Misericordia Hospital and The Nazareth Hospital, Philadelphia, Pa.

THEODORE H. DEDOLPH, D.D.S., M.S.D., F.A.C.D., Staff, St. Cloud Hospital, and Veterans Administration Hospital, Minnesota.

EDWARD J. DEGNAN, D.D.S., Staff Oral Surgeon, Veterans Administration Hospital, Bay Pines, Fla.

B. F. DEWEL, D.D.S., Orthodontist, Evanston, Ill. Editor, American Journal of Orthodontics.

REED O. DINGMAN, D.D.S., M.D., Professor and Head, Section of Plastic Surgery, University of Michigan Medical School, Ann Arbor.

E. LLOYD DUBRUL, D.D.S., M.S., Ph.D., Professor and Head, Department of Oral Anatomy, University of Illinois College of Dentistry, Chicago.

EUGENE R. ELSTROM, R.T., Chief X-Ray Technician, Illinois Eye and Ear Infirmary, Chicago.

SALVATORE J. ESPOSITO, A.B., D.D.S., Chief of Dental Service, Veterans Administration Hospital, Boston, Mass.

WILLIAM EVANS, D.D.S., M.S., Instructor, Ohio State University College of Dentistry (Oral Surgery). Chairman, Oral Surgery Department, St. Anthony Hospital. Chairman, Maxillofacial Department, Grant Hospital of Columbus. Oral Surgeon, University Hospital, Children's Hospital, St. Anthony Hospital, and Grant Hospital of Columbus.

VICTOR H. FRANK, D.D.S., Emeritus Attending Chief of Oral Surgery Department, Albert Einstein Medical Center. Emeritus Staff, Graduate Hospital, University of Pennsylvania, Philadelphia.

EDUARD G. FRIEDRICH, D.D.S., Formerly Professor of Oral Surgery, Northwestern University Dental School, Chicago, Ill.

GEORGE E. FULLER, JR., D.D.S., Professor and Chairman, Department of Oral Surgery, Emory University School of Dentistry, Atlanta, Ga.

ITALO H. A. GANDELMAN, D.D.S., Associate Professor of Oral Surgery, Faculdade de Odontologia da U. F. R. J., Rio de Janeiro, G. B. Brazil.

ROBERT J. GORLIN, D.D.S., M.S., Professor and Chairman, Department of Oral Pathology, University of Minnesota, Minneapolis.

JAMES GUGGENHEIMER, D.D.S., Departments of Oral Diagnosis and Oral Surgery, University of Pittsburgh School of Dental Medicine.

ROGER A. HARVEY, M.D., Head, Department of Radiology, University of Illinois College of Medicine, Chicago.

FREDERICK A. HENNY, D.D.S., Formerly Chief, Division of Dentistry and Oral Surgery, Henry Ford Hospital, Detroit, Mich.

MATTHEW J. HERTZ, D.D.S., Assistant Attendant in Prosthetics, Bronx-Lebanon Hospital, New York, N.Y.

DANIEL J. HOLLAND, D.M.D., Formerly Professor of Oral Surgery, Tufts University School of Dental Medicine, Boston, Mass.

PETER J. JANNETTA, M.D., Professor and Chairman, Department of Neurosurgery, University of Pittsburgh School of Medicine.

JOSEPH H. JOHNSON, D.D.S., Late Emeritus Professor of Oral Surgery, Faculty of Dentistry, University of Toronto.

SHREE C. JOSHI, M.S., D.O.M.S., Scientific Officer, Medical Division, Bhabha Atomic Research Center, Trombay, Bombay-85.

SAMUEL I. KAPLAN, D.D.S., Chief Oral Surgeon, Mount Sinai Hospital, Hartford, Conn.

V. H. KAZANJIAN, C.M.J., D.M.D., M.D., Formerly Professor of Plastic Surgery, Harvard University, Boston, Mass.

P. L. KHURANA, L.R.C.P.(Edin.), L.R.C.S.(Edin.), L.D.S., R.C.S.(Edin.), F.I.C.D.(U.S.A.), F.I.O.A.S., Hon. Professor, Maulana Azad Medical College. Hon. Dental Surgeon, Irwin Hospital, N. Rly. Central Hospital, Shroff's Charity Eye Hospital, Jawahar Lal Nehru Institute of Physical Medicine and Rehabilitation. Hon. Dental Surgeon to the President of India.

STUART N. KLINE, D.D.S., Associate Professor, Department of Surgery, Division of Oral Surgery, University of Miami School of Medicine. Chief, Oral Surgery Section, Miami Veterans Administration Hospital and Jackson Memorial Hospital, Miami, Fla.

W. B. KOUWENHOVEN, M.E., M.D.(Hon.), Johns Hopkins University School of Medicine; D.Sc.(Hon.), Syracuse University; Doktor Ingenieur, Karls Ruhe Technische Hochschule, Baden, Germany.

BRUNO W. KWAPIS, D.D.S., M.S., Professor and Chairman of Oral Surgery, Southern Illinois University School of Dental Medicine, Edwardsville.

DANIEL M. LASKIN, D.D.S., M.S., Professor and Head, Department of Oral and Maxillofacial Surgery, University of Illinois College of Dentistry, Chicago.

FRANCIS M. S. LEE, D.D.S., Professor and Head, Department of Oral Surgery and Oral Medicine, Faculty of Dentistry, University of Singapore.

T. A. LESNEY, D.C., U.S.N., Formerly Consultant-Instructor to Dental Training Programs, U.S. Naval Hospital, Portsmouth, Va.

JACK E. McCALLUM, M.D., Department of Neurological Surgery, University of Pittsburgh School of Medicine.

CHARLES F. McCANN, A.B., D.M.D., Chief of Oral Surgery Section, Veterans Administration Hospital, Boston, Mass.

FRANK M. McCARTHY, D.D.S., M.D., Professor and Chairman, Department of Anesthesiology, University of Southern California Dental School, Los Angeles.

A. E. McDONALD, D.D.S., Associate Professor, Department of Oral Surgery, University of Pittsburgh School of Dental Medicine.

STEPHEN B. MALLETT, D.M.D., Consultant in Oral Surgery, Veterans Administration Hospital, Boston, Mass.

MARIA JULIANA MALMSTROM, Dr. Odont., Instructor, Department of Oral Surgery, Institute of Dentistry, University of Helsinki, Finland.

LEO D. C. MARCH, L.D.S., R.C.S.(Eng.), F.I.O.A.S., F.A.C.D., Consultant and Associate Lecturer in Oral Surgery, University of the West Indies, Kingston, Jamaica. Chief of Oral Surgery Division, Kingston General Hospital, Jamaica.

IRVING MEYER, D.M.D., M.Sc., D.Sc., Research Professor of Oral Pathology, Tufts University School of Dental Medicine; Lecturer on Oral Pathology, Harvard University School of Dental Medicine, Boston, Mass.

SANFORD M. MOOSE, D.D.S., Clinical Professor of Oral Surgery, School of Dentistry, College of Physicians and Surgeons, University of the Pacific, Stockton, Calif.

JOE HALL MORRIS, D.D.S., Professor and Chairman, Department of Oral Surgery, University of Tennessee College of Dentistry, Memphis.

ROBERT L. MOSS, D.D.S., Chief, Oral Surgery Section, Veterans Administration Hospital, Phoenix, Ariz.

NORMAN R. NATHANSON, D.D.S., Chief of Oral Surgery, Framingham Union Hospital, Framingham, Mass.

PAUL NATVIG, D.D.S., M.D., Assistant Clinical Professor of Plastic and Reconstructive Surgery, Marquette University School of Medicine, Milwaukee, Wisc.

K. ODENHEIMER, D.D.S., Ph.D., Professor of Pathology (Oral), Louisiana State University School of Dentistry, New Orleans.

VALLE J. OIKARINEN, M.D., D.D.S., Department of Oral Surgery, Institute of Dentistry, University of Helsinki, Finland.

THEODORE R. PALADINO, D.D.S., Assistant Professor, Department of Oral Surgery, University of Pittsburgh School of Dental Medicine.

HAROLD J. PANUSKA, D.D.S., M.S.D., Staff, Department of Oral Surgery, Fairview Hospital, Methodist Hospital, and Memorial Hospital, Minneapolis, Minn.

JACK L. PECHERSKY, D.M.D., Assistant Professor of Pedodontics, University of Pittsburgh School of Dental Medicine.

OTTO C. PHILLIPS, M.D., Clinical Professor of Anesthesiology, University of Pittsburgh School of Medicine. Chief, Division of Anesthesiology, Western Pennsylvania Hospital, Pittsburgh.

ROBIN M. RANKOW, D.D.S., M.D., Assistant Clinical Professor of Anatomy, College of Physicians and Surgeons, Columbia University, New York, N.Y.

GUILLERMO RASPALL, D.D.S., M.D., Chairman, Department of Oral and Maxillofacial Surgery, Hospital de la Cruz Roja, Barcelona, Spain.

H. SERRANO ROA, D.D.S., Chief of Estomatology, Roosevelt Hospital, Guatemala.

SHELDON ROVIN, D.D.S., M.S., Dean, School of Dentistry, University of Washington, Seattle.

NORMAN L. ROWE, F.D.S.R.C.S., L.R.C.P., M.R.C.S., L.M.S.S.A., H.D.D.R.C.S., Consultant, Oral Surgery Department, The Westminster Hospital and The Institute of Dental Surgery, London.

H. CLAYTON SATO, D.D.S., M.D., Assistant Professor and Head of Dentistry and Oral Surgery, The Tokyo Jikeikai University School of Medicine.

WILLIAM G. SHAFER, B.S., D.D.S., M.S., Distinguished Professor and Chairman, Department of Oral Pathology, Indiana University-Purdue University School of Dentistry, Indianapolis.

ROBERT B. SHIRA, D.D.S., Dean, Tufts University School of Dental Medicine, Boston, Mass.

HARRY SICHER, M.D., D.Sc., Late Emeritus Professor of Anatomy and Histology, Loyola University School of Dentistry, Chicago, Ill.

N. P. J. B. SIEVERINK, D.D.S., Professor of Oral Surgery, Catholic University Dental School. Staff, Department of Oral Surgery, St. Radboud Hospital, Catholic University, Nijmegen, Holland.

N. H. SMITH, M.D.S., Senior Lecturer, Department of Oral Medicine and Oral Surgery, Faculty of Dentistry, The University of Sydney, Australia.

LAKANA SRIVIROJANA, D.D.S., Assistant Professor, Department of Oral Surgery, School of Dentistry (Pratum Wan), Mahidol University, Bangkok, Thailand.

EDWARD C. STAFNE, D.D.S., Emeritus Chief of Dental Radiography, Mayo Clinic, Rochester, Minn.

CHARLES W. SUMMERS, D.D.S., Oral Surgeon, U.S. Army. Formerly Chief of Oral Surgery and Professional Training, U.S. Army Hospital, Ft. Carson, Colo.

CHEVKET O. TAGAY, Late Professor and Director, Maxillo-Dental Surgery Clinic, Dental Faculty of the University of Istanbul, Turkey.

RICHARD W. TIECKE, B.S., D.D.S., M.S., Professor, Department of Oral Pathology, University of Illinois, Chicago.

RICHARD G. TOPAZIAN, D.D.S., Professor and Head, Department of Oral and Maxillofacial Surgery, School of Dental Medicine, University of Connecticut Health Center, Farmington.

PORUS S. TURNER, M.D.S., Scientific Officer, Dental Services, Bhabha Atomic Research Centre, Trombay, Bombay-85.

CHARLES A. WALDRON, D.D.S., M.S.D., Professor of Oral Pathology, School of Dentistry, Emory University, Atlanta, Ga.

ROBERT V. WALKER, D.D.S., Professor and Chairman, Division of Oral Surgery, The University of Texas Southwestern Medical School at Dallas.

KJELL WALLENIUS, M.D., L.D.S., Professor and Head, Department of Oral Surgery, University of Lund School of Dentistry, Malmo, Sweden.

JERROLD I. WASSERMAN, D.D.S., Assistant Adjunct in Periodontics, Bronx-Lebanon Hospital, New York, N.Y.

SAM WEINSTEIN, D.D.S., Formerly Chairman, Department of Orthodontics, University of Nebraska. Now Professor, Orthodontics Department, University of Connecticut Health Center, Hartford.

MAXWELL M. WINTROBE, B.A., M.D., B.Sc.(Med.), PhD., Professor of Internal Medicine, University of Utah College of Medicine, Salt Lake City.

CONTENTS

Volume II

CHAPTER 18

FRACTURES OF THE FACIAL BONES
AND THEIR TREATMENT

FIRST AID FOR JAW CASUALTIES

The four most important measures in emergency treatment of injuries of the face and jaws are: (1) control of hemorrhage; (2) clearance and maintenance of airway for respiration; (3) control of shock; (4) stabilization of parts.

CONTROL OF HEMORRHAGE

In order to save life, a rather rapid and hurried examination should be made, the examiner remembering that casualties frequently have multiple wounds and that hemorrhage must be brought under control promptly. Arterial hemorrhage being the most serious, it should be arrested at once by digital pressure, if possible, until more effective means can be applied. In the extremities, bleeding from dangerous wounds can be brought under control by the use of a tourniquet, but wounds of the face and neck require other procedures.

One must be familiar with the most effective points for the application of pressure to control hemorrhage of the head and neck. With gauze and bandages, pressure can be applied over these areas and bleeding controlled until a clamp or ligature is applied to the injured vessel. Hemorrhage from the external carotid artery and its branches may be temporarily controlled by digital pressure applied along the anterior margin of the sternocleidomastoid muscle at the hyoid bone.

The pulsation should be located and sufficient pressure applied inwardly and slightly posteriorly to compress the lumen of the vessel, thereby minimizing the loss of blood until terminal bleeders can be controlled. Hemorrhage from any branch of the external maxillary artery can be reduced by compressing the vessel where it crosses the lower border of the mandible in the facial notch just anterior to the angle. The most effective point at which to compress the superficial temporal artery is where this artery crosses the zygomatic process of the temporal bone just anterior to the ear. The lingual artery can be compressed to some extent by deep pressure under the angle of the mandible or, in severe cases, by compression of the external carotid artery. Pulling the tongue forward over the teeth may be effective and, in cases of loss of a portion of the mandible, the dorsum of the tongue can be compressed between the thumb and fingers. Hemorrhage from soft tissues should be cared for with sutures when possible, and excessive bleeding from the bone can be controlled by tissue or gauze held over the part under moderate tension (suture tension if available, digital tension in a grave emergency). It may be necessary to pack gauze into the wounds to check inaccessible bleeders, either suturing it into place or bandaging it in position under pressure. The prime object is to conserve the individual's blood supply, prevent shock, and better prepare these serious cases for transportation to the hospital, where more exacting measures can be instituted to save life.

MAINTENANCE OF AIRWAY FOR RESPIRATION

Severe injuries of the face and jaws frequently interfere with respiration. Establishing a patent airway should be the first consideration of treatment. Fragments of bone, fractured teeth, fillings, broken dentures, particles of clothing and other foreign material as well as soft tissue and blood often drop into the posterior part of the mouth and throat. All too frequently these foreign bodies are aspirated. The patient is confused, fearful, choking, or unconscious and his reflexes and reactions are dangerously disturbed. Obstructions must be removed immediately, and the fractured bones or disorganized tissues should be adjusted so as to assure an adequate airway. After all foreign bodies have been removed from the mouth, and the tongue has been pulled forward and held in this position, attention should be given to the immediate control of bone fragments and soft tissues which may drop back into the throat. Fractured superior maxillary bones must be adjusted anteriorly to avoid blocking the nasal and oral airway by posterior displacement. Gauze pads which are properly placed between the posterior teeth may give temporary support; however, extraoral anterior traction may be necessary to accomplish a satisfactory result.

As mentioned, the tongue falling backward because of loss of its attachments to the mandible will block the airway. A suture placed through the tip of the tongue may be necessary to control this factor. The ligature can be controlled by the patient or fastened to clothing or to a facial dressing for extraoral traction.

The transportation of a patient with a wound of the face or jaws is a very serious problem. Many patients have been placed in an ambulance while still alive but have died before arriving at the hospital as a result of respiratory failure caused by an unfavorable position. When possible, patients with face and jaw injuries should not be transported lying down. Their respiration is less restricted in a sitting position. If they must be taken in an ambulance or on a stretcher in a reclining position, they should not be on their backs, since this position favors the collapse of tissues into the pharynx. The patients should be placed downward, in a prone position, or well over on one side. This will help keep the air passages free and will allow mucus and blood which collect in the throat to be expelled.

Tracheostomy (Tracheotomy): Indications and Emergency Technique

The purpose of a tracheostomy is to prevent asphyxia by making an opening in the trachea to insure that air flow is not blocked by an obstruction in the pharynx or larynx.

In patients with an irremovable inhaled foreign body, acute edema of the larynx, wounds and trauma of the larynx itself, and compound comminuted fractures of one or more of the facial bones, e.g., maxilla, mandible, zygomas and nasal bones, which block the airway, an immediate tracheostomy is indicated.

The symptoms and signs of obstructive laryngeal dyspnea that call for a tracheostomy are restlessness, anxious facies, ashy cyanosis, rapid, shallow breathing, and indrawing of the soft tissue of the suprasternal notch, supraclavicular fossae, intercostal spaces and epigastrium. In very young children, indrawing of the sternum may be present.

Jackson and Jackson[87] stressed the indrawing at the suprasternal notch as the most important diagnostic sign of obstructive laryngeal dyspnea. This sign is not present in other types of dyspnea. In such cases not a moment should be lost in giving the patient relief, as death may rapidly follow.

One may be called upon to perform the emergency tracheostomy at the site of the accident or on the floor with a pen knife or with whatever sharp instrument happens to be at hand, without regard to asepsis. This operation consists essentially in cutting down on the trachea without regard to hemorrhage, and, with the finger in a pool of blood, incising the trachea and introducing the tracheotomy tube, if available—if not, some makeshift tube is introduced—and then arresting the hemorrhage.

When an "elective" tracheostomy can be performed, this is the treatment of choice.

In emergency admissions of patients with severe facial fractures and with respiratory embarrassment, if the tracheostomy cannot be accomplished under local anesthesia, it is wise to consider the insertion of an endotracheal tube in the conscious patient. First spray the throat with 4 per cent Xylocaine solution and then proceed with inhalation anesthesia using nitrous oxide and oxygen and one of the halogenated agents. Barbiturates are not administered intravenously because of the accentuation of a possible shock status and its alteration of blood volume.

For detailed information on the emergency tracheostomy, see Figures 25–8 to 25–10 and study pages 1549 to 1554 in Chapter 25. The use of the emergency cricothyrotomy trocar tube is also described there.

CONTROL OF SHOCK

Shock in facial injuries is uncommon except when it is secondary to severe hemorrhage or is associated with a concomitant injury. Whenever it is present, shock must be treated immediately and adequately. The reader is referred to pages 1541 and 1542 in Chapter 25 for a discussion of this vital subject.

STABILIZATION OF PARTS

Once temporary control of the first three dangerous problems in order to maintain the patient's life has been secured, consideration can be given to stabilization of the bone fragments and displaced soft tissues. Conservation of tissue is of utmost importance. Bone fragments that have any possible periosteal attachment should be preserved because they may live and form a nucleus for new bone growth. They can form a bridge across the gap in the bone and help to form new bone, whereas if everything is removed, there will be a gap that cannot be filled by nature and that will require months of bone grafting and hospitalization so that the space can be filled surgically. Likewise, all the mucous membrane and skin that can be saved is extremely useful to suture over torn ends after thorough debridement. Whatever fixation can be accomplished as a first aid measure is important and helpful in order to prevent recurrence of hemorrhage and to maintain a free airway. This stabilization of parts is also of extreme importance to the patient in reduction of pain and discomfort.

Pain. The patient's pain may require the administration of analgesic drugs. If respiratory difficulty is present, morphine should not be used. Analgesics other than acetylsalicylic acid are contraindicated if facial trauma is associated with central nervous system injury. Partial immobilization and support with an appropriate head bandage may help to relieve pain.

The first several critical hours through which the patient must pass are greatly influenced by the first aid treatment he receives. Application of these four major emergency measures is of the utmost importance.

ASSESSMENT OF THE PATIENT WITH HEAD INJURY

PETER J. JANNETTA, M.D.,
AND JACK E. McCALLUM, M.D.

The oral surgeon is the dental specialist most likely to be involved in the care of the head-injured patient. He must constantly be aware that the forces which cause facial injuries are the same as those which cause injuries to the brain and cervical spinal cord. Any patient with facial trauma must be examined for concomitant head and neck trauma. Mechanisms of head, neck and facial injury include blunt trauma, penetrating trauma and pendular motion of the head and neck, with or without associated blows to the head and face.

Blunt trauma may be associated with varying degrees of facial or soft-tissue injury, but these are not reliable indicators of the extent of underlying brain injury. The external appearance of penetrating wounds and the presence of skull fracture often belie the severity of related central nervous system damage.

It is, therefore, necessary to search for other indicators of the presence and severity of intracranial and intraspinal trauma. The methods for collecting this information differ little from those used to assess any acutely ill patient. The history and physical examination are of primary importance, and these are supplemented by various laboratory, radiographic and special diagnostic studies.

It is of supreme importance that a baseline be established with an accurate initial assessment of neurologic function. Then, subsequent change can be recorded and acted upon. Without such a baseline, the patient's neurologic status can deteriorate insidiously, putting him at great risk before proper therapy is started.

HISTORY

The history of a head injury is based on questions common to any medical evaluation. The age and handedness of the patient are most helpful, if such knowledge is available. The exact mechanism, timing and circumstances of the injury should be established as accurately as possible. These data are augmented by specific questions dealing with central nervous system function and integrity.

The age of the patient is the background against which future diagnostic, therapeutic and prognostic decisions are made. The type and severity of head injuries vary greatly with age. Approximately 75 per cent of head injuries in preschool-age children are due to falls, with most of the rest due to automobile accidents. In school-age children, falls account for only 39 per cent of the injuries, with automobile accidents, bicycle accidents and sports accidents accounting for the rest, in about equal proportion.[101] In adults, automobiles become a primary cause of head injury, accounting for approximately two thirds of the total.[196] With advancing age, falls again become prominent. Age also plays a major part in prognosis. In general, younger patients can recover from more severe head injuries than can older patients.

A second general question concerns the circumstances of the injury. The mechanism of injury is important in determining (a) the type of head injury; (b) the extent of head injury; and (c) the likelihood and type of associated injuries. Automobile accidents are the most common cause of major trauma in the United States, and 60 to 70 per cent of all automobile injuries involve central nervous system (CNS) trauma.[196] Severe automobile accidents are particularly likely to involve structures of the central nervous system. Seventy per cent of all automobile fatalities involve severe injuries to the brain or spinal cord.[196] This type of injury is usually associated with multiple trauma. Approximately 75 per cent of automobile injuries involve two or more systems.[71] Therefore, the patient involved in an automobile accident is likely to have a head injury, it is frequently severe, and it is usually associated with multiple-system trauma.

Falls, the next most common type of injury, are largely problems of the very old and the very young. Other common mechanisms of head injury are sports injuries, industrial accidents and civilian gunshot wounds.

Special features of the history of a head injury include loss of consciousness, amnesia, the occurrence of convulsions, nausea, vomiting, dizziness and headache.

The history of decreasing level of consciousness is perhaps the most useful information to be gained about a head-injured adult. Loss of consciousness in head trauma implies dysfunction of the brain-stem reticular formation. This may occur immediately from a concussive blow or at a later time from brain-stem compression due to an expanding intracranial mass lesion. Thus, the immediate loss of consciousness after head trauma implies that a sufficient force has been applied to the head to cause the brain stem to malfunction. It is generally accepted that the longer the period of unconsciousness, the greater the force applied must have been.

An indicator as useful as loss of consciousness is progression of consciousness. Immediate loss of consciousness followed by return to normal or near normal has already been identified as evidence of significant force applied to the brain. Besides the immediate, primary effect on the brain stem, such force may lead to delayed formation of a mass lesion. Progression of consciousness may follow one of three courses. Immediate loss of consciousness with rapid complete recovery, characteristic of cerebral concussion, has been described. Immediate and prolonged coma is the opposite extreme and may signify direct brain-stem injury, diffuse cerebral injury, rapid development of an intracranial mass lesion or any combination of these. The patient with a concussion should be observed. The immediately comatose patient must be observed, and he should have special diagnostic studies if his state of consciousness improves after resuscitative measures or rapid administration of intravenous osmotic agents or both. Finally, there are those patients who have an initial loss of consciousness and recover partly, or who are merely dazed and proceed to increasing irritability, drowsiness and lethargy. This type of patient has two problems. Concussion is the first process and is, of itself, benign. Subsequent deterioration may be evidence of an expanding mass lesion causing brain-stem compression. A declining level of consciousness at any point in the course of a head-injured patient should suggest expanding mass and should force the clinician to consultation and further studies. Children, especially those under 1 year of age, can sustain much greater trauma to the head without immediate loss of consciousness than can adults. Declining level of consciousness in the child thus assumes a much greater significance, because early loss of consciousness as an indicator of the severity of injury has been lost.

Retrograde and anterograde types of amnesia are closely related to duration of unconsciousness, both physiologically and prognostically. Approximately 80 per cent of patients with post-traumatic unconsciousness will have retrograde amnesia for a period preceding their injury.

Mild headache is a common symptom of head injury. It is said that the severity and duration of headache are unrelated to the severity of the head injury. Yet, in our experience, severe headache in the acutely head-injured patient is a cause of serious worry to the attending physician. A developing, acute epidural hematoma may cause severe headache, as may a fracture involving the foramen magnum. Vomiting is ubiquitous in minor head injuries. Eighty-five per cent of children from ages 2 to 12 with head injuries experience vomiting as do approximately 20 per cent of adults. Vomiting is, however, unusual in severely head-injured patients.

PHYSICAL EXAMINATION

The tendency to concentrate on the most obvious injury in a multiply injured patient is universal and may be disastrous. A thorough general physical examination can be carried out in a short period of time while emergency procedures are being undertaken, but it must be done systematically, and the neurologic examination should be performed last in the head-injured patient.

Vital Signs. Respiration is of first priority in the care of the traumatized patient. The examiner must be aware of potential obstruction at the upper airway, which is common in the head-injured patient. Intraoral bleeding in an unconscious patient may lead to fatal aspiration. Extensive facial fractures or lacerations can lead to edema and obstruction at the pharynx. Expanding hematoma in the neck may cause tracheal obstruction.

Lower airway obstruction may take a variety of forms. The most obvious are open chest injury and flail chest. Both require stabilization prior to the undertaking of any further diagnostic or therapeutic measures. Pneumothorax should be sought and treated. The mere presence of fractured ribs when positive pressure ventilation is contemplated indicates the use of a chest tube as prophylaxis against the development of pneumothorax.

Pulmonary parenchymal problems common in the traumatized patient include aspiration, pulmonary contusions and, especially, pulmonary edema.

Brief apnea following a concussion is the rule, but it is transient and is seldom observed by any but those immediately present at the time of injury. Cheyne-Stokes respirations are characteristic of diffuse bilateral hemispheric disease and are occasionally seen after head injury. Central neurogenic hyperventilation suggests a lesion of the midbrain tegmentum and is a sustained, rhythmic pattern similar to Kussmaul's respirations. Apneusis is a rhythmic breathing pattern characterized by apneic periods in inspiration and is seen with lesions of the mid and caudal basis pons. Ataxic respirations are nonrhythmic, are disorganized and suggest impending failure of the medullary respiratory center. The failure of respiratory movements of the intercostal muscles suggests a cervical cord injury. Each of these patterns suggests a serious and probably life-threatening injury to the central nervous system.

Hypotension and tachycardia are characteristic of hypovolemia and are seldom, if ever, directly attributable to head injury. This pattern compels the clinician to find the source of blood loss. There are two exceptions to this generalization. Infants may lose a significant portion of their blood volume intracranially, or from a scalp laceration. Adults and older children generally do not. Tachycardia and hypertension going on to hypotension may occur in the terminal stages of transtentorial herniation, but they are then associated with the other abnormalities of that syndrome.

Sequentially increasing hypertension and bradycardia are the classic findings associated with increased intracranial pressure. They may be absent, be transiently present or progress as the level of unconsciousness declines in a patient with an expanding lesion. These abnormalities are much less likely to occur with a supratentorial mass lesion than with a posterior fossa mass, but their presence compels immediate medical or surgical efforts to lower intracranial pressure. Because they are late signs of impending brainstem failure, they are unreliable criteria of deterioration in most patients.

Systemic Review. SKIN. Examination of the skin may furnish clues to sites of injury, adequacy of oxygenation, blood loss and traumatic epiphenomena such as petechiae about the neck, axillae and upper chest, which are useful in diagnosing fat emboli.

HEAD AND NECK. Examination of the head may reveal lacerations and abrasions and may suggest underlying depressed or penetrating head wounds. With the exception of threat to the airway, orofacial injuries assume secondary or tertiary priority in the immediate management of traumatized patients.

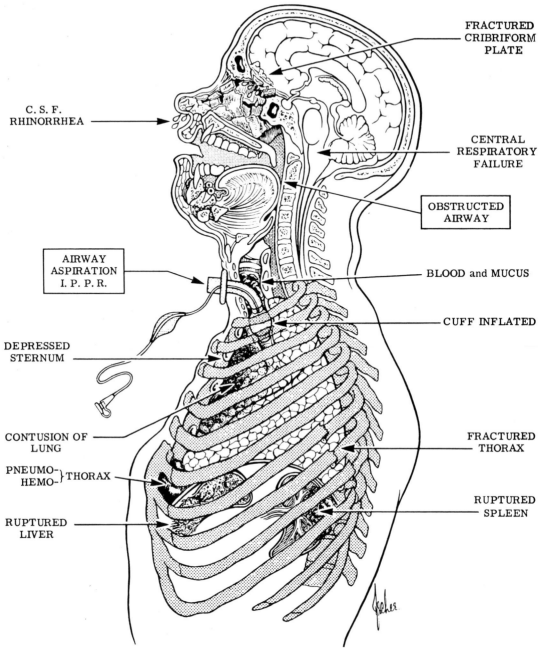

FRACTURED CRIBRIFORM PLATE

C. S. F. RHINORRHEA

CENTRAL RESPIRATORY FAILURE

OBSTRUCTED AIRWAY

AIRWAY ASPIRATION I. P. P. R.

BLOOD and MUCUS

CUFF INFLATED

DEPRESSED STERNUM

CONTUSION OF LUNG

FRACTURED THORAX

PNEUMO-HEMO-}THORAX

RUPTURED SPLEEN

RUPTURED LIVER

Figure 18–1 Some of the clinical and pathologic features that may be observed following a severe traffic accident. In rare instances the diaphragm may be ruptured and the viscera forced upward into the thorax. In the box *Airway* refers to the necessity of maintaining the airway. *Aspiration* emphasizes the importance of keeping all tracheostomy tubes sucked out at all times. *I. P. P. R.* relates to *intermittent positive pressure respiration,* or, in effect, the coupling of the patient's tracheostomy tube to a mechanical respirator delivering oxygenated air under positive pressure—a necessary requirement when the respiratory center in the brain stem is damaged, or the thoracic cage is ineffective because of multiple rib fractures around the costosternal junction, creating the so-called "floating sternum." (From Rowe, N. L., and Killey, H. C.: Fractures of the Facial Skeleton, Edinburgh, Churchill Livingstone, 1968.)

Neck injuries, on the other hand, may be of critical importance. They may be divided into injuries threatening the airway (which have already been dealt with), vascular injuries, injuries to the cervical spinal cord and other soft-tissue injuries.

The neck should be examined for contusions suggestive of local trauma. If there is, at any time, a question of cervical cord trauma, one should log-roll the patient to the supine position, place sand bags on either side of his head, and tape his forehead to a stretcher in a neutral position until lateral cervical spine films can either confirm or deny the suspicion. The index of suspicion of cervical cord injury with head injury should always be high, especially in the comatose patient, whose neurologic findings may be masked. In general, if the head injury is severe enough to warrant skull roentgenograms, cervical spine films should also be taken.

EYES. Injuries to the eye and adnexa may be multiple, but these will be discussed only as they apply to the emergency evaluation of the head-injured patient. An isolated periorbital ecchymosis ("raccoon eye") may be caused by local trauma to the eye or may represent extravasated blood from a fracture of the floor of the anterior fossa, and should lead to a search for anosmia and cerebrospinal fluid (CSF) rhinorrhea. Subconjunctival hemorrhage may reflect frontal or anterior basilar skull fracture. Papilledema from increased intracranial pressure is rare in the first few hours after head injury, even if the pressure is quite high. Retinal and optic disc hemorrhages, however, are not rare and should be looked for and recorded. The eyes of the comatose patient should be protected as soon as they have been examined.

EARS. Blood, cerebrospinal fluid or a mixture of these (giving the familiar "doublering" sign) coming from the ear is evidence of basilar skull fracture. Blood behind the eardrum and a retroaural ecchymosis (Battle's sign) are, similarly, indicators of basilar fracture.

NOSE. Cerebrospinal fluid rhinorrhea is evidence of an open basilar skull fracture. Recent evidence suggests that the spinal fluid leak will stop sooner, with a corresponding decrease in the risk of infection, if frontal and nasal fractures are reduced early.

TRUNK AND EXTREMITIES. The chest, heart, abdomen and extremities may also be subject to injury in the head-injured patient. Fractures or soft-tissue injury may sequester huge volumes of blood. Hemopneumothorax, lung contusion, cardiac contusion, or ruptured intra-abdominal and pelvic solid or hollow organs may all be life-threatening and may be occult in the patient with head injury.

NEUROLOGIC EXAMINATION

Mental Status. Evaluation of the state of consciousness in a head-injured patient is the most important consideration in establishing a baseline of neurologic function and noting early deviations from that baseline. A pa-

tient's initial status must be carefully evaluated in this regard. The use of such terms as coma, stupor, obtundation and confusion is not desirable in recording level of consciousness. These terms mean different things to different observers and may even mean different things to the same observer at different times. Since deviation from the baseline state of consciousness is so critical in evaluating the severity and progression of head injury, a clear description of clinical status is preferable to an ambiguous label.

Answers to the following questions, ranked from greatest to least functional disturbance, should be recorded for each patient:

1. Does the patient respond to painful stimuli?
2. Is the response decerebrate, decorticate or purposeful?
3. Is the response symmetrical?
4. Does the patient move spontaneously?
5. Does he move in response to verbal stimuli?
6. Will he follow commands?
7. Is he oriented to time, place and situation?
8. Can he handle mathematical problems and abstraction in keeping with his educational background?
9. Is the patient's behavior appropriate to the situation?

Only by repeatedly asking and recording the answers to these questions can the examiner determine the patient's condition within the spectrum of unresponsiveness to normal and the course that his state of consciousness is taking. Early changes in the state of consciousness include confusion when there was none before, disorientation when the patient was previously oriented, development of urinary or fecal incontinence in the patient who was continent, and agitation or lack of cooperation in a patient who was previously calm and cooperative.

Cranial Nerves. OLFACTORY NERVE (I). Although seldom routinely tested in the traumatized patient, the olfactory nerve is frequently damaged in head-injured patients.

OPTIC NERVE (II). Lesions of the visual system may occur anywhere from the retina through the optic nerve, chiasma, tracts and calcarine cortex of the occipital lobes.[114] Although lesions have been described in each of these areas, the retina and optic nerves are the most common sites of injury. Visual lesions occur in 1 to 5 per cent of head injuries, with about half of these resulting in permanent deficit.

OCULOMOTOR NERVES (III, IV, VI).   For practical purposes, injuries to the oculomotor system can be divided into (*a*) those involving the extraocular muscles in the orbit; (*b*) those involving the nerves or nuclei directly; and (*c*) secondary damage from increased intracranial pressure. The first group can be distinguished by association with local orbital trauma and failure to conform to usual neurogenic deficit. The restriction in movement of the globes is most often in direct upward or downward gaze, a situation not seen with damage to cranial nerves III, IV or VI. The third and fourth cranial nerves may be considered together because the fourth nerve is rarely injured without third nerve involvement.

Pupillary constriction is a function of third nerve parasympathetic fibers and is probably the most widely known sign of head injury. These fibers are the most sensitive to direct trauma and to pressure and usually cease to function before the somatic motor fibers are affected. Damage to these fibers leads to pupillary dilatation, and failure of reaction to light. In evaluation of pupillary inequality, one other less common possibility must be borne in mind. Sympathetic fibers arise in the neck, pass to the head in the carotid sheath, and innervate pupillary dilators. Constriction of the pupil on the side of the lesion, together with the ptosis and anhidrosis of Horner's syndrome, results from damage to these fibers. Thus, unilateral pupillary constriction from a cervical soft-tissue or thoracic spinal injury is occasionally misinterpreted as contralateral pupillary dilatation.

The somatic motor function of the third and fourth nerves serves to move the eye medially, superiorly, inferiorly and rotationally. The third nerve also supplies the elevator of the lid. Direct injury to the third nerve occurs rarely and is associated with frontal and local orbital trauma. The patient usually shows a stable or improving level of consciousness and stable vital signs. The onset of oculomotor paralysis is immediate, and the deficit is stable rather than delayed and progressive. These latter factors serve to distinguish the direct trauma cases from the more ominous paralyses due to pressure.

The same deficits in third nerve function that occur secondary to direct trauma may be seen secondary to increased intracranial pressure. As the medial temporal lobe is forced through the tentorial notch, the third nerve is trapped between the brain tissue and the unyielding fibrous tent. Progressive third nerve palsy thus combines with the decreasing level of consciousness and altered vital signs as the hallmarks of the immediately life-threatening injury.

ABDUCENS NERVE (VI).   This nerve serves to move the globe laterally. It is affected in approximately 3 per cent of head injuries.[154] As with the third nerve, the damage may be direct or indirect. Fracture of the petrous portion of the temporal bone may cause unilateral damage to the sixth, seventh and eighth nerves. Trauma at the apex of the orbit may cause unilateral damage to the second, third, fourth and sixth nerves. Like the third nerve, the sixth may be damaged by increased intracranial pressure. The damage may be unilateral or bilateral and, unlike third nerve paralysis, has little lateralizing value.

TRIGEMINAL NERVE (V).   The vast majority of injuries to the fifth nerve occur extracranially. Unilateral hypoesthesia or anesthesia over the forehead suggests trauma at the supraorbital foramen. The same findings over the malar eminence suggest trauma at the infraorbital foramen. Both are associated with orbital fractures.

FACIAL NERVE (VII).   Failure to move the muscles of facial expression on one side may result from damage to the contralateral motor strip, its projections to the internal capsule, the facial muscles or the ipsilateral seventh nerve itself. In the first two cases, it is most often associated with paresis of other muscle groups on the same side. Failure to wrinkle the forehead on the side of weakness is the usual, but not infallible, method of distinguishing a peripheral from a central lesion. Immediate peripheral seventh nerve palsies are usually the result of fractures of the petrous portion of the temporal bone traversing the facial canal. These injuries may be associated with sixth and eighth nerve malfunction as well has hemotympanum or cerebrospinal fluid otorrhea.

COCHLEAR VESTIBULAR NERVE (VIII). The eighth nerve is anatomically and physiologically two nerves, the cochlear and the vestibular. Hearing loss with head injuries occurs in 8 per cent of cases. It may result from damage to the cochlea itself with fractures of the middle cranial fossa, or fractures of the petrous temporal bone and internal auditory canal which damage the nerve.

Vestibular nerve injuries are common, poorly understood and difficult to differentiate from posterior fossa lesions. Nystagmus is the hallmark of these injuries and tends to be associated with vertigo in peripheral but not brain-stem lesions. Positional nystagmus may be present in up to 25 per cent of head-injured patients, and it is usually self-limited.[114]

GLOSSOPHARYNGEAL, VAGUS, SPINAL ACCESSORY AND HYPOGLOSSAL NERVES (IX, X, XI, XII). Damage to the lower four cranial nerves is rare and most often associated with fatal penetrating injuries or extensive fractures of the floor of the posterior fossa.[123] Paralysis of the tongue, trapezius, sternomastoid, larynx and palate result from these injuries.

Motor System. Disorders of motor function from nervous system lesions are disorders of groups of muscles. Monoparesis is usually due to nerve root or peripheral nerve injury. Paraparesis is the hallmark of spinal cord injury. Rarely, it can result from vertex injuries to the head, but spinal cord injuries should be considered and ruled out first. Quadriparesis may occur with severe head injury, but flaccid quadriparesis implies cervical cord injury until proved otherwise.

Hemiparesis, or weakness of one side of the body, may arise in several ways. Lateral hemisection of the cervical spinal cord may cause hemiparesis, but this is very unusual and is not associated with facial weakness or other abnormalities of brain function, such as decreased level of consciousness. Direct trauma to the cerebral hemisphere or corticospinal tracts in the brain stem may cause hemiparesis. These are severe injuries usually associated with disorders of consciousness and require special diagnostic studies. As with the third nerve, the motor system may be damaged by transtentorial herniation of the medial temporal lobe into the tentorial notch. If the medial temporal lobe is wedged into this passage, the cerebral peduncles, which lie exposed on the surface of the midbrain, can be damaged in two ways. If the peduncle is subject to direct pressure from the temporal lobe, contralateral hemiparesis may occur because the motor tracts cross lower down in the medulla. If the midbrain is forced to the opposite side, the peduncle may be lacerated by the edge of the tentorium. Hemiparesis in this case will be ipsilateral to the herniating brain. This may occur in 5 to 15 per cent of cases. In either case, the patient's cardiorespiratory function is in imminent danger, and immediate efforts to reduce the intracranial pressure are required.

Sensory Function. Abnormalities of sensory function are difficult to measure in head-injured patients except as responses to noxious stimuli, as mentioned previously and to be discussed under Reflexes. The decrease in state of consciousness and associated motor lesions cause difficulty in valid interpretation of findings.

Cerebellum. Traumatic mass lesions in the posterior fossa are unusual and are notoriously difficult to diagnose. Jamieson found posterior fossa hematomas in 2.5 per cent of his cases of subdural hematoma.[88] Ataxia of gait and nystagmus are common findings in patients with minimally or moderately severe head injuries and cannot be interpreted as firm evidence of a posterior fossa clot. Alterations of respiratory function and rising blood pressure out of proportion to decreasing level of consciousness should suggest posterior fossa lesions, especially in the presence of occipital bone fracture.

Reflexes. Absent deep tendon reflexes associated with muscular hypotonia are evidence of lower motor neuron disease and direct the attention of the examiner to the spinal cord and peripheral nerves. Hypoactive reflexes may accompany the decreased responsiveness of patients with concussion. Hyperactive reflexes suggest anxiety or an upper motor neuron lesion. Decerebrate rigidity implies brain-stem damage and may occur as a result of direct concussive damage or indirect compression from an expanding mass lesion.

A series of reflexes may be used to establish the highest level of functional integrity of the central nervous system in the comatose patient. The ciliospinal reflex is ipsilateral pupillary dilatation in response to a painful stimulus applied to the upper trunk. It is mediated through sensory nerves to the spinal cord and relayed from the upper thoracic cord through the superior cervical ganglion to the sympathetic nerves about the carotid arteries to the pupil. An intact reflex implies intact central nervous system function to the upper thoracic spinal cord. An intact corneal reflex implies functional integrity to the midpontine level. Intact oculocephalic or oculovestibular reflexes imply function to the upper midbrain.

Skull Fractures. Fractures of the cranial vault or the base of the skull may be open or closed. A closed fracture, which may be linear or comminuted, may be important, first, as an indicator of force applied to the head; second, because of its location; and third, whether or not the fracture is depressed below the normal plane of the skull. Even a nondepressed linear fracture implies significant force applied to the skull and suggests hospitalization and observation. Location is important because of underlying vascular structures that may be torn by the force which caused the fracture. The areas of greatest danger are (a) the temporal fossa, where the middle meningeal artery may be torn, and (b) areas overlying the dural venous sinuses, which may be torn or separated from the skull. It has been the consensus for many years that a skull fracture which is depressed more than the thickness of the skull ought to be elevated because of the threat of underlying brain atrophy. Recent evidence shows that much of the underlying brain atrophy is due to the initial force of injury, and there is little difference in the development of atrophy, seizures or neurologic deficit if depressed skull fractures are not elevated. This is still a controversial area, and closed depressed fractures of any significance are usually surgically treated. Open depressed skull fractures must be operated upon on an emergency basis because of the threat of retention of contaminated material in and below the lips of the fracture and subsequent infection.

SYNTHESIS

With the preceding historical, physical and neurologic findings, and radiologic findings as discussed here, one can make a tentative decision concerning whether a lesion of the central nervous system exists, where it is, what it is likely to be, what needs to be done about it, and when treatment should be started.

Intracranial traumatic lesions, as already suggested, are of several types. Concussion is a term reserved for head injuries causing brief loss of consciousness, short periods of retrograde amnesia and, often, vomiting. Focal neurologic deficits are not seen. Skull fracture may or may not be present. Full recovery may be expected in the absence of associated injury, and the only treatment required is observation.

Brain contusion is both a clinical and pathologic entity. Clinically, the patient has a prolonged period of unconsciousness and often has motor or cranial nerve deficits. X-ray films may show fracture or may reveal normal findings. Pathologically, the brain has

multiple punctate hemorrhages and edema. This edema may cause shift of the brain and compression of brain-stem structures vital to consciousness, cardiovascular function and respiration. Contusions may be operatively treated if they are in the frontal or temporal pole. Patients with compression of the medulla from focal contusions may have life and function saved by resection of the edematous brain. Patients with widespread brain contusion, however, have a poor prognosis; only 5 per cent of them return to their premorbid status.

Mass lesions secondary to trauma may be due to edema, as in contusions, to local hemorrhage, or to a combination of the two. Epidural hematomas most often occur in the temporal fossa but may also occur over the superior sagittal or lateral venous sinuses. They are often accompanied by the immediate loss of consciousness characteristic of concussion, with subsequent return of the level of consciousness toward normal. This is the classic "lucid interval." Examination during this period may reveal only minor behavioral abnormalities, such as inappropriate behavior or difficulty with mathematical problems. Motor and cranial nerve deficits are often absent. X-ray films may be normal but often show fractures crossing the middle meningeal artery or a major venous sinus. As intracranial bleeding progresses, the patient undergoes rapid deterioration, with a progressively decreasing level of consciousness and other signs of transtentorial or cerebellar herniation and secondary brain-stem compression. The ironic aspect of this condition is that the direct brain injury is small and the prognosis is excellent if the bleeding is diagnosed and controlled early. This currently occurs in only slightly over half of the patients with epidural hematomas.

Acute subdural hematomas result from direct injury to the cerebral cortex and its veins. Because of the underlying brain contusion, removal of the blood clot yields disappointing results similar to those in brain contusion. These patients are often unconscious from the time of injury and frequently have focal motor or cranial nerve deficits. Skull films may be normal or may show fractures.

Chronic subdural hematoma is often a late sequela of head trauma. These patients present with headaches, depressed level of consciousness and varying neurologic deficits occurring from weeks to several months after head trauma. This diagnosis should be suspected in any patient with alteration of consciousness or with a focal neurologic deficit in whom suspicion of prior head trauma exists.

CONCLUSION

A high index of suspicion of intracranial or cervical spinal trauma must be maintained in dealing with patients who have orofacial injuries. Orderly history and physical examination and minimal radiologic studies will allow the clinician to decide whether or not an injury to the central nervous system exists, is a threat to life, or is likely to become such a threat. Appropriate decisions regarding observation, consultation, and special diagnostic and operative procedures can then be made.

FACIAL SOFT-TISSUE WOUNDS

The simplest wound is known as an *incised wound;* the edges are clean-cut as if made by a sharp instrument, such as a piece of glass or sharp metal, and there is no loss of tissue. In *lacerated wounds* the tissues are torn apart, and the edges are irregular and frayed. *Contused wounds* are those in which there is crushing of the tissue, which may result in devitalization. The crushed tissue, which dies and sloughs off, is lost as well as that which may have been torn away at the time of injury. *Abrasions* are wounds that are raw, slowly bleeding surfaces caused by a forceful sliding contact of the skin with a rough surface which scrapes or grinds off the epidermis.

Nearly all lacerated and abraded wounds are infected or become infected by the foreign material carried into the wound on the object which caused the injury, or by dirt from the skin or from the ground. The ordinary pyogenic organisms are always present.

PROPHYLACTIC ANTIBIOTIC THERAPY*

Since all accidental wounds are assumed to be contaminated, the advisability of instituting antibiotic therapy at the onset of treat-

*Reprinted with permission from Committee on Trauma, American College of Surgeons: Early Care of the Injured Patient, p. 36. Philadelphia, W. B. Saunders Co., 1972.

ment must be considered in each instance. The following general principles should be kept in mind:

1. Foremost, a history of sensitivity or drug idiosyncrasy is sought. When the patient gives a clear history of sensitivity reaction to one or more antibiotics, it is well to consider an effective antibiotic which has not been previously used or to which the patient is known not to be sensitive.
2. Almost all patients with extensive wounds should be given antibiotics, preferably aqueous penicillin G and preferably intravenously, as part of their preoperative resuscitation. This becomes more important when primary treatment has been delayed or is likely to be delayed.
3. Minor wounds of the face, not including the buccal cavity, usually do not require antibiotics.
4. However, minor wounds in patients with diabetes, extensive vascular disease, or debilitating conditions of any origin, require antibiotic therapy.
5. Visceral injuries of the abdomen or chest require large doses of antibiotics.
6. Patients with massive wounds which afford ideal sites for anaerobic growth (see sections on Tetanus and on Clostridial Myositis) should receive large doses of aqueous penicillin G and one of the tetracyclines intravenously, as soon after injury as possible; these should be continued until the danger of this type of infection is over.
7. Animal bites, and especially human bites, even when the wounds are small, require antibiotic therapy. At the present time, penicillin is the agent of choice.
8. All patients who have been subjected to excessive or extensive radiation should receive antibiotics.
9. Antibiotic therapy should be continued for at least 5 days after all clinical evidence of infection has disappeared. When there is no evidence of infection following administration of prophylactics, the antibiotic may be continued until wound healing is advanced.
10. It is advisable to begin prophylactic antibiotic therapy prior to initiating operative procedures on traumatized patients so that an antibacterial blood level of the antibiotic agent will be

present in the tissues and body cavities before and throughout the operation.

11. Cultures should be taken at the time of operation from all contaminated areas so that if resulting infection develops, a more intelligent approach to specific antibiotic therapy will be possible. (Study Chapter 8, "Antibiotic Therapy.")

SPECIAL PROPHYLACTIC MEASURES*

TETANUS

This severe and dreaded infectious complication of traumatic wounds could be almost completely eliminated by universal active immunization during childhood. Tetanus is caused by the anaerobic organism *Clostridium tetani* and its toxins and is characterized by local convulsive spasm of the voluntary muscles and a tendency toward episodes of respiratory arrest. It may occur as a complication in either large or small wounds including lacerations, open fractures, burns, abrasions, and even hypodermic injections. However, the fact that approximately one-third of the patients seen with active tetanus either have no obvious wound or have wounds considered to be insignificant by the patient or his physician emphasizes the problem of tetanus prophylaxis following unknown or minimal wounds and suggests that the disease will never be eliminated until universal active immunization has been achieved.

General Principles of Tetanus Prophylaxis

Individual Consideration of Each Patient. For each patient with a wound, the attending physician must determine individually what is required for adequate prophylaxis against tetanus.

Surgical Debridement. Regardless of the active immunization status of the patient, meticulous surgical care, including removal of all devitalized tissue and foreign bodies, should be provided immediately for all wounds. Such

---

*Reprinted with permission from Committee on Trauma, American College of Surgeons: Early Care of the Injured Patient, pp. 37–41. Philadelphia, W. B. Saunders Co., 1972.

care is as essential for the prevention of tetanus as it is for other types of wound infection.

Active Immunization. Tetanus toxoid is the simplest, surest, and cheapest immunologic agent available. Immunization should be started in infancy with DPT shots, sometime between 2 and 6 months of age. Two to three doses given intramuscularly 1 month apart followed by a booster at 12 months is the usual method of immunization. Another booster is administered when the child is 5 or 6 years old, usually when he begins to attend school. Booster injections of tetanus toxoid should be given periodically, but the time schedule has not been definitely established since several studies to determine the need for tetanus boosters are still in progress. Basic active immunization with adsorbed toxoid requires three injections. A booster of adsorbed toxoid is indicated 10 years after the third injection or 10 years after an intervening wound booster.

Each patient with a wound should receive adsorbed tetanus toxoid intramuscularly at the time of injury, either as an initial immunizing dose or as a booster for previous immunization, *unless* he has received a booster or has completed his initial immunization series within the past 5 years. As the antigen concentration varies in different products, specific information on the volume of a single dose is provided on the label of the package.

Passive Immunization. Whether or not passive immunization with homologous (human) tetanus immune globulin should be provided must be decided individually for each patient. The characteristics of the wound, the conditions under which it was incurred, and the previous active immunization status of the patient must be considered. In those patients without previous active (toxoid) immunization, passive immunization is indicated. In the past it was traditionally administered with equine or bovine antitoxin in a dose of 3000 to 10,000 units. Because of the danger and frequency of allergic reactions, as well as the rapid elimination of the antitoxin, and the incidence of delayed serum sickness following the use of equine or bovine antitoxin, passive immunization with these agents has been discouraged and should be discontinued. Instead the safer human tetanus immune globulin (Hypertet) is recommended by intramuscular injection. It should *never* be given *intravenously*. This product (Hypertet) has a much longer half-life of protection of approximately 30 days.

Patient Record. Every wounded patient should be given a written record of the immunization provided and should be instructed to carry the record at all times and, if indicated, to complete his active immunization. For precise tetanus prophylaxis, an accurate and immediately available history regarding previous active immunization against tetanus is required.

Antibiotic Prophylaxis. The value of antibiotic agents in the prophylaxis of tetanus remains questionable. There is no doubt that *Clostridium tetani* is sensitive *in vitro* to penicillin and tetracycline, as well as other antibiotics, but there seems to be some difficulty in delivering an adequate dose of antibiotics to the susceptible bacteria before they liberate toxin. The tetanus-prone wound characteristically has a decreased blood supply and contains necrotic tissue which may prevent high antibiotic blood levels from reaching the infecting bacteria. It is recommended that antibiotic therapy not be relied upon as

adequate prophylactic therapy in the place of immunization. In large necrotic wounds, particularly those in which debridement has been delayed or compromised, penicillin and tetracycline have often been employed as prophylaxis against other types of wound infection which may occur, as well as for prophylactic action against tetanus.

Specific Measures for Previously Immunized Patients (Table 18–1)

When the patient has been actively immunized within the past 10 years:

1. To the great majority give 0.5 ml. of adsorbed tetanus toxoid as a booster unless it is *certain* that the patient has received a booster within the previous 5 *years.*
2. To those with severe, neglected, or old (more than 24 hours) tetanus-prone wounds, give 0.5 cc. of adsorbed toxoid

Table 18–1 *Prophylactic Treatment of Tetanus**

TYPE OF WOUND	PATIENT NOT IMMUNIZED OR PARTIALLY IMMUNIZED	PATIENT COMPLETELY IMMUNIZED TIME SINCE LAST BOOSTER DOSE		
		1† to 5 years	5 to 10 years	10 years +
Clean minor	Begin or complete immunization per schedule; tetanus toxoid, 0.5 cc.	None.	Tetanus toxoid, 0.5 cc.	Tetanus toxoid, 0.5 cc.
Clean major or tetanus-prone	In one arm: Human tetanus immune globulin, 250 mg.‡ In the other arm: Tetanus toxoid, 0.5 cc.; complete immunization per schedule.‡	Tetanus toxoid, 0.5 cc.	Tetanus toxoid, 0.5 cc.	In one arm: Tetanus toxoid, 0.5 cc.‡ In the other arm: Human tetanus immune globulin, 250 mg.‡
Tetanus-prone, delayed or incomplete debridement	In one arm: Human tetanus immune globulin, 500 mg.‡ In the other arm: Tetanus toxoid, 0.5 cc.; complete immunization per schedule thereafter.‡ Antibiotic therapy.	Tetanus toxoid, 0.5 cc.	Tetanus toxoid, 0.5 cc. Antibiotic therapy.	In one arm: Tetanus toxoid, 0.5 cc.‡ In the other arm: Human tetanus immune globulin, 500 mg.‡ Antibiotic therapy.

*Reprinted with permission from Committee on Trauma, American College of Surgeons: Early Care of the Injured Patient, p. 39. Philadelphia, W. B. Saunders Co., 1972.

†No prophylactic immunization is required if patient has had a booster within the previous year.

‡Use different syringes, needles and sites.

Note: With different preparations of toxoid, the volume of a single booster dose should be modified as stated on the package label.

unless it is *certain* that a booster was received within the previous *year*.

When the patient received active immunization more than 10 years previously and has not received a booster within the past 5 years (some authorities advise 6 rather than 10 years, particularly for patients with severe, neglected, or old tetanus-prone wounds such as may be sustained by military personnel in combat):

1. To the great majority give a dose of 0.5 cc. of adsorbed tetanus toxoid.
2. To those with wounds which indicate an overwhelming possibility that tetanus might develop:
   a. Give 0.5 cc. of adsorbed tetanus toxoid, and
   b. Give 250 units of tetanus immune globulin (human), using different syringes, needles, and sites of injection.
   c. In severe, neglected, or old wounds, inject 500 units of tetanus immune globulin (human).
   d. Consider providing oxytetracycline or penicillin prophylactically.

Treatment for Patients Not Previously Immunized

With clean minor wounds, in which tetanus is most unlikely, give 0.5 cc. of adsorbed tetanus toxoid (initial immunizing dose).

With all other wounds:

1. Give 0.5 cc. of adsorbed tetanus toxoid (initial immunizing dose).
2. Give 250 units of tetanus immune globulin (human). The dose should be increased to 500 units in severe or neglected wounds.
3. Consider providing oxytetracycline or penicillin prophylactically.

Equine or Bovine Antitoxin. Do *not* administer heterologous antitoxin (equine) except when tetanus immune globulin (human) is not available within 24 hours and ONLY if the possibility of tetanus outweighs the danger of reaction to heterologous tetanus antitoxin. Before using such antitoxin, question the patient for a history of allergy and test for sensitivity. If the patient is sensitive to heterologous antitoxin, do not use it because the danger of anaphylaxis probably outweighs the danger of tetanus; rely on penicillin or oxytetracycline. Do not attempt desensitization because it is not worthwhile. If the patient is not sensitive to equine tetanus antitoxin and

if the decision is made to administer it for passive immunization, give at least 3000 units.

CLOSTRIDIAL MYOSITIS (GAS GANGRENE)

Types of Wounds with Increased Risk

Clostridial myositis is most likely to develop in wounds which have the following characteristics:

1. Extensive laceration or devitalization of muscle such as occurs in compound fractures and injuries from high-velocity missiles.
2. Impairment of the main blood supply by the injury, a tourniquet, a tight cast, or delayed thrombosis.
3. Gross contamination by foreign bodies such as soil and clothing.
4. Delayed treatment.
5. Inadequate treatment such as incomplete debridement or lack of immobilization.

Prevention

Surgery. The most effective means of preventing gas gangrene continues to be early and adequate operation which includes wide incision, thorough debridement of all devitalized and potentially devitalized tissues, removal of contaminating dirt and all foreign bodies, and effective drainage as required. Adequate debridement is especially important in irregular deep wounds in which there are loculations and recesses which favor anaerobic bacterial growth. Dead and devitalized tissue and foreign bodies must be removed at the time of initial operation. In war wounds, in wounds incurred in mass disasters, and in all wounds in which there has been some trauma to the soft tissues, this thorough debridement should be coupled with delayed suture of the wound. The wound should be left open from 4 to 7 days following the debridement, and then delayed suture should be accomplished if the wound has remained clean.

Antibiotic. Antibiotic therapy is of some prophylactic value when combined with proper surgical procedures, but experimental and clinical experience affirms this principle and indicates that antibiotic therapy alone cannot be relied upon to prevent the occurrence of clostridial myositis. The tetracyclines are the most effective agents against the clostridial organisms.

Antitoxin. Prophylactic administration of gas gangrene antitoxin at the time of injury or shortly thereafter is not recommended. The evidence indicates that it has been of little or no practical value in the prevention of clinical gas gangrene. Many physicians, however, continue to give it at the time of injury despite evidence of its ineffectiveness.

Hyperbaric Oxygen Therapy. Hyperbaric oxygen therapy remains experimental and unproven as a prophylactic therapeutic measure in gas gangrene. The experimental evidence indicates that it has little value without adequate surgical debridement. It has been used more effectively in some instances in the treatment of established clostridial infections.

OCCURRENCE OF FACIAL BONE FRACTURES

Measurements of the occurrence of fractures among civilians indicate that the nasal bones are the most frequently fractured bones of the face. In many of these fractures there is little displacement, and frequently the patient never seeks treatment.

The mandible is the second most frequently fractured bone of the face and the tenth most frequently fractured bone in the whole body. Seldom are these fractures undetected and untreated, mainly because of the marked discomfort which is experienced by the patient.

The zygomatic bone is the third most frequently fractured osseous structure of the face. Here again, unless there is marked de-

formity, interference with mastication, diplopia, or numbness in the cheek, many of these fractures are unrecognized and untreated.

The maxilla is the fourth most frequently fractured bone of the facial skeleton. As a general rule, severe extraoral trauma is required to fracture the maxilla. A frequent fracture of the maxilla is one of the tuberosity of the alveolar process that occurs at the time of the extraction of molar teeth. In some cases a large segment of the maxilla containing one or more molar teeth, the floor of the maxillary sinus, and the tuberosity are fractured when attempting to remove one of the maxillary molars.

Fractures of the zygomatic arch are fifth in order of frequency. The depressed segments frequently prohibit the mandible from opening by obstructing the downward movement of the coronoid process. Otherwise they are frequently overlooked unless a local depression in the skin overlying the fracture area is noted.

ETIOLOGY OF FRACTURES

Fractures of the mandible and maxilla may be due to trauma or a pathologic process.

Traumatic Fractures. These may be caused by external violence, such as a blow by a fist or a club, by automobile or industrial accidents, by falls, by gunshot wounds, or by trauma during the extraction of teeth, especially when elevators are used for the removal of impacted teeth (Fig. 18–2). Fractures of the maxillary alveolar process and tuber-

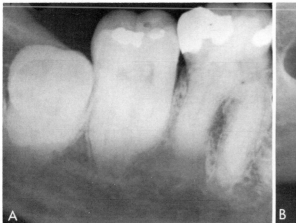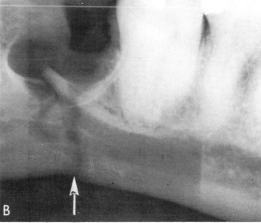

Figure 18–2 Fracture of the mandible resulting from insufficient removal of osseous tissue around the unerupted third molar before the application of the elevator to remove the tooth.

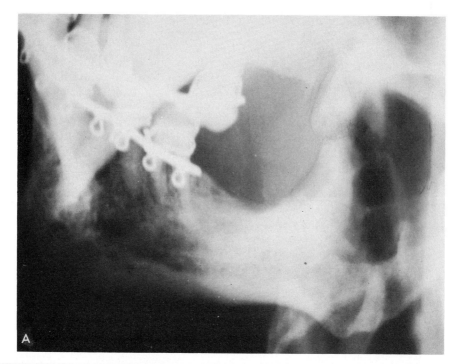

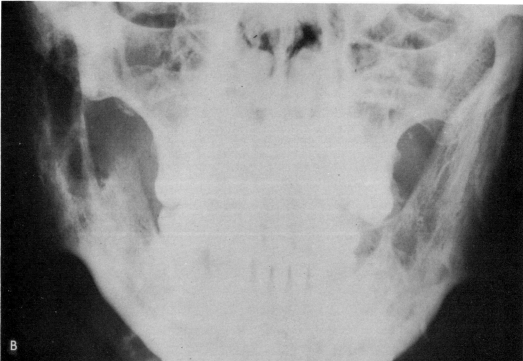

Figure 18–3 *A*, Oblique radiograph of the right ramus of the mandible. The large radiolucent area was the result of loss of bone due to metastatic carcinoma. Note the pathologic fracture of the coronoid process. *B*, Posteroanterior radiograph showing that the neck of the condyle was also fractured.

The splints attached to the necks of the maxillary and mandibular teeth had a few intermaxillary elastics stretched between them. These were *not applied to immobilize* the mandible, but to permit the patient to open and close his mouth and to masticate in normal occlusion. Otherwise, the mandible would swing to the right, out of occlusion, when the mouth was closed.

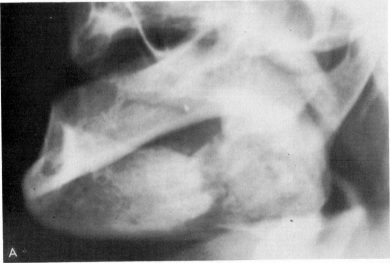

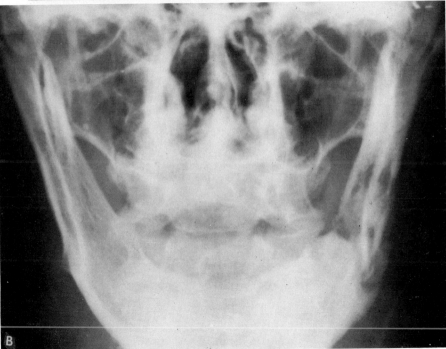

Figure 18-4 *A*, Carcinoma that metastasized from the cervix to the throat and then to the angle of the edentulous mandible, causing this pathologic fracture. *B*, Posteroanterior radiograph showing metastatic lesions and the overriding of the ramus.

osities occur more often than do fractures of the mandible during extractions.

Pathologic Fractures. These may be due to cysts, benign or malignant bone tumors, osteogenesis imperfecta, osteomyelitis, osteomalacia, generalized bone atrophy or osteoporosis, or necrosis (Figs. 18–3 and 18–4). Because of the extensive destruction of the body of the bone by these pathologic processes, fractures may occur spontaneously during talking, yawning or eating.

CLASSIFICATION OF FRACTURES

Fractures of the mandible and maxilla and zygomatic bone may be single, multiple, simple, compound, comminuted, complicated or impacted. (See pages 1226 to 1228 for a detailed classification of fractures of the maxilla.)

Single Fractures. These are fractures in which the bone is fractured in only one place. Such fractures are unilateral. They are rather uncommon on the mandible. When seen on

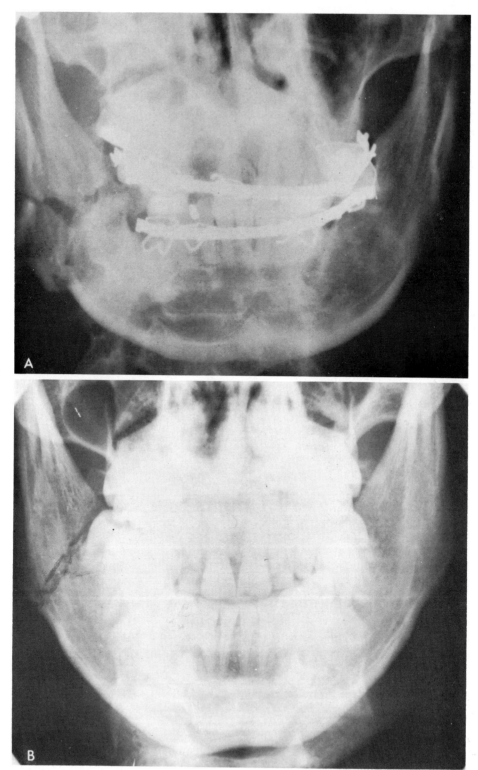

Figure 18–5   Examples of fractures through the angle formed by the junction of the vertical ramus and the horizontal ramus (body or corpus) of the mandible. Note the frequency with which a third molar is in the line of fracture. We do not extract these teeth unless it proves to be necessary. (See Teeth in the Line of Fracture.)

(Figure 18–5 continued on opposite page)

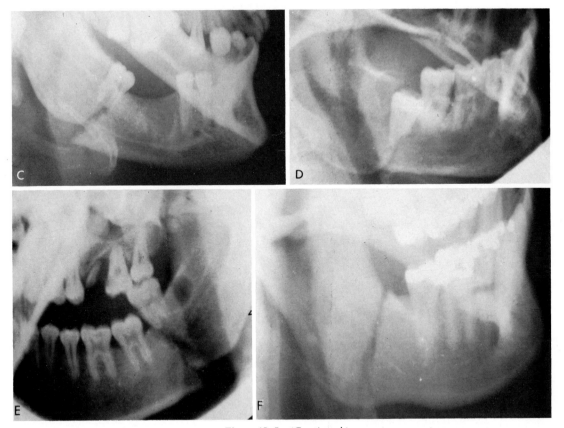

Figure 18–5 *(Continued.)*

(Figure 18–5 continued on following page)

the mandible, they are most frequently at the following locations: through the angle formed by the vertical ramus and the body, especially if an unerupted third molar is present; through the mental foramen; or through the neck of the condyle. In the maxilla they are usually seen in the tuberosity area or in the anterior alveolar maxillary ridge.

Multiple Fractures. Multiple fractures are those in which the bone is fractured in two or more places. Multiple fractures are generally bilateral. This is the type of fracture most frequently seen. It occurs in both the mandible and the maxilla.

If the fracture occurs through the neck of the condyle on one side, there is usually a fracture through the mental foramen on the contralateral side. If it occurs through the mental foramen on one side, it may occur through the angle formed by the ramus and body on the other side, or through the neck of the condyle.

Multiple fractures may also be unilateral,

the bone being fractured into several segments on one side only.

Simple Fractures. These are fractures in which the broken osseous structure is not in contact with the secretions of the oral cavity, or in which the broken osseous structure does not communicate with the oral cavity or external surface of the face through a laceration in the investing soft tissues.

Simple fractures are most frequently found as fractures of the ramus of the mandible, occurring anywhere on the ramus between the condyle and the angle formed by the ramus and the body of the mandible.

Compound Fractures. These are fractures in which the broken osseous structure communicates with the oral cavity or external surface of the face through a laceration in the oral mucosa or in the skin. These fractures generally occur anterior to the angle formed by the vertical ramus with the horizontal ramus (body of the mandible).

Comminuted Fractures. These are frac-

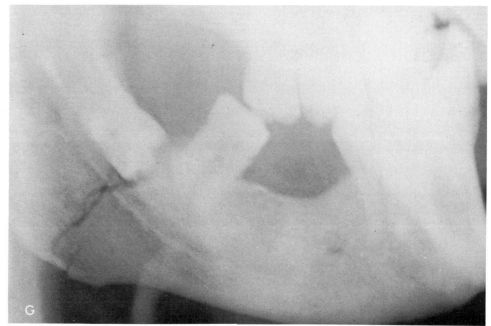

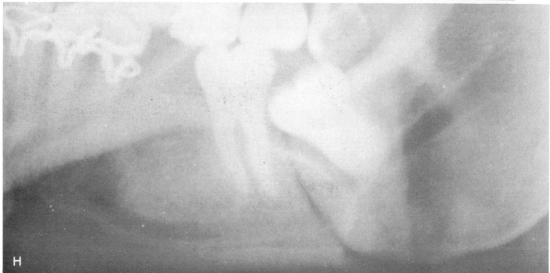

Figure 18–5 *(Continued.)*

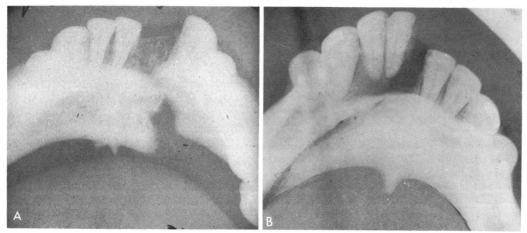

Figure 18–6 Examples of fractures of the symphysis of the mandible.

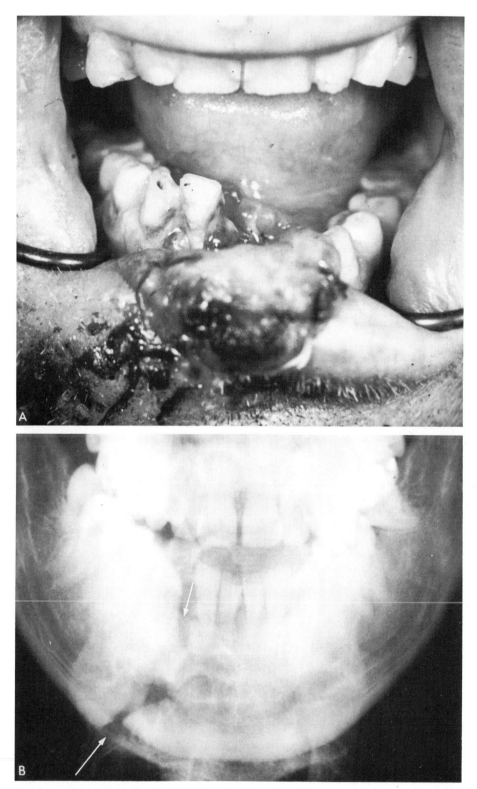

Figure 18-7   Laceration of the lower lip and a compound comminuted fracture of the symphysis with displacement of the segment.

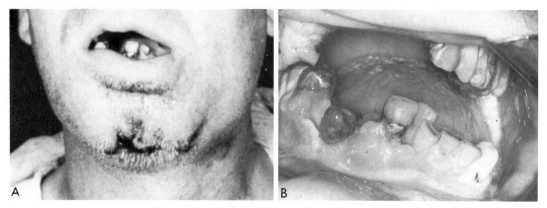

Figure 18–8   Laceration of skin over the symphysis and a segmental fracture.

tures in which the bone is broken up or segmented into several pieces or fragments, or in which the bone is shattered. They usually occur in the region of the symphysis of the mandible or in the anterior maxilla.

Complicated Fractures.   These are cases in which there are fractures of both the maxilla and the mandible, or in which the maxilla or the mandible is edentulous. Marked displacement of the compound comminuted osseous fragments of either or both the maxilla and mandible, with extensive trauma of the investing and covering soft tissues, always presents many problems.

Fracture cases with associated head injuries, such as fracture of the skull, also present complications. In every case of fracture of the mandible or maxilla, the possibility of an associated fracture of the skull should be ruled out before treatment is undertaken.

Complex fractures of the middle third of the face, the upper jaw, and associated structures generally involve the nasal bones and sinus cavities, the lacrimal bones and orbital walls, and even the floor or lateral walls of the cranial cavity.

In these cases there are the complications of respiratory obstruction, disturbance of vision, obstruction of the nasolacrimal ducts and most probably neurologic complications. It is necessary in these cases that the combined knowledge and skill of the neurosurgeon, otolaryngologist, ophthalmologist, plastic surgeon and oral surgeon be applied in the treatment.

FRACTURE AREA FREQUENCY

Maxilla.   The most common fracture of the maxilla is segmental fracture of the al-

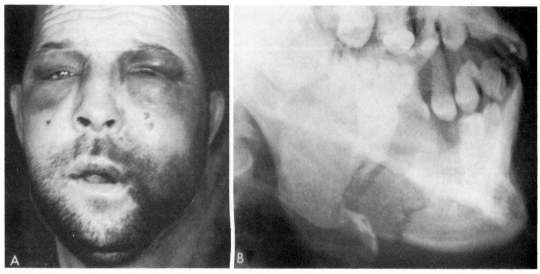

Figure 18–9   *A,* Patient "beat up" by thugs. *B,* He had sustained a comminuted fracture of the left body of the mandible, through the mental foramen area and the third molar.

veolar process, especially in the tuberosity region. This occurs most frequently in association with the extraction of teeth in the tuberosity area, through use of excessive force. It may involve one or more teeth, and it often involves all three molars and the floor of the maxillary sinus.

Next in order of frequency is segmental fracture of the anterior maxilla with the teeth contained therein, followed by transverse fractures through both maxillary sinuses and the nasal cavity. (Transverse fractures are most frequently associated with fractures of the nasal bones.) And fourth are compound comminuted fractures of the maxilla and its palatine process, associated with nasal bone fractures and unilateral or bilateral depressed fractures of the zygomatic bone.

Mandible. In the order of occurrence, fractures of the mandible may occur in the following places: through the angle of the mandible, especially through the unerupted or impacted lower third molar area; through the mental foramen; through the neck of the condyle; through the symphysis (from cuspid to cuspid); through the horizontal ramus (body) of the mandible, between the cuspid and the angle of the mandible; through the ramus, between the sigmoid notch and the angle; and through the coronoid process. There may be, finally, a fracture of a segment out of the mandible without the continuity of the horizontal ramus (body) being interrupted. This occurs with anterior blows that may fracture the alveolar process and six anterior teeth or that "punch out" a segment of the mandible.

FRACTURE LINES OF THE LOWER JAW

VALLE J. OIKARINEN, D.M. SC., D.D.S., AND
MARIA MALMSTRÖM, DR. ODONT.

Orthopantomography, the method of curved layer tomography, is especially suitable for roentgenography of jaw fractures. Since 1958, an orthopantomogram has been taken in every case of maxillofacial injury treated at the Oral Surgery Department of the University Dental Clinic of Helsinki. In obscure cases the orthopantomogram was verified by a three-dimensional picture.[130, 131, 132, 133]

During the 10-year period from 1958 to 1967 we treated a total of 1284 jaw fracture patients.[129] This discussion relates to only part of them, but some of the statistical data presented here are based on the whole series.

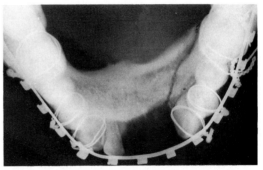

Figure 18-10   Another example of an oblique fracture of the anterior region of the mandible. The lower anterior teeth were knocked out by the blow that produced the fracture. (See Figure 18-26C, which illustrates a longer fracture of this type.)

In the 660 mandibular fracture cases, there were a total of 1114 fracture sites. This makes an average of 1.7 fractures per patient. Fracture lines were drawn from the orthopantomograms and arranged in groups according to the cause of the trauma.

The mandibular fractures of the males, a total of 589 cases, are presented in Figure 18-11 and in Table 18-2. A total of 119 fracture lines, collected from 71 cases of mandibular fracture in females, are presented in Figure 18-12. Figure 18-13 shows 23 fracture lines drawn from orthopantomograms of mandibular fractures in 12 children less than 10 years old.

Even though it may be true that no two fractures are exactly alike, the diagrams show that the majority of the fracture lines are situated in the so-called weak areas of the mandible, for example, the subcondylar, angular and canine tooth regions.[79] There seems to be a still more specific distribution dependent upon the mechanism of the trauma.

As seen in the orthopantomograms, the direction of the subcondylar fracture lines displayed considerable variety. The majority of the subcondylar fractures were located low on the neck of the condyloid process, especially in cases due to fights. In traffic accidents, there seemed to be fracture lines nearer the head of the condyle. The fracture lines were frequently directed obliquely downward, and in many of the cases due to fights the slope was very steep, nearly vertical. Nearly all of the fracture lines in the region of the angle passed downward and backward from the region of the third molar towards the mandibular angle.

The body fractures were not always paral-

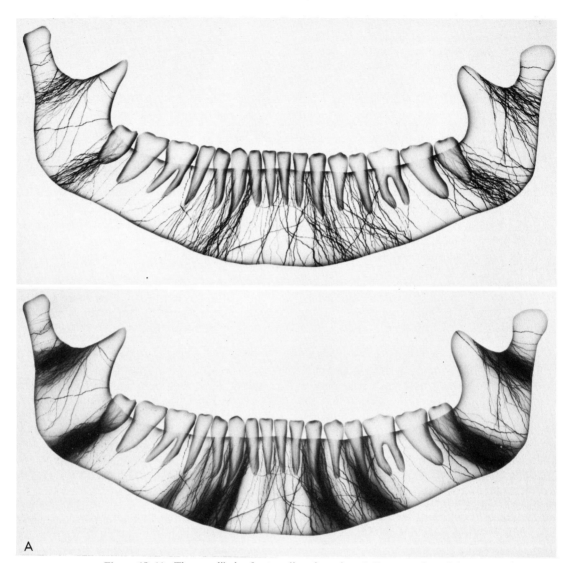

Figure 18–11   The mandibular fracture lines in males. *A*, Fractures from fights.

(Figure 18–11 continued on opposite page)

lel with the axes of the teeth. Most of the fracture lines of the body ran obliquely downward and backward to the base of the mandi-

Table 18–2   *Causes of Mandibular Fractures in 589 Males*

	CASES	FRACTURE LINES
Fights	225	365
Traffic accidents	170	308
Accidents at work	93	156
Other causes (falls, athletic injuries, etc.)	101	166
Total	589	995

ble. The fracture lines beginning at the alveolar region of the canines and incisors, for example, ran as far as the lower edge, below the bicuspids. Some fractures were vertically oriented or passed from the alveoli obliquely downward towards the midline.

When the orthopantomograms were divided into sections it was possible to assess statistically the frequency of fracture lines in different parts of the mandible, both overall and according to the mechanism of the trauma.

If all the fracture lines in the mandibular body are added up as shown in Figure 18–14,

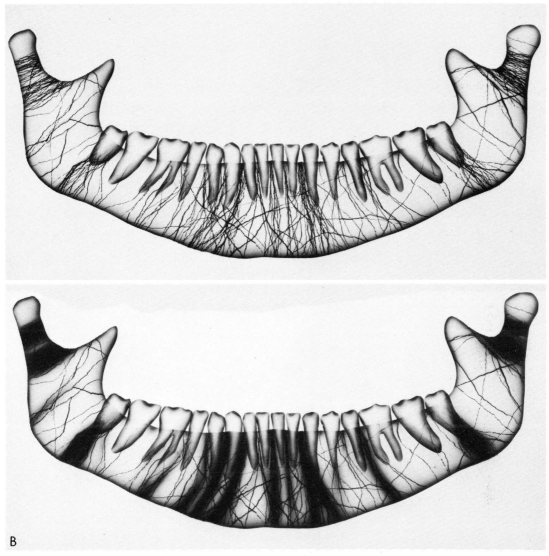

B

Figure 18–11   (*Continued.*)   *B,* Fractures from traffic accidents.

(Figure 18–11 continued on following page)

it appears that the frequency in this region only slightly exceeds the frequency in the subcondylar region (33.4 per cent against 32.9 per cent). Body fractures were most frequent in the region of the canine teeth. The majority of these fractures were unilateral. Bilateral subcondylar fractures almost always occurred in conjunction with other fractures, usually with lateral body fractures. Traffic accidents were the cause of subcondylar fractures in 37 per cent, fights in 25 per cent.

Fractures of the angle were found in 17.3 per cent of the patients, and 78.9 per cent of the angle fractures were single fractures (Fig. 18–15). Fractures involving only the supporting bone of the teeth were found in 6.7 per cent. Most alveolar fracture lines were in the region of the anterior teeth. Ramal fractures were infrequent, occurring in only 5.4 per cent (Fig. 18–16). Midline fractures likewise were rare (2.9 per cent), and in over half the cases were associated with other mandibular fractures.

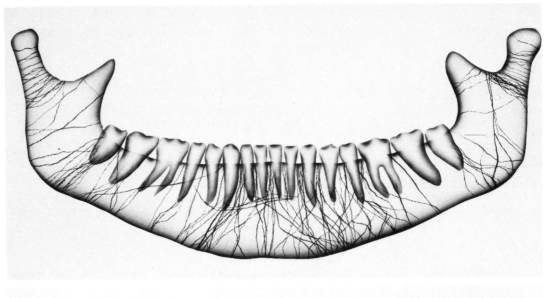

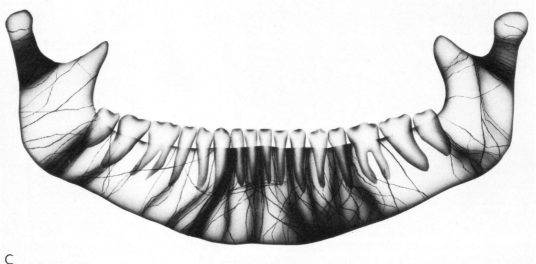

C

Figure 18–11 (*Continued.*) *C,* Fractures from accidents at work.

(*Figure 18–11 continued on opposite page*)

When all the cases are considered, the frequency of fracture lines in the left side of the mandible exceeds the frequency in the right side by about 10 per cent.

DIAGNOSIS OF FRACTURES

In diagnosing fractures of the mandible, maxilla, zygomatic bone, zygomatic arch, and nasal bones, the following sources of information should be utilized: history, symptoms, visual examination, digital examination, radio-graphic examination, and classification of the fracture or fractures.

Symptoms, Oral and Digital Examination. Fractures of the mandible and maxilla exhibit the symptoms described in the paragraphs below.

Malocclusion of the teeth may be markedly incorrect for the individual patient, or the alignment of the teeth may be abnormally irregular. This condition is usually associated with a history of trauma, such as a blow, an accident, or a fall.

Fragments may be moved individually, as discovered by manipulation.

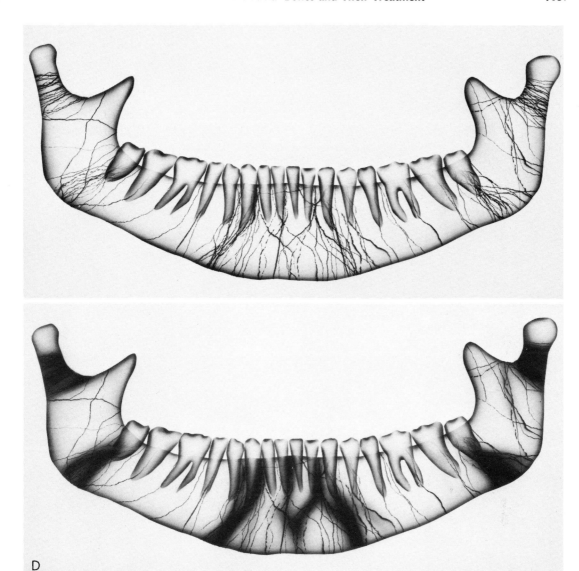

Figure 18-11 (*Continued.*) *D,* Fractures from other causes. (*Top illustrations,* From Oikarinen, V. J., and Malmström, M.: Jaw fractures. Suom. Hammaslääk. Toim., *65*:95, 1969.)

Crepitation—grating noises when the fractured ends rub together during the movements of mastication, talking or swallowing, or when they are manipulated—is present.

There is evidence of impaired function, such as inability to chew food.

The patient complains of tenderness and pain on movement of the jaw, as in eating and talking.

Movements of occlusal and incisal surfaces of teeth are observed when the patient opens and closes his mouth, or abnormal movements of the jaws and teeth occur in the fracture area when closing and opening the mouth.

Facial deformity is present, especially with fractures of the maxilla or zygomatic bone.

There are swelling and discoloration of overlying soft tissues. This is not always associated with fractures but should arouse suspicion.

Ecchymosis of the soft tissues about the jaws or the neck or about the orbital cavity is observed. This is frequently seen with a fracture of the zygomatic or nasal bones.

There is numbness of the lower lip or cheek.

Diplopia is usually indicative of a change in position of the globe due to changes in the shape of the orbit following displaced fractures of the bones forming the orbital walls.

Most fractures of the facial bones involve suture lines, particularly around the orbit, and

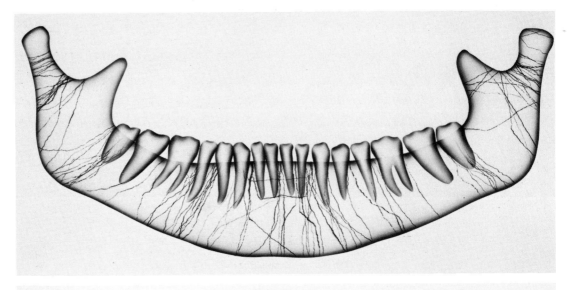

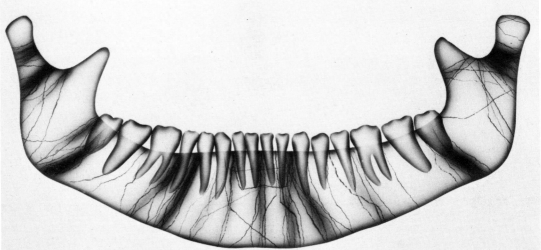

Figure 18–12   The mandibular fracture lines in females. (From Oikarinen, V. J., and Malmström, M.: Jaw fractures. Suom. Hammaslääk. Toim., *65*:95, 1969.)

consequently a typical pattern of palpable irregularity can usually be identified.

The bony contours of the nose and facial bones can be readily palpated externally and comparisons can be made between the two sides. With the examining finger inside the mouth, the contours of the alveolar processes of the upper and lower jaws can be identified and compared.

Interference with motions of the mandible may be the result of impingement on the coronoid process by the medially displaced zygomatic arch.

Abnormal mobility of the mandible may be indicative of fractures of the body, the ramus, or the condylar processes.

After inquiring into all subjective symptoms of fracture, and noting the objective symptoms, the x-ray examination is made.

Radiographic Examination.   The Committee on Trauma of the American College of Surgeons makes the following observations on roentgenographic examination for facial injuries:

"It is unwise to rush the patient to the x-ray department until a possible concomitant major injury (skull or cervical spine), which would make movement of the patient hazardous, has been evaluated. Complete roentgenograms should be obtained, however, when the patient's condition permits. Special views must be obtained for accurate diagnosis of

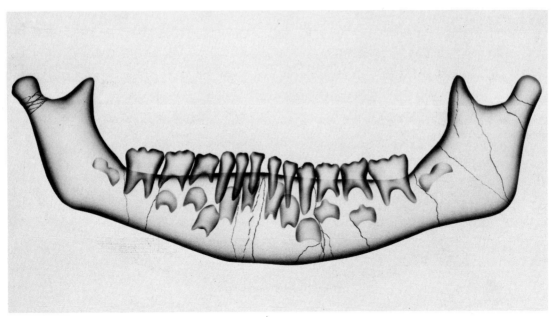

Figure 18–13 The mandibular fracture lines in children. (From Oikarinen, V. J., and Malmström, M.: Jaw fractures. Suom. Hammaslääk. Toim., *65*:95, 1969.)

facial bone injuries. In spite of proper roentgenograms, fractures of thin bones, such as the maxilla, ethmoid, and nasal bones, can be missed because of superimposition of shadows. **Usually, the bony injury is more severe than is indicated by roentgenographic examination.**

"The following roentgenographic views are recommended:

1. Lower jaw: lateral, oblique, and posteroanterior. Include additional views of the condyles.
2. Nasal bones: lateral views taken with soft tissue technique.
3. Facial bones of the central third of the face: stereo-Waters' view with horizontal shift; submento-occipital view to show zygomatic arches in relief; stereoscopic views to clarify superimposed bony shadows; tomography when necessary

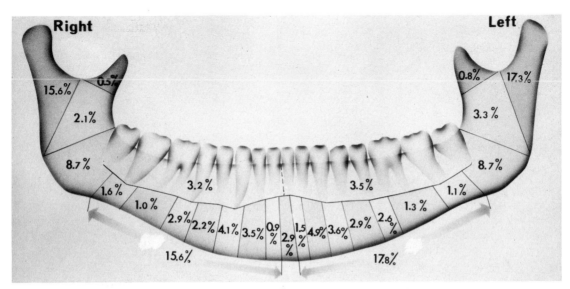

Figure 18–14 Frequency of fractures in various anatomic regions of the mandible. (Adapted from Oikarinen, V. J., and Malmström, M.: Jaw fractures. Suom. Hammaslääk. Toim., *65*:95, 1969.)

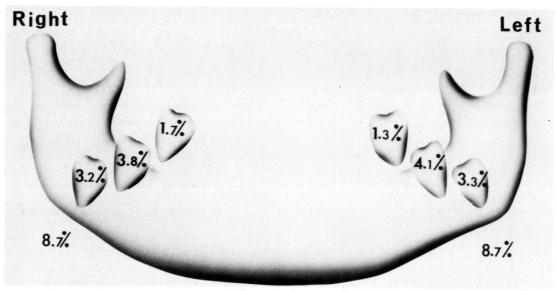

Figure 18–15   Frequency of angular fractures, depending on the positions of "wisdom" teeth.

to clarify orbital floor and condylar fractures.

"In viewing the roentgenogram, the principal things to look for are: (*a*) comparative size of the antra, (*b*) discontinuity of the antral wall, (*c*) clouding of one or both antra, indicating fracture with hemorrhage, (*d*) irregularity of the floor of the orbit, (*e*) irregularity of the orbital rim, (*f*) difference in distance between the coronoid and malar bones, (*g*)

fracture of the zygomatic arch, and (*h*) separation of the frontomalar suture line."*

Specifically, the radiographic examination should include several different views. Right

---

*Committee on Trauma, American College of Surgeons: Early Care of the Injured Patient, p. 114. Philadelphia, W. B. Saunders Co., 1972. Reprinted by permission.

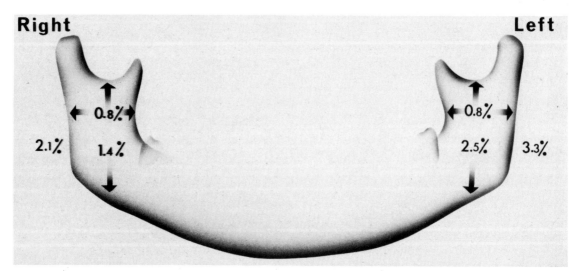

Figure 18–16   Ramal fractures, divided into vertical and horizontal groups.

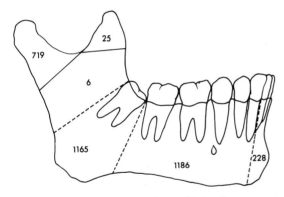

Figure 18-17 A survey of mandibular fractures at Bellevue Hospital from 1948 to 1974. (Courtesy of David E. Kelly, D.D.S., Assistant Professor, Oral Surgery, University of North Carolina, Chapel Hill.)

and left lateral (oblique) views of the mandible (see Figure 17–23 for technique) will reveal fractures in the ramus, at the angle, and in the body of the mandible up to the mental foramen area. A panoramic radiograph is most helpful and should be taken whenever the equipment is available.

The mandible in *PA* (posteroanterior) projection (see Figure 17–22) reveals any lateral or medial displacement of fractures of the ramus or body of the mandible (horizontal ramus) or fractures of the symphysis, *although intraoral periapical and occlusal views should always be taken of the mandible and teeth also* (see Figures 18–18, 18–19, 18–33, 18–34 and 18–118).

Fractures of the necks of the condyles may be shown or suspected from the *PA* view of the mandible (Fig. 17–22). However, an *AP* (anteroposterior) Towne projection (Fig. 17–20) or a reverse *PA* Towne projection (Fig. 17–21) are much better views to reveal fractures and displacement of the necks of the condyles.

The zygomatic bones and zygomatic arches are best shown by the *AP* Towne position (see Figure 17–19). The individual zygomatic arches, however, are usually best visualized in separate radiographs using the technique shown in Figures 17–11, 17–24, and 17–25.

Fractures of the maxilla, zygomatic, nasal, vomer and perpendicular plate of the ethmoid are best shown by the *PA* (Waters') view of the skull (see Figure 17–13). Additional information can be obtained from the basal view technique shown in Figure 17–12. In addition, an intraoral maxillary occlusal radiograph and periapical radiographs should be taken (Figs. 18–18 and 18–19).

The reader is urged at this point to review Chapter 17, "Roentgen Anatomy of the Facial Bones and Jaws."

TREATMENT PLANNING FOR FRACTURE MANAGEMENT

General Considerations. When the patient's physical condition so indicates, the necessary consultations should be obtained, such as those of an internist, neurosurgeon, ophthalmologist, otolaryngologist, or plastic surgeon.

These patients have often been in a severe accident and have had a severe mental and physical shock, possibly including other fractures or internal injuries. In severe injuries the operative procedures used to reduce fractures are delayed until the patient recovers sufficiently, and only emergency work is done first.

Brain damage, injuries to the chest and abdomen, cervical spine injuries, and major fractures take priority in treatment. Remember, however, that *the sooner fractures are reduced, the better the end result.* In the average fracture case without major complications, if circumstances permit, fractures of the jaws should receive definitive treatment within the first 24 hours after injury. The patient is immediately more comfortable after the bones have been stabilized, and the chances of infection are reduced. The time for specific operative procedures and the type of anesthesia to be used are problems which are the joint concern of the oral surgeon, medical and surgical consultants and the anesthesiologist.

After the patient's condition has been stabilized, the work of fracture management can begin. The examiner must consider the extent of injury to the soft tissues such as cheeks, lips, muscles, mucosa, tongue and other parts. He must also consider how much displacement has occurred and the kind of deformity produced. By making a thorough examination, he must determine: (a) the number, locations and types of fractures; (b) the position of the fragments and their relationships to each other; (c) the number of teeth present, their condition and their distribution; (d) the action of muscular pull on the various fragments (see below and Figures 18–20 to 18–25). *This examination must be done carefully.*

In fractures of the multiple bones compris-

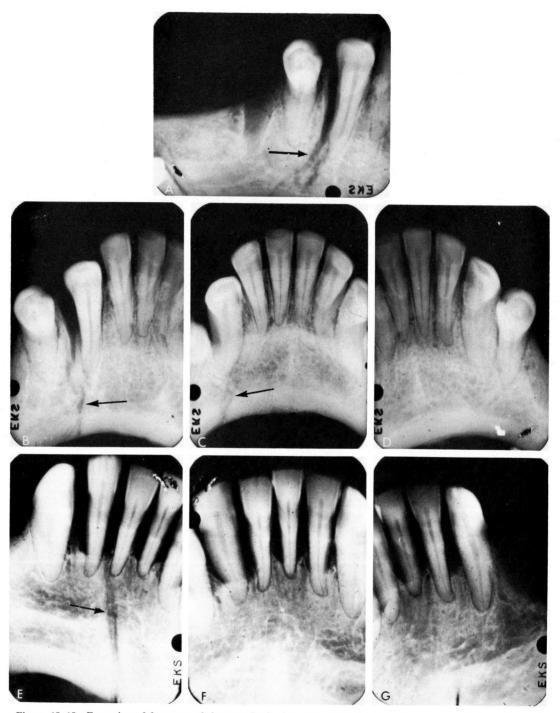

Figure 18–18 Examples of fractures of the symphysis that were not evident on the posteroanterior radiographs. Both periapical and occlusal views should *always* be taken when making a radiographic survey of the mandible to discover fractures.

(Figure 18–18 continued on opposite page)

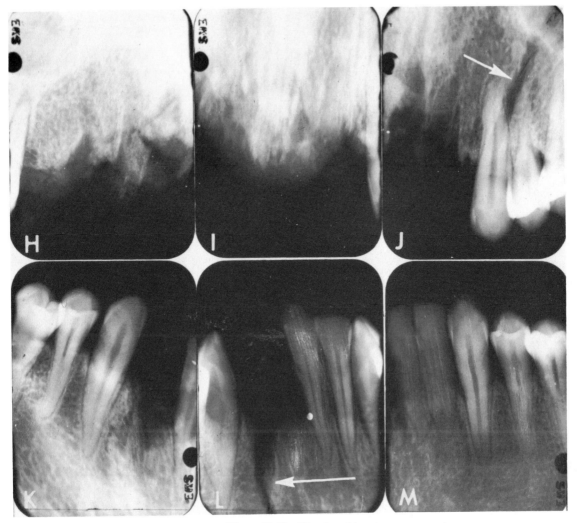

Figure 18–18   *(Continued.)*

ing the fragments of the middle third of the face, displacement is produced by the trauma itself and not by the pull of attached muscles, except for the buccinator and the masseter on the zygomatic arch. On the other hand, in mandibular fractures, the fragments can be displaced by the action of the very powerful muscles of mastication. Consequently, in reduction of fractures of the middle third of the face, the displaced bones are returned to their original position and held in place against the minimal elasticity of the soft tissues of the face and against the force of gravity, while in reduction and fixation of the mandibular fractures, appropriate splinting must be applied to counteract the pull of the powerful muscles of mastication.

ANESTHESIA FOR REDUCTION AND IMMOBILIZATION OF FRACTURES OF THE FACIAL BONES

OTTO C. PHILLIPS, M.D.

General Management. Vital signs (blood pressure, pulse, respiration) should be monitored for all patients treated for fractures of the facial bones. It is also wise to have a needle or catheter in a vein with an intravenous infusion running. Adverse reactions can occur with any type of drug or anesthesia. In addition, the trauma associated with reduction of a fracture can lead to reflex autonomic nervous system responses, impingement on the airway, or bleeding. The proposed precautions can help the attendants to

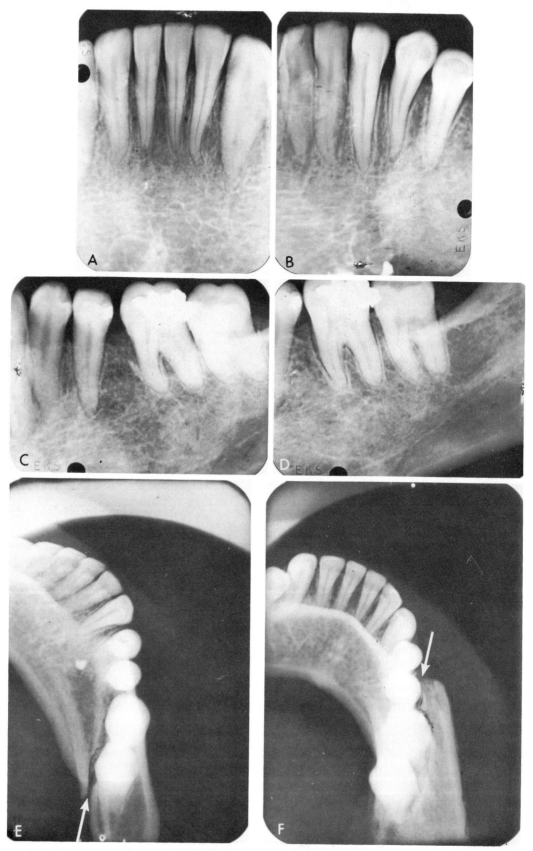

Figure 18–19   *See opposite page for legend.*

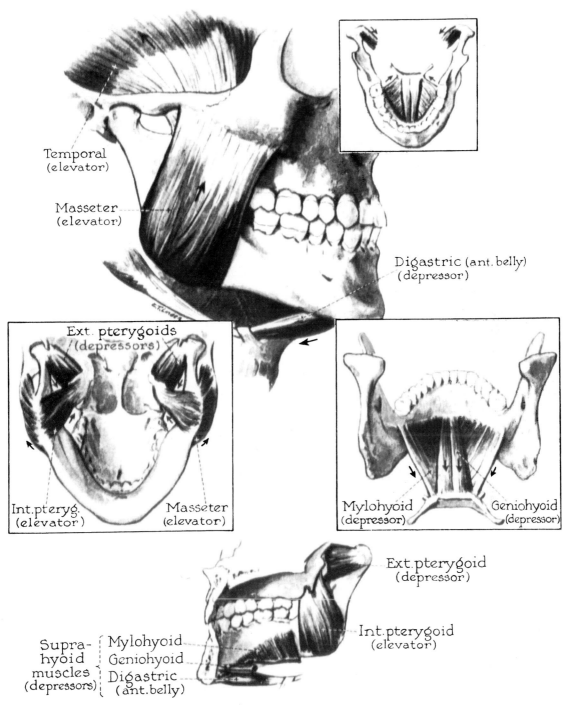

Figure 18–20 Muscles of the mandible. (From Massler, M., and Schour, I.: Atlas of the Mouth and Adjacent Parts in Health and Disease. Chicago, American Dental Association.)

Figure 18–19 The series of intraoral periapical radiographs (*A* to *D*) does not disclose the slightest sign of the oblique fracture that is clearly seen in the occlusal films (*E* and *F*) that were slightly altered by changing the central x-ray when the radiographs were made. This clearly demonstrates the necessity for taking a complete variety of both intraoral and extraoral views. Findings in the latter films were also negative in this case. The type of fracture shown here is well illustrated by the drawing in Figure 18–26C.

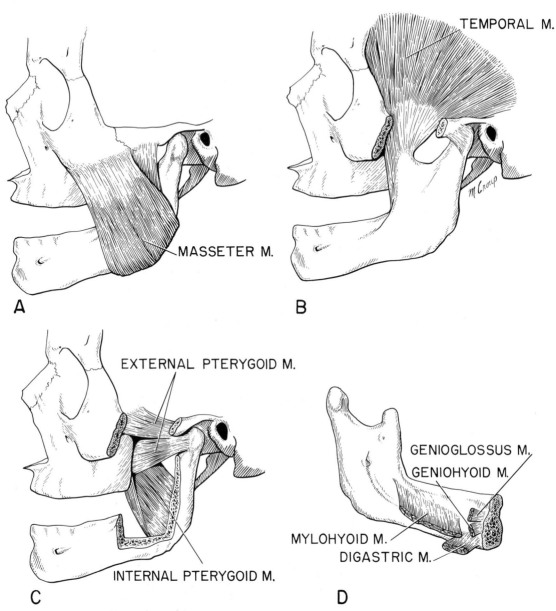

Figure 18–21 Muscular pull on various parts of the mandible and maxilla.

apprehend quickly any problem, and treatment can be instituted promptly.

Regional Anesthesia. Nerve blocks and local infiltration may offer adequate anesthesia and are frequently used. The attendant should be aware of the maximum safe dosage of the drug used and restrict his dose to this amount. Most reactions to local anesthetics are related to overdose; this may lead to central nervous system and cardiovascular complications and may accentuate systemic problems already existing. Regional anesthetic techniques are usually not adequate for re-

duction of fractures of the maxilla or for compound comminuted fractures of the mandible with a marked displacement.

General Anesthesia. Just as consideration of the patient's total physical condition is important in planning treatment of facial fractures, it is even more important before proceeding with general anesthesia. Little may be accomplished if fractures are successfully reduced with the aid of general anesthetic agents which in turn accentuate hypotension resulting from a bleeding viscus, or if positive-pressure breathing leads to a tension

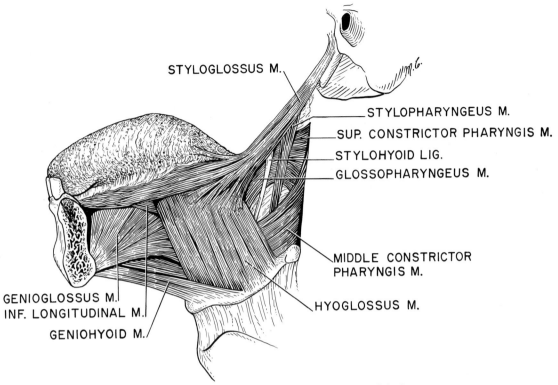

STYLOGLOSSUS M.

STYLOPHARYNGEUS M.

SUP. CONSTRICTOR PHARYNGIS M.

STYLOHYOID LIG.

GLOSSOPHARYNGEUS M.

MIDDLE CONSTRICTOR
PHARYNGIS M.

HYOGLOSSUS M.

GENIOGLOSSUS M.
INF. LONGITUDINAL M.

GENIOHYOID M.

Figure 18–22 Muscular pull on various sections of the jaw.

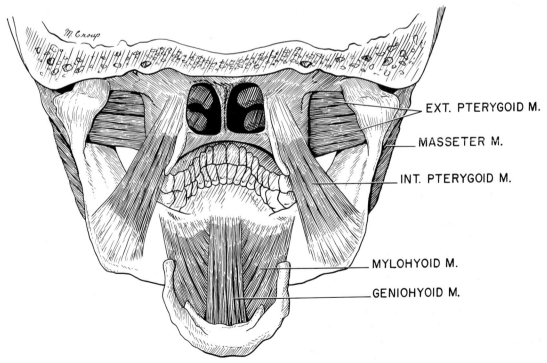

EXT. PTERYGOID M.

MASSETER M.

INT. PTERYGOID M.

MYLOHYOID M.

GENIOHYOID M.

Figure 18–23 Muscular pull on various parts of the jaw.

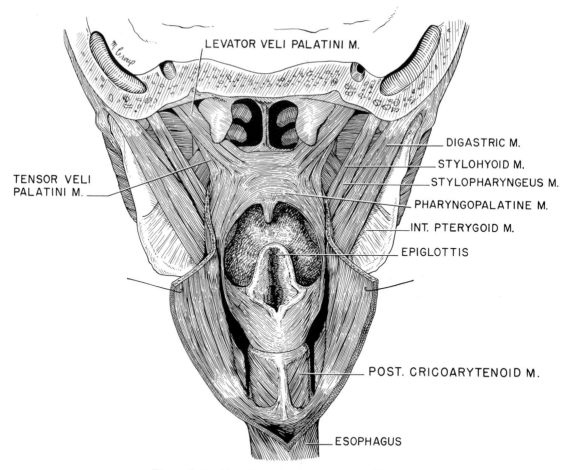

LEVATOR VELI PALATINI M.

DIGASTRIC M.

STYLOHYOID M.

STYLOPHARYNGEUS M.

PHARYNGOPALATINE M.

TENSOR VELI
PALATINI M.

INT. PTERYGOID M.

EPIGLOTTIS

POST. CRICOARYTENOID M.

ESOPHAGUS

Figure 18–24   Muscular pull on various parts of the jaw.

pneumothorax associated with a fractured rib. Just as general anesthesia affects the whole patient, the total effect of anesthesia on the patient must be considered.

Again, a patent airway is the first consideration in the emergency care of these patients; it is also the first consideration when preparing for general anesthesia for definitive treatment. It is often wise to insure an adequate airway by inserting a cuffed endotracheal tube under topical anesthesia before systemic drugs are given either intravenously or by inhalation. Otherwise, with induction of general anesthesia in these patients, partial obstruction may become complete and a previously good airway may become obstructed. When possible, the type of tube and the route of placement are adapted to the needs of the surgeon and a position is chosen that will least interfere with his work. A nasotracheal tube is usually chosen for treatment of fractures of the mandible, while an orotracheal

tube is preferable for fractures of the maxilla alone or for combinations of mandibular, nasal, and zygomatic bone fractures. If undue pressure or manipulation is anticipated, an anode tube (coiled wire embedded in rubber) offers the most secure airway.

A cuffed tracheostomy may be indicated when there are extensive trauma and edema of the neck causing preoperative impairment of the airway, or when these problems are extensive enough that an endotracheal tube would be necessary for many hours or even days beyond the termination of the operative procedure. Inhalation anesthesia machines and equipment can be adapted to most current tracheostomy tubes for institution and maintenance of anesthesia or for support of respirations.

The choice and selection of anesthetic drugs is not nearly as important as the establishment and maintenance of an airway. The insertion of an endotracheal tube under

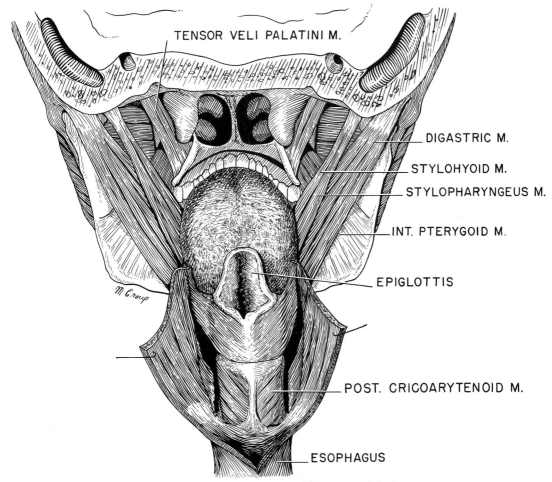

TENSOR VELI PALATINI M.

DIGASTRIC M.

STYLOHYOID M.

STYLOPHARYNGEUS M.

INT. PTERYGOID M.

EPIGLOTTIS

POST. CRICOARYTENOID M.

ESOPHAGUS

Figure 18–25 Muscular pull on various parts of the jaw.

topical anesthesia in a patient already severely traumatized is obviously not very comfortable. Once the proper position of the tube is assured, therefore, an intravenous barbiturate (Pentothal, Surital) can be injected into the existing intravenous infusion in a dose adequate to produce unconsciousness. Anesthesia can then be maintained with inhalation agents (nitrous oxide, halothane) and/or intravenous narcotics, and supplemented with a muscle relaxant (succinylcholine, curare).

TEETH IN THE LINE OF FRACTURE

The question of the retention of teeth in the line of fracture is one which, so far as the author is concerned, must be decided for each individual case. As a general rule, however, it is the author's policy to retain the teeth in the line of fracture as long as the teeth can serve some purpose in the reduction and immobilization of the fracture. The author has saved many teeth that were in the line of fracture, particularly bicuspids and anterior teeth. Simply because a tooth is in the line of fracture does not prove that this tooth will become a source of infection. It is true that a good percentage of posterior teeth do become sources of infection, but a much smaller percentage of anterior teeth become sources of infection. In Figure 18–40 the molar was removed at the end of 4 weeks, but the bicuspids were retained permanently.

TEETH ON THE FRACTURE LINE IN THE JAWS

Ricardo Cuestas Carnero, Prof. Dr. med.

One aspect of the treatment of jaw fractures that is still controversial concerns the teeth within the fracture area.

In spite of the positive assertions in which such outstanding authors as Clark, Ivy, Maurel, Reichembach and Thoma have prescribed the extraction of teeth approximating the fracture line, I must disagree with them, at least in part, as have Archer, Brachmann, Eudokimow, Guralnick, Kole, Kruger, Rowe and others who decide each case on its merits. My opinions are based on my experiences with 72 cases of maxillary and mandibular factures at surgical clinics and the second oral surgery course at the Córdoba National University in Argentina; in the Department of Oral Surgery, Córdoba Hospital; and in my private practice. In addition, I find that Müller has reported on 989 cases at the Halle Clinic,[126] Eudokimow (mentioned by Müller) on 314, and Dechaume and associates on 130.[39]

Fundamentally, I do not agree with the routine extraction of teeth within the fracture area. There should be a thorough study of their vitality, condition and location. The advantages of conservation should be weighed in each case against the disadvantages, and the decision based on the optimal future result in the jaw.

By way of introducing concepts and definitions, I should mention that, just as Lucas Gonzalez does,[61] I call the pieces into which the bone is divided as a consequence of the fracture "fragments of fracture"; the extremes next to the injury are then "fractured bone ends." The "fracture lines" are the radiographic images of the different edges that form the fractured bone ends. The "fractured area" is composed of the surfaces of the fractured bone ends, the blood collected among them, the teeth approximating the fracture line, and involved structures (the periosteum, the neurovascular bundle and the surrounding soft tissues). (See Figure 18–26A).

Teeth are often related to at least one of the surfaces of a fractured jaw bone and are therefore involved in the fracture area. Because of the resorption of bone ends, they become part of the healing site itself. Like Ackermann and Pompians-Miniac,[1] we can discuss both the advantages and the disadvantages of the presence of teeth in a fracture area.

The disadvantages are those involving pathologic processes. These unfavorable effects include allowing the entrance of microorganisms, or the movement of pre-existing ones from the periapical area (e.g., in chronic gingivitis), into the fracture area. This finally produces infection in the area, thus delaying the healing.

However, the presence of teeth may also be advantageous in preventing shifting and sliding of fragments of fracture. This is true particularly in fractures of the angle, where a tooth may act as a pin between two fragments. (See Figure 18–26B.) Additionally, the isolated tooth in a fragment of fracture can help to maintain the patient's occlusion, which ultimately may permit complete restoration of function.

My tendency is toward conservative treatment in most cases in which teeth related to the fractured area are concerned. My procedure is based on certain conditions.

First, I think that the only danger that exists when we leave a tooth in the fracture area is infection, and I believe that the therapeutic means we have today enable us to prevent and fight against infection.

Second, I believe it is potentially more dangerous to extract a tooth and allow wide communication of the fracture area with the oral cavity, even if the tooth is nonvital, whether as a consequence of trauma or of a pre-existing pathologic process. In those cases, endodontic and other treatments may overcome the problems inherent in retention of a nonvital tooth.

Third, I do not agree with the authors that advise the "prophylactic extraction" of teeth with several roots because of the difficulties in treating these endodontically. Specialists in this field have been able to obtain noteworthy results even in these cases.

Fourth, I also disagree with those who apply "prophylactic extraction" based on the "traumatic injury" suffered by the dental pulp, because I have observed that the dental pulp sometimes recovers from this injury. Even when it fails to survive, it usually remains without producing any infection during the period of time it takes the fracture to heal, after which endodontic treatment may be carried out.

Fifth, I have had the opportunity of observing patients treated by colleagues who insist on extraction and have noted that their luxation of the tooth, particularly in the

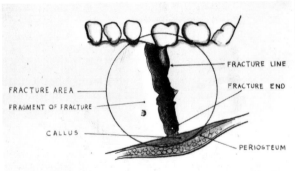

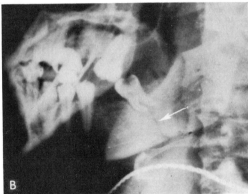

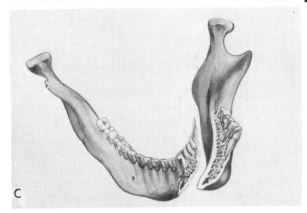

Figure 18–26   Teeth on the fracture line in the mandible. *A* to *C*, See text for details. *D*, Fracture of the mandible, with the second bicuspid on the line of fracture. *E*, Six months after removal of the splints. The second bicuspid is normal and vital. *F*, Fracture through the angle of the mandible, with the third molar on the line of fracture. *G*, Eight months after removal of the splints. Note that the third molar roots that were partially formed in *F* are now completely formed and the tooth is vital.

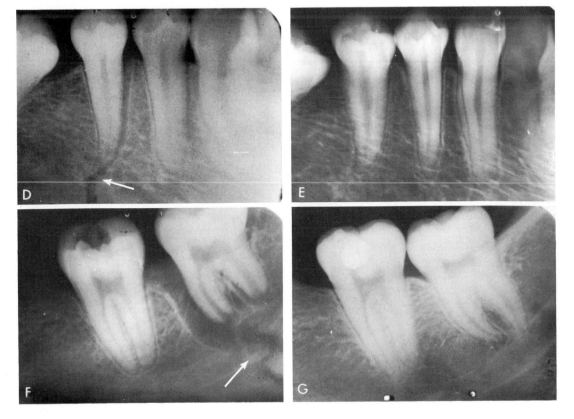

region of the mandibular third molar, resulted in the displacement of the posterior fragment. This forces the surgeon to use extraoral means of treatment or intraosseous wire fixation.

Sixth, the space left by the extracted tooth may be the starting point of an imperfection in the immobilization of the fragments, or it may produce secondary displacements, which are sometimes difficult to correct. The fracture lines are not always vertical, and they may even be horizontal in many cases.

The part of the fracture line that affects the external cortex of bone may also be related to a tooth, while the inner line may be related to another tooth or other teeth. (See Figure 18–26C.) These latter teeth may also have injuries or periapical lesions that are in the fracture area.

If we follow the counsel of those who advise extraction because "the naked root allows infection to reach the interfragmentary area," we may then find that we must extract a good number of teeth from bony segments in comminuted fractures of the jaw. This results in the loss of much bone. Among the consequences we must not forget the prosthetic future of the patient, as we considerably diminish the height of his alveolar ridges.

Seventh, in some cases I might accept the advice of the French authors who indicate a delayed extraction when the callus is being established, in order to produce an "osseous crystallization."[1] This procedure must not be routine and must be used only when the problem cannot be resolved by one of the means already mentioned.

Eighth, I must point out that the so-called pathologic fractures—i.e., those produced when there is a predisposing cause—are not considered here, since special problems arise.

Ninth, I accept extraction when the teeth involved are hopelessly mobile or otherwise complicate reduction of the fracture, for example, those with advanced periodontal disease. Only teeth decidedly useless for the fixation and stabilization procedures should be extracted. I must emphasize that in some cases, teeth that have been displaced have been replaced because they would be very useful for the recovery of occlusion or to guide in the future reconstruction of alveolar ridges.

Tenth, though it may be deduced by the points already discussed, I want to emphasize that the teeth that do remain, even those in the fracture area, may in many cases bring about the use of easier methods, thus making it possible even to avoid surgical intervention and its risks, troublesome postoperative complications and prolonged hospitalization of the patient.

In Figure 18–26D to G two cases are presented that will reinforce my stance.

In conclusion, teeth related to the fracture area must be preserved under the following conditions:

1. Long-term radiographic follow-up must always be performed, with special attention to monitoring the pulp's vitality, its evolution if it is a growing element or its contribution to periapical infection if it dies. In the latter case endodontic treatment is indicated.

2. Antibiotic treatment, without exception, must be carried out, since this is an area in which the constant menace of oral sepsis exists. Most jaw fractures cause a tearing of the oral mucous membrane, thus opening an access for penetration of saliva through the wound to the fracture area itself. This is why we disagree with those who have recommended retention of teeth on the fracture line without simultaneous antibiotic therapy.*

3. Strict oral hygiene for all patients must be enforced, particularly during the immobilization period. This must be taken into account, since the majority of patients have had very poor hygienic habits.

4. Every tooth that can be proved to be vital must be preserved, while radiographic vigilance and restoration of damaged crowns are simultaneously carried out.

5. If, after a reasonable amount of time, a tooth is proved to be nonvital, endodontic therapy must be instituted.

6. Radiographic examination should also be used to follow those teeth that had already undergone endodontic treatment prior to fracture, thus guarding against periapical infections.

7. For teeth with pre-existing periapical infection, endodontic treatment must be started as soon as the immobilization

---

*AUTHOR'S NOTE: However, it must be noted that the extraction of teeth also permits the invasion of bacteria into the alveolus, and the routine postextraction use of antibiotics is not universally accepted as necessary or desirable unless there are specific indications. (See Chapter 8.)

procedures will allow it. As a last resort, delayed extraction may be utilized.

8. When the apical third of the tooth is fractured, we advise conservation of the tooth, with endodontic treatment and apicoectomy, if indicated, after healing of the fracture.

TREATMENT OF MANDIBULAR FRACTURES

As explained earlier, fractures of the mandible may be single or multiple, unilateral or bilateral. Figures 18–27 to 18–29 illustrate some of the types and locations of fractures

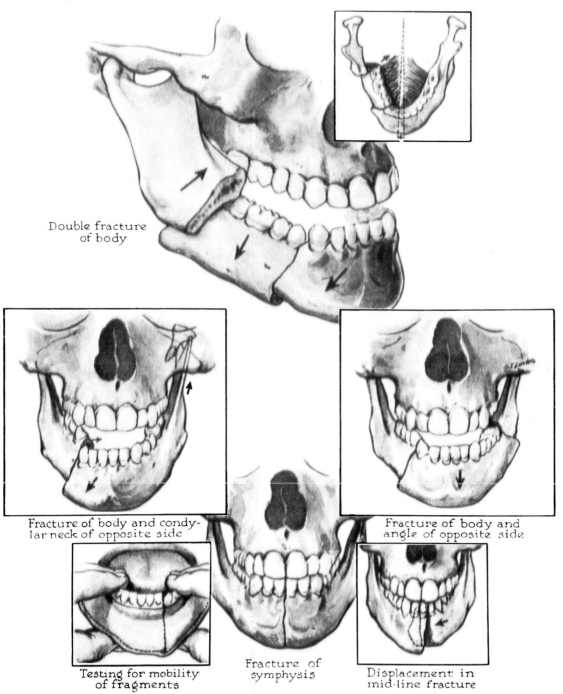

Double fracture of body

Fracture of body and condy- lar neck of opposite side

Fracture of body and angle of opposite side

Testing for mobility of fragments

Fracture of symphysis

Displacement in mid-line fracture

Figure 18–27   Multiple fractures of the mandible. (From Massler, M., and Schour, I.: Atlas of the Mouth and Adjacent Parts in Health and Disease. Chicago, American Dental Association.)

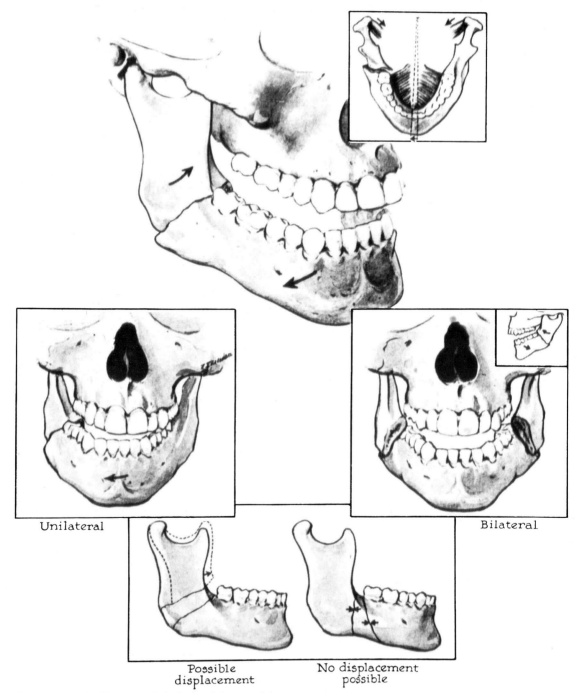

Figure 18–28   Fractures of the body of the mandible. (From Massler, M., and Schour, I.: Atlas of the Mouth and Adjacent Parts in Health and Disease. Chicago, American Dental Association.)

of the mandible. The methods of treatment of these fractures are discussed in the following sections.

ARCH BARS AND INTERMAXILLARY ELASTICS

This method involves attaching prepared and contoured metal splints, such as the Je- lenko, Winter or Erich, to the necks of both maxillary and mandibular teeth by wires, and then reducing the fracture or fractures and bringing the teeth into normal occlusion by the gradual and steady pull of intermaxillary elas- tics attached to the splints in each jaw. Wher- ever it can be used, it is the treatment of choice.

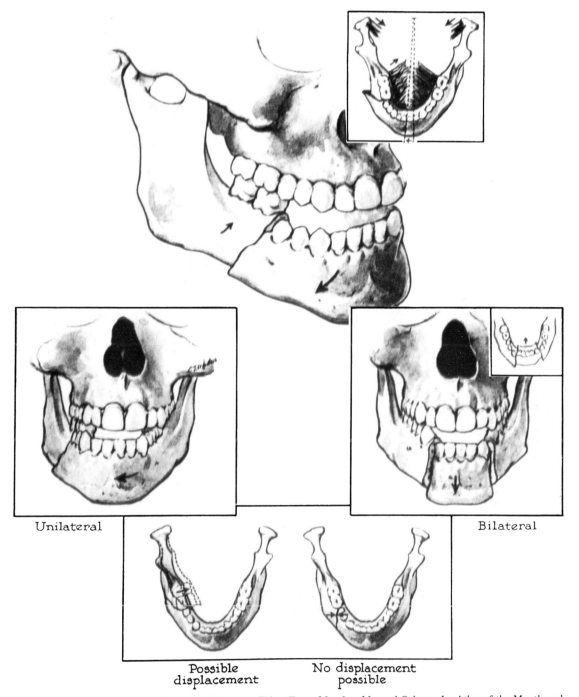

Unilateral   Bilateral

Possible   No displacement
displacement   possible

Figure 18–29 Fractures of the angle of the mandible. (From Massler, M., and Schour, I.: Atlas of the Mouth and Adjacent Parts in Health and Disease. Chicago, American Dental Association.)

Arch Bars Wired to the Teeth. One of the dangers in the application of Jelenko, Winter or Erich splints (see Figure 18–30) is that when these splints are attached to the anterior teeth for reduction of fractures of the symphysis (see Figure 18–31) and intermaxillary elastics are stretched between the maxillary and mandibular splint, the anterior teeth may be extruded by the pull of the intermaxillary elastics, particularly if the splints have been wired to the maxillary or the mandibular central and lateral incisors. The reason for the extrusion is that the anterior teeth do not occlude as do the posterior teeth, nor do they normally strike edge to edge, and so they slide by each other. The technique illustrated

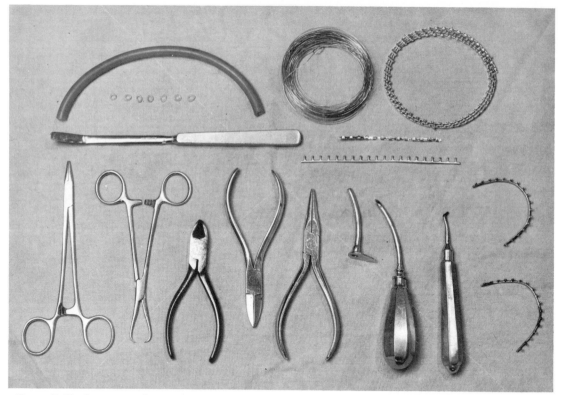

Figure 18–30 Instruments frequently used in immobilization of fractures.

Top row: Rubber tubing and rubber bands cut from it; roll of wire; roll of splint material.

Middle row: Batson Carmody elevator for reduction of a depressed fracture of the zygomatic arch; Erich and Winter arch bars before contouring.

Bottom row: Needle holder used to twist wires; towel clip used in some cases to grasp depressed fractures of the zygomatic arch through the skin and to elevate them; wire cutters; flat-nose and pointed-nose pliers for tightening wires and bending them into the interproximal spaces; cannula and trocar for use in circumferential wiring; band pusher to force wires beneath the cingulum on anterior teeth; contoured Jelenko splints.

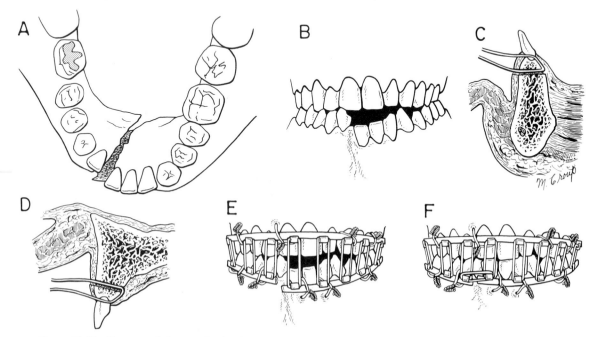

Figure 18–31 Fracture of the symphysis, showing wiring of splints to the maxilla and mandible and application of intermaxillary elastics. Note that the splints in the anterior maxillary and mandibular regions, *C* and *D*, are *wired to bone!* See text for details of technique.

1076

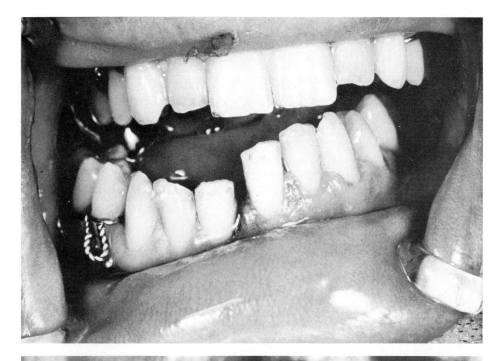

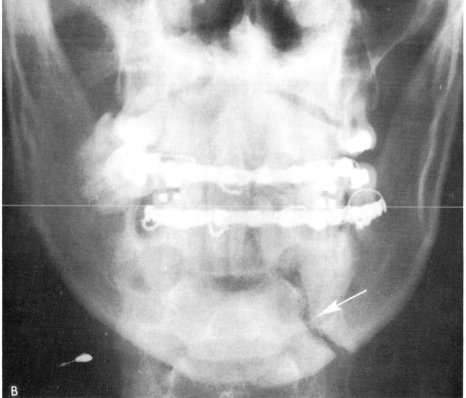

Figure 18–32 Compound fracture of the symphysis of the mandible.

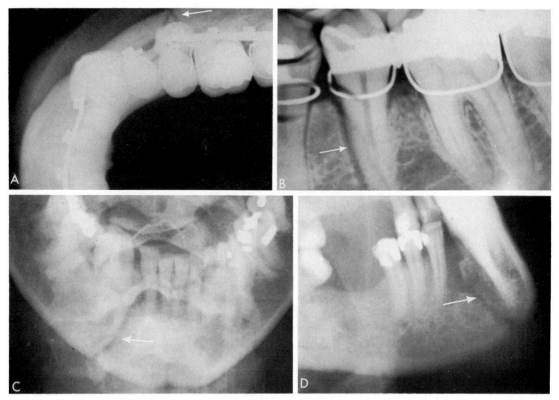

Figure 18–33 *A,* Occlusal radiograph of a simple fracture of the mandible between the bicuspids and through the mental foramen. Splints are wired to the teeth on either side of the fracture line. (For further information on treatment, see Arch Bars and Intermaxillary Elastics.)

B, Periapical radiograph showing the downward and anterior displacement of the distal fragment along the mesial surface of the root of the second bicuspid. We do not remove teeth in the line of fracture unless there is a very specific reason. (See Teeth in the Line of Fracture.)

C, Another example of a fracture of the anterior mandible shown in a posteroanterior radiographic view.

D, Oblique radiograph reveals fracture line in another case.

(Figure 18–33 continued on opposite page)

in Figure 18–31 will prevent this extrusion of the maxillary or mandibular anterior teeth, particularly in those cases in which anterior pull is needed because of a fracture through the symphysis. The fracture line extends between the mandibular right central and lateral incisors (Fig. 18–31*A*), and the left side of the mandible has been pulled downward and inward by the action of the mylohyoid, the anterior belly of the digastricus, the geniohyoid and genioglossus muscles (Fig. 18–31*B*). In such a case, of course, it is necessary to bring the left fragment forward and upward, which means that traction must extend in this direction between the maxillary anterior teeth and the mandibular anterior teeth. In order to prevent extrusion of these teeth, after the splints are wired to the necks of the teeth, in addition to the usual wires which are passed around the necks of the teeth, over the splint, and twisted and turned upward, another

splint retention wire should be added using the method described below.

A spear-point bur whose cutting point is larger than the shank is used to drill a hole 1 cm. above the gingival line through the mucoperiosteal membrane, the labial cortex, the cancellous bone and out through the lingual cortical plate. A wire is now passed through this hole from the labial to the lingual side, brought back through the interproximal space and then twisted over the maxillary splint. This is shown in Figure 18–31*D*. Exactly the same procedure is carried out on the mandible between the central incisors approximately 1 cm. from the gingival line. This hole is drilled through the interseptal bone between the necks of the teeth, as described above. A wire is threaded as shown in Figure 18–31*C*. Figure 18–28*E* shows the wires after they have passed through the soft tissues and bony structure and then have been twisted

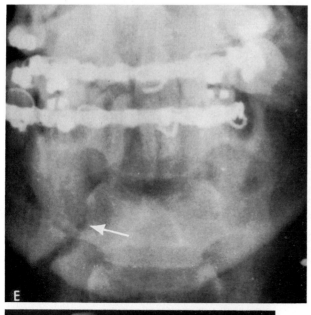

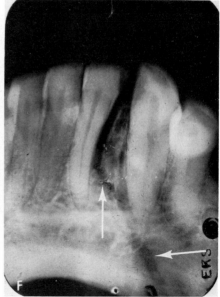

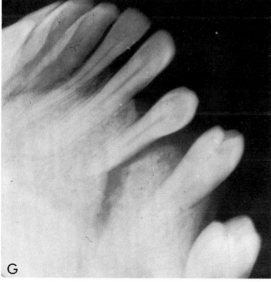

Figure 18–33 *(Continued.)*

E, Another fracture reduced by intermaxillary elastic traction between splints wired to the necks of the teeth in each arch.

F, Periapical view of the fracture shown in *E.*

G, Semiocclusal radiograph of a fracture between the mandibular cuspid and first bicuspid. Tooth in the line of fracture is not extracted. Note that in this case the apex is covered with bone. Even if it were not, we would not remove this tooth.

over the splint in both the mandible and the maxilla. The intermaxillary elastics are shown stretched between the two splints in Figure 18–31*E.* The fracture reduction is shown in Figure 18–31*F.* At the same time the intermaxillary traction is applied, lateral traction is applied between the splints by passing a rubber band across the splint as shown in Figure 18–31*F.* One or more of these small rubber ligatures can be inserted in this manner to bring about the reduction of the lateral displacement between the fragments.

WIRE SUPPORT OF ARCH BARS. When the space between the roots of the maxillary anterior teeth is too small to permit drilling through the alveolar process without damaging the roots of these teeth, then the maxillary arch bar is suspended by a stainless steel wire threaded through a hole in the anterior nasal spine. If this spine is inadequate, the maxillary arch bar is supported with stainless steel wires which have been passed through holes made through the bony margins of the pyriform apertures.

When the space between the mandibular roots is too narrow to permit drilling a hole from the labial to the lingual side without damaging the roots of the mandibular incisors, then the anterior portion of the mandibular arch bar should be immobilized by a

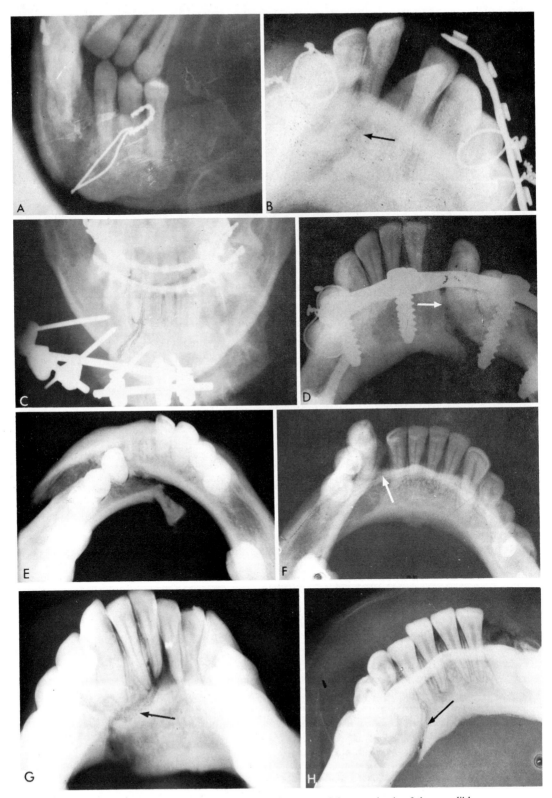

Figure 18–34   Examples of treatment of fractures of the symphysis of the mandible.

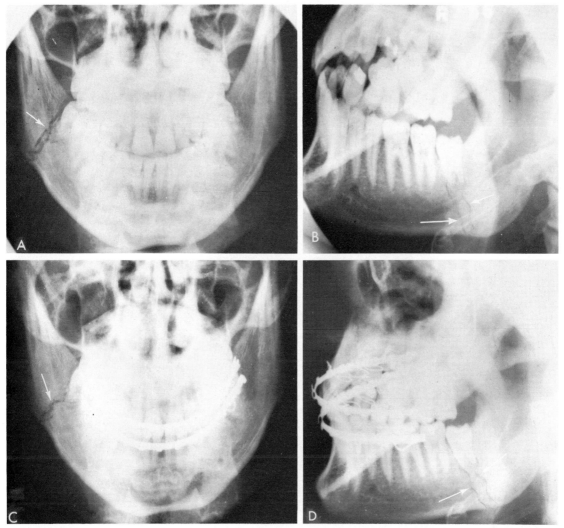

Figure 18–35 *A,* Posteroanterior radiograph of a unilateral simple fracture of the mandible through the region of the partially erupted third molar.

B, Oblique radiograph of the same area.

C and *D,* Fracture stabilized with splints. (See Arch Bars and Intermaxillary Elastics.)

An explanation of the double radiolucent lines is included in the legend for Figure 18–40*D.*

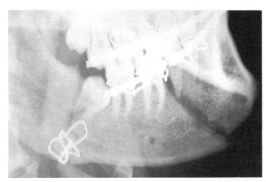

Figure 18–36 Treatment of a compound unilateral double fracture of the left body and angle of the mandible.

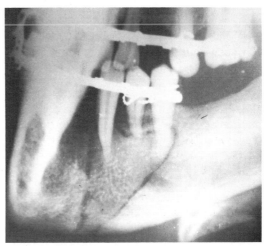

Figure 18–37 Unusual unilateral simple fracture of the body of the mandible, with fracture segments in good alignment.

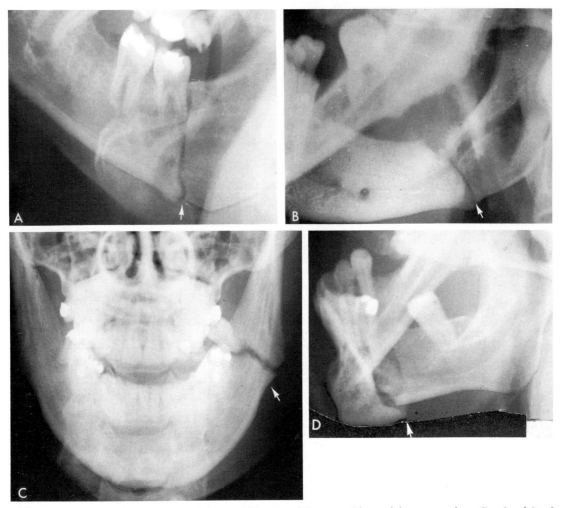

Figure 18–38 Examples of fractures of the mandible. (*E* and *F* are two views of the same patient; *G* to *I* and *J* to *L* are views of two other patients.)

(*Figure 18–38 continued on opposite page*)

mandibular circumferential wire over the arch bar.

Stout's Multiple Loop Wiring. In the place of commercial splints, the Stout method of forming wire loops on both maxillary and mandibular teeth over which intermaxillary elastics can be placed is also a satisfactory method.

Continuous multiple loop interdental wiring is a simple and effective method of satisfying the requirements of intermaxillary elastic fixation. The desirable qualities of a good continuous interdental wiring procedure might include simplicity in technique, minimum instrumentation and the formation of well-shaped, uniformly sized eyelets for elastic rubber band attachment.

On the basis of clinical experience, Kwapis[104] designed an instrument to meet these requirements (see Figure 18–41). The wire ligature carrier and loop former is a modification of a standard needle holder. With this instrument, it is possible for the operator to grasp the wire ligature and pass it between teeth (Fig. 18–41*A*), to hold the wire loop and, with several rotary motions (Fig. 18–41*B*), to create uniform-shaped eyelets (Fig. 18–41*C*) for the placement of intermaxillary elastic traction (Fig. 18–41*D*).

This method of wiring for reduction and fixation of fractures was developed for two reasons: to secure the maximal anchorage for traction and retention and to apply the required treatment as rapidly as possible.

(*Text continued on page 1087*)

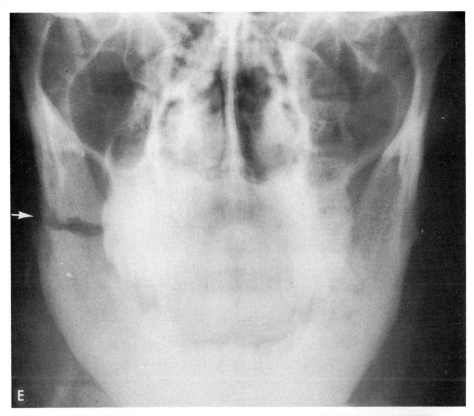

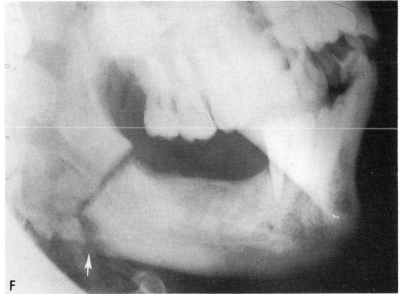

Figure 18–38 *(Continued.)*

(Figure 18–38 continued on following page)

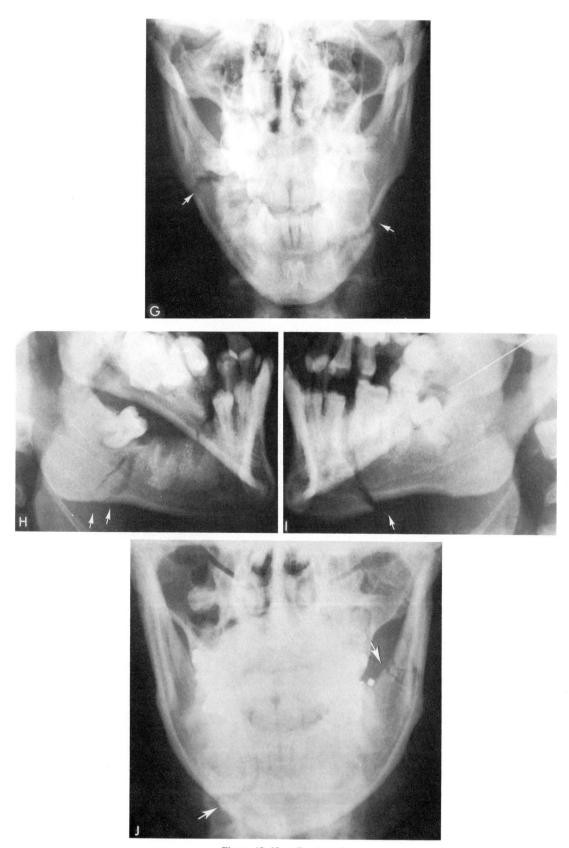

Figure 18-38 *(Continued.)*

(Figure 18-38 continued on opposite page)

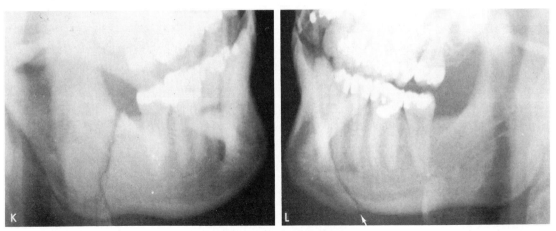

Figure 18–38   *(Continued.)*

Photographic Case Report

SINGLE COMPOUND FRACTURE OF THE MANDIBLE

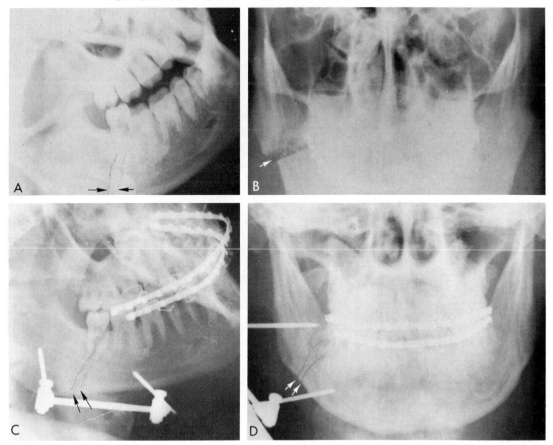

Figure 18–39   *A*, Fracture of the left angle of the mandible through third molar, fracturing the mesial root. Vertical ramus is pulled superiorly and laterally. *B*, Splints applied and occlusion established, but the posterior fragment is still mobile and is in distraction. *C*, Fragments are put into perfect apposition by the insertion of single pins in each fragment that are held together by a connecting bar. *D*, Perfect alignment. After healing, the third molar was extracted.

BILATERAL COMPOUND FRACTURES OF THE MANDIBLE

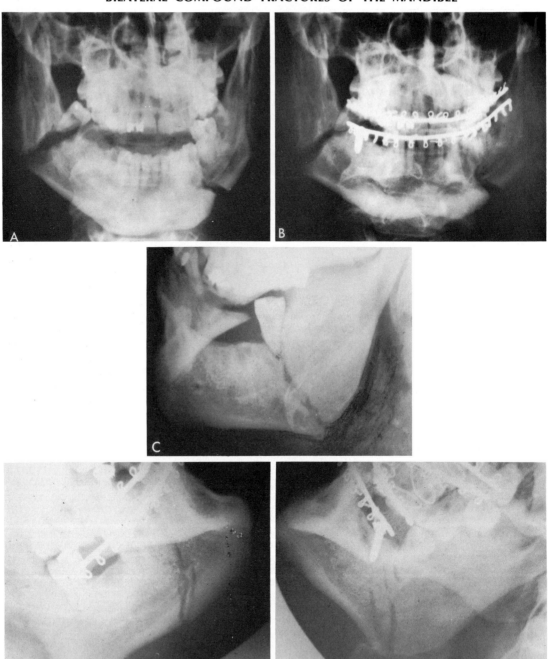

Figure 18–40 *A*, Bilateral compound fracture of the mandible of 6 days' duration. Note the wide separation of the parts due to the combined downward and backward pull of the depressor muscles of the mandible as a result of the prolonged delay in reducing this bilateral fracture. This case also illustrates the typical lines of fracture seen in a large percentage of fractures of the mandible, *e.g.,* through the angle formed by the vertical and horizontal rami and through the third molar socket on the left side; and then between the bicuspids and mental foramen on the right side. In every case of mandibular fracture the possibility of bilateral fractures must be investigated. Not infrequently, fractures of the neck of the condyle are overlooked.

B, There was a good distribution of maxillary and mandibular teeth except in the lower left horizontal ramus (body) of the mandible. There was nothing distal to the lower left first bicuspid except the loose third molar. In order to anchor the Jelenko splint in the molar area a Vitallium screw was inserted into the second molar area. Jelenko splints were wired to the necks of the maxillary and mandibular teeth, and intermaxillary elastics were applied, bringing the teeth into the patient's normal occlusion. As the depressed anterior fragment was pulled up, the mandibular third molar

          (Legend continued on opposite page)

Stainless steel wire (0.16 inch or 0.4064 mm.) is used.

For a stable and satisfactory fixation, we shall consider the application of a single wire with multiple loops to four teeth, from the first molar to the canine. This will require a wire about 9 or 10 inches (about 23 or 25 cm.) in length to engage the four teeth, form three loops, and have the necessary length for twisting the ends together. If more teeth are to be included, a longer wire will be necessary.

TECHNIQUE AND APPLICATION. The wire is first threaded through the interproximal space between the first and secondary molars, from the lingual aspect. The wire is pulled through buccally and forward, along the buccal surface of the teeth as far forward as the lateral incisor, allowing sufficient length for the final twisting of the ends at the mesiolabial angle of the canine. The long lingual end is threaded through the interproximal space mesial to the first molar, passing gingivally to the wire lying along the buccal surface of the teeth. The long end is bent back on itself and is threaded through the same interproximal space, forming a loop encircling the short buccal strand. At this point

the end of the lead wire, gauge 8 and about 2 in. (about 5 cm.) long, is inserted in the loop and held parallel with the buccal wire and in contact with the buccal aspect of the teeth. The lingual wire is now pulled tight, giving the loop its proper form, size, and correct relation to the buccal wire and the teeth. The lingual wire is then threaded through the next interproximal space (between the premolars), passing above the buccal wire and the lead wire; the end again is returned through the same interproximal space, forming the second loop (encircling the lead wire and buccal strand). In the same manner the next loop is made between the first premolar and the canine and the lingual end drawn tight so that the lead wire is held rigidly against the buccal surfaces of the teeth. The lingual wire is now threaded through the interproximal space between the canine and lateral incisor and again drawn tight. Pull is exerted forward (mesially) on the buccal wire, with the same tension as on the other end. This will draw all the loops up to their proper position and give them the desired uniform size. The lead wire is now removed by rotating it slightly and moving it forward. This is easily done by grasping the anterior end with pliers or the fingers.

(Text continued on page 1090)

Figure 18-40 *(Continued.)* came into contact with its opposing member in the maxilla, and this in turn stopped the posterior fragment, thus reducing and immobilizing, to some extent, the fracture. It is apparent here that the apposition of the parts is not ideal, although a satisfactory result was obtained. Today these spaces would be closed by the insertion of a Roger Anderson pin on either side of each fracture and the fragments held in contact with a connecting bar locked to each pin.

C, A left lateral jaw radiograph of the patient in *A* reveals the upward position of the fractured vertical ramus. This view does not reveal the true separation of these fragments because of the overlapping of the fragments resulting from the oblique direction of the x-rays necessary to secure a lateral jaw radiograph. It is also apparent from this radiograph that the only attachment the third molar has is to the distal portion of the alveolar process. This tooth cannot be used to attach a splint, but it may be of help in depressing the posterior fragment at the time of reduction. This patient was treated prior to the introduction of extraoral skeletal fixation.

D, The right reduced side of the fractured mandible shown in *A*. In this particular case the bicuspid teeth were permanently retained, as has been noted. Both of these fractures are on an oblique plane, and so two lines appear on the radiographs, creating the illusion that there are multiple fractures present. (The reader is referred to a fine article by Eli Olech: Fracture lines in the mandible, comparison of radiographic and anatomic findings. Dent. Radiogr. Photogr., *28*(2), 1955.)

E, Lateral radiograph showing the extent to which the posterior fragment was repositioned. It also shows the Vitallium screw that was inserted up to the head and to which the Jelenko splint is attached. A hole smaller in diameter than the screw is first drilled through the cortical bone, with the patient's mouth opened as far as possible. It is impossible to insert the screw vertically because the screwdriver must clear the upper anterior teeth. The farther posteriorly the screw is inserted, the greater the angle at which the screw must, of necessity, be inserted.

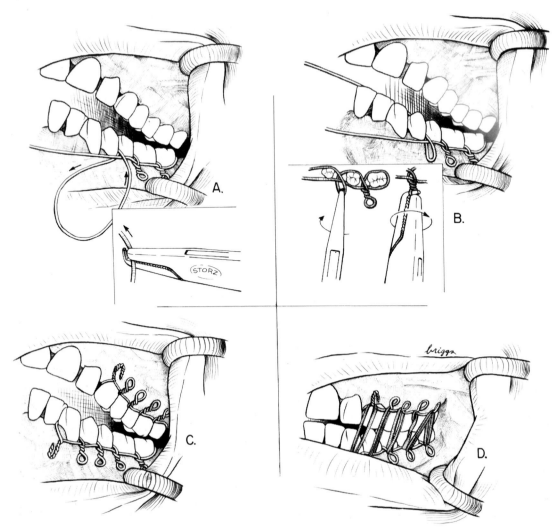

Figure 18–41 Technique for creating eyelets for placement of intermaxillary elastic traction. (From Kwapis, B. S.: Wire ligature carrier for continuous interdental wiring of fractured jaws. J.A.D.A., *69*:700 [Dec.], 1964.)

Case Report No. 1

INTERMAXILLARY ELASTIC TRACTION FOR TREATMENT OF A UNILATERAL FRACTURE OF THE MANDIBLE

This male patient, aged 21, had a unilateral displaced subcondylar fracture of the mandible. Only the right posterior teeth were in occlusion. The posterior fragment was pulled up and the rest of the mandible was pulled down and slightly to the left. Simple intermaxillary fixation, such as is illustrated in Figures 18–43 and 18–44, was the method of treatment.

Operation. General anesthesia was used with this patient. Sufficient relaxation of the jaw elimin-

ated the need for a mouth prop during most of the operation. A suture was passed through the tip of the tongue and tied loosely, and the ends of the suture were clamped with a hemostat. This was done to keep the tongue from falling back into the pharynx and obstructing the airway.

Jelenko splints were contoured to the labial and buccal surfaces of the necks of the maxillary and mandibular teeth. Doubled stainless steel wires were passed about the necks of the upper first bicuspids and molars with the aid of dental floss. The upper splint was then placed in position with the wires emerging from the mesial of the wired teeth placed above the splint and those emerging from the distal below the splint. The splint was retained in position by twisting each pair of wires together. The wires were then cut to a suitable length and their ends bent into the embrasures.

In the lower jaw, wires were passed around the necks of the first bicuspids and first molars and the lower splint was fixed in position in the same manner as described for the upper splint. Intermaxillary rubber bands, cut from fresh rubber tubing, were hooked on the upper and lower splints so as to bring the teeth into occlusion and bring the fragments into apposition and proper alignment.

The suture through the tongue was not removed until the patient had fully recovered from the anesthetic. The patient was returned to his room in good condition.

Postoperative Course. Five weeks later the splints were removed. (In young patients, and where there is a minimum of separation of the fractured parts with no complications, prolonged immobilization is not necessary.)

Photographic Case Report

UNILATERAL COMPOUND FRACTURE OF THE MANDIBLE

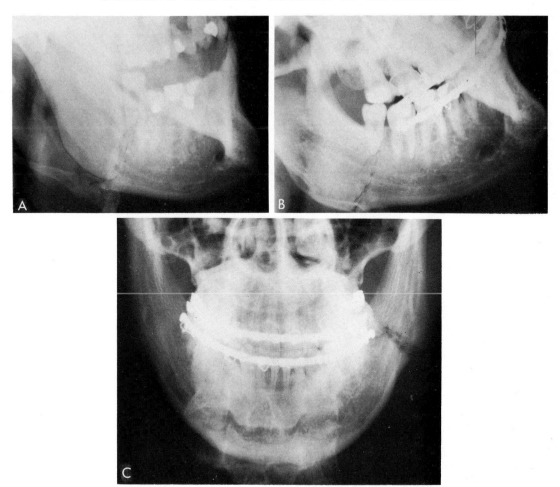

Figure 18–42 *A*, In this unilateral fracture the third molar was contained in the posterior fragment and was surprisingly firm. The anterior fragment was pulled down and the posterior pulled forward and upward. *B*, Fracture reduced and stabilized by intermaxillary elastics. *C*, This view shows good alignment and apposition. In this case it was not necessary to use extraoral pin fixation to reduce and immobilize the fragments.

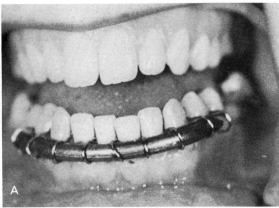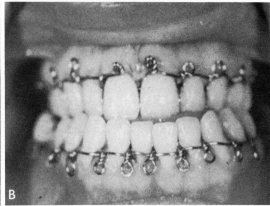

Figure 18–43 *A*, Interproximal wires are shown here after they have been passed around the soft lead wire to form loops. *B*, The lead wire removed and loops twisted; see text for details of technique.

The ends are now grasped with pliers and twisted a few times to stabilize the wire and to bring the twisted portion to rest on the mesiofacial angle of the canine. The posterior loop is grasped with smooth-beak pliers and twisted three-fourths of a turn, which will place the loop in a horizontal position, bringing the buccal wire slightly into the embrasure. The other loops are treated in the same manner. This adapts the wire well around each tooth. Starting again with the twisted ends, they are given the final adjustment; twisting is continued until the wire fits the mesiolabial angle snugly. The excess twisted ends are cut off and neatly adapted against the mesial aspects of the tooth as well as into the embrasure. On occasion these twisted ends can be carefully adjusted and used as an additional hook. The next adjustment of the loops is accomplished by giving each one an additional half turn, which gives the wire the

final adjustment around each tooth, carries the buccal wire closer into the embrasure, and secures the loops in their proper position. The final adjustment of the loops is to bend them gingivally so that they are in light contact with the gingiva and can be used as hooks for rubber traction. Then, by use of small elastic bands, both intramaxillary and

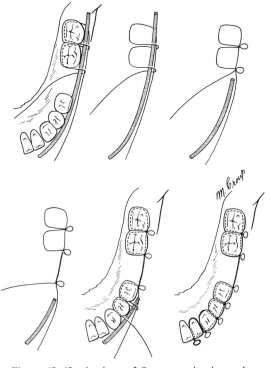

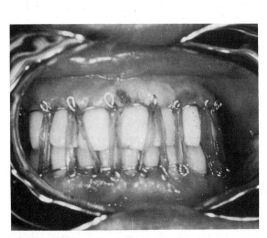

Figure 18–44 Intermaxillary elastics in place over wire loops (see Figure 18–43).

Figure 18–45 A piece of 8 gauge wire is used, as shown here, to help form loops of uniform size. Method of applying Stout multiple loop wiring when a tooth is missing is depicted.

intermaxillary traction and fixation can be obtained as desired. The requirements of stable anchorage with a broad base involving a number of teeth have been fulfilled. Application of the wire can be quickly accomplished and manipulation of the parts reduced to a minimum.

Edentulous portions. If edentulous areas are encountered, the formation of loops can be interrupted and the wire twisted to bridge the spaces. The twisted wire strand that bridges the space assists the stabilization of the teeth in that arch and provides points of anchorage for intermaxillary elastic bands (see Figure 18–45).

INTERMAXILLARY LIGATION WITH WIRES

The reduction of mandibular fractures by either intermaxillary ligation with stainless steel wires or horizontal wiring has a limited field of usefulness.

A fracture which is several days old with marked displacement is difficult to reduce by these methods. The intermaxillary elastics cannot be excelled in this respect. An additional objection to wiring is the fact that the wires gradually loosen and have to be repeatedly tightened or immobility is lost. In contrast, intermaxillary elastics, which are changed approximately every two weeks, provide positive and continuous immobilization of the fragments, and hold the patient's teeth in their normal occlusion.

CAST METAL OR PLASTIC SPLINTS

The author's limited experience with cast metal or acrylic splints constructed for the reduction and immobilization of fractures of the mandible has been uniformly poor. However, the excellent results that our British friends have obtained with cast splints proves the method is good but the author's technique

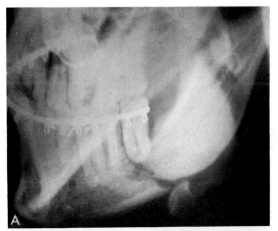

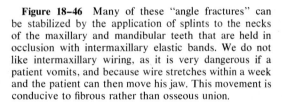

Figure 18–46 Many of these "angle fractures" can be stabilized by the application of splints to the necks of the maxillary and mandibular teeth that are held in occlusion with intermaxillary elastic bands. We do not like intermaxillary wiring, as it is very dangerous if a patient vomits, and because wire stretches within a week and the patient can then move his jaw. This movement is conducive to fibrous rather than osseous union.

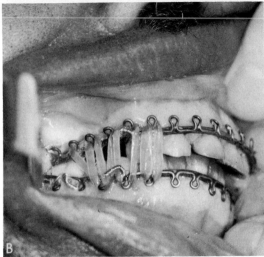

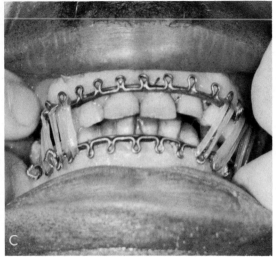

Figure 18–47 This type of splint is very satisfactory when treating linear fractures of the mandible with no displacement of the segments.

A, Split acrylic splint. Note the splint button and the wires through the missing tooth space on the right.

B, Splint locked around the mandibular teeth by wiring the two halves of the button together. The wires through the missing tooth area are also tightened. A wire through the molar interproximal spaces and around the splint also strengthens and locks the splint more securely.

C, Note that the occlusal and incisal surfaces of the teeth are exposed, so that there is no interference with normal occlusion.

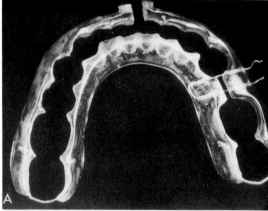

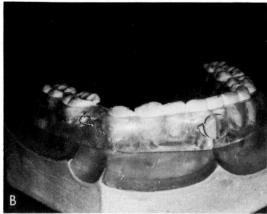

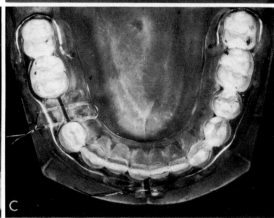

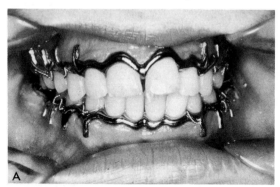

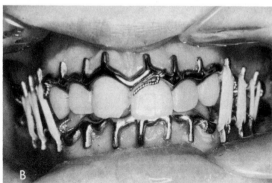

Figure 18–48   Examples of cast metal splints for mandibular fractures with minimal displacement of the fragment.

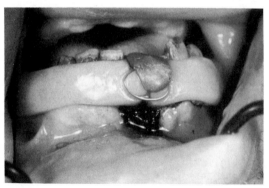

Figure 18–49   Acrylic splint for reducing and immobilizing a simple fracture through the symphysis. Two teeth with attached alveolar bone were knocked out.

1092

was bad. For this reason Chapter 19 by Irby on cast and acrylic splints follows. The author at present uses only the split acrylic or metal splint for stabilization of the fractured segments of a mandible after the original reducing and immobilizing splints have been removed. This is necessary in some cases in which there has been loss of bone and a bone graft is to be carried out after all local infection has subsided.

Split splints are also necessary as part of the treatment of fractures of the maxilla through the palate. These splints are constructed so that the occlusal surfaces are exposed and normal occlusion is not interfered with (see Figure 18–47).

CIRCUMFERENTIAL WIRING

Fixation of fractures by circumferential wiring has found its greatest use in fractures of the edentulous mandible. The procedure of passing wires around the body of the mandible and securing the fragments by fastening the wires over the patient's denture, or a prefabricated splint, works well in an occasional case. However, there are definite disadvantages associated with this type of fracture management. One disadvantage is that if the wires are placed sufficiently close to the fracture ends to effect accurate reduction, there is a tendency for the wire to pull through the fracture defect.

The chief disadvantage in the use of circumferential wiring, however, stems from the fact that most fractures of the endentulous mandible occur in older persons or in persons in whom the alveolar process has undergone extensive resorption for some other reason. In the presence of the swelling which accompanies displaced fractures of the mandible, the adherent tissues over the ridge become submerged and the ridge is therefore lower than the surrounding tissues. This makes the placing of a denture or splint impracticable. The insertion of circumferential wiring causes additional soft tissue trauma in areas already traumatized, and new trauma to uninjured areas resulting in new and additional swelling.

To summarize, the chief value of circumferential wiring is in cases of simple undisplaced fractures of the edentulous mandible, and in cases in which the edentulous mandible has a prominent alveolar process and the fracture is accompanied by only minor swelling. The author prefers extraoral pin fixation because it is less traumatic and gives more accurate end results.

Geriatric Complications in Circumferential Wiring*

EDWARD J. DEGNAN, D.D.S.

The management of mandibular fractures of edentulous, older patients has always been a problem. This is true not only because of mandibular atrophy often seen in the geriatric patient, but also because of the associated pathologic entities common to this age group. What would be an excellent treatment plan for a fracture in a young person might show a significant increase in surgical and possibly anesthetic morbidity if used for the same type of fracture in the elderly. (Read Chapter 15, "Oral Surgery and the Geriatric Patient.")

The following avenues of therapy are available, and all have been used with varying degrees of success: oral open reduction with or without splints by use of direct bone wiring; extraoral reduction with or without splints by use of direct bone wiring; extraoral reduction with splints and bone graft; extraoral reduction with splints and bone plate; extraoral skeletal pin or screw fixation devices and the peri-cortical clamp. These are discussed in this chapter by others.

Course of Therapy. In judging which of these courses of treatment to follow, it is essential to weigh the possible complications of geriatric fracture surgery against the feasibility and questionable necessity of anatomical reduction. Medical, surgical and dental factors must be considered in such a manner that a patient's welfare is evaluated in its totality rather than as an isolated facial fracture.

Physical and Mental Health. A patient whose cardiorespiratory status is compromised by organic disease is not a prime candidate for a procedure requiring a general an-

*Adapted from Degnan, E. J.: Mandibular fracture in the geriatric patient: problems in treatment planning. Report of a case. J. Oral Surg., 28:438 (June), 1970. Copyright by the American Dental Association. Reprinted by permission.

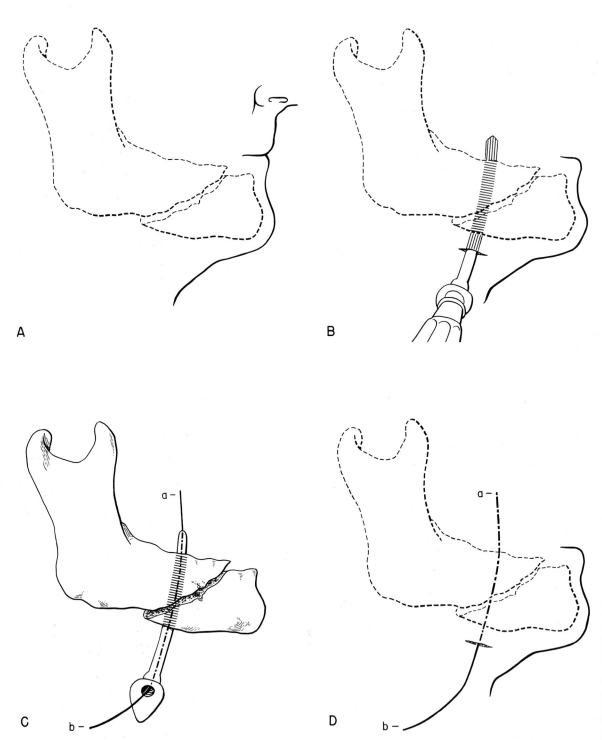

A

B

C   a –
           b –

D   a –
           b –

Figure 18–50   Circumferential wiring of a unilateral fracture of an edentulous mandible. *A*, Oblique fracture of eden-tulous mandible through the mental foramen. *B*, Trocar and cannula are passed through the ½-inch incision in the skin, and contact with the lingual cortical bone is achieved. *C*, Trocar is removed and a wire is passed upward through the cannula. *D*, Cannula is withdrawn, leaving the wire along the lingual cortical plate.

(Figure 18–50 continued on opposite page)

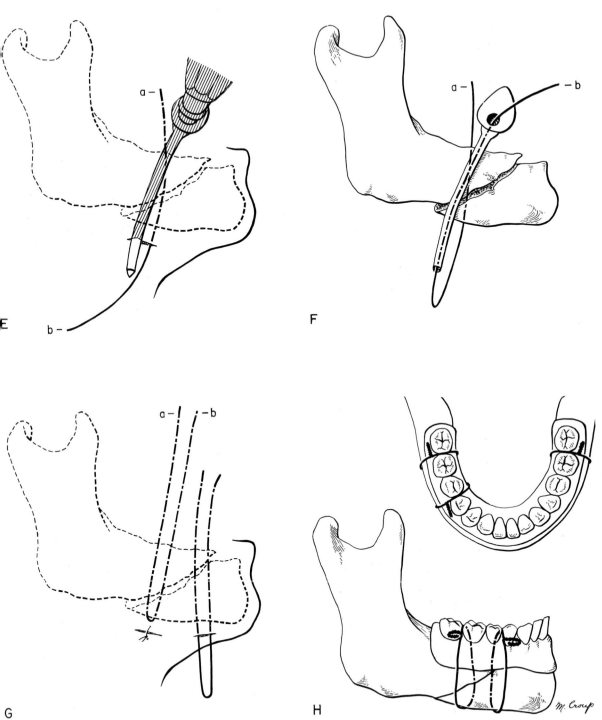

Figure 18–50 *(Continued.) E,* Trocar and cannula are passed down from the mouth in contact with the buccal cortical plate, and the cannula emerges from the original incision. *F,* Trocar is removed, and the inferior end *(b)* of the wire is passed upward through the cannula, emerging into the oral cavity. *G,* The cannula is withdrawn and the wire drawn taut into position. The procedure is repeated on the opposite side of the fracture. *H,* The ends of the wire in the oral cavity are twisted together over the denture so that reduction of the fracture is attained. *Note:* For additional stabilization, a circumferential wire is placed around the mandible and the denture in the molar region of the opposite side.

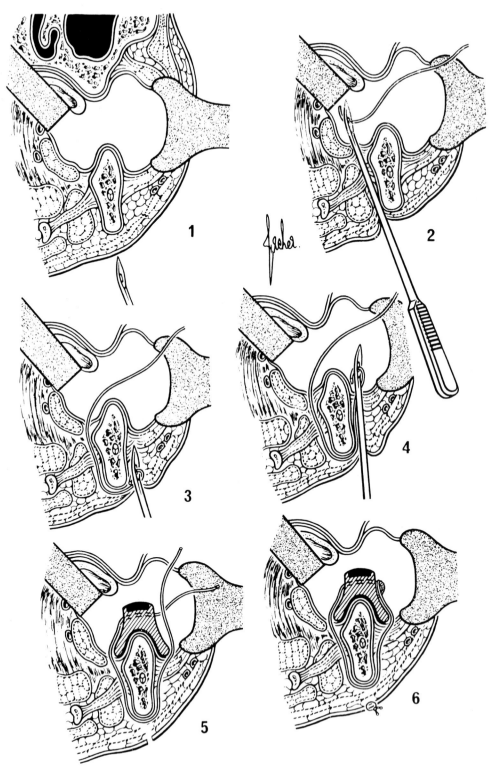

Figure 18–51   The instrument used to insert these circumferential wires is the Obwegeser awl. (From Rowe, N. L., and Killey, H. C.: Fractures of the Facial Skeleton. Edinburgh, Churchill Livingstone, 1968.)

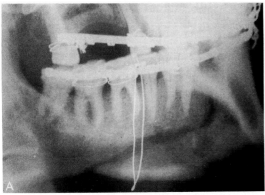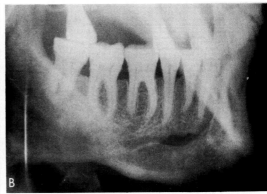

Figure 18–52 *A,* Circumferential wiring of a long, splitting fracture of the mandible below the apices of the teeth. The mandible is further stabilized and the teeth held in normal occlusion by means of intermaxillary elastic band fixation between mandibular and maxillary splints, as illustrated. *B,* Healed fracture site.

esthetic. In such cases, the treatment of choice should be altered for treatment that will result in an adequate reduction. Functional results can be expected using local anesthesia with premedication. By not aspiring to an exact anatomic repair, potential problems with general anesthesia can be eliminated.

The tolerance of the elderly patient to intermaxillary immobilization is variable. In some instances there is no cooperation or accommodation during this period of 6 to 8 weeks. Therefore, it is wise to evaluate carefully the ability of a patient to cooperate prior to completing a treatment plan.

Bone Physiology and Repair. The main causes of nonunion are infection, excessive mobility of the parts, soft tissue in the fracture line and a decrease in the regenerative capacity of the patient. Whether it be hard or soft tissue repair, the regenerative capacity of elderly patients is decreased. Because of difficulty in minimizing mobility in the fractured edentulous mandible, the possibility for a nonunion is always present and often becomes a clinical reality. If there is absolutely no mobility or shearing force at the fracture site, there will be few cartilage cells deposited and, possibly, no eventual invasion by osteoblasts with subsequent bone formation. Conversely, if there is excessive mobility at the fracture site, no cartilage cells will form, and the best one can hope for is a fibrous

union (pseudarthrosis). In many instances this fibrous union is in itself covered by cartilage (nearthrosis). The absence of osseous union, while most undesirable, is not catastrophic in the edentulous patient. Dentures can function adequately in the presence of nearthrosis or pseudarthrosis.*

The Atrophic Mandible. When the atrophic mandible is fractured, the following technical problems can arise. If splints are to be made, it is difficult to approximate and hold the mandible in an accurately reduced manner while an impression is being taken. Regardless of the type of direct bone wiring, one can only approximate, not fix, the fractured segments of a pipe-stem mandible.

Excessive mobility of the redundant oral mucosa associated with atrophy further mitigates against an accurate impression.

Vitallium bone plates are limited in their use because of the reduced distance from the floor of the alveolar canal to the inferior border of the mandible.

Damage to the neurovascular bundle from wire ligatures or screws is also possible. This trauma may be followed by a transitory paresthesia, which is often a cause of anxiety.

Case Report No. 2 documents the complications that arose in a simple bilateral mandibular fracture.

---

*AUTHOR'S NOTE: These are very exceptional cases.

REDUCTION OF A MANDIBULAR FRACTURE IN AN EDENTULOUS JAW

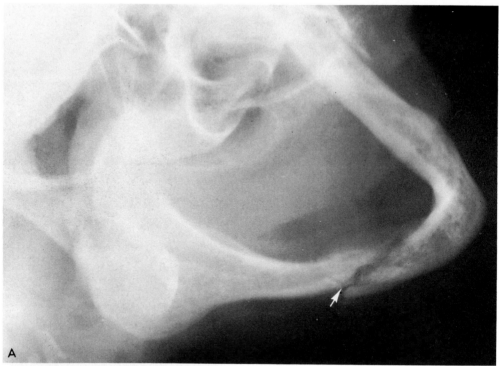

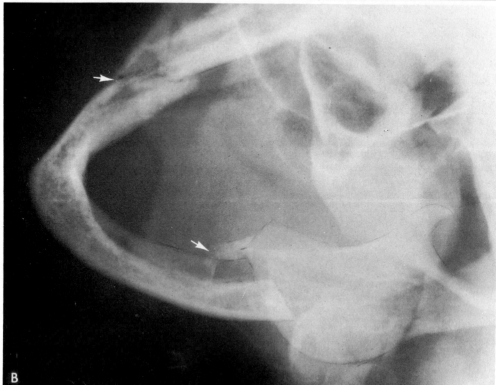

Figure 18–53 Right and left oblique radiographs of bilateral fractures of an edentulous mandible.
A, Oblique fracture through the left mental foramen.
B, Comminuted fracture through the right angle area.

(Figure 18–53 continued on opposite page)

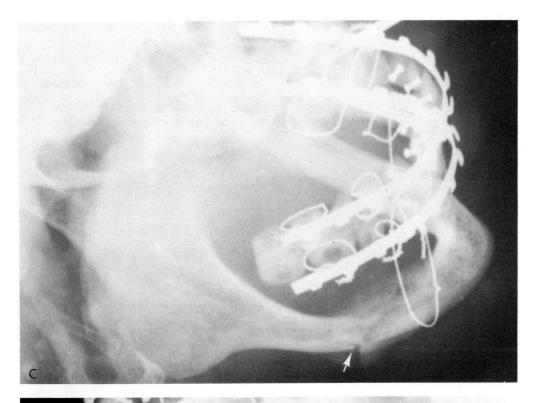

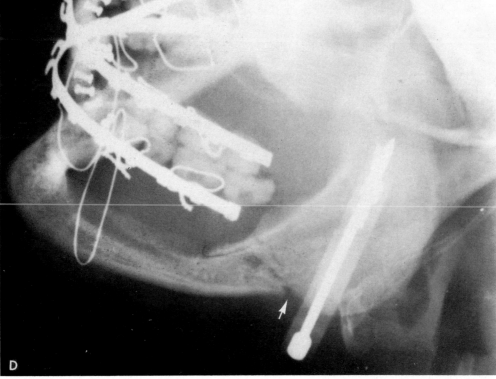

Figure 18–53   *(Continued.)* C and D, Patient's full dentures with splints wired to the necks of the teeth were inserted. The mandibular denture was fixed to the mandible by circumferential wire. The maxillary denture was fixed to the maxilla by the insertion of pins through the labial flange into the maxilla. Next, intermaxillary elastics were placed from the maxillary splint to the mandibular splint. (In *D* a plastic and metal hair curler is superimposed over the vertical ramus.)

(Figure 18–53 continued on following page)

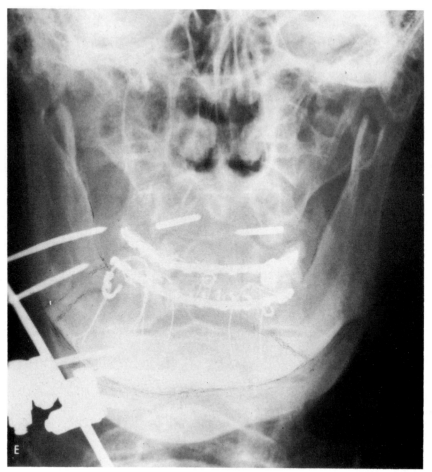

Figure 18–53 *(Continued.)* As can be seen in the posteroanterior radiograph in *E,* both fractures have been reduced and immobilized by this technique. (There are limitations in the use of this technique, which are noted in the text and are demonstrated in Case Report No. 2 and Figures 18–54 to 18–59.)

Case Report No. 2

BILATERAL FRACTURE OF AN ATROPHIC (PIPE-STEM) MANDIBLE*

EDWARD J. DEGNAN, D.D.S.

A 67-year-old edentulous man was admitted to the hospital. The patient stated that he "fell during a blackout and broke his jaw." A radiograph taken at the time showed a fracture of the left body of the mandible with minimal displacement and a fracture through the right body of the mandible with slight upriding of the proximal fragment. There was considerable atrophy of the mandible with little or no alveolar bone present (Fig. 18–54).

The patient's history and physical examination revealed that he had had multiple attacks of cerebrovascular ischemia secondary to arterio-sclerotic heart disease but demonstrated no gross abnor-

malities other than blood pressure at 150/100. There was no evidence of mucosal lacerations. A slight step deformity could be felt along the superior surface of the right side of the mandible. Results of laboratory studies, which included complete blood cell count, urinalysis, fasting blood sugar, blood urea nitrogen, and liver function were all within normal limits.

---

*Adapted from Degnan, E. J.: Mandibular fracture in the geriatric patient: problems in treatment planning. Report of a case. J. Oral Surg., *28*:438 (June), 1970. Copyright by the American Dental Association. Reprinted by permission.

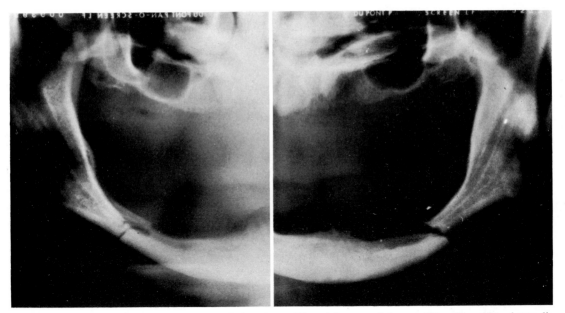

Figure 18–54 Panoramic radiograph on admission shows bilateral fracture of the mandible with only moderate displacement on the right side.

The treatment plan consisted of bilateral oral open reductions and fixation of the fragments with direct bone wiring and immobilization of the jaw using the patient's dentures as fracture splints.

After evaluation and clearance by the medical service, the patient was taken to the operating room two weeks after admission. Anesthesia was induced with thiopental sodium and maintained with a thiopental sodium–nitrous oxide combination. A 3-cm. incision was made, extending from the right retromolar pad anterior to a point in line with the mental foramen, along the superior border of the mandible. A mucoperiosteal flap was developed buccally and lingually which allowed easy visualization of the fracture line. The proximal fragment was displaced superior and medial to the distal

fragment. The pipe-stem thickness of the atrophic mandible was noted. Bur holes were placed at least 5 mm. from the fracture line. Stainless steel wire (24-gauge) was threaded through the bur holes and tightened, thus effecting an adequate reduction. The cut end of the steel ligature was adapted close to the inferior lateral border of the mandible, and the oral mucosa was closed with No. 0000 chromic gut sutures. A similar incision was carried out in the left side of the mandible.

After the elevation of the mucoperiosteal flap, the fracture line was visualized. No displacement was seen, and mobility was minimal. It was felt that direct bone wiring was not needed, and, if placed, would only serve to distract the fracture line.

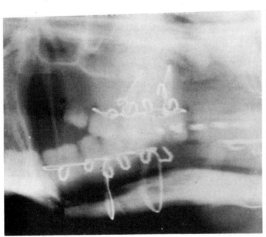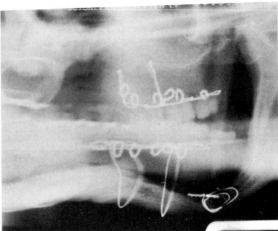

Figure 18–55 Panoramic radiograph 24 hours postoperatively shows increased displacement of fractures.

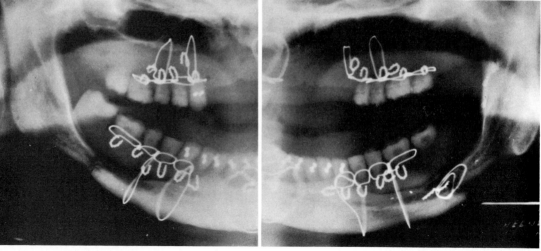

Figure 18–56 Panoramic radiograph taken 24 hours after insertion of corrective acrylic wedge.

By use of a technic previously described,[40] the denture splints were fixed to the maxilla and mandible. When the patient was fully recovered from the general anesthesia and the danger of postoperative emesis was minimized, elastic traction was initiated. This immobilization was supported by a headcap with chin suspension from a bandage.

After the patient had been immobilized for 24 hours, a postreduction radiograph (Fig. 18–55) showed increased bilateral displacement at both fracture sites. Both elastics and headcap were immediately removed. The prosthodontist fabricated an acrylic wedge, which was wired to the mandibular denture to reduce and prevent further displacement of the mandible. After 24 hours, another radiograph (Fig. 18–56) was taken, which

showed a correction of the displacement on the left side and maintenance of adequate alignment on the right side. The patient was discharged from the hospital 10 days after surgery to be followed on an outpatient basis.

Two weeks later the patient returned to the outpatient clinic. He stated that, while turning his head the night before, "something slipped out of place and was very painful." A radiograph (Fig. 18–57) showed gross displacement of the fracture on the left side but no definite change on the right side. He was readmitted to the hospital for secondary repair of the left mandibular fracture.

The old splints were removed and new splints were constructed that were keyed to reduce the possibility of splint displacement during the period of immobilization. The patient was scheduled for

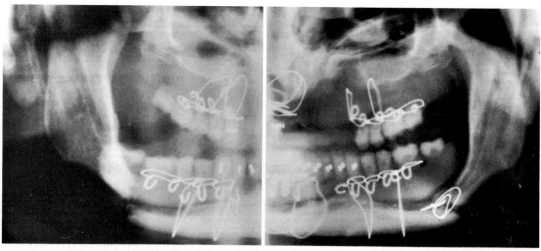

Figure 18–57 Panoramic radiograph shows displacement of fracture of the left side of the mandible caused by the patient's turning his head during period of immobilization.

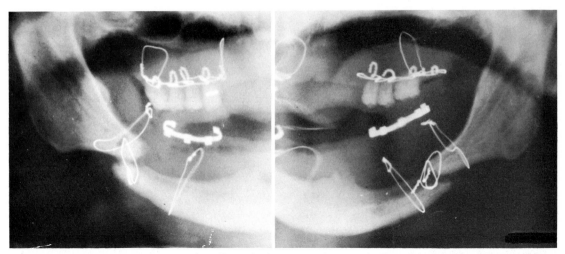

Figure 18–58　Postoperative panoramic radiograph after extraoral open reduction of the left side of the mandible.

definitive oral surgery, but because of cardiovascular difficulty the night before the operation, surgery was canceled.

After medical clearance, the patient was scheduled for surgery a week later. During intubation in the operating room, the patient had a prolonged hypotensive episode, and surgery was canceled. After a period of absolute bed rest and further cardiac studies, he was again taken to surgery 2 weeks later, when he was anesthetized without event. An extraoral open reduction was done on the left side by use of direct bone wiring. The keyed splints were inserted and ligated to the maxilla and mandible. A repeat postoperative radiograph (Fig. 18–58) showed adequate approximation of the fracture. Elastic traction was started 24 hours after surgery. The patient did well in the postoperative period, and he was discharged to the outpatient clinic. At the time of discharge, there was complete bilateral paresthesia in the region anterior to both mental foramens.

Six weeks later clinical union was evident and the splints were removed. A radiograph (Fig. 18–59) taken 6 months later showed osseous bridging and remodeling of the mandible at both fracture sites. There was no paresthesia, and the patient was scheduled for denture construction.

DISCUSSION

Reflection on this case provokes the following questions for discussion. Was this patient overtreated? Was too little consideration given to the degree of mandibular atrophy in treatment plan-

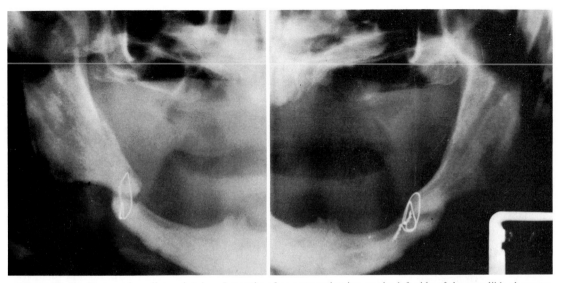

Figure 18–59　Panoramic radiograph taken 5 months after open reduction on the left side of the mandible shows osseous bridging and remodeling of the mandible at the fracture site.

ning? Would it have been better after the hypotensive episode in surgery not to have selected a procedure that required a general anesthetic? Probably the most important question is: Was too little consideration given to this patient's age and general health in choice of therapy?

Perhaps, after the severe hypotensive episode during intubation in the operating room, every effort should have been directed toward a surgical procedure that could have been done under local anesthesia, supplemented by effective premedication.

Because of the lack of bulk in the body of the mandible, it was impossible to make a denture splint the flanges of which would be adequate to give good stabilization. The right proximal fragment was already displaced, and any denture splints constructed would not reflect an accurate vertical dimension.

If the sole primary procedure done on this patient after admittance was an oral open reduction of the right side of the mandible under local anesthesia, real benefits would have been realized. A

general anesthetic for a patient with cardiovascular disease would have been eliminated. If the patient had been maintained on a high-protein, high-caloric, liquid diet, it is possible that the intermaxillary immobilization of denture splints could have been avoided. This would have eliminated displacement of the fracture that occurred when splints were first inserted.

Summary. Any treatment for facial trauma must take into consideration the whole patient, not just an isolated facial bone. It often takes more diagnostic acumen to know when not to operate and to recognize the indications for conservative patient management. This is a cautious approach that should be considered in the treatment of elderly patients.*

---

*Author's note: These are excellent and pertinent comments made by Dr. Degnan. My personal preference of treatment for these pipe-stem jaw fractures is illustrated in other case reports in this chapter.

EXTRAORAL SKELETAL PIN FIXATION*

Unfortunately, the application of this mode of treatment requires more skill and experience to achieve satisfactory results than any other method, and as a result its use has been limited. It requires time and care to develop the skill necessary to obtain the excellent results which this method is capable of producing.

Indications for Extraoral Skeletal Fixation. Extraoral skeletal fixation is used in *edentulous* mandibles in which there is marked displacement of the fragments or overriding of the fragments, or in which the fracture line is through the angle of the mandible, or in those cases in which the patient's dentures are not satisfactory for circumferential wiring (see Figure 18–71), and in particular in those mandibles that are very atrophic—the so-called pipe-stem mandibles (see preceding section).

External skeletal fixation is used in *dentulous* mandibles in which there are only a few remaining teeth, worthless because of advanced caries or periodontoclasia; in conjunction with intermaxillary elastic reduction

and immobilization to control a posterior fragment in which there are no teeth (see Figure 18–72); in those cases in which it is impractical from a psychic standpoint to hold the jaws closed for a long period of time, and for mentally deficient patients who are institutionalized; in those patients with excessive or pernicious vomiting, as is seen occasionally during pregnancy. External skeletal fixation is also used in fractures with loss of bone substance as a result of the accident itself or as a result of a pathologic condition. External fixation will hold the parts in their normal relationship to each other until a bone graft is subsequently inserted.

The use of extraoral skeletal fixation is excellent for the treatment of a bilateral compound comminuted fracture of the mandible for a patient whose only remaining mandibular teeth are lower anterior teeth and the maxilla is edentulous.

Insertion of Pins. Fuller sectioned a number of mandibles to determine the areas that would offer the extraskeletal fixation pin its greatest support.[55] (See Figure 18–61.) In considering the best bony support offered to the individual pin it was found that pins should take full advantage of the lingual cortical bone. Thus, pins should be placed just through this plate. If a pin is short of the lingual plate the labial cortical bone acts as a fulcrum and the pin is soon loosened. Greater stability can

---

*The most frequently used extraoral pin fixation splint is the Roger Anderson, small size, for facial bone fractures (Arista Surgical Company, New York).

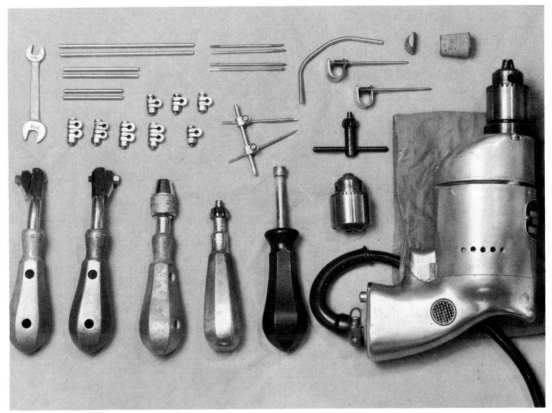

Figure 18–60 Extraoral skeletal pin fixation equipment: Roger Anderson pins, connectors, bars, pin vise, socket wrench, adjusting handles and electric drill geared down to 500 r.p.m.

be offered a pin if it is placed at a 20-degree angle to the bone. This allows the pin to rest in a greater area of supporting cortical bone than if placed at a right angle to bone. Pins nearest the fracture line should be placed at least ½ inch from, and angled away from, the line of fracture.

In applying this investigation to the common fracture sites of the mandible the areas of pin placement described below were determined to be best.

In fractures through the third molar region, one of the posterior pins should be placed in the retromolar area, and the other 6 mm. above the lower border of the vertical ramus. The anterior pin unit should be placed in the body posterior to the mental foramen and approximately 6 mm. above the lower border of the bone (Fig. 18–62).

In fractures through the ramus, from the retromolar area through the angle, the posterior pin unit should be placed in the ramus. The anterior pin of this unit gains adequate support in the inferior half of the anterior border. The posterior pin of this unit should be placed in the upper third of the posterior border. The anterior pin unit should be placed in the body of the mandible. The best position for the pins of this unit is approximately 6 mm. above the lower border of the mandible (Fig. 18–62).

Fractures through the ramus, from the sigmoid notch to the angle of the mandible, are the most difficult to treat from the standpoint of gaining adequate pin support by bone. These fractures can be treated best by a single pin unit. The anterior pin should be placed in the lower half of the anterior border of the ramus. The posterior pin should be placed in the upper third of the posterior border of the ramus (Fig. 18–63).

In fractures through the ramus, from the anterior to the posterior border, the anterior pin unit should be placed in the lower half of the anterior border. This unit should be placed so that its superior pin is situated in the superior fragment and its inferior pin in the inferior fragment. The single pin unit in

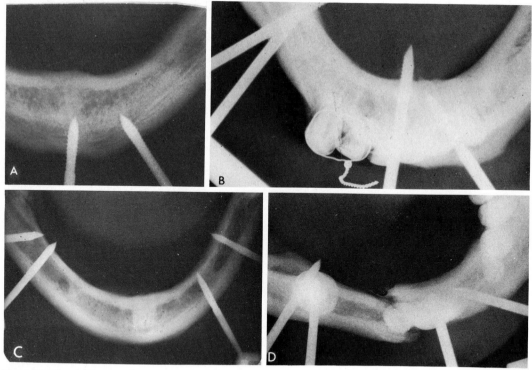

Figure 18–61   *A*, Pins too close and too shallow. *B*, Pins too close and too deep. *C*, Pins inserted correctly, just into or slightly through the lingual cortex. Angles and spacing are good. *D*, Distal pins too close.

this type of fracture is adequate for reduction (Fig. 18–63).

In fractures through the neck of the condyle, it was found that the upper third of the head of the condyle offered adequate support for a pin. The fixation pin in the ramus proper should be placed in the lower half of the anterior border of the ramus (Fig. 18–63).

In fractures of the symphysis, pin units should be placed one on either side of the fracture line. If possible, the units should be situated anterior to the mental foramen region

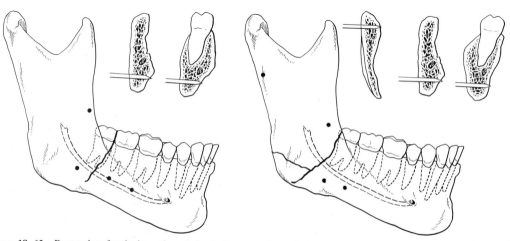

Figure 18–62   Best points for the insertion of pins in fractures through the third molar region. (See text for explanation.)

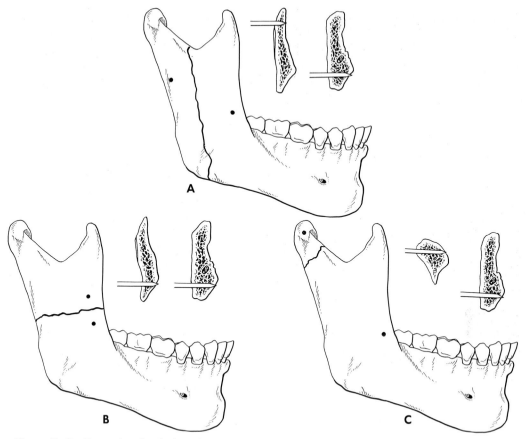

Figure 18–63   Best points for the insertion of pins in fractures of the ramus. (See text for explanation.)

as this provides the greatest area of support in the mandible. The pins should be placed approximately 6 mm. above the lower border of the bone (Fig. 18–64).

In fractures through the mental foramen

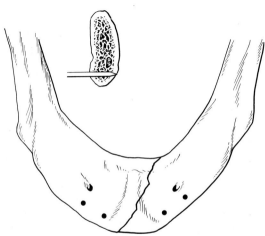

Figure 18–64   Insertion of pins for fractures of the symphysis of the mandible. (See text for explanation.)

region, the pin units should be placed one on either side of the fracture line, care being used not to approximate the line of fracture by the pins. The best position for the pins is approximately 6 mm. above the lower border of the mandible (Fig. 18–65).

In fractures of the body, as in fractures of the mental foramen area, pin units are placed one on either side of the line of fracture. The pins should be placed approximately 6 mm. above the lower border of the mandible (Fig. 18–65).

A Study of the Acute Changes in Bone Following Insertion of Extraoral Skeletal Fixation Pins at Varying Speeds.   The histologic response and thermal changes in bone from drilling were studied by Thompson[182] in order to provide basic information needed to determine whether aseptic thermal necrosis, one of the attributed causes of loosening of extraskeletal pins, can be controlled.

Two types of studies were performed. The first was accomplished by drilling extraskeletal pins at speeds of 125, 250, 500, 1000, and

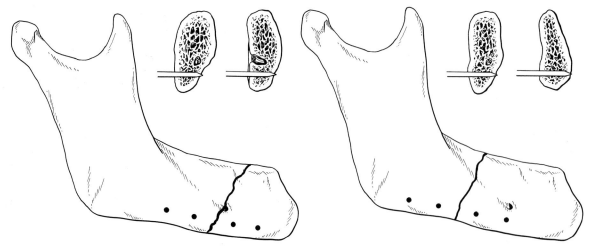

Figure 18–65   Insertion of pins for fractures of the body of the mandible. (See text for explanation.)

2000 r.p.m., and studying histologically the response of the bone to these drill speeds. In the second, the effect of the various speeds on the temperature of the pin immediately following drilling, and of the neighboring bone during drilling, were determined.

The acute histologic reactions in bone were hyperemia, degeneration of osteocytes,

(Text continued on page 1112)

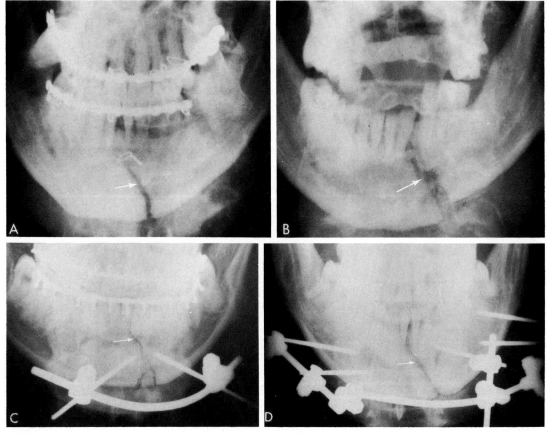

Figure 18–66   Examples of fracture lines in the anterior mandible, symphysis region, and some methods of fixation.

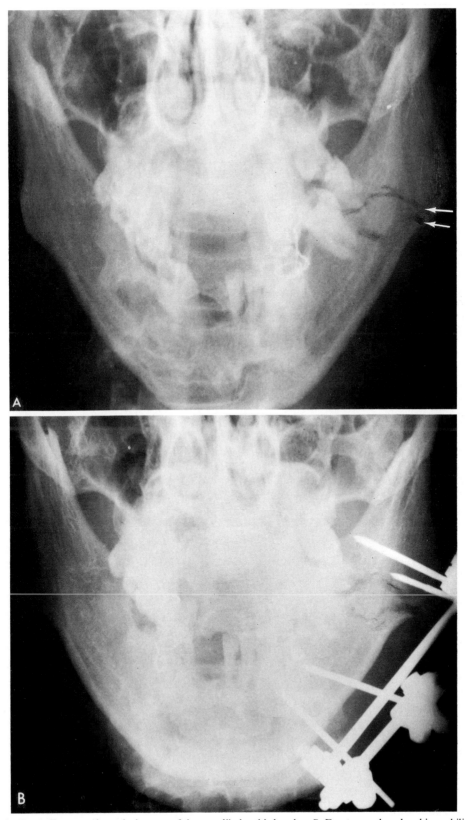

Figure 18–67 *A,* Fracture through the area of the mandibular third molar. *B,* Fracture reduced and immobilized with an extraoral skeletal pin fixation appliance.

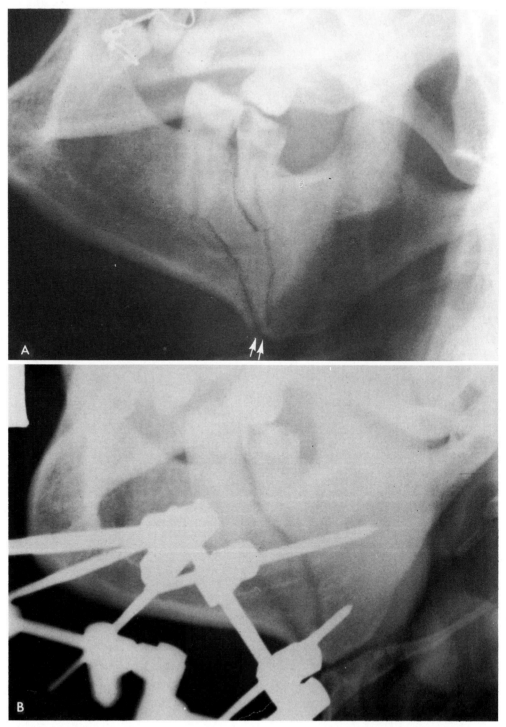

Figure 18–68 *A*, Fracture through the area of the mandibular third molar. *B*, Fracture immobilized by extraoral skeletal pin fixation units.

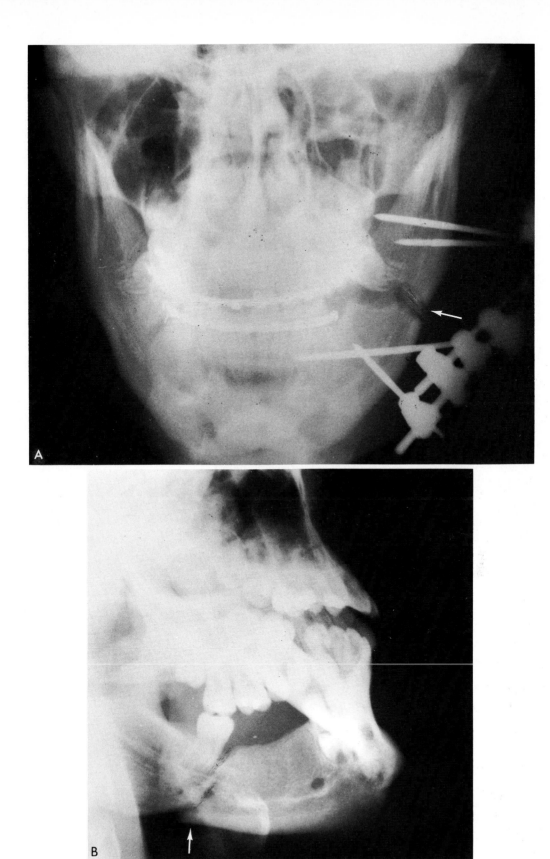

Figure 18–69 *A* and *B*, Fracture through the area of the mandibular third molar. The fracture was reduced and immobilized by splints wired to the maxillary and mandibular teeth, which were held in occlusion with intermaxillary elastic bands. The angle fracture was immobilized with an extraoral skeletal pin fixation unit.

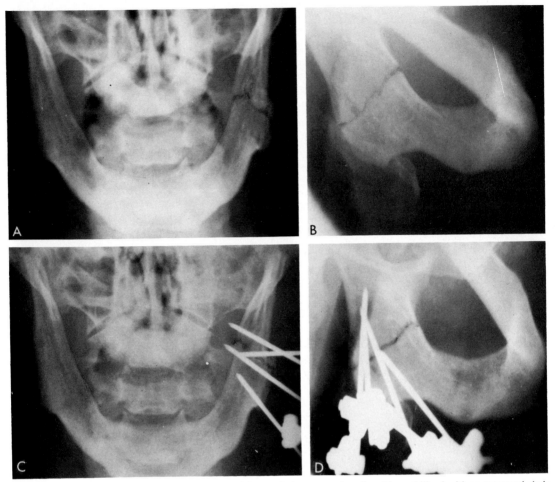

Figure 18–70   A transverse unilateral fracture of the vertical ramus reduced and immobilized with an extraoral skeletal pin fixation unit.

change in bone stainability, and tears and fragmentation of the bone edges around the drill holes. These reactions increased in severity with increasing drill speed, and were more pronounced at 72 hours following the operation than at either 24 or 48 hours.

Thermal changes in the external and internal portions of the pins were slight. Thermal changes in the bone, however, increased with the increase in drill speeds, ranging from 38.3° to over 65.5° C.

The various drill speeds studied were evaluated on the basis of the histologic reactions, thermal changes, mechanical effects, ease of

Figure 18–71   *A,* Unilateral fracture of the dentulous mandible without teeth in the posterior fragment. *B,* Frac-Sur units are placed in each segment, and a manipulating handle is attached to each Frac-Sur unit as shown. *C,* The manipulating handles are grasped, one in each hand, and the fracture reduced and stabilized with the connecting bar. *D,* Splints are attached to the maxillary and mandibular teeth (or Stout wiring can be used). Intermaxillary elastics are placed to bring the teeth into normal occlusion. It may be necessary to loosen the connecting bar so as to permit the rubber bands to pull the mandibular teeth into normal occlusion with the maxillary teeth. Then the connecting bar is tightened. Radiographs are taken to check the fracture alignment. If necessary, additional adjustments can be made. At the end of 10 days the intermaxillary rubber bands are taken off, and at the end of 6 weeks the extraoral pin fixation appliance can also be removed.

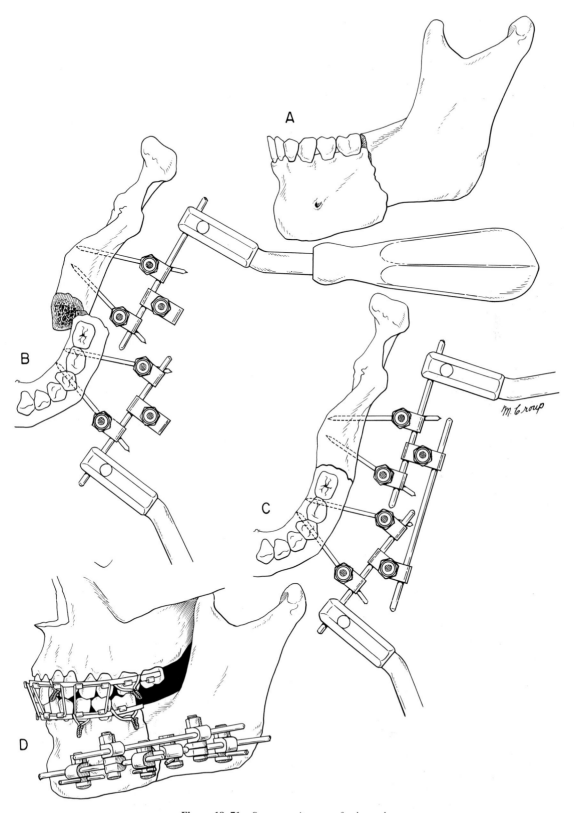

Figure 18–71 *See opposite page for legend.*

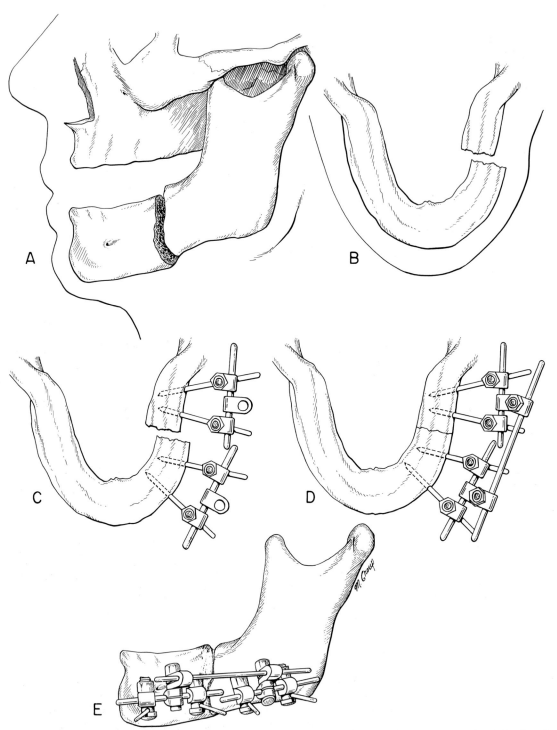

Figure 18–72 Use of Roger Anderson appliance with supplementary intraoral wiring for reduction and fixation of a fractured edentulous mandible. *A,* Lateral view of fracture. *B,* Occlusal view of fracture. *C,* Two pins inserted with slight convergence on each side of fracture line and connected by short connecting bars to form two separate units. Each unit is called a Frac-Sur unit. *D,* Longer connecting bar (which will immobilize the fracture when locked into position) is placed to connect Frac-Sur units but is not locked into position. Fracture is reduced by correctly affixing bone surfaces by manipulation, and long connecting bar is locked firmly into position. Normally this is sufficient to fix the fracture. *E,* However, in some fractures there will be bowing at the fracture line due to excessive muscle pull that places too great a strain on the pins. This is not uncommon in fractures around the third molar area with anteromedial upward displacement of the distal fragment. In such a case supplementary fixation is indicated.

(Figure 18–72 continued on opposite page)

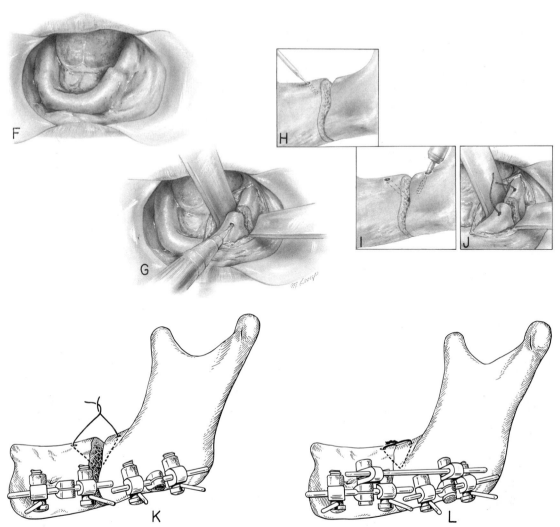

Figure 18–72 *(Continued.)* Occasionally an unreduced fracture of an edentulous mandible of 10 or more days' duration is seen that will have displacement of the fracture segments due to muscle pull and early fibrous healing. *G* to *I,* Buccal and lingual flaps are reflected, fibrous tissue is curetted from between the bone segments, and converging holes are drilled into both fragments. Spear-point drills are used. If necessary, holes can be enlarged and with a crosscut fissure bur. *J,* Stainless steel wire (0.020) is passed through the drill holes. The ends of the wire are twisted together at the same time that the extraoral skeletal fixation unit is adjusted, until the fractured ends are in contact. *L,* Then the excess twisted wire is cut off and turned down into the buccal fold, and the connecting bar of the extraoral pin fixation unit is tightened. The oral incision is then closed, covering the wire.

penetration of bone, and steadiness of application in order to determine a drill speed which would be desirable in clinical use, and which would produce minimal histologic and thermal changes in bone. This evaluation suggested such a desirable speed to be in the neighborhood of 500 r.p.m. with the power drill.* This speed produced a minimal histo-

logic response and thermal change in bone, yet was fast enough to prevent fragmentation and an irregular pin hole margin. It also provided ease of penetration of bone. The power drill provided steady application of the pin.

Although this study has indicated a desirable drill speed to be 500 r.p.m. with the power drill, it does not, by any means, rule out the possibility that aseptic thermal necrosis could develop from its use. A further

*Black & Decker electric drill geared down to 500 r.p.m.

BILATERAL FRACTURE OF THE MANDIBLE

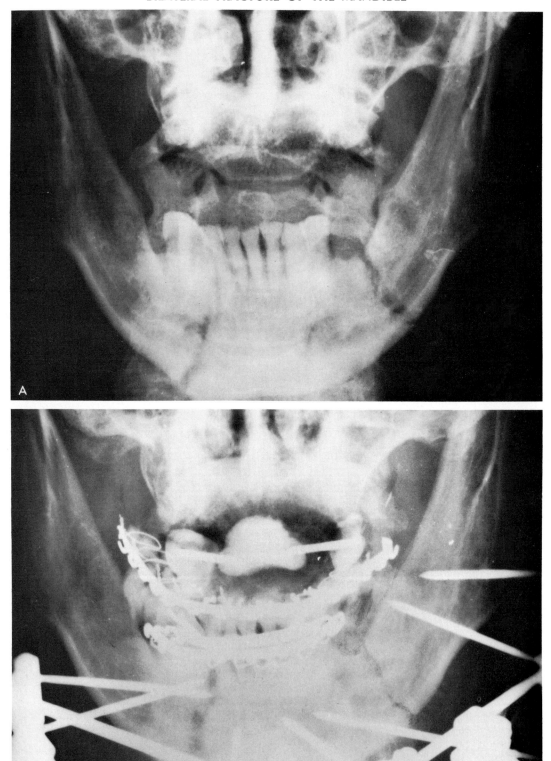

Figure 18–73   Treatment of a bilateral fracture of the dentulous mandible of a patient with an edentulous maxilla.

(Figure 18–73 continued on opposite page)

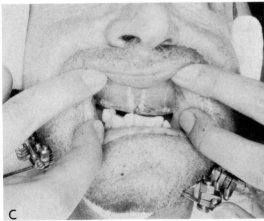

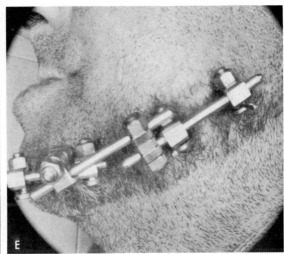

Figure 18–73   *(Continued.)*

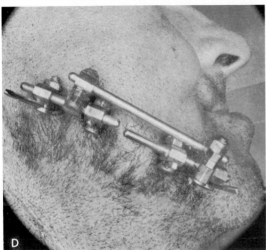

study of the reaction of bone to drilling at long intervals of time at different speeds may possibly show whether aseptic thermal necrosis could be prevented by using this drill speed.

The method of application of the Roger Anderson Frac-Sur appliances is described in Figures 18–71, 18–72, and 18–150, and their legends. The technique for application of the Stader splint is described in Chapter 22, pages 1455 to 1459. Also see Figures 18–115 to 18–117 and their legends.

BIPHASE EXTERNAL SKELETAL FIXATION
JOE HALL MORRIS, D.D.S.

Although abuse of external skeletal fixation at the close of World War II almost gave it a "kiss of death," it is another useful modality of treatment for complicated fractures of the mandible, as attested to by over 25 years of successful utilization.

As stated in 1949, success of the technique is dependent upon:
1. Correct application
2. An indicated situation
3. A properly trained surgeon
4. Utilization of biomechanically sound equipment and technology.

When one concedes that there have been failures with external skeletal fixation, it is appropriate to be equally honest and intellectually objective in pointing out that other modalities have an equal or higher failure rate when all factors, such as specificity of indication, proper technique and the use of appropriate equipment, are considered in true perspective.

Biphase external skeletal fixation refers to a specific modality employing a mechanical splint (Fig. 18–81) for a short period of time
(Text continued on page 1128)

BILATERAL FRACTURES OF AN EDENTULOUS MANDIBLE

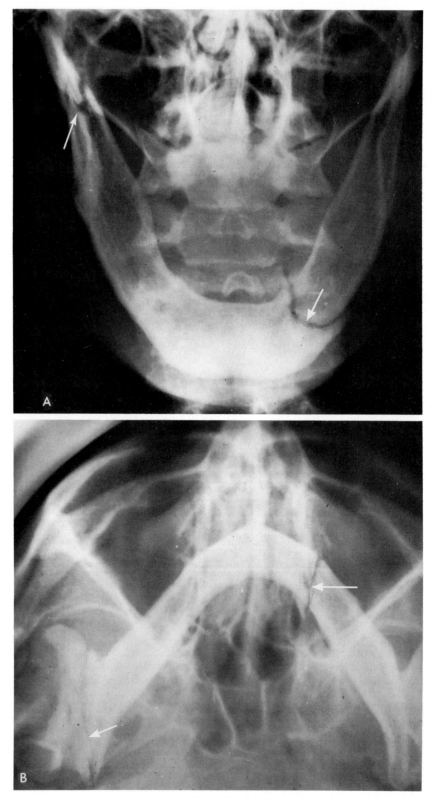

Figure 18–74

(Figure 18–74 continued on opposite page)

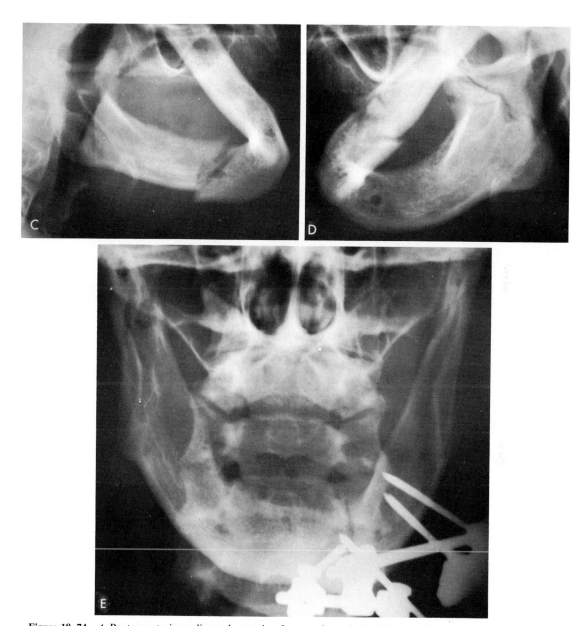

Figure 18–74 *A*, Posteroanterior radiograph reveals a fracture through the right mental foramen and a semitransverse fracture high on the left vertical ramus just below the sigmoid mandibular notch, which includes the coronoid process in this segment.

B, Basal view shows no lateral displacement of the fractures.

C, Left oblique film shows slight elevation of the left proximal fragment and depression of the distal one.

D, No superior or inferior displacement of these fractures of the vertical ramus.

E, Posteroanterior view of the reduction and immobilization of the right segments with extraoral skeletal pin (Roger Anderson) fixation.

(Figure 18–74 continued on following page)

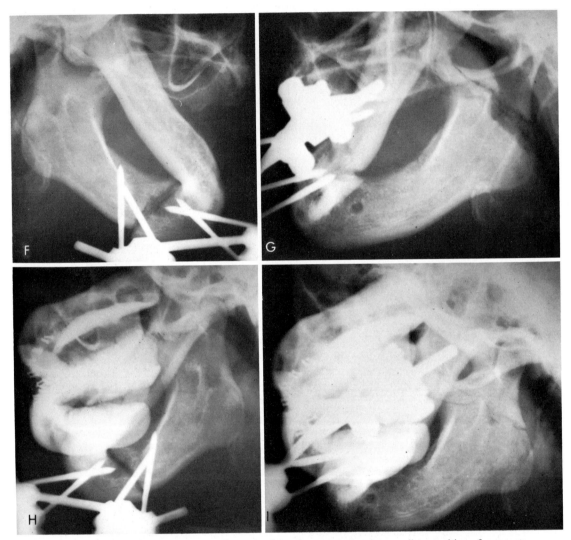

Figure 18–74   *(Continued.) F,* Oblique radiograph of the same area, showing excellent position of segments.
G, Right oblique radiograph of the horizontal body and vertical rami. Fragments still in normal alignment.
H, Patient was able to wear and use his dentures, with a soft diet for the first three weeks.
I, Four weeks postoperatively the right ramus fractures are healing.
J, Posteroanterior view showing normal intermaxillary space still maintained 4 weeks postoperatively. Splints are not removed for at least 8 weeks.

(Figure 18–74 continued on opposite page)

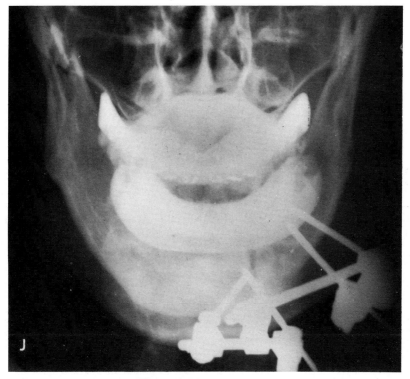

Figure 18–74   *(Continued.)*

Photographic Case Report

UNILATERAL FRACTURE OF AN EDENTULOUS MANDIBLE

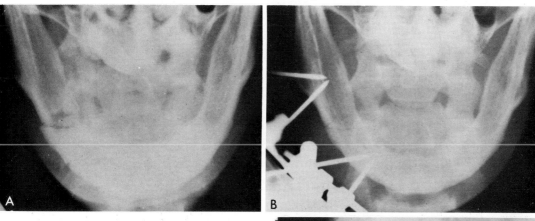

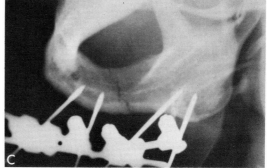

Figure 18–75   Unilateral fracture of an edentulous mandible reduced and stabilized with extraoral skeletal pin fixation.

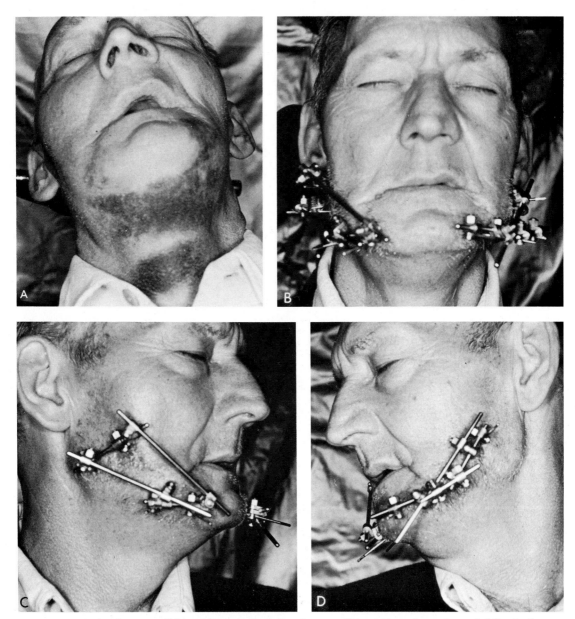

Figure 18–76　Another case of bilateral fracture of an edentulous mandible. *A*, Extensive ecchymosis following hemorrhage from the fracture site. *B* to *H*, Stabilization, as previously described.

(Figure 18–76 continued on opposite page)

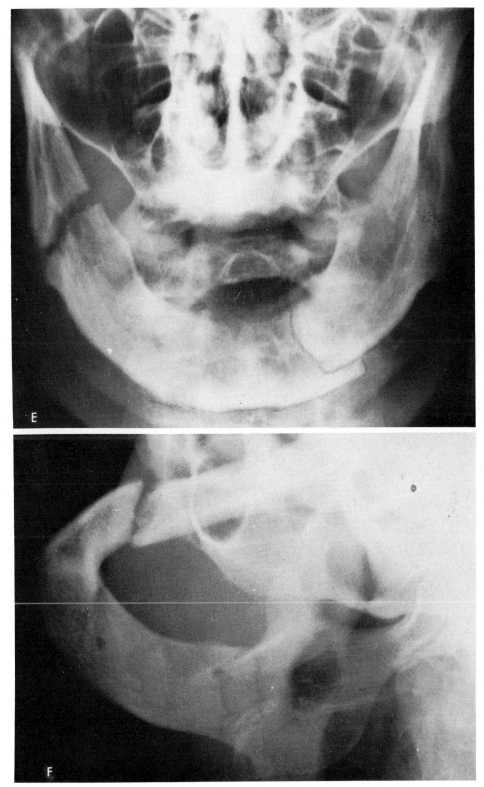

Figure 18–76   *(Continued.)*

(Figure 18–76 continued on following page)

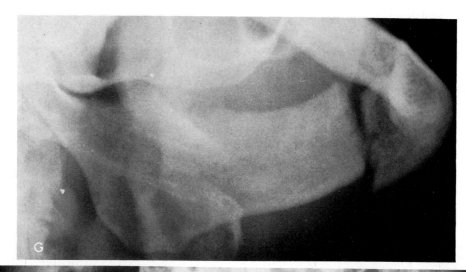

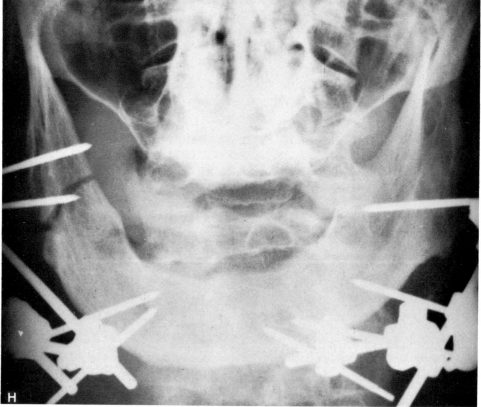

Figure 18–76   *(Continued.)*

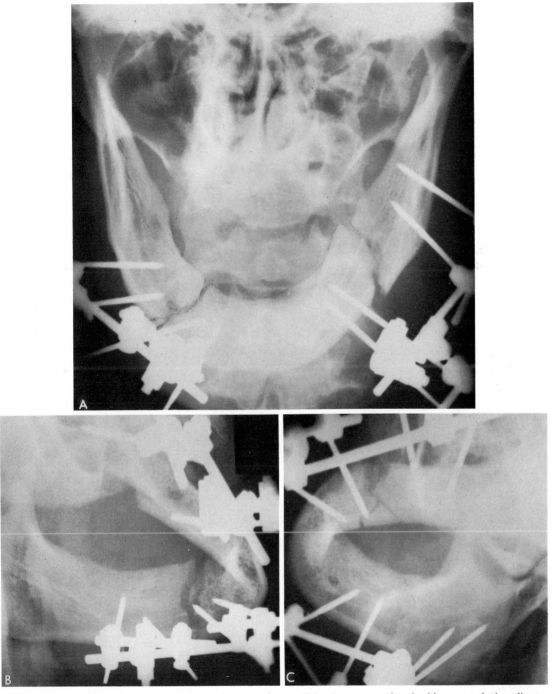

Figure 18–77　Typical bilateral fracture of an edentulous mandible. Fractures reduced with extraoral pin splints.

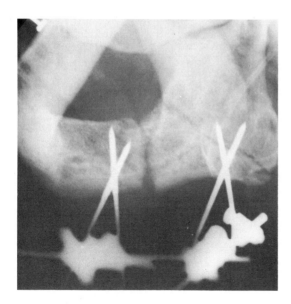

Figure 18–78 Edentulous mandible with unusual double fracture combination on one side only. Fracture segments were in good position; all that was required in this case was immobilization by extraoral skeletal pin fixation.

Photographic Case Report

UNILATERAL FRACTURE OF AN EDENTULOUS MANDIBLE

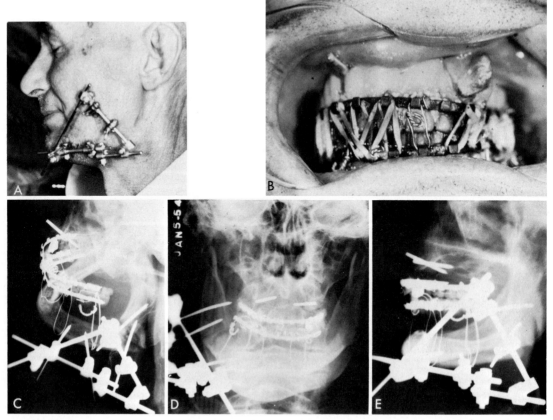

Figure 18–79 *A*, Unilateral fracture through the angle, reduced with a combination of methods. There was considerable displacement and the fracture was a week old. The extraoral skeletal pin fixation appliance was inserted so that the unit forms a triangle, the strongest form. *B*, The maxillary denture was pinned to the maxilla. One pin here is shown exposed; the other is covered with compound. *C*, The lower denture was devoid of a labial flange so that pinning this denture to the mandible was impossible; instead, circumferential wiring was used.

BILATERAL COMPOUND FRACTURE OF THE MANDIBLE

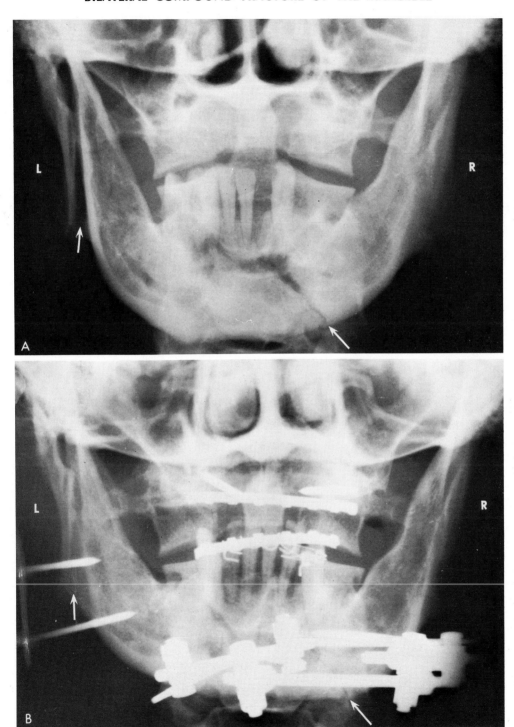

Figure 18–80 *A,* Vertical fracture through the ramus with lateral displacement and a second oblique fracture through the symphysis. Maxilla was edentulous, and patient's denture was lost in the accident. *B,* An acrylic maxillary bite block was made and a splint attached to its buccal and labial surfaces. This unit was then pinned to the maxilla. Next the mandibular symphysis fracture was reduced with Frac-Sur units, a splint was wired to the mandibular teeth, and intermaxillary rubber bands were placed. Then the vertical fracture in the ramus was reduced with a single Frac-Sur unit.

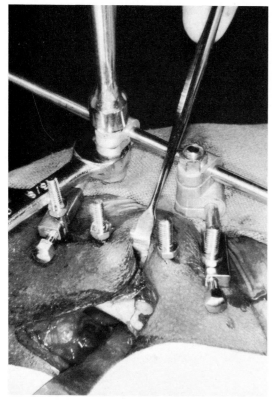

Figure 18–81 Biphase external skeletal fixation. The primary (mechanical) splint, attached to one of two special bone screws inserted through the skin into each of the fragments of the fractured mandible, is being locked into position to hold the open reduction of the fracture in appropriate alignment and apposition.

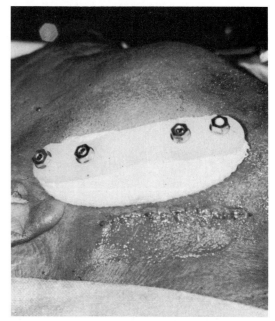

Figure 18–82 The compact, resilient acrylic bar attached to the machine thread end of the bone screws takes the place of the cumbersome, but adjustable, primary splint.

in the operating room to hold the fragments in correct alignment and apposition until the secondary plastic splint (Fig. 18–82) can be securely affixed to the specially designed bone screws (Fig. 18–83). The bone screws have been placed in the fragments of a fractured mandible via skin incisions and pre-drilled holes in the bone.

A broad, general indication for the use of biphase external skeletal fixation for fractures of the mandible exists in the edentulous or essentially edentulous patient who also has an ample mass and quality of mandibular bone to accept the bone screws. The term "essentially edentulous" is used to mean that any existing teeth are inadequate in either number, condition or position to permit effective alignment of fragments and immobilization by interdental wiring or elastics.

Technique. Although the procedure is probably done more frequently under general anesthesia, it may be performed quite successfully under local anesthesia with adjunctive sedation. Success with external fixation

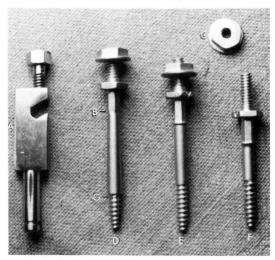

Figure 18–83 *A*, Screw clamp with precision fitting for the hexagonal throat of the bone screw. *B*, Hexagonal throat of special bone screws. *C*, Washer-faced lock nut for securing plastic bar to the machine thread end of the bone screws. *D*, Ramus bone screw with definite 1/64-inch shoulder at *G*. *E*, Long body screw. *F*, Short body screw, with the only difference in dimension being in the unthreaded screw shank for the purpose of accommodating different thicknesses of soft tissue.

is more assured when it is combined with open reduction, but there are situations in which the blind application of external skeletal fixation is effective. Case Report No. 3, describing the operative procedure in detail, represents such a useful application and will permit pertinent technical comments to be made.

Case Report No. 3

BLIND APPLICATION OF BIPHASE EXTERNAL SKELETAL FIXATION
JOE HALL MORRIS, D.D.S.

Patient. This 27-year-old, well-developed and well-nourished female, in otherwise generally good physical condition, had received a single blow to the lower portion of her face, approximately 4 hours prior to being seen in the emergency room. Her chief complaints were pain in the area of the angle of the mandible and inability to get her teeth to close together properly.

Examination. Pertinent observations from examination, along with radiographic findings, revealed that the patient was wearing an anterior flangeless full maxillary denture (Fig. 18–84), which was designed to occlude with a full complement of mandibular natural teeth, with the exception of the mandibular left first molar and mandibular right third molar, which were absent. A single oblique fracture extending from between the mandibular second and third molars, diagonally to the angle of the mandible, existed on the left side (Fig. 18–85). An unfavorable relationship between muscle pull and fracture plane had elevated the mandibular third molar and posterior fragment

superiorly, preventing the patient from bringing the teeth into proper occlusion. An unstable mediolateral relationship involving the natural mandibular third molar against the artificial denture above also existed. The patient was in moderate pain with minimal swelling and considerable trismus.

The patient's history, physical examination and laboratory findings indicated that she was able to undergo a general endotracheal anesthetic.

The patient was informed of the advantages of biphase external skeletal fixation—primarily comfort and convenience, along with ease of taking nu-

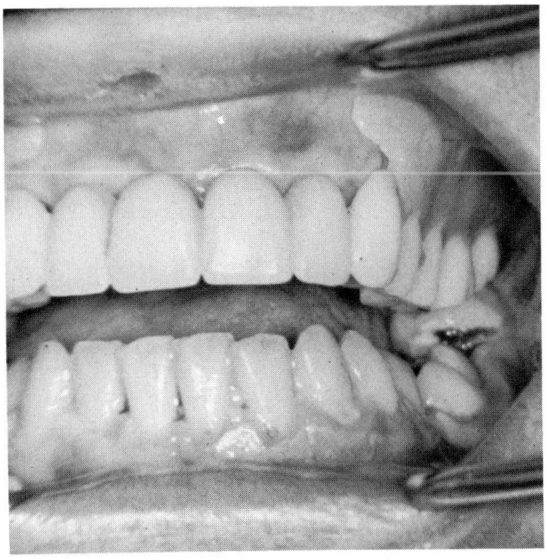

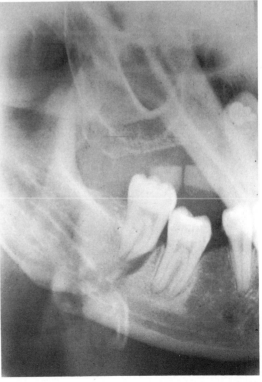

Figure 18–84 Flangeless full upper denture occluding with full complement of lower natural teeth. Fracture was anterior to the lower third molar and caused superior displacement, preventing the patient from closing in centric occlusion.

Figure 18–85 Radiograph of fracture situation in biphase external skeletal fixation may be used as an effective modality of treatment. Note unstable relationship of the lower third molar and posterior fragment with respect to the maxillary artificial denture.

trition—as opposed to a subfacially suspended denture with interarch immobilization.

The quasi-disadvantage of a neat external appliance and the minimal scarring resulting from the procedure were also discussed with the patient.

Operative Note. The single fracture, along with the opportunity for promptness of treatment and the ability to register the natural occlusion against the artificial denture, made it feasible to attempt a blind application of the external splint.

The patient was placed in a supine position, and anesthesia was established with a combination of intravenous and inhalation agents. Nasoendotracheal ventilation was employed.

The patient's skin was scrubbed with surgical soap and the field prepared with an antimicrobial preparative solution. Along with conventional surgical draping, a sterile Vi-drape was used to enhance the surgical field by making such pertinent anatomic landmarks as the corner of mouth, ala of nose and lobe of ear visible for orientation.

Since the angle of the mandible was involved, some compromise was exercised in the usual rotation of the head to the opposite side. This rotation was minimized. (If the head is rotated in an extreme manner to facilitate access, and a screw is

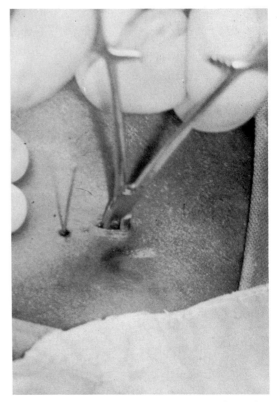

Figure 18–87 A small, straight hemostat is used to make a blunt dissection down to the bony surface. It is important that periosteum be stripped from the bone prior to attempting to drill the pilot holes.

placed without appreciation for this feature, there will be a "piling up" of the soft tissues above the screw when the head is returned to its normal position.)

A Keith needle (Fig. 18–86) was introduced through the skin to confirm precisely the position of the fracture plane in relation to the overlying skin. Two per cent lidocaine, 0.5 cc., with epinephrine (1:100,000) was injected into the skin and underlying soft tissues precisely at the screw sites to facilitate hemostasis. Following a delay of 7 minutes for hemostatic activity to become effective, a skin-only incision was made $\frac{3}{8}$ inch in length, compatible with Langer's lines. This initial incision was placed posterior to the Keith needle and at the lower border of the mandible, in such a manner as to permit a screw to be positioned in the bone without "fracturing out" the inferior or posterior border, or entering the fracture plane.

With a small, straight hemostat, the subcutaneous tissue, fascia, muscle and periosteum were bluntly dissected to develop a single pathway down to the bone (Fig. 18–87). Care was exercised to produce a neat, unragged, single passage from skin to bone. (It is important that the periosteum be definitely stripped from the bone at the site of drilling.)

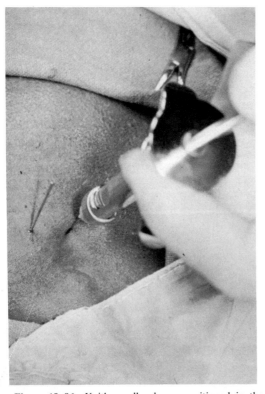

Figure 18–86 Keith needle shown positioned in the fracture plane to facilitate location of the external skeletal bone screws in a closed (or "blind") application. Anesthetic (2 per cent lidocaine with epinephrine, 1:100,000) is infiltrated at the actual screw site prior to making the small skin incision.

A ⁵/₆₄-inch, stainless steel twist drill was passively introduced into the lips of the incision and the point seated on periosteum-free bone. To prevent soft-tissue entanglement into the flutes of the drill point, an infant's nasal speculum (Fig. 18–88) was carefully positioned in the wound, with its blades parallel to the drill, for retraction of the soft tissue in such a way as to prevent trauma to adjacent nerve and vessel structure and fouling of the drill flutes (Fig. 18–89). The nasal speculum was kept in place by the assistant until the special cobalt-chromium (Vitallium) bone screw was positioned in the pilot hole (Fig. 18–90). (Compare Alternate Technique in text.)

The technique of individual screw insertion was repeated until two screws were appropriately located in each fragment.

One screw clamp of the primary splint was carefully positioned below the hexagonal table of the anterior mean screw. The other screw clamp was similarly positioned on the hexagonal shaft of the posterior mean screw, and both clamps were firmly locked with light instrument torque (Fig. 18–91). (This locking of the primary splint to the bone screws must be firmly and rigidly accomplished, but care must also be exercised not to tighten the system excessively or else the appliance will be damaged.)

At this time, attention was directed intraorally, where the denture was placed in position and, by manipulation, mandibular teeth were brought into occlusion with the denture. The lower third molar, in occlusion with the upper denture, held the pos-

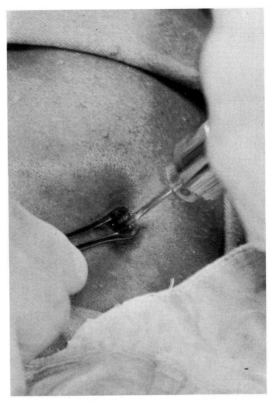

Figure 18–89 The nasal speculum not only protects the skin and subcutaneous structures but also prevents soft tissue from being introduced into the pilot hole and reaming it to oversize, which is the cause of a loose screw. It also prevents soft tissue from being carried into the pilot hole with the threads of the bone screw, which results in a wet screw.

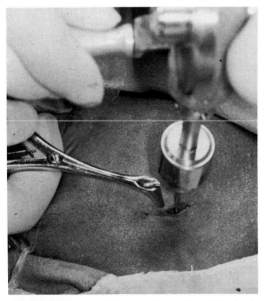

Figure 18–88 The drill point is positioned in the incision so that it exits without distorting the tissue. An infant's nasal speculum is then positioned to serve as a retractor and to prevent entanglement of soft tissue in the flutes of the drill.

terior fragment in an acceptable vertical position. Its precarious mediolateral position was aligned by manipulation, and the two rod clamps of the primary splint were tightened, using an antitorque wrench to prevent displacement as the mechanical splint became finally locked.

The distance between the two extreme screws was ascertained, and the take-apart mold was adjusted to accommodate this measurement (Fig. 18–92). Autopolymerizing denture acrylic was mixed in the ratio of 1 cc. of liquid to 3 cc. of powder. For this particular splint, 4 cc. of liquid were combined with 12 cc. of powder. After 3 minutes of *bench curing,* the putty-like mass was thoroughly kneaded and pressed into the lubricated take-apart mold (Fig. 18–93). After a minute's delay, the still-pliable plastic bar was carefully removed from the take-apart mold without deforming its shape. The plastic bar (while still in this plastic putty-like condition) was pressed onto the machine threads of the bone screws. Good adaptation and negative impression of the hexagonal table were insured by using the tamping end of the antitorque wrench, which has a small hole in the

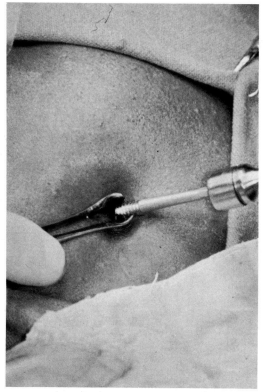

Figure 18–90 The predrilled pilot hole is more easily found when the assistant keeps the nasal speculum in position until the bone screw is introduced into the hole.

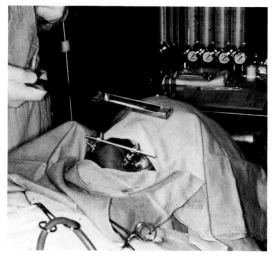

Figure 18–92 The take-apart mold in the surgeon's right hand has been adjusted in length to permit the formation of a plastic bar incorporating the four bone screws.

end of its handle to facilitate this operation (Fig. 18–94).

(This tamping contribution of the instrument facilitates adaptation of the acrylic bar to the screw without overly thinning the bar and, at the same time, leaves an appropriate protrusion of the threaded screws through the acrylic for placement of the lock nuts. If the span of the bar is lengthy, or if for any other reason there is likelihood that the acrylic will touch the skin, provision is made to prevent this with a wet sponge. The bar must definitely not actually contact soft tissue, since the heat of polymerization will be damaging to the tissue. However, if there is any air space between the soft tissue and acrylic, or if a wet sponge is between the soft tissue and acrylic bar, sufficient protection will be afforded. There is ample mass in the screws and the primary splint to dissipate all the heat of polymerization, so that there is no appreciable change in temperature carried through the screws to the tissue.)

The washer-faced nuts were then placed on the machine-threaded end of the bone screws and twisted only to a position slightly less than flush with the end of the screw. The final tightening to secure each nut flush with the end of the machine

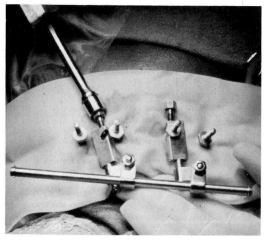

Figure 18–91 Screw clamp of primary splint being attached to one of the two screws in each fragment of the fractured mandible.

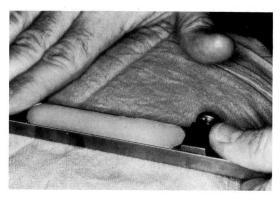

Figure 18–93 Autopolymerizing acrylic is pressed into the shape of a bar while it is still of a putty-like consistency. It is removed from the take-apart mold while it is in this pliable state.

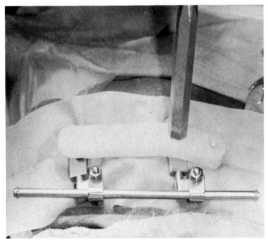

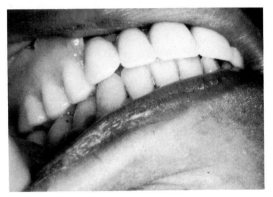

Figure 18–95 View of the patient's occlusion of natural lower teeth against upper denture during the period of biphase external skeletal fixation. Fixation in this manner permitted the patient to partake of a soft diet throughout her period of convalescence.

Figure 18–94 While still pliable, the plastic bar can be placed on the machine threads of the bone screws, even though the long axes of the screws are not parallel. A hole in the handle of the wrench facilitates adapting the plastic around the machine threads and down onto the hexagonal table, leaving an appropriate number of threads protruding through the plastic to accommodate the washer-faced lock nut, which is tightened only after the acrylic has polymerized.

thread was accomplished after the heat of polymerization had dissipated, which took from 3 to 5 minutes. (To overtighten the lock nut while the acrylic is soft is to invite a weakness in the splint, due to an excessive thinning of the bar at this site. This manifests itself by protrusion of machine threads past the head of the lock nut. Once autopolymerization has begun, heat dissipation and cooling may be sped up by the use of sloppy, wet sponge applications.)

When the bar had returned to room temperature, a rigid, resilient, light and uncumbersome connector held the mandible in the desired position for the fragments to heal. The primary or mechanical splint was then removed in reverse order from its application; that is, the rod clamps were first unlocked, after which the screw clamps were released and removed from the throats of the bone screws. For the first 24 hours a 4-inch by 4-inch gauze sponge was wrapped around the screw base to form a simple airscreen-type dressing (see Figure 18–82).

Good occlusion of the natural lower dentition against the full artificial denture was achieved and maintained without inner arch immobilization (Fig. 18–95). The patient received a full liquid diet for the first few days and then proceeded to a soft, "nonchewing"-type diet.

After a period of 5 weeks, the acrylic bar between the two mean screws was sectioned with a No. 703 tapering fissure bur. Consolidation was adequate, and the splint was removed without the support of any anesthesia, first by removal of the washer-faced lock nuts, and then by the notching of the acrylic above and below each machine-threaded portion of the individual bone screws. These notches were actually deep grooves made with a No. 703 fissure bur. A No. 34S elevator, placed in the grooves and rotated, fractured the acrylic from the screws and permitted the screwdriver to be attached to the hexagonal tables for removal by counter-rotation. Assuring the patient that there would be a slight sensation of pressure was all that was needed to effect an uneventful removal of the screws. All screws were firmly seated at the time of removal and required a counter-torque equivalent to that used to place the screws.

A very slight oozing of blood from each screw site was readily controlled with a 2-inch by 2-inch sponge and pressure, after which each screw site was painted with 2 per cent methylene blue, and a light dressing was applied for 48 hours.

Alternate Technique. An alternate technical approach to preventing soft-tissue entanglement into the flutes of the drill point (compare technique in Case Report No. 3) is to use a 10 gauge needle, cut off to a length of 2 inches, as a tube speculum. There may be some advantage in alignment which facilitates the screw in exiting through the lips of the incision without soft-tissue distortion (see Figure 18–97), but there is the occasional disadvantage of locating the pilot hole after the speculum is removed, which of course, is necessary.

The tube speculum technique offers an additional advantage, in that the drill may be placed in the chuck in such a manner that its point will project through the tube to a length equal to that of the threaded portion of the bone screw (Fig. 18–96). The hand drill, armed in this fashion, is helpful in indicating to the surgeon the thickness of the mandible at this particular location.

For drilling in the body of the mandible where two cortices exist (see Figure 18–99), a ³⁄₃₂-inch drill is employed. For drilling in a thin ascending ramus, or at the angle of the mandible where the two cortices fuse into one plate (see Figure 18–98), a ⁵⁄₆₄-inch drill is employed. Although not mandatory to the procedure, the use of surgical stainless steel, specially tempered twist drills and hand drilling has merit.

A properly positioned bone screw will exit from the lips of the incision with the surrounding tissues remaining passive and undis-

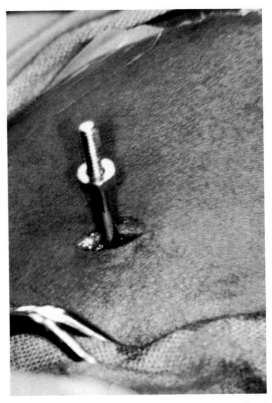

Figure 18–97 A properly placed bone screw will exit from the lips of the incision without distorting the soft tissue.

torted (Fig. 18–97). The hexagonal table of the screw will be near, but not impinging on, the soft tissues. The screw point will be well into, or better still have penetrated, the lingual plate. With regard to the inferior border, posterior border and fracture plane, the screw should be no closer than ¹⁄₂ inch, preferably ⁹⁄₁₆ inch, to such an edge. In the case of adjacency to the fracture plane, appropriate consideration is given to the obliqueness of the fracture. In general, but not mandatorily, screws are not placed closer to each other than ³⁄₈ inch.

The distance between screws in the same fragment is not critical, with the exception that they can be placed too close together. A space of from ¹⁄₂ to ⁵⁄₈ inch between the screws in the same fragment is quite generally acceptable as a minimum, whereas 1, 2 or even more inches may separate the screws as a maximum. The space between screws separated by the fracture plane is dictated by such factors as obliqueness of the plane and comminution and fragmentation of the bone, with a minimum distance falling in the range of 1 to 1¹⁄₄ inches.

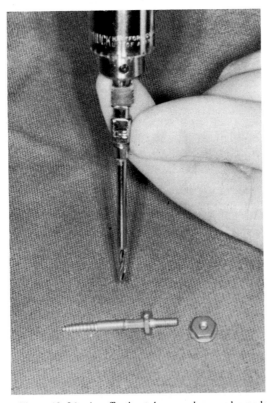

Figure 18–96 An effective tube speculum can be made by cutting a 10 gauge needle to a length of 2 inches. This type of speculum has the advantage of permitting the twist drill to be placed in the chuck in such a manner that the point of the drill protrudes through the speculum for a distance equal to the threaded portion of the bone screw. By noting the distance between the beaks of the chuck and the top of the speculum while drilling, one may ascertain the thickness of the mandible.

When placed in their functional position, the bone screws can be identified as *mean* and *extreme* screws. Those screws adjacent to the fracture plane are considered the mean screws. Those screws in a fragment with a screw between them and the fracture plane are designated extreme screws.

Two lengths of body screws are available (see Figure 18–249). The threaded portion is the same dimension on both screws. The difference in overall length results from a longer or shorter unthreaded cylindrical shaft to accommodate individual difference in musculature, edema and hematoma, which may vary from patient to patient.

One length of ramus screw is available. It differs from the body screws in that its threaded portion is shorter and a distinct shoulder has been developed at the termination of its threads. This remarkably enhances its stability in the compromised anatomic relationship with a single bony cortex in this region (Figs. 18–98, 18–99).

All screws have a hexagonal portion of the shaft just below the hexagonal table to facilitate a positive no-skid attachment of the screw to the primary mechanical splint. The hexagonal throat of the screw shaft fits pre-

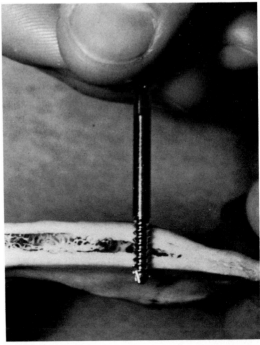

Figure 18–99 Screws placed in the body of the mandible have the benefit of two cortical plates. This greatly enhances the mechanical advantage and biomechanical stability of a screw placed in this position.

cisely into the slot of the screw clamp in such a way that minimal twisting of the set screw tends to seat the screw into the base of the slot securely, and virtually eliminates rotation.

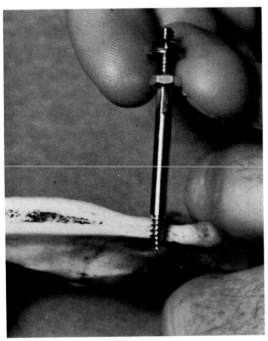

Figure 18–98 The inferior border of this dry specimen of a mandible has been planed off to the level at which screws are placed in the mandible. The single cortex of the ramus portion of the mandible requires a screw with shorter threads and with a distinct shoulder to enhance stability.

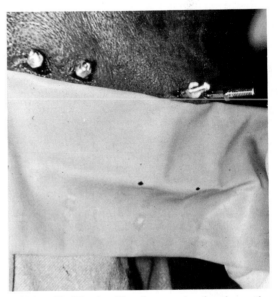

Figure 18–100 A rubber dam may be placed over the bone screws to isolate the adjacent tissues prior to intraoral work to establish occlusion. Contamination of the incisions at the screw sites is thus reduced.

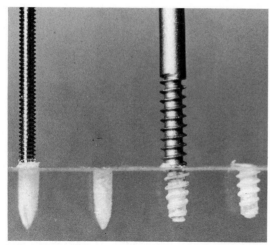

Figure 18–101 An artificial "mock-up" to illustrate the increased mechanical advantage and thread viability gained by using coarse lag-type threads of a bi-phase screw (on the right), twisted into a predrilled hole, as opposed to the pyramidal-pointed, machine-threaded Kirschner wire-type pin (on the left), which destroys any threading capability as it reams its own hole.

In some situations, one may wish to isolate the four screws with a sterile rubber dam, prior to making the application of the primary splint (Fig. 18–100).

Advantages. Biphase splints utilized as in Case Report No. 3 may be expected to retain their biomechanical stability routinely for periods in excess of 6 or 8 weeks. Numerous situations may be cited in which the splint has remained effective and stable for periods in excess of 9 months.

It appears that one of the truly significant differences accounting for exceptionally long periods of biomechanical stability with bi-phase external skeletal fixation relates to thread design of the screws and the technique of their placement. Early bone pins amounted to pyramidal-pointed, machine-threaded Kirschner wires of about 3/32-inch outside diameter with shallow threads of from 36 to 40 per inch. The pyramidal point drilled a hole in bone very close to the diameter of the Kirschner wire. The fine machine threads reamed the hole to this size and destroyed the true threading effect (Fig. 18–101). The bi-phase screw utilizes a lag-type thread (wood-screw thread), which is a coarse, deep thread. Only 20 threads per inch are turned on to a shaft of 1/8 inch in diameter. A screw is thus developed with a minor diameter of 3/32 inch and a major diameter of 1/8 inch. A predrilled pilot hole of 3/32 inch permits the screw to cut

viable threads into the bone cleanly. These threads offer remarkable surface area resistance, so that forces that would loosen a poorly developed machine-threaded pin can be resisted (Fig. 18–101).

OPEN REDUCTION

In this method the bone ends are surgically exposed either intraorally or extraorally, holes are drilled through the ends, and then a wire is threaded through the holes and twisted together, thus bringing the broken ends into direct apposition and immobilizing them. Two holes should be placed one above the other in the ends of each fragment. Two wires are passed through the holes crossing the wires as they pass from the upper hole in one fragment to the lower hole in the other so that they form an X before they are tightened (see Figure 18–102 and other forms of bare wiring in Figures 18–103 to 18–108).

Some oral surgeons prefer to use a bone plate to immobilize the fragments. A long plate with three or four holes will provide much better immobilization than the short plates with only two holes.

Since the introduction of external skeletal fixation, the author has found it less frequently necessary to use the open reduction method, except in cases of fibrous union (see Figures 18–255, 18–256, 18–261 and accompanying text).

LATERAL COMPRESSION
Stuart N. Kline, D.D.S.

Axial compression techniques, as exemplified by the use of various compression plates, have for many years been used by orthopedic and general surgeons in long bone fractures with notable success. However, axial compression is most effective for transverse fractures, and its efficacy diminishes in direct relationship to the degree of obliquity of the fracture. In long oblique fractures, compression plating may actually produce overriding of the fracture fragments (Fig. 18–109).

Since the vast majority of traumatic fractures of the mandible are to a greater or lesser degree oblique, lateral compression should be considered as a treatment method.

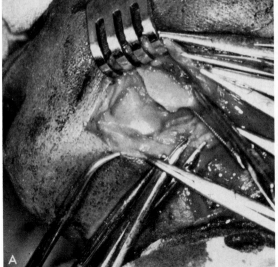

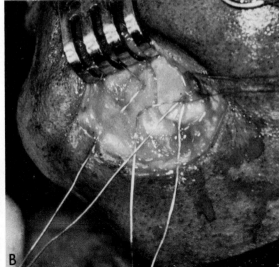

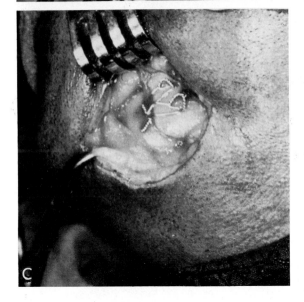

Figure 18–102   Extraoral open reduction of a unilateral fracture of an edentulous mandible by direct wiring.

As provided by the Peri-Cortical Clamp System,* lateral compression achieves marrow-to-marrow apposition of the fragments and rigid fixation and stabilization at the fracture site, thus leading to early consolidation of the fracture.

In experimental work on rhesus monkeys, the animals were first rendered edentulous and then, at an appropriate later date, bilateral fractures of the mandible were surgically created. One side was repaired with the Peri-Cortical Clamp and the opposite side by another method. The symphysis was divided,

so that neither type of internal fixation would influence the opposite side. No intermaxillary fixation was utilized.

Tetracycline fluorescent studies and histologic sections revealed bony union as early as 3 weeks at the fracture site repaired with the Peri-Cortical Clamp. Bony union occurred significantly later on the opposite side and in the symphyseal region.

Clinical experiences with the Peri-Cortical Clamp System utilizing lateral compression have confirmed the results of the experimental work. The basic goals of fracture fixation—anatomic reduction, bony union at the fracture site and early return of normal function—have been accomplished.

In the edentulous patient with a fractured

---

*Arnold Sampson, M.D., Pittsburgh, Pa., invented and designed the Peri-Cortical Clamp System.

(Text continued on page 1141)

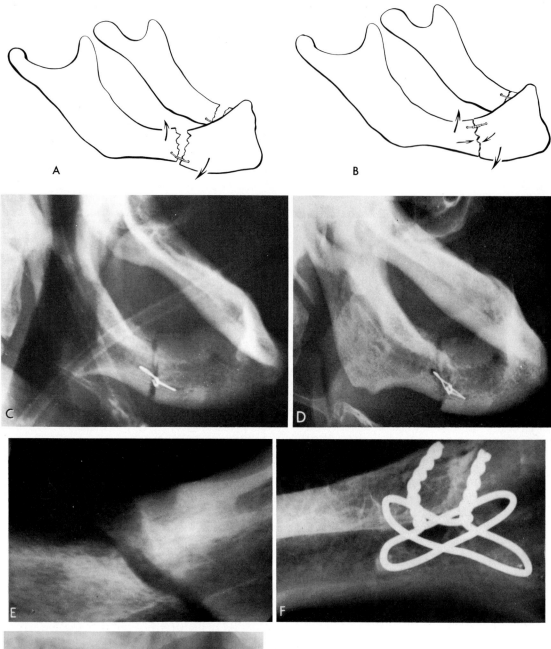

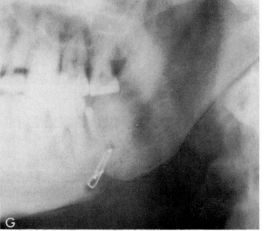

Figure 18–103 Incorrect and correct placement of interosseous wire for the reduction of fractures of the edentulous mandible. *A*, With this incorrect kind of wiring, the fragments have a tendency to separate because of the pull of the muscles attached to them. *B*, When the wiring is near the crest of the alveolar ridge, the pull of the muscles tends even to enhance the reduction accomplished by the correct wiring.

C to *G*, These radiographs illustrate that even in wide mandibles a single wire across the middle of the fracture, from the inferior to the superior cortical bone, will not prevent downward movement of the anterior segment.

(*A* and *B*, From Dingman, R. O., and Natvig, P.: Surgery of Facial Fractures. Philadelphia, W. B. Saunders Co., 1964.)

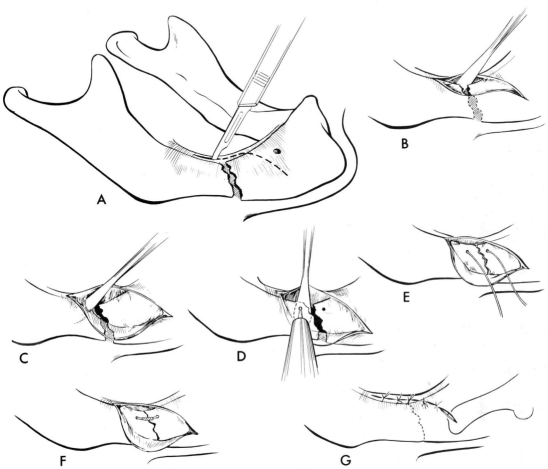

Figure 18–104 Steps in intraoral open reduction for fracture of the body of the mandible. *A,* An incision is made along the crest of the alveolar ridge and downward and forward, anterior to the site of the fracture. The flap should be large enough to give adequate covering to the fracture site after reduction, and designed so that the suture line does not lie directly over the line of fracture of the bone. *B,* The periosteum is elevated from the medial surface of the bone with a sharp elevator. *C,* The periosteum is stripped from the lateral surface sufficiently to expose the site of the fracture and to permit instrumentation without damage to the tissues. *D,* Bur holes are drilled on each side of the fracture site 5 mm. below the crest of the alveolar ridge and 5 mm. from the fractured margin. *E,* A stainless steel wire is passed through the bur holes, both ends appearing upon the lateral surface of the bone. The loop of wire on the medial surface should be flattened against the bone. *F,* The wires are twisted clockwise to fix the fragments in position securely. The ends of the wires are cut off. The remaining twisted end is bent and inserted into one of the bur holes. The wire should be flattened against the bone surface to avoid irritation from an overriding denture. *G,* A single layer closure of the mucoperiosteum is made with silk or absorbable sutures. The wire may have to be removed if it interferes with the wearing of an artificial denture (From Dingman, R. O., and Natvig, P.: Surgery of Facial Fractures. Philadelphia, W. B. Saunders Co., 1964.)

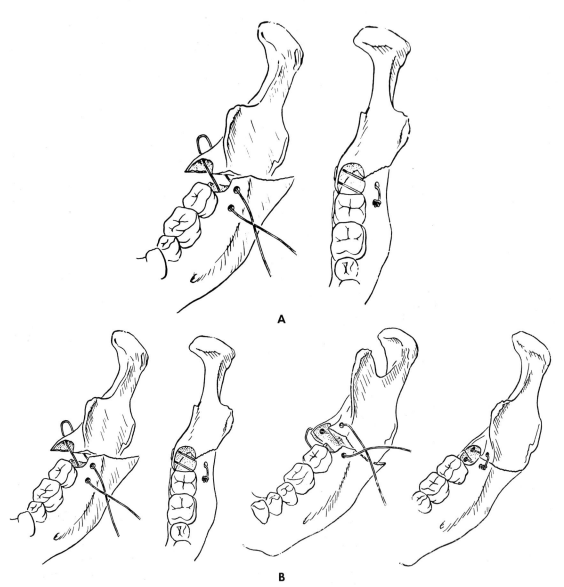

Figure 18–105 *A*, Method of upper border wiring used to correct the upward and medial displacement of the edentulous posterior fragment following fracture through the socket of the third molar.

B, Method of upper border wiring for the correction of upward displacement of the edentulous posterior fragment following fracture through the socket of the third molar. The horizontal mattress-type wire provides optimal stability, but in many cases, a simple loop through the buccal plate and bone is adequate. (From Rowe, N. L., and Killey, H. C.: Fractures of the Facial Skeleton. Edinburgh, Churchill Livingstone, 1968.)

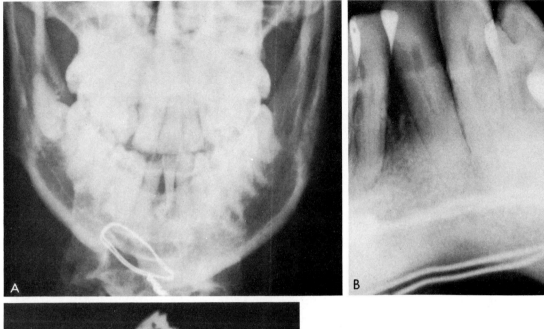

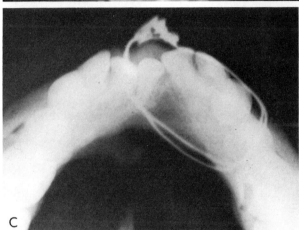

Figure 18–106   Several views of a healed fracture of the symphysis of the mandible in which the fracture was wired.

mandible repaired by the Peri-Cortical Clamp System no intermaxillary fixation is necessary.

In the edentulous patient the teeth should first be placed in proper occlusion by an occlusal wafer, interdental fixation or the method of choice of the individual surgeon, and then the Peri-Cortical Clamp should be applied. This patient's jaws may be mobilized as early as 3 weeks or less after fixation. (See Figures 18–110 and 18–111.)

Advantages of the Peri-Cortical Clamp System are:

1. Ease of application.
2. Elimination of intermaxillary fixation in the edentulous patient.

3. Early mobilization in the patient with dentition, avoiding problems of temporomandibular ankylosis, nutrition and oral hygiene.
4. Decrease in patient discomfort.

Removal of the Peri-Cortical Clamp is indicated after fracture healing has occurred in certain cases: (a) in anterior fractures of the body or symphysis when cosmetic considerations suggest removal; and (b) in those edentulous patients whose dentures no longer fit well because of the clamp. Since fracture healing is almost exclusively endosteal utilizing the Peri-Cortical Clamp, removal is simple and can usually be done under local anesthesia.

(*Text continued on page 1146*)

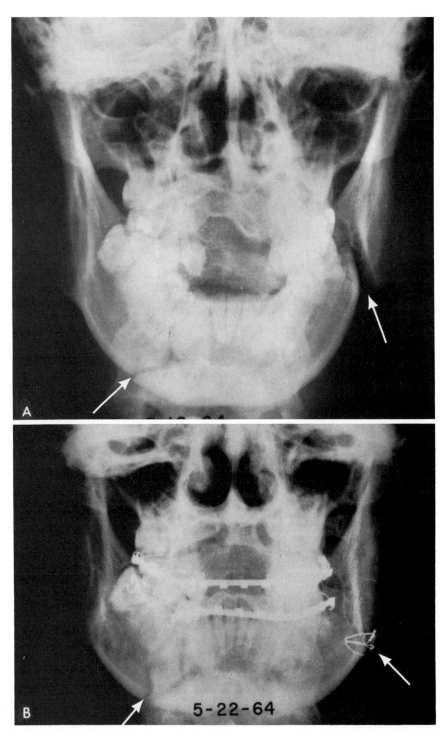

Figure 18–107   *A*, Bilateral fracture of the mandible. A linear fracture of the symphysis with no displacement of the fragments and a compound fracture through the angle with lateral displacement of the ramus.

B, Fracture at the angle treated by open reduction and wiring of the fragments. Intermaxillary elastic bands between the maxillary and mandibular splints were used to hold the fragments in normal occlusion. No additional stabilization was required for the simple linear fracture of the symphysis.

C, Left oblique radiograph after open reduction and wiring of the fracture through the angle of the mandible.

(Figure 18–107 continued on opposite page)

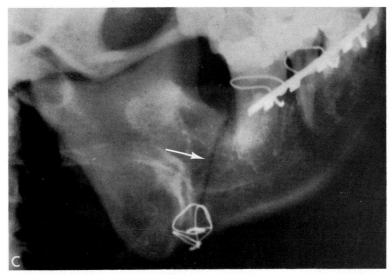

Figure 18-107   *(Continued.)*

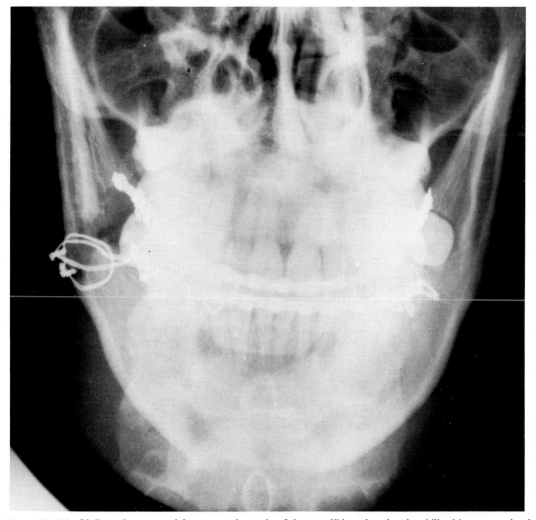

Figure 18-108   Unilateral compound fracture at the angle of the mandible reduced and stabilized by open reduction and wiring. The usual intermaxillary fixation, as previously described, is a necessary part of the treatment.

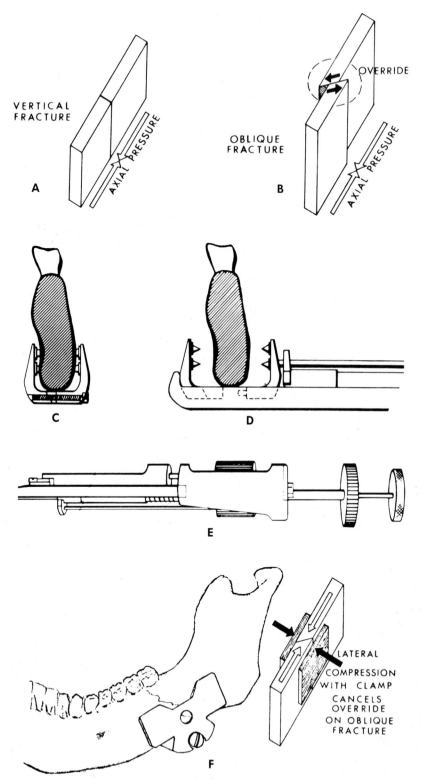

Figure 18–109 *A*, Vertical fracture: axial compression does not produce overriding. *B*, Oblique fracture: axial compression produces overriding. *C* and *D*, Maintenance of compressive force with screw. *E*, Inserter with compression knob. *F*, Oblique fracture: lateral compression prevents overriding.

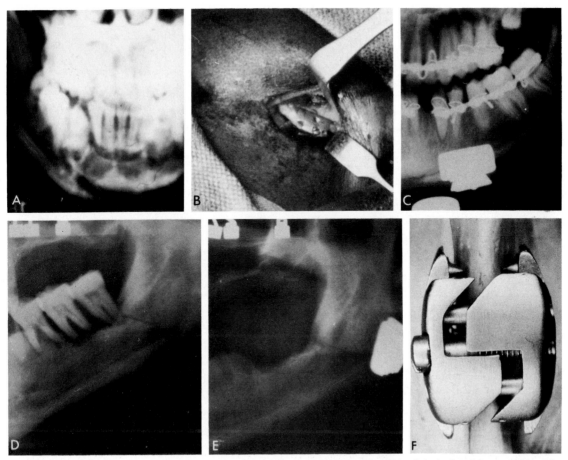

Figure 18–110 *A* to *C*, Treatment of a dentulous patient. *A*, Longitudinal fracture of the body of the mandible with lateral displacement of the posterior fragment. *B*, Fracture area exposed with the compression clamps in place (see *F*). *C*, Oblique radiograph showing reduced and immobilized fracture with clamp in position. It is necessary in dentulous patients to attach splints to the necks of the maxillary and mandibular teeth and to place intermaxillary elastics between the splints to bring the teeth into normal occlusion and then to hold them in occlusion when the clamps are applied.

D to *F*, Treatment of an edentulous patient. *D*, Fracture through the angle of the mandible. Note the extremely advanced destruction of alveolar bone due to periodontoclasia, which necessitated the extraction of these teeth. *E*, Fracture reduced and immobilized with a clamp. *F*, Inferior view of a clamp on an anatomic specimen of the mandible.

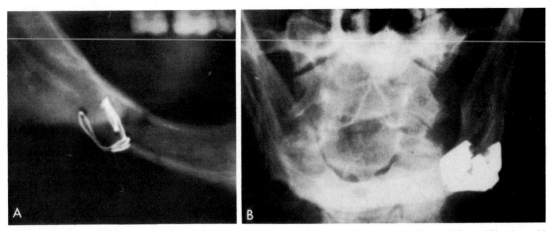

Figure 18–111 *A*, Nonunion with a draining extraoral sinus due to inadequate reduction and immobilization with open reduction wiring of the fragments. *B*, After removal of wires and necrotic bone, the fracture was reduced and immobilized with a bone clamp. Healing was uneventful.

SIMPLE BILATERAL FRACTURE OF THE MANDIBLE

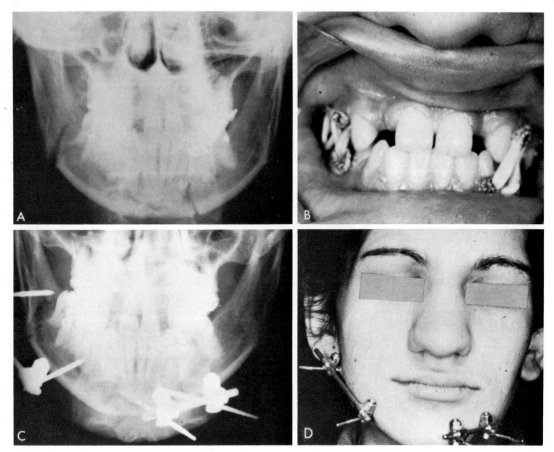

Figure 18–112 *A,* Simple bilateral fracture of the mandible through the molar socket (right) and between the left cuspid and first bicuspid. *B,* Occlusion has been established by intermaxillary elastics between wire knobs. In *A,* the fracture lines are separated at the inferior border. *C,* Single pins inserted on either side of each fracture; the pins are pulled together and held with connecting bars. *D,* Extraoral pin fixation for each fracture.

Case Report No. 4

TREATMENT OF OSTEOMYELITIS AND NONUNION OF MANDIBLE WITH MALOCCLUSION, AS PART OF GENERAL REHABILITATION OF PATIENT WITH COMPLETE LEFT HEMIPLEGIA AND PARTIAL PARESIS OF RIGHT LOWER EXTREMITY*

Past History. The history of this patient, both unusual and fascinating, has a direct bearing upon the oral surgical treatment which was later instituted. It will, therefore, be quite complete.

This patient sought the advice of a physician because of a feeling of fullness, accompanied by some difficulty in swallowing, in his oropharynx. He was advised that his tonsils were enlarged and should be removed. Upon the removal of the right tonsil, it was noted that a tumor was present in the

*The Department of Physical Medicine is to be highly complimented for the thorough and highly efficient manner in which they proceeded with the rehabilitation of this patient. Case report prepared by W. B. Irby, as an Oral Surgery Resident, Veterans Administration Hospital, Pittsburgh, Pa.

tissues of the throat posterior to the tonsillar bed. Acting on the advice of his two brothers, who were physicians, this patient went to New York for treatment. During the biopsy of this tumor, in the oncologist's office, a severe hemorrhage occurred which necessitated an emergency tracheostomy and packing of the throat. He was immediately admitted to the hospital, where he remained for 10 days. Three months later he returned to New York City and underwent an operation for the removal of the tumor of the pharynx. This tumor proved to be a schwannoma. A record of the operation performed follows.

Findings. There was a 4 by 5 by 4 cm. encapsulated tumor mass in the right pterygomaxillary space. This mass lay just anterior to the vagus nerve, medial and posterior to the hypoglossal nerve and posterior to the internal carotid artery and had displaced the internal carotid artery medially. It was attached to the internal carotid artery at one point which was thought to be the point where the previous punch biopsy had been taken.

Procedure. After the patient had been anesthetized and the neck and right face draped in a sterile field, a U-shaped incision was outlined in the right upper neck extending from just below the mentum of the mandible down along the upper border of the anterior belly of the digastric muscle and over the upper border of the posterior belly of the digastric muscle back to just below the mastoid process. The upper skin flap was then raised to the angle of the mandible. The mandibular branch of the facial nerve was protected after being identified. Dissection was then carried down anterior to the border of the sternocleidomastoid muscle. The hypoglossal nerve was identified. The external carotid artery was identified and ligated with tantalum wire and the internal carotid artery identified. The tumor mass bulged posterior to the posterior belly of the digastric muscle and lateral to the internal carotid artery and posterior to the hypoglossal nerve. The surface of the tumor mass was identified by blunt and sharp dissection after dividing several small veins. The hypoglossal nerve was identified, protected and retracted downward. The posterior belly of the digastric muscle was transected and the muscle retracted to the side and the tumor mass more adequately mobilized. By blunt finger dissection, the tumor mass was freed up laterally and posteriorly. Medially, there was attachment along a large vessel, and during finger dissection very brisk arterial bleeding was encountered. It was thought that a tear had been made in the internal carotid artery. With digital pressure the bleeding was controlled and the tumor mass was shelled out by blunt dissection. It appeared to be attached to the vagus nerve posteriorly, but by sharp dissection it was removed from the surface of the vagus nerve. During the rapid dissection and removal of the tumor which followed the bleeding, the hypoglossal nerve was inadvertently torn. After the tumor mass had been removed, the bleeding point was identified as the tear in the internal carotid artery. The tear measured about 1 cm. in length. The wound was packed to control the bleeding. The mandible, which had been sectioned, was then approximated with 2 criss-crossing stainless steel sutures. Subcutaneous tissues of the wound were then approximated with interrupted chromic No. 0 catgut sutures, the pack being brought out through a Penrose drain in the middle portion of the wound. The skin was closed with interrupted Dermalon sutures. The patient withstood the procedure well and received 1500 cc. of blood.

Note: In order to more readily mobilize the tumor mass, it was deemed necessary to transect the mandible. Therefore, in the region of the right first molar, the mandible was transected with a Stryker saw in a V-type incision, so that one fragment of the mandible was notched and the other tapered. Four holes were then drilled in the mandible, two on either side of the line of incision, and the wires were inserted and twisted for stability.

Six days after the operation, while the packing of the wound was being exchanged, the patient suffered a severe hemorrhage which necessitated ligation of the right common carotid artery. Following this, he went into a state of semi-coma and showed an apparent complete paralysis of the four extremities. He received a series of stellate ganglion blocks, a course of heparin for 10 days and daily injections of Etamon which were later discontinued because they produced diarrhea. Beginning 5 weeks after ligation, he was able to sit up and to control his sphincters, but had to be fed. The paralysis appeared to be generally lessening and the patient had acquired good motion of the right upper extremity. He could also move slightly the fingers of his left hand and bend his toes on the right side. There was some return of function of the left knee. He was transferred to the Physical Medicine Service, Veterans Administration Hospital, Aspinwall, Pennsylvania, for the purpose of rehabilitation.

Physical Findings. Examination upon admission to this hospital, 6 weeks after ligation of the common carotid, revealed a bedfast, white male, age 52, well-developed and poorly nourished. He was pleasant and eager to cooperate. He appeared rather anxious and apprehensive. His speech was relevant and coherent but conversation was difficult because of a speech defect caused by paralysis and atrophy of the right muscles of the tongue. His voice was hoarse and he could only whisper because of residual paralysis of his right vocal cords. He did not appear unduly depressed. Sensorium was clear. There was no apparent memory impairment. Intelligence was impossible to evaluate. Insight and judgment were not considered impaired. There was marked hypertrophy of the right lower side of the face with an unhealed draining incision at the angle of the right mandible (Fig. 18–113*A*). There was a healed scar at the site of the common right carotid artery. Another healed scar appeared midline in the neck over the trachea

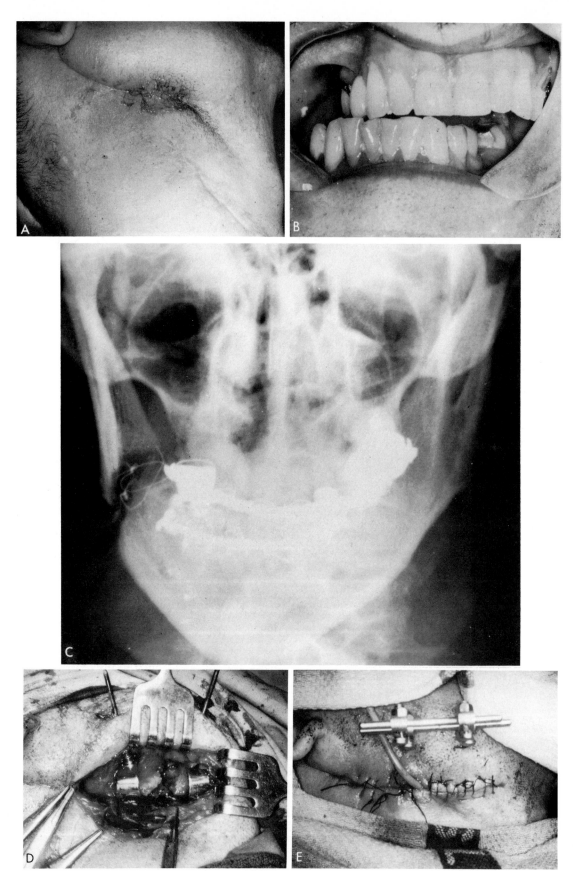

Figure 18–113 Treatment of osteomyelitis and nonunion of the mandible. (See Case Report No. 4 for details.)

(*Figure 18–113 continued on opposite page*)

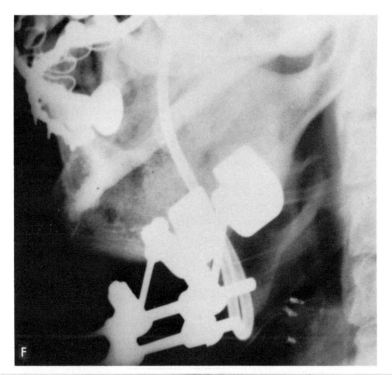

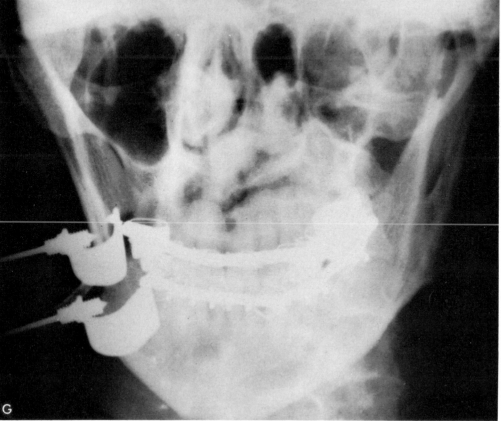

Figure 18–113 *(Continued.)*

(Figure 18–113 continued on following page)

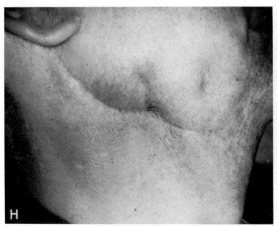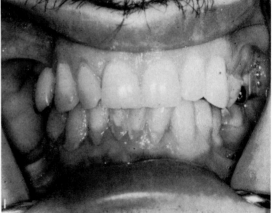

Figure 18–113   *(Continued.)*

(tracheostomy). The pupils were in myosis, equal and regular, and reacted briskly to light and accommodation. Fundi examination was not feasible. There was considerable atrophy of the muscles of the tongue on the right side with resulting paralysis. It was impossible to examine the throat at a deep level. He had difficulty in swallowing and drooled saliva. There were moist rales at both lung bases posteriorly. The heart appeared moderately enlarged downward and to the left. The pulse missed occasional beats. Peripheral vessels were moderately sclerosed. Blood pressure was 172/88. Neurologically, the patient was bedfast, with complete left hemiplegia and partial paresis of the right lower extremity. Muscle tone was poor throughout. The left upper extremity was flabby and was held in a semi-cast. There were weak flexion motions of the left fingers and a bilateral foot drop. Sensory functions were impossible to ascertain. The deep reflexes were hypoactive in the upper extremities, absent in the lower extremities. Examination of the cutaneous reflexes showed that the

right plantar was absent and there was a fanning of the left toes. Involved cranial nerves were as follows: VII, right central paresis; IX, right paralysis, dysarthria and dysphagia; XII, right paralysis. Urinary and rectal sphincters apparently were controlled at this time.

Oral Examination. Examination revealed a scar extending from below the lobe of the right ear, along the lower border of the body of the right mandible as far forward as the cuspid region. A fistula was evident opposite the molar area on this side from which oozed thick white pus. There appeared to be considerable contracture of the incision line, particularly in the region of the fistula. Intraoral examination disclosed that the molar and first premolar teeth were missing on the mandibular right side. The remainder of the teeth were in excellent condition. Attempts to occlude the teeth revealed a severe deviation of the mandible toward the right side (Fig. 18–113B). Digital and visual examination disclosed evidence of a nonunion of the mandible, with the posterior fragment elevated

Figure 18–114   Use of Thoma clamp for skeletal fixation of fracture. This is useful for potentially infected sites where insertion of pins into healthy bone may introduce infection. *A*, Diagram showing fracture and site of incision under body of mandible. *B*, Clamps without screws are placed on bone. *C*, The external end of the screw, which has a sharp point, is then passed from the inside of the incision out through the cheek at a point opposite the threaded portion of the clamp. Another technique of placing the screw involves the use of a stab incision through the cheek and insertion of the screw from the external surface. However, since the screw is much wider than the attached pin, too large an incision must be made, and the author prefers the former technique even though there must be somewhat wider retraction of the extraoral incision. *D*, Screw threaded into clamp and tightened so that clamp becomes firmly engaged to mandible. Incision closed (actually this is not done until fracture is reduced and fixed). Also, the threaded portion of the screw does not usually project as far externally as shown here but is completely covered with soft tissues. *E*, Pins and clamp in place. *F*, Fracture reduced and fixed with two short connecting bars. Extra rigidity in prevention of rotational torque is obtained by using two bars instead of one. *G*, Incision closed with rubber dam drain inserted or, *H*, with irrigation tube inserted. Use of tube or drain depends upon individual circumstances.

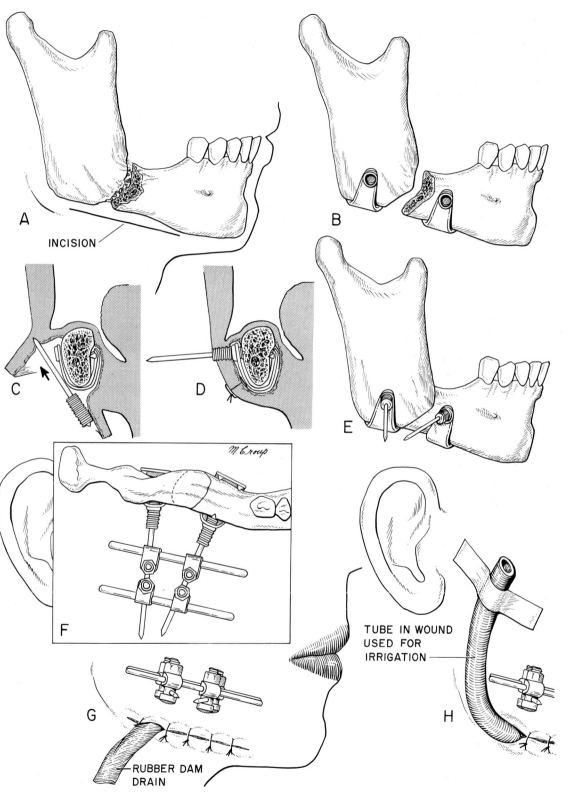

A INCISION

B

C

D

E

F *M. Croup*

G RUBBER DAM DRAIN

H TUBE IN WOUND USED FOR IRRIGATION

Figure 18–114 *See opposite page for legend.*

upward and forward. The right side of the tongue appeared to have undergone considerable atrophic changes.

Radiographic examination showed an area of rarefaction of the body of the right mandible located in the molar area. There was approximately 2 cm. distance between the bone ends, and the posterior fragment was upward and forward from its normal position. A radiopaque object which appeared to be coiled wire of fine gauge was seen in the rarefied area between the bone ends (Fig. 18–113C).

Laboratory Findings. All test results were within normal limits.

Opinions of Consultants. This patient was placed on the physical medicine service for a program of rehabilitation. Consultation requests were sent to the Neurologic, E.N.T., Plastic and Oral Surgery services.

The E.N.T. Department decided upon and scheduled an operation for the closure of a tracheal fistula.

The Plastic Service reported that it was the opinion of this group that the case was not a surgical case at the present time.

The Oral Surgery Department reported that the presence of a localized osteomyelitis and soft tissue infection, accompanied by a nonunion of the mandible, constituted a serious threat to the rehabilitation of this patient and that an attempt should be made to correct this condition. A treatment outline was formulated and an operation was to be scheduled as soon as the Physical Medicine Department deemed it advisable.

Treatment and Progress. *September 11.* The patient underwent an operation for closure of the tracheal fistula performed by the E.N.T. Department.

September 29. The patient was much more active. He attempted to feed himself and sat on the side of his bed dangling his feet. At this point the patient was attending Physical Therapy Clinic twice daily, and showed considerably more incoordination than was first apparent.

October 8. Patient showed considerable return of power in upper extremities. Progress was termed satisfactory.

October 24. Impressions were taken of upper and lower arches and stone models were constructed.

October 26. Cast arch bars were wired to the teeth of the upper and lower arch. The patient was scheduled for surgery October 29.

Operation. Under intravenous and nasoendotracheal anesthesia the patient was prepared and the operative field was draped with sterile drapes. The patient's teeth were occluded and secured in this position by intermaxillary stainless steel wires applied to previously placed cast dental splints. A portion of the operative scar extending approximately 1½ inches medially and 1½ inches laterally to the draining sinus was excised. An elliptical incision was made about the sinus tract, and the sinus tract, which extended to the fracture, was excised. The remainder of the skin incision was then carried down through scar tissue approximately ¾ inch thick to the lower border of the mandible. The underlying portion of the mandible was exposed and freed by blunt dissection with periosteal elevators. The distal fragment of the mandible was found to be retracted upward. The necrotic tissue about the bone fragments was removed by curettes and the necrotic bone removed with bone files. Two pieces of what appeared to be tantalum wire were removed with the necrotic tissue near the fracture site. The ends of the bone fragments were then scarified with a small gouge and mallet. A Thoma bone clamp was applied to each fragment approximately ½ inch from the fracture. The locking pin of each bone clamp was brought out through the skin and tightened (Fig. 18–113D and G). The bone fragments were then manipulated manually and were held fixed in reduced position by two Roger Anderson bars applied to the projecting locking pins of the Thoma bone clamps. A No. 10 French urethral catheter was placed at the fracture site and fixed to the skin with one black silk suture (Fig. 18–113E and F). Bleeding was controlled by the use of a Bovie unit and by 000 chromic ties. The subcutaneous tissue was closed with 000 chromic catgut sutures and the skin was closed with 0000 black silk sutures. The intermaxillary wires, previously applied to the dental splints, were removed. The patient was taken from the operating room in good condition.

Study Figure 18–114 for the technique used in this case.

Postoperative Notes. *October 29.* Orders included penicillin, 100,000 units every 3 hours, and Demerol, 100 mg. every 3 hours when required. The patient's head was to be kept turned to the right, and rubber intermaxillary ligatures were to be placed as soon as patient recovered.

October 29, 12 A.M. Patient was sleeping but could be readily aroused, and was quite clear in answering questions. Intermaxillary rubber bands were placed. Blood pressure was 148/96, and chest was clear.

At this time, orders included a liquid diet. The patient was to be turned frequently (with care being taken not to change head position) and catheterized every 8 hours when required.

October 30. More bands were placed to swing mandible to right. Continuous irrigations were begun through catheter. (Solution contained 500,000 units penicillin.)

November 4. Purulent drainage still persisted around catheter. Irrigations were made through catheter using 10,000 units. Bacitracin in 10 cc. water four times a day; sutures were removed.

November 12. Irrigations were continued. An area of erythema was evident on right side of neck which was probably due to continuous moisture and local sensitivity to antibiotics.

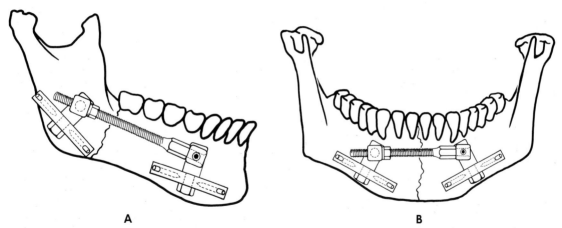

A   **B**

Figure 18–115 *A,* Stader splint applied to reduce and immobilize the posterior fragment. This fragment is generally displaced lingually and upward, overriding the anterior fragment, or it is displaced bucally and upward, overriding the anterior fragment. The treatment in these cases is as follows: (*1*) Place the pin bars in position. (*2*) Attach splints to the maxillary and mandibular teeth. (*3*) Apply intermaxillary elastics to bring the teeth into normal occlusion. (*4*) Attach the connecting bar to the pin bars so that the units may be manipulated. (*5*) Adjust the connecting bar so as to reduce and immobilize the posterior fragment. (*6*) Do not remove the elastics for approximately 4 weeks in the average case. (*7*) If, after several days, the occlusion is still normal, the splints can be removed from the teeth. (*8*) At the end of 6 weeks loosen the connecting bar and test for union by digitally attempting to move the fragment. If satisfactory union is present, the Stader splint can be removed. If not, tighten the connecting bar.

B, In this type of fracture there may be no displacement. All that is required is immobilization, which may be obtained by the application of the Stader splint, as illustrated in *A.* The Frac-Sur Roger Anderson external fixation appliance may also be used when there is no displacement. When there is marked displacement, however, the Stader splint is indicated.

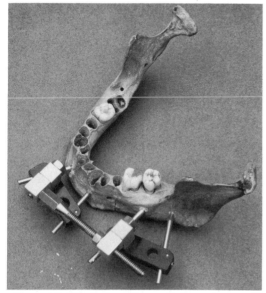

Figure 18–116 Stader splint applied on a dry mandible.

November 13. Rubber ligatures were changed, and the drainage lessened considerably.

November 18. Drainage completely ceased.

November 20. A slight amount of serous drainage was noted. Irrigations through a polyvinyl tube were started using a Bacitracin solution. Rubber intermaxillary ligatures were replaced by wire ligatures due to attempts of patient to open mouth.

November 26. Drainage completely ceased. At this point, the patient was being seen daily by the hygienist for cleansing of mouth.

January 3. The patient was now ambulatory with the aid of crutches and drop foot braces. He was not using body braces. Oral splints were removed.

February 11. The pins were removed from the bone clamp. A slight amount of pus was seen around the pins.

February 13. There was no discharge from the pin sites. Extraoral x-rays showed evidence of bony union of the mandible. No movement was evident clinically.

March 10. The site of the former drainage continued healthy and dry (Fig. 18–113*H*). The pa-

UNILATERAL COMPOUND COMMINUTED FRACTURE OF THE MANDIBLE

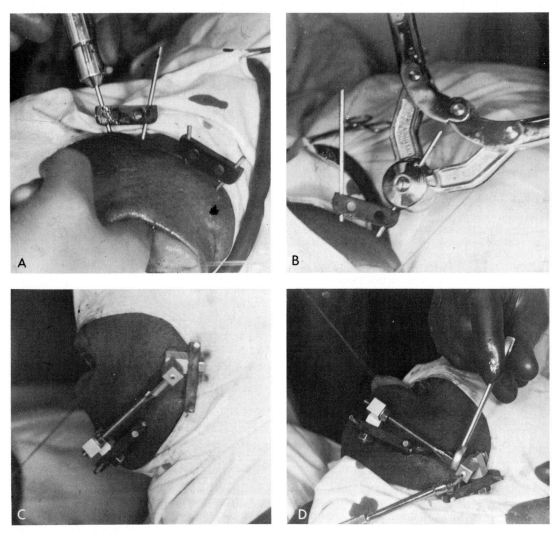

Figure 18–117 Application of the Stader splint for reduction of a unilateral fracture of an edentulous mandible.

A, A pin bar is placed on either side of the fracture. (Be careful not to place the pins too close to the fracture.) The assistant places his finger in the mouth and alongside the lingual surface of the mandible to support the mandible while the pins are inserted with the drill.

B, The pins are then cut off with the pin bar cutter.

C, The fracture is reduced and immobilized.

D, The Stader connecting bar is attached, and the overriding fragments are reduced to normal alignment. Then all nuts and set screws are tightened to hold the fragments in place.

tient was now taking all types of food, his teeth were in normal occlusion (Fig. 18–113*I*) and he was walking with a cane. He was placed on a 45-day furlough, to be recalled for a revision of his scar and the removal of the bone clamps.

April 21. The patient returned complaining of pain in the right side of his jaw. Examination re-vealed that one of the bone clamps had become loose and was gravitating through the skin.

April 23. The bone clamps were removed under local anesthesia and a catheter drain inserted for irrigation.

May 3. The incision was healed. Patient discharged.

Case Report No. 5

TREATMENT OF MARKED OVERRIDING OF MANDIBULAR FRACTURE WITH STADER EXTRAORAL APPLIANCE

Patient. This male patient, aged 54, was attaching a chain to a tractor from a truck when the truck backed into him, striking his lower jaw and left ear. The patient stated that his external ear was torn and hung on by only a small pedicle. He was treated at another hospital, where his ear was sutured and a bandage applied. He was transferred to Eye and Ear Hospital with a head bandage in place (Fig. 18–118*A* and *B*).

Examination. This revealed a well-developed, well-nourished white man in acute distress from a unilateral fracture of the left mandible in the mental foramen area with marked overriding of the fragments. Intraoral examination revealed a partially edentulous maxilla and mandible, poor oral hygiene and partial trismus. There was marked edema and ecchymosis of the anterior portion of the ridge, mucobuccal fold and floor of the mouth. The chin was displaced to the right.

The pupils reacted to light and accommodation, and there were no gross disturbances in vision. There was a laceration of the left ear. Examination of the nose was negative.

Laboratory Findings. The results were all within normal limits.

X-ray Examination. This confirmed a fracture of the right mandible in the bicuspid region. The fragments lapped each other for a distance of about 1 inch (Fig. 18–118*C*) and the posterior fragment was pulled laterally. No other fractures of the facial bones or skull were found.

Course. The head bandage was removed and replaced with a mastoid dressing. The patient was scheduled for reduction of the fracture by the application of a Stader splint.

Operation. Under general anesthesia, the fracture line was located by digital palpation. The lower portion of the mandible, and the fracture line, were outlined with tincture of iodine; locations for pin insertions on either side of the fracture line were marked with dots of iodine. A pin was coated with petrolatum and placed in the electric drill. The skin was pierced by the pin and the cortex contacted, then the pin drilled into the mandible at the points marked. Two pins were placed through the pin bar in the left fragment of the mandible and two in the right. The connecting bar was then placed between the pin bars and bolted into place. The threaded connecting bar was turned to distract the overriding fragments and then turned in the opposite direction so as to bring the fractured ends together. The units were then locked with a wrench.

The patient was taken from the operating room in good condition.

Postoperative Course. The patient received 400,000 units of penicillin every 24 hours with routine postoperative orders. The patient had marked edema and ecchymosis for several days.

Radiographs taken on the tenth postoperative day showed the mandibular fragments, after application of the Stader splint, in satisfactory position. See Figure 18–118*D* and *E*.

The edema continued to subside, and the patient was discharged from the hospital on the fourteenth postoperative day, to be followed at the office.

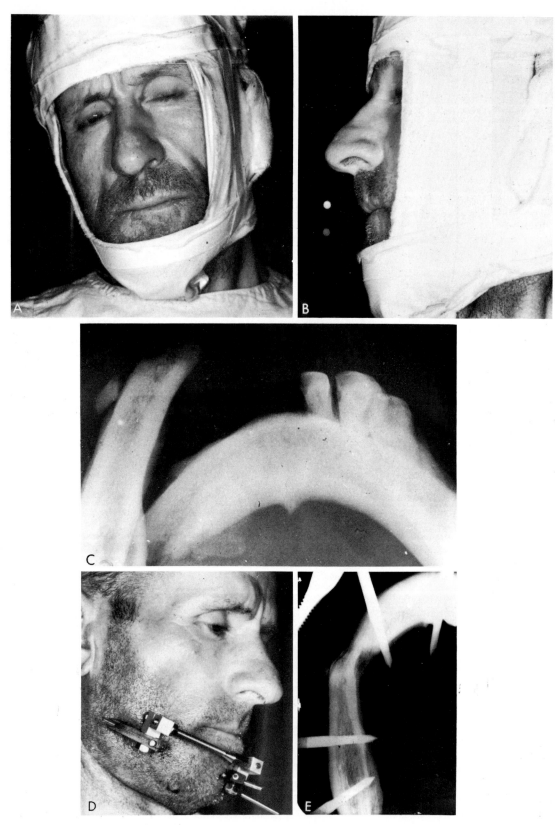

Figure 18–118   *See opposite page for legend.*

FRACTURES OF THE NECK OF THE CONDYLE

There is no indication for open reduction of subcondylar fractures. Numerous surveys, and at least one animal experiment, have shown conclusively that the conservative or "closed method" of treating these fractures, unilateral or bilateral, has resulted in complication-free, very satisfactory end results.

On the contrary, meddlesome surgery in the form of open reduction frequently results in trismus or ankylosis, or sterile or suppurative resorption of the condyle. It has been reported that it is necessary occasionally to remove a fractured and displaced condyle because it obstructed mandibular movement. The author has never seen this situation.

Treatment. These fractures, unilateral or bilateral (see Figure 18–119), are treated best by the simple process of holding the teeth in their normal occlusion by intermaxillary elastics attached to splints. In edentulous cases the dentures are then attached to the maxilla and mandible as shown in Figure 18–132 and held in their normal occlusion by intermaxillary elastics.

When one or both of the dentures have been destroyed or lost at the time of the accident, then acrylic bite plates are made up arbitrarily to establish the correct intermaxillary relationship and the jaws are immobilized, as shown in Figures 18–130 or 18–132.

If the dentures are serviceable, splints are wired to the necks of the maxillary and mandibular teeth. The mandibular splint is pinned to the mandible if there is a wide labial flange on the denture; otherwise it is wired to the mandible by circumferential wiring. The upper denture is inserted and held in position by pins as shown in Figures 18–130, 18–132 and 18–150, or by a stainless steel wire passed through a hole drilled in the base of the nasal septum and then twisted around the maxillary splint. The overriding of the fracture of the neck of the condyle is reduced by placing elastic traction in the form of rubber bands between the maxillary and mandibular splints.

In the author's experience the less manipulation of fractures of the neck of the condyle, the better the end result. This applies to cases in which the head of the condyle is still in the mandibular fossa or to those in which the head has been dislocated from the mandibular fossa.

For additional information on this subject read the next section, Mandibular Fractures in Children.

(Text continued on page 1174)

Figure 18–118   See Case Report No. 5. *A* and *B*, Appearance of patient on admission to our hospital. This bulky bandage and adhesive-type Barton bandage with ear dressing had produced more overriding of the fragments than the accident because of the back traction of the bandage around the neck (see *C*).

C, Radiograph showing fracture of right mandible with overriding of fragments.

D, Patient 2 days after operation, showing extraoral appliance in place which was used first to distract the fragments, correcting the override, and then to bring them into apposition and to maintain fragments in alignment.

E, Occlusal radiograph showing alignment of fractures 6 weeks after reduction and fixation with the extraoral Stader splint.

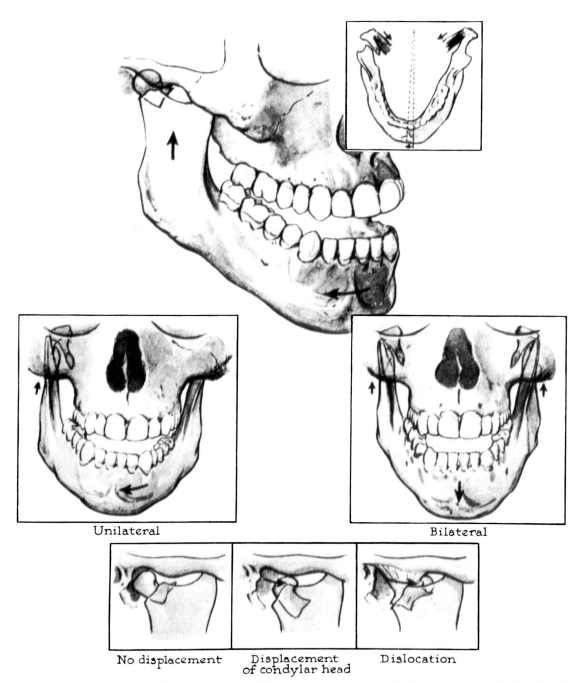

Unilateral   Bilateral

No displacement   Displacement   Dislocation
                      of condylar head

Figure 18–119   Fractures of the neck of the condyle. (From Massler, M., and Schour, I.: Atlas of the Mouth and Adjacent Parts in Health and Disease. Chicago, American Dental Association.)

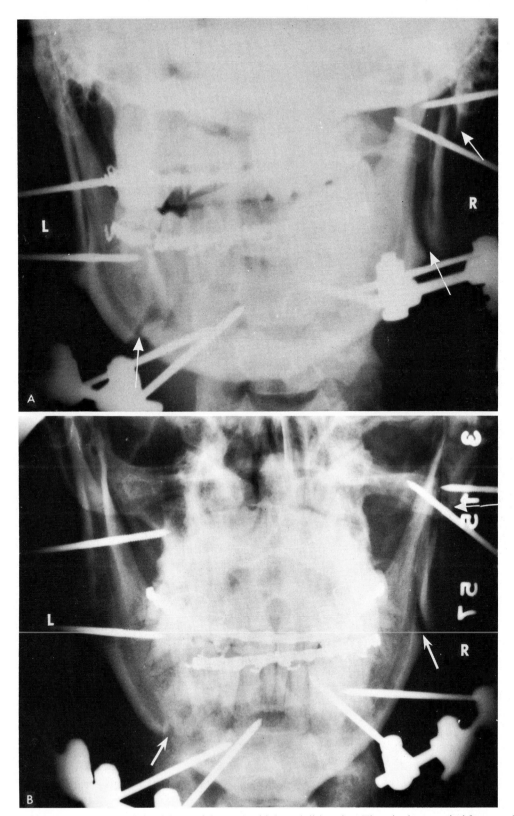

Figure 18–120 *A,* Fracture of the right condylar neck with lateral dislocation. There is also a vertical fracture of the ramus from the sigmoid notch through the inferior border, and this segment is laterally displaced. In addition, there is a fracture of the left body (horizontal ramus) in the bicuspid area. Splints are wired to the necks of the teeth in both arches. Extraoral pin fixation splints are in place and ready to be locked once the teeth are brought into normal occlusion by the intermaxillary elastics. *B,* Fractures are reduced and immobilized.

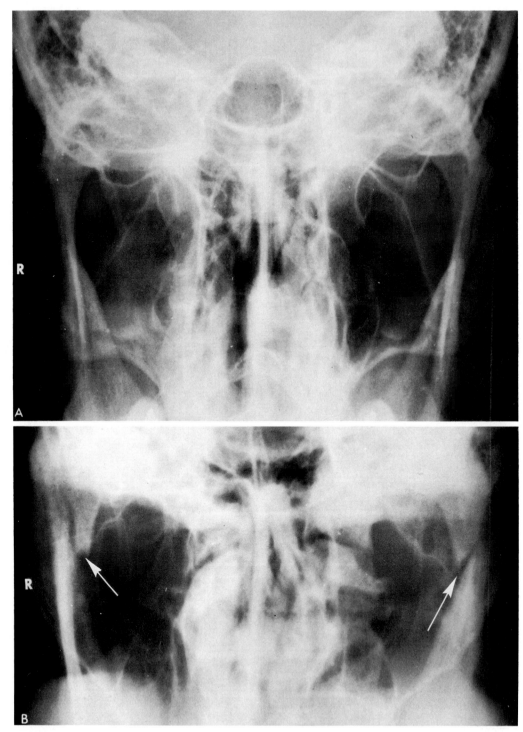

Figure 18–121 *A,* Radiograph of the normal bilateral necks of the mandibular condyles as shown by the antero-posterior (AP) Towne projection technique. Right and left sides are reversed in this position as compared with the Waters' projection.

B, Accident patient in whom both condylar necks were fractured. The right is dislocated medially, but there is only minor medial displacement in the left. (See also Figure 18–191.)

(Figure 18–121 continued on opposite page)

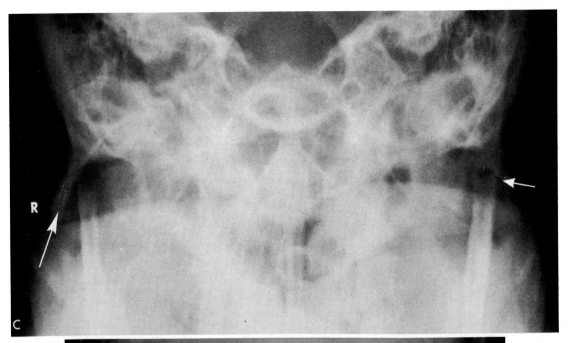

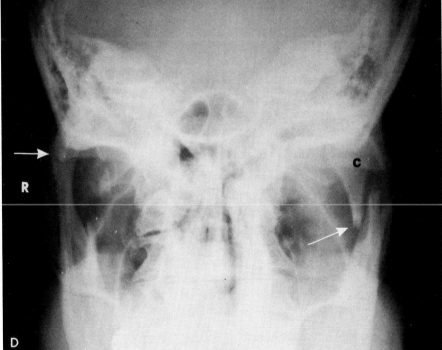

Figure 18–121 *(Continued.)*
C, Lateral displacement of the right fractured condylar neck. Fracture of the left condylar neck, no displacement.
D, Lateral deviation of the right fractured condylar neck. Fracture of the left condylar neck with medial displacement.

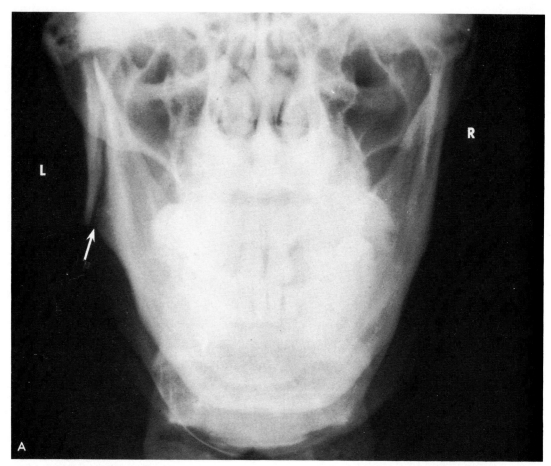

Figure 18–122 *A*, Third case of a vertical fracture of the left ramus. *B*, and *C*, This single fracture was treated first by bringing the maxillary and mandibular teeth into occlusion, that being the primary objective in fracture treatment, and by holding them there with intermaxillary continuous traction with small rubber bands. Finally, the extraoral skeletal pin fixation units were inserted into each segment and manipulated to bring the fractured vertical segment of the ramus into apposition with the rest of the ramus. Then these fragments were tightly held in apposition by locking the connecting bar between the two units, one in the small segment and the other in the body of the mandible.

(Figure 18–122 continued on opposite page)

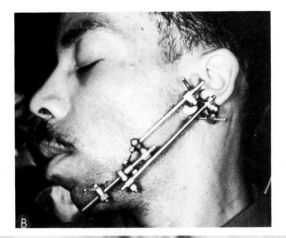

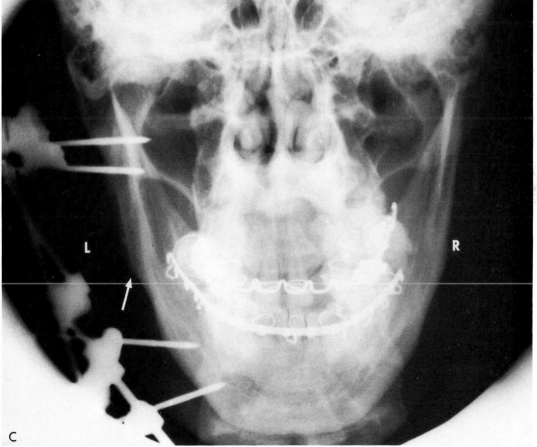

Figure 18–122 *(Continued.)*

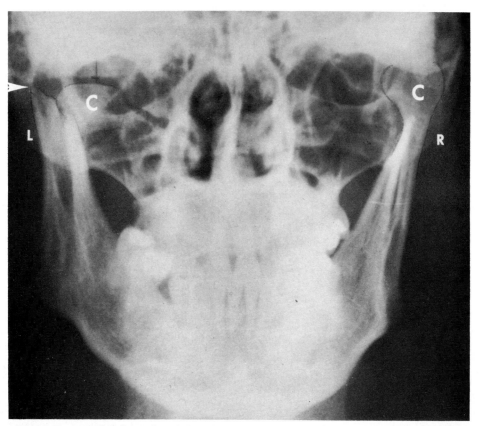

Figure 18–123 Gross medial dislocation of the left condyle. This does not alter the usual conservative treatment. Open reduction is *not indicated* except when the displaced condyle interferes with normal masticatory movements. Only in these cases is it removed. (See Condylectomy in Chapter 25.)

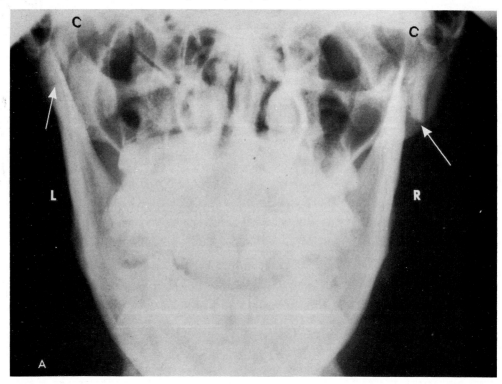

Figure 18–124

(Figure 18–124 continued on opposite page)

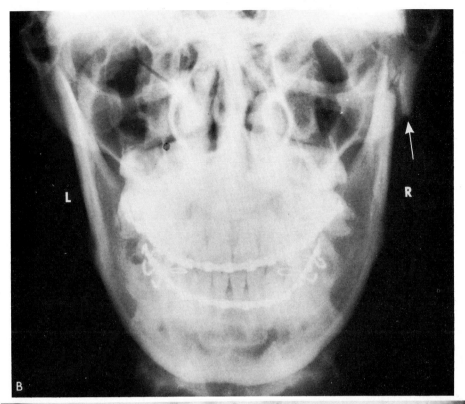

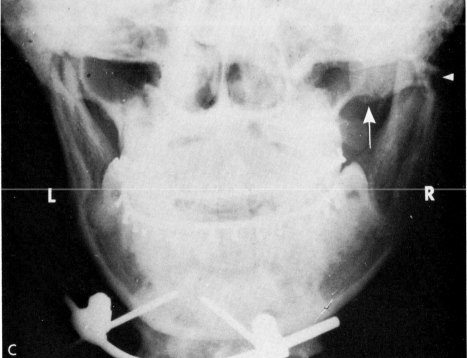

Figure 18–124 *(Continued.)*

Figure 18–124 Three cases of condylar neck fractures.

A, Bilateral fractures with medial dislocation of the left condyle and lateral displacement of the right condyle.

B, Immobilization with splints wired to maxillary and mandibular teeth and with intermaxillary rubber bands between the splints. No attempt is made to reposition the medially dislocated right condyle.

C, In this case there is also a left linear fracture of the mandibular symphysis (reduced by a Frac-Sur unit). The right condylar head is dislocated medially and the neck laterally inclined. The jaws were immobilized as previously described.

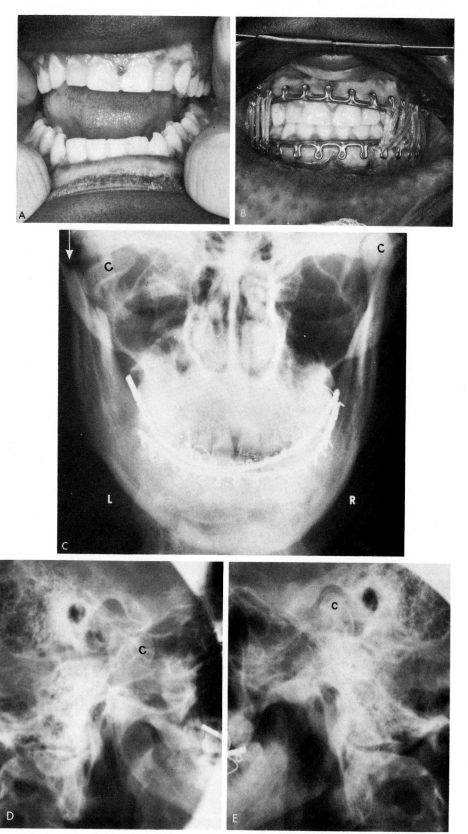

Figure 18–125 *A,* Unilateral preocclusion of the posterior teeth in a patient with a history of trauma is an axiomatic sign of a fracture of the condylar neck on that side. This was confirmed by the radiograph (*C*), which shows a medial dislocation of the condyle. *B,* Fracture immobilized. *D,* Note the vacant glenoid fossa and the head of the condyle, labeled *c. E,* Right condyle in normal closed position.

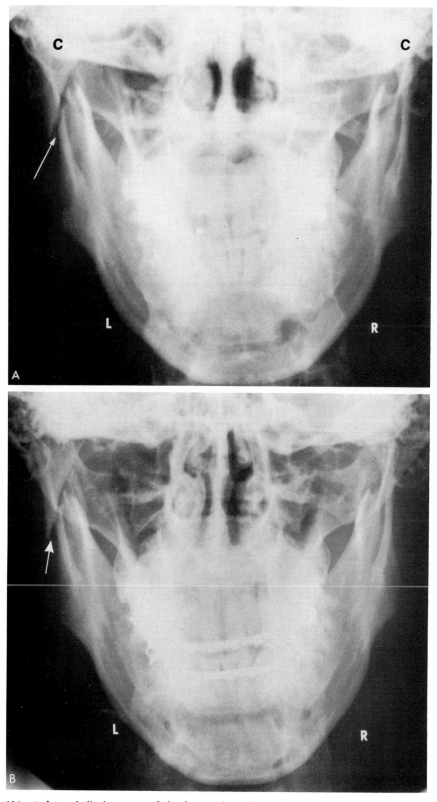

Figure 18–126 *A,* Lateral displacement of the fractured condylar neck. *B,* Fracture immobilized, as previously described.

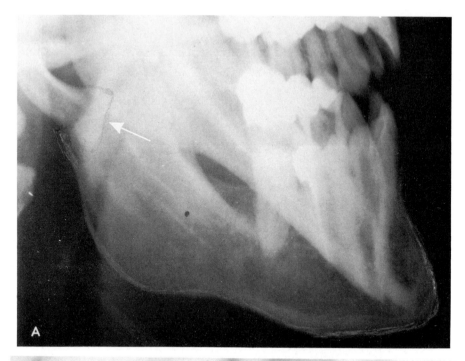

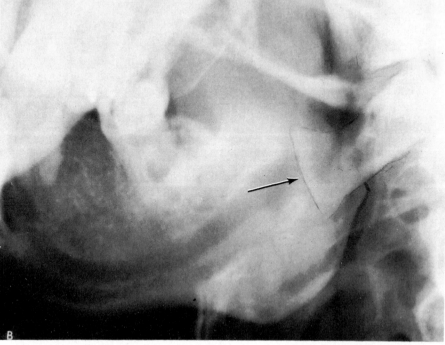

Figure 18–127   Five oblique radiographs of subcondylar fractures: *A,* Fractures of the neck moved anteriorly, superiorly and medially. *B,* Condyle and neck are dislocated medially. This can be suspected on oblique films because of the enlarged radiographic image distorted by the increased distance of the condyle from its radiographic film. (Shadow of an object increases in size as it nears the source of light, or in this case, radiation.)

(Figure 18–127 continued on opposite page)

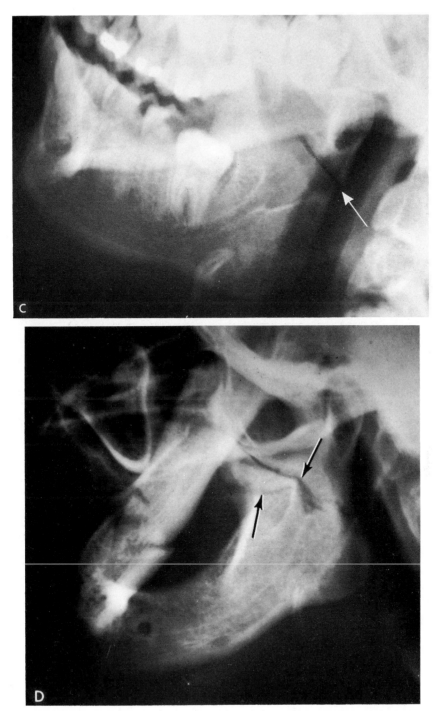

Figure 18–127 *(Continued.)*   *C*, Displacement and rotation of the condylar head. *D*, Fracture of the coronoid process and an angular fracture of the vertical ramus through the anterior area of the sigmoid notch downward and posteriorly some distance below the condylar neck.

(Figure 18–127 continued on following page)

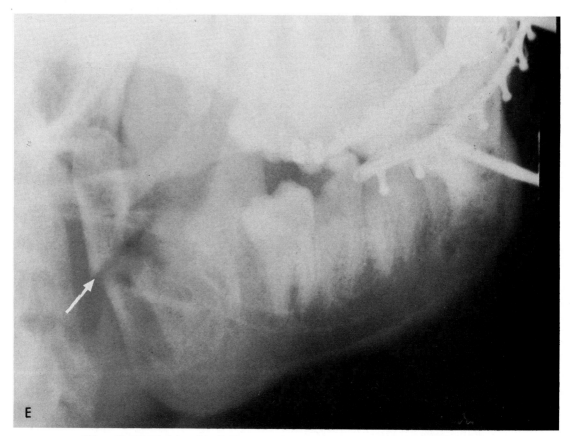

Figure 18–127 *(Continued.)*   *E,* Fracture of the condylar neck with minor displacement.

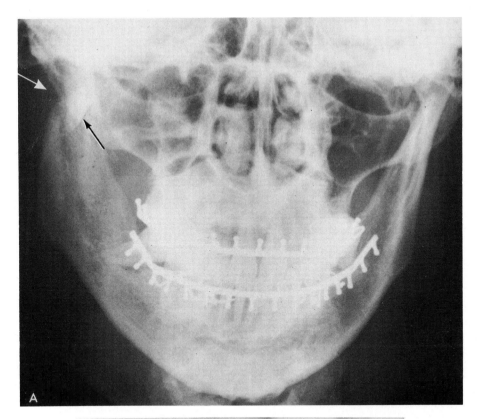

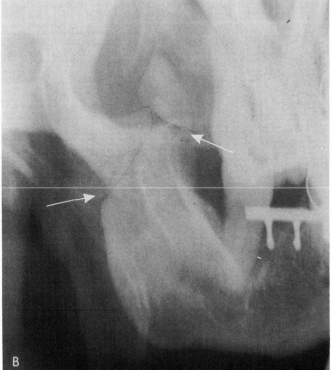

Figure 18–128 *A*, Subcondylar and coronoid process fractures. *B*, Oblique radiographic view. Maxilla and mandible immobilized, as described and here illustrated, during healing process.

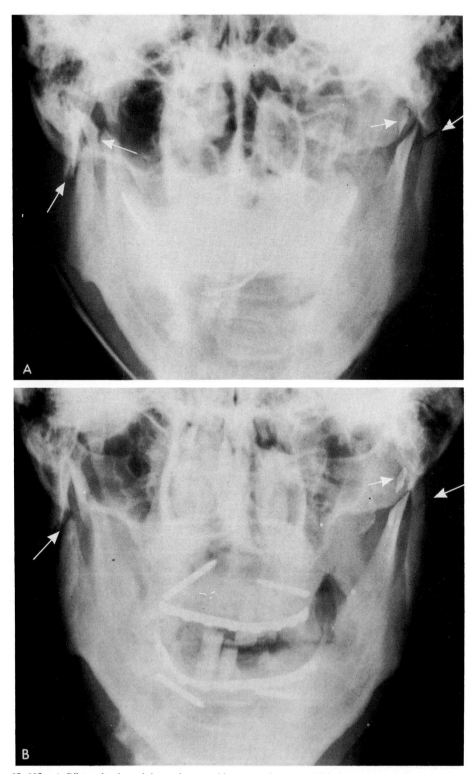

Figure 18–129 *A,* Bilateral subcondylar and coronoid process fractures. This is a rare occurrence.

B, Patient was partially edentulous and wore partial dentures. These were fixed to both jaws by pins, and intermaxillary fixation was carried out as usual.

(Figure 18–129 continued on opposite page)

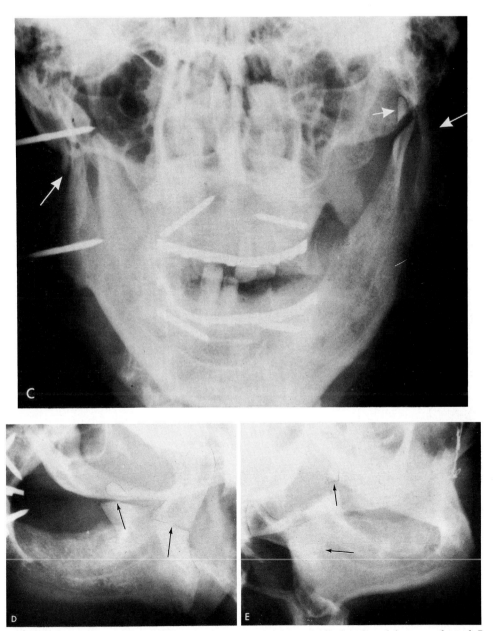

Figure 18–129   *(Continued.) C,* Extraoral pin fixation of the large, laterally displaced condyle was performed. *D* and *E,* Right and left oblique radiographs of the fractures. Note in *E* the single wire that had been strung between the maxillary and mandibular teeth at the emergency room where the patient was first treated.

CONSERVATIVE TREATMENT OF FRACTURE OF NECK OF LEFT MANDIBULAR CONDYLE

Patient. A woman had a fracture of the neck of the left condyle of the mandible, as revealed by posteroanterior radiographs. (See Figure 18–126A.) The right molars were the only teeth which met when the patient brought her teeth into occlusion.

The patient was prepared for an operation, which was reduction of a fractured neck of the condyle of the mandible by the application of Jelenko splints and intermaxillary rubber bands.

Operation. The patient was anesthetized. The lips were coated with petrolatum jelly to prevent cracking or injury. The Molt mouth gag was inserted to hold the jaws open. The oropharyngeal partition was placed to keep blood and saliva out of the pharynx. These partitions were changed when they became saturated with blood and mucus. A No. 2 catgut suture was passed through the tip of the tongue. The suture was tied and clamped with a hemostat. This was done to control the tongue and to keep it from slipping back into the pharynx and blocking respiration.

One of the Jelenko splints was adapted to conform to the gingival curvature of the labial and buccal surfaces of the maxillary teeth. The mandibular splint was adapted in a similar manner. With the aid of dental floss, doubled steel wires were passed beneath the free gingiva, going through the embrasures from buccal to lingual and out to the buccal. The following teeth were wired in this manner: maxillary and mandibular right and left first bicuspid and molars.

The mesial wires were bent up and the distal wires down. The splint was retained in position by twisting each pair of wires together. The wires were then cut to a suitable length and the ends bent into embrasures.

In the lower jaw the splints were attached in the manner described. The intermaxillary rubber bands were then hooked on to the upper and lower splints with the desired traction secured. The teeth were slowly brought into the patient's normal occlusion, thus insuring the immobilization of the fractured segments of the mandible. (See Figure 18–126B.) The patient was removed from the operating room in good condition.

MANDIBULAR FRACTURES IN CHILDREN

SUBCONDYLAR FRACTURES

In children, fractures of the mandible are usually through the symphysis or are subcondylar. The author is opposed to open reduction of subcondylar fractures in children or adults.

Rowe states: "It is the rich vascular nature of the condyle with its thin covering shell and high osteogenic potential that influences the sequel of events after trauma directed along the long axis of the condylar neck, especially in patients of this age group. However, a crushing injury at any time during childhood is liable to produce ankylosis, particularly when this incident is combined with cerebral injuries resulting in a period of prolonged unconsciousness when the mandible is left relatively immobile.

"The severe disruption of the growth center produced by such injuries restricts the treatment that ensures early mobility, prevents ankylosis, and preserves the growth potential that remains. Thus, careful observation with a view to the surgical correction of residual deformity at a later date is necessary.

*Any attempt at open reduction will serve only to aggravate the situation.**

"Most of the condylar injuries sustained in childhood are a greenstick-type of angulation of the condylar neck, with or without dislocation from the glenoid fossa.[157] Experiments by Walker[189] on the *Macaca rhesus* monkey, and by Boyne[17] using tetracycline labeling of newly formed bone, have demonstrated that resorption and remodelling of the displaced condyle take place with resumption of a more vertical mediolateral orientation, and preservation of the growth center.

"This research is substantiated clinically by Blevins and Gores,[13] Rakower and others,[145] Kaplan and Mark,[92] MacLennan and Simpson,[116] and Rowe and Killey.[159] *It is time to state unequivocally that there is no indication for open reduction and transosseous wiring in the case of condylar fractures in children unless there is a mechanical interference with mandibular movement.** A conservative policy offers the best chance of

(Text continued on page 1185)

---

*Author's note: Italics mine.

Photographic Case Report

BILATERAL SUBCONDYLAR FRACTURE OF THE MANDIBLE IN AN EDENTULOUS PATIENT

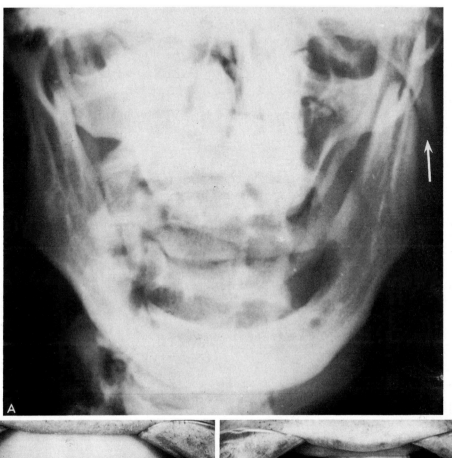

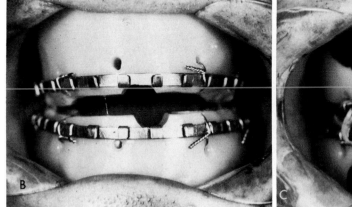 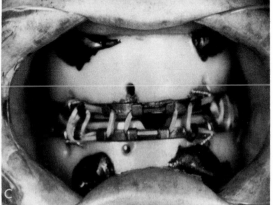

Figure 18–130 *A,* Unilateral subcondylar fracture in an edentulous patient who lost both his dentures at the time of his auto accident. Impressions were taken, models made, wax bite blocks on base plates were fitted in his mouth, and the intermaxillary space necessary was established on the wax bite blocks.

B, These were converted into acrylic, to which were attached splints; these splinted blocks were then placed in the mouth. Here the open bite may be seen that had been built in to compensate for the right intermaxillary space closure that was expected to result from the overriding of the fragments as the masseter and temporalis muscles pulled up on the mandible.

C, The bite blocks were pinned to the maxilla and mandible. The exposed ends of the pins were covered with green compound. Intermaxillary elastics were placed and the open bite gradually closed. When the fracture healed, the intermaxillary space was excellent, and new dentures functioned very well.

1175

UNILATERAL SUBCONDYLAR FRACTURE

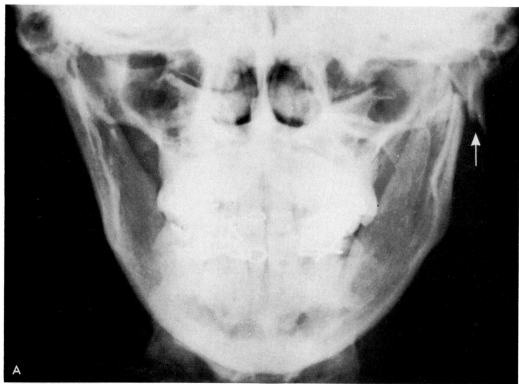

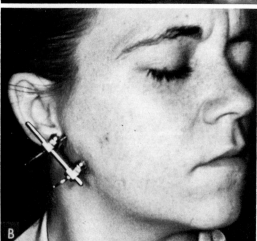

Figure 18–131 *A*, Right subcondylar fracture, with lateral displacement of the neck. *B*, Fractures immobilized with extraoral pin fixation. This is rarely indicated.

(Figure 18–131 continued on opposite page)

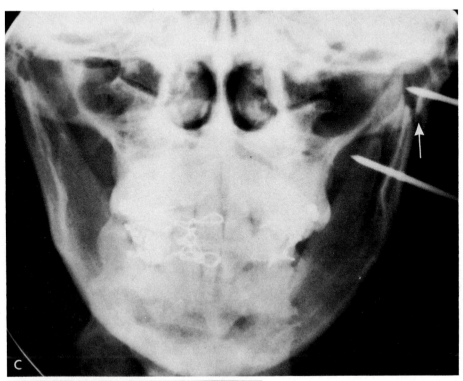

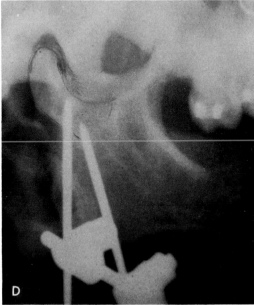

Figure 18–131 *(Continued.) C,* Inter-maxillary immobilization with rubber bands over wire loops on both maxillary and mandibular teeth. *D,* Oblique radio-graph of the temporomandibular joint with pin fixation.

UNILATERAL SUBCONDYLAR FRACTURE: DENTULOUS MANDIBLE, EDENTULOUS MAXILLA

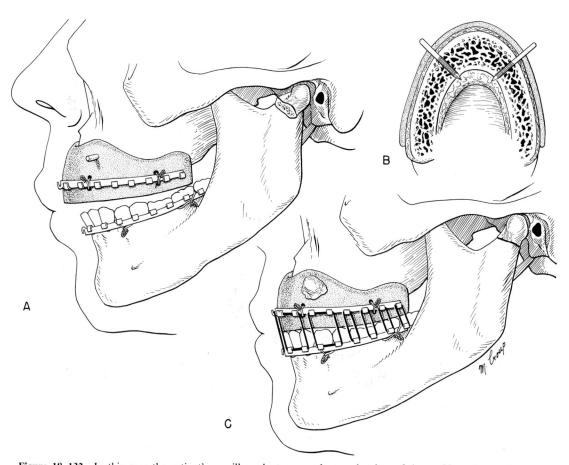

Figure 18–132 In this case the patient's maxillary denture was lost at the time of the accident. Impressions were taken, stone models made, wax bite taken and models mounted on a straight line articulator. The bite was then opened on the fractured side to conform to the uninjured side, and the maxillary stone model was reset to the new bite. The wax bite rim and base plate were finished in acrylic. Splints were wired to the acrylic bite block (or attached by quick-curing acrylic) and to the mandibular teeth.

A, The acrylic bite block is pinned to the maxilla by drilling a Roger Anderson pin with an electric drill through the labial flange in each cuspid region as is shown in the cross section (*B*). The excess portion of each pin is cut off to within 5/16 inch of the labial flange with a pin cutter or by safe-sided carborundum discs. This permits the eventual removal of these pins with a hand vise. *C*, The pin ends are covered with soft compound, which is then chilled. This protects the lip. Intermaxillary elastics are placed to close the bite, thus reducing and immobilizing the fracture. In many cases better apposition is secured by pinning the fracture, in addition to the technique just described. See Figure 18–131 for an example of the reduction of a subcondylar fracture with Roger Anderson pins in addition to intermaxillary fixation with elastics.

Figure 18–133 *A*, Unilateral fracture of the left condylar neck with dislocation in an edentulous patient.

B, Dentures were inserted after pins were introduced into the right and left zygomas and body of the mandible, as previously described. Upward hand pressure beneath the chin was exerted to bring the dentures into normal occlusion, and then right and left connecting bars between the pins in the maxilla and mandible were locked.

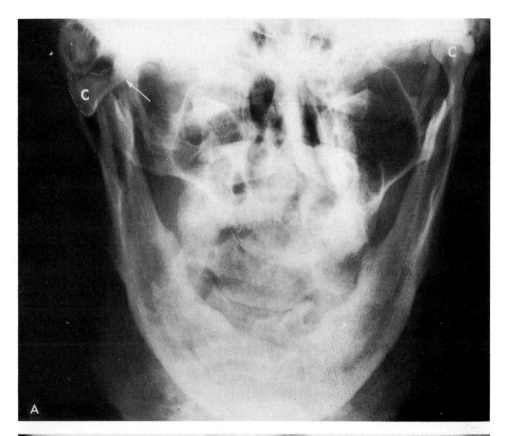

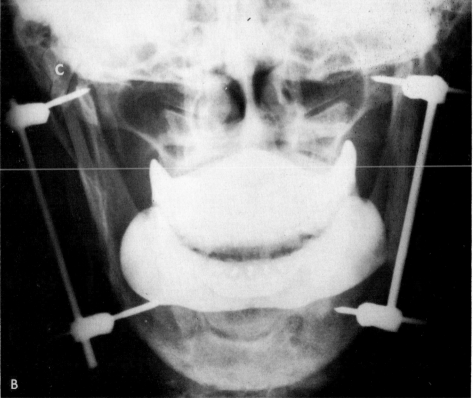

Figure 18–133   *See opposite page for legend.*

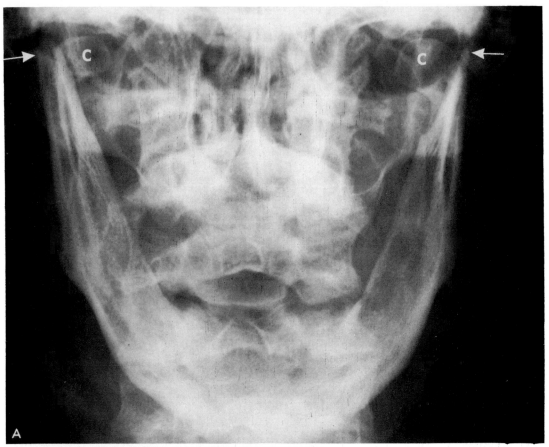

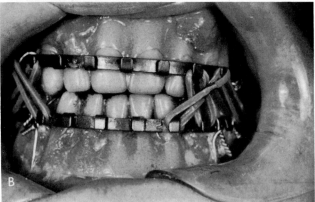

Figure 18–134 *A,* Bilateral fractures of the condylar necks with medial dislocation in an edentulous patient. *B,* The patient still had her dentures. The lower denture, which was devoid of a flange to pin to the mandible, was held in place by circumferential wires, as previously described. The maxillary denture was pinned to the maxilla. The bilateral open bite was closed by intermaxillary rubber bands, and the preaccident intermaxillary space was reestablished. She did not need new dentures when the fractures healed.

Figure 18–135 *A,* Healed site 1 year after fracture of the condylar neck with medial dislocation.
B, Oblique radiograph of healed condyle that was medially dislocated. Patient has practically normal masticatory function and no complaints.

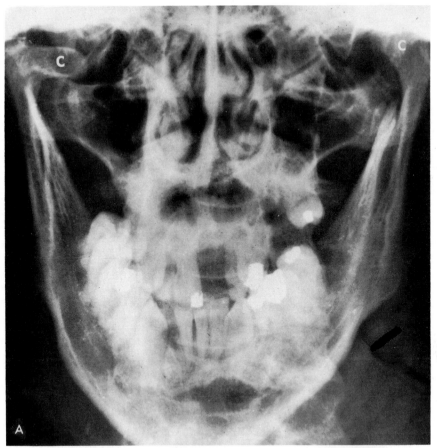

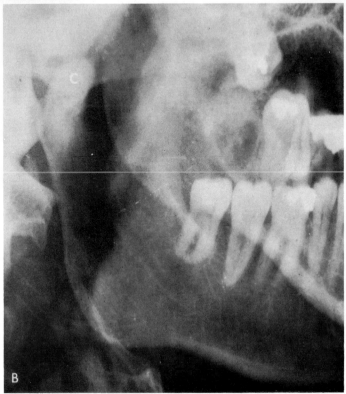

Figure 18–135 *See opposite page for legend.*

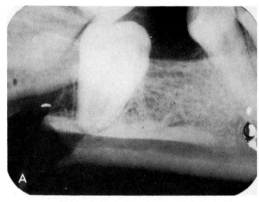

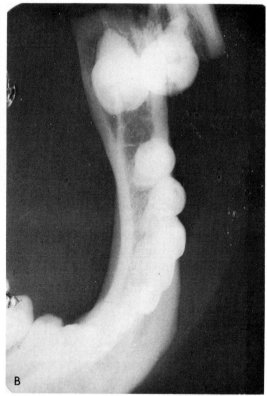

Figure 18–136 These fractures of the neck of the condyle were 6 weeks old when this patient came in for treatment. *A,* Periapical view shows the buccal overlapping of the posterior fragment. *B,* Occlusal radiograph dramatically shows the overriding and early osseous union.

C, Intraorally the fragments were easily separated with a chisel. Before this was done a Stader splint was placed spanning the fracture site. After the segments were freed, and by rotation of the threaded connecting bar, the fragments were separated, as shown in this posteroanterior radiograph. Also note the partially healed neck of the condyle that was manually refractured. *D,* The threaded connecting bar was manipulated to line up the fragments and then closed in order to bring the fragments into apposition. *E,* Healing in the new position.

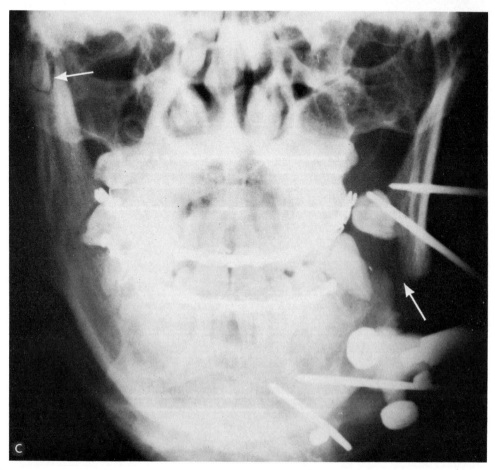

1182

(Figure 18–136 continued on opposite page.)

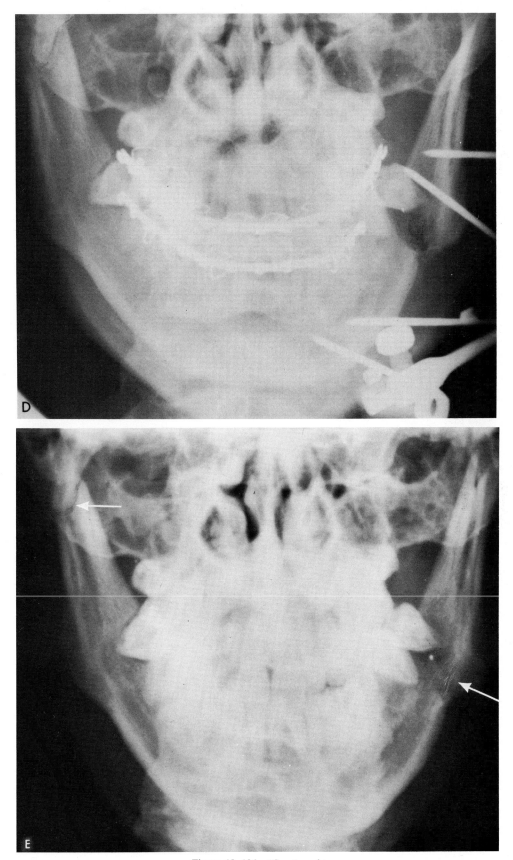

Figure 18–136 *(Continued.)*

SUBCONDYLAR FRACTURE WITH MEDIAL DISLOCATION

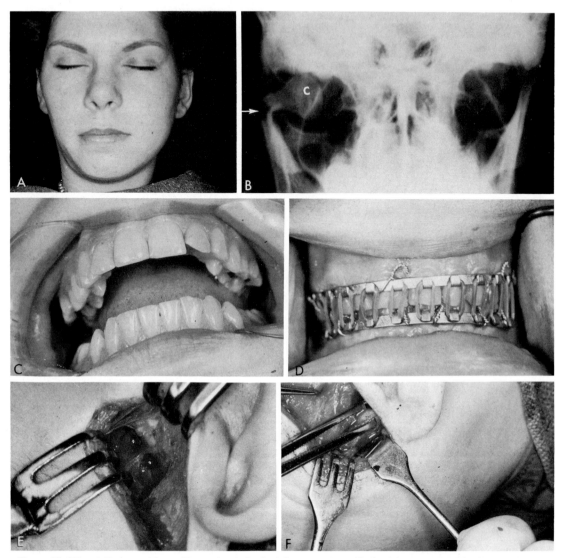

Figure 18–137 *A*, Patient with swelling and pain in the left temporomandibular joint area. Swelling is not a frequent symptom following a subcondylar fracture. *B*, Fracture of condyle and neck with medial dislocation. *C*, Left molars striking prematurely. In addition, the patient could not open her mouth any more than is shown in this photo. We did not recognize the reason and believed it was due to the edema and trauma. *D*, Maxilla and mandible immobilized in normal occlusion. On removal of the splints 6 weeks later, the patient could not open her mouth any more than she could pre-operatively, as shown in *C*. It was obvious that the dislocated condyle was in some way interfering with her ability to open her mouth wide. It was decided to remove the condyle. *E*, Empty glenoid fossa exposed. *F*, With considerable difficulty the condyle was located and removed.

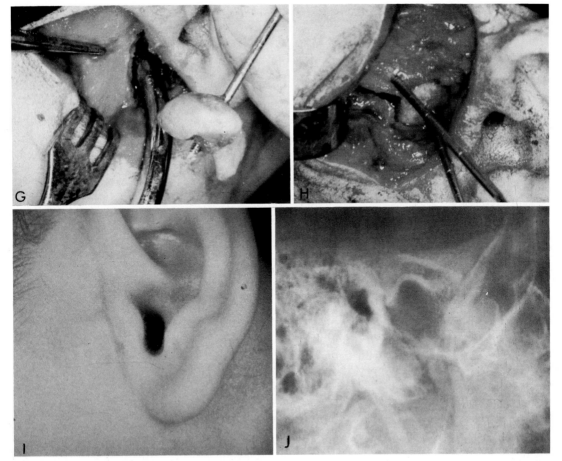

Figure 18–137 *(Continued.)*
G, We decided to replace the condyle and pin and wire it in place to see if it would heal. *H,* A pin was placed in the head of the condyle and another in the eminentia articularis; they were locked together with the connecting bar. *I,* Normal healing followed, with no swelling, pain or drainage. Joint functioned normally, and no radiographs were taken when the splints were removed. Patient left town, but kept in touch with us and returned for a final check-up 9 months later. *J,* Much to our surprise, when the usual radiographs were taken at this site, we could not see a condyle or neck anywhere in the area. This radiograph of the temporomandibular joint area, void of a condyle, indicated to us that there must have been aseptic necrosis of the condyle and condylar neck. But where was the small wire that had been inserted? The patient had a full range of masticatory movement with slight deviation of the mandible when she opened her mouth, but she was very satisfied with the results.

obtaining a morphologically and functionally acceptable condyle."*

Walker summarizes the results of his animal experimental work on traumatic fracture dislocations of the condyle as follows:

"A thorough understanding of the potential for repair and possible uninterrupted and continued mandibular growth following traumatic fracture dislocations of the condyle in the young child is a requisite for anyone concerned with management of this type of injury. An unequivocal description of either of the above consequences of condylar fractures

_____
*From Rowe, N. L.: Fractures of the jaws in children. J. Oral Surg., 27:505, 1969. Copyright by the American Dental Association. Reprinted by permission.

in the child is difficult to find. Such lack of documentation of the optimum treatment for a not-uncommon mandibular fracture in the child predicated the initiation of a pilot animal study to observe what happened in young macaca rhesus monkeys over an 18-month follow-up of similar fracture dislocations produced in them.

"The original eight young animals had fracture dislocations produced either unilaterally or bilaterally. One half of the animals had the fracture dislocations reduced and maintained via stainless steel interosseous wire fixation, and the remaining animal condyles were left in a medial and anterior position ('conservative treatment'). No immobilization of the jaws was maintained. Over an 18-month

Photographic Case Report

DELAYED SURGICAL-OCCLUSAL TREATMENT OF BILATERAL SUBCONDYLAR FRACTURE

M. E. Robinson, D.D.S., and E. Rowe, D.D.S.

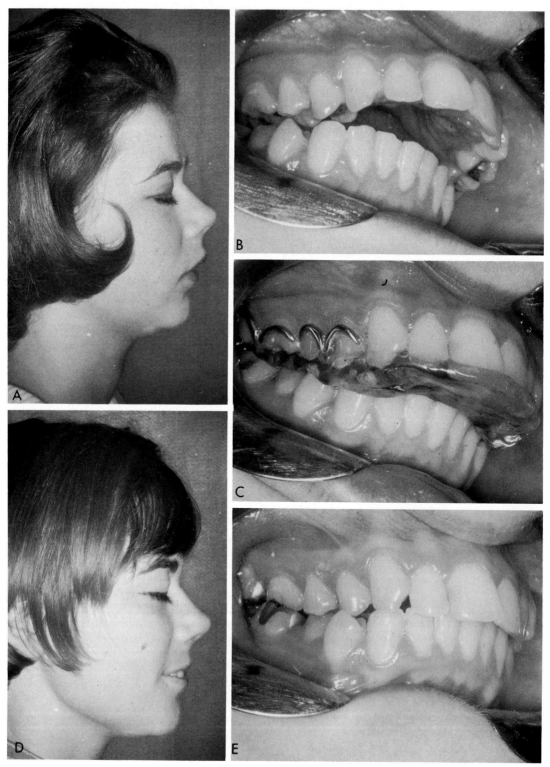

Figure 18–138   *See opposite page for legend.*

follow-up there was remarkably little difference in the overall dimensions of the jaw, and at the time of sacrifice of the animals, it was demonstrated by x-ray and clinical examination that all condyles were in a relatively normal position and had a normal appearance with only minor qualifications. Occlusion in all animals was good and there was no open bite at the incisor areas.

"Eight additional young animals have been followed after the production of fracture dislocations in them. These animals have had the 'advantage' of a two week period of jaw immobilization via intermaxillary wiring techniques following their fractures. It is apparent that these animals likewise do fairly well in reestablishing the condyle in a normal position, and growth likewise is not seriously retarded. However,...it is a great deal slower.

"It would appear at this time that the reestablishment of function through mobilization of the jaw as early as possible following fracture would be the optimum course to follow in treatment. At least it does not seem to jeopardize the overall result.

"The timing of jaw mobilization is predicated on the ability to achieve proper occlusion and function, the degree of pain with function, and blocking of the mandible by the fragments (a different consideration altogether where, generally, an open reduction is indicated to relieve such a situation). The earlier this mobilization can be achieved consistent with the above, probably the more favorable can the prognosis be made for acceptable repair and continued growth."[189]

The author treats subcondylar fractures in children by immobilization of the mandible for 1 to 3 weeks depending on the child's age. Younger children (1 to 3 years old) need a shorter time of immobilization. Even when 2 to 3 weeks of immobilization is used, we carefully check the occlusion for 3 days following the removal of immobilization. If the

bite opens, it is too early to remove the immobilization and it is replaced. The same test is applied to teenagers and adults. The technique is illustrated and described in Figures 18–139, 18–140 and 18–142.

It would appear from Walker's report that immobilization in these cases is not necessary in young children. Kaplan[92] published a report of an 18-month-old child who suffered bilateral subcondylar fractures plus a fracture of the symphysis; he treated only the fracture of the symphysis with no immobilization of the mandible. He reports[91] 3 years later that the patient has perfect occlusion and normal development of the mandible. The author is reducing the time of immobilization in these cases and will stop entirely when someone demonstrates that immobilization for subcondylar fractures is not necessary in 6- to 10-year-old children.

Doane[43] reports a very rare case in which a blow to the chin of a 13-year-old girl drove the right mandibular condyle up through the articular fossa into the middle cranial fossa. The original roentgenographic examination failed to reveal this situation. When treatment failed to correct the malocclusion, additional roentgenograms were taken. If both condylar heads are not visualized on the original roentgenograms, additional studies at various angles should be made to rule out this possibility before treatment is instituted.

FRACTURES IN THE BODY OF THE MANDIBLE

In my opinion, extraoral pin fixation is the best way to handle mandibular fractures in children. This technique may be used as the only method of reduction and immobilization or as an adjunctive treatment. The only precaution is to be certain that the pins are in-

(Text continued on page 1195)

Figure 18–138 *A*, Right lateral view of patient shows retruded position of mandible due to untreated bilateral fractures of the condylar necks with displacement sustained 6 months earlier. *B*, Patient's occlusion shows retruded open bite deformity. *C*, Photograph taken 19 months after injury shows maxillary occlusal splint in position; relief of pain was obtained by use of the splint. *D*, Right profile of patient approximately 2 years after surgery shows improved appearance. Note absence of obvious submandibular scar on neck. *E*, Patient's occlusion shows improvement achieved by surgical-occlusal treatment. Note that fractured lower right molar has been restored.
(From Robinson, M. E., and Rowe, E.: Delayed surgical-occlusal treatment of malocclusion and pain from displaced subcondylar fractures: Report of case. J.A.D.A., *83*:639 [Sept.], 1971.)

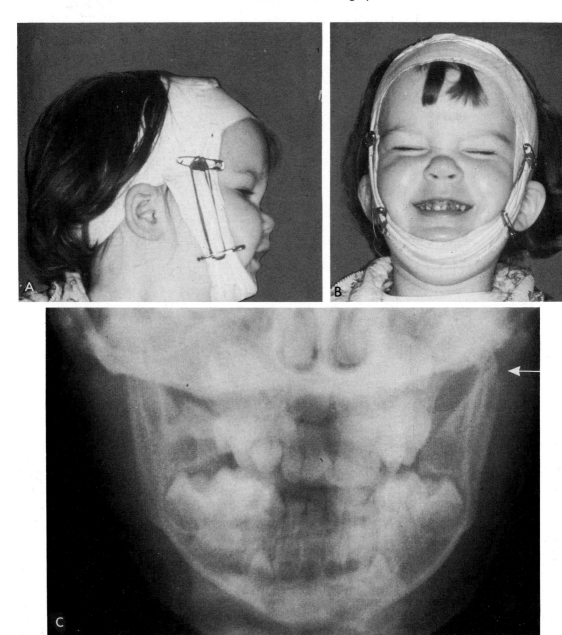

Figure 18-139 This 20-month-old girl fell down the stairs and fractured the neck of the left condyle, which was dislocated medially (*C* and *D*). There was marked displacement resulting in gross malocclusion. *A*, Avertin basal anesthetic and infiltrated local anesthetic were used, and stainless steel wire loops were twisted around the necks of each of the 16 deciduous teeth. Then by manual manipulation normal occlusion of the maxillary and mandibular teeth was obtained. Small elastic bands cut from rubber tubing were placed between the maxillary and mandibular wire loops to help hold the teeth in occlusion. It was anticipated that excessive traction on the 12 anterior teeth would pull these teeth out of their sockets. To prevent this the elastics selected were of such a size that when placed between the anterior teeth they were *not* stretched. However, an attempt to separate the jaws would stretch the elastic. Between the first deciduous molars, the only molars in position, the elastics were under tension because here there could not be any dislodgment of these teeth, the occlusal surfaces being in contact. To supplement the immobilization, extraoral traction on the symphysis was obtained by the modified Barton bandage. *B*, Anterior view of same patient. *C* and *D*, Posteroanterior and basal radiographs. *Note:* Today this patient would be treated as shown in Figures 18-140 and 18-142.

(Figure 18-139 continued on opposite page)

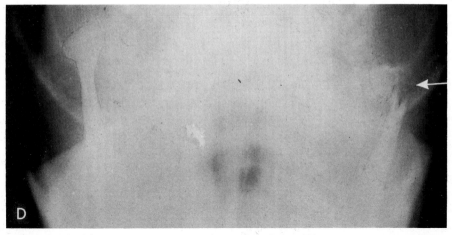

Figure 18–139   *(Continued.)*
   I disagree with those surgeons who insist on performing open reduction of fractures of the condyle, and especially so in the young. Concerning this age group, Rowe states:
   "The severe disruption of the growth center (condyle) produced by such injuries restricts the treatment that ensures early mobility, prevents ankylosis, and preserves the growth potential that remains.
   "Any attempt at open reduction will serve only to aggravate the situation.
   "It is time to state unequivocally that there is no indication for open reduction and transosseous wiring in the case of condylar fractures in children unless there is a mechanical interference with mandibular movement. A conservative policy offers the best chance of obtaining a morphologically and functionally acceptable condyle."[158]

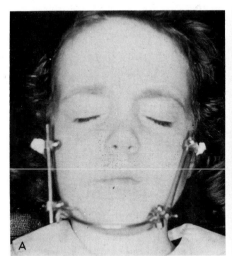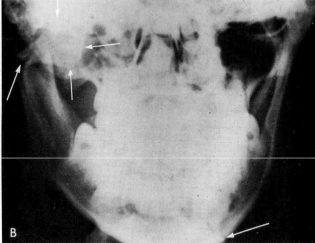

Figure 18–140   *A,* Eight-year-old girl with a fracture of the right condylar neck with medial dislocation and a mandibular linear fracture between the central and lateral incisors. (See posteroanterior radiograph, *B.*) There was advanced caries in the deciduous molars that were present. Treatment was the immobilization of the anterior fracture by inserting one pin on either side of the fracture and then reducing the fracture and holding it stable by a connecting bar. Next the permanent molars and anterior teeth were brought into normal occlusion and held there by connecting bars between each zygoma and the mandibular pins, as shown in *A.*

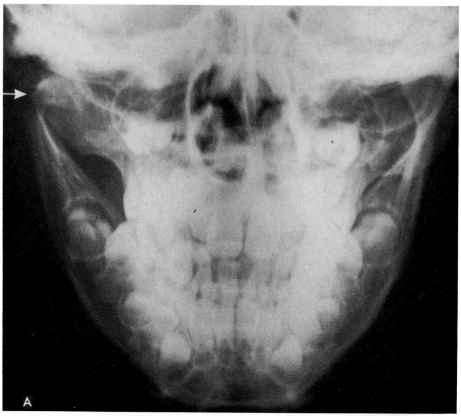

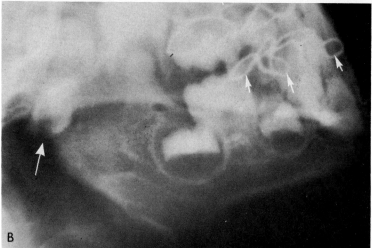

Figure 18–141   *A,* Another example of a fracture of the condylar neck with medial dislocation, this one in a 5-year-old male. *B,* The deciduous teeth have roots that are sufficiently long so that wire loops (see arrows) can be attached to the necks of the maxillary and mandibular posterior teeth and intermaxillary rubber bands placed. Note the rotated dislocated condyle in this oblique radiograph of the left mandible. *C,* Right oblique radiograph shows a few of the wire loops (see arrows) around the necks of the maxillary and mandibular molars and cuspids. Small rubber bands (orthodontia) are then stretched from over the maxillary to the mandibular wire loops. These are easily cut to permit removal in case of vomiting. In fact, we do not place so many rubber bands that the patient cannot separate his jaws if necessary.

(Figure 18–141 continued on opposite page)

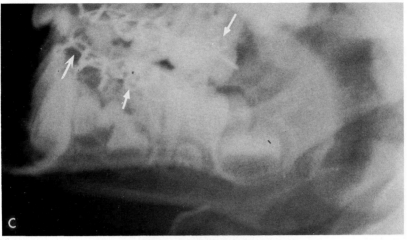

Figure 18–141 *(Continued.)*

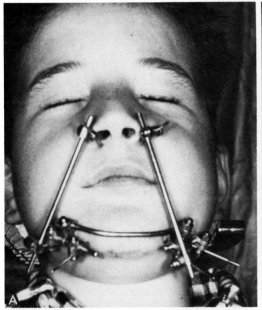

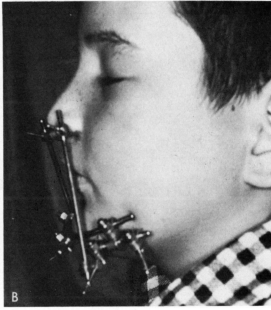

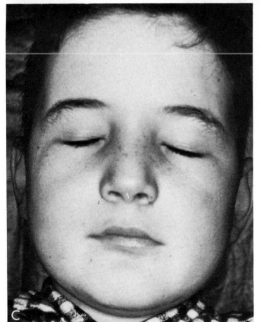

Figure 18–142 Radiographs of this case have been lost. *A,* This 9-year-old boy had a fracture of the right condylar neck with medial displacement and a second fracture through the lateral incisor region of the symphysis. The treatment of the mandibular symphysis is shown in *A* and *B.* Intermaxillary fixation for the subcondylar fracture could not be achieved by wiring or splinting the posterior teeth because of early loss of the 6-year mandibular molars and because of the partially erupted bicuspids, which obviously could not be used. Use of posterior pins in the body of the mandible and the zygoma with the connecting bar, as previously shown, would have increased the amount of "hardware." So this unusual application for immobilizing the mandible in occlusion with the maxilla was used. *C,* Note in this facial postoperative view that there is no scarring as a result of the pins passing through the skin.

SUBCONDYLAR FRACTURE OF THE MANDIBLE IN A 6-YEAR-OLD PATIENT

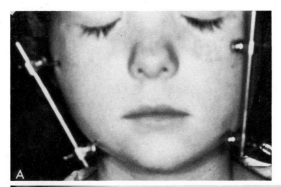

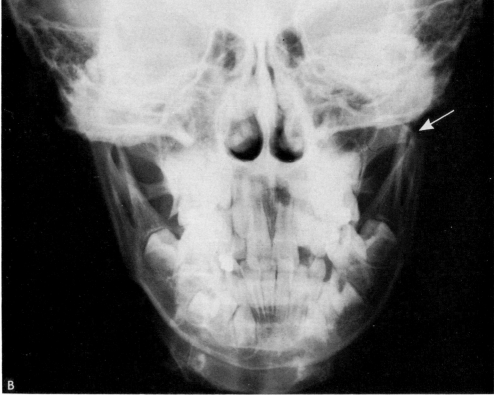

Figure 18–143 *A,* Six-year-old girl with a subcondylar fracture. (See *B, C* and *D.*) The mandibular deciduous molars had been extracted and the first permanent molars had not erupted sufficiently to permit wiring. The anterior teeth were loose. Under general anesthesia single pins were inserted in each zygoma and in the right and left horizontal rami. Then the teeth were brought into normal occlusion and held there while intermaxillary connecting bars were locked onto the pins, thus immobilizing the mandible to the maxilla during the healing period of 4 to 5 weeks.

B, Right subcondylar fracture in which the condyle was dislocated medially at a right angle to the ramus. *C,* Mandible immobilized in normal occlusion by locking a connecting bar between bilateral pins in the zygomas and body of the mandible. *D,* Note that the mandibular pins are inserted below the succedaneous teeth. The foreshortened angle of this x-ray exposure makes the pin appear closer to the second molar crypt than it actually was. The author also uses this method to immobilize a transverse fracture of the maxilla.

(Figure 18–143 continued on opposite page)

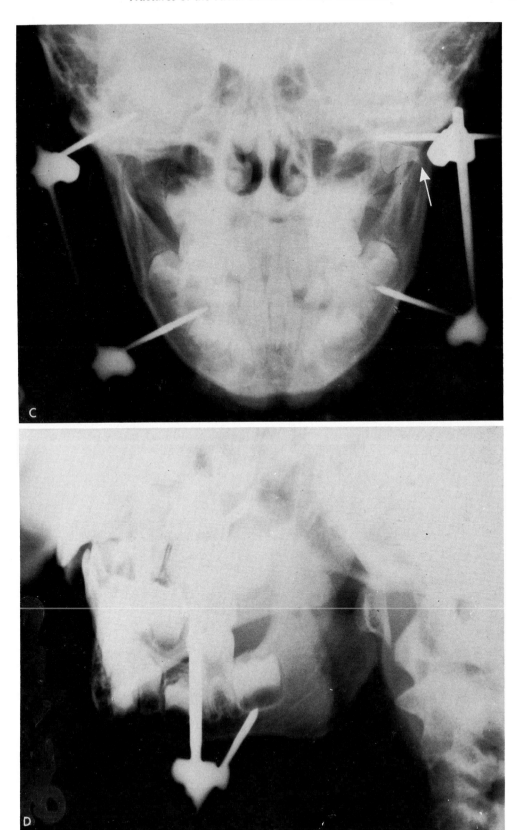

Figure 18–143 *(Continued.)*

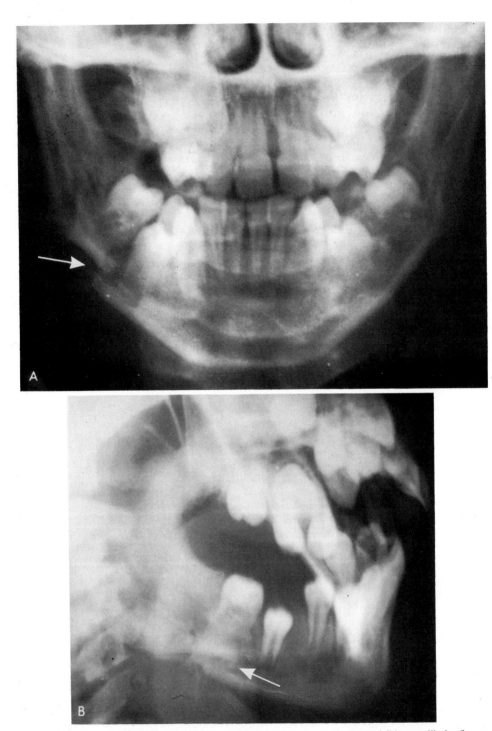

Figure 18-144   *A,* Fracture of the body of the mandible mesial to the erupting, nonvisible mandibular first molar in an 8-year-old boy. The posterior mandible was pulled superiorly and the anterior mandible inferiorly. *B,* The mandible was split longitudinally, as shown in this oblique lateral radiograph.

(Figure 18-144 continued on opposite page)

Figure 18–144 *(Continued.) C,* An examination of the radiographs will prove to the reader that intermaxillary fixation was not possible; nor was the construction of an acrylic splint and circumferential wiring of the splint over the fracture site, as shown in Figure 18–149, logical. The indicated treatment is shown in *C:* extraoral skeletal fixation with *double connecting* bars, necessitated by the displacement of the fractures. It is always appreciated by patients if they can open and close their jaws for talking, eating and drinking. Even in those cases in which we use intermaxillary fixation in conjunction with extraoral pin fixation, it is not usually necessary to continue the intermaxillary fixation for more than 2 weeks. The pin fixation is quite adequate for the remainder of the healing process.

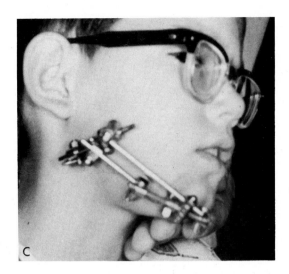

serted below the tooth buds. A careful study of the radiographs, allowing for the usual distortion in lateral jaw radiographs, will indicate the best areas for pin insertion. In addi-

tion, keeping the insertion point no higher than 1/4 inch from the inferior border of the mandible will avoid the tooth buds or apices of erupted teeth.

(Text continued on page 1199)

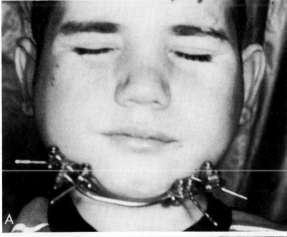

Figure 18–145 *A,* Ten-year-old boy with an oblique fracture through the symphysis. *B,* Note the lack of posterior teeth. Fracture reduced and stabilized with extraoral skeletal fixation. The right mandibular central incisor was loose and displaced labially. It was repositioned and wired. It was not necessary to do a root canal filling. *C,* Postoperative appearance five weeks later.

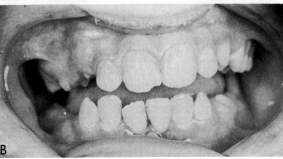

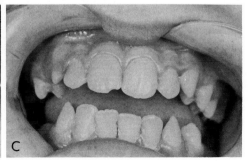

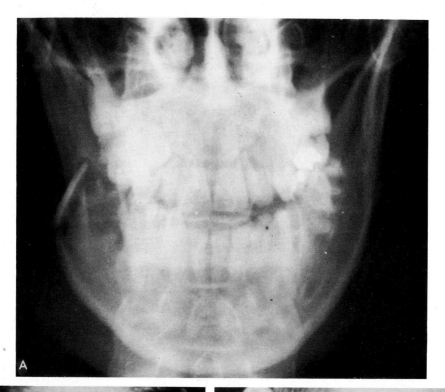

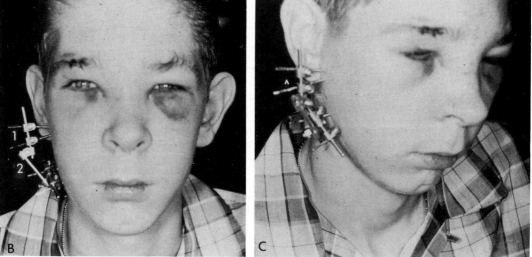

Figure 18–146 *A*, Compound comminuted fracture of the angle of the ramus and body of the mandible in a 10-year-old male. Intermaxillary fixation, as previously described, with rubber bands between maxillary and mandibular splints, brought the teeth into occlusion. *B* and *C*, Then extraoral skeletal fixation pin units were placed (*1*) in the vertical ramus and (*2*) in the body of the mandible. In 2 weeks the intermaxillary elastics were removed. The splints are not removed from the teeth until the elastics can be left off for 72 hours without the bite opening even a millimeter. Then the oral splints can be removed for the rest of the healing process, which in this case was 7 weeks. The time of fixation of fractures of the facial bones cannot be arbitrarily set for all fractures. Most authors I read state that they use a shorter period of immobilization than I do. Frankly, my patients do not heal that rapidly. Too early removal results in nonhealing fibrous union and open bites.

If I err, it is in *overimmobilization* rather than underimmobilization.

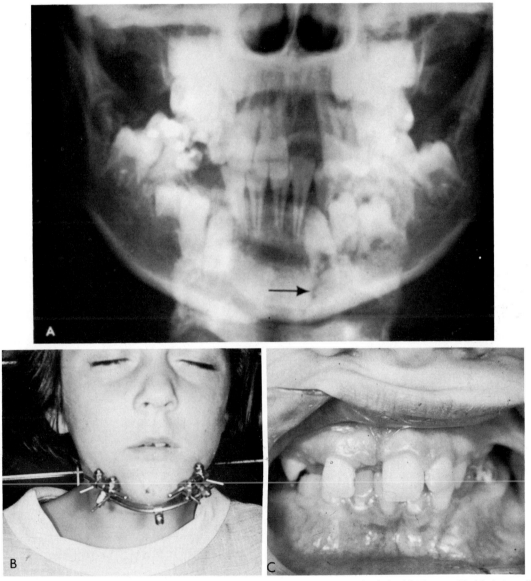

Figure 18–147   *A*, Posteroanterior radiograph of a linear fracture of the symphysis in this 6-year-old girl. As usually seen in fractures of the mandible, the fracture line passes through the crypt of the partially formed permanent cuspid. *We do not disturb these teeth.* (See Teeth in the Line of Fracture, this chapter.) *B*, Fracture stabilized with extraoral skeletal pin fixation. No additional support is needed. *C*, Postoperative appearance 4 weeks later.

BILATERAL COMPOUND FRACTURE OF THE SYMPHYSIS OF THE MANDIBLE

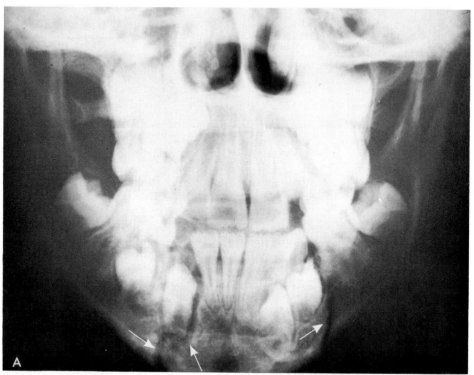

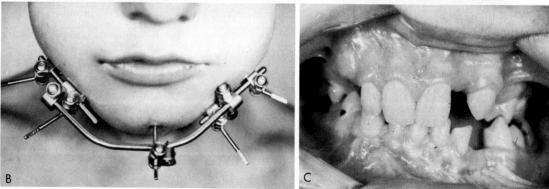

Figure 18–148 *A*, Bilateral mandibular fracture through the areas of the unerupted cuspids and bicuspids.

B, Treated with extraoral skeletal fixation. The central fragment of the symphysis of the mandible was driven lingually by the trauma. To move it anteriorly into normal position, it was necessary to insert a pin (the center one) into this fragment to which was attached elastic traction from the pin to the connecting bar. When the fragment was in normal contour with the right and left bodies of the mandible, the traction was removed, the connecting bar was loosened at each pin fixation unit, and medial pressure was applied to the right and left bodies of the mandible until both were in contact with the central segment. At this time the connecting bar was locked at both right and left pin fixation units. No intermaxillary fixation was used.

C, Postoperative appearance 5 weeks later.

Case Report No. 7

CIRCUMFERENTIAL WIRING OF A COMPOUND COMMINUTED FRACTURE OF THE MANDIBLE IN A CHILD

Patient. A 5-year-old girl, while sledding, had run under the rear end of a parked automobile and struck the left side of her jaw. There was severe pain and swelling of the left mandibular region. She was admitted to another hospital where reduction and fixation of her fractured mandible was attempted by intermaxillary wiring. This not only was a failure, but the broken segments were further separated (see Figure 18–149).

Examination. This revealed a well-developed, well-nourished white girl. The pupils were round and equal and reacted to light and accommodation. The ears and nose were normal. The left side of the face over the mandible was swollen and very tender. Several brass wires were dangling from the deciduous teeth.

Laboratory Examination. All findings were within normal limits.

X-ray Report. The x-ray revealed a unilateral compound comminuted fracture of the body of the mandible in the region of the left cuspid and molars. The second deciduous molar was missing. A triangular segment of bone was below the partially formed bicuspids. There was displacement of the fragments (Figure 18–149C and D).

Operation. Under Avertin anesthesia, after selecting the proper size of impression tray for the mandible, the tray was filled with warm impression compound and was inserted into the mouth. After removing the lower tray, the impression of the upper arch was taken in the same manner. The patient was taken from the operating room in good condition.

From the impressions taken, models were made.

The lower model was cut at the fracture sites and then mounted in occlusion with the upper model, a clear acrylic splint covering the occlusal, lingual, buccal and labial surfaces of the mandibular teeth.

The patient was again scheduled for an operation for reduction of the fracture and application of a splint by circumferential wiring.

Under Avertin anesthesia, tincture of Merthiolate was used to sterilize the area around the oral cavity, and the lips were coated with petrolatum. Four grooves about 2 mm. deep were cut into the occlusal surface of the splint to retain the wires (Fig. 18–149F). The acrylic splint, which had been prepared the day before, was inserted in the mouth to check its fit. It was discovered that the lingual surface of the carious crown of the lower right second deciduous molar had to be removed in order for the splint to be properly adapted. This portion of the crown was removed with long flat-nosed pliers and the sharp edges were smoothed with a revolving stone in the dental engine. Then the splint was inserted and held in place. The skin was prepared and the splint was now attached to the mandible by circumferential wiring (Fig. 18–149H and I). The reader is referred to Figures 18–50 and 18–51 for the details of this technique.

The patient was taken from the operating room in good condition.

Postoperative Course. The patient was placed on a liquid diet and given 1500 cc. of fluids daily. An infrared lamp was used for 30 minutes 4 times a day.

The patient experienced surprisingly little edema or trismus, and was discharged on the fifth

(Text continued on page 1203)

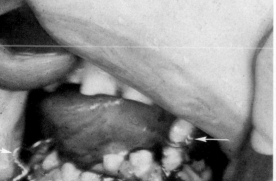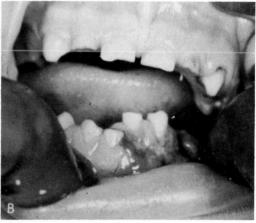

Figure 18–149 *A,* An attempt was made by the referring dentist to treat this 5-year-old girl's multiple compound sagittal and segmental fractures of the left body of the mandible and symphysis by intermaxillary wiring of the jaws (see arrows). One wire pulled off the maxillary tooth to which it was attached, and the other pulled the mandibular fracture up and partially extracted the upper cuspid. Note the elevated anterior fragment.

B, The maxillary cuspid was pushed back into its alveolus. Note the elevated anterior fragment.

(Figure 18–149 continued on following page)

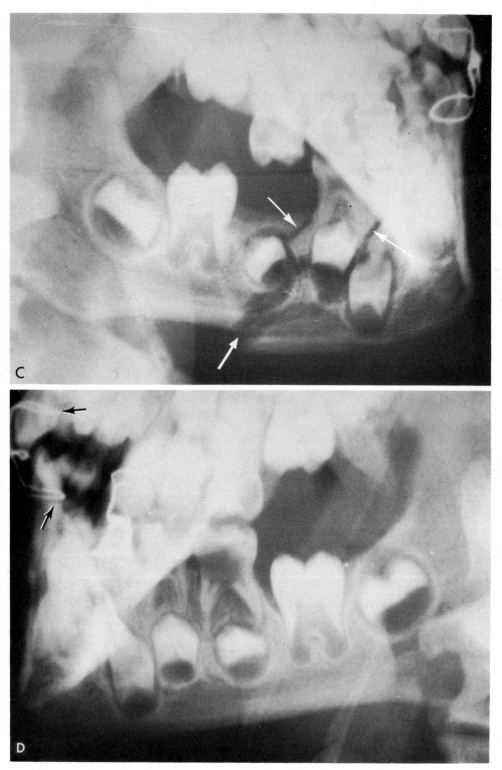

Figure 18–149   *(Continued.)*   *C,* Note fracture lines. *D,* Right body of the mandible is intact. Note how the intermaxillary direct wiring has elevated the fracture.

(Figure 18–149 continued on opposite page)

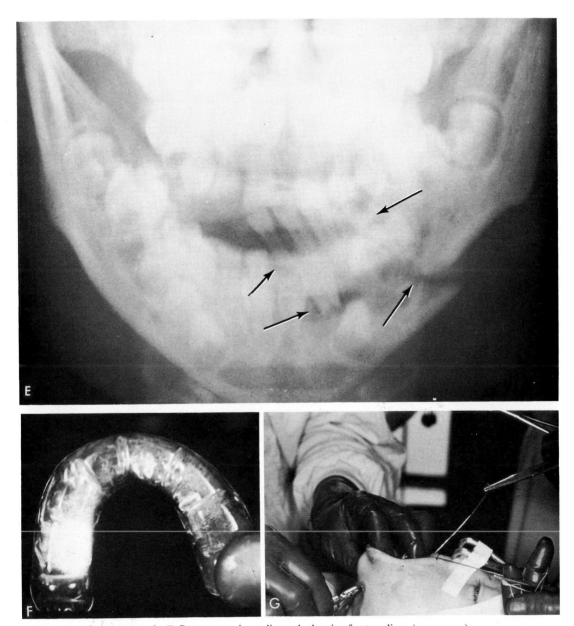

Figure 18–149 *(Continued.) E,* Posteroanterior radiograph showing fracture lines (see arrows).

F, Impression was taken of the mandible and poured. The stone model was cut at the fracture line and mounted on an articulator in normal occlusion with the maxillary teeth. With the model fixed in this position, an acrylic splint, shown here, was made.

G, By circumferential wiring of the splint over the occlusal surfaces of the mandibular teeth, the fragments were pulled into their original occlusal plane.

(Figure 18–149 continued on following page)

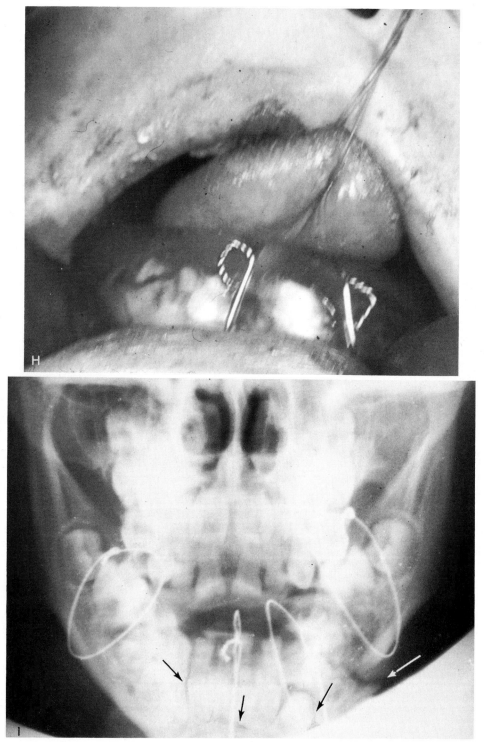

Figure 18–149 *(Continued.)*   *H,* Splint wired into position. *I,* Radiograph showing the circumferential wiring and the apposition of the fragments. (See Case Report No. 7.)

postoperative day for further office treatments. Radiographs taken at this time revealed the fragments in good apposition.

The patient was readmitted 6 weeks later and taken to the operating room, where the acrylic splint was removed under Avertin anesthesia.

After removal of the splint and circumferential wiring, subcutaneous abscesses developed at these sites. These were treated with hot dressings and an infrared lamp. The abscesses ruptured and drained. The edema and induration subsided.

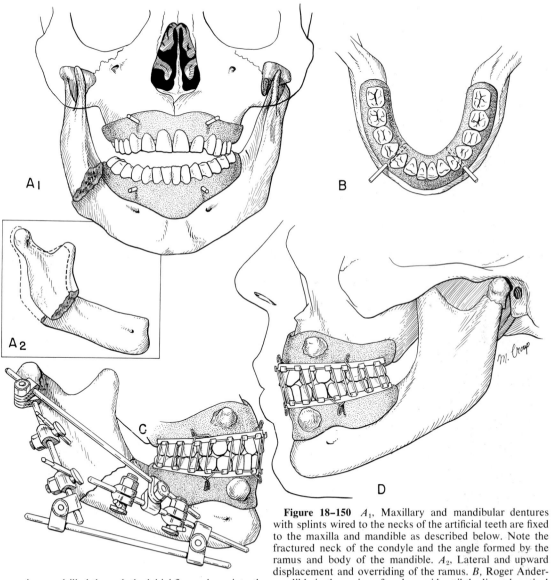

Figure 18–150 A_1, Maxillary and mandibular dentures with splints wired to the necks of the artificial teeth are fixed to the maxilla and mandible as described below. Note the fractured neck of the condyle and the angle formed by the ramus and body of the mandible. A_2, Lateral and upward displacement and overriding of the ramus. B, Roger Anderson pins are drilled through the labial flange down into the mandible in the region of each cuspid until the lingual cortical plate is reached. The maxillary denture is attached to the maxilla in a similar manner. C, The protruding ends of the pins are cut off ¼ inch from the denture flange and are covered with compound. The maxilla and mandible are held in their normal relationship by intermaxillary elastics between splints that are wired to the dentures. Actually these splints are wired to the dentures before the dentures are fixed to the maxilla and mandible. For the sake of clarity the splints were not shown in sketches A and B. After the maxilla and mandible are fixed, Roger Anderson pins are inserted into the ramus and body of the mandible and Frac-Sur units are assembled on the pins. By manipulation of these units the segments are moved into normal apposition and fixed in position by a triangular arrangement of connecting bars. D, Fractured neck of the condyle is in good position.

COMBINED METHODS OF FACIAL FRACTURE TREATMENT

In many cases of fractures of the facial bones a combination of methods is necessary to reduce and immobilize the fractures. In Figure 18–150 there is a bilateral fracture of an edentulous mandible in which one fracture is through the angle and the other through the neck of the condyle. In this particular case the patient's dentures were not broken.

The dentures were fixed to the maxilla and mandible by drilling Roger Anderson pins through the labial flanges of both dentures and through the labial and lingual cortical plates. Then the pins were cut off, leaving enough protruding through the labial flange so that the pins could subsequently be grasped by a hand drill and removed. That portion of the pin which protruded from the denture was covered with modeling compound to protect the lips. Next, by means of intermaxillary elastics stretched between splints which had been previously wired to the necks of the artificial teeth of the denture, the correct relationship was established between the maxilla and the mandible. This also reduced the overriding of the fracture of the neck of the condyle.

The remaining fracture through the angle of the ramus and the body of the mandible was then reduced and stabilized by the application of Roger Anderson Frac-Sur appliances. See x-ray of this case in Figure 18–151. Similar kinds of combined treatment are illustrated in Figures 18–152 to 18–166.

TREATMENT OF MAXILLARY FRACTURES

Fractures of the maxilla may be divided into three general classifications: (1) Segmental fractures of the alveolar process (Le Fort I). In this type of fracture the teeth are detached from the main body of the maxilla and

(Text continued on page 1209)

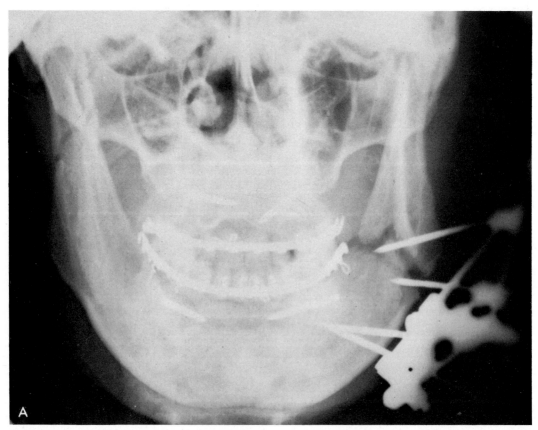

Figure 18–151   *A,* This bilateral fracture through the right angle and left vertical ramus has been treated as shown in Figure 18–150. The left fracture has not been displaced and is immobilized by the insertion of the pterygoid muscles.

(Figure 18–151 continued on opposite page)

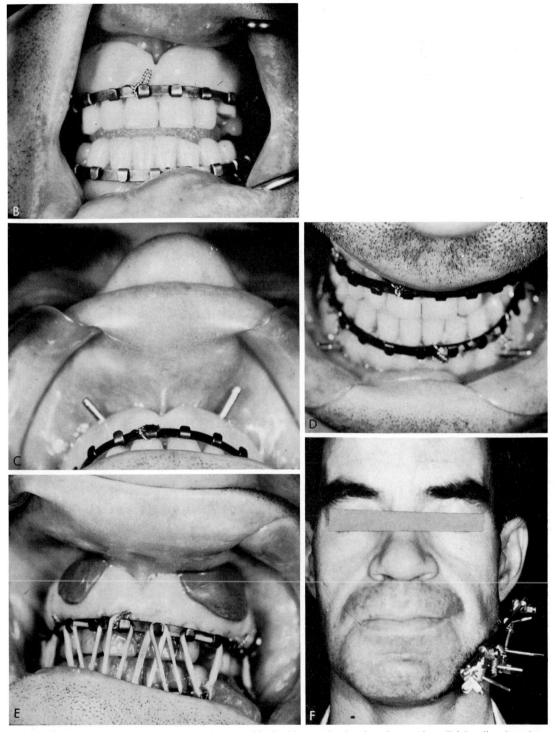

Figure 18–151 (*Continued.*) *B,* The resulting open bite in this completely edentulous patient. Erich splints have been wired to the necks of the artificial teeth.

C, The maxillary denture is now fixed to the maxilla by drilling Roger Anderson pins through the labial flange and on through the alveolar ridge. The ends of the pins can be seen protruding through the labial flange of the denture.

D, The mandibular denture is now fixed to the mandible in the same manner as the maxillary denture was fixed to the maxilla. The ends of the pins can be seen protruding through the flange of the mandibular denture.

E, The ends of all four pins are covered with compound to protect the lips. Intermaxillary elastics are now placed to reduce and immobilize the fracture of the neck of the condyle.

F, The fracture through the angle is reduced and fixed with Frac-Sur units as illustrated. See radiograph in *A.*

BILATERAL COMPOUND FRACTURE OF THE MANDIBLE

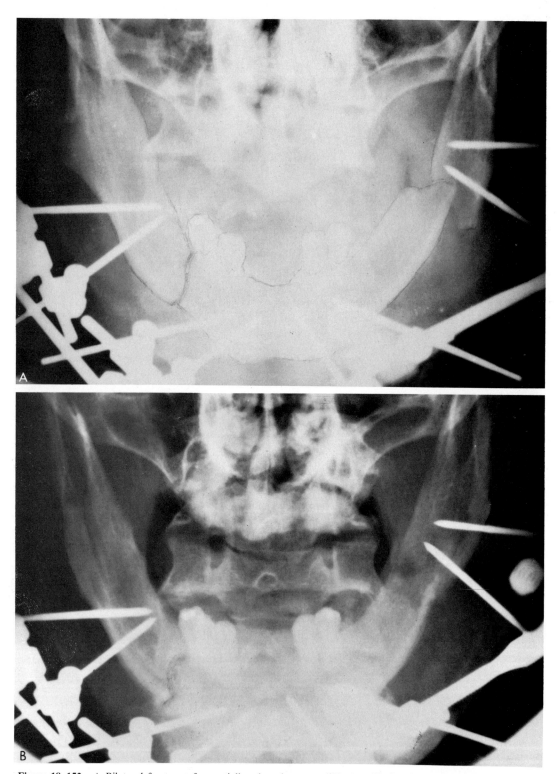

Figure 18–152 *A*, Bilateral fracture of a partially edentulous mandible (maxilla is edentulous), with Frac-Sur units reducing and stabilizing the fracture through the mental foramen on the right side. A Stader splint was applied to the left side, and it is apparent that good reduction was not achieved. The Stader splint was adjusted so that the excellent alignment seen in *B* was secured.

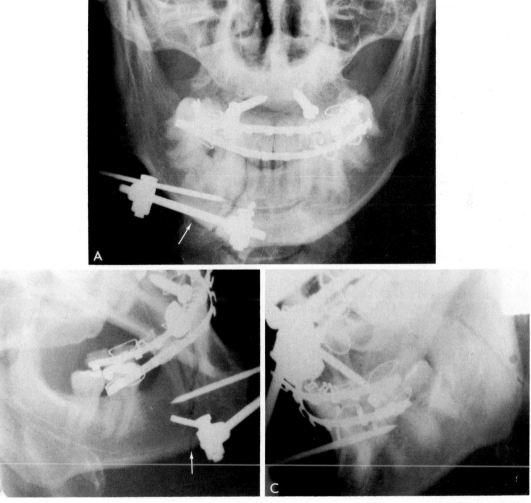

Figure 18–153 *A* and *B*, Fracture of the anterior mandible between the lateral incisor and cuspid. This fracture was reduced and immobilized by the following method: A splint was wired to the full maxillary denture, which was then inserted and attached to the maxilla by screws through the labial flange. The fracture in the symphysis was immobilized by Roger Anderson pins locked together. A splint was then wired to the mandibular teeth. Elastic bands were placed between the maxillary and mandibular splints to hold the teeth in normal occlusion and to immobilize the transverse fracture through the sigmoid notch and posterior border of the vertical ramus, shown in *C*. In the oblique view of the mandible (*B*) the anterior reduced fracture is seen. The distortion by the angle of the x-rays accounts for the incorrect relationship of the pins to the fracture line. Actually, of course, a pin is inserted on either side of the fracture line.

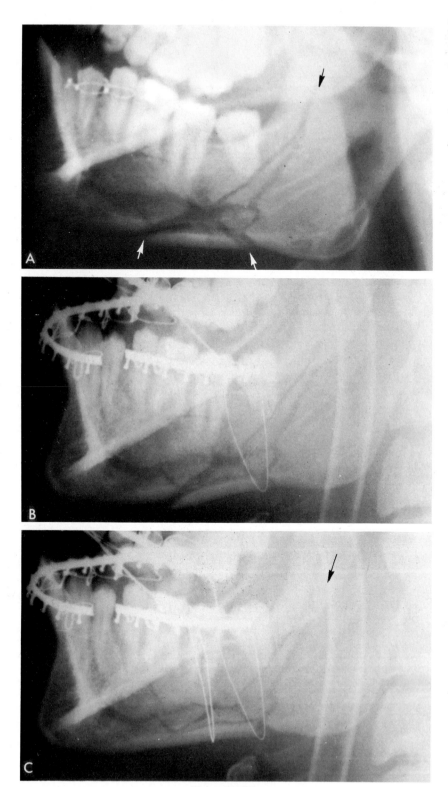

Figure 18–154

(Figure 18–154 continued on opposite page)

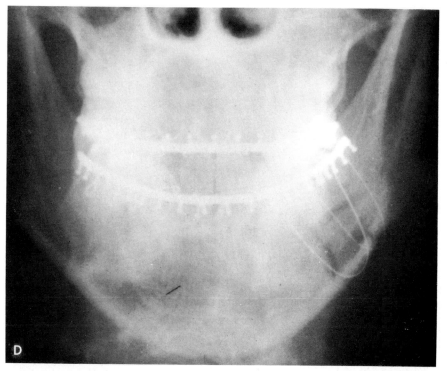

Figure 18–154 *(Continued.)*

Figure 18–154 *A,* Oblique radiograph of an 18-year-old white male who was water skiing and was hit on the right side of the lower jaw by a beer bottle, intentionally thrown by a man who was fishing in another boat. There was no loss of consciousness. The patient was seen in the emergency room; a laceration over the fracture site was sutured, and temporary wires were applied across the fracture site (bicuspids). Note the multiple linear horizontal fracture lines.

B to *D,* Treatment was subsequently performed in the operating room, under nasotracheal anesthesia. Splints were wired to the maxillary teeth (*D*), and a split splint (*B*) at the fracture site was wired to the mandibular teeth. The linear fractures were pulled into apposition with circumferential wires. The mandible was further stabilized and the teeth held in normal occlusion by intermaxillary fixation with elastic bands. The mandibular bicuspids in the line of fracture *were not extracted* at this time or later. (Radiographs and history courtesy of Anson G. Hoyt, D.D.S., and Leon Reisner, Jr., D.D.S., Red Bank, N.J.)

usually still contained within the fractured bone of the alveolus (see Figures 18–167*A,* *D,* and *F* and 18–172). (2) Unilateral or bilateral fractures of the maxilla, separating the body of the maxilla from the facial skeleton (Le Fort II). These fractures may extend through the body of the maxilla down the midline of the hard palate through the floor of the orbit and into the nasal cavity (see Figure 18–167*C, E, G* and *H*). (3) Fractures involving the maxilla in which the entire maxilla and one or more of the facial bones (usually the zygomatic bone) are completely separated from the craniofacial skeleton (Le Fort III).

FRACTURES OF THE ALVEOLAR PROCESS WITH TEETH OR SEGMENTS OF THE MAXILLA

Small alveolar segments with teeth are treated as shown in Figures 18–172 and 18–

173, and the treatment of a large segment is illustrated in Figure 18–167*D.*

Larger segments of the maxilla containing a reasonable number of teeth are best treated by taking an impression of both the maxillary and mandibular teeth, cutting the upper stone model and articulating it correctly with the lower teeth, plastering the portions of the upper model together in this position, then constructing a cast or acrylic splint as shown in Figure 18–47. It is necessary that this be done as soon as possible after injury, as it will be difficult to move this segment after 48 hours.

Most of these larger segments are driven downward so that it will be necessary to pull and push the segment up. This is done by applying a Winter, Jelenko or Erich splint to the lower teeth and incorporating hooks in the upper splints to which intermaxillary elastics are applied on that side or area of the maxilla

(Text continued on page 1217)

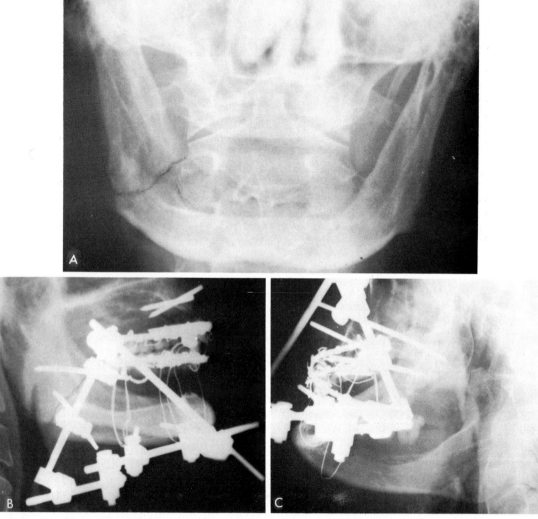

Figure 18–155 *A,* Unilateral fracture through the angle in an edentulous mandible. The ramus was pulled medially and superiorly by the temporalis and external pterygoid muscles. The rest of the mandible was pulled inferiorly, thus altering the intermaxillary relationships.

B, The ramus was correctly positioned by the manipulation of the extraoral pin fixation units, as illustrated in Figure 18–72, and partially fixed in position, but before final locking the patient's dentures were inserted. The mandibular denture was fixed to the mandible by circumferential wiring, and the maxillary denture was pinned to the maxilla, as shown in *B* and *C.* Intermaxillary elastics were placed to bring the mandibular denture into normal occlusion with the maxillary denture. Then the extraoral pin fixation units were completely tightened.

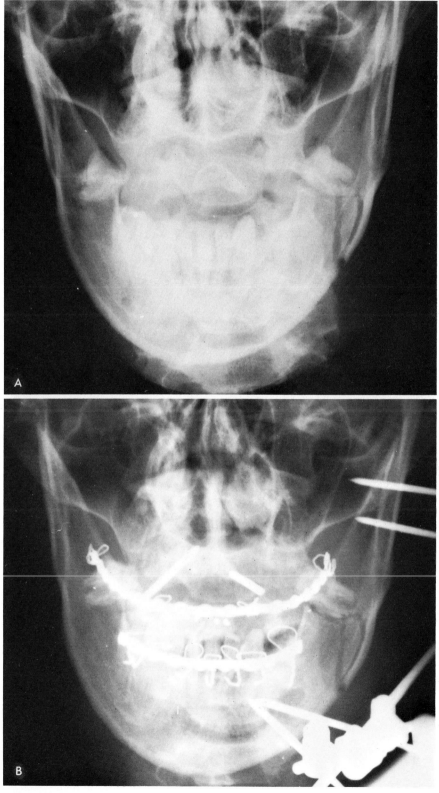

Figure 18–156 *A*, Patient with an edentulous maxilla having a linear fracture of the right body of the edentulous mandible.
B, Fracture reduced and immobilized as illustrated.

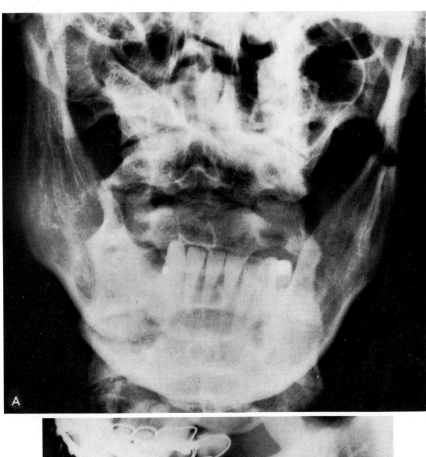

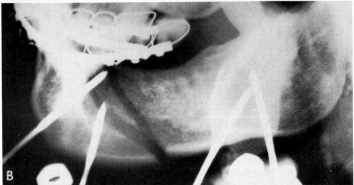

Figure 18–157   Fractures of the right ramus and left body of the mandible, treated as previously described. It is of interest to note that the transverse fracture was reduced and stabilized by the simple process of closing the open inter-maxillary space when the intermaxillary elastics pulled the mandible up, so that the mandibular teeth were in normal occlusion with the maxillary denture.

(Figure 18–157 continued on opposite page)

Figure 18–158   *A*, Unilateral comminuted fracture of the right horizontal ramus of an edentulous mandible. Note the upward and medial position of the posterior fragment and the overriding. (See Figure 18–115 for method of treatment.)
   B, Fracture reduced and immobilized by means of a Stader splint, a very excellent method of treatment when there is overriding of the fragments. (See also Figure 18–118 for another case.)
   C, Oblique view. *D*, Oblique view after reduction.

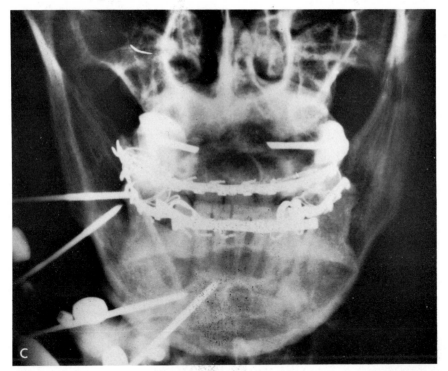

Figure 18–157 *(Continued.)*

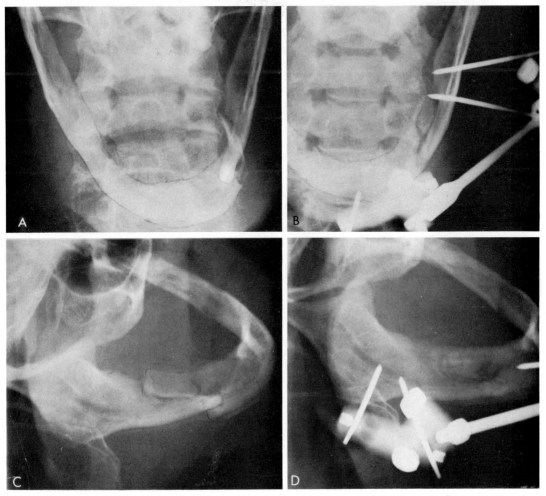

Figure 18–158 *See opposite page for legend.*

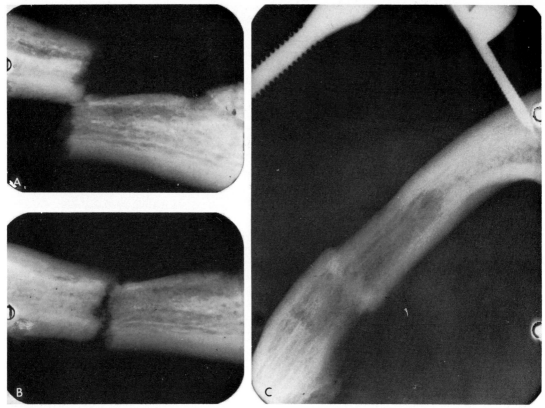

Figure 18--159 *A*, Unilateral fracture of an edentulous mandible with upward displacement of the posterior fragment. *B*, Fracture reduced. *C*, Occlusal view showing a portion of the Stader splint by which the fracture was reduced and immobilized.

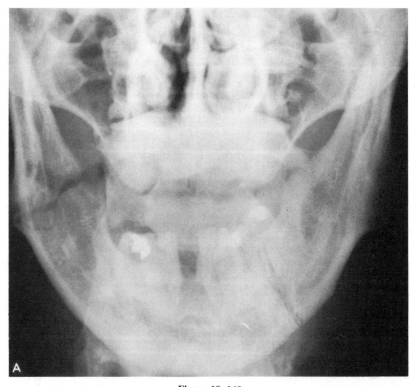

Figure 18–160

(Figure 18–160 continued on opposite page)

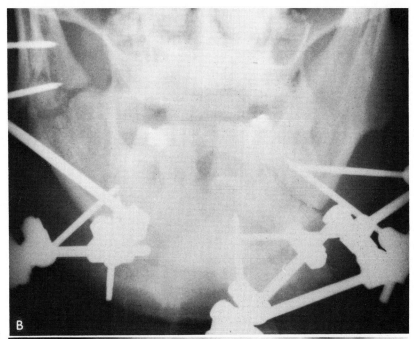

Figure 18–160 Bilateral fracture of a partially edentulous mandible. The fractures were in good alignment because of the minimal trauma that produced them and because the patient was seen within 3 hours after the injury, before the downward muscle pull had existed long enough to cause movement of the fragments. Therefore, the slight alteration that did exist in the intermaxillary space was easily corrected when the fractures were fixed with the bilateral pin fixation units, and it was not necessary to fix the mandible to the maxillary denture, as shown previously.

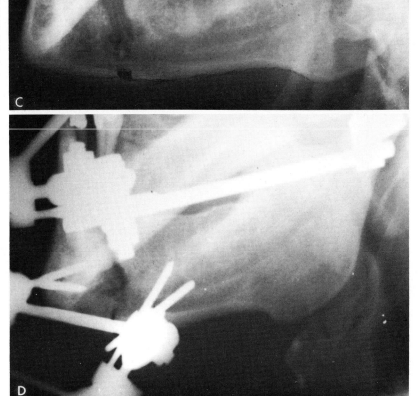

Figure 18–160 *(Continued.)*

1215

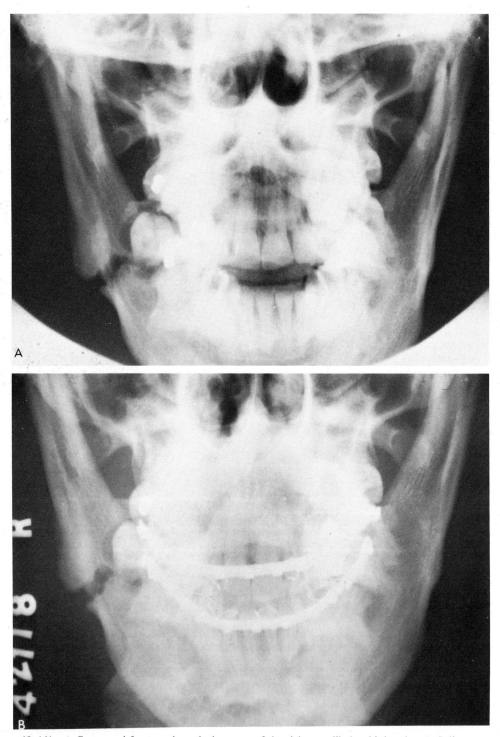

Figure 18–161 *A,* Compound fracture through the crypt of the right mandibular third molar. *B,* Splints were wired to the maxillary and mandibular teeth and intermaxillary elastics placed between them. The partially formed, mesially impacted third molar was removed.

(Figure 18–161 continued on opposite page)

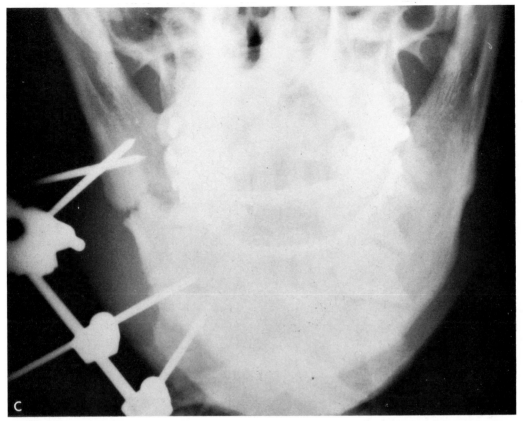

Figure 18–161 *(Continued.)* C, The laterally displaced fractured ramus was repositioned and fixed in place with an extraoral pin fixation unit.

which is still attached to the skull. The lower teeth, creating upward pressure against the depressed teeth, will force these teeth and their investing bone up to their normal relationship. In some cases it will be necessary to apply extraoral traction by means of a head-chin bandage with elastic traction as shown and described in Figure 18–139. Once the fragment is moved up, the split splint can be applied to bring the fragments together laterally, thus closing the gap in the ridge and palate.

TRANSVERSE (HORIZONTAL) FRACTURES OF THE MAXILLA

In transverse maxillary fractures the lines of separation may be through the maxillary sinuses and the floor of the nasal cavity as shown in Figure 18–167C, or they may be through the orbital cavity, sinuses and nasal cavities. In these cases there is usually considerable comminution and fracture of the nasal bones as well.

In transverse fractures of the maxilla, in which the maxilla was driven backward and downward as illustrated in Figure 18–174A, we generally find the bite to be opened because the posterior maxillary teeth are in contact prematurely with the posterior mandibular teeth. If the fracture is seen immediately after the accident, the fracture can be reduced by the application of splints to the necks of the teeth as illustrated in Figure 18–174B, which will bring the maxillary fragment anteriorly into normal occlusion with the mandible. However, the weight of the mandible plus its attached soft structures drags the fractured segment of the maxilla downward. It is necessary that upward traction be applied on the mandible which in turn forces the fractured segment of the maxilla back up into its former relationship with the facial bones.

In the past, it has been customary to pro-
(Text continued on page 1222)

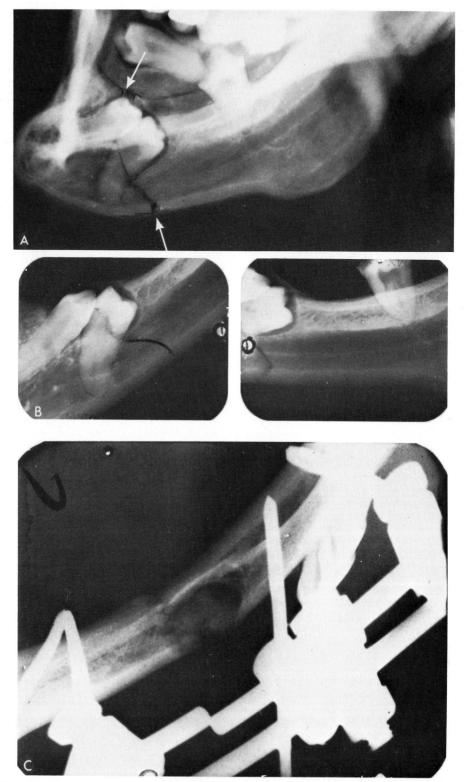

Figure 18–162 *A*, Impacted, unerupted right mandibular first and second bicuspids were the site of this simple fracture. *B*, Periapical radiographs furnish additional information concerning the location of the impacted teeth.

C, Before excision of the impacted teeth, with a minimum of bone removal, extraoral skeletal pin fixation units were inserted on either side of the fracture. The occlusal radiograph confirms the perfect alignment of the buccal and lingual cortical plates.

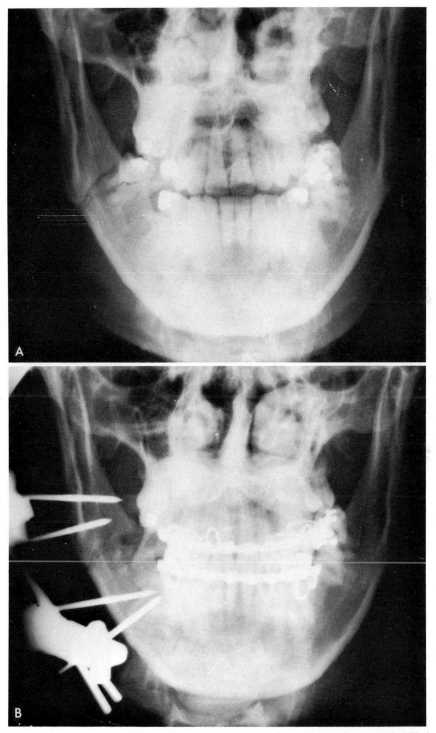

Figure 18–163 *A,* Simple fracture through the mandibular third molar area that split the tooth. This is a reason for its removal.

B, Before removal of the tooth, splints are applied to the necks of the maxillary and mandibular teeth, intermaxillary elastics are placed between the splints, and extraoral pin units are inserted. The intermaxillary fixation can be removed in about 2 weeks and the extraoral pin units after 4 weeks more. During this time the patient is on a soft diet.

COMMINUTED FRACTURE OF THE MANDIBLE IN A 12-YEAR-OLD BOY

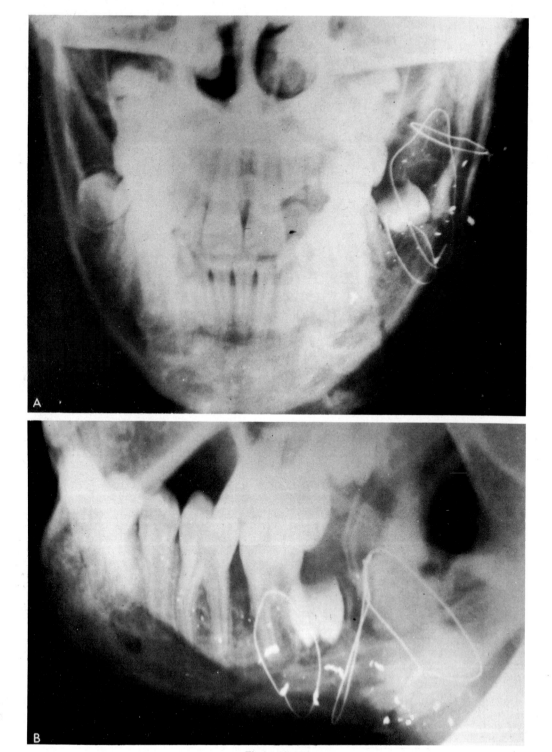

Figure 18–164

(Figure 18–164 continued on opposite page)

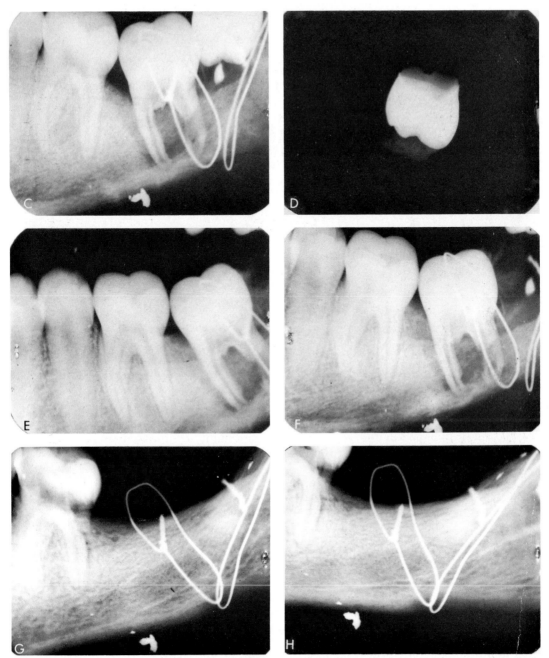

Figure 18–164 *(Continued.)* Compound comminuted fracture of the mandible in a 12-year-old boy accidentally shot in the face by his father while hunting in the woods. The bullet struck the mandible and fragmented, shattering the body of the mandible and ramus and blowing the cheek apart (see *I*).

A, Posteroanterior radiograph taken after reduction of the fractures by circumferential wiring. It is obvious that the bone fragment containing the crown of the partially formed third molar was inadvertently replaced upside down in the "jigsaw puzzle" of bone fragments blown around in this mass of lacerated tissue, in which structures could be identified only as bone or soft tissue.

B, Postoperative oblique radiograph of the mandible.

C, Eight weeks later.

D, Third molar crown removed.

E and *F*, Ten weeks later. The second molar was extracted, since there was buccal drainage of pus and the tooth had become mobile.

G and *H*, Ten months following the injury. The wires were not visible or troublesome and so were left in place.

(Figure 18–164 continued on following page)

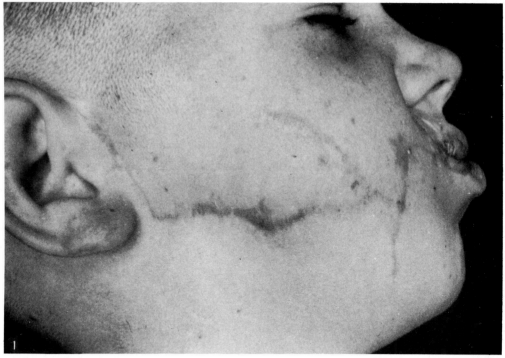

Figure 18–164   *(Continued.)*   *1*, Scars of the cheek and corner of the mouth after healing of original wounds but before surgical revision.

duce this upward traction by the use of head caps or head frames of various construction. (See later in chapter for these techniques.) Hooks extend from these plaster of paris head caps or frames to which elastic bands are attached to either pins in the mandible or cups over the symphysis. A much simpler, better, more comfortable, and more accurate method of bringing about this pressure is illustrated in Figure 18–174*C*. In this particular case, a fracture unit has been inserted in both the right and left body of the mandible and one in each zygomatic bone. Rubber bands are now stretched between the units in the zygomatic bones and mandible. These bands produce traction that moves the mandible and its attached maxillary fragment up-

ward until the fracture of the maxilla has been reduced. Once this has been accomplished, the mandible and maxilla are fixed together as a unit, by means of the connecting bar shown in Figure 18–174*D*. The intermaxillary rubber bands are now discarded.

It can be readily seen that this simple and comfortable method of cranial fixation (as compared to plaster head caps, surgical strapping headgear, Barton bandages, and so on) is a very efficient way to reduce the separation of the maxilla from the skull. Once the reduction has been accomplished (a matter of hours), long connecting bars are substituted for the rubber bands and are locked in place. This prevents movement of the fractured segment.

(Text continued on page 1232)

Figure 18–165   *A,* Compound comminuted fracture of the mandible in an adult who was accidentally shot by a fellow hunter.

B, There was not enough bone left to fill the void in the body of the mandible produced by the trauma, so a rib graft was inserted. Further immobilization was supplied by maxillary and mandibular splints and intermaxillary fixation with elastic bands. (Regretfully, the name of the oral surgeon who supplied these radiographs has been mislaid.)

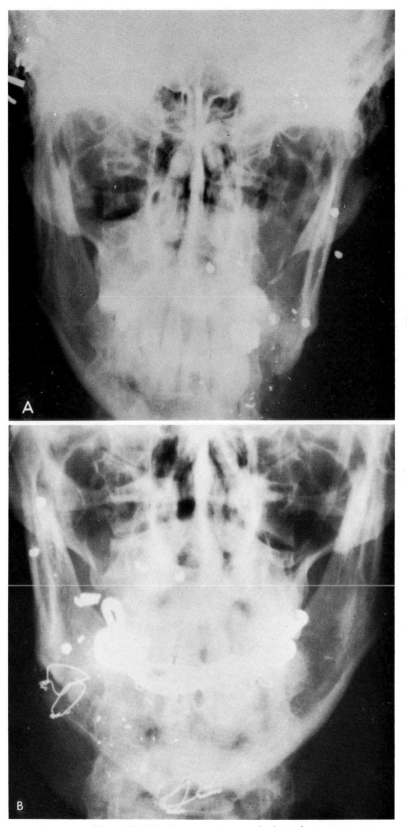

Figure 18–165 *See opposite page for legend.*

COMMINUTED FRACTURE OF THE MANDIBLE AND SEVERED PAROTID DUCT

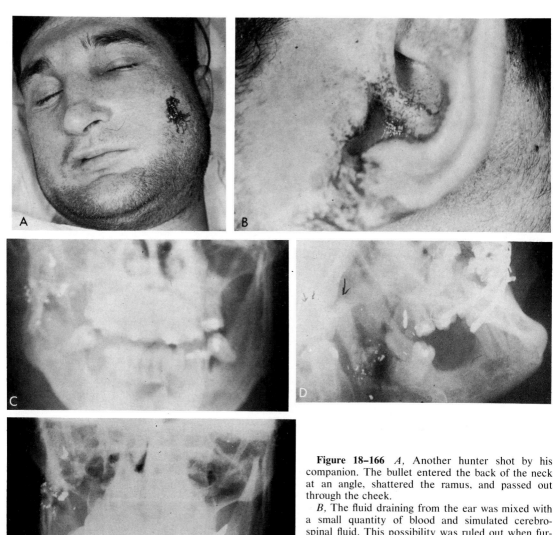

Figure 18–166 *A,* Another hunter shot by his companion. The bullet entered the back of the neck at an angle, shattered the ramus, and passed out through the cheek.

B, The fluid draining from the ear was mixed with a small quantity of blood and simulated cerebrospinal fluid. This possibility was ruled out when further examination revealed a severed parotid duct. The treatment of a cut duct and fractures is described in Figures 14–27 to 14–31.

C, D and *E,* Pre- and postoperative treatment radiographs.

(Figure 18–166 continued on opposite page)

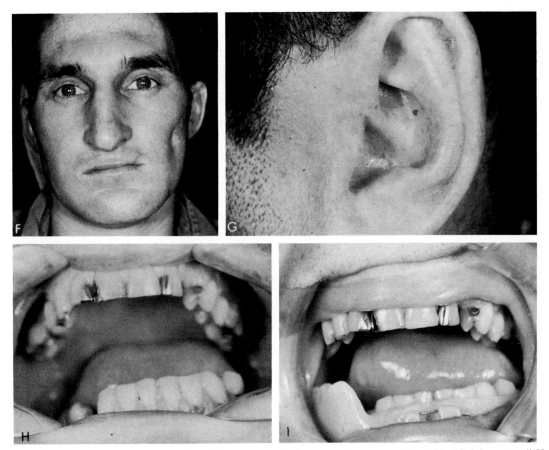

Figure 18-166 *(Continued.)* *F*, Final facial appearance. Patient was not concerned about his "tied-down scar." He was glad to be alive.

G, Drainage of saliva from the ear ceased as soon as the patency of the parotid duct was established. (See Figures 14-27 to 14-31.)

H, After splints were removed there was a slight swing of the mandible to the left on opening the mouth.

I, A split splint with a buccal superior flange was attached to the lower teeth, as illustrated. In 3 weeks this "training splint" resulted in unilateral muscle development that compensated for the slight loss of bone in the right vertical ramus, so that on opening and closing the mouth, the teeth met in normal occlusion.

(For an example of treatment of a severe mandibular gunshot wound with a head frame, see Figure 18-198.)

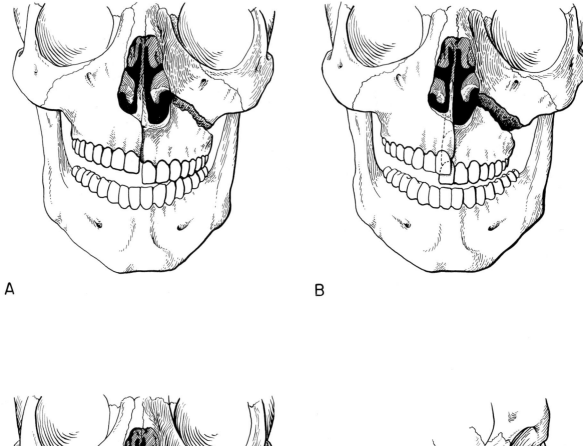

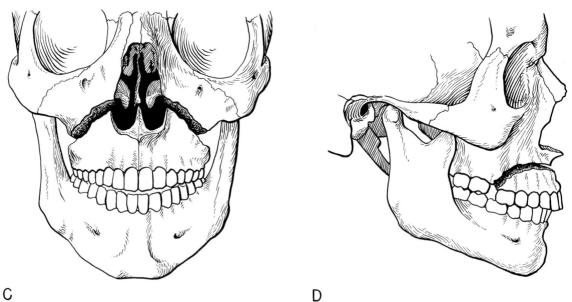

Figure 18–167 Fractures of the maxilla. *A,* Unilateral fracture with downward displacement. *B,* Unilateral fracture with downward and inward displacement. *C,* Bilateral horizontal fracture with downward displacement. *D,* Large anterior segmental fracture with downward and forward displacement.

(Figure 18–167 continued on opposite page)

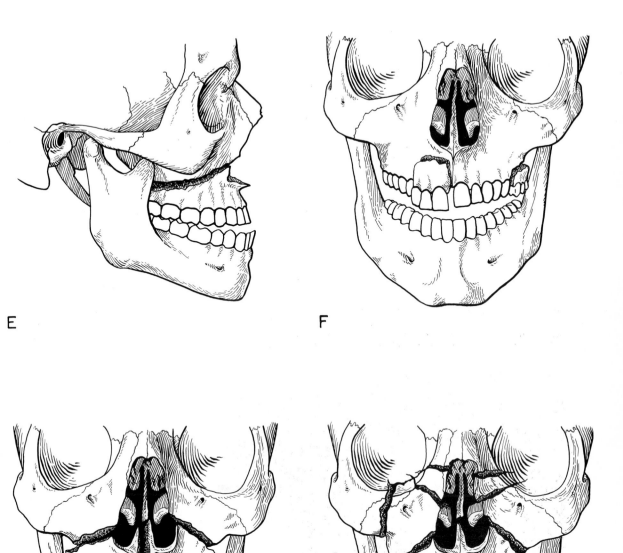

E

F

G

H

Figure 18–167 *(Continued.)* *E*, Transverse (horizontal) fracture with downward and backward displacement. *F*, Anterior small segmental fracture with downward displacement. Posterior segmental fractures usually involve the floor of the maxillary sinus. *G*, Bilateral horizontal fracture with median fracture through palatal suture. *H*, Bilateral fracture with comminution of bones of upper part of face.

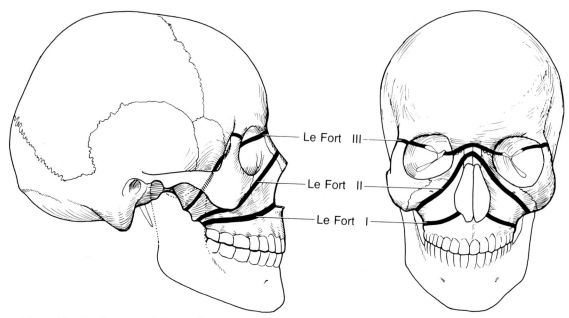

Figure 18–168 Fractures of the maxilla. Mobility of the maxilla when pushing or pulling on the anterior alveolar process indicates a fracture of the maxilla. In a Le Fort III fracture, the whole of each infraorbital rim moves with the maxilla. In a Le Fort II fracture, only the medial section of each infraorbital rim moves with the maxilla. In a Le Fort I fracture, the whole orbital complex remains stable. (From Committee on Trauma, American College of Surgeons: Early Care of the Injured Patient. Philadelphia, W. B. Saunders Co., 1972.)

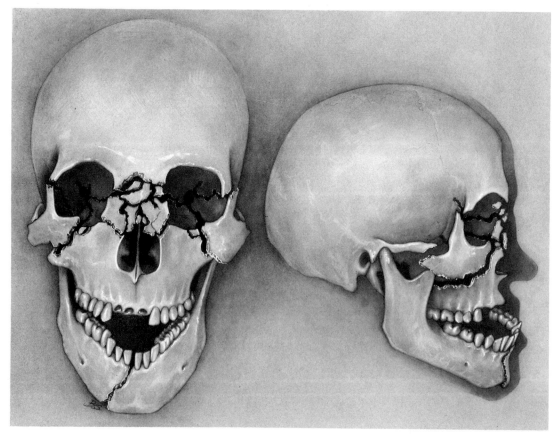

Figure 18–169 Fracture-dislocation of the upper portion of the facial skeleton, fracture of the symphysis, and missing anterior teeth. (See treatment in Figure 18–192.)

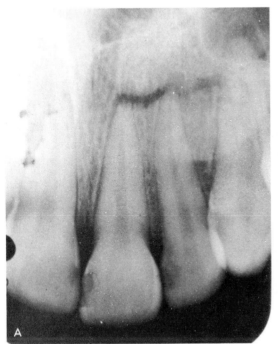

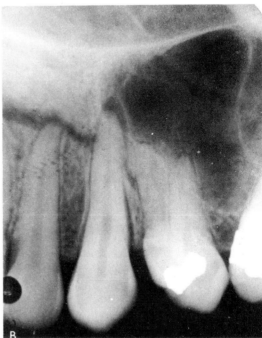

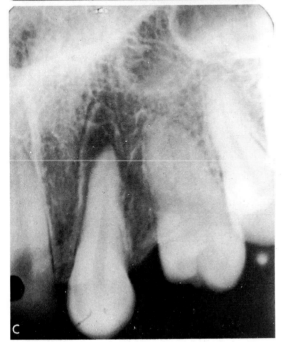

Figure 18–170 Linear fractures of the maxilla, unless there is gross displacement, are very hard to visualize on extraoral radiographs. It is imperative to include periapical films in the examination, such as those shown in *A* and *B*. The cuspid tooth in *C* is partially dislodged from its alveolus.

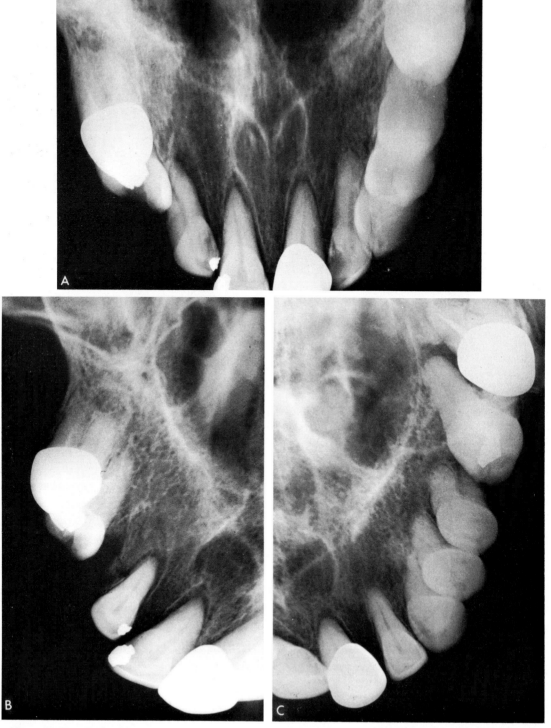

Figure 18–171 Occlusal intraoral radiographs of the maxilla for the detection of linear fractures. The four maxillary incisors were very loose, but this was due to the partial avulsion of these teeth from their alveoli. No linear fractures were seen in this survey.

FRACTURE OF A SEGMENT OF THE ANTERIOR MAXILLA

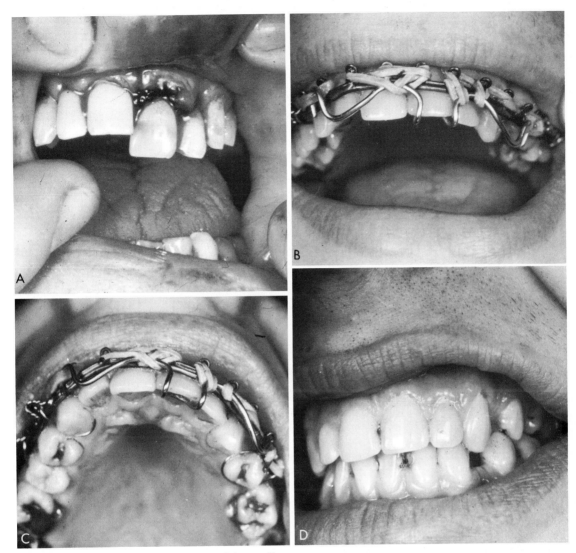

Figure 18–172 A fracture of a segment of the maxilla.

A, A fairly frequent fracture is illustrated here, in which from two to four anterior teeth and their investing alveolar processes are fractured as a unit from the rest of the maxilla. A satisfactory method of treatment is illustrated in this case.

B, A Jelenko splint is contoured to the gingival line of the maxillary teeth and then wired to the necks of every maxillary tooth except those contained in the fractured segment. Then a stainless steel wire crib is contoured to fit over the incisal edges of the teeth. This is connected to the Jelenko splint by appropriately sized elastic bands. These elastics gradually reduce the fractured segment and immobilize it.

C, This occlusal view shows the manner in which the wire crib is contoured. A new crib with curved wire arms or extensions to which the elastics are attached must be contoured to fit the particular patient under treatment. It must be contoured so as not to interfere with occlusion.

D, End result of the treatment.

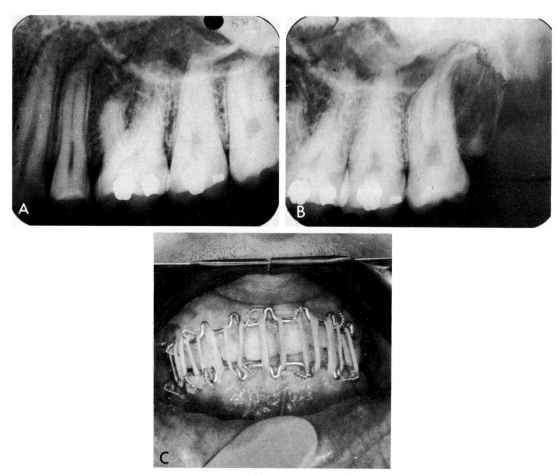

Figure 18–173 *A* and *B,* Unilateral fracture of the right maxilla through the maxillary sinus, palate and tuberosity. Fragment contains the second premolar, first, second and third molars. *C,* Fracture reduced and immobilized by splints wired to each arch and intermaxillary rubber bands.

INTERNAL WIRE SUSPENSION

This technique has a limited field of usefulness and is illustrated in Figures 18–185 and 18–186. Note that in these cases the mandible is intact and there is good dentition in both jaws. This makes it possible to bring the fractured maxilla, which has been driven downward and backward, forward by means of intermaxillary elastic traction using the intact mandible as the fixed point. Then the mandible is pulled upward with the attached maxilla, by craniomaxillary wire suspension.

Unfortunately some surgeons are treating multiple facial fractures in which there are subcondylar and other fractures of the mandible, plus transverse fractures of the maxilla, nasal and zygomatic bones, by direct wiring and craniomaxillary suspension. Many of these cases have a very poor cosmetic end result. This is because craniomaxillary suspension in these cases pulls the fractured bones not only upward, but *backward.* What is indicated in these cases is not to elevate the fractures but to bring them *forward.* This can only be obtained, in these cases, by pulling the fragments upward and *forward* by attachment to a skeletal head frame such as those described and illustrated later in this chapter.

(Text continued on page 1250)

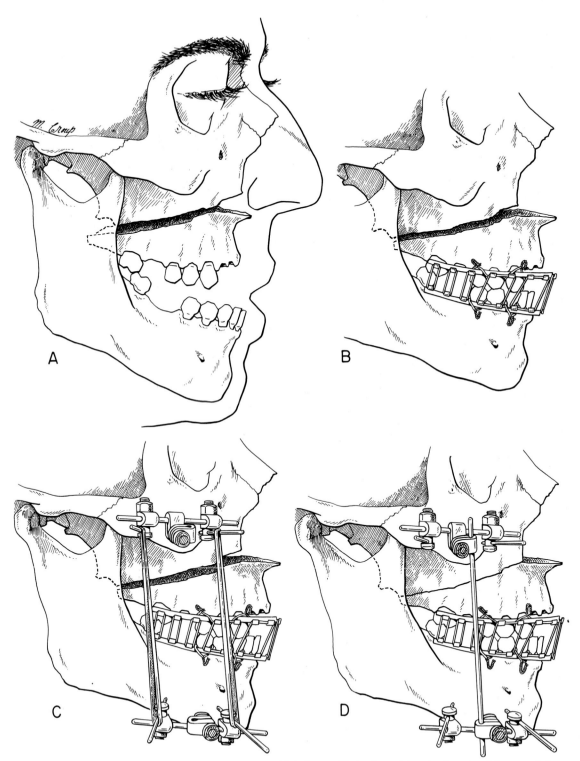

Figure 18–174 Transverse fracture of the maxilla, in which the maxilla has been driven backward and downward. See test for explanation.

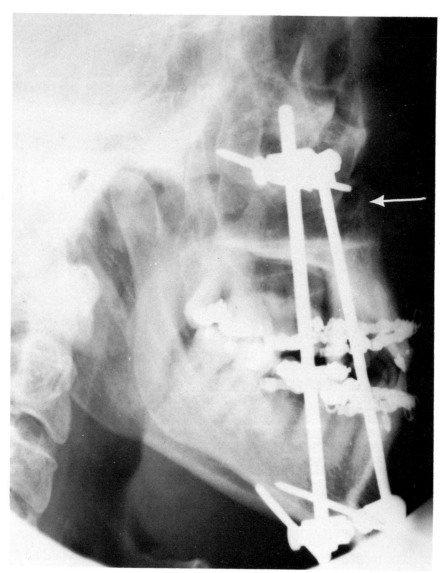

Figure 18-175   Le Fort I fracture of the maxilla, reduced in the same manner as that described in the legend of Figure 18-187.

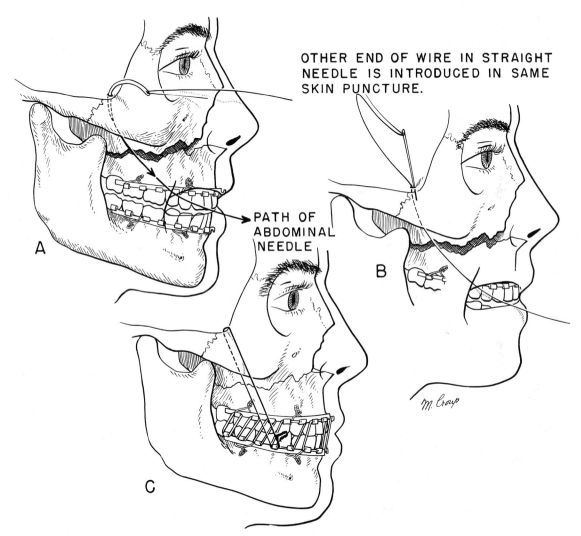

OTHER END OF WIRE IN STRAIGHT
NEEDLE IS INTRODUCED IN SAME
SKIN PUNCTURE.

PATH OF
ABDOMINAL
NEEDLE

A

B

C

Figure 18–176 A method for the treatment of a horizontal fracture of the maxilla is shown here. Obviously, both zygomatic arches must be intact. The author prefers the method shown in Figure 18–174.

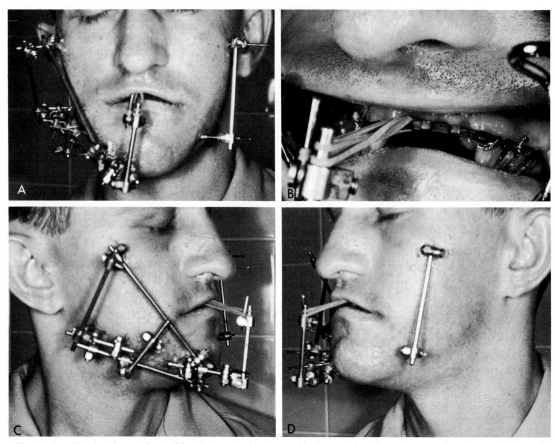

Figure 18–177 Another patient with a Le Fort I fracture, with the maxilla driven downward and posteriorly, and a fracture of the right body of the mandible. Note how frequently Le Fort I patients have had their maxillary anterior teeth knocked out. The treatment in this case was as follows: *(1)* Reduction and fixation of the fracture in the body of the mandible with extraoral skeletal fixation units *(A and B)*. *(2)* Maxillary and mandibular splints were then wired to the necks of the remaining maxillary and mandibular teeth. *(3)* Traction was produced by means of rubber bands from the maxillary splint to an extension bar from the pin fixation unit *(B to D)* to bring this fractured segment anteriorly and downward. *(4)* When the maxilla was in its original location, intermaxillary rubber bands were applied to bring the teeth into occlusion *(B)*. *(5)* The articulated maxilla and mandible were then pulled up as a unit to close the fracture gap between the fractured maxilla and the osseous areas from which it was torn loose.

Figure 18–179 Le Fort II fracture of the maxilla. Note the fracture points. This patient was referred to us after having received the treatment shown in this radiograph because the maxilla was still retruded and only the posterior teeth were in contact, resulting in an open bite. The suspension wire obviously pulled the maxilla up and back, compounding the original displacement. Treatment now required removal of the wire and intermaxillary fixation and anterior traction by means of a head frame until a normal maxillary-mandibular relationship was attained. Intermaxillary elastic traction (small rubber bands) was then used until the teeth in both jaws were in normal occlusion. Next, by traction, the mandible and maxilla were moved upward as a unit into apposition with the frontal and zygomatic bones and were locked into this position with intermaxillary rods between pin fixation units. (See Figures 18–191 to 18–193 and 18–195.)

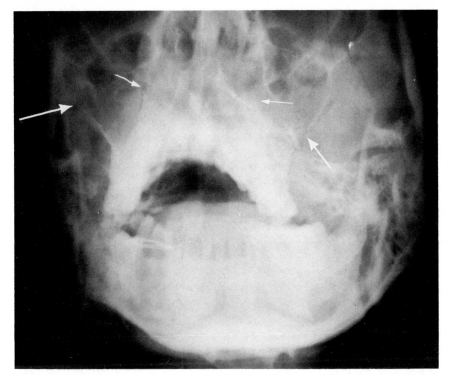

Figure 18–178 Posteroanterior radiograph of a transverse fracture (Le Fort II) of the maxilla with gross lateral and downward displacement. Note the relationship of the maxilla to the nonfractured mandible. The treatment will be demonstrated in following cases.

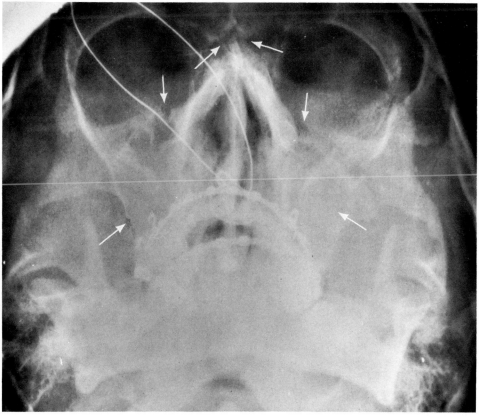

Figure 18–179 *See opposite page for legend.*

CORRECTION OF MALUNION OF A TRANSVERSE FRACTURE OF THE MAXILLA AND BILATERAL FRACTURES OF THE MANDIBLE

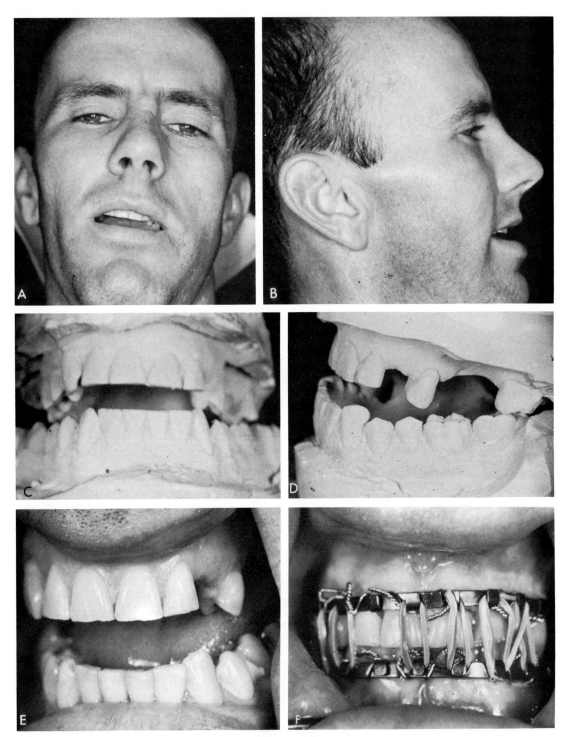

Figure 18–180

(Figure 18–180 continued on opposite page)

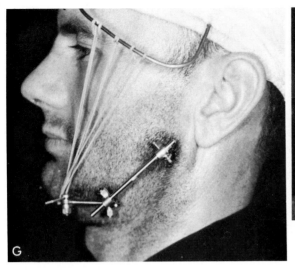

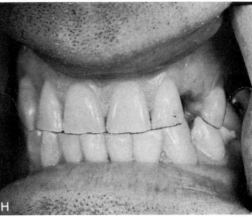

Figure 18–180   *A* and *B*, This patient came in 10 weeks after an automobile accident. He had been discharged from another hospital as "cured." *B*, It is obvious that the patient cannot bring his lips together normally, and the open bite shown in *C* to *E* shows why. Only the posterior teeth are in contact. Examination revealed: (1) a partially healed transverse fracture of the maxilla; (2) fracture through the left angle of the mandible and a right subcondylar fracture. The maxilla was refractured, with the method shown in Figure 18–204. The left angle of the mandible was refractured and the ends freshened intraorally. Manual manipulation fractured the subcondylar union, if any had taken place. In *F* and *G* are shown the methods of reduction and stabilization restoring normal occlusion and facial contour. Bilateral traction from the plaster head cap was used for the maxillary fracture, and angle fracture was immobilized with extraoral pin fixation. *H*, Final results.

Photographic Case Report

UNILATERAL FRACTURE OF THE MAXILLA

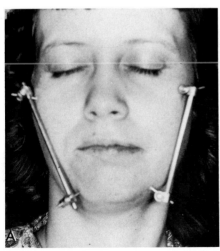

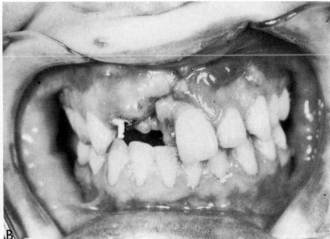

Figure 18–181   Segmental unilateral fracture of the left maxilla reduced and immobilized by (*A*) placing single pins in each zygomatic bone and in the horizontal rami (body of mandible), and (*B*) passing rubber bands over each set of pins. This brings the mandibular teeth into articulation with the left maxilla (which had been displaced downward and backward), gradually forcing it back into contact with the right maxilla and the zygoma. When this is accomplished, then solid bars are substituted for the rubber bands and locked into position. Frac-Sur units and pins are used. This is the type of fracture shown in Figure 18–167*A*.

TRANSVERSE COMPOUND FRACTURE OF THE MAXILLA

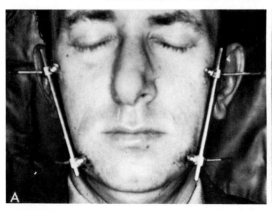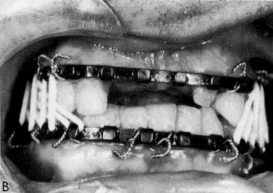

Figure 18–182 This 7-day-old transverse fracture of the maxilla was the type shown in Figure 18–167*E*. It was treated as described for the case illustrated in Figure 18–181, except that splints and intermaxillary elastics were needed to secure perfect occlusion. Then extraoral traction was applied, and then fixation.

TRANSVERSE FRACTURE OF THE MAXILLA AND A BILATERAL FRACTURE OF THE EDENTULOUS MANDIBLE

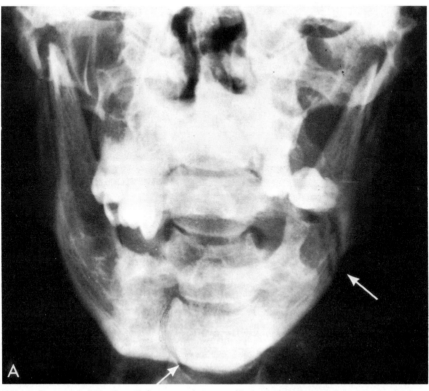

Figure 18–183 *A,* Transverse (Le Fort I) fracture of the maxilla, anterior teeth knocked out (see *E*), and a bilateral fracture of the mandible, which is edentulous except for a third molar in the line of fracture at the angle; there is also a right subcondylar fracture and one in the symphysis. *B,* Fractures reduced and stabilized. *Note:* pins in each zygomatic bone. Frac-Sur units in mandible reducing mandibular fractures, connecting bar, elastic traction, mandibular denture pinned to the mandible. *C,* Rubber band traction pulling maxilla-mandible unit up into contact with cranial bones. *D,* Connecting bars between zygomas locked when the fracture line between the maxilla and cranial bones is closed. **E,** Mandibular denture pinned to mandible, pins cut off ¼ inch from denture flange (so they can be locked in the pin vise and

(*Figure 18–183 continued on opposite page.*)

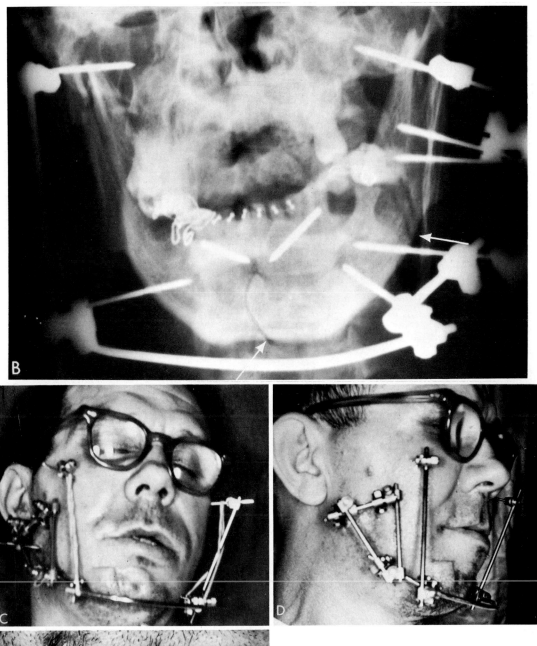

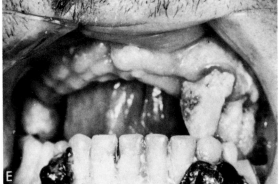

Figure 18–183 (*Continued.*) removed when treatment of the case is completed), and extruding ends covered with black compound to protect the lips.

TRANSVERSE FRACTURE OF THE MAXILLA AND A COMPOUND FRACTURE OF THE SYMPHYSIS

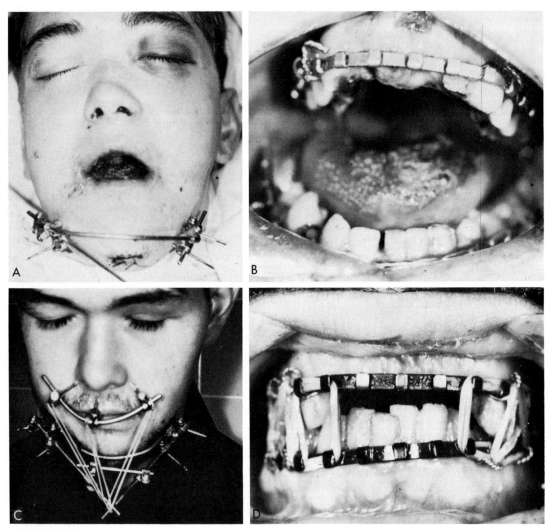

Figure 18–184 Transverse maxillary fracture, as shown in Figure 18–167*E*, and an oblique fracture through the mandibular symphysis. *A*, Mandibular fracture reduced and stabilized with Frac-Sur units. *B*, Splints attached to maxillary and mandibular teeth. *C*, Frac-Sur pins inserted into anterior maxillary fragment and pulled down and forward as illustrated. *D*, Final normal alignment of fractures and restoration of occlusion.

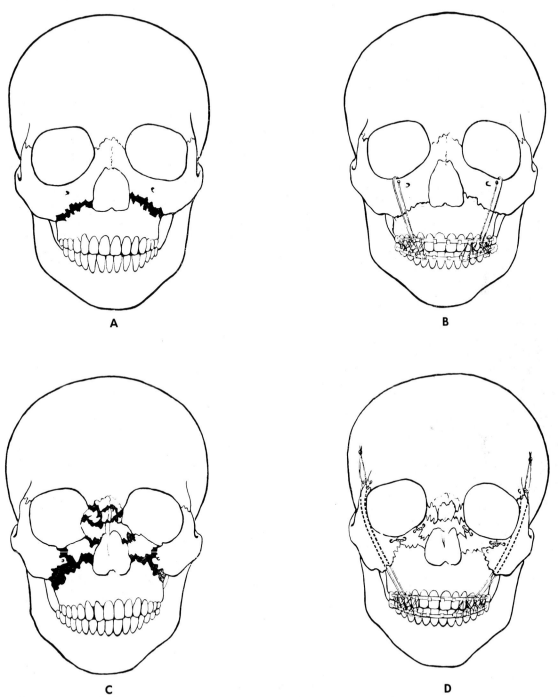

Figure 18–185   *A*, Transverse maxillary fracture (Le Fort I). *B*, Treatment by intermaxillary rubber band traction with arch bars and internal wire suspension from the infraorbital rim. *C*, Pyramidal type maxillary fracture (Le Fort II) associated with extensive comminution of the nasal, lacrimal and ethmoid areas. *D*, Correction by intermaxillary fixation, craniomaxillary suspension, and interosseous wiring of fragments in the infraorbital region. (From Dingman, R. O., and Natvig, P.: Surgery of Facial Fractures. Philadelphia, W. B. Saunders Co., 1964.)

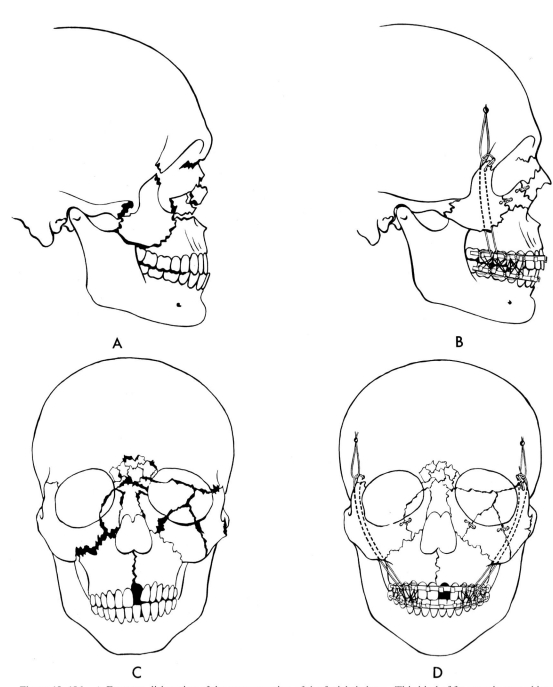

Figure 18–186 *A*, Fracture-dislocation of the upper portion of the facial skeleton. This kind of fracture is caused by a blow above the level of the nasal spine and results in compound comminuted fractures of the zygomatic, nasal, lacrimal and ethmoid areas, with fracture of the maxilla. *B*, Reduction and interosseous wire fixation of multiple bone fragments, and craniomaxillary suspension with internal wire fixation. *C*, Diagram of multiple fractures of the middle third of the face, including maxilla, left zygoma, nasal, lacrimal and ethmoid bones, with involvement of the frontal sinus. *D*, Treatment by intermaxillary arch bar fixation, open reduction, and interosseous wire fixation of the fragments of the infraorbital bones, elevation of nasal and frontal bone fractures, fixation of fracture at the zygomaticofrontal suture line on left, and craniomaxillary internal wire suspension. (From Dingman, R. O., and Natvig, P.: Surgery of Facial Fractures. Philadelphia, W. B. Saunders Co., 1964.)

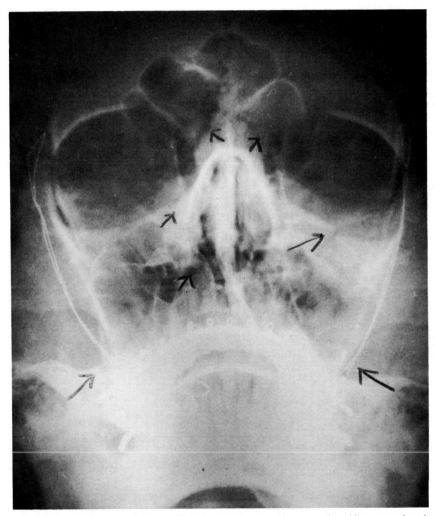

Figure 18–187   Le Fort III fracture of the maxilla. First the fractured jaws are placed into normal occlusion by means of intermaxillary elastic rubber bands placed over splints on the maxillary and mandibular teeth. When this traction has closed the fracture space in the maxilla, the maxilla is moved up to close the fracture space with wires from the lateral orbital rim, as described in Figure 18–188.

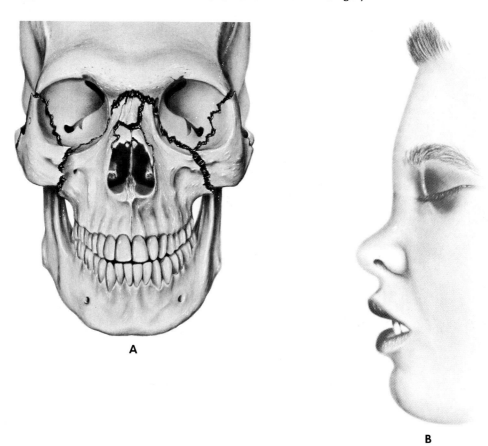

A

B

Figure 18–188   *A*, Severe trauma to the middle third of the face may result in complete craniofacial dislocation. The facial bones are broken loose from their articulations at the base of the skull. This fracture with craniofacial disjunction is associated frequently with fractures of the cribriform plate, causing lacerations of the dura and cerebrospinal rhinorrhea. Many or all of the facial bones may be involved with comminution and downward and posterior displacement. The fractured segments may be supported only by soft-tissue attachments.

B, Fractures due to trauma to the nasal region may result in craniofacial dislocation (Le Fort III fracture), with a comminution of the nasal bones, septum, ethmoid and sphenoid causing a dish-face profile.

C, Reduction and internal wire fixation require identification of the fractures and an orderly plan for reduction and fixation to adjacent solid structures. The immediately adjacent solid structure is usually the zygomatic process of the frontal bone. Fractures at the zygomaticofrontal suture are fixed securely with interosseous stainless steel wires. The drill holes are placed at the anterior edge of the orbital rim and pass posteriorly into the temporal fossa. Both ends of the wire are passed posteriorly and twisted so that the knot will be behind the orbital rim where the wire can be cut off and pressed against the bone firmly. In this location the twisted cut end of the wire will not cause irritation to the soft tissues.

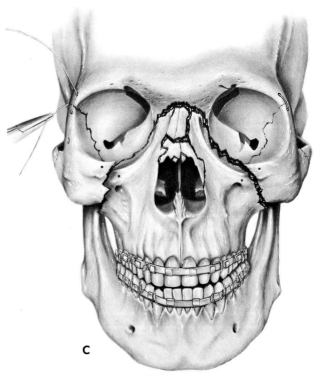

C

(*Figure 18–188 continued on opposite page*)

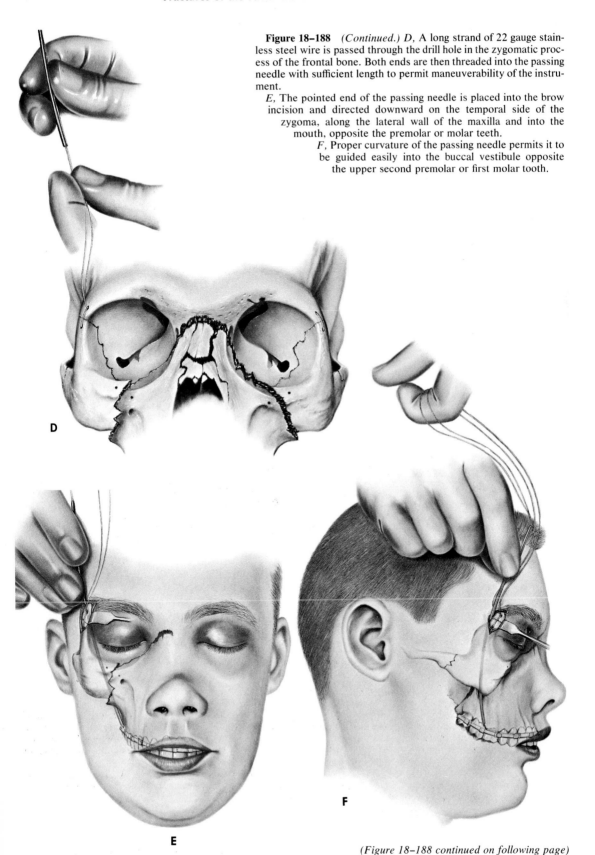

Figure 18–188 *(Continued.) D,* A long strand of 22 gauge stainless steel wire is passed through the drill hole in the zygomatic process of the frontal bone. Both ends are then threaded into the passing needle with sufficient length to permit maneuverability of the instrument.

E, The pointed end of the passing needle is placed into the brow incision and directed downward on the temporal side of the zygoma, along the lateral wall of the maxilla and into the mouth, opposite the premolar or molar teeth.

F, Proper curvature of the passing needle permits it to be guided easily into the buccal vestibule opposite the upper second premolar or first molar tooth.

(Figure 18–188 continued on following page)

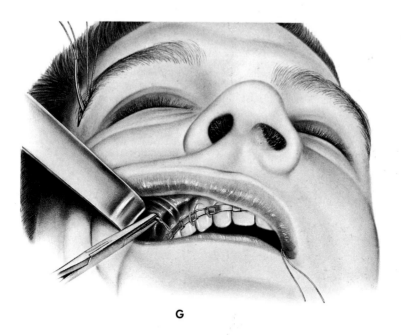

G

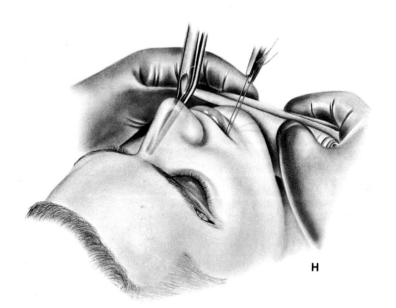

H

Figure 18–188 (*Continued.*) *G*, As the beveled end of the passing needle comes into the mouth through the buccal mucosa, the end is grasped with a hemostat and pulled through into the mouth. The wires are pulled down and rest at the corner of the mouth. Precautions are taken to avoid buckling or bending of the wire at the site of the drill hole in the frontal bone. After the long wires that are to be used for craniofacial suspension have been brought out through the mouth, the teeth are brought into occlusion and fixed by intermaxillary rubber band traction.

H, When the teeth are in occlusion, an assistant exerts firm traction against the inferior border of the mandible to produce upward force. Simultaneous traction on the anterior maxilla and on the nasal bone structures by means of an Asch forceps will permit the facial bones to come into proper position.

(*Figure 18–188 continued on opposite page*)

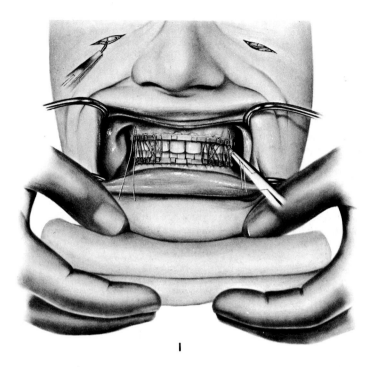

I

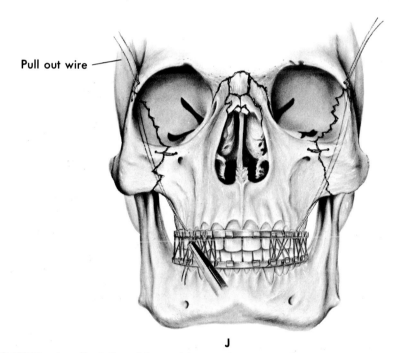

Pull out wire —

J

Figure 18–188 (*Continued.*)   *I*, One of the cranial suspension wires is passed on the inner surface of the upper arch bar in the premolar region, and the other is brought out on the outer surface of the bar. When satisfactory positioning of the total bony complex has been established, pressure is maintained against the mandible and the cranial suspension wires are twisted securely against the arch bar.

J, Craniofacial suspension supplemented with interosseous wire fixation at the infraorbital areas and at the zygomatico-frontal sutures gives positive fixation at the fracture sites. The intact mandible and normal dental occlusal relations provide a guide for reduction of fractures in the middle third of the face. Pull-out wires in the forehead region simplify the removal of the cranial suspension wires. At the end of the period of fixation, which is usually 4 or 5 weeks, the long wires are cut as they emerge through the oral mucosa. Tension on the pull-out wires permits easy removal. The small interosseous wires cause no reaction and are not removed.

(From Dingman, R. O., and Natvig, P.: Surgery of Facial Fractures. Philadelphia, W. B. Saunders Co., 1964.)

INTERNAL WIRING OF MAXILLARY-ZYGOMATIC FRACTURES

JAMES L. BRADLEY, D.D.S., M.S.D., M.Sc.,
AND GERALD H. BONETTE, D.D.S.

The fixation problem for fractures of the maxilla and zygoma has not yet been solved. Any method, in a given case, has both advantages and disadvantages. In our opinion, the advantages of internal wiring considerably outweigh the disadvantages. The advantages are:

1. Ease of application.
2. Smaller armamentarium.
3. Simplified postoperative care.
4. No need for extraoral appliances.
5. The patient is more comfortable and can carry on his normal routine earlier.

The disadvantages are:

1. Scarring.
2. Occlusion must be established at time of surgery, as readjustments are usually difficult or impossible.
3. Some dentists object to leaving small wires in place permanently. (We feel that this is not a justifiable objection.)
4. The Lesney and Adams type of fixation wiring may produce an objectionable tension backward and upward with no support for the anterior portion of the maxilla. This may require supplemental procedures.

In our hands, internal wiring has proved to be a valuable adjunct to standard techniques for handling fractures. Methods first described by Adams,[2] Thoma,[181] and Lesney[110] have been modified slightly for use with both pyramidal and horizontal types of transverse fractures of the maxilla. Results have been gratifying.

Patient. A young woman, involved in an automobile accident, sustained facial lacerations (Fig. 18–189A) and fractures of both the left maxilla and zygoma. She received emergency treatment at a civilian hospital and was transferred to the naval hospital 9 days later. Oral examination revealed downward and backward displacement of the fractured segment, a depressed left zygoma, and a subcondylar fracture of the left mandible with medial displacement of the fractured head. X-ray examination revealed a comminuted fracture of the left zygoma with a compression of the maxillary sinus, and a comminuted fracture of the left mandible (Fig. 18–189B).

Operation. The following procedure was performed 11 days after the accident. Pentothal sodium, nitrous oxide-oxygen endotracheal anesthesia with Anectine was administered, and an incision about 3/8-inch long was made at the left eyebrow. By blunt dissection, the zygomaticofrontal sutures were exposed and 2 holes were drilled in each segment. The zygoma was elevated and reduced by transosseous wiring with .020 stainless steel wire (Fig. 18–189C). Another wire was then passed from the frontal process of the frontal bone down below the zygomatic arch and secured to the arch bar. A third wire was passed over the right zygoma to the arch bar (Fig. 18–189D). The fractured segment was then reduced upward into position and elastic traction was applied. The left maxillary sinus was packed with iodoform gauze to hold the zygoma in place.

Postoperative Course. For 3 weeks following the operation, the patient was given 300,000 units of procaine penicillin twice a day, kept on a liquid diet, and seen daily for postoperative treatments.

Six weeks after the first procedure the same type of anesthesia was administered, and the wires were cut and loosened from the arch bar. The wire on the right side was pulled out and the incision over the left eyebrow was closed with three interrupted sutures.

Both arch bars were removed the next day and the patient was placed on a normal diet and allowed to go home.

Figure 18–189 *A*, Preoperative clinical photograph. *B*, Preoperative x-ray examination. *C*, X-ray examination showing reduction of fracture and wiring of zygoma. *D*, X-ray examination recording position of the arch bars and the suspension wires. (See Case Report No. 8.)

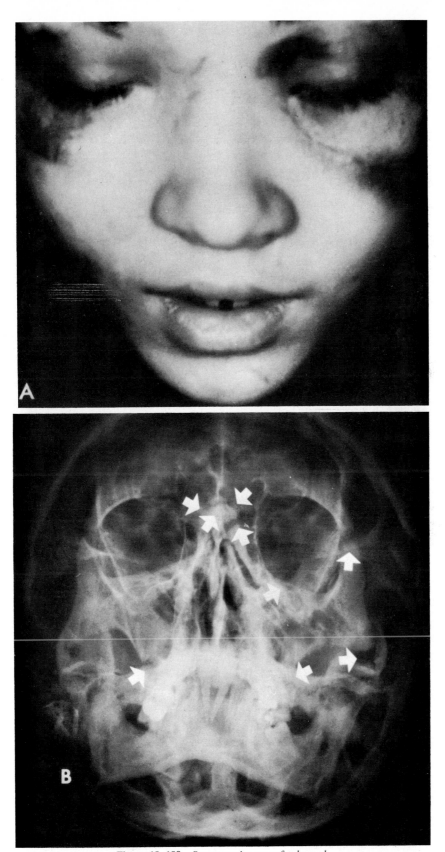

Figure 18–189   *See opposite page for legend.*

(Figure 18–189 continued on following page)

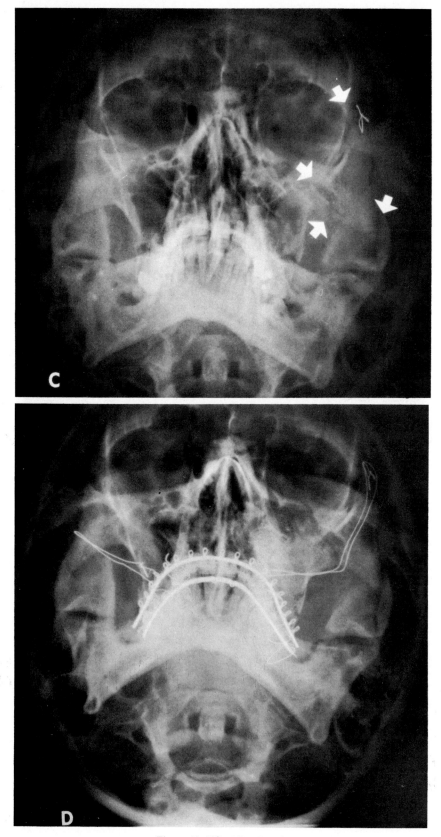

Figure 18–189 *(Continued.)*

TRANSVERSE (HORIZONTAL) AND VERTICAL FRACTURES OF THE MAXILLA

In addition to a transverse fracture of the maxilla, the palate also may be split. In other words, the patient has a vertical fracture as well as a transverse fracture of the maxilla. This situation is illustrated in Figure 18–190*A*. Split splints are attached to the maxillary teeth as illustrated in Figure 18–190*D;* over the split splints are stretched rubber bands from right to left, and bands are passed between the bicuspids and between the molars. It may be possible to snap the rubber bands between contact points; if this is not possible, then the rubber bands extend up over the contact points. The traction exerted

by these rubber bands will bring the two portions of the maxilla together. When this happens, the split splints are joined by means of a small piece of splint material which is wired to the splints. Intermaxillary elastics are placed as shown in Figure 18–190*C*. If the maxilla is not brought forward into normal occlusion by such a procedure, then the intermaxillary elastics are removed and overhead traction is applied as shown in Figure 18–190*D*. When overhead traction brings the maxilla far enough forward that the intermaxillary elastics bring the teeth into normal occlusion, the overhead traction is discontinued. Next, the fractured maxilla is moved into contact with the facial bones. This is accomplished (as shown in Figure 18–190*E*) by

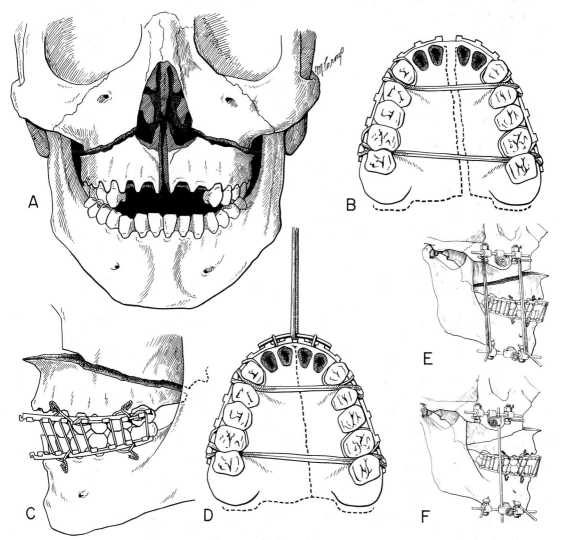

Figure 18–190   Transverse (horizontal) and vertical fractures of the maxilla. See text for explanation. (Also see Figure 18–167.)

placing intermaxillary elastics between the fracture units bilaterally in the zygomas and in the mandible, and stretching rubber bands over the units. Once this reduction has been accomplished, the mandible is fixed to the maxilla, as shown in Figure 18–190F, by locking a connecting bar between the respective fracture units. This holds the fractured segments in contact with the rest of the facial bone.

MAXILLARY FRACTURES WITH NASAL FRACTURES

When there are nasal fractures in addition to maxillary fractures, these fractures are treated as described on pages 1318 to 1323. The head is free for the application of the Kazanjian nasal fracture splint, either the simple or the suspension type. Or the Crawford head frame, as described on pages 1256 to 1260, may be applied and both the mandibular pins (there is no need for zygomatic bone pins if the Crawford head frame is used) and the nasal fracture appliance can be suspended from this head frame.

If there is downward and lateral displacement of the maxilla, the head frame should be used as the anchor for upward and lateral traction until intermaxillary traction can be applied. Once the teeth are in occlusion, then upward traction for cranial fixation is applied by means of rubber bands between bilateral pins in the mandible and the head frame.

THE PLASTER OF PARIS HEAD CAP

Indications. The plaster of paris head cap has a very limited field of usefulness. Where *minor* extrafacial traction or support is needed for the relatively short period of time of a week or 10 days, such as is needed in the treatment of some nasal or zygomatic bone fractures, this can be provided by the application of a plaster of paris head cap. To obtain the best cosmetic end result in the treatment of fractures of these bones, they must in many cases be *held up and out.* Direct wiring of depressed fractures of the zygomatic bone holds the bone up but does not hold it out. There is a flattened appearance to this area of the face unless the zygomatic bone is held out during the healing process. The same is true with fractured nasal bones.

Technique. A wire clothes hanger is opened up and then contoured into a circle so as to surround the patient's head, leaving a projecting loop in the region of the left depressed zygoma.

The ring is made large enough to allow approximately $1/4$ inch between the wire and the patient's head around the whole circumference. A stockinet cap is placed over the patient's hair. Both the operator and the assistant wear gloves because of the drying effect of the plaster. A 4-inch wide plaster bandage roll is removed from its paper wrapper and immersed in a pail of cold water. The roll is held in the water until the bubbling subsides. The loose end of the roll is held in place by the assistant, as the operator encircles the head, until four layers of bandage are placed. The metal ring is then positioned over these layers, and a plaster bandage is applied over the ring and across the crown of the head. With his free hand the assistant follows the course of the plaster roll, smoothing out the wrinkles with his fingers and liberal applications of water. The plaster which now holds the metal ring in position encircles the head—over the temples, over the frontal eminence, and below the occipital protuberance, which keeps the cast from sliding forward. Advantage is taken of all the natural undercuts of the skull to anchor the plaster cast firmly. The ears are left completely free because of the severe pain which results from pressure on them.

The bandage is also carried over the median line of the head anteroposteriorly, leaving two free spaces on either side to allow ventilation. After the bandage is placed, the edges of the stockinet cap are turned up and another layer of plaster bandage is wound over it to hold it in place.

As the plaster hardens, the patient will feel some heat. After the setting is complete, two rubber bands are stretched from the wire loop to the Frac-Sur unit in the zygomatic bone or it is attached to the support for depressed nasal bones (see Figures 18–182, 18–222 and 18–231 for examples).

THE SKELETAL HEAD FRAME

T. A. LESNEY, D.C., U.S.N.

In the management of fractures of facial bones, when it becomes necessary to use an extraoral point of fixation from which traction can be applied for the purpose of reducing

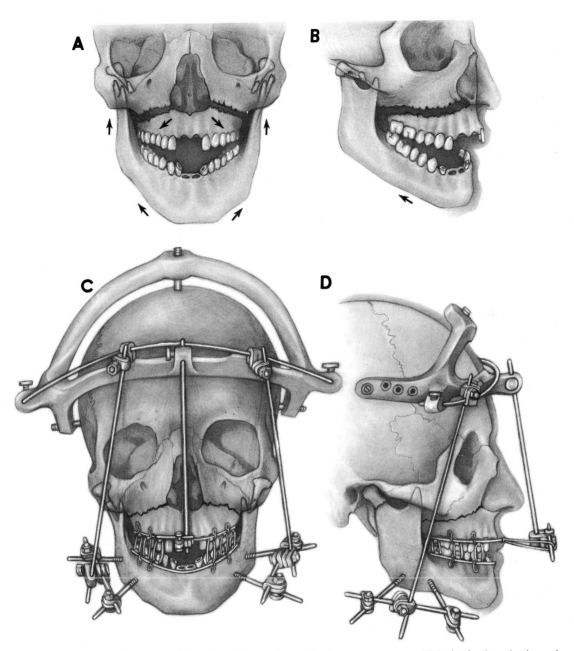

Figure 18–191   Use of the skeletal head frame in one of the author's cases, as an essential device for the reduction and immobilization of a transverse fracture of the maxilla and bilateral subcondylar fractures of the mandible and the restoration of a *normal facial contour*.

A and *B*, This patient was thrown against the dashboard in an automobile accident, producing a transverse fracture of the maxilla with *downward* and *backward* displacement of the maxilla and the loss of anterior teeth in both the maxilla and mandible. Bilateral subcondylar fractures of the mandible with medial displacement also resulted when the symphysis struck the dashboard. Suspension of the maxilla by wires from the zygomatic arch or lateral orbital rim would elevate the maxilla but in a *retracted* position and would also hold the mandible in a retruded position when the mandibular teeth were brought into occlusion with the maxillary arch. In this situation extraoral traction from a head frame is absolutely necessary.

C and *D*, A Crawford head frame provides a fixed extraoral point from which anterior and superior traction can be exerted by elastic traction until normal contact of the maxilla with the other facial bones is established, bringing with it the patient's mandible, restoring his normal profile. Fixation by rods attached by connectors between the head frame and Roger Anderson units, immobilizes the fractures during healing.

and immobilizing the fractured bones, the plaster head cap has been commonly used to provide that extraoral point of fixation.

The surgeons who have extensively used the plaster head cap are well acquainted with its shortcomings. It is never rigidly stable, and at best it will certainly move in direct proportion to the movements of the scalp.

Despite the use of felt pads or sponge rubber over prominent bony areas of the skull, it is common to obtain pressure necrosis in one or more areas under plaster head caps. The more felt or rubber used in relief areas over bony prominences, the less stable is the plaster head cap.

In hot weather the plaster head cap can be extremely uncomfortable. During wartime duty in the tropics, Navy oral surgeons frequently found the plaster head cap intolerable in many cases. Constant perspiration and unbearable scalp itch often preceded fungus infection or infection secondary to scratching, and the head caps had to be removed.

Many patients are reluctant to have any of their hair cut off in preparation for the installation of a plaster head cap.

The most effective type of plaster head cap, extending well under the mastoids to take advantage of the undercuts, can be bulky and relatively heavy.

A plaster head cap cannot be used in cases in which there are lacerations or abrasions of the scalp associated with fractures of the face.

Many patients with facial injuries also have broken legs or abdominal injuries which make them bedfast. Plaster head caps are contraindicated in these cases, for when the patient moves his head, greater irritation to the scalp is noted. The skeletal head frame is designed so that the head may rest comfortably on a pillow.

Osteomyelitis of the skull has been noted following use of the plaster head cap. Plastic surgery to replace de-epithelized areas of scalp after use of the plaster head cap has been necessary.

In an attempt to overcome the disadvantages and to provide the necessary extraoral point of fixation frequently required in the management of maxillofacial fractures, a skeletal head frame was devised in the Navy Dental Corps to meet the urgency presented in the management of war injuries. Captain M. J. Crawford, D. C., U.S.N.,[33] devised and introduced a lightweight aluminum head frame which is comfortably and rigidly re-

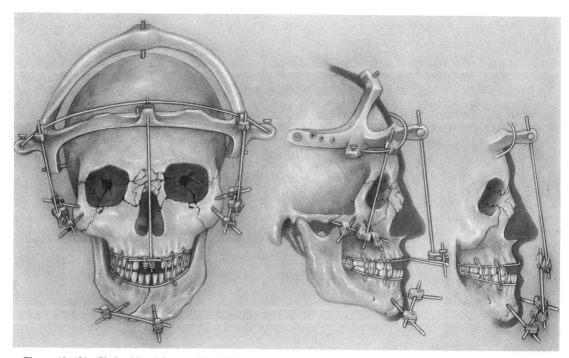

Figure 18–192 Skeletal head frame with additional applications for the reduction and immobilization of fractures of the facial bones. (See Figure 18–169 for original fractures and displacement.)

tained in position by three skeletal pins attached against, but not into, the cortical plate of the skull. This head frame can be quickly and easily installed in the dental office under aseptic conditions and with local anesthesia to the skin under the skeletal pins. The scalp is incised to permit the entry of the skeletal

pin, and the success of the installation is dependent upon direct contact of the pin and bone, with no interposition of tissue. Retention is insured by the distribution of the three skeletal pins along the head frame in such a manner as to take advantage of the normal undercuts of skull contour. The appliance is

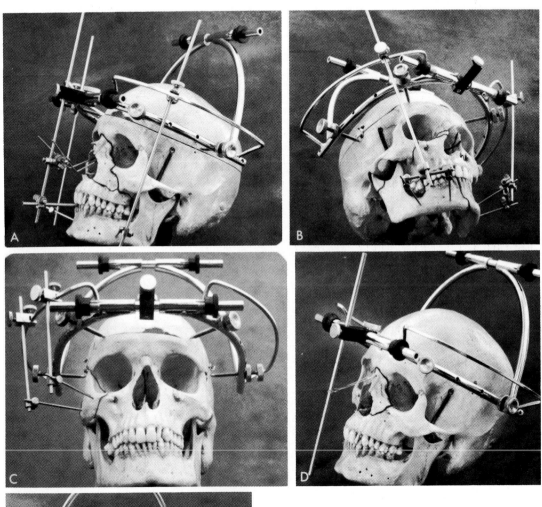

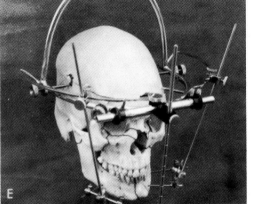

Figure 18-193 Irby Extra-Cranial Fixation Appliance for the reduction and immobilization of various fractures of the facial bones. (Courtesy of W. B. Irby, D.D.S.)

not retained by burrowing into bone in the manner of Crutchfield tongs or the Roger Anderson pins.

This appliance has been used extensively at the National Naval Medical Center with no untoward results, by Captain Theodore A. Lesney, D.C., U.S.N., Chief of the Oral Surgery Service, and by the author of this text with most excellent results. Some of the benefits observed are the following: (a) The head frame provides a rigid stability beyond comparison with any other methods previously used. (b) The design of the head frame is such as to permit the use of almost any variety of orthopedic appliances and a wide choice of direction from which the traction may be applied. (c) This aluminum head frame is more than 50 per cent lighter in weight than the majority of plaster head caps in use today. (d) It is possible, with rigid regard for asepsis, to remove only sufficient hair at the site of pin installation.

Over an appreciable series of cases it has been noted that: (1) There was no clinical or roentgenographic evidence of bone resorption at the site of pin adaptation to cortical bone of the skull. (2) The appliance has been retained for as long as 12 weeks without requiring any adjusting of the pins. (3) If the patient complains of a "crushing sensation," the skeletal head frame has been installed with entirely too much, and unnecessary, traction. The appliance can be well used fully within the patient's physiologically tolerable limits.

(4) Patients have often vigorously jarred the head frame against their hospital beds without either loosening the head frame or damaging the skull bones. (5) At no time has osteomyelitis of the skull been experienced with the use of this appliance by the authors of this article and text.

There is a current trend in specialty practice to use fewer skeletal fixation appliances and to use them less frequently in the management of jaw fractures. Open reduction techniques and a better capability for aborting secondary infection, or in managing it should this be a complication, have been developed and are being practiced. Nevertheless, there remains the occasional case that can best be managed through the use of skeletal-pin traction and immobilization. Furthermore, the surgeon who has the added benefit of knowledge and experience with skeletal appliances is better prepared to manage complex facial fractures.

Figures 18–197, 18–199 and 18–200 illustrate the head frame in several practical cases treated at large naval hospitals.

Crawford,[33] Charest,[26] Irby[86] and halo head frames have been found to be indispensable in the treatment of many combinations of fractures of the facial bones and are shown in Figures 18–193 to 18–196. The head frame is a most important contribution to fracture management and should be used much more extensively than it is.

Case Report No. 9

REDUCTION OF MULTIPLE COMPLEX FRACTURES OF THE MAXILLA AND MANDIBLE USING THE HALO HEAD FRAME AS AN ESSENTIAL PART OF THE TREATMENT*

Harold J. Panuska, D.D.S., M.S.D.,
and Theodore H. Dedolph, D.D.S., M.S.D.

A 19-year-old man was admitted to the hospital for treatment of multiple facial injuries. Palpation of the facial bones revealed a fractured mandible to the left of the symphysis. There was a displacement of the right and left infraorbital margins. The maxilla was comminuted and impacted. There was a separation at the midline of the palate. The maxilla appeared to be free of the cranial base. The lower anterior teeth were fractured off and displaced distally.

Operative Procedures. After open and closed reduction of the fractured mandible and maxilla

had been performed and facial lacerations had been sutured, the halo head frame was applied. (See Figure 18–194.)

The mandible was reduced manually and an arch bar was applied to the remaining teeth with 25 gauge stainless steel wire. The maxilla was

*Adapted from Panuska, H. J., and Dedolph, T. H.: Extraoral traction with halo head frame for complex facial fractures. J. Oral Surg., 23:212–221 (May), 1965. Copyright by the American Dental Association. Reprinted by permission.

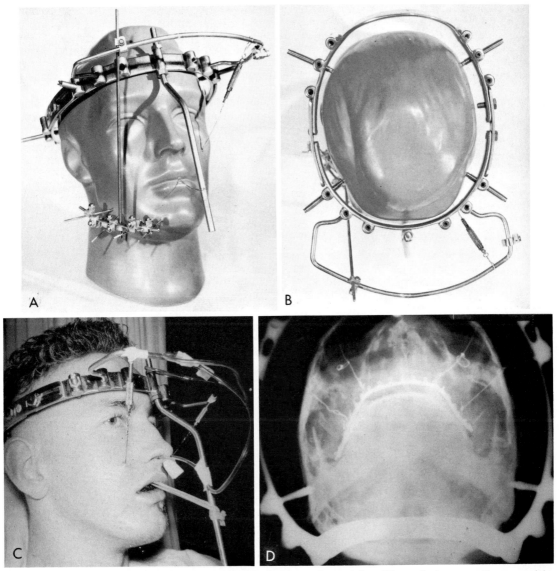

Figure 18–194 *A*, Halo head frame with transfacial wire suspension on left and Roger Anderson appliances on right and maxillary traction bar in center. *B*, Top view showing pins inserted and anterior rod fixation points. *C* and *D*, See Case Report No. 9. (*A* and *B*, Courtesy of the Journal of Oral Surgery.)

found to be fractured in several places forming a pyramid fracture, midline fracture and comminution on the right maxillary sinus floor. The arch bar then was secured to the remaining teeth to stabilize the fragmented maxilla into a block.

The right sinus cavity was evacuated and examined. The floor of the orbit was fractured. The medial wall of the nasal cavity was fractured. The lateral wall and inferior walls of the sinus were comminuted.

The fractured bones were reduced with finger pressure, the right tuberosity was brought into position, and the right zygomatic maxillary process was brought into position with the remaining max-

illary bones. A 1-inch Vaseline gauze packing was placed into the antrum. Transfacial wires then were passed through the cheeks bilaterally and secured to the mandibular arch bar.

The teeth were brought into occlusion with elastic bands. The halo head frame* then was affixed to the skull, and the transfacial wires were at-

---

*AUTHOR'S NOTE: The halo head frame is readily available in most medical centers. It is used by orthopedic surgeons, and the conversion items are easily produced from welding rods and available odds and ends.

tached. The anterior traction bar was placed on the head frame and a penrose drain was placed from the anterior maxillary arch bar to the traction bar exerting traction on the maxilla in a forward-downward direction. The transfacial wires transmitted pressure in an upward and forward direction.

The right nasal cavity was packed with 1-inch gauze to control bleeding and to contain the sinus wall. The patient then was returned to the intensive care unit in good condition.

Postoperative Course. The patient was discharged from the hospital on the tenth postoperative day. His postoperative course continued without complication; traction was maintained on the maxilla until reduction was complete. The halo head frame was kept intact for 5 weeks. No infection was evident at the site of insertion of the pins. The head frame was removed at the end of this period. Intermaxillary fixation was maintained for 1 week after the head frame was removed. The fractures healed well. The patient was referred for dental care and prosthetic replacement of the missing teeth after removal of the arch bars.

DELAYED TREATMENT OF MAXILLARY FRACTURES

Frequently patients with fractures of the maxilla sustain other injuries which make it necessary to delay definitive treatment. When this happens, it is not unusual that we obtain such a case for treatment from 1 to 2 weeks after the original injury. This means that healing has already started and fibrous union, at the least, is present. In such a case, intermaxillary elastics are not sufficient. It is necessary to employ extraoral traction by means of an overhead bed frame, as illustrated in Figure 18–203.

The weights applied usually start at 3 lb. for about 1 hour, at which time the weight is stepped up to 4 lb. for another hour and 5 lb. for another hour. Then, if movement has not started, the weight is increased to 6 or 7 lb. However, the patient must be carefully observed to make certain that once the movement starts, it is not carried on too fast because it is possible to over-reduce such fragments. The patient is able to tell when there is movement, and once the maxilla starts to move, then the weights are reduced so that there is a gradual reduction of the displacement. The traction is removed at meal time and generally for 6 to 8 hours at night. From time to time, the movement is checked by removing the weights and having the patient attempt to bring the teeth into occlusion.

(Text continued on page 1272)

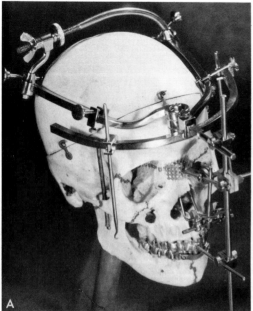
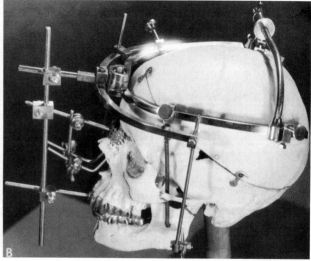

Figure 18–195 A head frame designed by André Charest, D.D.S., of Quebec.

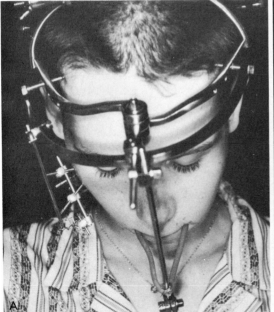

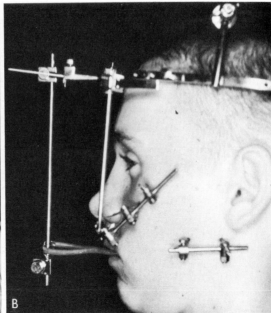

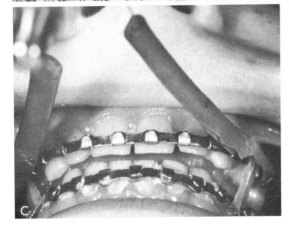

Figure 18–196　Charest head frame reducing and stabilizing a depressed fracture of the zygoma, a Le Fort I transverse fracture of the maxilla with downward and posterior displacement, and a unilateral fracture of the mandible.

Figure 18–197　Aluminum skeletal head frame with an assortment of orthopedic appliances used in managing multiple fractures of facial bones: pyramidal maxillary fracture with detachment of maxilla from cranial base; compounded fracture of the mandible at both mental ► foramina and simple fracture at the necks of both condyles; insufficient remaining teeth to provide wholly adequate intraoral immobilization by interdental wiring. (Courtesy of T. A. Lesney, D.C., U.S.N.)

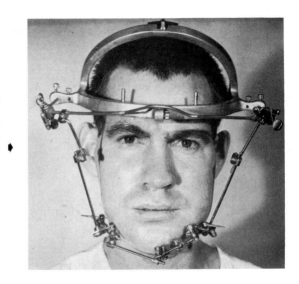

COMPOUND COMMINUTED FRACTURES OF THE MANDIBLE TREATED WITH A HEAD FRAME

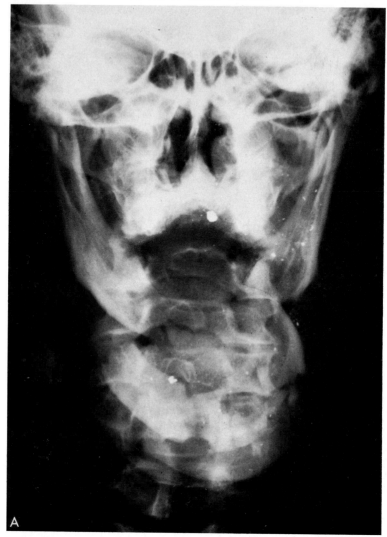

Figure 18–198 *A*, Gunshot wound. Multiple fractures of the mandible, loss of anterior portion of the maxilla.
B, Diagram made from radiograph shown in *A*.
C, Lateral head radiograph. Note position of symphysis.

(Figure 18–198 continued on opposite page)

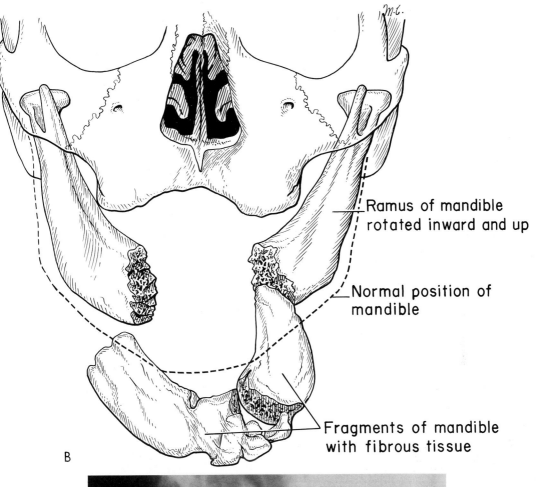

Ramus of mandible
rotated inward and up

Normal position of
mandible

Fragments of mandible
with fibrous tissue

B

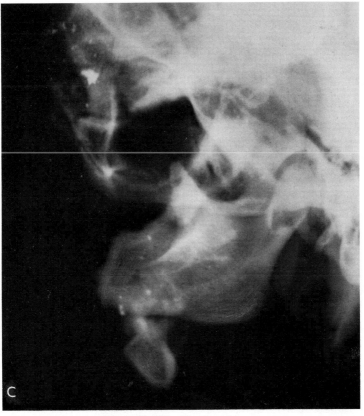

C

Figure 18–198 *(Continued.)*

(Figure 18–198 continued on following page)

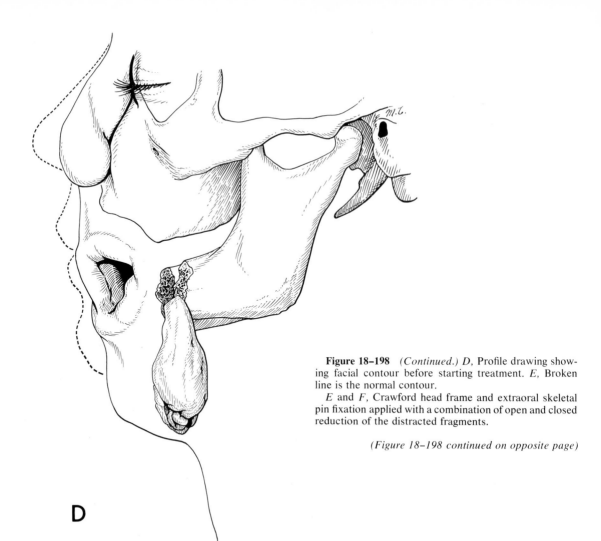

D

Figure 18-198 *(Continued.) D*, Profile drawing showing facial contour before starting treatment. *E*, Broken line is the normal contour.

E and *F*, Crawford head frame and extraoral skeletal pin fixation applied with a combination of open and closed reduction of the distracted fragments.

(Figure 18-198 continued on opposite page)

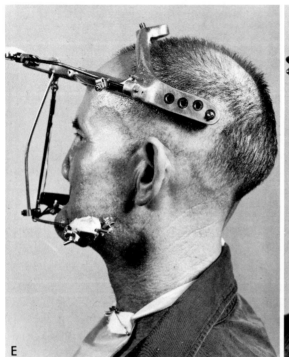

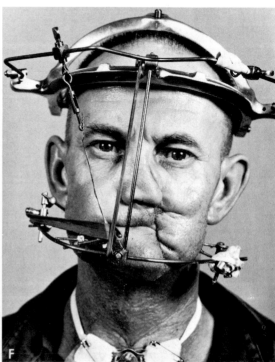

E

F

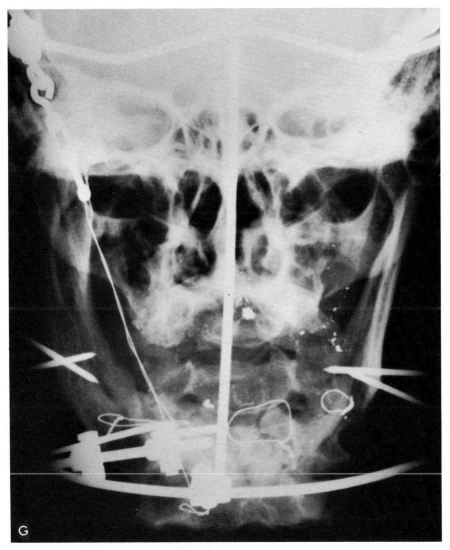

Figure 18–198 *(Continued.)* *G* and *H,* Radiograph and drawing show wires inserted when fragments were freed at the open reduction. Skin was closed and the pins inserted and extraoral traction was applied by elastic traction from the Crawford head frame, pulling the fragments up to their normal position.

I, Scar tissue resulting from the excessive trauma.

(Figure 18–198 continued on following page)

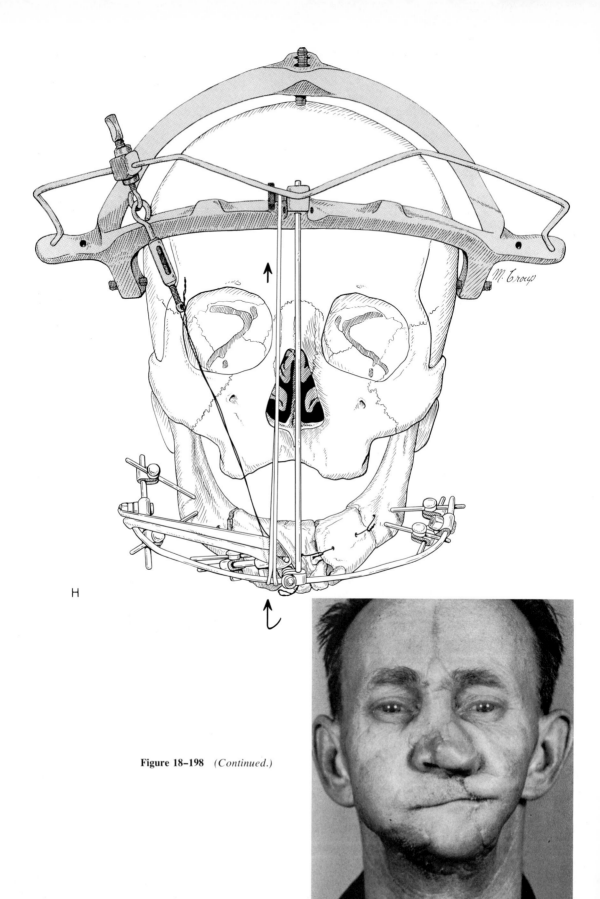

H

Figure 18–198 *(Continued.)*

I

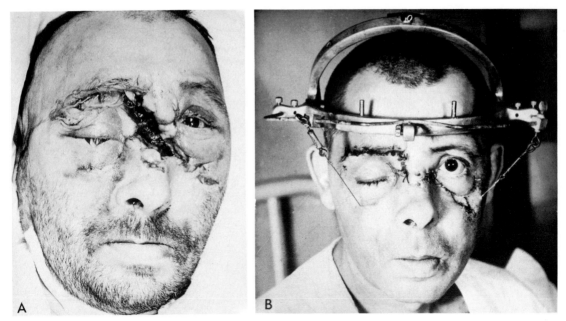

Figure 18–199 *A*, Before treatment. Because of swelling and edema over the right eye, a plaster head cap could not be used. Wound is 5 days old and had to be approximated immediately so that any healing at all would take place.

B, After treatment. The maxillary teeth are placed in normal occlusion by means of splints wired to the necks of the patient's maxillary and mandibular teeth, between which intermaxillary elastics are stretched to realign and maintain the correct occlusion. (Courtesy of T. A. Lesney, D.C., U.S.N.)

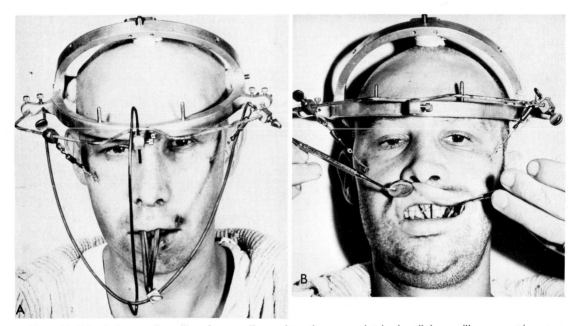

Figure 18–200 *A*, Impacted maxillary fracture. Forward traction was maintained until the maxilla came out in proper position 48 hours later. The normal occlusion was maintained with intermaxillary fixation.

B, Maxilla in proper position. An upper acrylic splint was used as an attachment for the maxillary traction wires to the Crawford head frame and also for the attachment of intermaxillary elastic traction to hold the maxillary and mandibular teeth in normal occlusion during healing. (Courtesy of T. A. Lesney, D.C., U.S.N.)

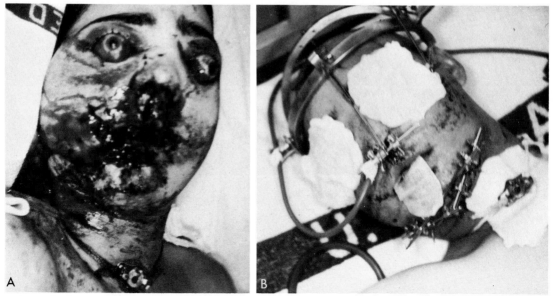

Figure 18–201 *A*, Macerated maxilla, nasal bones, zygomatic bones and mandible. Both optic nerves were severed. *B*, Crawford head frame supporting Frac-Sur units that are reducing and stabilizing the zygomatic bones, nasal bones and maxilla. Frac-Sur unit reducing and immobilizing fractured mandible.

Photographic Case Report

COMPOUND COMMINUTED FRACTURE OF MANDIBLE, BILATERAL SUBCONDYLAR FRACTURES, TRANSVERSE FRACTURE OF MAXILLA, AND DEPRESSED FRACTURE OF THE ZYGOMATIC BONE

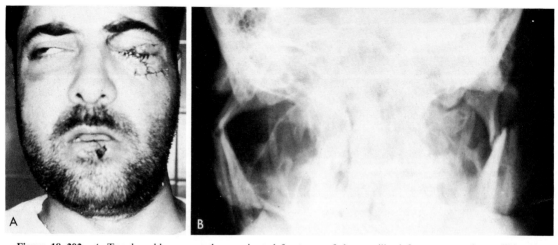

Figure 18–202 *A*, Ten-day-old compound comminuted fractures of the maxilla, left zygoma and mandible. Note open mouth, the result of the maxilla's being driven downward and backward. *B*, Posteroanterior view of the mandible and zygomas. Note fracture through the symphysis and interior maxillary, bilateral subcondylar, and left zygomatic bones. (See *E* for a better view of fractured maxilla and left zygoma.) *C*, Bilateral subcondylar fracture with displacement is shown clearly in this anteroposterior Towne projection radiograph. *D*, The improved position of the subcondylar

(Figure 18–202 continued on opposite page)

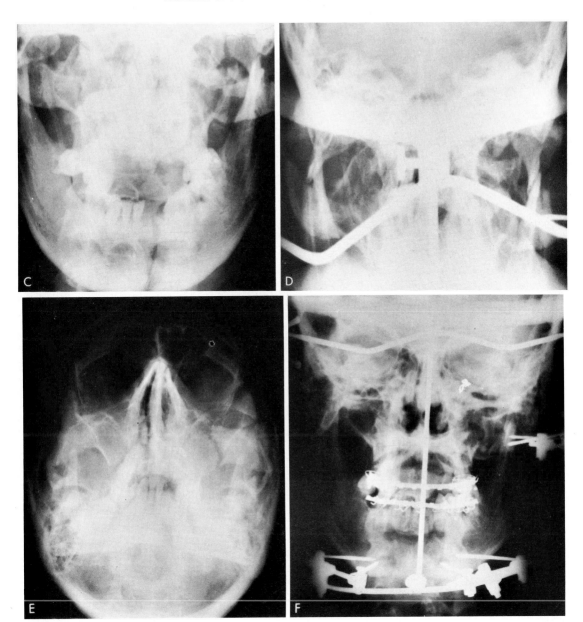

Figure 18–202   (*Continued.*)
fractures is shown in this view. A portion of the Crawford head frame and the Frac-Sur unit in the left fractured zygoma are also shown. *E*, This Waters' view of the maxilla and zygomas clearly shows both maxillary sinuses filled with blood (normal sinuses show up dark — blood makes sinuses opaque), fracture lines through both lateral walls and a comminuted fracture of the left zygoma. *F*, This posteroanterior projection of the mandible shows Crawford head frame, splints wired to remaining maxillary and mandibular teeth, Frac-Sur unit in left zygoma, and two Frac-Sur units and connecting bar in the mandible. *G*, *H* and *I*, These views illustrate the extraoral appliances used in conjunction with the intraoral splints and intramaxillary elastics used in the treatment of these multiple fractures.

    Treatment: The steps followed included:

    1. Frac-Sur splints were inserted in the mandible to reduce and immobilize the fracture of the symphysis. A Frac-Sur unit was also inserted in the left zygoma, and splints were wired to the remaining maxillary and mandibular teeth at this time. No intermaxillary elastics were used at this time.

    2. The maxillary splint was attached to an overhead traction bed frame, as shown by the middle traction rope of Figure 18–203. Weights were increased until the maxillary segments moved upward and forward and were over their articulating members in the mandible. This required 8 lb. of weight and 48 hours.

    3. When this position was reached, intermaxillary rubber bands inserted between the maxillary and mandibular splints restored normal occlusion in 24 hours.

(*Figure 18–202 continued on following page*)

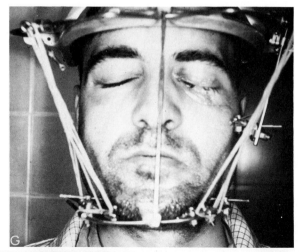

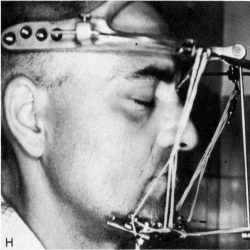
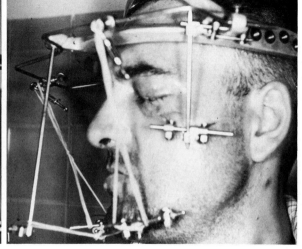

Figure 18–202 *(Continued.)*
4. Now overhead traction was attached to the maxilla-mandible unit to restore normal profile. This took 12 hours.
5. The Crawford head frame was attached to the skull. Upward traction by bilateral rubber bands moved the maxilla-mandible unit up to normal contact with cranial bones. At the same time anterior rubber band traction from the midline rod to the Frac-Sur units in the mandible maintained the patient's normal profile. And last, the fractured and displaced left lateral zygoma was pressed back into position, elevated and maintained in position by the Frac-Sur unit attached to the Crawford head frame (see *G* and *I*).

Figure 18–203 The fractures actually present in one of our cases, and the combination of methods used to treat them.
A, Both zygomatic bones were fractured and driven downward and inward. The nasal bones were fractured. The maxilla was fractured horizontally and vertically and driven downward and backward. There was a transverse fracture of the mandible, with overriding and loss of anterior teeth.
B, The fracture line extended through the palate, and a nasal-oral fistula was present.
C, The two halves of the maxilla were approximated by stainless steel wire threaded around the necks of the molars and twisted together. Then an Erich splint was wired to the necks of the maxillary teeth, and a stainless steel wire was attached to this bar and in turn made ready for attachment to overhead traction, as seen in *D.*
D, Frac-Sur units were placed in each zygomatic bone. A Stader splint was attached to the fractured mandible, and these fragments were reduced and stabilized. Then an Erich splint was attached to the remaining mandibular teeth ready for intermaxillary elastics when the maxilla was drawn forward, so that gradually the maxillary and mandibular teeth would be drawn into occlusion. Extraoral traction was applied as illustrated to bring the zygomatic bones out and permit the maxilla to be drawn forward and then upward. When these fragments were in correct superior-inferior position, then the gaps were closed by elastic traction (rubber bands) between the Stader splint pin blocks in the mandible and each Frac-Sur unit in the zygomatic bones. This pulled all the facial bones up into contact with the skull. The rubber bands were then removed and connecting bars between the various pin fixation units and a cranial head frame, as illustrated in Figures 18–191, 18–192, and 18–195 to 18–197, were used.

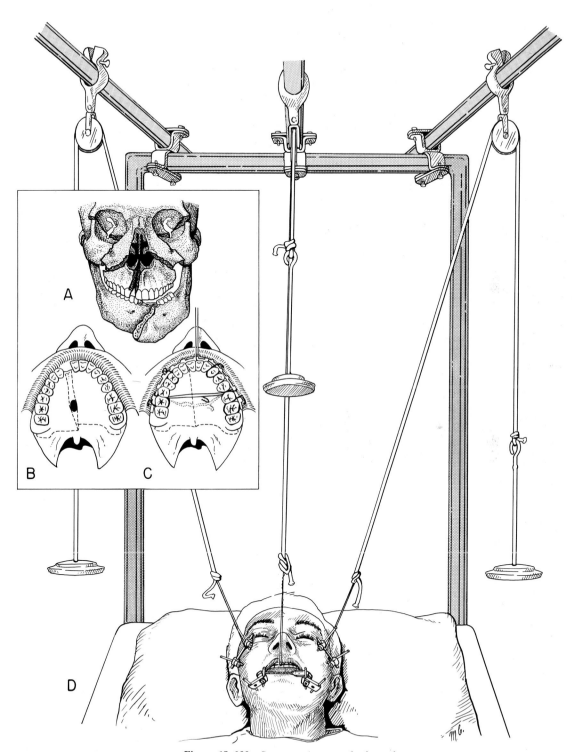

Figure 18–203 *See opposite page for legend.*

We can then determine how much more movement is necessary. When movement has started, it is also possible, particularly if there are no fractures of the mandible, to use inter-maxillary traction between splints attached to the maxillary and the mandibular teeth as an additional aid in guiding the maxilla into proper occlusion with the mandibular teeth. Once the patient's normal occlusion has been established, the overhead traction is discontinued and the mandible is fixed to the maxilla as has just been described.

Treatment of Malpositioned Healed Maxillary Fractures. Occasionally, a patient presents for treatment in whom osseous union has already taken place. In this case, the maxilla must be refractured. This is carried out in the manner illustrated in Figure 18–204. A tray filled with soft, high-temperature fusing compound is forced well up over the crowns of the maxillary teeth and the labial and buccal cortical plates of bone. After the compound has been thoroughly chilled with ice water and the patient is anesthetized, the maxilla is refractured by sharp mallet blows on a round stick (a piece of broomstick being ideal) in the direction shown in Figure 18–204D. Once the maxilla has been refractured, a splint is wired to the maxillary teeth and extraoral traction is applied by means of weights on an overhead bed frame as shown in Figure 18–204E. When proper intermaxillary relationship is established by this method, the teeth are brought into normal occlusion by means of intermaxillary elastics between the maxillary splint and the splint

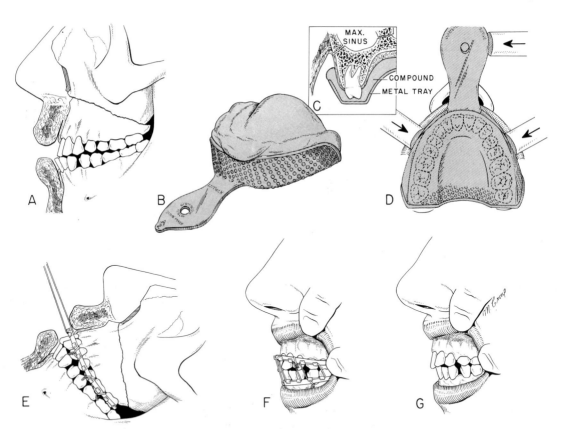

Figure 18–204   The treatment of malunion of a horizontal fracture of the maxilla. *A,* The fracture has healed with the maxilla in a retruded position. *B,* A tray is filled with soft, high-temperature fusing compound. *C,* This tray is forced up well over the crowns of the maxillary teeth and labial and cortical plates. *D,* After the compound is thoroughly chilled with ice water and the patient is anesthetized, the maxilla is refractured by sharp mallet blows on a round stick in the directions shown. *E,* A splint is wired to the maxillary teeth, and extraoral traction is applied by means of weights on an overhead bed frame. *F,* Once the maxilla is brought forward, the teeth are brought into normal occlusion by means of intermaxillary elastics between the maxillary splint and a mandibular splint, and they are held in this position during healing. *G,* The final result showing normal occlusion.

which has been applied to the mandibular teeth. Immobilization is then obtained by placing pins in the zygomatic bone and in the body of the mandible and connecting an inter-maxillary connecting rod as previously illustrated and described.

MAXILLARY FRACTURES IN CHILDREN

Transverse or segmental fractures of the maxilla in children are treated in the same manner as those in adults already discussed.

Rarely, however, is there a transverse max-

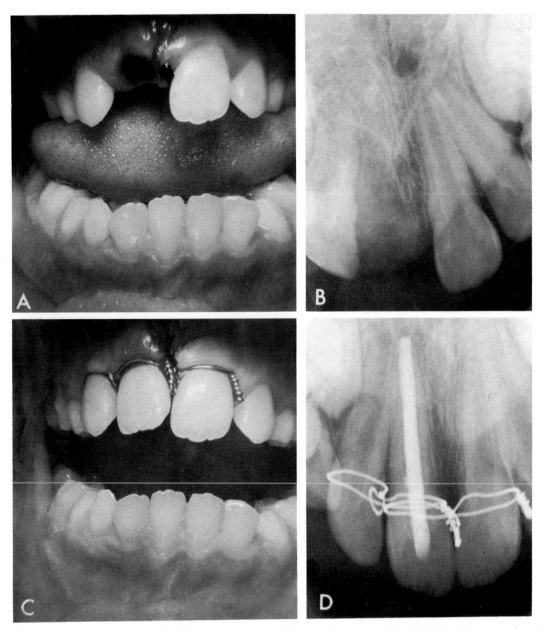

Figure 18–205 Reimplantation of a right permanent central incisor that was completely dislodged by trauma in a 9-year-old boy. *A*, Right central incisor alveolus. *B*, Roentgenogram of the alveolus. No fractured bone noted. *C*, Reimplanted tooth wired into position. The tooth should be held in this position for 3 to 6 months. *D*, Roentgenogram showing root canal filling and wire splint. Unfortunately, many of these roots eventually resorb. (Courtesy of Paul M. Burbank, D.M.D.)

illary fracture in children. The usual maxillary fracture involves the anterior maxillary alveolar process and teeth. Frequently, the anterior teeth are knocked out. If they have not been lost, they should be cleaned, washed in 70 per cent alcohol, replaced and supported by a splint and wire cradle as illustrated in Figure 18–172*A* to *D*. Root canal therapy is done when teeth are firmly reattached. (See also Chapter 6.) Some dentists treat and fill the root canals before replantation and wiring in position. This is illustrated in Figure 18–205. The same technique is used when the teeth are loose and the alveolar process is shattered. The process is digitally molded back around the teeth, and the mucosa, if torn, is sutured from the labial to the lingual side between the necks of the teeth, and the teeth are wired and supported with a cradle. Root canal therapy is performed later if necessary. As was illustrated and described in Chapter 2, in teeth with partially formed roots seldom is it necessary to fill the root canals if the teeth are promptly replanted.

FRACTURES OF THE ZYGOMATIC BONE AND ZYGOMATIC ARCH

The early reduction of fractures of the zygomatic bone or zygomatic arch is in most cases a relatively simple procedure. On the other hand, the late correction, once fibrosis has formed, is not only a difficult procedure, but most frequently an unsuccessful one. Delay in these cases thus results in a facial deformity, which to many people is a most serious disability.

After-Effects of Unreduced or Poorly Reduced Fractures. Failure to reduce a fracture of the zygomatic bone or zygomatic arch, or poor reduction of such a fracture, may result in (*a*) facial deformity because of asymmetry of facial contour; (*b*) limitation of masticatory movements of the mandible, particularly a restriction of the opening movement of the mandible; (*c*) visual disturbances; (*d*) paranasal disease and anesthesia of the cheek.

Delay in Treatment. Most frequently these patients suffer from head injuries which

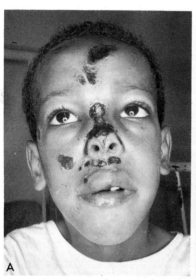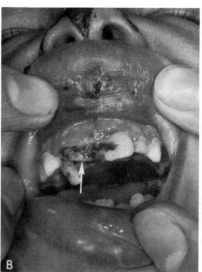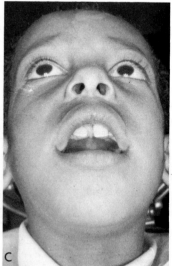

Figure 18–206 *A*, Trauma to the face and anterior maxillary ridge was caused by a bicycle tumble, during which the permanent maxillary central incisor and its labial bone were driven superiorly to the position shown in *B*. *B*, The incisal edge of the incisor was just visible (see arrow). Strangely, the permanent left maxillary central incisor was only slightly loose. The deciduous right lateral incisor was only attached to the lingual gingival tissue and so was removed. The right central incisor was brought down slowly with forceps until it was in alignment with the left central incisor. When the slight bleeding produced had stopped, soft cement was applied over the labial and distal surfaces of the anterior teeth from cuspid to cuspid. Wires had previously been placed around the necks of the deciduous cuspids and the labial ends twisted into loops. The cement covered these loops and when hardened kept this labial splint in position. The patient was restricted first to a liquid diet and then to a soft diet. *C*, Healing was uneventful and the splint was removed in 10 days.

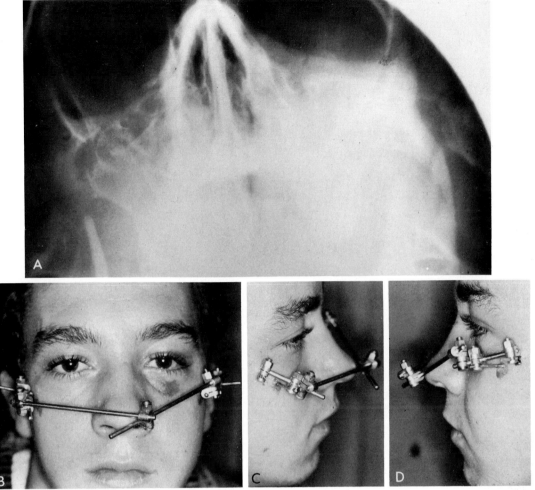

Figure 18–207   Reduction and stabilization of the depressed zygomatic fracture in a 12-year-old male. (See text for the technique used in treatment of these fractures.)

make neurologic observation mandatory for at least several days. However, the neurosurgeon must understand the importance of treatment as early as possible in these cases.

Causes of Fractures.   Zygomatic bone fractures usually result from trauma, such as direct violence, automobile accidents, blows and falls.

Signs and Symptoms of Zygomatic Arch Fracture.   The most common subjective symptom is the patients' complaint that since having received a blow to the side of the head, they have had difficulty in opening their jaws. They report that "something seems to catch" as they try to open their mouths. If the injury is several days old and the traumatic swelling has subsided, a definite depression of one or two fingers' width along the arch is visible and is readily felt.

Signs and Symptoms of Zygomatic Bone Fracture.   The signs and symptoms of a fracture of the zygoma, in order of frequency, are:

1. Periorbital swelling and ecchymosis.
2. Local tenderness on palpation.
3. A depression beneath the eye and alongside the face resulting in facial deformity. This is not noticeable in the early days of the injury, because of the swelling.
4. Pain.
5. Marked reduction of the space between the coronoid process of the ramus and the zygoma on the injured side as compared by simultaneous digital exploration with the index finger of this space on both sides of the maxilla. When the fracture involves the max-

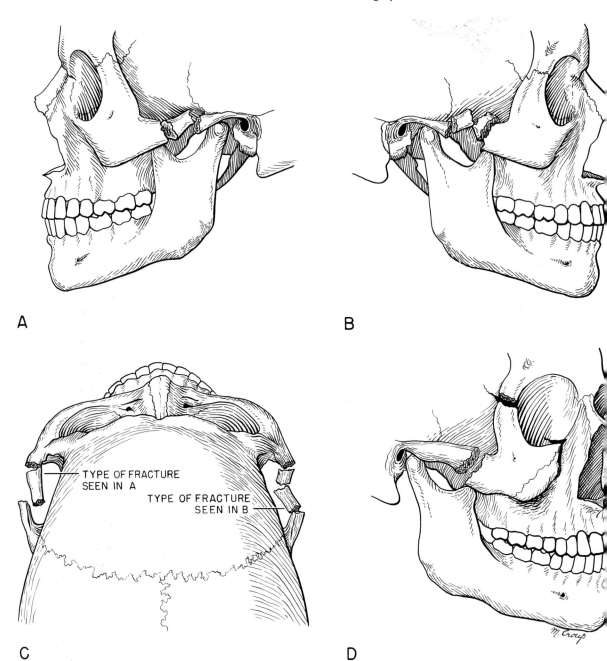

A

B

C

TYPE OF FRACTURE
SEEN IN A

TYPE OF FRACTURE
SEEN IN B

D

M. Croup

Figure 18–208 Fractures of the zygomatic bone and zygomatic arch. *A,* Fracture of the zygomatic arch. *B,* Comminuted fracture of the zygomatic arch. *C,* Superior view of skull showing the fractures of the zygomatic process as illustrated in *A* and *B*. Bilateral fractures of the zygomatic arches are rare. *D,* Fracture of the zygomatic bone at the suture lines and at the infraorbital foramen, with a downward and inward displacement along a fracture of the lateral wall of the maxillary sinus. Bilateral fractures of the zygomatic bones are frequently associated with crushing injuries of the face.

Figure 18–210 Two cases of fractures of the zygomatic arch. Compare the right arch with the left fractured arch. See Figure 18–214 for the technique of reducing these minor fractures.

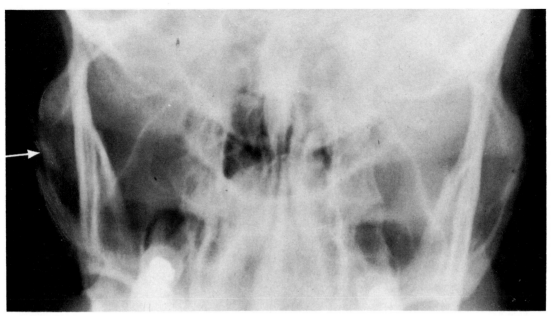

Figure 18-209   Segmental fracture in the middle of the zygomatic arch.

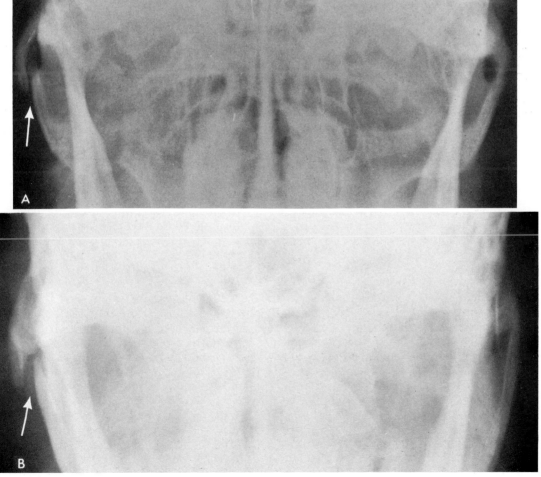

Figure 18-210   *See opposite page for legend.*

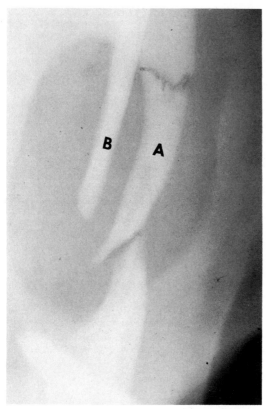

Figure 18-211 Segmental fracture of the zygomatic arch. This radiograph is the result of an excellent technique originated by George Fuller, D.D.S. See Figure 17-24 for the procedure, which makes use of an occlusal film and a dental x-ray machine.

Note that this is the only technique that clearly shows the relationship of the arch *(A)* with the coronoid process *(B)* of the vertical ramus.

illary site, a distinct ridge can be felt along the maxilla by the index finger when measuring the space between the coronoid process and the zygomatic process of the maxilla.

6. Epistaxis. While many facial injuries also produce nose bleeding, the frequent cause is rupturing of the antral mucous membrane by the depressed zygomatic fracture, with subsequent bleeding into the antrum and then through the ostium maxillae into the nasal cavity. Posterior-anterior head radiographs reveal the presence of blood or blood clots in the maxillary sinus on the involved side.

7. Numbness below the eye, ranging from a tingling, burning sensation (paresthesia) to a profound numbness. This depends, of course, on the extent to which the anterior-superior alveolar nerve or the infraorbital nerve has been injured by the displaced infraorbital ridge or the bony floor of the orbital cavity.

8. Conjunctival hemorrhage.

9. Visual disturbances such as diplopia or blurred vision.

10. Drooping of the face and lip.

11. Headache.

12. Difficulty in opening the mouth. This is most frequently seen in fractures of the zygomatic arch. Seldom does a depressed fracture of the zygomatic bone interfere with masticatory movements of the mandible.

13. Dizziness.

14. Mobility or crepitus. This is rather difficult to produce in the usual case. In early fractures there is too much swelling; after the swelling leaves, the granulation tissue prevents the mobility necessary to produce crepitus.

Associated Injuries. Other injuries may be associated with a fracture of the zygomatic bone or zygomatic arch. In order of their occurrence these are as follows: local contusions and lacerations, cerebral concussion, fracture of the mandible, fracture of the nasal bones, and fracture of the maxilla.

TREATMENT

The earlier the treatment, the better the end result. In addition, the more simple methods of reduction are unsatisfactory when too much time has elaspsed between injury and treatment. Specifically, to accomplish the best results, these fractures should be treated immediately if there is no marked swelling, or at most within 72 hours of injury. This does not mean that these fractures cannot be treated successfully after 72 hours, but they are definitely more difficult then, and will require, in many cases, extraoral traction to hold the fractured zygoma in place.

Treatment of the Fractured Zygomatic Arch. The most common fracture is that of the arch. In practically all these cases there is a marked limitation in the patient's ability to open his mouth widely. This is because the coronoid process on the injured side comes in contact with the depressed bony fragments of the zygomatic arch, thus mechanically preventing the complete opening of the lower jaw. This, in my opinion, is best treated by

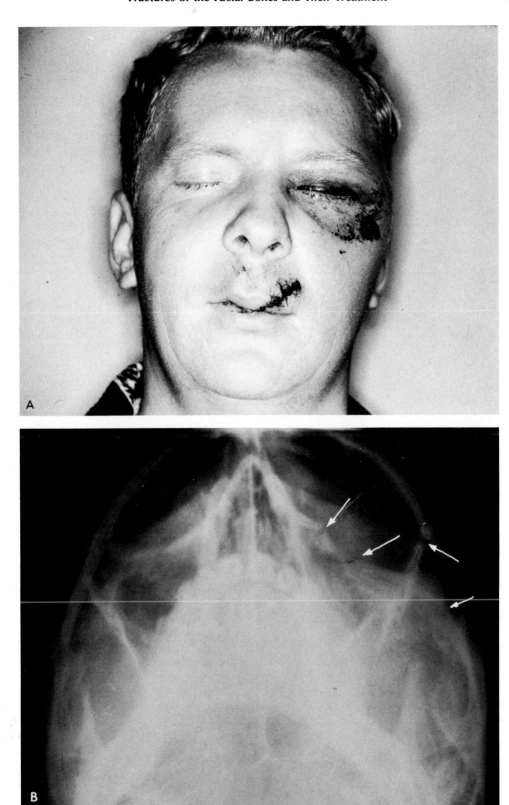

Figure 18–212 *A*, Severe edema from a depressed fracture of the zygoma. *B*, Fracture points are shown in this radiograph.

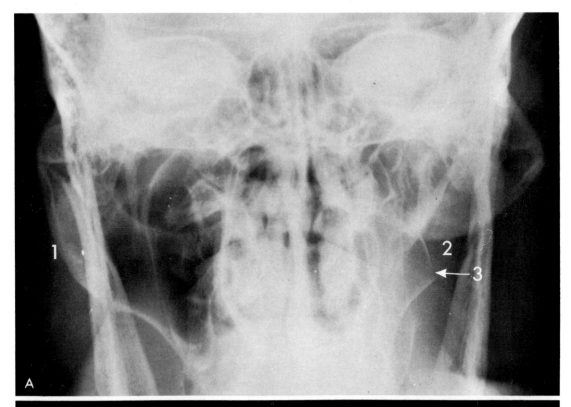

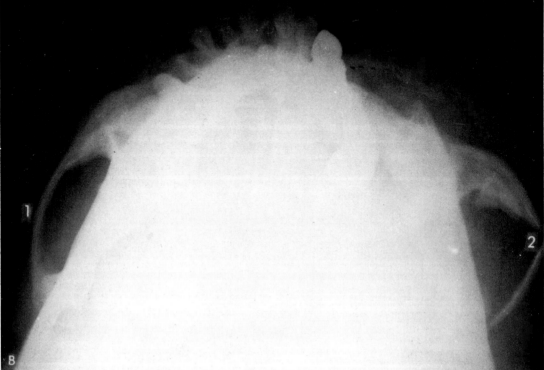

Figure 18–213 *A,* Comparison of the left zygoma (*1*) with the right zygoma (*2*) will demonstrate a case in which gross inward displacement has occurred. Note the buckled lateral wall of the maxillary sinus pointed out by the arrow at *3*. Compare this with the lateral wall of the maxillary sinus on the other side.

B, Basal radiograph that is deliberately underexposed to prevent "burning out" the image of the thin bone which makes up the zygomatic arch. This gives the examiner additional information about the contours of the arches.

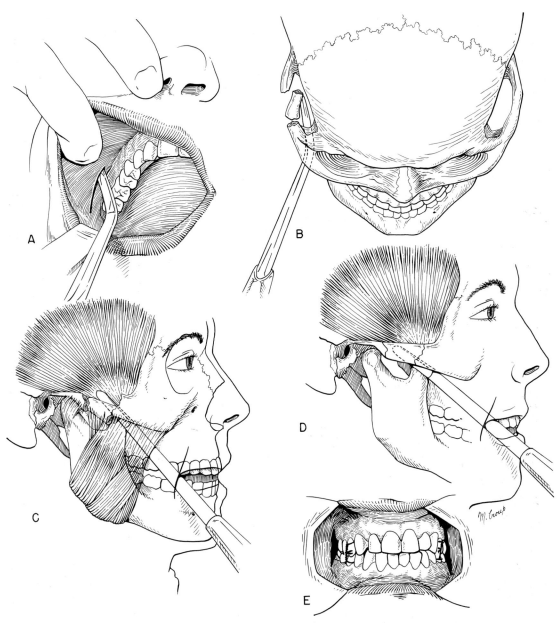

Figure 18–214   Reduction of a fracture of the zygomatic arch.

the Carmody-Batson method by the intraoral route.

TECHNIQUE.   Anesthesia may be local or general. If local anesthesia is elected, the tissues in the pterygomaxillary fossa and oral mucosa must be anesthetized by a so-called "high zygomatic injection."

The oral cavity is prepared by the use of cleansing agents to reduce the oral flora, and the oral mucosa, tongue, and teeth are scrubbed with germicidal agents, such as tincture of benzalkonium (Zephiran) chloride. An incision 1 inch long is made in the mucobuccal fold distal to the zygomatic process of the maxilla (see Figure 18–214A).

The Carmody-Batson elevator is inserted in this incision, and it should be passed upward and backward until the tip is beneath the depressed zygomatic arch (see Figure 18–214B). The heel of the elevator is moved into contact with the lateral wall of the maxilla. This point will be the fulcrum when levering the depressed fragments back into position (see Figure 18–214C).

With proper manipulation of the tip of the elevator the depressed fragment or fragments are located and elevated back into position. Crepitus is heard when these fragments are moved into position (see Figure 18–214D). The realignment of this fracture removes the mechanical obstruction to downward passage of the coronoid process of the mandible when the patient opens his mouth, thus permitting normal masticatory movements again.

However, movements of the lower jaw should be prevented for fear of dislodging the fragments by the pull of the masseter muscle. This muscle consists of a superficial and a deep set of fibers, with the outer or superficial the stronger of the two. It has its origin in the tendinous aponeurosis on the zygomatic process of the maxillary bone and also on the anterior two-thirds of the inferior border of the zygomatic arch. The superficial muscle fibers extend downward and backward, and insert into the outer surface of the ramus in the region of the angle of the mandible. The deep fibers, the smaller portion of the muscle, arise from the entire undersurface of the zygomatic arch. These fibers extend downward and forward and are inserted into the upper and outer portions of the *ramus* and the outer surface of the *coronoid process*.

The author has seen fractures of the zygomatic arch that were reduced, and then the patient was permitted to use his mandible as before the accident. Shortly thereafter the patient again experienced limitation of movement of the mandible that was incorrectly attributed to trismus or injury of the temporomandibular joint. Examination revealed that limitation of movements of the mandible again was caused by the downward deflection of the zygomatic arch by the inner or deep fibers of the masseter muscle during the contraction of this muscle during mastication. It is true that following reduction of many simple fractures of the zygomatic arch, the fragments remain in position in spite of movements of the mandible. The author believes, however, in immobilization of the mandible in these cases for at least 2 weeks and for a longer period of time when the zygomatic bone is involved.

As already stated, when these fractures are reduced early, in the great majority of cases the fragments will remain in position. However, if they do not remain in position, it will be necessary to use some form of extraoral fixation such as the Frac-Sur unit alone or in combination with a traction rod in a plaster of paris head cap (see page 1254 for application method).

Treatment of the Fractured Zygomatic Bone. Practically all fractures of the zygomatic bone are depressed multiple fractures in that there is usually a fracture at or near each of its points of articulation: namely, (*a*) along the lateral orbital ridge where the zygoma articulates with the frontal; (*b*) through the zygomatic process of the temporal bone; (*c*) through the maxilla along the anterior maxillary sinus wall; and (*d*) through the infraorbital foramen.

The author uses, as a rule, one of the techniques described below.

EXTRAORAL TRACTION. A Frac-Sur unit (two converging pins, bar and lock nuts) is inserted through the skin into the depressed zygoma. Then the operator elevates and posi-

(*Text continued on page 1287*)

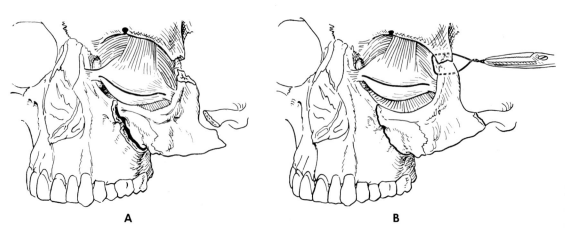

| A | B |

Figure 18–215 *A*, Bony displacement of the zygomatic bone. *B*, Wiring of the fracture sites. (From Rowe, N. L., and Killey, H. C.: Fractures of the Facial Skeleton. Edinburgh, Churchill Livingstone, 1968.)

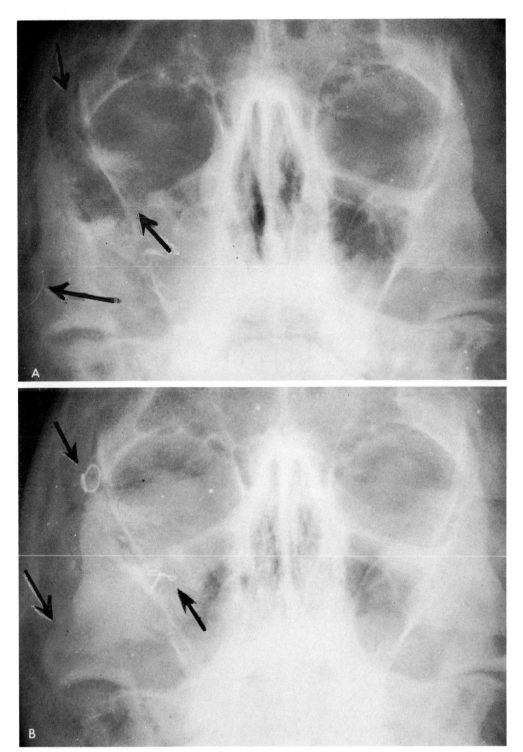

Figure 18–216 *A*, Fractured zygoma. *B*, Reduction with wiring.

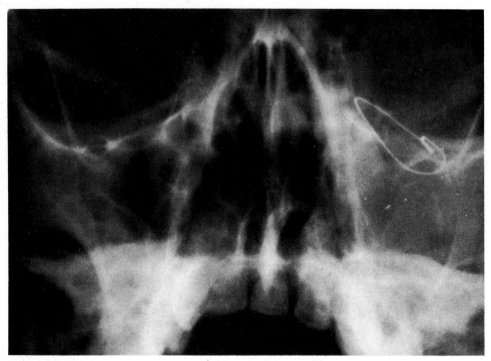

Figure 18–217   In this case the lower orbital rim was severely comminuted, which made it necessary to insert the retaining wire as illustrated here.

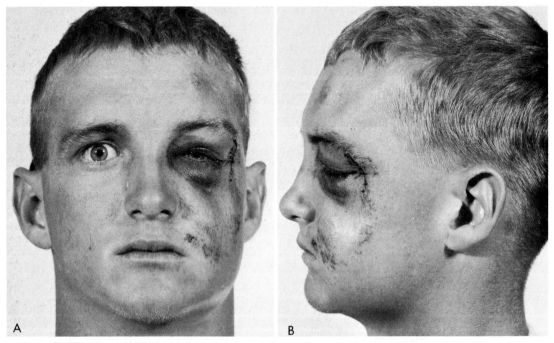

Figure 18–218   Depressed fracture of the zygoma and floor of the orbit. Note the alteration in the ocular level due to the marked downward and medial displacement of the zygoma.

Figure 18–219 Inadequate treatment (by wiring alone) of the fracture sites of this patient's zygoma has left the patient with diplopia and an unsightly depression of the right side of his face. The lowering of the right eye because the zygoma was not elevated and the possible need of a graft in the floor of the orbital cavity are quite evident. See Blowout Fractures of the Orbital Floor, following this section.

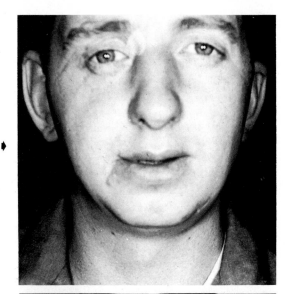

Figure 18–220 *A*, Depressed zygomatic fracture. The edema has practically all disappeared, and the depression in this area of the face is very apparent. Wiring the orbital rim fracture sites will not restore the normal facial contour. This can only be accomplished by moving the zygoma *laterally* as well as *superiorly*. This will require extraoral traction on the zygoma. Otherwise, depending on the extent of the lowering of the floor of the orbit, the patient may develop diplopia in addition to the facial depression, as was true in the case illustrated in Figure 18–219, in which wiring only of the fracture sites was done.

B, Radiograph with fracture sites identified.

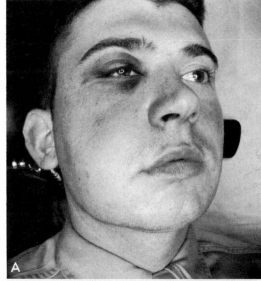

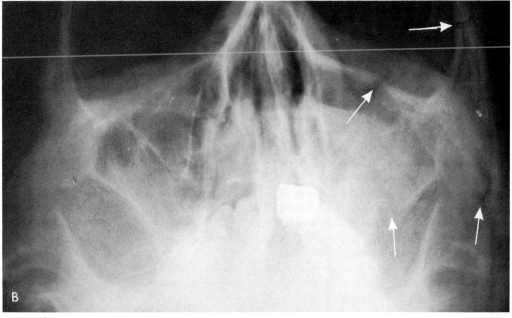

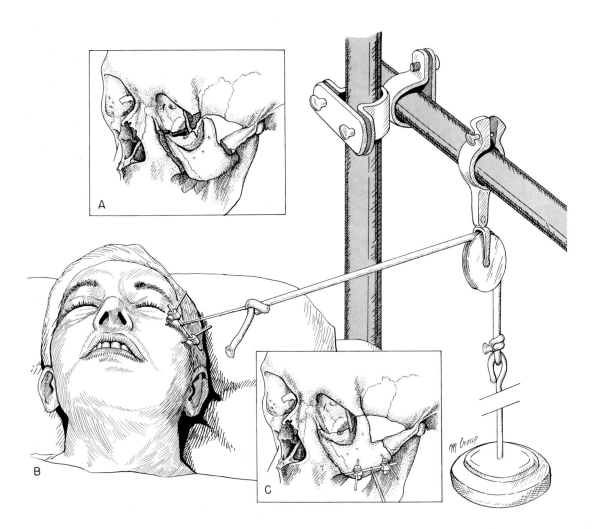

Figure 18–221 The traction method for reduction of a depressed fracture of the zygomatic bone.

A, The zygomatic bone has been driven downward and inward.

B, A Roger Anderson Frac-Sur unit is inserted in the zygomatic bone, and traction is applied as illustrated. The weight is gradually increased until movement takes place and the deformity is corrected. The patient must be seen frequently during the day to prevent overreduction. The traction is removed at night. The traction can be applied in any direction by adjustment of the position of the pulley.

C, The zygomatic bone back in normal position.

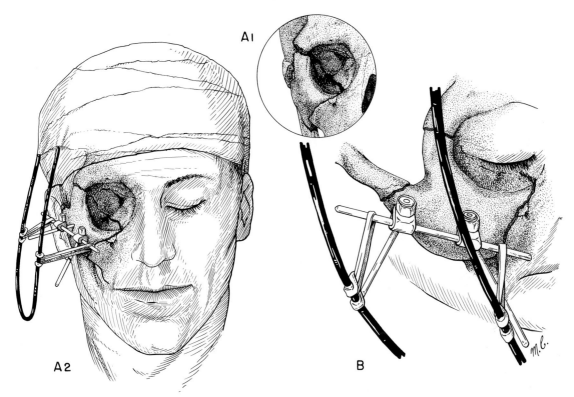

Figure 18–222 A method of treatment of depressed fractures of the zygomatic bone in ambulatory patients is illustrated here. Elastic bands are attached from the Frac-Sur unit to the wire extensions from the plaster of paris head cast or from a head frame. Any required number of bands may be attached, and the U-shaped heavy wire extension bar permits a variety of directions of pull, *e.g.,* up or down, more traction anteriorly than posteriorly, producing a rotation, and so on. In fractures over 5 days old, use the traction as shown in Figure 18–203 or in Figure 18–221. Once the fragment is moved into its normal position, it can be held there during healing by the plaster head cap or a head frame. This is a very satisfactory method of treatment.

tions the fractured zygoma by grasping the connecting rod between the pins. If this is done early, the zygoma may stay put. If not, then it should be treated as shown in Figure 18–222. If fibrosis has formed at the fracture points, because of a delay of 1 or 2 weeks, then it is necessary to use extraoral elastic traction attached to appropriately placed bars extending from a plaster of paris head cap.

In these fractures there is a depressed infraorbital ridge, and the zygomatic bone is driven down part way into the maxillary sinus.

INTRAMAXILLARY SINUS MANIPULATION. In the second method where the zygomatic bone, infraorbital ridge and orbital floor are comminuted, a mucoperiosteal flap is turned back along the multiple depressed fragments of the wall of the maxillary sinus, and a blunt curved instrument such as a medium or large curved urethral sound is passed into the maxillary sinus beneath the depressed zygoma; then by a lifting pressure upward and outward an attempt is made to reposition the fragments. Correct repositioning of the zygomatic bone is essential to correct diplopia.

SUPPORT OF ZYGOMATIC BONE AND ORBITAL FLOOR FROM WTHIN THE MAXILLARY SINUS. Packing the antrum with iodoform gauze is not a completely satisfactory way to hold the zygoma in position. Because of the high incidence of sinus infection and antro-oral fistula, there has been less tendency to resort to the packing of the maxillary sinus for support of the orbital contents, according to Fickling.[51]

Another method which Commander Arthur Turville, D.C., U.S.N.,[183] and others have

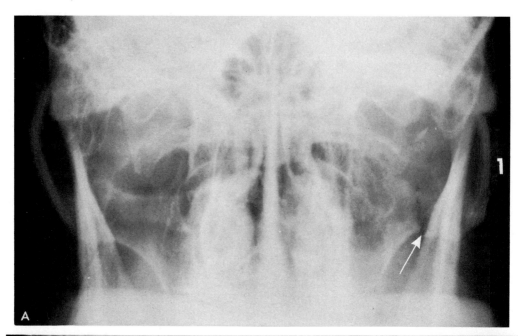

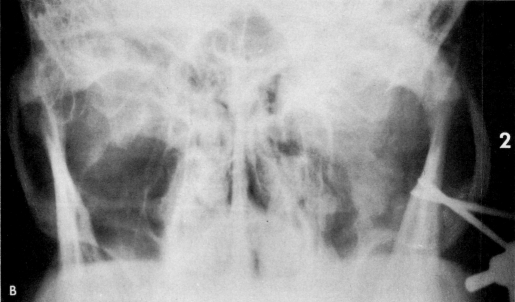

Figure 18–223 *A*, This depressed fracture of the zygoma was treated as illustrated in Figure 18–222. *B*, The extent of the correction of depressed zygoma can be seen by comparing the arch (*1*) in *A* and the arch (*2*) in *B*.

C to *G*, Technique for the insertion of Frac-Sur skeletal pin fixation in the zygoma. *C*, Pins inserted. *D*, Connecting bar locked over the pins. *E*, Rubber bands are stretched from the connecting bar at the lock nut positions to the wire extension from the plaster of paris head cap, as shown in Figure 18–222, or one of the head frames shown in Figures 18–191 to 18–195. *F* and *G*, Extent of correction with reduction of pin fixation.

(*Figure 18–223 continued on opposite page*)

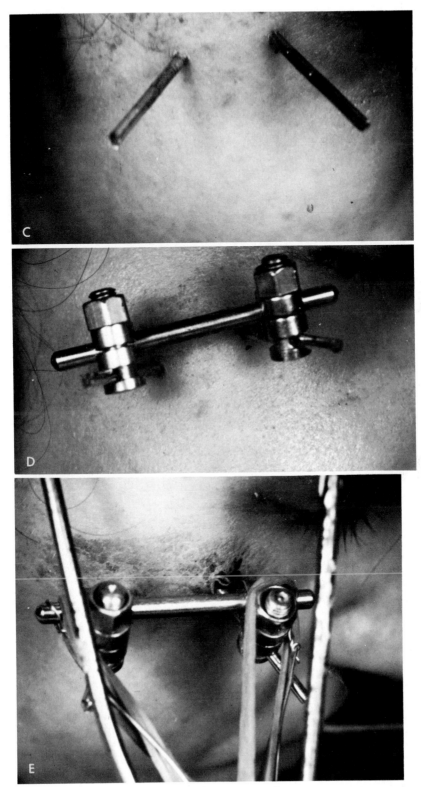

Figure 18–223   *(Continued.)*

(Figure 18–223 continued on following page)

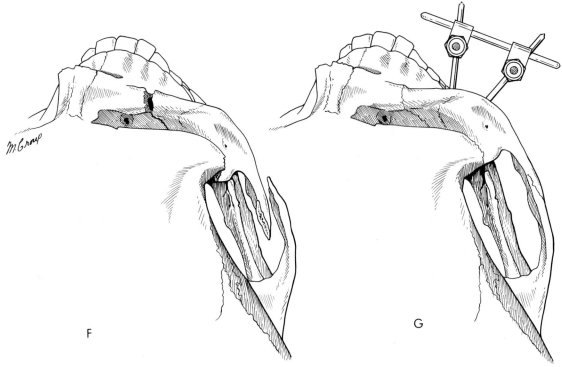

F

G

Figure 18–223 *(Continued.)*

used with considerable success in treating comminuted depressed fractures of the walls of the maxillary sinus and floor of the orbital cavity, alone or in conjunction with a depressed fracture of the zygoma, is to introduce a No. 16, 30 cc. Foley urethral catheter into the maxillary sinus, either through an opening high in the canine fossa or through the nasal cavity beneath the inferior turbinate. Blood clots are sucked out and the catheter is inserted and inflated with sterile water. The catheter is inflated by wiring it to the adapter tip of a 10 cc. syringe. When the catheter is inflated to the point where the fragments are elevated to their normal or near normal position, it is tied off near its entrance point in the sinus and excess tubing is cut off.

In some cases this procedure is in itself sufficient to elevate not only the smaller fragments but the zygoma as well to a satisfactory position. In others the above method is used in conjunction with either direct manual manipulation or with extraoral traction as has already been described.

OPEN REDUCTION. This involves wiring the fragments at the lateral orbital rim (zygomatico-frontal suture line) and, in some cases, also along the infraorbital rim. Satisfactory results can be obtained if there has not been too much medial displacement. In these

cases, to restore normal facial contour it is necessary to insert a Frac-Sur unit in the zygomatic bone and apply traction as shown in Figure 18–221. This combination of methods gives excellent results.

BLOWOUT FRACTURES OF THE ORBITAL FLOOR

T. WILLIAM EVANS, D.D.S., M.D.

The term blowout fracture of the floor of the orbit refers to a specific clinical entity. There are two types of blowout fractures: the pure type and the impure type. The pure blowout fracture can be defined as a disruption of the orbital floor without involvement of the orbital rim; the impure type involves the orbital rim, *i.e.,* there is a concomitant midfacial fracture. A blowout fracture is almost always accompanied by herniation and incarceration of the periorbital soft tissue into the subjacent maxillary sinus, which results in various clinical signs and symptoms.

The incidence of blowout fracture of the orbital floor is increasing every year, as evidenced by the attention it is receiving in the current literature. The reason for this is two-

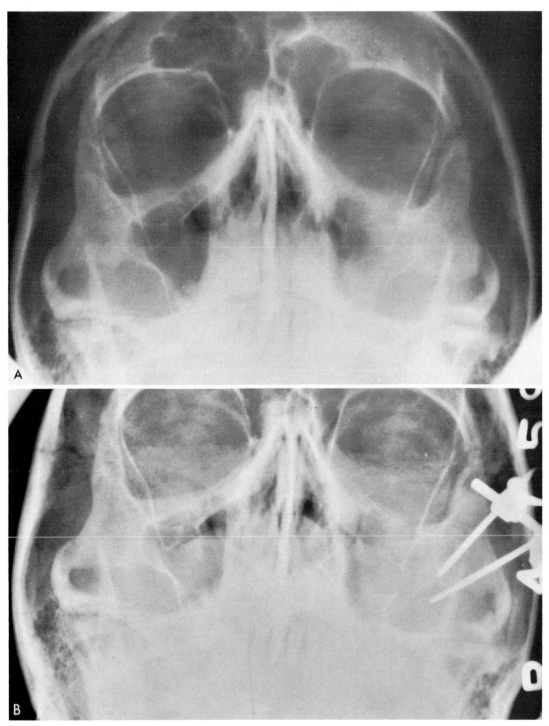

Figure 18–224 *A,* Another fractured zygoma. *B,* Zygoma reduced and immobilized with a pin fixation unit and traction.

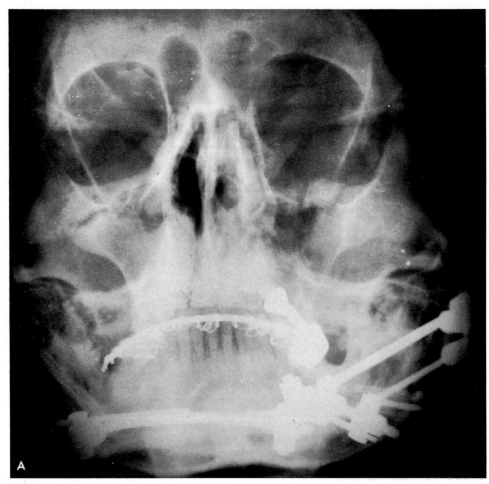

Figure 18–225 Treatment of multiple fractures of the zygoma, maxilla and mandible. The maxillary and mandibular teeth were brought into occlusion by intermaxillary elastics stretched between the splints attached to the maxillary and mandibular teeth. At the same time the fragments of the fractures of the mandible were brought into apposition by means of the extraoral skeletal fixation appliances. A cranial fixation frame was attached to the skull and by means of the extension rods from it attached to the maxilla and zygoma, these bones were moved into position. (See Figures 18–191 and 18–192.)

(Figure 18–225 continued on opposite page)

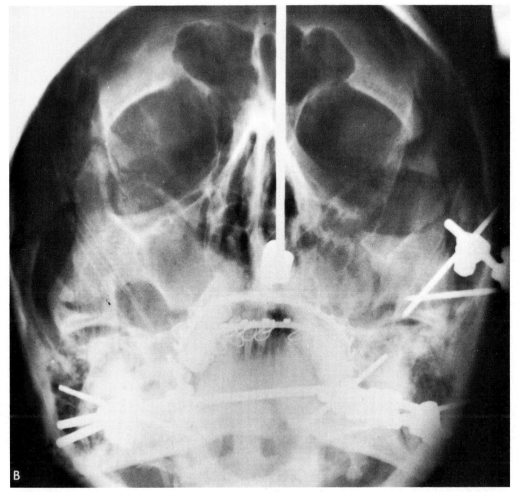

Figure 18–225 *(Continued.)*

fold: (1) a higher incidence of maxillofacial trauma from the use of seatbelts (in the older literature the prime etiologic factor in blow-out fracture was the human fist, but recently a series has been reported in which automobile accidents were the cause of 50 per cent of blowout fractures), and (2) a higher index of suspicion by clinicians.

It is of prime importance for clinicians who see maxillofacial trauma in the emergency room to be acquainted with the evaluation and treatment of blowout fractures. The ophthalmology literature is full of case reports of the late treatment of undiagnosed blowout fractures. Late treatment is usually unsatisfactory because of the extensive fibrous scarring and periorbital tissue atrophy which results from an untreated blowout fracture. Satisfactory treatment of blowout frac-

tures can only be accomplished when they are diagnosed early.

Mechanism and Anatomy. The orbital cavity is cone-shaped. Sudden pressure applied over the orbital soft tissue pushes the orbital contents backward into the narrower part of the orbit, like a piston in a cylinder (Fig. 18–233*A*). This produces a rapid rise in intraorbital pressure, which is transmitted to the bony orbital walls, causing a pure blowout fracture.

The orbit has two weak areas: the orbital plate of the ethmoid bone, called the lamina papyracea (a plate of paper), and the orbital floor overlying the maxillary sinus. Experimental orbital blowout fractures which have been produced in cadavers suggest that 80 per cent of pure blowout fractures occur in the posterior orbital floor immediately an-

(Text continued on page 1305)

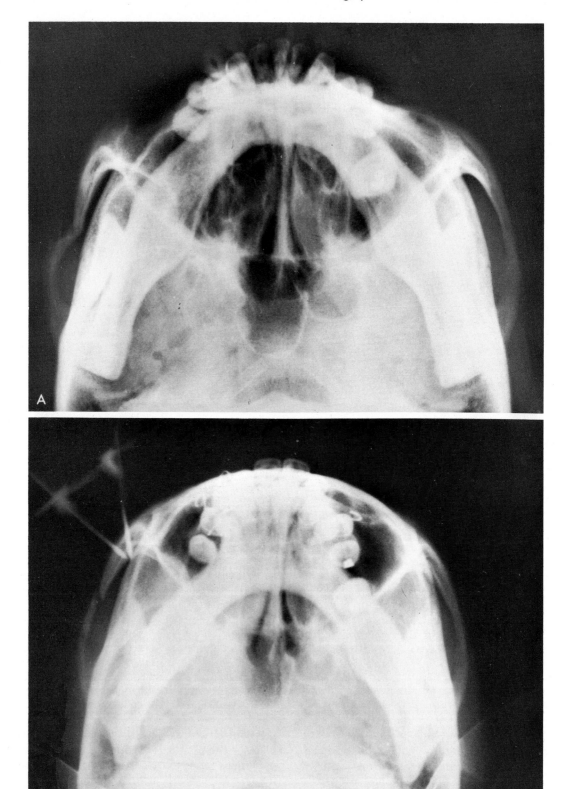

Figure 18–226 *A,* Another example of a fractured and depressed zygoma. *B,* It was reduced and immobilized as previously described. The extraoral traction is not shown on these radiographs.

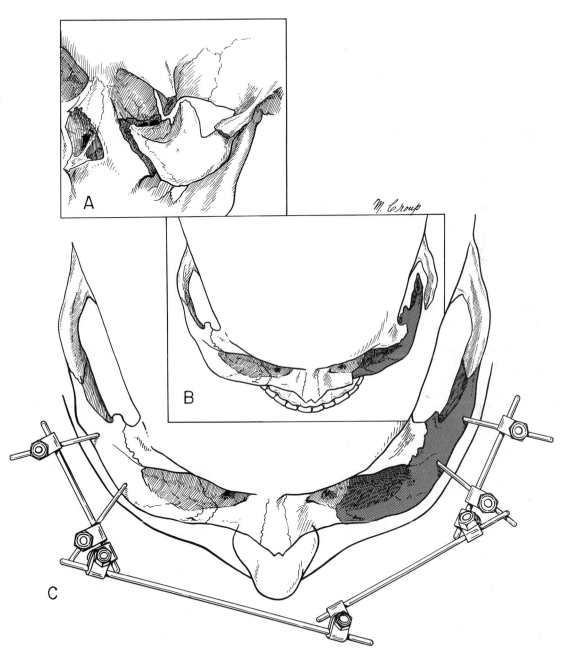

Figure 18–227 Technique used in the treatment of a fractured and depressed zygoma such as that shown in Figure 18–228. This is a more exact and comfortable method of support than is suspension from a plaster of paris head cap.

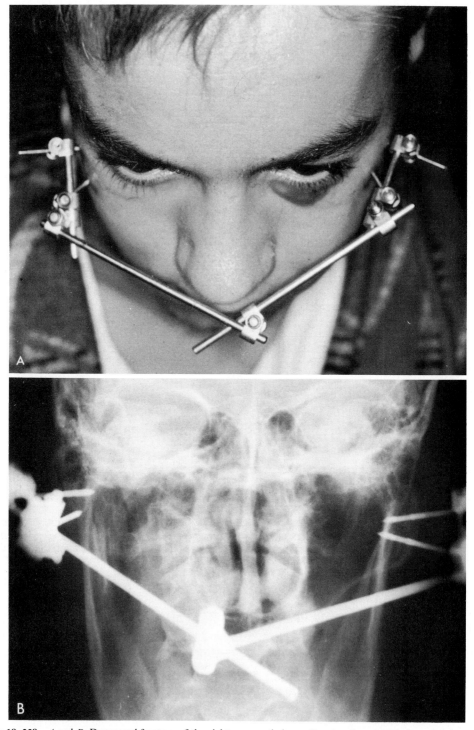

Figure 18–228 *A* and *B*, Depressed fracture of the right zygomatic bone. Fractured zygomatic bone has been reduced and is supported in normal position by suspending it from a skeletal pin fixation (Frac-Sur) unit in the opposite zygomatic bone. (See Figure 18–227.)

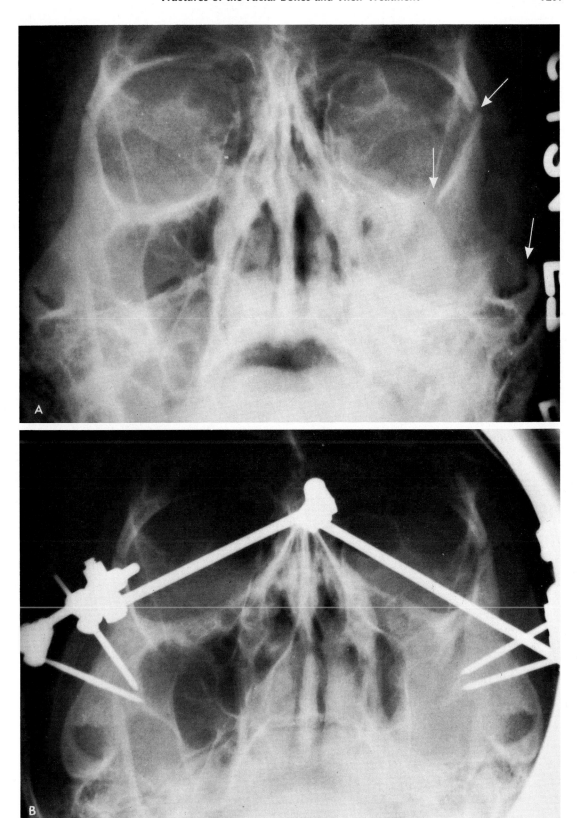

Figure 18–229   *A,* Another case of a fractured and depressed zygoma. *B,* It has been reduced and is supported in its position by a skeletal pin fixation unit in the opposite zygoma, which is healthy and sound.

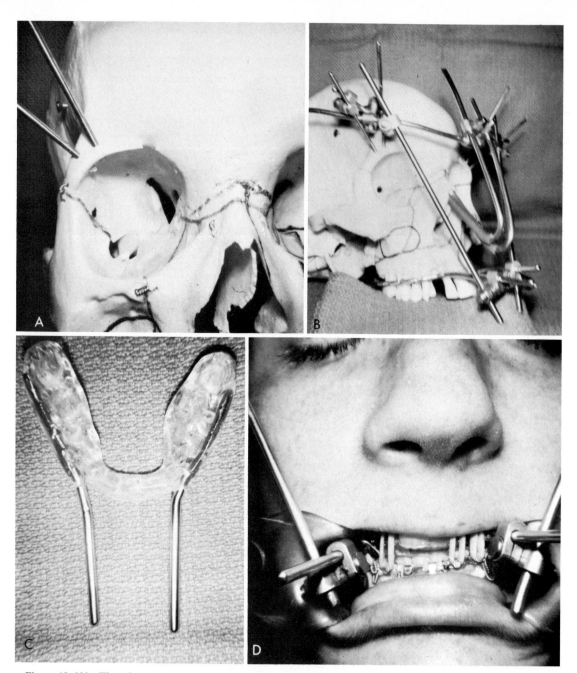

Figure 18–230 The advantages of the supraorbital pin head frame technique are the same as those for any cranial fixation unit: it is simple and safe. The lacrimal gland is slightly punctured, which causes no problem. The necessary equipment (Roger Anderson skeletal pin fixation units) is always at hand.

A, As may be seen, it is strong and is not as bulky as the head (cranial) frame or plaster of paris head cap. *B* to *D,* Use of this technique for the treatment of a Le Fort I fracture (*B* additionally shows a "nasal fracture.") *E* to *G,* These pins will support any facial bones, including the nasal and zygomatic bones, and are excellent for Le Fort III fractures. *H,* The rubber-covered extension rods, used to support a fractured nose in conjunction with a Le Fort II or III fracture, are excellent if there is cerebrospinal rhinorrhea. Packing the nose to maintain the fragments is contraindicated when there is drainage of cerebrospinal fluid. The fractured nose can be reduced and immobilized with these pins suspended from the supraorbital head frame drainage. *I,* Waters' position radiograph of a treated case of a Le Fort I fracture of the maxilla and a fracture of the mandible in an edentulous patient. Splints were wired to the denture teeth. The mandibular fracture was one that was ideal for circumferential wiring over the denture. The mandibular and maxillary dentures were brought into occlusion, and with traction from the supraorbital head frame pulling up the mandible, which in turn exerted pressure on the maxilla, the Le Fort I fracture was reduced and immobilized. *Note:* The right suspension rod, duplicate of the left, was cut off when this radiograph was made. *J,* Lateral head radiograph of a dentulous patient with a Le Fort I fracture of the maxilla and no fracture of the mandible. Treatment is the same as previously described except obviously no treatment of the mandible was required. (Courtesy of T. William Evans, D.D.S., M.D.)

(Figure 18–230 continued on opposite page)

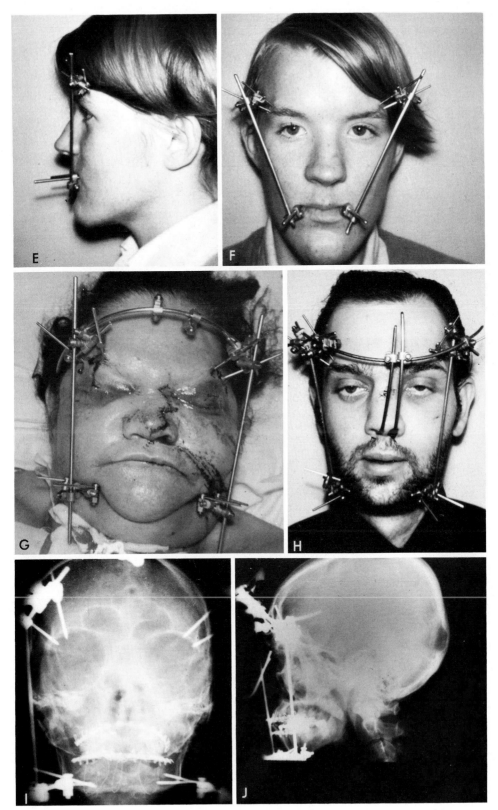

Figure 18–230 *(Continued.)*

UNILATERAL COMPOUND FRACTURE OF AN EDENTULOUS MANDIBLE, AND A DEPRESSED FRACTURE OF THE LEFT ZYGOMATIC BONE

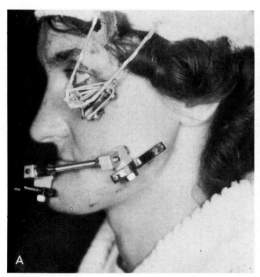 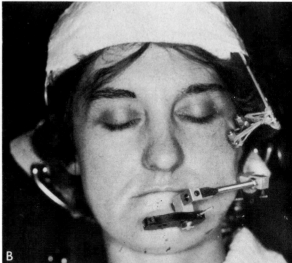

Figure 18–231 *A*, Treatment of a depressed fracture of the left zygomatic bone and a unilateral fracture of an edentulous mandible with marked overriding and lateral displacement of the fragments. (See *C* and *D*.) This lateral view illustrates the various directions of force that can be secured by elastic traction from the Frac-Sur unit to the wire extension. Those depressed zygomas that are not reduced shortly after the accident will not stay in their normal positions unless they are held there by traction. Furthermore, these fractures are difficult to reduce if treatment is delayed. Because of the facial edema that accompanies the trauma, these fractures are frequently missed until the edema disappears and the flattened, depressed appearance of the face is apparent.

B, This case was treated, as illustrated, by the application of a Stader splint to reduce and immobilize the fractured mandible. (See *E* and *F*.) Then a Roger Anderson Frac-Sur unit was inserted in the depressed zygoma. The unit was attached with elastic bands to a heavy wire loop extending downward and outward from a plaster head cap. When the zygoma is elevated into position, as determined by observation, palpation and roentgenograms, stainless steel wires are substituted for the elastic bands to maintain the position of the zygomatic bone. No felt or sponge rubber strips were used under the head cap. The hair acts as a cushion for the head cap.

C, Unilateral fracture of the edentulous mandible, with marked lingual and superior displacement of the posterior fragment and overriding of the fragments. In addition, there was a depressed fracture of the zygoma. Note the break in continuity of the left lateral wall of the left maxillary sinus.

D, Mandibular fracture reduced and the fragments fixed in position, and the zygoma elevated to its normal position.

E and *F*, Oblique radiographs before and after reduction and immobilization of the fracture of the mandible.

(Figure 18–231 continued on opposite page)

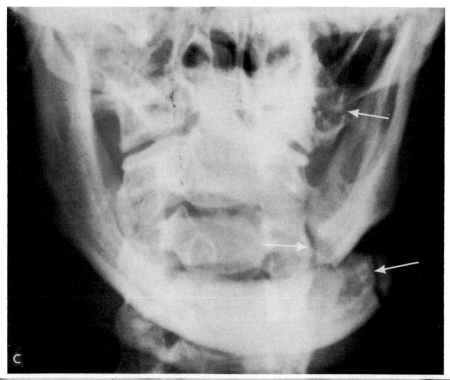

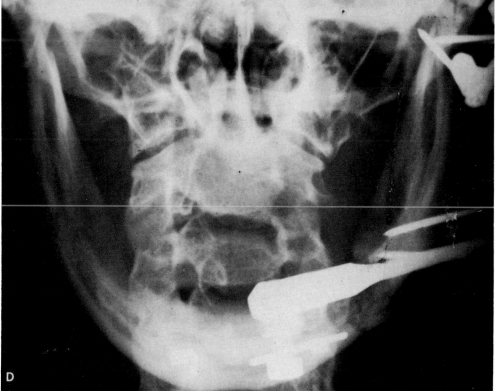

Figure 18-231   *(Continued.)*

(Figure 18-231 continued on following page)

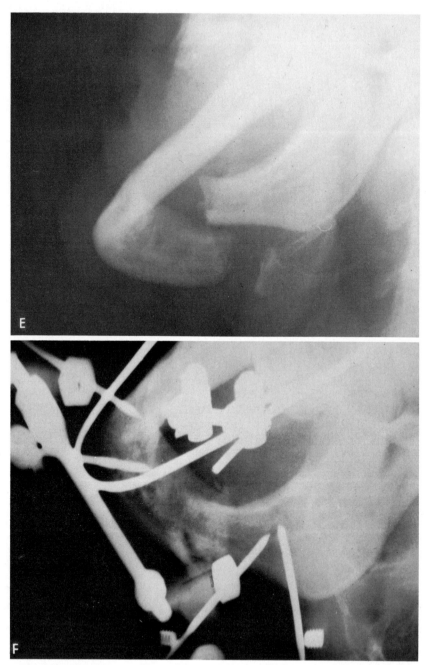

Figure 18–231 *(Continued.)*

Photographic Case Report

MULTIPLE COMPOUND COMMINUTED FRACTURES OF THE MAXILLA, ZYGOMATIC BONE, ZYGOMATIC ARCH AND MANDIBLE

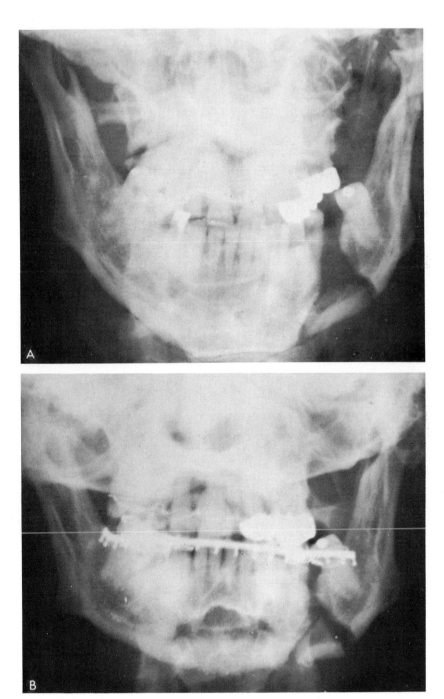

Figure 18–232

(Figure 18–232 continued on following page)

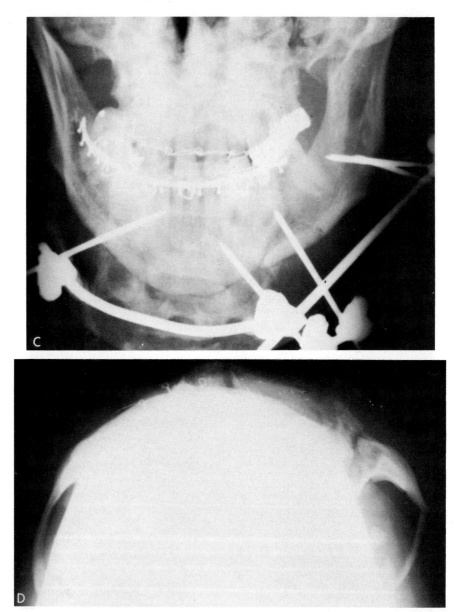

Figure 18–232 *A,* Multiple compound comminuted fractures of the maxilla, zygoma, floor of orbit, zygomatic arch, nose and mandible. (See *D* and *E* for zygoma and zygomatic arch, nose, orbit and maxillary fracture.) *B,* Patient was treated, as shown here, in another hospital, and then referred for more definitive treatment. *C,* Mandibular fractures reduced and stabilized with Frac-Sur appliances and intermaxillary elastics. *D,* The crushing blow has buckled and fractured the zygomatic arch and driven the zygoma laterally and medially. (The usual position of fractured zygomas is downward and medially.) *E,* The transverse fracture of the maxilla, blood in both sinuses, comminuted infraorbital ridge and laterally displaced zygoma are clearly shown here. *F,* All fractures are reduced and stabilized. To reduce the maxillary, zygomatic bone and zygomatic arch fractures, an operating room cap was placed on the patient's head and reinforced with adhesive tape. Then rubber bands were pinned to the cap on both sides and stretched down to and over the pins in the Frac-Sur units. On the left side a compound slab was heated slightly and contoured, then placed beneath the rubber bands. This pressure reduced the zygoma and zygomatic arch and maxillary fractures as shown in this radiograph.

(Figure 18–232 continued on following page)

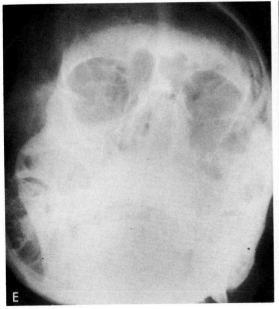 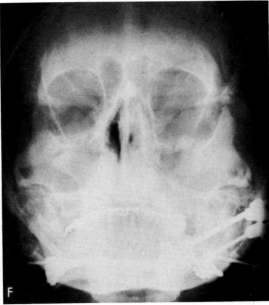

Figure 18–232 *(Continued.)*

terior to the inferior orbital fissure and medial to the infraorbital groove (Fig. 18–233*B*). The remaining 20 per cent involve the lamina papyracea.

It is interesting to note that this area of greatest incidence of fracture is not the thinnest area of the orbital walls. Measurements of the thickness of the orbital walls show that the thinnest areas are the floor of the infraor-

bital groove and the orbital plate of the ethmoid. It is believed that the orbital floor fractures more easily because it lies directly below the geometric orbital axis and extends backward and upward in an inclined plane, receiving the brunt of the increased intraorbital pressure. The infraorbital groove is usually not involved because it receives support from the infraorbital vessels and nerves. The

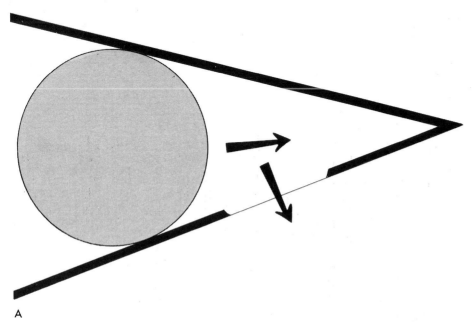

A

Figure 18–233 *A*, Mechanism of blowout fracture (piston in a cylinder).

(Figure 18–233 continued on following page)

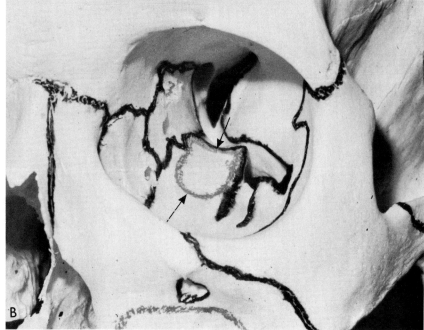

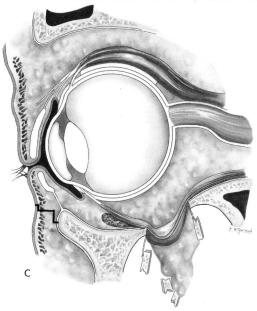

Figure 18–233 *(Continued.)* B, Anatomy of orbit. The outlined area of incidence of most blowout fractures is between the arrows.

C, Blowout fracture with impingement of infraorbital structures (infraorbital fat, inferior rectus muscle and branch of third nerve to inferior oblique muscle). The suspensory ligament is not shown.

(Figure 18–233 continued on opposite page)

lamina papyracea receives support from the bony partitions of the ethmoidal air cells.

The loss of bony floor support predisposes to herniation and incarceration of the orbital soft tissue into the maxillary sinus. These tissues include the ruptured periosteum (periorbita), Tenon's capsule (Lockwood's suspensory ligament), periorbital fat, the inferior rectus muscle, the inferior division of the third cranial nerve, which supplies the infe-

rior oblique muscle, and possibly the inferior oblique muscle (Fig. 18–233C).

Diagnosis. The typical physical findings of blowout fractures are the result of the herniation and incarceration of the orbital soft tissue. These signs (Fig. 18–233D to F), which may not become manifest until 24 hours after the trauma, are as follows:

1. Periorbital edema and ecchymosis ("black eye")—this is usually the first

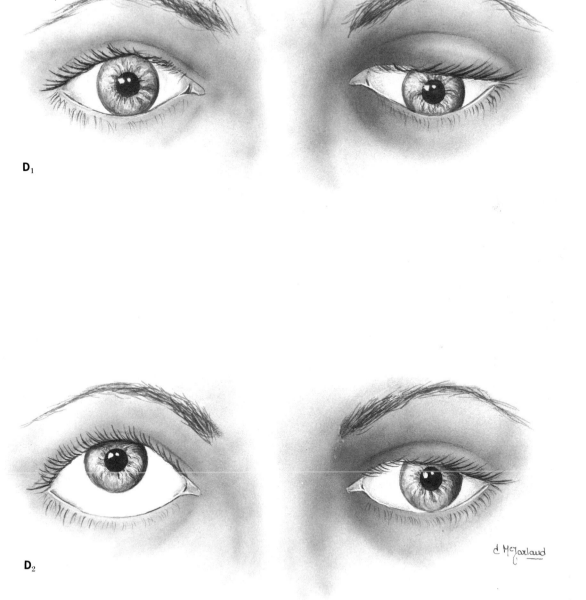

D₁

D₂

Figure 18–233 *(Continued.)*   *D*, Clinical signs: patient looking straight ahead (*D₁*) and looking up (*D₂*).

(Figure 18–233 continued on following page)

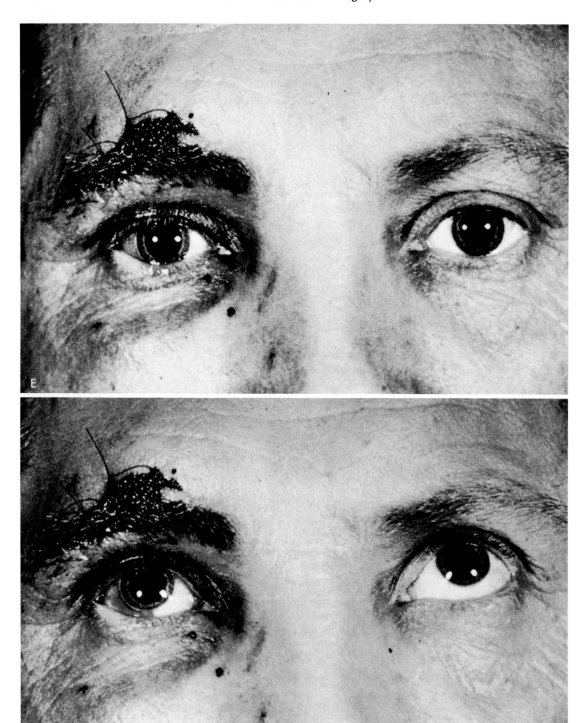

Figure 18–233 *(Continued.)* *E*, Clinical appearance of patient looking straight ahead. *F*, Clinical appearance of patient looking up.

(Figure 18–233 continued on opposite page)

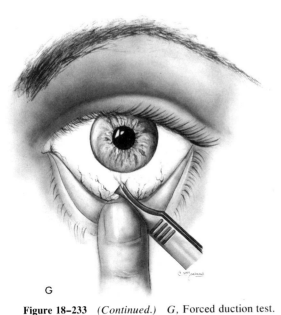

G

Figure 18–233 *(Continued.)* G, Forced duction test.

(Figure 18–233 continued on following page)

and sometimes the only clinical sign; when this is present one should entertain a strong suspicion of blowout fracture of the orbital floor.

2. Decreased vertical oculorotary movements—caused by the entrapment of the inferior rectus muscle, the nerve to the inferior oblique muscle and possibly the inferior oblique muscle. There is restriction in upward and possibly downward gaze of the affected eye.

3. Enophthalmos of the globe—the eye recedes downward and backward, mainly because of the lack of support from the herniated orbital fat.

4. Ptosis of the upper eyelid—the eyelid droops because of the enophthalmos (really pseudoptosis).

5. Vertical diplopia (double vision), especially in upward gaze—this is the result of deviation of the visual axis of the two eyes secondary to decreased vertical oculorotary movement and to enophthalmos. It may be secondary to periorbital edema or hematoma.

6. Infraorbital anesthesia—the least consistent sign because the blowout usually occurs medial to the infraorbital nerve.

These clinical signs may or may not be present with an orbital blowout fracture. Two procedures may be performed to help estab-

Table 18–3   *Clinical Signs of Blowout Fracture*

1. Periorbital edema and ecchymosis ("black eye")
2. Decreased vertical oculorotary movements
3. Enophthalmos of globe
4. Ptosis of upper eyelid
5. Vertical diplopia
6. Infraorbital anesthesia

lish the diagnosis: the forced duction test and radiographic examination.

The forced duction test consists of grasping the tendon of the inferior rectus muscle through the topically anesthetized conjunctiva with a small tooth forceps (Adson forceps) (Fig. 18–233G). The ocular globe cannot be rotated upward when entrapment of the inferior rectus is present.

Radiologic examination is an essential part of the diagnostic procedure and should be routinely performed on any patient with a history of trauma to the eye or an evident "black eye," even with the absence of other clinical signs. The most useful projections are the Waters' view and anteroposterior laminograms of the orbits (Fig. 18–190H). If the following radiographic signs are present, a blowout fracture should be strongly suspected:

1. Cloudy maxillary sinus—due to hematoma formation.

2. "Hanging drop" sign—opacification caused by the herniated orbital soft tissues and bony fragments.

3. Bone fragments in the maxillary sinus—which can be demonstrated as white lines if the edges of the fragments are parallel to the x-ray beam or as a gray density if they are not parallel to the beam.

4. Obliteration of the infraorbital foramen—due to superimposition of the herniated orbital soft tissue and bone fragments.

5. Increased thickness of the involved orbital floor—due to the inflammatory reaction in the area.

6. Emphysema of the involved orbit—due to entrance of air from the subjacent maxillary sinus.

Table 18–4   *Radiologic Signs of Blowout Fracture*

1. Cloudy maxillary sinus
2. "Hanging drop" sign
3. Bone fragments in the maxillary sinus
4. Obliterated infraorbital foramen
5. Increased thickness of orbital floor
6. Orbital emphysema

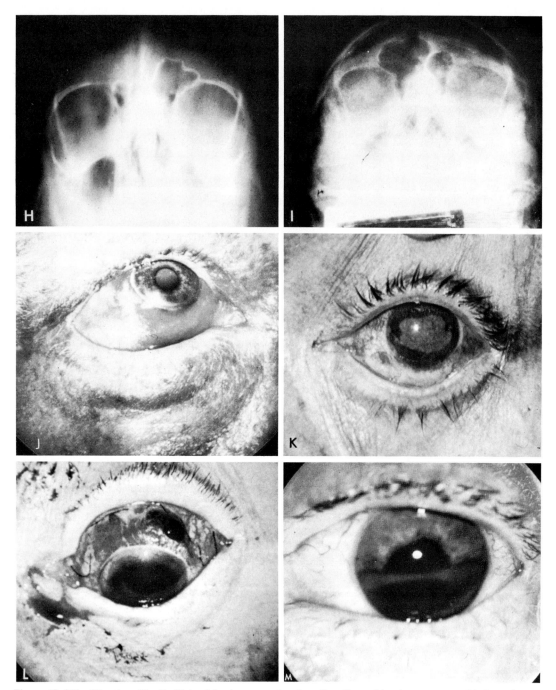

Oral and Maxillofacial Surgery

Figure 18–233 *(Continued.)* *H*, Waters' laminogram showing all radiographic signs except orbital emphysema. *I*, Waters' laminogram showing all radiographic signs except orbital emphysema. *J* to *M*, Ocular injuries associated with blowout fracture. *J*, Subconjunctival hemorrhage. *K*, Corneal abrasion or ulcer. *L*, Ruptured globe. *M*, Hyphema.

(Figure 18–233 continued on opposite page)

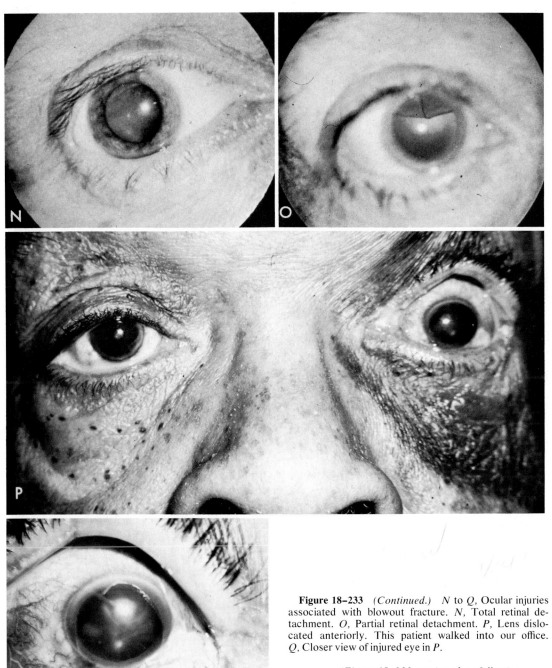

Figure 18–233 *(Continued.)* *N* to *Q*, Ocular injuries associated with blowout fracture. *N*, Total retinal detachment. *O*, Partial retinal detachment. *P*, Lens dislocated anteriorly. This patient walked into our office. *Q*, Closer view of injured eye in *P*.

(Figure 18–233 continued on following page)

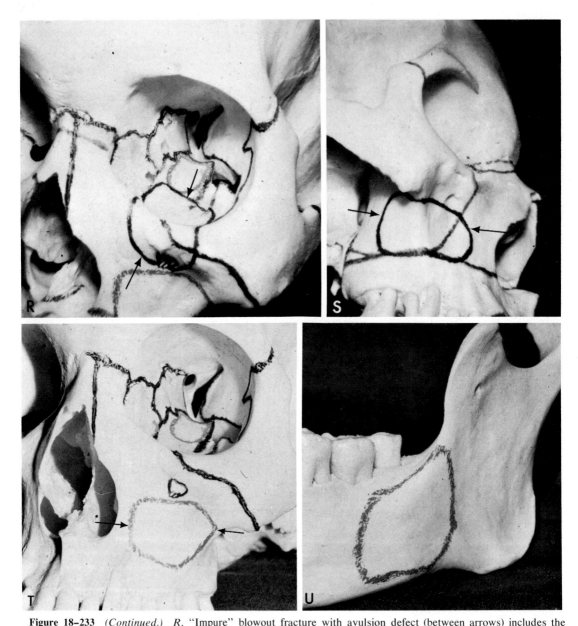

Figure 18–233 *(Continued.)* *R,* "Impure" blowout fracture with avulsion defect (between arrows) includes the rim and orbital floor. An "impure" blowout fracture is actually a fractured zygomatic complex with a concomitant blowout fracture.

S, Donor site of bone (between arrows) to repair an "impure" blowout fracture with avulsion defect of the orbit on the opposite side of the face. The posterior portion of the graft is used as the anterior maxilla; the anterior portion is used as the orbital floor.

T, Donor site of bone to repair a "pure" blowout fracture (between arrows).

U, Another possible donor site if the maxilla is crushed.

(Figure 18–233 continued on opposite page)

Many times these radiographic signs will be masked by a completely opaque maxillary sinus from hemorrhage or from pre-existing sinus disease. This is especially true when there is a concomitant midfacial fracture, *i.e.,* an impure blowout fracture. Visualization in this case is facilitated by needle evacuation of blood and introduction of air into the max-illary sinus. Another technique that may be utilized for a more precise radiologic diagnosis is the injection of radiopaque material along the orbital floor.

Once the diagnosis has been made, the earliest operation consistent with the patient's general condition is indicated. Correction after 12 to 15 days is usually followed by an

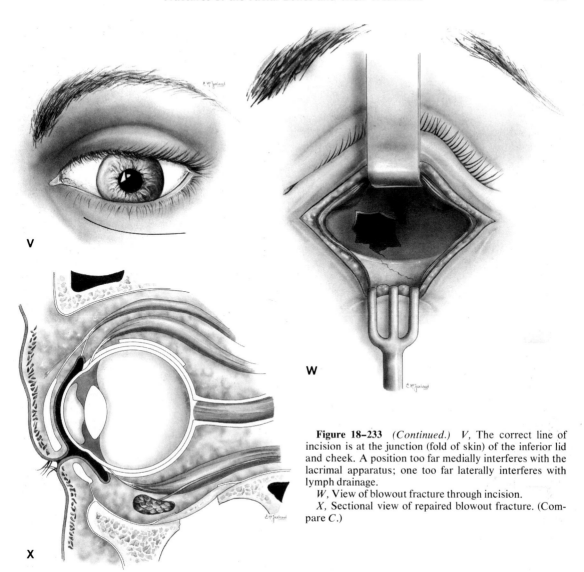

Figure 18–233 *(Continued.)* *V*, The correct line of incision is at the junction (fold of skin) of the inferior lid and cheek. A position too far medially interferes with the lacrimal apparatus; one too far laterally interferes with lymph drainage.

W, View of blowout fracture through incision.

X, Sectional view of repaired blowout fracture. (Compare *C*.)

unsatisfactory operative result. One word of caution: this type of fracture is often complicated by injury to the globe itself (Fig. 18–233*J* to *Q*). In this era of public awareness to iatrogenic injury, any ocular complication should be determined preoperatively. This requires a complete examination by an ophthalmologist.

Treatment. The indication for surgery for correction of orbital blowout fractures is the establishment of the diagnosis, whether or not there are clinical signs. In the past, the patients with asymptomatic blowout fracture diagnosed only by radiographs were treated conservatively with fairly good results. To those who did develop complications, though,

it was difficult to restore satisfactory ocular function. It seems that the ordeal of the surgery is much less than the possible complications that may occur if the fracture is not treated.

If the blowout fracture is of the impure type, the concomitant midfacial fracture should be reduced first. Many times this will be sufficient to treat the blowout fracture adequately. In order to prevent further impingement of the herniated periorbita, the reduction should be performed only with direct visualization of the orbital floor via either the transantral or infraorbital approach. The presence of an impure blowout fracture is a definite contraindication to blind reduction of the concomitant fracture, such as a zygomatic complex fracture. (In my opinion all zygomatic complex fractures should be reduced with the surgeon simultaneously observing the fracture line in the orbital floor via the transantral or infraorbital approach.)

Often after reduction of the concomitant midfacial fracture there is a defect in the orbital floor and orbital rim from avulsion of bone (Fig. 18–233R). This can be repaired with a bone graft from the lateral maxillary wall of the unfractured side, utilizing the zygomatic buttress as the infraorbital rim, the posterior maxillary wall of the graft as the anterior maxillary wall and the anterior maxillary wall of the graft as the orbital floor (Fig. 18–233S).

The methods of approach to treating the pure blowout fracture are the transantral approach, with use of a sinus pack to elevate and support the herniated periorbita; the infraorbital approach, with use of an implant; or both approaches simultaneously. It has been well proven that the infraorbital approach is the method of choice. The advantages of the infraorbital approach are the re-establishment of the continuity of the orbital floor, the separation of the antral from the orbital cavity, the assurance of adequate eye mobility and the prevention of restricting adhesions. It also allows for direct observation of the desired height and position of the new orbital floor. The transantral approach should be used in conjunction with the infraorbital approach when there is concomitant midfacial fracture (impure blowout fracture) or when there is chronic sinusitis requiring debridement and antibiotic pack.

Many materials have been employed as implants in orbital floor fractures. The ideal material should fit certain criteria: (1) it should be tolerated by the patient, (2) it should prevent adhesions to the orbital capsule, (3) it should be strong enough to support the orbital contents, (4) it should be easily obtained at the time of surgery, and (5) it should not require stabilization, which is difficult in this area. In the past 10 years the use of alloplastic material such as Silastic or Teflon has become very popular, but these are not without shortcomings. In the case of a blowout fracture there is a source of contamination from the maxillary sinus and the placement of an alloplastic material in a contaminated area could be dangerous. It has been proved many times that autogenous bone is the material of choice for filling any

bony defect,* especially in a contaminated area (it is felt that the bone revascularizes and is permeated by the systemically administered antibiotic, thus resisting bacterial invasion).

The most popular sources of autogenous bone have been the crest of the ilium or rib. The major disadvantages for using these sites are the increased discomfort for the patient, longer preambulatory time, leading to an increased incidence of postoperative complications, and, probably most important, the fact that these sources entail a major operation not within the realm of the oral surgeon. An alternate method that eliminates these disadvantages is the utilization of bone from the anterior maxillary wall or lateral surface of the ramus of the mandible. These areas are easily accessible and leave no residual deformity or disability (Fig. 18–233T and U).

The decision of where to obtain the graft for the pure blowout fracture is determined by the necessity of a transantral approach. If this approach is necessary, the graft can easily be taken from the anterior maxillary wall in the area in which the sinus is to be entered. If a transantral approach is not required, the graft may be taken from either the anterior maxillary wall or the lateral surface of the mandible, as the operator desires.

The infraorbital approach to the orbital floor requires precise technique for satisfactory postoperative results. The incision is made in the natural skin fold at the junction of the lower lid with the cheek (Fig. 18–233V). Care must be taken not to extend the incision too far medially, where it may interfere with the nerve supply to the "lacrimal pump," nor too far laterally, where it may interfere with the lateral orbital lymphatic channels, which will cause persistent lid edema. The orbicularis oculi muscle is separated at a point slightly inferior to the skin incision, and the dissection is carried inferiorly to the anterior part of the orbital rim, with care not to penetrate the septum orbital, which is an extension of the periosteum to the inferior tarsal plate. This undermining dissection helps assure an invisible scar and prevents postoperative vertical shortening of the lower lid from scar retraction.

The periosteum is incised and elevated from the orbital floor, exposing the fracture

---

*See Chapter 23, "Transplantation and Grafting Procedures in Oral Surgery."

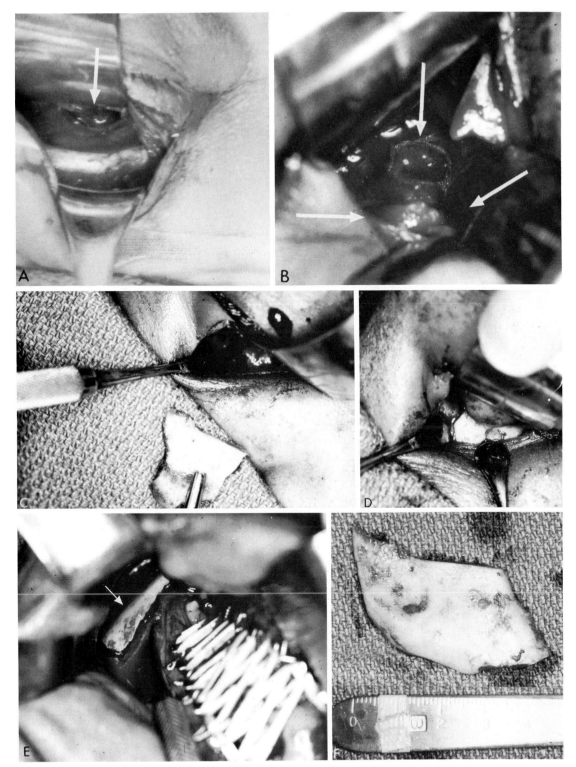

Figure 18–234   *A*, Clinical case of typical "pure" blowout fracture with entrapment of infraorbital contents.
B, Clinical case of "impure" blowout fracture with avulsion defect of orbital rim and orbital floor.
C, Repair of avulsion defect of "impure" blowout fracture with bone carved to repair anterior maxillary wall, infraorbital rim and orbital floor.
D, Avulsion defect of "impure" blowout fracture repaired.
E, One possible donor site for bone graft, the buccal cortical plate of the angle and body of the mandible.
F, Buccal cortical plate of the angle and body of the mandible removed and ready to carve to shape.

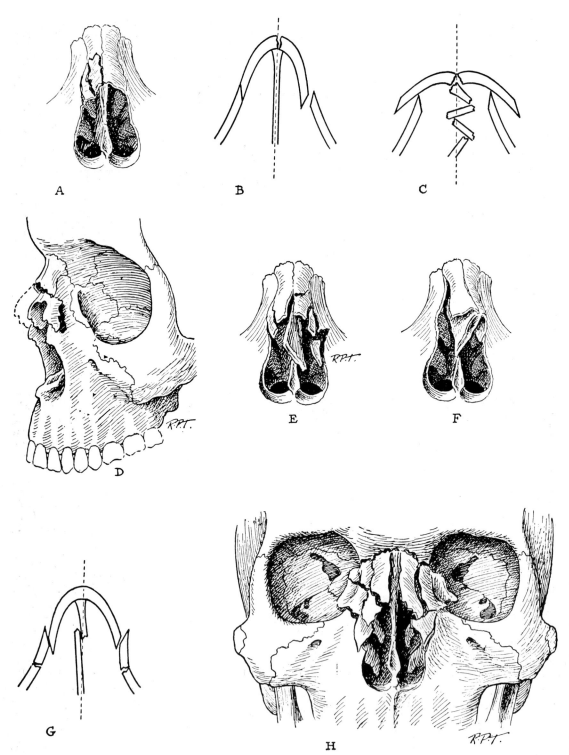

Figure 18-235 Various types of fractures of the nasal bones. *A* and *B*, Depressed fracture of one nasal bone. *C*, Open-book type of fracture seen in children. *D*, Fracture of the nasal bones at the junction of the thick upper and thin lower portions, *E*, Comminuted fracture. *F* and *G*, Fracture-dislocation. *H*, Comminuted fracture of the nasal bones involving the frontal processes of the maxilla. (From Kazanjian and Converse: The Surgical Treatment of Facial Injuries. The Williams & Wilkins Co., Baltimore, 1959.)

and herniated orbital contents. Careful gentle traction will deliver the herniated periorbital structures (Fig. 18–233W). A retractor maintains elevation of these contents while the graft is being placed. Damage to the optic nerve is improbable because of its high position, but retraction must be done with care.

The bone graft is shaped with scissors and placed over the defect. If the fracture extends into the infraorbital groove and canal, a **U**-shaped portion of bone should be cut from the posterior aspect of the implant to prevent infraorbital nerve impingement. The periosteum is sutured, and the wound is closed in layers (Fig. 18–233X).

In conclusion, I would like to emphasize the importance of early diagnosis obtainable from a high index of suspicion. Every patient with facial trauma should be examined for evidence of a blowout fracture of the orbital floor. Treatment of these fractures should be instituted as early as possible to restore the normal anatomic structure and physiologic function of the orbit. Examples from clinical cases are shown in Figure 18–234A to F.

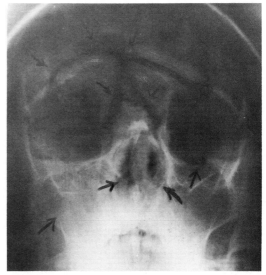

Figure 18–236 Posteroanterior (Waters' position) radiograph of multiple facial bone fractures, Le Fort III.

FRACTURES OF THE NASAL BONES

The type of fracture depends upon the direction of the blow to the nose. Injury di-

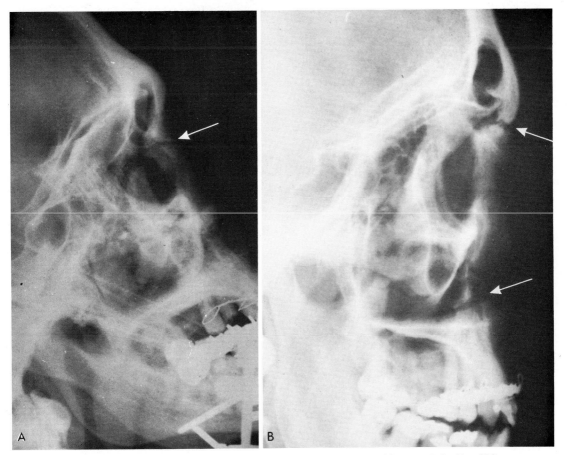

Figure 18–237 *A,* Le Fort III fractures. Lateral head radiograph. Note nasal fracture. *B,* Le Fort II fracture.

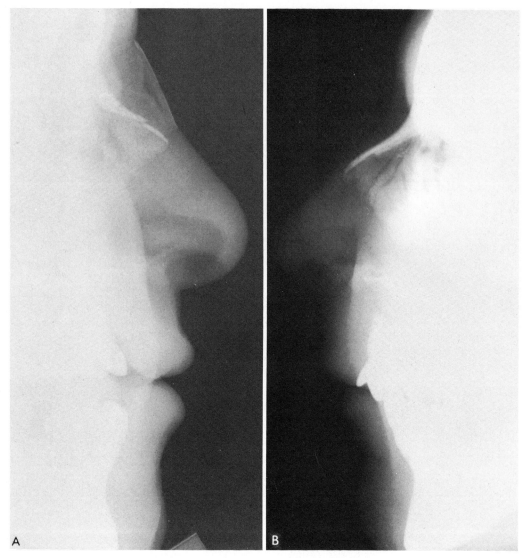

A   B

Figure 18–238   Two examples of nasal fractures.

rectly on the bridge of the nose results in squashing injury with much comminution. These injuries are very frequently associated with transverse, vertical or multiple fractures of the maxilla, particularly if the blow is directly downward on the dorsum of the nose. Lateral trauma usually fractures the nasal bones close to their attachment to the frontal and maxillary bones. These are seldom associated with fractures of the maxilla.

In both of these fractures there is involvement and deformity of the nasal septum because of either displacement or actual fracture. In the squashing type of fracture, the frontal process of the maxillary bones and the perpendicular plate of the ethmoid and vomer

are usually fractured in addition to the nasal bones.

The oral surgeon should ask the cooperation of the rhinologist in treating these complicated nasal fractures.

TREATMENT OF SIMPLE NASAL FRACTURES

A periosteal elevator wrapped with gauze and covered with petrolatum is introduced into the nostril. With upward pressure the fractured bones are lifted and with finger pressure manipulated back into position. If hemorrhage continues, the nose should be packed with petrolatum gauze for 24 hours. If possible, the fragments should be replaced within a few hours of injury before swelling masks the deformity and interferes with reduction. An external splint is now applied to maintain the bones in position. If a splint is not used, a deformity will be the result.

Simple Nasal Fracture Splint. Kazanjian and Converse describe an excellent splint as follows: "A piece of flat soft metal (gauge 22, tin) shaped like an hourglass is bent so that the lower part conforms to the general shape of the nose and the upper part rests flat against the forehead. This piece of metal serves as a tray for a small quantity of dental compound. The splint is adjusted, and because it is molded to the nose, an equalized pressure is established on all sides. The entire appliance is retained by strips of adhesive tape passing across the forehead at the top, and over the cheeks beneath the eyes at the bottom of the appliance (see Figure 18–244). Only moderate pressure need be exerted; the splint or dressing is not disturbed for at least two days. At the termination of this period, the nose is free from inflammation and edema. This method is not as positive as the following one, but may be utilized as an emergency measure in the absence of a suitable splint."*

Kazanjian Nasal Fracture Splint. This splint was designed to deliver the desired amount of continuous force against the lateral aspects of the nose at any select point (see Figure 18–245A to J).

The splint consists of an oblong metal frame; the lower surface is supplied with a round bar about 1/4 inch thick. The frame is embedded in dental compound spread over the forehead. The frame and compound are held in place securely with the aid of adhesive tape passed around the head (Figure 18–245E). The horizontal bar of the splint is not covered with dental compound but is left open for the attachment of a universal joint which can be passed freely along the bar and then held in place either to the right or to the left of the median line (Figure 18–245F and H). A vertical bar is attached to this joint, the lower end consisting of a flat base covered with soft dental compound pressed against the side of the nose. Elastic bands are employed to exert pressure against the side of the nose; gentle pressure should be applied, for the splint is used only to maintain the fractured bones in their corrected position.

COMMINUTED NASAL FRACTURES*

V. H. Kazanjian
and J. M. Converse

Comminuted fractures are generally characterized by marked flattening of the nasal bridge; the bones may be elevated into a satisfactory position if treated while the various fragments are still loose. Additional support is required for a few days to immobilize the fragments in the corrected positions. For this purpose, it is often necessary to pack the nasal cavity with petrolatum gauze strips; if the packing interferes with proper drainage, other methods must be employed to permit free drainage.

Suspension Methods. A wire appliance is employed by Kazanjian and Converse[93] as an internal support to elevate and immobilize the comminuted fragments of a nasal fracture. No. 14 gauge wire, 2 inches long, is bent to form a U. Small metal hooks are soldered to one of the arms of the U. A small piece of dental compound is softened and added to the smooth arm of the U-wire (Figure 18–245G). This is then introduced into the nose, well up under the comminuted nasal bones, and pressed against the displaced fragments, in order that the soft plastic dental compound may mold itself to the inner surface of the nose. The mold and wire are then removed, and after trimming the surplus compound, it is again inserted into the nose. A bar (10 gauge wire) with a hook on its lower end is extended from the forehead to the nose, and is retained by the cranial fixation appliance already described (Figure 18–245A to E). A small elastic band connects the intranasal and extranasal attachments (Figure 18–245G). The force exerted by the elastic is slight, merely enough to hold the bone fragments in position.

(Text continued on page 1323)

---

*Reprinted with permission from Kazanjian, V. H., and Converse, J. M.: The Surgical Treatment of Facial Injuries. 2nd ed. Baltimore, The Williams & Wilkins Co., 1959.

*Reprinted with permission from Kazanjian, V. H., and Convese, J. M.: The Surgical Treatment of Facial Injuries. 2nd ed. Baltimore, The Williams & Wilkins Co., 1959.

Photographic Case Report

TREATMENT OF NASAL FRACTURE WITH ALUMINUM SPLINT
Guillermo Raspall, D.D.S., M.D.

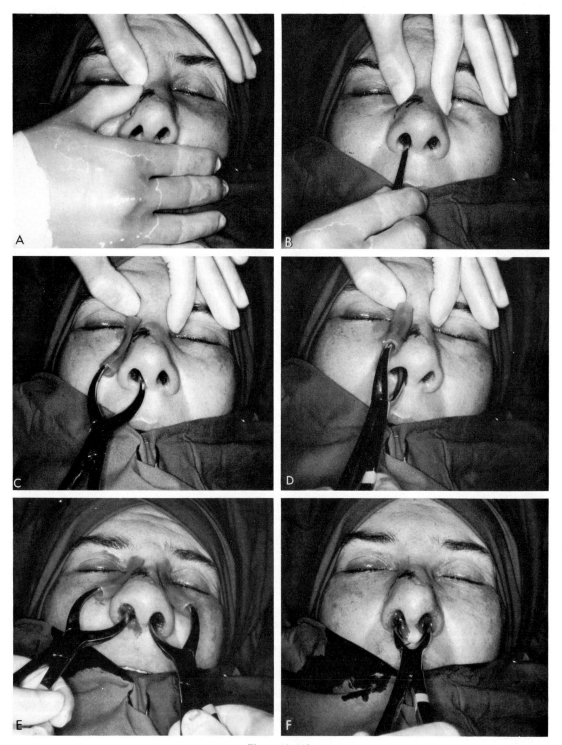

Figure 18–239

(Figure 18–239 continued on opposite page)

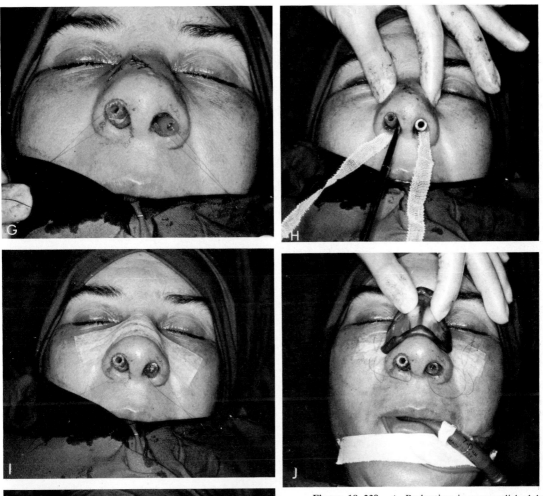

Figure 18–239 *A,* Reduction is accomplished by digital manipulation with thumb pressure.

B, Upward and forward elevation with an instrument manipulated under the nasal bones by one hand; the other hand molds the bones from the outside.

C, Reduction with Walsham's forceps. The unpadded blade is inserted into the nose, and the frontal process of the maxilla and the nasal bone are gripped between this blade and the padded blade, which is placed externally on the skin overlying the bone. Anterior traction and medial rotation are shown.

D, Lateral rotation and anterior traction.

E, Reduction with Walsham's forceps used simultaneously in both sides.

F, The septal cartilage is replaced accurately in the vomerine and maxillary grooves with an Asch septal forceps.

G, After reduction, small soft rubber draining tubes are placed in the floor of the nose to provide aeration of the nasopharynx.

H, Intranasal packs are inserted into the nasal cavity firmly for internal support of the structures during the course of healing.

I, Steri-Strips are placed externally molding the nose.

J, Nasal splint of thin aluminum is lined with dental impression compound or black gutta percha and fitted.

K, Fixation is effected by an elastic bandage (Elastoplast).

TREATMENT OF NASAL FRACTURE WITH WIRE AND LEAD PLATES
Guillermo Raspall, D.D.S., M.D.

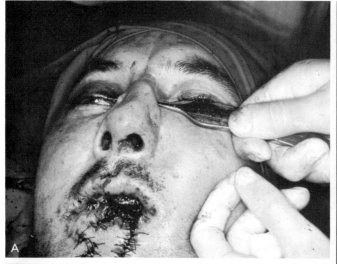

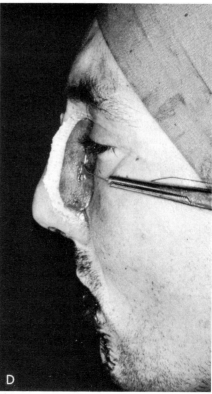

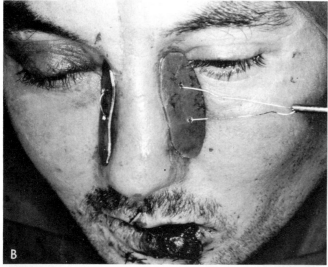

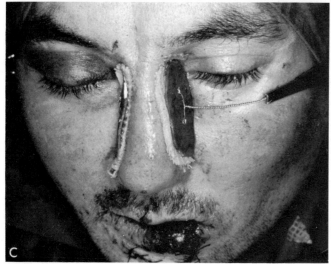

Figure 18–240 *A,* When the nasal fragments are unstable, or in the case of a depressed naso-ethmoid type of fracture, a horizontal mattress suture of 30 gauge stainless steel wire transfixes and stabilizes the comminuted nasal fragments and septum.

B to *D,* The wire is ligated over two oval lead plates of 2-mm. thickness and sized approximately 2 cm. by 1.5 cm. Tulle gras or absorbent rolled cotton is placed between the skin and the lead plates before the wires are tied together. The realigned fragments and lacerated nasal mucosa are additionally supported by an intranasal petrolatum gauze packing.

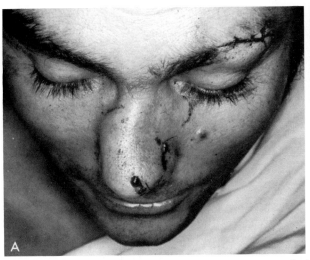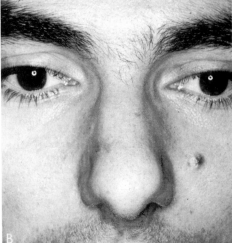

Figure 18–241 *A*, Preoperative appearance with laterally displaced nasal fracture. *B*, Postoperative appearance. (Courtesy of Guillermo Raspall, D.D.S., M.D.)

REPAIR OF FRACTURES*

LLOYD E. CHURCH

Irrespective of its mode of formation, bone, when fully developed, differs from other connective tissue in several respects. It is relatively cell-poor. The cells present are either widely separated from one another in lacunar spaces as osteocytes, or they are distributed as a single layer of cells upon the bone surfaces, where they constitute either the periosteal or endosteal layer.

*Adapted from Church, L. E.: Repair of fractures. Rev. Belg. Med. Dent., *14*:425–429, 1959.

When a bone is injured, the endosteal and periosteal cells respond by changing to large, rounded or cuboidal shaped cells, as mitotic figures appear. These cells are capable of producing the intercellular matrix of bone and they produce phosphatase which plays an important role in bringing about the deposition of bone salts. Thus the embryological sequences of bone formation are re-established.

From the time a bone is fractured until complete functional and anatomical restoration has been accomplished, one may observe morphological changes of a reparative nature. Although the processes by which a fractured bone is restored to normal are continuous, it

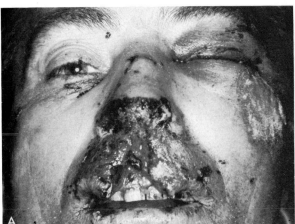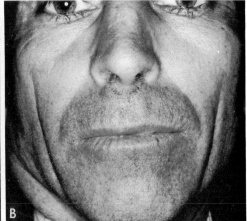

Figure 18–242 *A*, Preoperative appearance with depressed nasal fracture. *B*, Postoperative appearance. (Courtesy of Guillermo Raspall, D.D.S., M.D.)

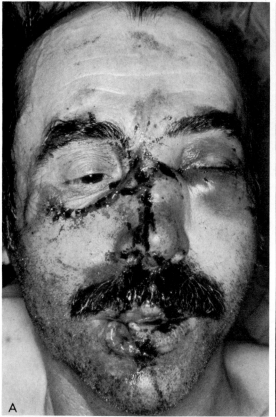

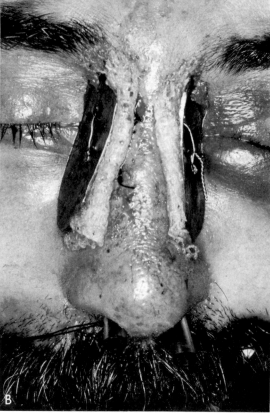

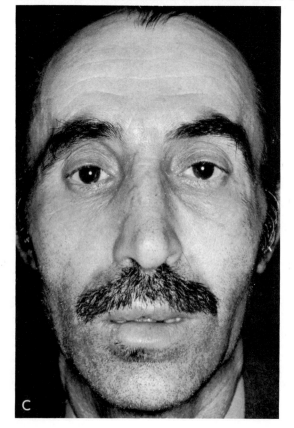

Figure 18–243   *A,* Preoperative appearance with depressed and unstable nasal fracture.
   B, Reduction and fixation with the through-and-through method shown in Figure 18–240.
   C, Postoperative appearance. (Courtesy of Guillermo Raspall, D.D.S., M.D.)

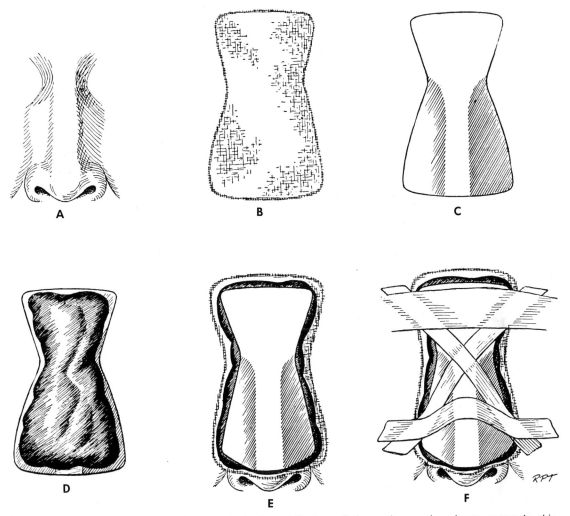

Figure 18–244 Nasal splint. *A,* The nose. *B,* A piece of lint is applied over the nose in order to protect the skin. *C,* A piece of tin splint, gauge 22, is cut and shaped. *D,* Softened dental compound is spread over the tin splint. *E,* Splint applied to nose. *F,* Splint retained with adhesive tape. (From Kazanjian and Converse: The Surgical Treatment of Facial Injuries. 2nd ed. Baltimore, The Williams & Wilkins Co., 1959.)

is convenient to discuss them in four stages, depending on the length of time since injury.

STAGE I: TRAUMA

Simultaneously with the occurrence of a fracture, the soft tissues within and around the bone are injured. The periosteum is torn or detached from the outer surface of the cortex. The endosteum is stripped from the surfaces of the marrow spaces, and this tissue is disrupted. Blood vessels and capillaries in all the adjacent soft tissues, as well as within the intraosseous vascular channels, are disrupted.

Such an injury results in the production of a hematoma, surrounding the ends of the fractured bone. At the same time there is hyperemia, extravasation of the edema fluid, and beginning inflammatory cell infiltration. Fibrin is formed at the periphery of the hematoma beneath the detached periosteum, and between the ends of the fractured bone. The injured parts are thus joined together by a loose-meshed, fibrinous framework, which serves as a scaffold upon which subsequent granulation tissue may grow. In a fracture, the detachment and displacement of the periosteum are greater at the point of fracture

(Text continued on page 1329)

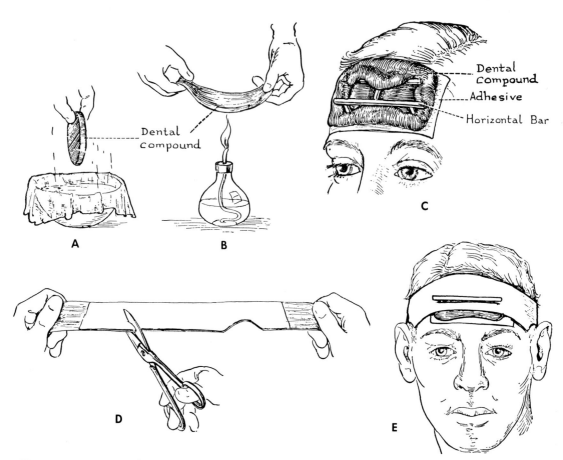

Figure 18–245 Method of application of the Kazanjian splint. *A*, Dental compound is softened in hot water. *B*, Dental compound is passed over an open flame to make it more adherent. *C*, The frame of the splint is embedded into the dental compound on the forehead, leaving the horizontal bar exposed. *D*, Method of preparing adhesive tape to be placed around the head. *E*, Adhesive tape anchoring the frame of the splint on the forehead. A plaster bandage may be used to hold the frame in position.

F, This splint is anchored to the forehead as shown in *E* and *G*. It consists of a metal frame (*1*), and a horizontal bar (*2*), to which is attached a joint (*3*). The arm (*4*) is held by the joint and may be placed in the desired position by varying the position of the joint (*3*).

G, U-splint for suspension of comminuted nasal bones. (*1*) Softened compound is placed over one branch of the splint. This branch is then introduced into the nasal cavity and molded to the under-surface of the nasal bridge. (*2*), Suspension and elevation of the comminuted bony bridge is obtained by elastic traction with the appliance shown in *F*.

H, The skin of the nose is protected by adhesive (*1*); a small pad of compound has been molded to the nose after being placed over the pad of the arm (*2*); the joint (*3*) is placed in the position best suited for the case. Elastic pressure is exerted between the frame (*4*) and the arm (*5*). *I*, To protect the nose from excessive pressure the stop (*6*) may be applied. Note alternate position of elastic band. *J*, Lateral view of the appliance.

(From Kazanjian and Converse: The Surgical Treatment of Facial Injuries. 2nd ed. Baltimore, The Williams & Wilkins Co., 1959.)

(Figure 18–245 continued on opposite page)

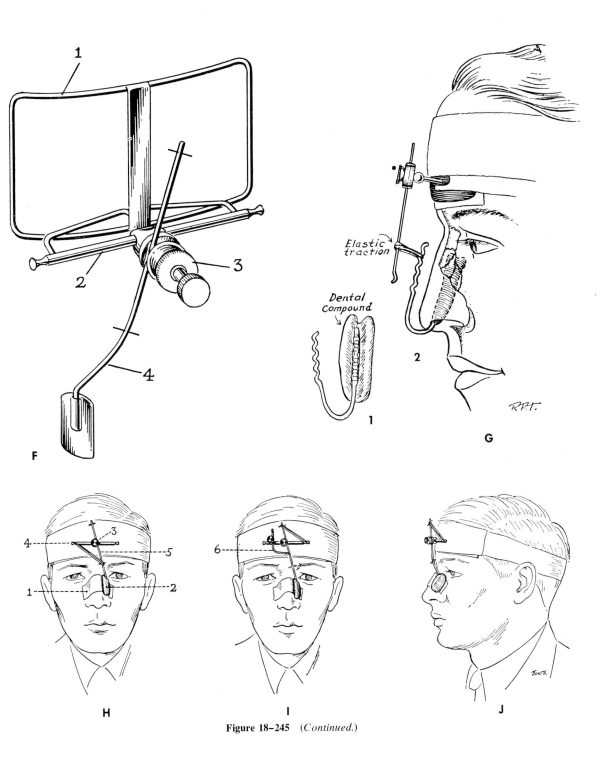

Figure 18–245 (*Continued.*)

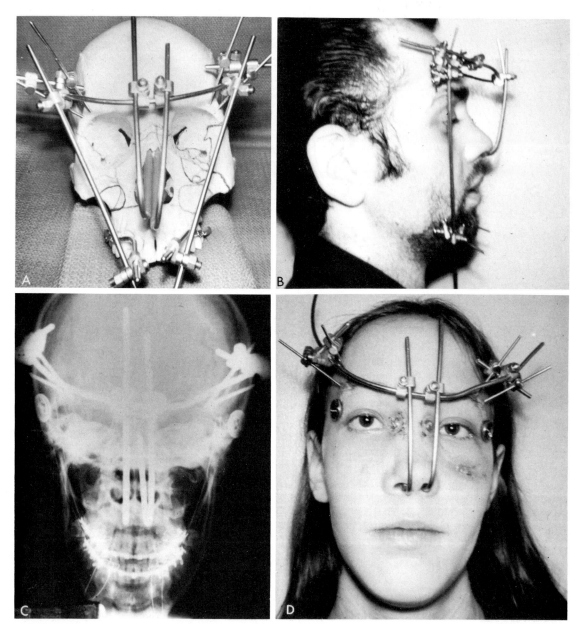

Figure 18–246 *A,* Supraorbital pin head frame with nasal supports. This head frame is the same as that described in Figure 18–230, but this photograph shows how nasal fractures as well as fractures of the maxilla would be supported.

B, Patient treated for a nasal fracture and fractures of the mandible and maxilla, as described in Figure 18–230.

C, Radiograph of a fractured nose during treatment. In addition the fractured portion of the maxilla (Le Fort I) is held in apposition with the superior portion of the maxilla by wires from the lateral orbital rim (see buttons in *D* and *E*). The maxillary and mandibular teeth are held in correct occlusion during healing by intermaxillary elastics.

F, Severely traumatized patient with multiple fractures of nasal and temporal bones and cerebrospinal rhinorrhea treated as shown in *D* and *E*. (Courtesy of T. William Evans, D.D.S., M.D.)

(Figure 18–246 continued on opposite page)

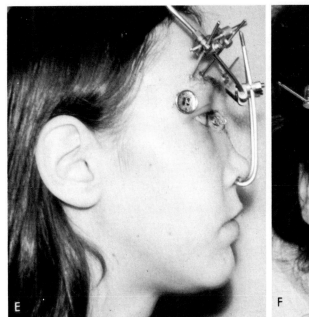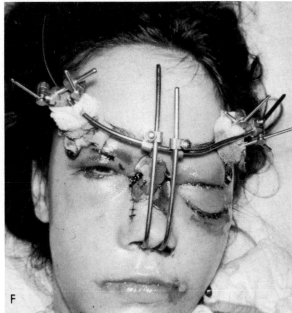

Figure 18–246   *(Continued.)*

than they are at more distant levels. Thus the area of hemorrhage and exudation early assumes a fusiform shape which is usually maintained throughout the process of healing.

STAGE II: ORGANIZATION

During the first 24 to 48 hours after injury, the inflammatory and exudative changes increase. Leukocytes appear in large numbers. The tissues become swollen and indurated from the extravasation of blood and edema fluid. Fibrin precipitation increases steadily. These cellular alterations represent the earliest stages of repair. The fibrin clot between the ends of the fractured bone undergoes organization, followed by proliferation of connective tissue cells, and budding of capillary endothelium to form granulation tissue. In addition to the numerous polymorphonuclear leukocytes that are present during the early stages, one now observes increasing numbers of mononuclear phagocytes, apparently phagocytizing necrotic cells and tissue debris.

Up to this point the healing and repair of a fracture and any soft tissue wound are similar. In each case collagenous fibrils are deposited between proliferating connective tissue cells. In the fracture, such fibrillar ground substance is obscured by deposition of a homogeneous hyaline matrix. The appearance of this specialized intercellular matrix constitutes the first demonstrable evidence of bone formation.

Due to the peculiar origin and distribution of the blood supply of bone, extensive necrosis may be present. Following injury such necrosis will be evidenced by empty lacunar spaces in the bone, adjacent to the fracture line. These areas of bone necrosis involve a few millimeters to a centimeter or so on either side of the point of injury. The rate of resorption of this devitalized bone varies in every case.

STAGE III: UNION BY CALLUS FORMATION

By the end of the first week, the process of intramembranous bone formation is present in most fractures. While new and indistinct bars of homogenous osteoid matrix are being deposited between the proliferating cells, connective tissue cells assume the shape and function of osteoblasts. They align themselves in solid rows along one border of each new bar of matrix, and apparently aid in the formation of new matrix. Some of these cells become surrounded by their own matrix, and thus become osteocytes.

New osseous tissue is laid down beneath the detached periosteum to form a tubular sleeve of external callus. This may be subdivided into bridging and buttressing callus. It

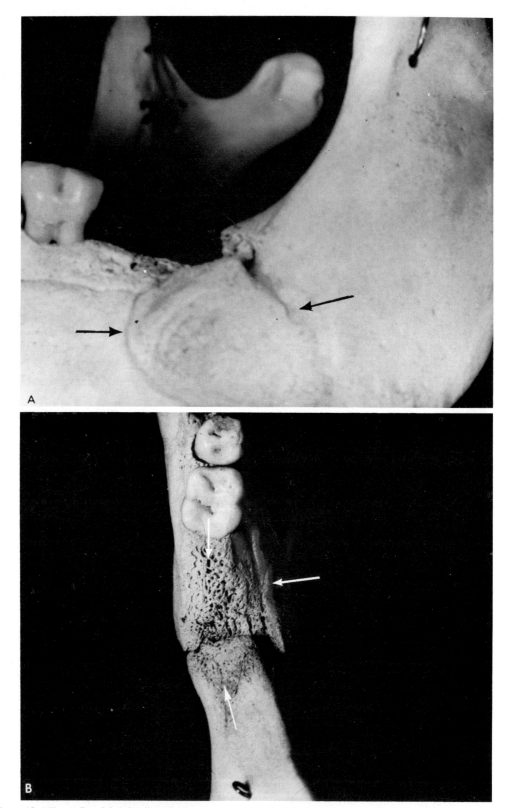

Figure 18–247 *A*, Provisional callus (between arrows; see also *B*), thrown out as nature's splint to keep the ends of the bone in apposition while healing takes place. It is absorbed after union is complete. *B*, Note the marked increase in the vascularity of the bone on either side of the fracture line.

is also deposited in the medullary canal near the ends of the fractured bone as endosteal callus. Gradually, such osseous tissue grows inward from the periphery of the hematoma, and ultimately replaces it. At the widest part of the spindle overlying the actual site of fracture, cartilage is present. Whether osteogenic cells differentiate into cartilage or bone may depend on the vascular environment in which they differentiate. Therefore, if the environment is vascular they differentiate into osteoblasts, and form bone. If the environment is poor in vascularity, as in the center of the spindle-shaped clot, they differentiate into chondroblasts, and form cartilage. However, age, health, and local factors also influence the capacity of an individual to produce cartilage.

The appearance of cartilage in the callus is most prominent in fractures of long bones with displacement or large defects. Here the cartilage serves as a quick, temporary filling material for later replacement and bridging of the defect by new bone. Small drill holes and thin saw cuts produce relatively little cartilage, and are repaired chiefly by growth of connective tissue cells and osteoblasts from one surface to another. Long bones, formed as cartilage models in fetal life, more commonly produce cartilage in a fracture callus. Flat bones, formed by intramembranous ossification, usually heal without the appearance of cartilage. Regeneration of bone and filling of defects, as in the calvarium, usually fail in adult life.

New bone does not form at random within the callus, but grows by extension of periosteal and endosteal new bone toward the fracture gap, enveloping and replacing the fibrocartilaginous callus.

It appears that cartilage has an active, rather than passive, influence in osteogenesis, possibly through the mechanisms of induction.

STAGE IV: REARRANGEMENT OF THE CALLUS, BONY UNION AND RECONSTRUCTION

In the average fracture, the callus attains its maximum size in 2 or 3 weeks. There is a progressive increase in its density, due to the continuous addition of new osseous tissue, and increased deposition of bone salts.

The external or subperiosteal callus is first formed largely of trabeculae that radiate transversely from the shaft of the bone. Between the ends of the fractured bone the initial callus has very little discernible structure. Rearrangement of this new bone takes place in subsequent weeks. This is accomplished by resorption of certain portions of the first trabeculae by osteoclastic action and addition of bone to other trabeculae by osteoblastic action and is determined largely by stresses and strains to which the callus is subjected. The original osseous structures are gradually resorbed, and firm attachments between the old and new bony parts are re-established. The amount of osseous tissue comprising a callus gradually diminishes. This process of adaptation continues for many months or years, leaving only the bone required for union of the fracture ends. This varies with the bone involved and the amount of motion present.

The shape of the callus and the volume of tissue required to bridge a fracture depend upon the amount of bone damage, and displacement. Healing time is directly proportional to the total volume of damaged bone, and the breadth of the fracture defect.

The local process and the systemic factors in bone repair are interdependent. The callus appears to hold the highest priority on all tissue-building material in transport, regardless of the general condition of the patient. Metabolic balance studies with nitrogen, phosphorus, potassium, sulfur, and other elements indicate that muscle tissue catabolism may supply many of the materials needed for building bone matrix. The body actually elects to catabolize muscle to meet the exigency of the moment, when there is need for rapid reconstruction of new bone.

The growing callus is calcified in the same way as are cartilage and bone in the normal skeleton.

There is wide variation in the time required for complete healing of fractures, and many factors influence the repair process. Interposition of soft tissue between fragments, infection, disturbance of nutrition, and impairment of blood supply all play an important part in healing of fractures. Adequate immobilization is one of the most important factors in promoting rapid and complete union. Failure in this will lead to tissue injury. In some cases the cartilaginous and bony callus is replaced by more yielding fibrous tissue which will not revert to bone. Occasionally a pseudoarthrosis results, complete with a joint cavity.

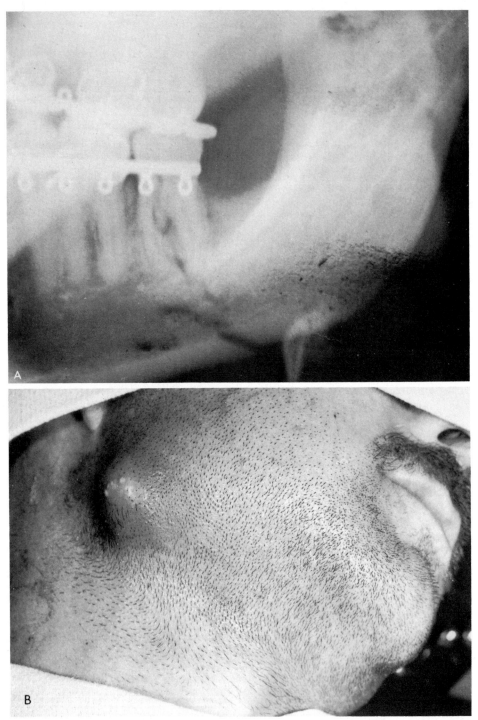

Figure 18–248 The reader is urged to review the discussion of infection in Chapter 10. *A,* A tooth in the line of fracture has become infected. This is not a frequent occurrence (see discussion of this subject earlier in this chapter). *B,* Well-circumscribed abscess almost ready to rupture and drain spontaneously. As pointed out in Chapter 10, an incision for drainage is preferable because this leaves only a small scar, which is much less noticeable than that which follows spontaneous rupture of the skin and drainage. In the latter case a healed pressure necrosis scar forms.

Discussion: Besides drainage, treatment must include extraction of the infected second molar, which has kept the ramus in its normal relationship with the body of the mandible. The posterior fragment, the ramus, must now be held in correct alignment, preferably by extraoral skeletal pin fixation, but alternatively by some other device.

The following basic rules seem amply justified in all fractures:

1. The fractured bone fragments should be placed in the most advantageous position at the earliest possible moment.
2. Once satisfactory alignment and close apposition have been obtained, the part should be immobilized.
3. Immobilization should be maintained until union has been established, or until it has been determined that healing has failed to take place, and that other therapeutic measures are required.

COMPLICATIONS OF FRACTURES

Infections. *Cellulitis* and *osteomyelitis* are the most frequent complications of fractures of the mandible and maxilla.

Since most fractures are compound fractures, infection may develop because of con-

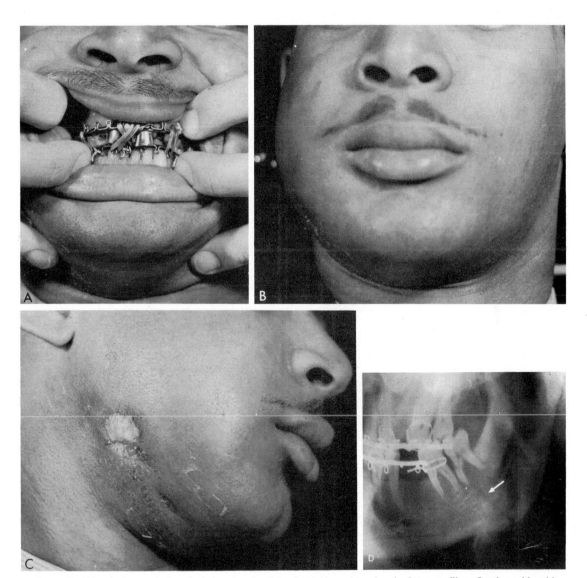

Figure 18–249 *A*, An exceptionally heavy application of anterior rubber bands. Intermaxillary fixation with rubber elastics in the area of the anterior teeth, as shown here, must be applied only when the *splints* are primarily carrying the pressure exerted by the elastics, *not the anterior teeth*. Otherwise these teeth will be withdrawn from their alveoli and possibly lost.

B, Edema due to infection. *C*, Spontaneous rupture of the abscess through the skin with a continuously draining fistula. *D*, Infected third molar in the line of fracture. This was extracted, and the posterior fragment was maintained in position during healing by extraoral skeletal pin fixation (Frac-Sur) units.

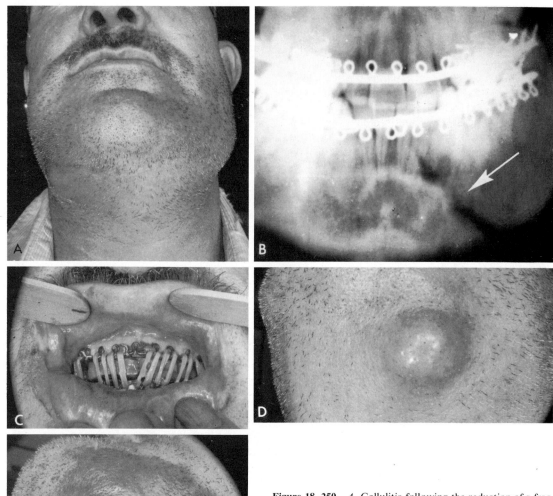

Figure 18–250 *A*, Cellulitis following the reduction of a fracture of the mandible (*B*) in the bicuspid area. *C*, Intermaxillary fixation. *D*, Swelling resolved, followed by this well-circumscribed and localized subcutaneous abscess. *E*, Incision and drainage.

tact with oral secretions or outside air. When infection occurs, establish drainage and administer penicillin and sulfonamides.

Since the mouth is the filthiest orifice of the body, it is surprising that more infections do not follow compound jaw fractures.

Although the time required for healing of various fractures of the jaws or facial bones cannot be predetermined in an individual case, experience has shown that for a certain type of fracture or fractures in a particular age group, sufficient healing should take place in a fairly constant number of weeks to permit

removal of the splints and moderate function. If this usual time has elapsed and the trial removal of the immobilizing device permits the bony segments to separate, then the splints are replaced for an additional week or more until union does occur. A complete physical examination with blood studies is ordered if these have not already been done to help determine a cause for the slow healing.

Suppuration at the fracture lines, of course, will delay healing. While the incidence of osteomyelitis in fracture cases is very low, it does occur and if present should be treated.

(*Text continued on page 1339*)

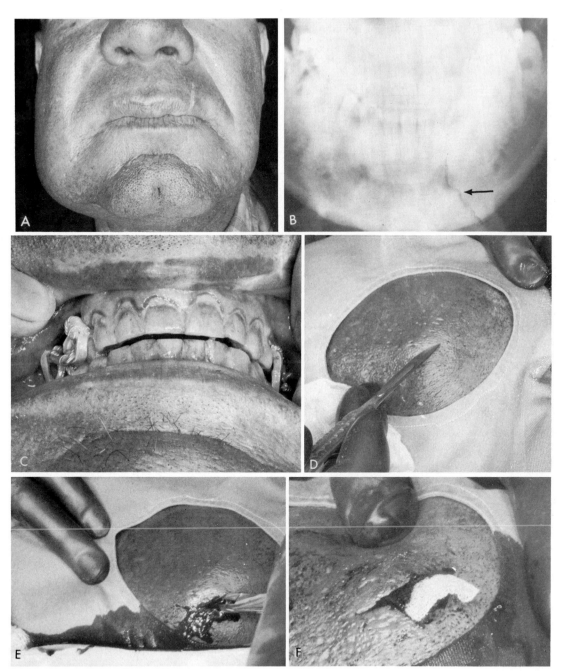

Figure 18–251 *A*, Cellulitis with edema as a result of infection from a simple linear fracture (*B*), with no separation of the fragments. *C*, Minimal fixation. *D*, Localization of pus. *E*, Incision and drainage. *F*, Iodoform gauze drain.

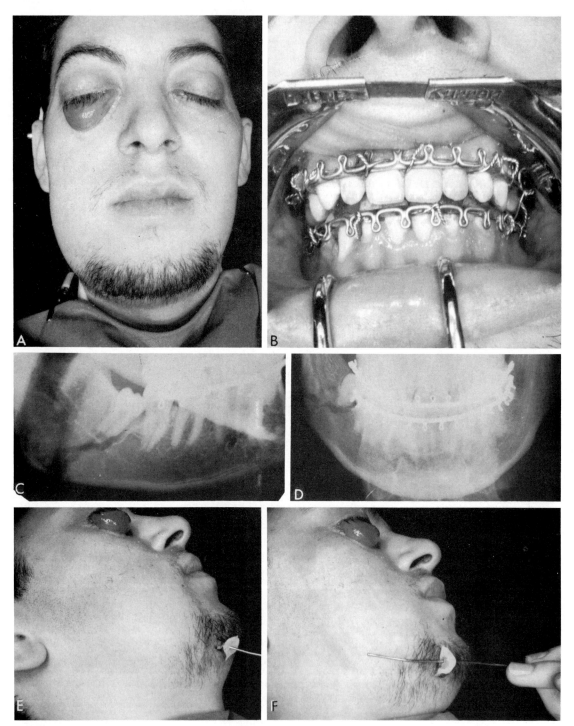

Figure 18–252 *A*, Extension of infection from a mandibular fracture (*C* and *D*) in the third molar area.

B, Intermaxillary fixation. (*Note:* We do not now use intermaxillary wiring for reasons already stated.)

C and *D*, Fracture line along the edge of the mesioangularly impacted third molar.

E, The interesting factors in this case were the lack of swelling other than a minimum, the extension of the infection to the orbital cavity, and the formation of a fistula that drained at the right lower border of the symphysis, as shown here. We inserted a probe easily to the origin of the fistula.

F, The rubber disc shows the depth to which the probe was easily inserted. Placed on the face, the tip of the probe reached the mandibular third molar area, the location of the fracture. Treatment included the removal of the impacted third molar and immobilization of the ramus by extraoral skeletal fixation. Intraoral drainage was adequate, and the infection subsided. This was in the ''preantibiotic'' days.

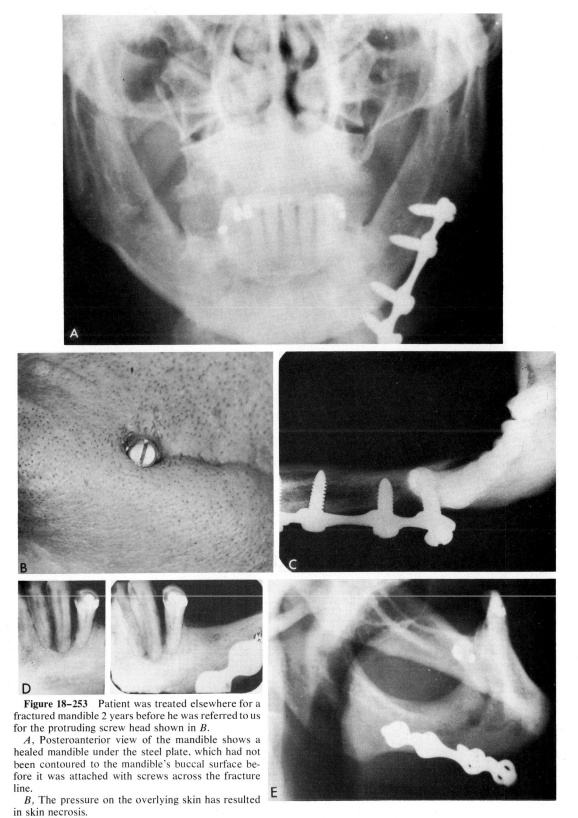

Figure 18–253   Patient was treated elsewhere for a fractured mandible 2 years before he was referred to us for the protruding screw head shown in *B*.

A, Posteroanterior view of the mandible shows a healed mandible under the steel plate, which had not been contoured to the mandible's buccal surface before it was attached with screws across the fracture line.

B, The pressure on the overlying skin has resulted in skin necrosis.

C to *E*, Additional radiographs, confirming the radiographic evidence in *A*. *Note:* Because of the distortions that occur in radiography, it is essential to take a variety of different views and angles to reduce to a minimum errors in interpretation.

Treatment: Removal of plate and closure of fistula.

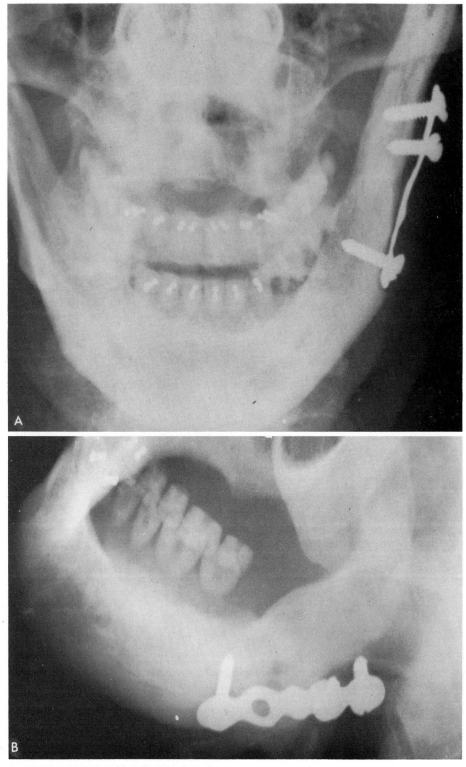

Figure 18–254 *A,* Another referred case, a patient whose fracture of the mandibular angle was "fixed" with a noncontoured steel bone plate. There is a draining fistula in the face. *B,* It is apparent from radiographs that the bone plate was not correctly lined up over the fracture line because one of the openings in the plate was over the fracture area and so only three screws could be inserted. It is surprising that the end result was this good. *Treatment:* Removal of screws and plate. Drainage then ceased.

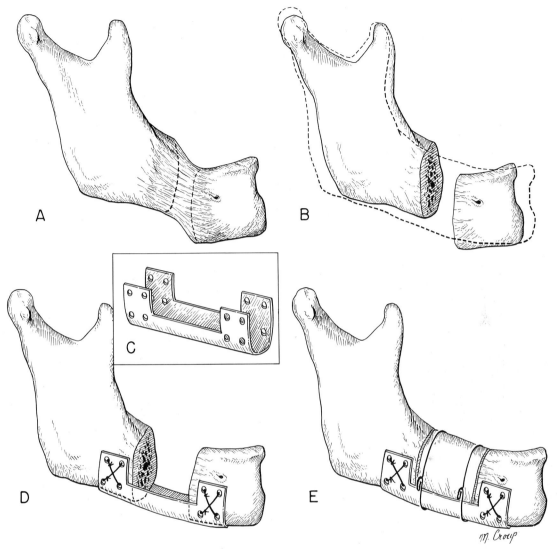

Figure 18–255   Treatment of a fibrous union of the mandible following the loss of bone substance because of a pathologic condition or trauma.

A, Fibrous union over rounded, eburnated ends of the mandible.

B, After extraoral exposure the cortical bone over the rounded ends is removed with the Stryker saw and the ends squared at the same time. The broken line shows the desired ultimate correct length and position of the fragments of the mandible.

C, A tantalum plate is cut and contoured as shown to form a trough.

D, The trough is adapted to the exposed bone ends and wired into position. It is also possible to screw this plate into position.

E, A segment of the crest of the ilium is cut and contoured to fit the space created and is placed in the trough, where it is held by circumferential wires. The wound is then closed.

If there is a tooth in the line of fracture and there is suppuration, the tooth should be extracted.

Injury to Nerves and Blood Vessels.   In mandibular fractures, numbness of the lower lip indicates that the contents of the mandibular canal (mandibular nerve and blood vessels) have been injured or severed. Normal sensation will usually return to the lip in time, except in cases of comminuted fractures. In an extensive comminuted fracture some bone is usually lost because of infection. However, *bone fragments should not be removed* until it is definitely proved that they are nonvital.

Malunion.   This means that the fractured segments have healed but not in correct ana-

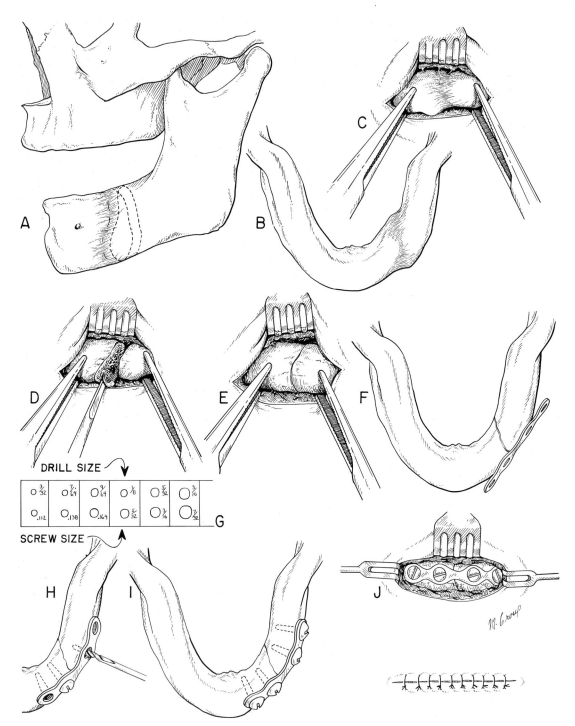

DRILL SIZE

| O $\frac{3}{32}$ | O $\frac{7}{64}$ | O $\frac{9}{64}$ | O $\frac{1}{8}$ | O $\frac{5}{32}$ | O $\frac{3}{16}$ |
| O .112 | O .138 | O .164 | O $\frac{5}{32}$ | O $\frac{3}{16}$ | O $\frac{7}{32}$ |

SCREW SIZE

Figure 18–256 Use of internal plate fixation in treatment of fibrous union of a fractured mandible. *A* and *B*, Drawing showing deformity of lateral surface of jaw in second molar area. Note lateral bulge in occlusal view as well as shortening of affected side. This deformity is obviously due to lateral anterior overriding of the proximal fragment (masseter and temporal muscle pull) and medial rotation of the distal fragment (mylohyoid muscle pull). Improperly reduced, there is now facial deformity and malocclusion. *C*, Fracture site exposed by extraoral incision. *D*, Mandible refractured and bone ends freshened and contoured with chisel and mallet. *E*, Fracture repositioned correctly. *F*, Sherman bone plate measured for size. *G*, Suitable screws must be selected for fastening the plate. As seen in the chart, the size of the

(Legend continued on opposite page.)

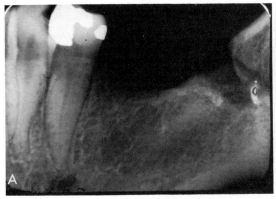 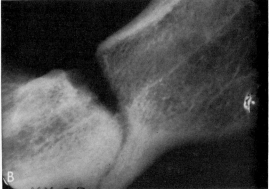

Figure 18–257 *A,* Incompletely healed fracture, cause unknown. Incomplete healing was probably due to an interposition of soft tissue between the fracture ends that was not removed at the time of reduction. We have seen voids this large that were bridged with bone when a fracture healed. *B,* The patient has normal sensation in his lip. An examination of the inferior alveolar canal in this periapical radiograph shows that the contents of the inferior alveolar canal must be contained for a short distance in the soft tissue within this space.

Treatment: In my opinion there was a possibility of injury to the neurovascular bundle if the soft tissue in this space was removed. Because of this possibility the patient did not want surgery; he was not concerned about the increased risk of a fracture. As a result, no operation was performed.

tomic relationship; the occlusal plane or occlusion is wrong. Treatment may necessitate refracturing and resetting if there is an extensive disturbance to the occlusion. Also it may necessitate the extraction of several judiciously chosen teeth and the construction of a dental prosthesis.

Fibrous Union. In the treatment of fibrous union open reduction permits, as a rule, better access for the removal of fibrous tissue from the fracture line and for the freshening of the fractured ends. This is particularly true in cases of several months' duration in which the fractured ends have become covered with cortical bone, or in cases in which there has been extensive loss of bone at the fracture site. Such a case is illustrated in Figure 18–255, in which a fibrous union of the mandible is treated and the contour of the mandible is restored by a bone graft at the same time.

In Figure 18–261 is shown the open reduction of a fibrous union of a fracture of an edentulous mandible.

Nonunion. This means that the fractured ends have not healed together. Nonunion may occur because (*a*) the fragments have not been held rigidly; (*b*) reduction of the fragments has been delayed too long; (*c*) appliances have been removed too soon; (*d*) soft tissue has become interposed between widely separated bony fragments; (*e*) an abscessed tooth was allowed to remain too long in the line of fracture; (*f*) good drainage was not established in the presence of osteomyelitis; or because of (*g*) diabetes or (*h*) syphilis.

TREATMENT OF NONUNION. The treatment is based on the reason for the nonunion. Every oral surgeon of any experience has seen many cases of fractured mandibles heal satisfactorily with an abscessed tooth in the line of fracture. When there is nonunion after a lapse of 6 to 8 weeks, and there is an abscessed tooth in the line of fracture, obviously the extraction of this tooth is indicated.

When all reasons for nonunion have been eliminated, and much more time has passed

Figure 18–256 *(Continued.)*
drill is slightly smaller than that of the screw to insure a snug fit and yet not create enough pressure to split the bone. The length of the screws must be such as to engage the lingual cortex or else the plate may bend or the screws loosen. Ideally there should be two screws on each side of the fracture line to eliminate rotational stress. *H,* The plate is contoured to the bone and one screw hole is drilled and the screw inserted. This helps fix the plate solidly to allow accurate drilling of the other holes. A hand drill is preferable to an engine drill, for there is less chance of producing thermal bone necrosis. *I,* The other holes are drilled and the screws inserted. *J,* Lateral view of plate and closure of incision in layers. See actual case illustrated in Figure 18–261.

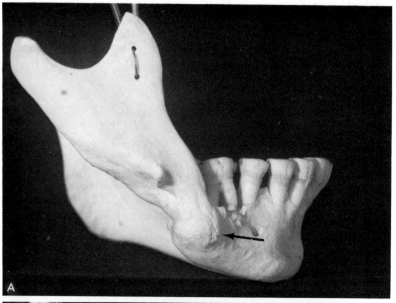

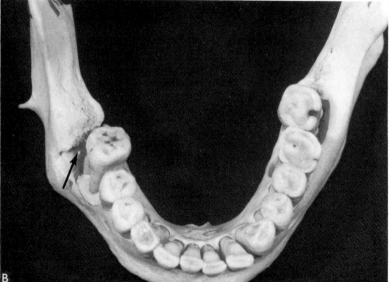

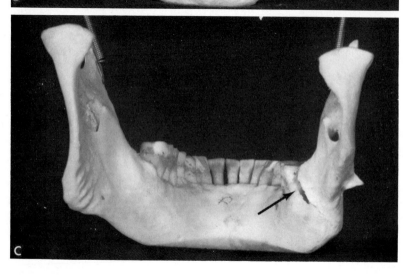

Figure 18–258 *A*, Anatomic specimen of what appears to have been a compound comminuted fracture of the angle of the mandible. In *B* and *C* can be seen a wide-open space in which there is no evidence of any osseous healing. One can surmise that there was chronic infection in this area. However, it did not interfere with osseous union in the lower third of the fracture.

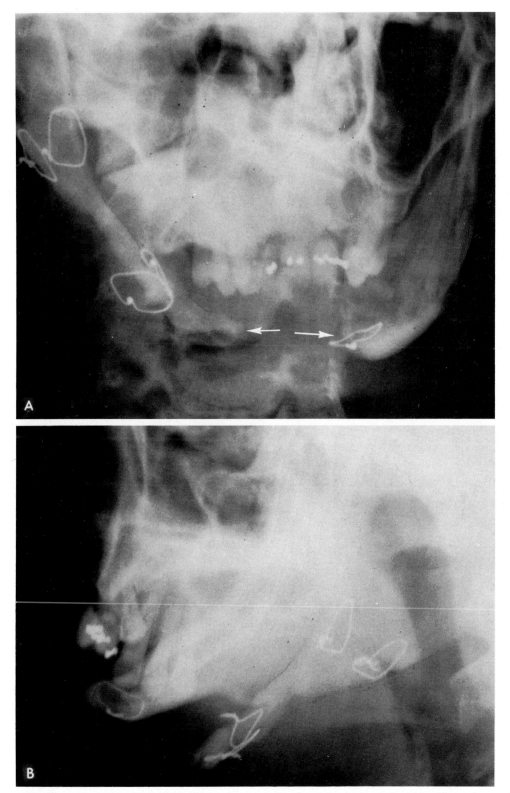

Figure 18–259 *A*, Extensive rib grafting had been done to replace lost bone 2 years before this radiograph was taken. Note the resorption of a major area of the anterior portion of the rib. *B*, Oblique radiograph shows this loss of the graft, which has steadily been increasing with time.

Note: This "melting away" of rib grafts has resulted in a decreasing use of these grafts to replace lost mandibular bone. (Read Chapter 23, "Transplantation and Grafting Procedures in Oral Surgery.")

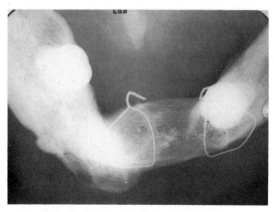

Figure 18–260   A graft from the crest of the ilium to the mandible with no sign of resorption after 5 years.

than is usually required for healing of the fracture of the type under treatment, then other measures must be considered.

One possibility is exposure of the fractured bony ends by the extraoral route, and careful removal of the fibrous tissue covering and separating the bony ends. Then a series of holes is drilled with spear-pointed drills into the exposed ends. This produces new channels through which blood may escape to form a hematoma and subsequently granulation tissue, and then perhaps a callus will form if the fragments are held rigid and the operation has been carried out under rigid asepsis.

Another method to be considered is bone grafting (see Chapter 23, "Transplantation and Grafting Procedures in Oral Surgery"). If

Photographic Case Report

OPEN REDUCTION OF A FRACTURED MANDIBLE WITH FIBROUS UNION

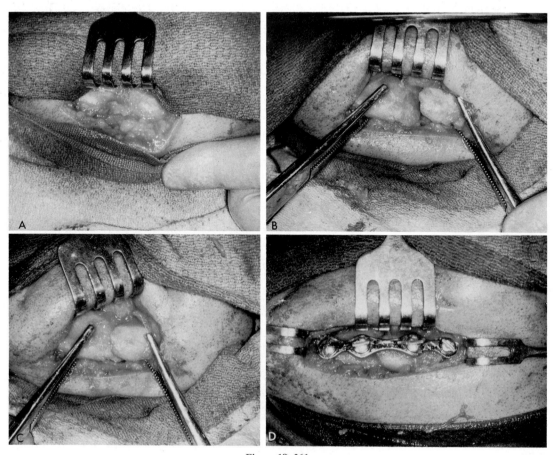

Figure 18–261

(Figure 18–261 continued on opposite page)

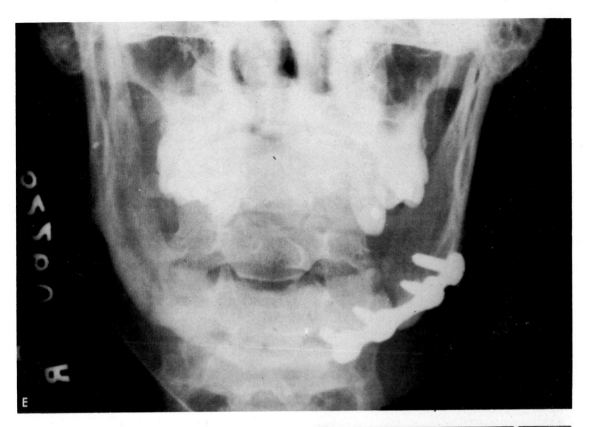

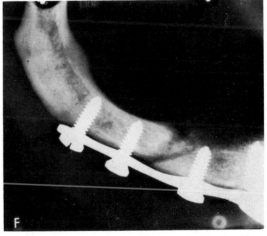

Figure 18–261 *A,* Exposure of fibrous union of the edentulous mandible. *B,* Fibrous tissue excised and the oblique ends of the fracture freshened so that there are many bleeding points. *C,* Fractured ends aligned. *D,* Fracture reduced and immobilized with a bone plate. *E,* Postoperative posteroanterior radiograph showing correct apposition of the parts. *F,* Occlusal x-ray film showing bone plate and screws for fixation of the fractured mandible shown in *E.*

there has been considerable loss of bone substance due to osteomyelitis, and wide separation of the bony ends, then bone grafting is indicated. Before attempting bone grafting, it must be definitely determined that no infection is present at the fracture site. Likewise extreme care must be exercised at the time of operation to prevent any communication from the operative site into the oral cavity. In either case it is practically certain that the bone graft will be lost.

Regardless of the method of bone grafting, careful thought must be devoted to planning both the operation and the method of immobilization. Reliance should not be placed on the fixation of the graft to maintain immobilization. Ideally, the maintenance of the teeth in normal occlusion by intermaxillary elastics will rigidly hold the fragments in position and prevent strain on the graft. When this is not possible, the ingenuity of the oral surgeon is required to bring about the necessary stability.

Case Report No. 10

BILATERAL FRACTURES OF BODY OF MANDIBLE WITH NONUNION OF RIGHT FRAGMENTS CORRECTED BY BONE GRAFT*

A 23-year-old man was referred to the oral surgery service for diagnosis and treatment of pain in the right mandible and inability to masticate food properly because his teeth did not occlude.

Three years ago the patient was struck across the face by a steel cable while having his automobile towed. The patient suffered bilateral fractures of the mandible, loss of his maxillary teeth, fracture of the left wrist and right index finger, and multiple lacerations of the face. The patient was treated at another hospital, where his mandibular fractures were reduced by extraoral open reduction with transosseous wiring.

Oral Examination. The maxilla was edentulous and the patient was wearing a full denture. Mandibular teeth present included those from the right lateral incisor to the left first molar. The centrals and the right lateral were quite mobile due to an extreme loss of alveolar bone in this area. Radiographic examination revealed a healed fracture of the left body of the mandible and a nonunited fracture of the right body with loss of bone between the parts, whose ends were rounded and covered with cortical bone. The left mandible was displaced medially and inferiorly, the right posterior fragment was displaced medially and superiorly (see Figure 18–262). Individual movements of the two fragments could be observed by applying manual pressure to each fragment separately. The area between the two fragments was filled with dense fibrous connective tissue.

Treatment. Under local anesthesia, the mandibular central incisors and the right lateral incisor were extracted, and an Erich arch bar was ligated to the remaining mandibular teeth. The patient's maxillary denture, with an Erich arch bar attached, was secured to the maxilla with Roger Anderson pins. Intermaxillary elastics were applied to move and maintain the left mandible in correct relationship to the maxilla. One week later, under local anesthesia, a Stader splint was applied to the right mandibular segments in order to distract the fragments into their normal relationship and maintain them in position (see Figure 18–262B). Over a period of 2 weeks, by properly adjusting the Stader splint, the fragments were moved, restoring the contour of the mandible. It was now apparent that approximately 5 cm. of bone had been lost from the body of the right mandible. It was decided to take a bone graft from the right iliac crest to repair this defect.

Procedure. The intermaxillary elastics were removed and under intravenous Pentothal and nasoendotracheal nitrous oxide-oxygen-ether anes-

thesia, with plastic and oral surgery teams working together, the face and right iliac crest area were prepared with tincture of green soap, ether, alcohol and Merthiolate. The operative fields were draped with sterile drapes. An incision was made 4 cm. below the inferior border of the right mandible, starting just anterior to the angle and ending at the symphysis. A flap was elevated superiorly, exposing the ends of the fragments. With a periosteal elevator, the periosteum was stripped back for approximately 3 cm. on the ends of the fragments. A segment of bone measuring approximately 5 cm. in length and 3 cm. in width was removed from the right iliac crest. The segment of bone was trimmed to the correct size and placed in the defect so that the cortex would be to the buccal side and the medullary portion to the lingual side. Two holes were drilled in the end of each fragment, and two holes were drilled on each end of the bone graft. Using 23 gauge stainless steel wire, the bone graft was secured in position by transosseous wiring. The soft tissues were replaced and the incision was closed with interrupted subcutaneous sutures using 5–0 white silk, and interrupted sutures on the skin surface using 6–0 black silk. A sterile dressing was applied over the incision. *Note:* This procedure was carried out with the Stader splint in position (see Figure 18–262C for postoperative x-ray). The patient tolerated the procedure well and returned to the ward in good condition.

Two days postoperatively the intermaxillary elastics were reapplied. Two days later slight movement was noted between the mandible and maxilla, and the elastics were supplemented by intermaxillary wires, since the wires would aid in immobilization.

Eight weeks postoperatively the intermaxillary wires and intraoral appliances were removed. Fourteen weeks postoperatively the Stader splint was removed. Radiographs taken at this time revealed a "take" of the graft and the fragments in satisfactory alignment. (See Figure 18–262D; Figure 18–262F shows the healed left fracture.)

The patient was discharged from the hospital at this time and was followed by periodic examinations as an outpatient. Over a period of 2 years the results have remained satisfactory.

---

*Case report prepared by Frank J. Moore, D.D.S., Oral Surgery Intern, Veterans Administration Hospital, Pittsburgh, Pa.

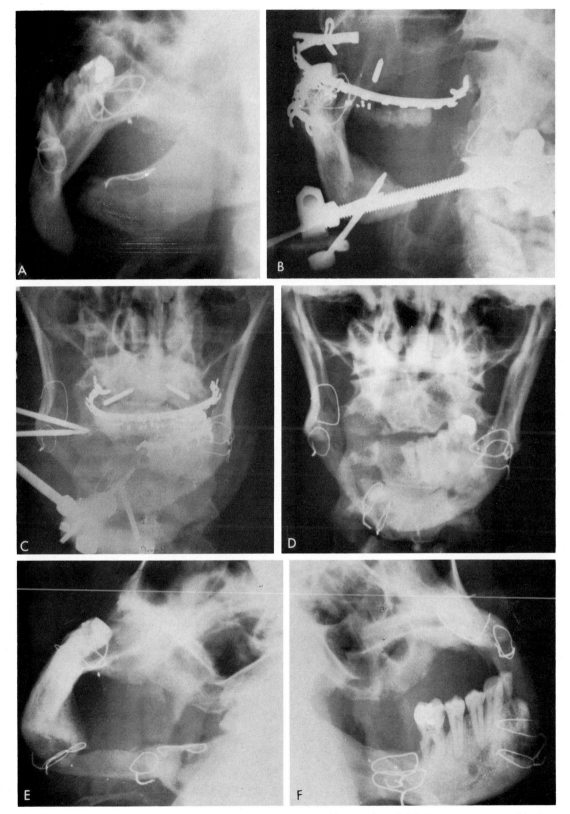

Figure 18–262 Bilateral fractures of the body of the mandible with nonunion of right fragments, corrected by bone graft. (See Case Report No. 10.)

TREATMENT OF MANDIBULAR NONUNION

Norman R. Nathanson, D.D.S.

Two characteristics of nonunion are osteo-porosis of the fragments or eburnation of the fractured ends with resulting pseudoarthrosis.

Callus formation, a growth process from the fractured bone ends, is essential for healing. The production of callus does not continue indefinitely. If the bone ends are close together, the calluses will meet and unite more rapidly than if they are far apart. If the bone ends are too far apart or if the fractured ends are in motion, the calluses will fail to meet, causing fibrous nonunion.

Nonunion accompanied by malunion may result in permanent functional disturbances affecting the mobility of the jaw and in malocclusion that detracts from the patient's appearance. In unilateral fractures, crossbite will occur if occlusion becomes deficient, which can be the cause of scar contraction.

If the length of the jaw is adequate, mandibular nonunion is treated by open operation. Scar tissue can thus be excised, which freshens the fractured bone ends and aids effective reduction and fixation. After the ends of the fragments are freshened, no shortening should occur through loss of tissue. Proper apposition, transosseous wiring, and some method of intermaxillary wiring are of the utmost importance. If a fracture has bone loss of over 0.5 cm. caused by osteomyelitis, comminution with loss of viable fragments, or extensive pathosis (such as neoplasm), a bone graft is indicated.

Radiographic evidence of nonunion is usually unmistakable. The bone ends soon appear rounded off and, after a lapse of time, a deposition of cortical bone can be seen at the edges of the fragments. When these changes occur, nothing but surgical interference will lead to osseous union.

A case of early nonunion caused by inadequate fixation is presented. It was treated by extraoral exposure of the fractured bone ends, careful removal of the fibrous tissue, transosseous and circumferential wiring, and intermaxillary fixation.

Patient. A 31-year-old housewife was admitted to the hospital suffering from a broken jaw. It had been caused by a blow from a fist a week earlier. She had not been knocked unconscious, but there had been some pain and bleeding. Examination showed mandibular swelling with marked tenderness on the left side over the mental and preauricular areas. Since there had been neither crepitus nor displacement, the occlusion was still normal.

X-ray examination revealed a fracture of the mandible posterior to the left second bicuspid (Figure 18–263A). There was also an undisplaced fracture of the subcondylar neck. The mandibular second molar occluded against the maxillary second molar, which helped maintain good position.

Treatment. Since the fragments were undis-turbed, simple intermaxillary fixation was considered adequate. The patient was placed on a regimen of antibiotics. The next day local anesthesia was administered, and the jaws were wired intraorally to arch bars which had been secured to upper and lower teeth. Intermaxillary wires were used for rigid immobilization and maintaining the teeth in proper occlusion. All fragments were in good position. The patient was discharged on her third hospital day.

The patient failed to keep her postoperative appointment and was not seen again until 6 months later. Her family revealed that during the interval she had been admitted to a State Hospital for psychiatric observation and therapy. Without the knowledge of the hospital staff, she had removed the arch bars 4 days after they had been placed in position.

The patient appeared healthy but complained of pain when eating solid food. There was asymmetry of the face and deviation of the mandible on motion (Fig. 18–263B). She was unable to bring her jaw into centric occlusion because of a marked disturbance of occlusion. Motion at the fracture site could be demonstrated by bimanual manipulation of the fragments.

Examination. A second x-ray examination not only showed that both the second bicuspid and second molar had been removed but that there was also a defect involving the inferior cortex and communication with the distal wall of the bicuspid socket (Fig. 18–263C). The molar had been removed previously because of caries, and the bicuspid had been extracted when the patient complained of pain 3 weeks before her second examination. There had been moderate loss of osseous structure indicating an early nonunion without appreciable loss of jaw length. The subcondylar neck fracture had healed satisfactorily in good position.

Because the patient had removed the arch bars 4 days after they had been placed in position, inadequate fixation had resulted in motion and nonunion. A lower splint was constructed. She was readmitted to the hospital and placed on a regimen of supportive and antibiotic therapy, using daily 2 cc. intramuscular injections of Combiotic.

Urinalysis, bleeding and clotting time, white and red blood cell counts, serum calcium and inorganic phosphorus examinations were all within normal limits. The hemoglobin concentration was 13.5 gms. Results of the Kahn test were negative, and chest radiographs were normal.

Operation. Two days after readmission, the patient was placed under general anesthesia. An incision was made below the border of the left mandible extending from just anterior to the angle to a point anterior to the mental foramen. Dissection was extended through the platysma muscle

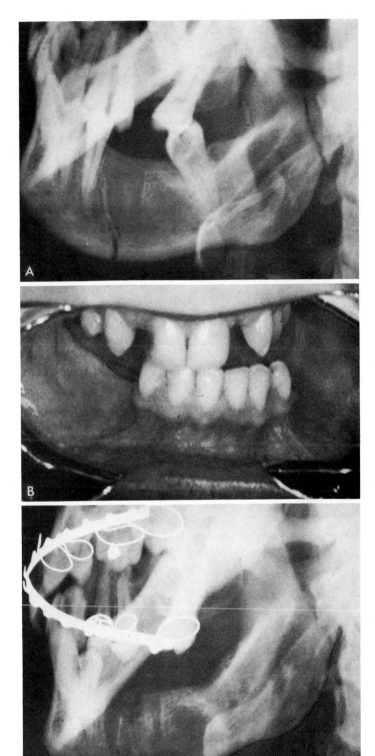

Figure 18–263 *A*, Lateral jaw radiograph made during patient's first examination shows fractured mandible. (See Case Report No. 11.) *B*, Clinical photograph taken 6 months after the injury shows marked deviation of the mandible. *C*, Lateral jaw radiograph made during patient's second examination reveals early nonunion.

(Figure 18–263 continued on following page)

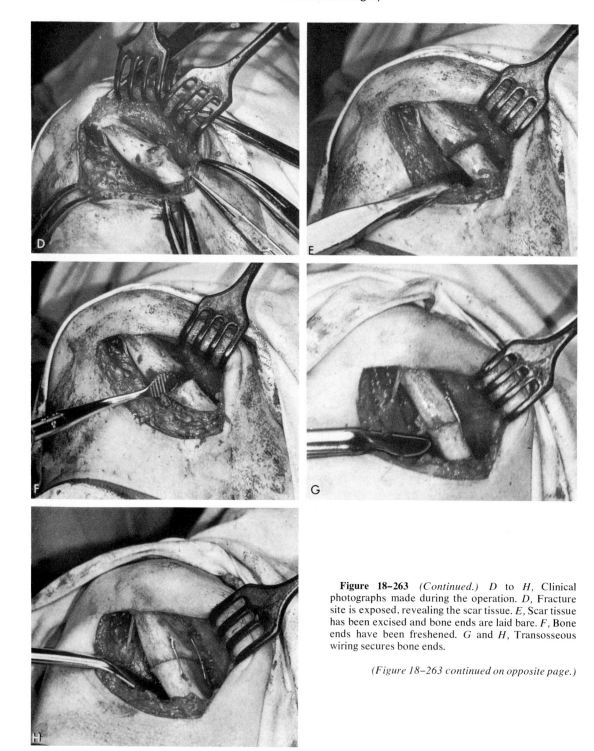

Figure 18–263 *(Continued.)* *D* to *H*, Clinical photographs made during the operation. *D*, Fracture site is exposed, revealing the scar tissue. *E*, Scar tissue has been excised and bone ends are laid bare. *F*, Bone ends have been freshened. *G* and *H*, Transosseous wiring secures bone ends.

(Figure 18–263 continued on opposite page.)

exposing the external maxillary artery and vein, which were clamped and tied with chromic 000 sutures. The periosteum was incised, stripped from the bone, and retractors inserted to expose the fracture site (Fig. 18–263*D*). Scar tissue, which had bridged the two fragments, was excised so that both bone ends were laid bare (Fig. 18–263*E*). The eburnated bone was removed from each segment with files until fresh bleeding was obtained (Fig. 18–263*F*). A number of small oblique holes,

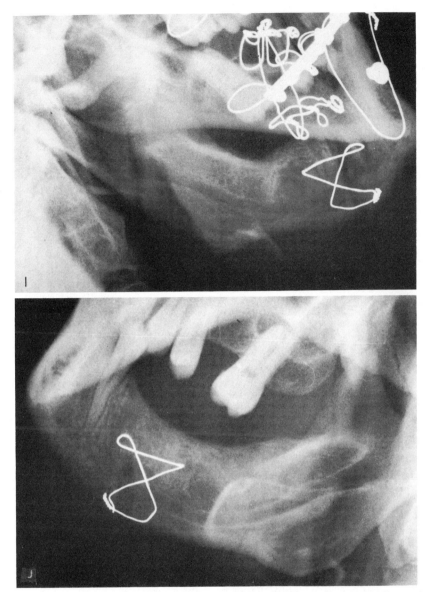

Figure 18–263 *(Continued.)* *I*, Lateral jaw radiograph made one day after the operation shows the fragments to be well aligned. *J*, Lateral jaw radiograph made 1 year after the operation shows a well-healed mandible.

some crossing the fracture line, were drilled into each fragment to facilitate bleeding. Two holes were then drilled in each fragment to receive the transosseous wires. Stainless steel wire was inserted, one end through each upper hole, crossed on the lingual surface and brought through the lower holes to the buccal surface. The fragments were held in good apposition while the wire was twisted until secure. This figure-of-eight wire was burnished against the lingual and buccal surfaces of the bone (Figs. 18–263*G* and *H*). With the periosteum replaced, the muscles were returned

and secured in their normal position with deep chromic sutures. Superficial structures were closed with chromic catgut sutures, and the skin was carefully brought together with a subcuticular 0.035 gauge stainless steel wire.

The acrylic splint was inserted. It had been made so that it fitted against the lingual aspects of the remaining teeth, with saddles resting on the edentulous portions of the mandible. The occlusal surface of the appliance contained a groove into which the upper molar fitted. This assisted in stabilizing the posterior fragment.

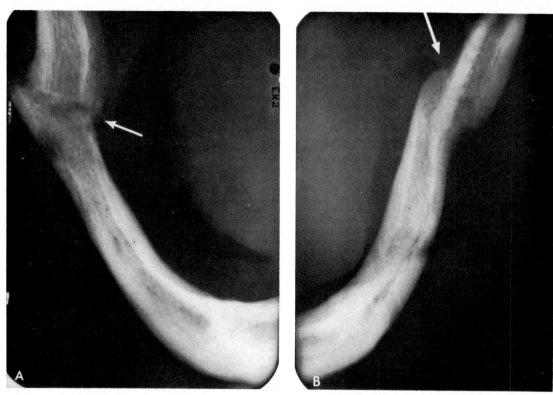

Figure 18–264 How nature compensates for man's failure to place the ends of fractures in ideal, "before-fracture," alignment and proceeds to develop osseous union anyway. While this may return the part to function, in the jaws there is the additional all-important requirement of function *with normal occlusion,* or the correct *intermaxillary space* and *jaw relationships* in edentulous mouths. There is also the requirement of cosmetics based on the necessity of restoration of symmetry in the healed facial bones. Note Figures 18–265, 18–266, and 18–267 for examples in which this objective, as well as normal function, was not achieved.

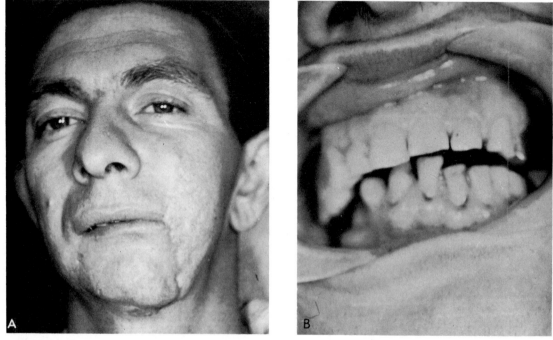

Figure 18–265 *A,* Loss of facial harmony. *B,* Loss of the normal occlusal relationship between the maxilla and the mandible. *Reason:* Incorrect alignment of the fractured segments of the mandible when healing took place.

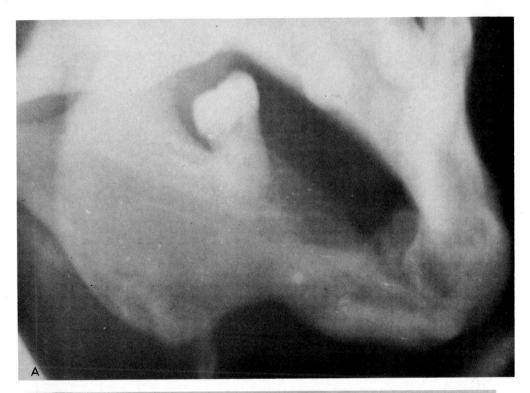

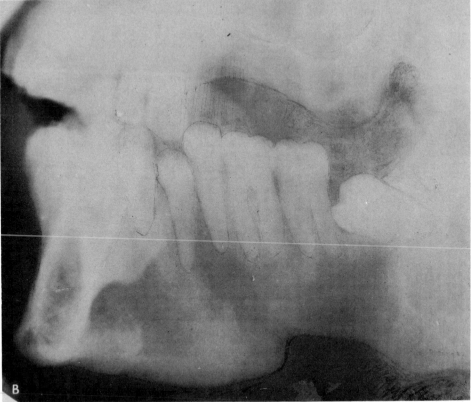

Figure 18–266 Two examples of the very poor end results from the use of Barton bandages to reduce and immobilize fractures of the mandible. Both cases were treated in another city. It is amazing that we still see cases of fractures of the mandible incorrectly treated with Barton bandages because the technique still appears in books and emergency manuals. Regretfully, the instructions in some emergency manuals are such that in many instances simple fractures are compounded, respiratory embarrassment results, or is increased, and fragments are displaced more than they were by the original trauma.

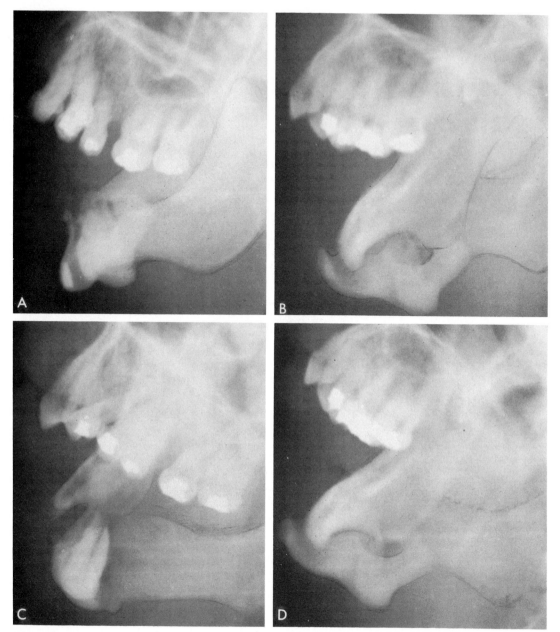

Figure 18–267   This compound comminuted fracture of the mandible was incorrectly treated elsewhere by a Barton bandage. Note malposition of the fragments and the fibrous union. *A,* Lateral jaw radiograph. *B* to *D,* Oblique, right and left radiographs.

The patient was so ashamed of her appearance with an "Andy Gump" jaw that she would not permit us to take photographs of her face.

A 6-inch piece of stainless steel wire having a Hagedorn needle attached to each end was used for the circumferential wiring. One needle was inserted through the skin, following the curvature of the bone to the inner surface of the jaw. By careful manipulation it was made to penetrate the mylohyoid muscle, so that it emerged in the gingiva just below the lingual flange of the splint. The other needle was inserted through the same hole in the skin and emerged on the buccal aspect of the appliance. Two circumferential wires were thus used to secure the splint—one in the first molar area, the other near the midline of the mandible. These wires were carefully pulled tightly around the bone and over the splint, securing it firmly. Immobilization was obtained by elastic traction from the maxillary arch bar to loops around the lower teeth and buttons on the splint. After application of a pressure bandage, the patient was taken from the operating room in good condition.

Postoperative Course. Except for the usual mild postsurgical traumatic edema and ecchymosis, the patient had a normal postoperative period, aided by penicillin therapy, cold compresses, bed rest, and adequate fluid intake. A lateral-jaw radiograph made the day after the operation showed the fragments to be well aligned (Fig. 18–263*I*). On the second day the elastics were replaced with wire ligatures to maintain a more rigid immobilization. Three days later the subcuticular wire was removed, and the wound was bridged and supported by collodion strips. The patient was discharged on the seventh hospital day.

Eight weeks after the operation all appliances were removed. A clinical examination 1 year later showed a solidly healed mandible in good function. X-ray examination verified this finding (Fig. 18–263*J*). The cosmetic results were also satisfactory.

Case Report No. 12

RIB GRAFT FOR CORRECTION OF MANDIBULAR DEFECT

CHARLES F. McCANN, D.M.D.,
STEPHEN P. MALLETT, D.M.D.,
AND SALVATORE J. ESPOSITO, D.D.S.

History. A 20-year-old white male was admitted with a large right mandibular defect. Twenty-two months prior to admission the patient had had open reduction of bilateral mandibular fractures. However, an infection had developed in the right fracture site, with subsequent loss of approximately 6 cm. of bone. One attempt to correct this by means of an iliac bone graft failed, resulting in

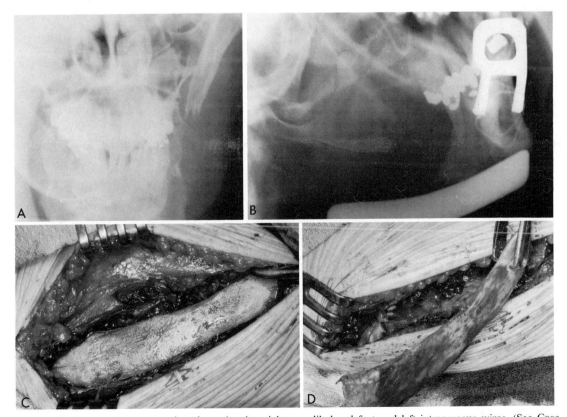

Figure 18–268 *A,* Posteroanterior view, showing right mandibular defect and left intraosseous wires. (See Case Report No. 12.) *B,* Right oblique view, showing defect, position of ramus and steel bar used in estimating amount of rib necessary to correct defect. *C,* Rib exposed and ready to be excised and removed. *D,* Rib cut through and being removed from its bed.

(Figure 18–268 continued on following page)

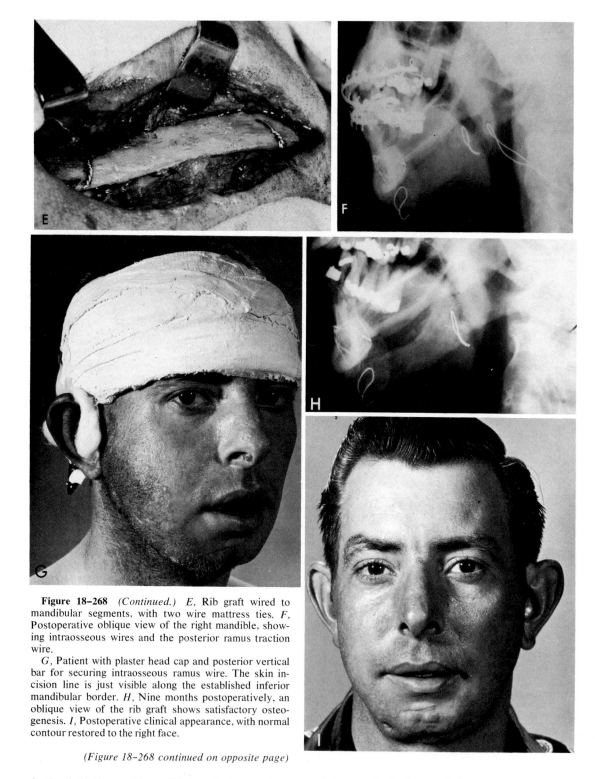

Figure 18–268 *(Continued.)* *E*, Rib graft wired to mandibular segments, with two wire mattress ties. *F*, Postoperative oblique view of the right mandible, showing intraosseous wires and the posterior ramus traction wire.

G, Patient with plaster head cap and posterior vertical bar for securing intraosseous ramus wire. The skin incision line is just visible along the established inferior mandibular border. *H*, Nine months postoperatively, an oblique view of the rib graft shows satisfactory osteogenesis. *I*, Postoperative clinical appearance, with normal contour restored to the right face.

(Figure 18–268 continued on opposite page)

further infection and loss of the graft. A second attempt was abandoned when a rather large orofacial tear was noted; this was surgically corrected, but no further attempt was made to correct the bony defect. At the time of this admission to our hospi- tal 17 months had passed since the second procedure, and except for surgical scars the soft tissue was now essentially normal.

Treatment. Following a complete physical examination, which revealed the patient to be a

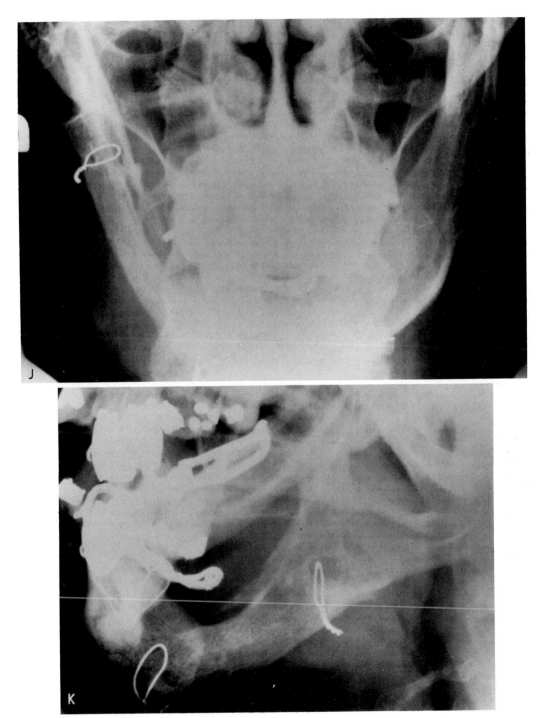

Figure 18–268 *(Continued.)* *J* and *K*, Ten-year follow-up films. *J*, Posteroanterior view. *K*, Oblique view. There is no evidence of "melting away" of the graft.

healthy male, extraction of the first and second right mandibular bicuspids was accomplished. Maxillary and mandibular arch bars were secured to the remaining teeth to be used after surgery in maintaining normal occlusal relationships. The pa-

tient was taken to the operating room, and under general anesthesia a 9-cm. segment of the seventh rib was secured by a physician from the chest service and subsequently prepared and wired into position by the oral surgeon. The anterior and posterior mandibular stumps had been prepared by removal of sufficient cortical bone to create fresh bleeding surfaces in apposition with the decorticated surfaces of the graft. An overlap of $1\frac{1}{2}$ cm. of rib was established and held in position by two intraosseous wire mattress sutures. A traction wire was also secured to the angle of the mandible, later to be used to guard against muscular pull on the ramus. A plaster headcap would later support a postauricular vertical metal bar used to secure the necessary posterior traction. Finally, the wound was closed in layers, with 00 catgut used subcutaneously and 0000 dermal interrupted ties used for the skin. A sterile dressing was placed over the wound and secured by means of a head roll. An in-

traoral examination revealed no mucosal lacerations. The patient was taken to the recovery room in good condition.

Subsequent Course. The patient did well following surgery, and all sutures were removed. Extraoral traction was continued 4 weeks more, and then the plaster head cap was removed and the posterior traction discontinued. X-ray films revealed the rib graft to be in satisfactory position and repeat films 8 months later further revealed a vital right mandible. A partial mandibular prosthesis was inserted 10 months postoperatively, and follow-up appointments revealed mandibular function to be satisfactory.

ORAL HYGIENE IN FRACTURE CASES

A sodium hypochlorite mouthwash should be used at least three times daily.

Table 18–5   *Soft Diet for Fracture Patients**

BREAKFAST
1 cup citrus fruit juice (*e.g.*, orange)
1 cup gruel (*e.g.*, oatmeal)
2 soft cooked eggs—2 minute
Milk
2 tablespoons cream
2 tablespoons sugar
Coffee or tea

DINNER
Cream soup (*e.g.*, cream of pea)
Finely ground meat (*e.g.*, beef)
Mashed potatoes and gravy
Pureed vegetable (*e.g.*, carrots)
Ice cream
Milk
4 tablespoons cream
1 tablespoon sugar
Coffee or tea

SUPPER
Cream soup (*e.g.*, tomato)
Finely ground meat (*e.g.*, chicken)
Mashed potatoes and gravy
Vegetable puree (*e.g.*, string beans)
Fruit puree (*e.g.*, peaches)
Milk
4 tablespoons cream
1 tablespoon sugar
Coffee or tea

BEDTIME FEEDING
Hi-pro supplement (6 ounces homogenized milk, 1 table-
    spoon skim milk powder, 1 tablespoon chocolate syrup)

*This diet is recommended by the Veterans Administration Hospital, Pittsburgh, in consultation with Miss S. Andersen, clinic dietitian.

The patient must use a toothbrush and toothpaste to the best of his ability.

Whenever possible, the patient should be given a thorough prophylaxis, including the scaling of the teeth, before reduction of the fracture.

The mouth should be thoroughly sprayed by the dentist at least three times a week with a good antiseptic solution.

DIET FOR PATIENTS WITH FRACTURED JAWS

Many of the treatment methods for patients with fractures of the facial bones interfere with mastication, and so provisions for a special diet must be made during the recovery period. Both the patient's comfort and nutritional needs must be considered.

Methods of Feeding. Patients with a fractured jaw may be fed through a drinking tube or straw, from a cup or bowl, by spoon feeding, or by nasopharyngeal or rectal feeding in exceptional cases. The diet must be either liquid or soft.

Liquid Diet. This is necessary in all cases in which the jaws are wired together. It should consist of fruit juices; milk or cream or malted milk or cocoa or chocolate; eggnog; meat juices or soups; cooked and thin cereals; canned baby foods; beverages of any sort except alcohol.

Soft Diet. This should consist of mashed potatoes or any soft-cooked vegetables; soft fresh or canned fruit; soft-boiled eggs; soft meats such as sweetbreads or brains; desserts such as ice cream, gelatin (Jello), rennet custard (Junket) and other custards.

Table 18–6   *Liquid Meals for Fracture Patients*

BREAKFAST
1 cup of fruit juice
½ cup of gruel
Milk
2 tablespoons cream
2 tablespoons sugar
Coffee or tea

10 A.M.
7 oz. Hi-pro

DINNER
Cream soup
1 cup fruit juice
7 oz. milk drink (*e.g.,* eggnog, made with a coddled egg)
Ice cream
Milk
2 tablespoons cream
1 tablespoon sugar
Coffee or tea

2 P.M.
7 oz. Hi-pro

SUPPER
Cream soup
1 cup of fruit juice
7 oz. milk drink (*e.g.,* milkshake)
Ice cream
Milk
1 tablespoon sugar
Coffee or tea

8 P.M.
7 oz. Hi-pro

Required Foods. The following foods must be taken each day: at least 1 quart of milk; a choice of fresh orange juice, 8 ounces of tomato juice, or fresh grapefruit juice; a quarter pound of butter; yolks of two raw or soft-boiled eggs; vegetables—strained and mashed canned vegetables (baby foods) such as spinach, carrots, parsnips, turnips, peas, string beans, corn, asparagus, beets, lima beans, summer squash, or others (one or two helpings daily of any of these vegetables; it is good to vary the choice so that each day's menu is different from that of the day before); cod liver oil—2 tablespoonfuls three times daily for an adult; one cake of yeast or three vitamin B complex tablets.

Optional Foods. These may be eaten raw or baked. They include ripe bananas, cereals, desserts, cheese, meats, fish and beverages.

Table 18–7   *Nutritional Values of Special Diets*

	RECOM-MENDED	SOFT DIET	LIQUID DIET
Calories	3000	3150	3244
Protein (gm.)	70	125	123
Fat (gm.)	—	170	140
Carbohydrate (gm.)	—	282	375
Calcium (gm.)	1.0	2.1	3.7
Phosphorus (gm.)			
Iron (gm.)	15	16	19.9
Vitamin A (I.U.)	5000	29,909	11,198
Ascorbic acid (mg.)	75	114	205
Thiamin (mg.)	1.5	1.52	3.3
Riboflavin (mg.)	2.0	3.7	7.0
Niacin (mg.)	15	17	23

REFERENCES

1. Ackermann, R., and Pompians-Miniac, L.: L'Urgence en Odonto-Stomatologie. Paris, Masson et Cie., 1964.
2. Adams, W. M.: Internal wiring fixation of facial fractures. Surgery, *12*:523 (Oct.), 1942.
3. Alling, C. C., and Davis, B. P., Jr.: Compound, comminuted, complex maxillofacial fractures. J. Oral Surg., *32*:415, 1974.
4. Anderson, M. F.: Blowout fractures: report of a series. J. Oral Surg., *22*:405 (Sept.), 1964.
5. Arentz, R. E., and Hayward, J. R.: Severe facial fractures in a hemophiliac: report of case. J. Oral Surg., *25*:359, 1967.
6. Atkin, W. O., and Johnson, E. C.: Facial fractures: incidence and diagnosis. J. Oral Surg., *28*:316, 1970. (Abstr.)
7. Austin, E. U.: Intraoral open reduction of mandibular fractures. J. Oral Surg., *24*:470, 1966.
8. Bailey, B. J., and Gaskil, R.: Management of fractures of the mandible. J. Oral Surg., *26*:213, 1968. (Abstr.)
9. Barak, J. P.: Anesthesia of the left side of the lower lip and the left half of the tongue following mandibular fracture. J. Oral Surg., *26*:423, 1968.
10. Beekler, D. M., and Walker, R. V.: Condyle fractures. J. Oral Surg., *27*:563, 1969.
11. Beke, A. L., *et al.*: Posttraumatic cervicofacial neuritis: report of case. J. Oral Surg., *23*:78, 1965.
12. Blair, A. E.: Teeth involved in the line of the mandibular fracture. J. Oral Surg., *25*:84, 1967.
13. Blevins, C., and Gores, R. J.: Fractures of the mandibular condyloid process: results of conservative treatment in 140 patients. J. Oral Surg., *19*:392, 1961.
14. Bonnette, G. H.: Experimental fractures of the mandible. J. Oral Surg., *27*:568, 1969.
15. Bosco, H. F.: Use of plaster of paris headcaps as part of the oral surgeon's armamentarium. J. Oral Surg., *24*:470, 1966.
16. Bowerman, J. E.: The superior orbital fissure syndrome complicating fractures of the facial skeleton. J. Oral Surg., *28*:635, 1970. (Abstr.)
17. Boyne, P. J.: Osseous repair and mandibular growth after subcondylar fractures. J. Oral Surg., *25*:300, 1967.
18. Branca, R. W.: Healing of zygomaticomaxillary complex fractures: a hypothesis concerning the induction mechanism in facial fractures. J. Oral Surg., *28*:735, 1970.

19. Briggs, R. M., and Wood-Smith, D.: A simple tech-nic for intermaxillary fixation. J. Oral Surg., 28:473, 1970. (Abstr.)

20. Brons, R., and Boering, G.: Fractures of the man-dibular body treated by stable internal fixation: a preliminary report. J. Oral Surg., 28:407, 1970.

21. Byrne, R. P., and Woodward, H. W.: Occult frac-ture of the odontoid process: report of case. J. Oral Surg., 30:684, 1972.

22. Caldwell, J. B.: Management of maxillary fractures. J. Oral Surg., 19:313, 1961.

23. Callins, J. F., et al.: Mandibular deformity asso-ciated with nonunion treated by vertical osteot-omy: report of case. J. Oral Surg., 29:817, 1971.

24. Cameron, J. R.: Complications in the treatment of fractures. J. Oral Surg., 23:14, 1965.

25. Capodanno, J. A.: Reconstruction of acutely trau-matized orbital floor. J. Oral Surg., 25:510, 1967.

26. Charest, A.: A new craniofacial immobilization device for use in maxillofacial surgery. Oral Surg., 15:15 (Jan.), 1962.

27. Choukas, N. C., et al.: Effects of surgically reduced fracture dislocations of mandibular condyles on facial growth in Macaca rhesus monkeys. J. Oral Surg., 28:113, 1970.

28. Church, L. E.: Repair of fractures. Rev. Belg. Med. Dent., 14:425, 1959.

29. Cohen, B. M., et al.: Management of comminuted mandibular fractures: report of case. J. Oral Surg., 26:537, 1968.

30. Committee on Trauma, American College of Surgeons: Early Care of the Injured Patient. Philadelphia, W. B. Saunders Co., 1972.

31. Converse, J. M.: Reconstructive Plastic Surgery. Vols. II and III, The Head and Neck. Philadel-phia, W. B. Saunders Co., 1964.

32. Converse, J. M., et al.: The conjunctival approach in orbital fractures. J. Oral Surg., 32:715, 1974. (Abstr.)

33. Crawford, M. J.: Appliances and attachments for treatment of upper jaw fractures. U.S. Nav. Med. Bull., 41:1151, 1943.

34. Crikelair, G. F., et al.: A critical look at the "blow-out" fracture. J. Oral Surg., 30:778, 1972. (Abstr.)

35. Crompton, M. R.: Visual lesions in closed head in-jury. Brain, 93:785, 1970.

36. Crosby, J. F., Jr., and Woodward, H. W.: Au-togenous bone graft for repair of nonunion of maxillary fracture: report of case. J. Oral Surg., 23:441, 1965.

37. Cutright, D. E., et al.: Fracture reduction using a biodegradable material, polylactic acid. J. Oral Surg., 29:393, 1971.

38. Dalitsch, W. W.: Maxillary-orbital fractures: im-proved treatment. J. Oral Surg., 27:830, 1969. (Abstr.)

39. Dechaume, M., Crepy, C., and Regnier, J. M.: Conduite à tenir au sujet des dents en rapport avec les foyers de fracture des maxillaires. Rev. Stomatol. Chir. Maxillofac., 58(9):512 (Sept.), 1957.

40. Degnan, E. J.: Mandibular fracture in the geriatric patient: problems in treatment planning: report of case. J. Oral Surg., 28:438 (June), 1970.

41. Dessner, L., and Holm, O. F.: Fracture-dislocation of the condyloid process in children. Svensk a Tandläk. Tidskr., 51:57 (Feb.), 1958.

42. Dingman, R. O., and Natvig, P.: Surgery of Facial Fractures. Philadelphia, W. B. Saunders Co., 1964.

43. Doane, H. F.: Dislocation of the right mandibular condyle into the middle cranial fossa. J. Oral Surg., 21:510 (Nov.), 1963.

44. Doneker, T. G., and Hiatt, W. R.: Buccal airway device: an aid in the postoperative management of patients with wire fixation of the jaw. J. Oral Surg., 24:318, 1966.

45. Ekholm, A.: Fractures of the condyloid process of the mandible. Suom. Hammaslääk. Toim., 57:1, 1961.

46. Eubanks, R. J.: Fractures of the neck of the condy-loid process. J. Oral Surg., 22:285, 1964.

47. Evans, J. N., and Fenton, P. J.: Blow-out fracture of the orbit. J. Oral Surg., 30:540, 1972. (Abstr.)

48. Everett, G., et al.: Blood volume changes asso-ciated with surgical treatment of fractures of the mandible. J. Oral Surg., 27:637, 1969.

49. Fein, S. J., et al.: Infection of the cervical spine as-sociated with a fracture of the mandible. J. Oral Surg., 27:145, 1969.

50. Ferraro, J. W., and Berggren, R. B.: A precise method for determination of the displacement in fractures of the midface. J. Oral Surg., 31:234, 1973. (Abstr.)

51. Fickling, B. W.: Long-term treatment for facial in-juries. J. Oral Surg., 22:142 (Mar.), 1964.

52. Foster, C. F., and Yound, W. G.: Tuberculous in-fection of a fractured mandible: report of case. J. Oral Surg., 28:686, 1970.

53. Fraser-Moodie, W.: Mr Gunning and his splint. J. Oral Surg., 28:636, 1970.

54. Fujino, T.: Experimental "blowout" fracture of the orbit. J. Oral Surg., 32:935, 1974. (Abstr.)

55. Fuller, G. E., Jr.: A study of the interosseous rela-tionship of the extraoral skeletal fixation pin in the mandible. Study in partial fulfillment of M.S. requirements, University of Pittsburgh, 1954.

56. Funkhouser, J., and Na Ayuthia, I.: Metastasizing basal cell carcinoma: case report. J. Oral Surg., 32:74, 1974. (Abstr.)

57. Gargiulo, E. A., et al.: Use of titanium mesh and autogenous bone marrow in the repair of non-united mandibular fracture: report of case and re-view of the literature. J. Oral Surg., 31:371, 1973.

58. Gelsinon, T., et al.: Correction of mandibular non-union and gross malocclusion: report of case. J. Oral Surg., 32:855, 1974.

59. Getter, L., et al.: A biodegradable intraosseous ap-pliance in the treatment of mandibular fractures. J. Oral Surg., 30:344, 1972.

60. Goldberg, J. R.: Use of splints questioned (Letter). J. Oral Surg., 31:326, 1973.

61. Gonzalez, L. I.: Cirugía Maxilo-Facial. Buenos Aires, Purinzón, 1958.

62. Grasso, A. M., et al.: Traumatic cyst of the mandi-ble: report of case. J. Oral Surg., 27:341, 1969.

63. Gustavson, E. H., and Strane, M. F.: Fractures of the medial wall of the orbit. J. Oral Surg., 32:75, 1974. (Abstr.)

64. Hagan, E. H., and Huelke, D. F.: Analysis of 319 case reports of mandibular fractures. J. Oral Surg., 19:83, 1961.

65. Hahn, G. W., and Corgill, D. A.: Mandibular frac-ture fixation with malleable metal mesh. J. Oral Surg., 27:180, 1969.

66. Hahn, G. W., and Corgill, D. A.: Surgical implant

replacement of the fractured displaced mandibular condyle: report of three cases. J. Oral Surg., 28:898, 1970.

67. Harding, R., and Herceg, S. J.: Simple method for reduction of fractures of zygoma. J. Oral Surg., 27:590, 1969. (Abstr.)

68. Harnisch, H.: Five-year statistics of jaw fractures. Zahnarztl. Prax, 10:126 (June), 1959.

69. Harrington, K. D., *et al.:* The use of methylmethacrylate as an adjunct in the internal fixation of malignant neoplasm fractures. J. Oral Surg., 31:567, 1973. (Abstr.)

70. Hazard, D. C.: Treatment of facial fractures. J. Oral Surg., 22:504, 1964.

71. Hekmatpanah, J.: The management of head trauma. Surg. Clin. North Am., 53(1):47, 1973.

72. Hendrix, J. H., Sanders, S. G., and Green, B.: Open reduction of mandibular condyle: a clinical and experimental study. Plastic & Reconstr. Surg., 23:283 (Mar.), 1959.

73. Hensler, J. D.: Transfer of metallic particles between the screwdriver and the screws and plate in treating mandibular fracture. J. Oral Surg., 23:86, 1965.

74. Herold, H. Z., and Tadmor, A.: Cartilage in the treatment of experimental bone defects. J. Oral Surg., 26:148, 1968. (Abstr.)

75. Heslop, I. H.: Complicated maxillofacial injuries. J. Oral Surg., 22:151, 1964.

76. Hinds, E. C., and Parnes, E. I.: Late management of condylar fractures by means of subcondylar osteotomy: reports of cases. J. Oral Surg., 24:54, 1966.

77. Hooley, J. R.: Reduction of mandibular fractures by intraoral inferior border wiring. J. Oral Surg., 27:87, 1969.

78. Hooley, J. R., and Freedman, G. L.: "Degloving" in treatment of fracture of the mandibular symphysis. J. Oral Surg., 25:236, 1967.

79. Huelke, D. F., and Burdi, A. R.: Location of mandibular fractures related to teeth and edentulous regions. J. Oral Surg., 22:396, 1964.

80. Huelke, D. F., and Harger, J. H.: Maxillofacial injuries: their nature and mechanisms of production. J. Oral Surg., 27:451, 1969.

81. Huelke, D. F., and Harger, J. H.: Mechanisms in the production of mandibular fractures: an experimental study. J. Oral Surg., 26:86, 1968.

82. Huelke, D. F., and Patrick, Z. M.: Mechanics in the production of mandibular fractures: strain-gauge measurements of impacts to the chin. J. Dent. Res., 43:437 (May-June), 1964.

83. Hughes, C. L.: Hemorrhagic bone cyst and pathologic fracture of mandible: report of case. J. Oral Surg., 27:345, 1969.

84. Hughes, C. L., and Gibson, D. H.: Heterogenous bone graft of nonunion of mandibular fracture: report of case. J. Oral Surg., 26:749, 1968.

85. Hunsuck, E. E.: A method of intraoral open reduction of fractured mandibles. J. Oral Surg., 25:533, 1967.

86. Irby, W. B., and Rast, W. C., Jr.: Extracranial fixation of the facial skeleton: review and report of case. J. Oral Surg., 27:900, 1969.

87. Jackson, C., and Jackson, C. L.: Bronchoesophagology. Philadelphia, W. B. Saunders Co., 1950.

88. Jamieson, K. G., and Yelland, J. D. N.: Surgically treated traumatic subdural hematomas. J. Neurosurg., 34:137, 1972.

89. Joy, E. D., Jr.: Nonunion of a mandibular fracture treated by sliding bone graft: report of case. J. Oral Surg., 25:356, 1967.

90. Joy, E. D., Jr., *et al.:* Facial elongation after treatment of horizontal fracture of the maxilla without vertical suspension. J. Oral Surg., 27:560, 1969.

91. Kaplan, S. I.: Personal communication.

92. Kaplan, S. I., and Mark, H. I.: Bilateral fractures of the mandibular condyles and fracture of the symphysis menti in an 18-month-old child. Two year preliminary report with a plea for conservative surgery. Oral Surg., 15:136 (Feb.), 1962.

93. Kazanjian, V. H., and Converse, J. M.: The Surgical Treatment of Facial Injuries. 2nd Ed. Baltimore, Williams & Wilkins Co., 1959.

94. Kennedy, J. W., and Kent, J. N.: False aneurysm and a partial facial paralysis secondary to mandibular fracture: report of case. J. Oral Surg., 28:854, 1970.

95. Kerr, H. R., Jr.: Subcondylar fractures of the mandible. J. Oral Surg., 24:367, 1966.

96. Khedroo, L. G.: External pin fixation for treatment of mandibular fractures: a reappraisal. J. Oral Surg., 28:101, 1970.

97. King, D. R.: Giant cell reparative granuloma associated with a pathologic fracture: report of case. J. Oral Surg., 26:203, 1968.

98. Kingsbury, B. C.: Alveolar fractures. J. Oral Surg., 27:530, 1969.

99. Kline, S. N.: Lateral compression in the treatment of mandibular fractures. J. Oral Surg., 31:182, 1973.

100. Kline, S. N., *et al.:* Use of autogenous bone from the symphysis for treatment of delayed union of the mandible: report of case. J. Oral Surg., 28:540, 1970.

101. Klonoff, H.: Head injuries in children. Am. J. Public Health, 61:2405, 1971.

102. Kufner, J.: A method of craniofacial suspension. J. Oral Surg., 28:260, 1970.

103. Kwapis, B. W.: Treatment of malar bone fractures. J. Oral Surg., 27:538, 1969.

104. Kwapis, B. W.: Wire ligature carrier for continuous interdental wiring of fractured jaws. J.A.D.A., 69:700 (Dec.), 1964.

105. Kwapis, B. W., *et al.:* Surgical correction of a malunited condylar fracture in a child. J. Oral Surg., 31:465, 1973.

106. Lancaster, L. L., Jr., *et al.:* Treatment of malunited fractures of the mandible and maxilla. J. Oral Surg., 28:310, 1970.

107. Lane, S. L.: The blow-out fracture. J. Oral Surg., 27:544, 1969.

108. Laros, G. S.: Fracture healing. J. Oral Surg., 32:872, 1974. (Abstr.)

109. Leonard, J. R., *et al.:* Condylectomy. J. Oral Surg., 26:678, 1968. (Abstr.)

110. Lesney, T. A.: Method of immobilizing a common type of maxillary fracture. J. Oral Surg., 11:49 (Jan.), 1953.

111. Lewis, J. M., *et al.:* Consideration of the intrinsic nerve supply of the eye in orbital fractures. J. Oral Surg., 28:707, 1970.

112. Lore, J. M., and Zingapan, E.: External traction for depressed facial fractures. J. Oral Surg., 30:779, 1972. (Abstr.)

113. McCleve, D. E., and Quickert, M. H.: Treatment of orbital floor fractures. J. Oral Surg., 24:183, 1966. (Abstr.)

114. McHugh, H. E.: *In* Caveness, W. F., and Walker, A. E.: Head Injury Conference Proceedings, pp. 97–105. Philadelphia, J. B. Lippincott, 1966.

115. Mackenzie, D. L., and Ray, K. R.: The Royal Berkshire Hospital "halo." J. Oral Surg., *29*:232, 1971. (Abstr.)

116. MacLennan, W. D., and Simpson, W.: Treatment of fractured mandibular condyle processes in children. Br. J. Plast. Surg., *18*:423, 1965.

117. Magnus, W. W., *et al.:* A conjunctival approach to repair of fracture of medial wall of orbit: report of case. J. Oral Surg., *29*:664, 1971.

118. Marano, P. D., *et al.:* Traumatic herniation of buccal fat pad into maxillary sinus: report of case. J. Oral Surg., *28*:531, 1970.

119. Messer, E. J.: A simplified method for fixation of the fractured mandibular condyle. J. Oral Surg., *30*:442, 1972.

120. Messer, E. J., *et al.:* Use of intraosseous metal appliances in fixation of mandibular fractures. J. Oral Surg., *25*:493, 1967.

121. Miller, G. R.: Blindness developing a few days after mid-facial fracture. J. Oral Surg., *27*:912, 1969. (Abstr.)

122. Miller, S. H., and Morris, W. J.: Current concepts in the diagnosis and management of fractures of the orbital floor. J. Oral Surg., *31*:231, 1973. (Abstr.)

123. Mohanty, S. K., Barrios, M., Fishbone, H., *et al.:* Irreversible injury of cranial nerves 9 through 12 (Collet-Sicard syndrome). J. Neurosurg., *38*:86, 1973.

124. Mohnac, A. M.: Maxillary osteotomy for the correction of malpositioned fractures: report of case. J. Oral Surg., *25*:460, 1967.

125. Moss, M., *et al.:* Open bite with superimposed bilateral mandibular fractures: report of case. J. Oral Surg., *22*:538, 1964.

126. Müller, W.: Zur frage des Versuches der Erhaltung der im Bruchspalt stehenden Zähne unter antibiotischem Schutz. Dtsch. Zahn. Mund. Kieferheilkd., *41*(9–10):360, 1964.

127. Muska, K.: Suspended fixation of the mandible. J. Oral Surg., *26*:172, 1968.

128. Norwich, I., Uys, B. C., Hertzenberg, L., Barnard, J. N., and Kaplan, S.: The treatment of fractures of the mandible by external pin fixation. South African M. J., *33*:979 (Nov.), 1959.

129. Oikarinen, V. J., and Malmström, M.: Jaw fractures. A roentgenological and statistical analysis of 1284 cases including a special study of the fracture lines in the mandible drawn from orthopantomograms in 660 cases. Suom. Hammaslääk. Toim, *65*:95, 1969 (in English).

130. Paatero, Y. V.: Stereoscopy in orthoradial pantomography of the jaws. Acta Radiol. (Stockh.), *51*:449, 1959.

131. Paatero, Y. V.: Orthoradial jaw pantomography. Ann. Med. Intern. Fenn., *48*:222, 1959.

132. Paatero, Y. V.: Pantomography in diagnostics of jaw fractures. Odont. T., *64*:30, 1956.

133. Paatero, Y. V.: Pantomography in theory and use. Acta Radiol. (Stockh.), *41*:321, 1954.

134. Panagopoulos, A. P., and Mansueto, M. D.: Treatment of fractures of the mandibular condyloid process in children. J. Oral Surg., *19*:355, 1961. (Abstr.)

135. Panuska, H. J., and Dedolph, T. H.: Extraoral traction with halo head frame for complex facial fractures. J. Oral Surg., *23*:212 (May), 1965.

136. Patzakis, M., *et al.:* The role of antibiotics in the management of open fractures. J. Oral Surg., *32*:871, 1974. (Abstr.)

137. Paul, J. K.: Continuous arch bar. J. Oral Surg., *26*:114, 1968.

138. Paul, J. K., and Acevedo, A.: Intraoral open reduction. J. Oral Surg., *26*:516, 1968.

139. Percy, E. C.: Orbital facial fracture. J. Oral Surg., *30*:539, 1972. (Abstr.)

140. Peters, P. B.: Sliding cortical mandibular grafts. J. Oral Surg., *27*:565, 1969.

141. Porritt, H. B., and Hanft, R. J.: Recognition of signs of intracranial injury in patients afflicted with facial trauma. Oral Surg., *15*:1038 (Sept.), 1962.

142. Prowler, J. R.: Immediate reconstruction of the orbital rim and floor. J. Oral Surg., *23*:5, 1965.

143. Quinn, J. H.: Open reduction and internal fixation of vertical maxillary fractures. J. Oral Surg., *26*:167, 1968.

144. Radulescu, M., and Milosescu, P.: Axial projection with an occlusal film in the radiographic diagnosis of fractures of nasal bones. J. Oral Surg., *27*:913, 1969. (Abstr.)

145. Rakower, W., Protzell, A., and Rosencrans, M.: Treatment of displaced condylar fractures in children: report of cases. J. Oral Surg., *19*:517, 1961.

146. Ricciardelli, L. A., *et al.:* External biphasic pins for fixation and immobilization of a mandibular bone graft: report of case. J. Oral Surg., *27*:362, 1969.

147. Ricker, O. L.: Technics of internal suspension of maxillary fractures. J. Oral Surg., *20*:108 (Mar.), 1962.

148. Ritchie-Russell, W.: *In* Brock, S. (Ed.): Injuries of the Brain and Spinal Cord and Their Coverings, p. 124. New York, Springer, 1960.

149. Robinson, M.: New onlay-inlay metal splint for the immobilization of mandibular fractures. J. Oral Surg., *19*:266, 1961. (Abstr.)

150. Robinson, M.: New onlay-inlay metal splint for the immobilization of mandibular fractures. Plastic & Reconstr. Surg., *25*:77–79 (Jan.), 1960.

151. Robinson, M., and Shuken, R.: L splint for immobilization of iliac bone grafts to the mandible. J. Oral Surg., *24*:10, 1966.

152. Robinson, M., *et al.:* Sleeve over interosseous wire to aid immobilization of jaw fractures. J. Oral Surg., *23*:183, 1965. (Abstr.)

153. Rontal, E., and Hohmann, A.: External fixation on facial fractures. J. Oral Surg., *32*:551, 1974. (Abstr.)

154. Rowbotham, G. F., and Clark, P. R. R.: *In* Rowbotham, G. F.: Acute Injuries of the Head, pp. 159–228. Baltimore, The Williams and Wilkins Co., 1964.

155. Rowe, N. L.: Fractures of the jaws in children. J. Oral Surg., *27*:497 (July), 1969.

156. Rowe, N. L.: Fractures of the facial skeleton in children. J. Oral Surg., *26*:505, 1968.

157. Rowe, N. L.: Mandibular joint lesions in infants and adults. Int. Dent. J., *10*:484 (Dec.), 1960.

158. Rowe, N. L.: Personal communication.

159. Rowe, N. L., and Killey, H. C.: Fractures of the Facial Skeleton. Edinburgh and London, E. S. Livingstone Ltd., 1968.

160. Sachs, R., *et al.:* Osteomyelitis following fixation of

a mandibular fracture with biphasic pins. J. Oral Surg., *21*:923, 1973.

161. Samuels, H. S., and Oatis, G. W.: The use of Kirschner wires in facial fractures: report of cases. J. Oral Surg., *28*:382, 1970.

162. Sazima, H. J.: The leg-face trauma syndrome: report of cases. J. Oral Surg., *28*:448, 1970.

163. Sazima, H. J.: Facial trauma treatment at a Marine Corps base. J. Oral Surg., *27*:858, 1969.

164. Schemmel, W. L.: Alloplastic implants in orbital floor fractures versus antral packing. J. Oral Surg., *25*:464, 1967.

165. Schweber, S. J., *et al.:* Healing of a fracture through a mandibular myxoma: report of case. J. Oral Surg., *27*:275, 1969.

166. Selman, A. J., *et al.:* Simplified removal of broken circumosseous wires. J. Oral Surg., *24*:321, 1966.

167. Sklans, S., *et al.:* Effect of diphenylhydantoin sodium on healing of experimentally produced fractures in rabbit mandibles. J. Oral Surg., *25*:310, 1967.

168. Sleeper, H. R., *et al.:* Intraoral subperiosteal circumferential wiring for fractures of the edentulous mandible: report of two cases. J. Oral Surg., *24*:351, 1966.

169. Smylski, P. T.: Closed transpalatal method of wiring a maxillary splint or denture. J. Oral Surg., *32*:551, 1974.

170. Stark, R. B.: Early versus late treatment of facial fractures. J. Oral Surg., *23*:471, 1965.

171. Steier, A., *et al.:* Effect of vitamin D2 and fluoride on experimental bone fracture healing in rats. J. Oral Surg., *26*:67, 1968. (Abstr.)

172. Stemmer, A. L.: Fixation of horizontal maxillary fractures. J. Oral Surg., *24*:471, 1966. (Abstr.)

173. Stemmer, A. L., *et al.:* Pteriomalar fracture, management and recognition. J. Oral Surg., *26*:357, 1968. (Abstr.)

174. Stewart, F.: Infection at a fracture site. J. Oral Surg., *23*:88, 1965.

175. Stoica, L., and Gall, C.: Apical resection in the conservative management of teeth in fracture foci. J. Oral Surg., *27*:912, 1969. (Abstr.)

176. Stoneman, W., *et al.:* A new approach to the radiologic evaluation of the mandible. J. Oral Surg., *25*:468, 1967. (Abstr.)

177. Stranc, M. F., and Gustavson, E. H.: Primary treatment of fractures of the orbital roof. J. Oral Surg., *31*:888, 1973. (Abstr.)

178. Sveinsson, E.: Pure "blow-out" fractures of the orbital floor. J. Oral Surg., *32*:76, 1974. (Abstr.)

179. Swenson, R. D.: Alternative treatments for depressed zygoma fracture. J. Oral Surg., *23*:179, 1965.

180. Taddeo, R. J., *et al.:* Management of facial bone fractures. J. Oral Surg., *28*:393, 1970. (Abstr.)

181. Thoma, K. H.: Oral Surgery. 4th ed. St. Louis, The C. V. Mosby Co., 1963.

182. Thompson, H. C., III: The histologic response from thermal changes in mandibular bone as the result of the drilling of skeletal pins through the cortices. Study in partial fulfillment of M. S. requirements, University of Pittsburgh, 1956.

183. Turville, A.: Personal communication.

184. Van de Mark, T. B., *et al.:* Pathologic fracture resulting from mandibular atrophy: report of two cases. J. Oral Surg., *28*:77, 1970. (Abstr.)

185. van Herk, W., and Hovinga, J.: Choice of treatment of orbital floor fractures as part of facial fractures. J. Oral Surg., *31*:600, 1973.

186. Van Zile, W. N.: Surgical reduction of fractures of the mandibular condyle. J. Oral Surg., *22*:461, 1964.

187. Van Zile, W. N., and Samuels, H. S.: Postoperative parotitis: a complication in a fracture of the maxilla. J. Oral Surg., *19*:219, 1961.

188. ViGario, G. D.: A radiological analysis of 35 cases of blow-out fractures of the orbit. J. Oral Surg., *26*:148, 1968. (Abstr.)

189. Walker, R. V.: Personal communication adapted from: Traumatic mandibular condylar fracture dislocations. Effect on growth in Macaca rhesus monkeys. Amer. J. Surg., *100*:850 (Dec.), 1960.

190. Ward, P. H., *et al.:* Clothesline avulsion of the maxilla. J. Oral Surg., *27*:831, 1969. (Abstr.)

191. Weber, D. D., *et al.:* Fracture of mandibular rami complicated by scleroderma: report of case. J. Oral Surg., *28*:860, 1970.

192. Wiesenbaugh, J. M., Jr.: Diagnostic evaluation of zygomatic complex fractures. J. Oral Surg., *28*:204, 1970.

193. Weisfeld, B.: Fracture of coronoid process. J. Oral Surg., *26*:485, 1968. (Abstr.)

194. Weiss, J. A.: Orbital blowout fracture: rationale of surgical technic. J. Oral Surg., *28*:231, 1970. (Abstr.)

195. Whinery, J. G.: An armed atraumatic wire for use in circumferential and internal wiring of fractured facial bones. J. Oral Surg., *26*:188, 1968.

196. White, J. C.: Care of the severely injured patient—neurosurgical injuries. J.A.M.A., *165*:1924, 1957.

197. Wilde, N. J.: Tolerance of the temporomandibular joint to fracture, dislocation and associated injury. J. Oral Surg., *19*:85, 1961. (Abstr.)

198. Wilder, L. R.: Blowout fractures of the orbit. J. Oral Surg., *27*:973, 1969. (Abstr.)

199. Williams, A. C.: Clarification ("A bullet lodged in the glenoid fossa." Oct. 1968 article). J. Oral Surg., *27*:86, 1969.

200. Williams, A. C., *et al.:* A bullet lodged in the glenoid fossa: report of case. J. Oral Surg., *26*:659 (Comments 661), 1968.

201. Wray, J. B., and Rogers, L. S.: Effect of hyperbaric oxygenation upon fracture healing in the rat. J. Oral Surg., *27*:673, 1969. (Abstr.)

202. York, B. V.: Management of mandibular fracture in 3-week-old infant: report of case. J. Oral Surg., *28*:857, 1970.

203. Zambito, R. F., and Laskin, D. M.: Follicular cyst of mandible associated with pathologic fracture: report of case. J. Oral Surg., *22*:449, 1964.

204. Zielinski, D. E.: Anesthesia of the mental nerve secondary to a condylar fracture: report of case. J. Oral Surg., *27*:227, 1969.

CHAPTER 19

CAST OR ACRYLIC SPLINTS—THEIR APPLICATION IN ORAL AND MAXILLOFACIAL SURGERY

WILLIAM B. IRBY, D.D.S., M.S.

The use of various types of splints* in the management of maxillary and mandibular fractures, in cosmetic and reconstructive surgery, and in a variety of other surgical procedures involving the oral cavity is not new. However, the employment of splints has remained a controversial question and has failed to receive the general acceptance which this extremely valuable adjunct to the field of oral surgery so richly deserves. As this chapter will be concerned primarily with the application of splints in regard to treatment of facial fractures, we shall first define the results desired. In brief, one should strive to develop a technique that will assure the most accurate and positive reduction and fixation of the fragments. One should also seek to achieve this result by the simplest method that will guarantee the desired end effect.

The following technique of constructing and applying splints is based upon experience derived from treating a large number of facial injuries over a period of time, including both World War II and the Korean conflict. During this time a conscientious effort was made to develop an approach to these cases that incorporated practicability of approach, simplicity in application, and the greatest chance of eliminating future complications. However-

er, it should be emphasized at this point in the discussion that each case is individual and should be approached as such. The use of splints, therefore, is merely a step in accomplishing the desired results. To this end, the dentist is admirably suited, owing to his knowledge of impression and laboratory techniques.

It should be stressed that the utilization of splints is applicable to both civilian and military practice and that the often-voiced complaint of many oral surgeons, to the effect that splint construction is costly and time-consuming, is without substantial grounds.

FRACTURE REDUCTION AND STABILIZATION WITHOUT SPLINTS

The most consistently used methods of reducing and stabilizing fractures without employing splints are (1) interdental wiring with the use of intermaxillary elastics; (2) arch bars with intermaxillary elastics; (3) pin fixation with or without intermaxillary fixation; and (4) circumferential wiring.

Interdental Wiring with Intermaxillary Elastics. This is by far the most commonly used method of treating jaw fractures throughout the United States and most of the world. A review of the literature leads to the conclusion that over 80 per cent of all fractures are treated by this method.

---

*Throughout this chapter the term "splint" refers to a cast or acrylic splint.

The forces involved in displacing and rotating fractures of the body of the mandible are such that less than an accurate reduction is often attained by this means. First, the muscles of the floor of the mouth tend to go into a state of contraction and to displace the fragments lingually with rotation. Second, the intermaxillary elastics, which must be placed on the buccal surface of the teeth, contribute an additional force that adds to the rotation. Therefore, rotated segments and separated fracture lines often occur (Fig. 19–1). Because of these factors and others, which will be mentioned later, it has become our policy to use this type of fixation only in the following cases:

1. In fractures occurring distal to the second molar of the mandible, including simple fractures of the neck of the condyle.
2. In simple, undisplaced fractures of the maxilla not involving the alveolus.
3. To serve as an emergency stabilization of fragments until definitive care may be accomplished.
4. In the treatment of patients whose general physical condition may be compromised, at least temporarily, by any more extensive therapy.

CAST OR ACRYLIC SPLINTS

Advantages. Splints that are properly designed and secured to each tooth tend to bind all the teeth into a single unit that will withstand strong intermaxillary traction without extruding the teeth.

Splints may be so designed and constructed that the teeth contained in each fragment may be accurately positioned to the splint, thus affording an accurate and stable reduction. This will be illustrated in detail by photographs.

The problem of fragment rotation due to muscle pull and intermaxillary elastics is eliminated.

Simple splints afford excellent and accurate stabilization of the mandible upon which an open reduction has been performed.

In more extensive injuries of the jaws necessitating a prolonged healing period or extensive reconstructive surgery, the utilization of a complex type of splint is beneficial to the health of the teeth and supporting tissues and assures the maintenance of the fragments in fixed position.

Splints can and should play an integral part in the treatment of deformities and in pathologic conditions of the jaws that necessitate extensive surgery. The reasons for this will be clarified in the discussion of special splints.

Splints may be so applied that simple fractures of the mandible or maxilla, occurring within the complement of teeth, are so firmly supported that intermaxillary fixation becomes unnecessary.

Splints serve as an excellent medium for applying traction to displaced bones, especially the maxilla.

Simple splints, especially those of acrylic material, may be easily and cheaply constructed.

Disadvantages. The more complex types of splints require accurate impression techniques and a skilled technician, which becomes costly and time-consuming. It should be emphasized that complex splints are necessary only in complicated or very extensive cases and that, when they are properly utilized, the effort is most worthwhile.

Splints that cover the lingual surface of the mandible or the palate do tend to accumulate

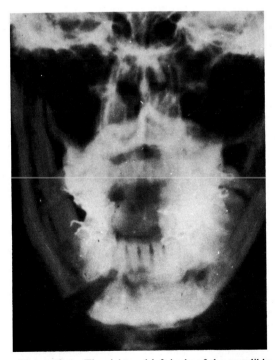

Figure 19–1 The right and left body of the mandible has responded to the combined action of intermaxillary elastics and pull of the mylohyoid muscle, resulting in rotation of the teeth to the lingual side of the alveolar ridge and separation of the fracture line.

debris. Following the application of hundreds of splints of this type, no undue gingival irritation or infection has ensued as long as the buccal surfaces of the teeth have been left uncovered and normal oral hygiene has been maintained.

Impression Technique. In general, it may be said that the same principles apply in securing impressions of the teeth in fractured jaws as apply to the taking of impressions for the construction of partial dentures or other reconstructive work. The teeth should be properly cleansed and any heavy calcareous deposits removed. After this, impressions of the jaws may be secured in alginate material with the regular tray if the fractures are simple. In an occasional and more complicated case, it may be necessary to construct a special tray. The author has found that orthodontia trays afford an excellent vehicle for the taking of impressions in severely comminuted fractures if the sides of the trays are trimmed down and perforated.

SIMPLE SPLINTS

Into this category fall relatively uncomplicated types of splints which may be easily constructed with an economical expenditure of time and money. They are (1) mandibular lingual splints of acrylic or metal, (2) palatal splints of acrylic or metal, and (3) cast labial arch bars or similar types of splints.

The construction and application of certain types of these splints is illustrated in Figures 19–2 to 19–10.

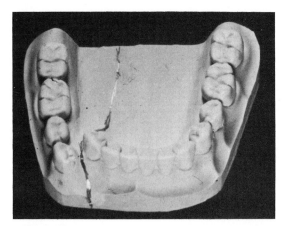

Figure 19–3 Hydrocal cast which has been made from an alginate impression of the dental arch. A pencil mark has been made to indicate the line along which the cast will be cut, utilizing a jeweler's saw with either a ribbon or spiral blade.

Clear acrylic material is preferred for these simple splints whenever practical because it affords the opportunity to observe the tissues under the splint. Additionally, it is much easier to place the holes accurately, and wiring of the splint to the teeth is simpler.

Root canal therapy, which frequently becomes a necessity in the treatment of traumatic injuries involving the anterior portion of the mandible or maxilla, may be initiated

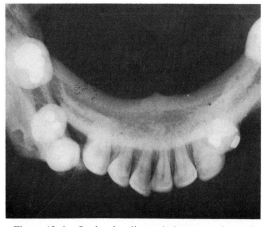

Figure 19–2 Occlusal radiograph demonstrating a displaced and overriding fracture of the anterior portion of the mandible.

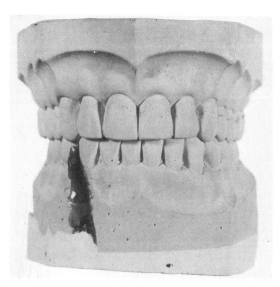

Figure 19–4 The two sections of the lower cast have been reassembled to occlude accurately with the teeth of the maxillary dentition. Sticky wax is used to hold the two segments in their correct relationship until the base is reinforced with plaster.

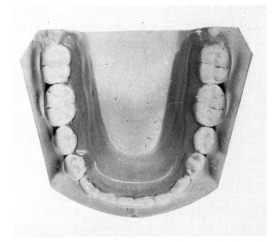

Figure 19–5 Two duplicate models are made from the reassembled lower cast. Upon one of these the outline of the proposed lingual splint is drawn and waxed, using two thicknesses of base plate wax.

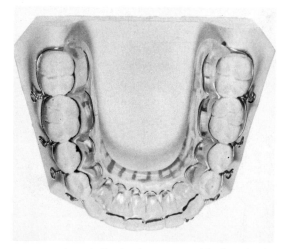

Figure 19–7 Splint has been prepared for insertion by placing a hole through the splint at each interproximal space opposite the cervical line of the tooth. A shallow trough is fashioned between each two holes to accommodate the wire, and a notch is made in the distal ends of the splint. After final polishing the splint is placed in the mouth, and the fracture is manually reduced and secured by wires around each tooth.

without removing the splint by simply boring a hole through the acrylic material.

The application of simple acrylic splints, as shown in Figure 19–8, has proved to be an effective and superior method for the accurate reduction and stabilization of displaced anterior teeth and fractures of the alveolus encountered so frequently in children.

Splints of acrylic material may be strengthened by incorporating a metal bar when it becomes necessary to span an edentulous space in the arch.

COMPLEX SPLINTS

This group of splints is reserved for the more severe or complicated types of facial fractures requiring prolonged fixation and possible restorative surgery. Teeth that are subjected to traction over long periods of time tend to migrate and extrude if not locked into a single unit, or units, by a rigid appliance. This fact is dramatically illustrated by Figure 19–11. Indications for splints of this group are shown in Figures 19–12 and 19–13.

Many variations of the complex splint exist, owing either to choice or necessity. In general, however, they may be grouped as follows:

1. Cast cap splints whose segments, or in which the splints of the opposing arches, may be united and secured by the use of a pin-and-slot appliance or by the screw-lock method.
2. Cast nonocclusal splints that are connected and fixed by the screw-lock method.
3. Cast labial splints that are designed to withstand heavy traction forces (Fig. 19–14).

The procedure of aligning and securing individual segments of the splint involving the

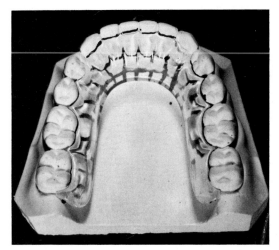

Figure 19–6 Mandibular lingual splint of clear acrylic is polished and replaced on the duplicate model. Clear acrylic is generally used because it facilitates the correct positioning of the holes and the passing of the wires.

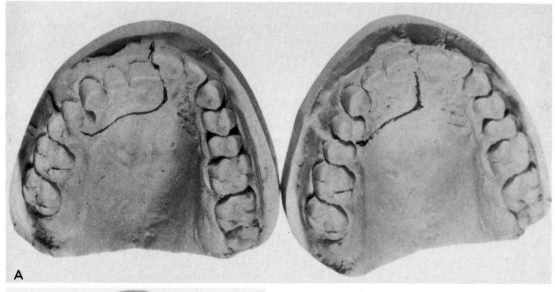

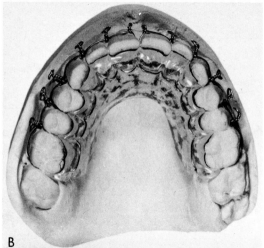

Figure 19–8 The management of an actual case involving a fracture of the alveolar process of the maxilla is illustrated. The cast on the left in *A* shows that the alveolar process has been fractured with a palatal displacement of the right central incisor, lateral incisor, cuspid and first premolar teeth. The cast on the right in *A* has been sectioned and reassembled with the teeth in their correct relationship. *B,* The completed splint wired in place as accomplished in the patient's mouth.

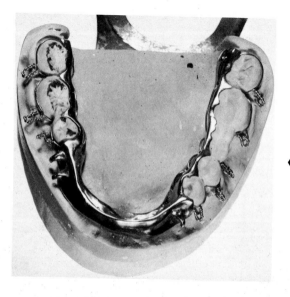

Figure 19–9 A cast lingual splint (Ticonium) that was utilized in the treatment of a comminuted fracture of the symphysis. This splint remained in the patient's mouth for 5 months, and for 3 of these months the patient attended an advanced school. Upon removal of the splint the gingival tissues were found to be healthy, and they regained a completely normal appearance within 1 week.

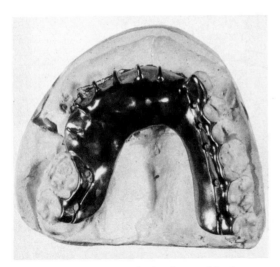

Figure 19-10 A cast palatal splint used in the treatment of a comminuted fracture of the maxilla with a collapsed arch. Splint is shown on the sectioned and reassembled model.

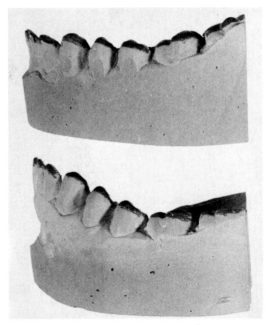

Figure 19-11 These models were made from the same mouth, but 3 months apart. The upper model shows the left side of the arch prior to the resection of the right side of the mandible because of a malignant tumor. The lower photograph illustrates the dramatic extrusion of the teeth after 3 months of intermaxillary traction between cast arch bars. It is well established that cast cap splints that are cemented into place will prevent this tooth migration to a marked degree.

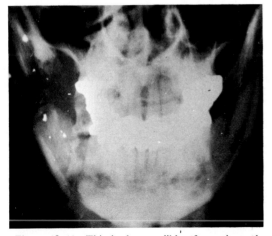

Figure 19-12 This is the mandible of a patient who suffered a shrapnel wound. Note that cast cap splints have been constructed in order to insure a firm fixation of the dental arch relationship that is atraumatic to the teeth and supporting tissues. This splint is designed to remain in place until bone grafting is completed.

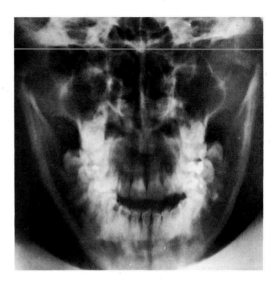

Figure 19-13 Posteroanterior radiograph of a mandible that illustrates the open bite sometimes experienced in cases of bilateral subcondylar fracture with displacement. Cast splints are often necessary in such cases to allow for the strong intermaxillary traction necessary to overcome spasm of the muscles of mastication.

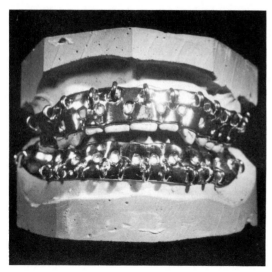

Figure 19–14   Heavy cast labial splint. This splint is of special value in cases in which powerful forward traction is necessary. A metal loop may be placed on the labial surface of the splint to afford a method of attachment for extraoral traction. The splint was used in an actual case of an old, fused fracture of the maxilla with displacement in which refracture and forward positioning were necessary.

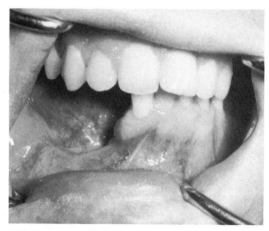

Figure 19–15   Clinical appearance of a patient who had undergone hemisection of the mandible 4 months previously. Cast cap splints will be constructed before a bone graft is inserted.

same arch, or of splints attached to the maxillary and mandibular teeth, may be accomplished in several ways. Figure 19–18 illustrates cast metal splints that are aligned and secured by the pin-and-slot method. This method is very effective in certain cases, while in many others the screw-and-connecting-bar method proves to be effective. Critics of the cast cap splints generally prefer the cast nonocclusal splint in the belief that a more accurate occlusal relationship is attained. This has not been the author's experience. Both types of splints have their indications and serve a definite purpose when used in carefully selected cases.

SPECIAL SPLINTS AS ADJUNCTS TO ORAL SURGICAL PROCEDURES

It has been emphasized repeatedly that both the general practitioner of dentistry and the specialist have the advantage of being able to utilize an almost unlimited variety of prostheses as adjuncts to surgical procedures. However, this opportunity has not been utilized to its fullest extent. These prosthetic appliances vary from the relatively simple types, designed to support and protect tissues after minor surgical procedures, to the more extensive types that are so necessary a part of the treatment plan in major surgical procedures for the mandible or maxilla. The list that follows includes some of the prostheses that have proved effective in planned surgical procedures for the oral and supporting structures:

1. Types of acrylic stents, designed to support and maintain tissues in their desired position after surgical techniques of ridge extension or muscle repositioning.

Figure 19–17   A splint of clear acrylic material that was inserted at the operating table after resection of the left body of the mandible. Two circumferential wires were utilized to stabilize the remaining portion of the mandible against the lower rim, while two Kirschner wires were passed through the upper portion of the labial flanges in the maxillary cuspid regions for fixation of the upper half of the splint. These splints remained in the mouth for 2 months during the healing phase. Upon removal, construction of a denture prosthesis was initiated.

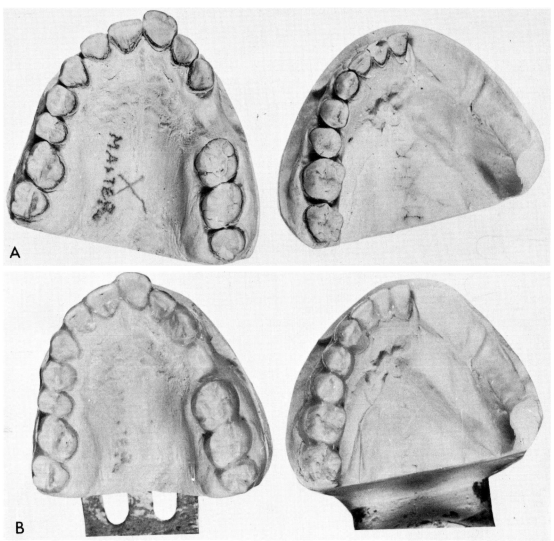

Figure 19-16 Hydrocal casts of the mouth of the patient shown in Figure 19-15. *A*, The cut models have been surveyed in preparation for waxing out undercuts. *B*, Undercuts have now been waxed out and the models are ready for duplication in casting investment material.

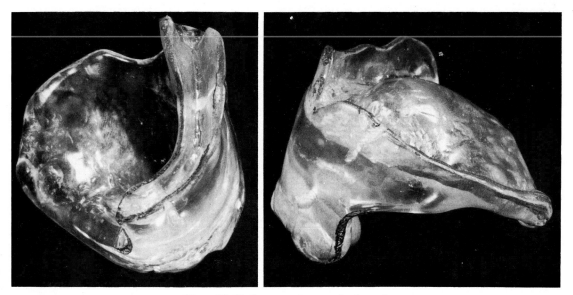

Figure 19-17 *See opposite page for legend.*

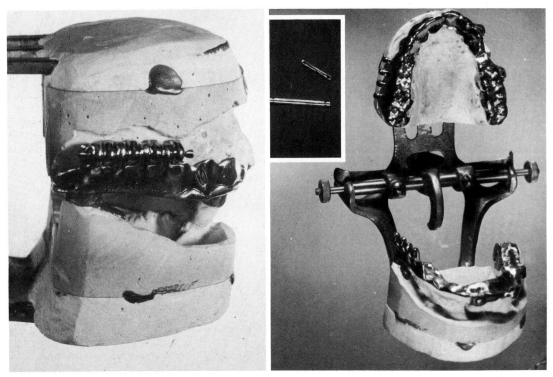

Figure 19–18   Cast splints that are ready for insertion. These splints will be cemented over the mandibular and maxillary teeth with black copper cement. The "pin and slot" method of establishing intermaxillary fixation was selected for use in this case. This may also be accomplished by the use of screws and a connecting bar.

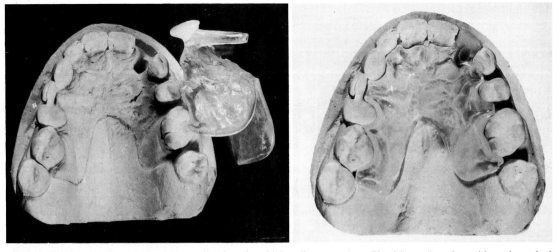

Figure 19–19   Another of the many applications in which splints may be utilized in conjunction with oral surgical procedures. The splint shown here is designed to accomplish decompression and healing of a maxillary radicular cyst.

2. The simple acrylic palatal splint, designed to be inserted immediately after surgery of the palate for conditions such as removal of impacted teeth or tori.

3. Simple acrylic splints for tissue support and protection after closure of naso-oral or antro-oral openings.

4. Properly planned and designed splints for immediate insertion after the removal of a portion of the palate or maxilla.

5. Splints designed to support and prevent deviation of the remaining portion of the mandible after a part has been resected (Fig. 19–17).

6. Splints that serve to maintain a constant opening when the decompression technique is used in the treatment of large cysts (Fig. 19–19).

PROPER SEQUENCE IN THE TREATMENT OF JAW FRACTURES COMPLICATED BY SEVERE ORAL OR LIP LACERATIONS

One of the objectives of this chapter is to stress the necessity of placing the various phases of treatment in their proper sequence. Importance of proper treatment sequence was dramatically demonstrated in the Korean conflict, where it was shown that one of the principal reasons for breakdown of wounds of the lips and surrounding tissues was the closure of these lesions prior to the reduction and fixation of the underlying jaw fractures.

In order to illustrate the proper sequence in the treatment of a maxillofacial injury, the following problem is presented.

HYPOTHETICAL CASE REPORT

Patient. A patient is admitted to the hospital with facial injuries suffered in an automobile accident. Clinical examination reveals no evidence of intracranial pressure or internal injury. Examination of the face and oral structures discloses the following complications:

1. Distortion of occlusal relationship, extreme mobility of entire maxilla, with a collapse of the right side toward the midline, and a separation between the mandibular central incisors, with a disruption of tooth alignment.

2. A severe tongue laceration.

3. Facial lacerations involving both lips (Figs. 19–20 to 19–24).

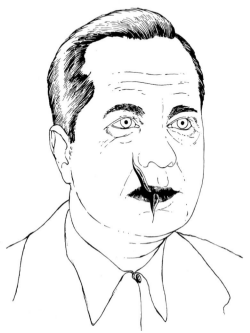

Figure 19–20 Appearance of the patient at the time of injury.

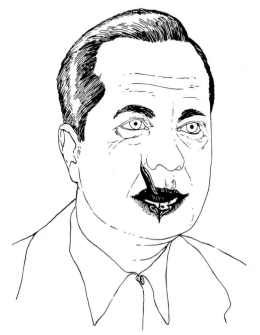

Figure 19–21 Alginate impressions are taken of the maxillary and mandibular arches.

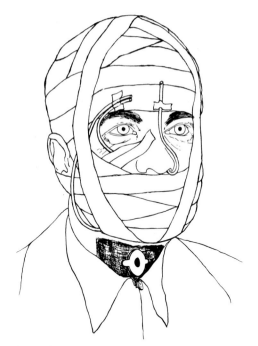

Figure 19–22 The fractures and facial lacerations are supported by a heavy gauze bandage. Tubes are incorporated into the bandage in order that the lacerations may be kept moist.

Radiographic Examination. Radiographs of the facial bones and skull taken on the operating table and interpreted while wet confirm the clinical diagnosis of (1) fracture, simple, symphysis of mandible; (2) fracture, comminuted, maxilla, with displaced fractures of the infraorbital rims; (3) fractures of nasal bones with lateral displacement; and (4) fracture of alveolus and palate with deviation of the right side toward the midline.

The management of this patient is best accomplished by dividing it into two phases, Immediate Treatment and Definitive Treatment.

Immediate Treatment.
1. *Tracheostomy.* This procedure receives first priority, because severe tongue lacerations consistently produce marked swelling after they are sutured. When complicated by a comminuted fracture of the maxilla, the possibility of respiratory embarrassment must be anticipated. Therefore, the first surgical procedure consists of the performance of a tracheostomy under local anesthesia.
2. The tongue laceration is next closed by deeply placed nontension sutures.
3. Alginate impressions are made of the dental arches (Fig. 19–21).
4. A nasogastric tube (Levin) is passed for feeding until the oral tissues heal.
5. The facial and lip wounds are thoroughly cleansed and covered by a heavy pressure

dressing into which two polyethylene tubes are inserted for irrigation (Fig. 19–22).
6. Antibiotics, analgesics, and necessary laboratory studies are ordered, and the patient is returned to the recovery room or ward. Surgery is scheduled for the next day.

Splint Construction. Models are prepared from the alginate impressions that were taken on the operating table. The procedures previously described and illustrated are accomplished, and acrylic splints are prepared for the mandibular and maxillary arch. Rapid-curing acrylic is utilized if time becomes an acute factor.

Definitive Treatment. Approximately 24 hours after admission to the hospital, the patient is again taken to surgery. A general anesthetic is administered through the tracheal opening. Upon removal of the dressing, it is found that considerable swelling of the facial tissues has occurred (Fig. 19–23), but the facial and lip wounds appear to be moist and healthy. Treatment is carried out in the following order:
1. The mandibular splint is inserted and the symphysis fracture is reduced and stabilized by the procedure previously described.
2. The maxillary fractures are reduced and stabilized to the palatal splint.
3. Intermaxillary elastics are applied, and the teeth of the opposing arches are brought into their proper occlusal relationship.
4. The face is thoroughly prepared and the patient redraped.

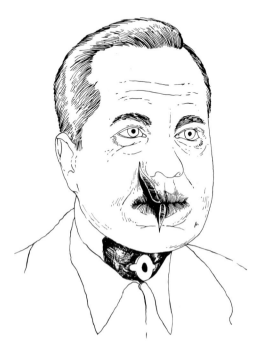

Figure 19–23 Appearance of patient approximately 24 hours after he was admitted to the hospital. Note that considerable facial and neck swelling has occurred.

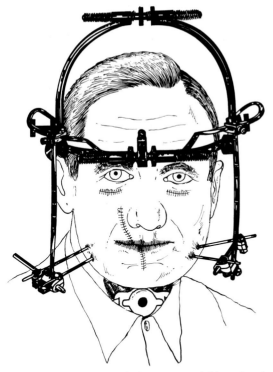

Figure 19-24 The surgical treatment of this patient is completed approximately 28 hours after admission to the hospital. Procedures consisted of reduction and stabilization of the fractures followed by careful suturing of the soft-tissue wounds. The vertical dimension of the face is established and secured by tightening the bolts holding the two vertical connecting rods. (Courtesy of the U.S. Army.)

5. Open reduction with transosseous wiring is performed on each infraorbital rim.
6. The nasal fractures are reduced and supported by passing a straight cutting-edge needle, to which is attached a stainless steel wire, through the fractured nasal bones. The wire is then threaded through two holes of a large flat button, reattached to the needle and passed back through the nasal bones. The two free ends of the wire are next threaded through holes of a second button on the opposite side of the nose and twisted until the buttons afford firm support to the fractures.

7. A Kirschner wire is passed through the bodies of the mandible below the first premolar teeth to serve as an attachment for stabilization of the comminuted maxilla.
8. The lip and facial lacerations are again cleansed and carefully sutured in layers, beginning with the mucosa.
9. A head frame is applied and secured by the use of four screws that engage the outer table of the skull (Fig. 19-24). This appliance, which has proved to be extremely effective in the treatment of severe midface fractures, especially those complicated by fractures of the condyle necks, has the distinct advantage of multiple holes for the insertion of the screws. This makes it possible to avoid skull defects and scalp lacerations. It has been repeatedly proved that this appliance is vastly superior to the plaster head cap because of stability, ease of appliance and comfort to the patient. In addition it is estimated that the rigid stabilization achieved by this appliance results in a reduction of approximately one third of the time required for healing of maxillary fractures of the severely comminuted type.
10. The correct vertical dimension of the face is next determined and stabilized by two metal connecting rods, as shown in Figure 19-24. Shortening of the face is a complication that is observed all too frequently in the treatment of severely comminuted fractures of the maxilla. Most techniques that are recommended for support of the fractured maxilla are designed to counteract the downward pull of the mandible and thus prevent lengthening of the face. The repeated act of swallowing must be considered, however, for it tends to produce an upward pressure with a resultant shortening of the face. In severe injuries of the midface, this shortening can result in a permanent disfigurement. Firm stabilization of the vertical dimension of the face by a method such as the one described above, therefore, becomes a necessity in such cases.

Discussion. The orderly and practical approach to complicated facial injuries, as briefly described in the preceding hypothetical case, has consistently resulted in satisfactory reduction of fractures, excellent cosmetic results and early completion of the case. It must be emphasized again that facial injuries occur in countless varieties and that each case requires alterations in treatment. However, the principles of proper sequence of approach remain constant, and when violated result in undesirable complications.

Note: No fracture of the jaw is treated in any manner without some alteration of occlusal relationship. Therefore, the case cannot be considered completed and the patient should not be discharged until an occlusal relationship study is made and an equilibration of the occlusion accomplished.

CHAPTER **20**

SEGMENTAL SURGERY IN THE TREATMENT OF DENTAL AND FACIAL DISHARMONY*

T. CRADOCK HENRY, F.D.S., L.R.C.P., M.R.C.S.
G. WREAKES, B.CH.D., F.D.S., D.ORTH.R.C.S.

Patients with marked skeletal disproportion and associated severe malocclusions have been successfully treated surgically for many years. The fact that less severe discrepancies and malocclusions can be similarly treated has not been widely appreciated until relatively recent times, despite the publication as long ago as 1921 by Cohn-Stock, describing the successful repositioning of anterior teeth.[3] Since then, sporadic accounts of a similar nature have appeared in the literature, but credit should probably be given to Wassmund in 1935 for establishing the treatment technique. However, probably because of poor anesthesia, inadequate immobilization, surgical complexity and relapse rate, this form of surgery did not receive wide acceptance at the time.

In postwar years, the more refined techniques that have been evolved, together with a more discriminating choice of patients, has enabled the oral surgeon to obtain positive results, virtually devoid of guesswork or risk.

References in the last 12 years are now so numerous that it is felt that a full bibliography would be out of place. However, a comprehensive résumé has been published by Barton and Rayne, and readers might be advised to refer to this article for further information.[1]

Segmental surgery is essentially the movement of groups of teeth and their investing bone to a new position without loss of dental vitality, an adequate blood supply being maintained by soft-tissue pedicles. While no precise terminology has yet been evolved to describe these surgical procedures, "segmental surgery" seems to be a most appropriate title. "Subapical osteotomy" or "ostectomy," although nominally correct, is open to misinterpretation, while "dentoalveolar surgery" is inaccurate, not least because basal bone may also be involved.

The segments that can be repositioned most usefully are the two labial segments and, less frequently, the upper buccal segments, to which passing reference will also be made. This type of surgery parallels certain orthodontic movements, the difference being that, in the latter, teeth are moved through the bone; in the former, teeth and bone are moved *in toto*. The facial changes in response to orthodontic therapy at the postpubertal stage are not gross and are confined to the immediate perioral area. Segmental surgery

---

applied to similar cases likewise produces localized facial improvement, but these may be made more radical by the use of associated procedures, as described later. Therefore, if facial harmony is being sought by segmental procedures alone, the anteroposterior and vertical relationship of the chin point should be correct, and the nose should be of acceptable size and shape.

It follows, therefore, that any disharmony in the immediate perioral area has to be assessed in relation to the face as a whole and the underlying malocclusion. The judgment of favorable facial harmony is complicated by its subjective character and by ethnic considerations, there being no absolute ideal.

Malocclusion, on the other hand, has been objectively analyzed for many years, but even here we rely on Edward Angle's concept of normality as a treatment goal. Since any improvement in the external esthetics of the perioral region must involve changes in the position of the underlying dental structures, it is worth considering the nature of malocclusion.

The denture develops on the underlying skeletal relationship, which is genetically determined; in other words, on the three-dimensional jaw relationship that exists in the absence of dentoalveolar structures. Dental development takes place from the skeletal base line into an environment determined by the tongue on the inside, together with the lips and cheeks on the outside. The shape and activity of these muscle masses determine the spatial relationship of the denture upon the underlying skeletal structures. If the skeletal base relationship and soft-tissue environment are correct, and the dental bases large enough to accommodate the teeth without crowding, then the classic Angle normal occlusion will be obtained. The malocclusions we see are due to the interaction of these etiologic factors.

Orthodontic treatment of a malocclusion out of the mixed dentition stage does not influence the basic skeletal relationship and is primarily induced dentoalveolar remodeling. Similarly, the form and shape of the soft tissue are not altered by the movement of components of the denture relative to the soft tissues, but favorable adaptive changes to the new tooth positions may occur and play an important part in the subsequent stability.

There are obviously similarities between orthodontic treatment and segmental surgery, and the fundamental differences are analyzed in Table 20–1. As can be seen, the main advantage of surgery is the expediency with which the result can be obtained, making the method particularly attractive to adult patients. However, the finesse of orthodontic treatment results is generally not available, and in many cases a combination of orthodontics and surgery is the ideal approach.

CASE ASSESSMENT AND TECHNIQUE

Ideally, patients should be seen jointly by the oral surgeon and orthodontist at an early stage of planning. This presupposes, of course, that the oral surgeon accepts that segmental movement is not the universal panacea of all malocclusions and that the orthodontist, on his side, accepts that his more difficult skeletally adverse cases can be helped by surgical intervention. This agreement makes it possible for the general practitioners to be confident that cases referred to either an orthodontist or an oral surgeon will receive a fair and balanced assessment, leading to optimal treatment.

A general discussion with a patient before any elective medical or dental procedure seems to be an obvious preliminary, and its importance in this field cannot be overstressed. For example, a patient who rejects the concept of orthodontic therapy may have to accept a compromise in treatment because of the technical limitations of surgical manipulation, and it is useful to be able to think within the correct parameters at the outset. When the viewpoint and motivation of the patient are known, a clinical assessment can be carried out, as discussed in the following section.

CLINICAL EXAMINATION

GENERAL AND EXTRAORAL

The patient is examined in profile and in full-face aspect. For this, he is seated in an upright position with the Frankfort plane parallel to the floor. The following points are then noted:

1. The vertical and anteroposterior relationship of the chin relative to the forehead (Fig. 20–1).
2. The size and shape of the nose (Fig. 20–2).

Table 20–1 *Surgical vs. Orthodontic Treatment of Dental and Facial Disharmony*

CONSIDERATION	SEGMENTAL SURGERY		ORTHODONTIC TREATMENT	
	Feasibility	*Comment*	*Feasibility*	*Comment*
Movement of groups of teeth	Yes—*in toto.*		Yes—often moved in subgroups for anchorage reasons.	
Treatment time	Short—6 weeks.		Medium-long—1–2 years.	
Direction of movement	Any dimension of space.		Any dimension of space.	Difficult in deep bite, as in Angle Class II, Division 2, malocclusions. Open-bite closure not always predictable—fairly lengthy retention. Overbite cannot be created. Anteroposterior movement of lower incisors limited.
Individual tooth movement	Possible.	Blood supply may be a problem and method only applicable to individual teeth.	Readily accomplished.	
Correction of rotations	Not possible.		Readily accomplished.	
Prepubertal age treatment	Possible.	Not generally advised because further growth may invalidate result.	Possible.	Growth at the pubertal growth spurt can be used to advantage.
Adult patients	Possible.	Short treatment time desirable.	Possible.	Longer treatment often not acceptable.
Closure of tooth spacing in the segment to be moved	Possible to a degree.	Midline diastemas may be closed by dividing the labial segment in the midline. Additional corticotomy.	Possible	Readily accomplished.
Reduction of tooth proclination in overjet reduction	Possible.	Rotate fragment during distal repositioning. If carried out to excess will carry cuspids to infraocclusion.	Possible.	Readily accomplished.

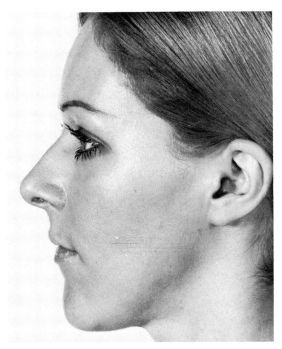

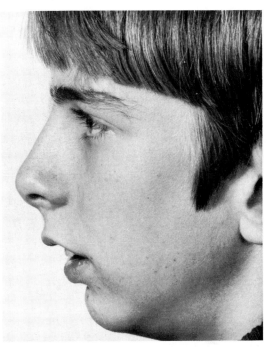

Figure 20-1 The correct anteroposterior chin position disguises the Angle Class III incisal relationship, but there is an excessive vertical chin prominence.

Figure 20-2 The retrusive chin position is very obvious in this case of Angle Class II, Division I, malocclusion, and the effect is heightened by the nose size.

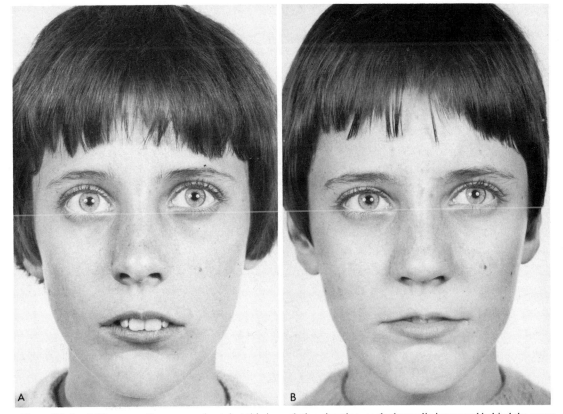

Figure 20-3 *A,* The upper lip appears short, but this is a relative situation, as the lower lip is trapped behind the upper incisors. *B,* After movement of the upper labial segment, the lips are almost in contact at rest, and the upper lip shortage is, therefore, in fact minimal.

3. The form and length of the lips—at rest, while swallowing and as a result of conscious effort (Fig. 20–3).

4. The presence or absence of compensatory actions to disguise the condition; for instance, in cases of mandibular retrusion, an attempt to improve the profile and facilitate lip apposition by forward posturing of the mandible. This type of habit can produce temporomandibular joint symptoms (Fig. 20–4).

5. The presence of abnormal speech patterns and whether these patterns have produced the dental problems or are only secondarily associated with them (Fig. 20–5).

INTRAORAL

The malocclusion associated with the adverse facial appearance is noted after intraoral examination. The state of the periodontal tissues is also noted, as well as carious lesions of the teeth. A poor gingival condition in the upper labial segment is not uncommon in cases such as that shown in Figure 20–6,

but it is likely to improve after treatment that facilitates lip apposition, because gingival dehydration is thus eliminated. The presence of teeth with a great deal of restoration may influence the choice of extractions necessary for treatment.

Consideration of these factors gives the operator an idea of the underlying fault, of the desirable corrections and of the limits of such corrections. For example, the patient shown before treatment in Figure 20–6 has an upper lip that is excessively short, and, as a result of treatment (Fig. 20–26), the lips can be sealed with little effort in the correct relationship to the upper incisors. However, they are still apart at rest, owing to a shortage of upper lip tissue, which is unaffected by repositioning the underlying dentoalveolar tissues. The patient should be told that, in this one respect, the result may be less than perfect.

Orthodontic movements are affected by changes in the collagenous elements of the periodontal ligament with or without bone deposition and resorption. This state of fluidity is induced by light pressures similar to those that may be exerted by aberrant soft

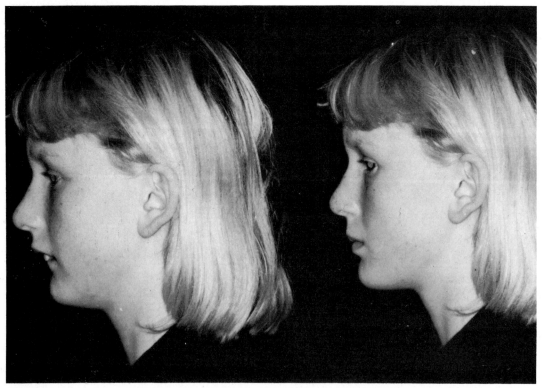

Figure 20–4   This Class II, Division 1, malocclusion with mandibular retrusion is disguised by forward mandibular posturing.

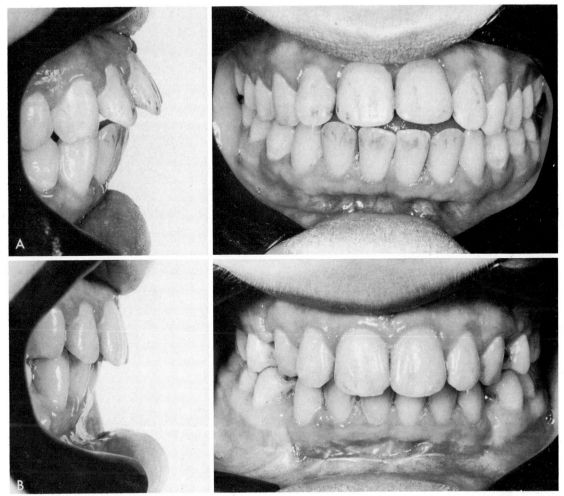

Figure 20–5 *A*, Mild sigmatism thought to be secondarily associated with the bimaxillary proclination. *B*, After surgical repositioning of the labial segments, the improved speech and absence of relapse confirms the original assessment.

tissue activity. Conversely, a successful orthodontic result is retained after treatment by the soft tissues exerting similar forces in a favorable direction.

Two examples may serve to illustrate this point. In a normal occlusion, the lower lip overlies the occlusal third of the labial aspect of the upper incisors. Orthodontic stability would be achieved if the lip, prior to treatment in a maxillary protrusive case, lay behind the upper incisors but lay as in a normal occlusion after treatment. An anterior open bite, nonskeletal in origin, associated with a sigmatic speech defect and therefore tongue thrusting, would be very suspicious for orthodontic stability, since this type of tongue activity is endogenous and unchanged by alteration of the dental environment.

Surgical movement of tooth-bearing segments does not involve the changes required in orthodontic movement, but it is analogous to the healing process of a fracture at a site remote from the crowns of the teeth. Our experience and that of others suggest that a certain license can be taken in surgical repositioning, but, wherever possible, the parameters of known orthodontic stability are observed.

ROENTGENOGRAPHIC EXAMINATION

Localized radiographs of the teeth are important for showing pathologic conditions in apical or periodontal regions. If surgical division between adjacent teeth is contemplated, then it is essential to know the amount of

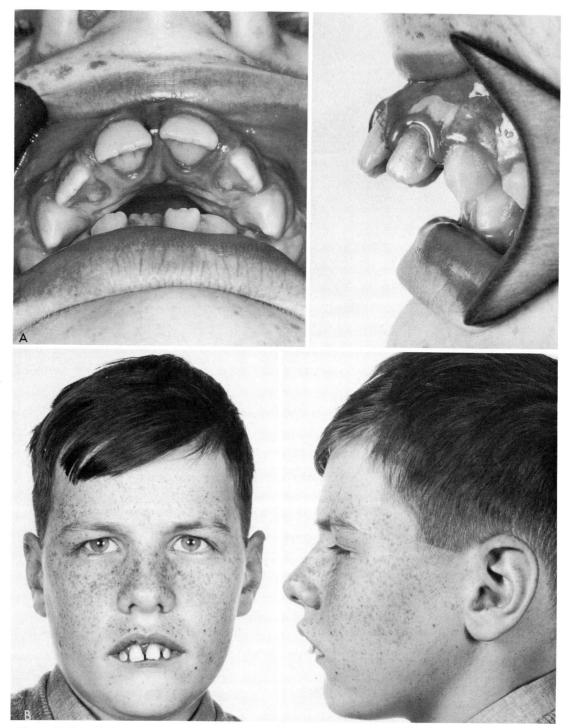

Figure 20–6   *A,* Severe Class II, Division 1, malocclusion with labial gingival hypertrophy and hyperemia. *B,* Facial views showing marked upper lip shortness.

bone available between the roots, as well as any abnormality in root form. It is also useful to know the locations of bony foramina, such as that of the mental foramen, and to be able to judge the approximate root length before making subapical ostectomy cuts. Because of the proximity of surgical division to the maxillary sinus in maxillary procedures, it is wise to obtain an occipitomental view if there is any suspicion of sinus infection in the patient's history.

Lateral skull films and their associated tracings provide valuable information. However, as with radiographs used for any other purpose, they should be used to corroborate a clinical diagnosis rather than be made the basis of the diagnosis. The value of cephalometrics in this field is well summarized by Moore.[10]

CLINICAL PHOTOGRAPHY

Photographs are invaluable for record purposes, and black-and-white photographs enlarged to life size have a specific place in the assessment and planning of the mild Angle Class III malocclusion. In the moderately severe case, in which one is in doubt about the choice between labial segment surgery and osteotomy of the ramus, the position of the chin postoperatively is often the deciding factor. This can be illustrated graphically by

sectioning the profile photograph along the occlusal plane and adjusting the mandible to the proposed degree of occlusal movement (Fig. 20–7). The accuracy of the simulation can be increased as follows:

1. A soft-tissue profile roentgenogram is obtained simultaneously with the hard-tissue film.
2. The occlusal plane, as derived from the hard-tissue film, is transferred to the soft-tissue film.
3. The profile photograph is enlarged to correspond to the soft-tissue profile size.
4. Superimposition of photograph and x-ray film allows the transfer of the occlusal plane.
5. The photograph can then be sectioned in the direction that operative movement would actually occur.

STUDY AND PLANNING MODELS

Although clinical photographic and cephalometric evaluation may have suggested what corrective change is desirable, the actual occlusion is the final arbiter of what can in fact be achieved. Study models make possible a three-dimensional consideration of the occlusion, and the manipulation of the models gives some idea of the possible corrective operative procedures. However, some years ago, one of us (G.W.) became dissatisfied

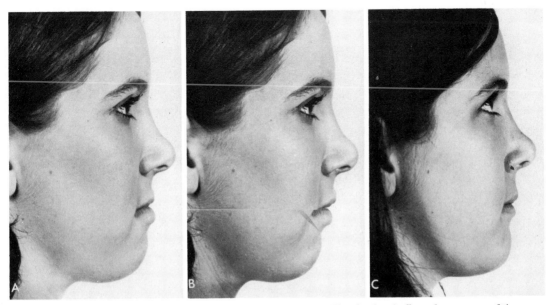

Figure 20–7 Mild Class III malocclusion. *A*, Before treatment. *B*, The simulated effect of osteotomy of the ramus, which would overcorrect the chin position. *C*, The result of lower segmental movement.

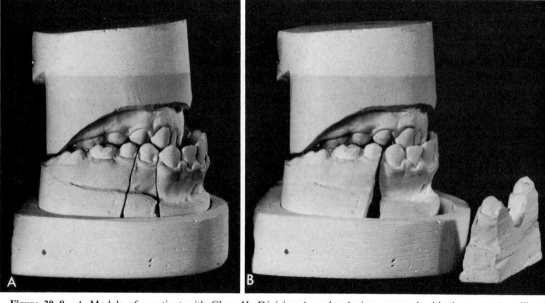

Figure 20–8   *A,* Models of a patient with Class II, Division 1, malocclusion mounted with the upper (maxillary) model on the lower arm of the articulator (not shown). *B,* Section removed and labial segment repositioned to simulate results of the operation.

with the conventional method of both mounting and manipulating the study casts; planning discrepancies seemed too frequent, probably because digital movement of the anterior segment did not simulate the operative maneuver. To overcome the problem of gravitational displacement, the method that follows was devised.

The base of the upper (maxillary) model is given a slight taper and the models are sealed in occlusion. The lower (mandibular) model is then attached to the upper arm of a plane-line articulator. Separating medium is applied to the base of the upper model, and it is seated into soft plaster covering the lower arm of the articulator. When this has set, the upper model is removed from the plaster base and sectioned mesial and distal to the first bicuspids (Fig. 20–8). The anterior and posterior components of the upper model are now returned, and the arm of the articulator is closed. The anterior segment can now be

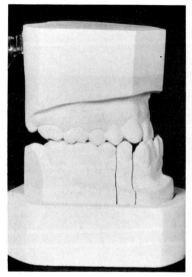
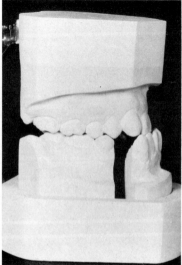
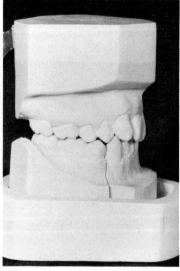

Figure 20–9   Models of a case of Class III malocclusion treated in a similar manner to that in Figure 20–8.

digitally repositioned in one plane without gravitational disturbance. This makes it possible to determine the amount of bone removal required for operation.

Simulated mandibular procedures do not present gravitational problems. The upper and lower models, therefore, can be mounted in a conventional position on the articulator arms (Fig. 20–9). A faulty diagnosis can also be shown in this way, for if the bicuspid space does not provide sufficient space to reduce the overjet completely, then the original condition is too gross for segmental surgery; or, alternatively perhaps, segmental movement should be applied to both jaws to gain the overall desired effect.

Wherever possible, the aim of our segmental surgery has been to reduce the segmental movement to one spatial plane and one linear direction. This has been done by orthodontic preparation, and it is on this premise that the planning technique we have described is based. The time for this preparatory work rarely exceeds 6 months, and the actual operative surgery time is reduced to a minimum. Since trauma and postoperative swelling are related to operating time, there are considerable advantages in this method.

IMMOBILIZATION

When the orthodontic preparation is complete, the method of immobilization at the time of operation can be considered. While it is true that almost any of the conventional methods of fixation—for instance, arch bars, fixed orthodontic appliances or acrylic splints—can be used, our personal preference

is for the cast metal cap splints (Fig. 20–10), because they offer such positive fixation and control. The splints are made in sections that are united at the time of operation by locking bars, these having been prefabricated in the laboratory to correspond to the final desired position.

Fixation is maintained for an average of 6 weeks, and the segment is tested for union prior to splint removal by unscrewing the locking bars and testing by digital pressure.

Surprisingly, patients tolerate the appearance of these splints extremely well and seem to prefer them to a less noticeable orthodontic appliance if this has to be worn for a longer period of time.

SURGICAL APPROACH

The osteotomy procedure may be carried out in either the maxilla or the mandible or in both jaws. Basically, this consists of the extraction of two bicuspids and the removal of a slot of bone as an extension of the socket, so that the tooth-bearing segment is mobilized and may be moved in a superior, inferior, anterior or posterior direction (Fig. 20–11). The segment is then moved to the desired posttreatment position and immobilized until union is complete.

When no distal movement is required, for example, to elevate or depress the lower anterior teeth in an axial direction, surgical division can be made between the first bicuspids and the cuspids without the extraction of a bicuspid. In the maxilla, cuspids may be removed instead of bicuspids, should this be advantageous in a particular case.

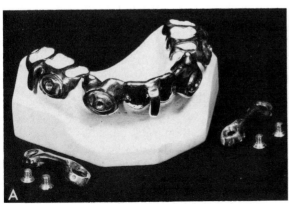 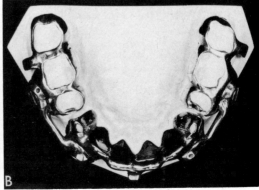

Figure 20–10 *A,* Cast cap splints, with locking bars removed. *B,* Occlusal view of the assembled splint units.

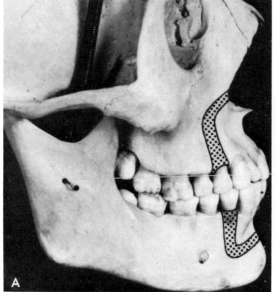
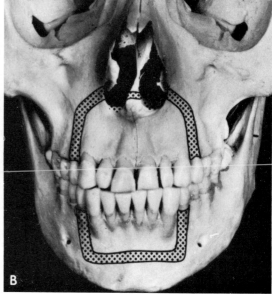
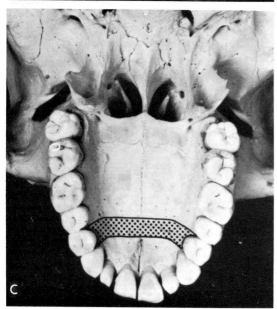

Figure 20–11 The maxillary and mandibular ostectomy sections demonstrated on a skull. *A,* Lateral view. *B,* Anterior view. *C,* Palatal view.

OPERATIVE TECHNIQUE

MAXILLARY LABIAL SEGMENT

Staging in Maxillary Surgery

In the maxilla it has been our custom to perform a two-stage operation, partly because this ensures better visibility with a more precise resection of palatal bone, and partly because the viability of the labial segment never appears in doubt. This clinical assessment seems to have been confirmed in recent animal studies carried out by Bell and Levy.

These authors showed that under simulated clinical conditions there was minimal histologic evidence of vascular ischemia when the labial segment was adequately pedicled to the labiobuccal mucoperiosteum. Moreover, in a two-stage procedure, waiting 3 weeks between the first and second stages allowed revascularization of the initially raised palatal flap to the underlying bone.[2]

From clinical experience we believe these findings to be correct, but on the two occasions when an interval of 3 weeks was left between the palatal and buccal ostectomy, we found difficulty in reducing the segment, owing to the firmness of the newly formed fibrous tissue. Revascularization almost certainly occurs in 15 days, and we would advise, if the two-stage operation is performed, that the second stage should not be delayed more than that time.

However, we have performed upper labial segment surgery in one stage and have found this to be satisfactory in regard to viability, although leaving an anterior palatal attachment for insurance purposes reduced both visibility and access. We therefore describe only the two-stage operation here.

Staged Operative Procedure

The patient's general condition is assessed, and blood is cross-matched as a precaution. However, at no time has transfusion ever been required, as blood loss with hypotension has not exceeded 250 ml. Antibiotic coverage is instituted, should there be evidence of recent upper respiratory infection. The cap splints are also tried on at this stage, to check that they fit satisfactorily.

Anesthesia.   Anesthesia is induced with intravenous thiopentone and suxamethonium and maintained through a nasal endotracheal tube, with the pharynx packed, and with use of nitrous oxide, oxygen and halothane.

We prefer hypotensive anesthesia, since the relatively bloodless field facilitates the surgery. In addition to posture, the two drugs commonly used are trimethaphan camphorsulfonate (Arfonad), 1:1000, administered by drip, or hexamethonium chloride by injection.

If hypotensive anesthesia either is not available or is contraindicated, vision at the operative site can be improved by local infiltration of 1:200,000 epinephrine into the soft tissues.

First Stage of Operation.   As already indicated, the first operation is confined to the palatal ostectomy, and it is, therefore, an advantage to position the patient on the operating table with the neck fully extended and a sandbag under the shoulders.

The surgeon either sits or stands behind the patient's head, with the assistant on the appropriate side. The endotracheal tube can be connected to the anesthetic apparatus in such a way that it does not impede access to the oral cavity.

The palatal mucoperiosteal incision skirts the incisive foramen and then continues in a line adjacent to the necks of the teeth as far as the second molar region (Fig. 20–12). The

flap is then elevated; this exposes most of the hard palate but leaves the posterior palatine arteries intact. It can often be packed neatly out of the way; otherwise, it is retracted by an assistant (Fig. 20–13B).

If the 4/4 teeth are to be extracted, this is done, and measured horizontal markings are carried across the palatal bone to the determined width. The amount of bone to be removed will have been estimated on the model preoperatively. This will vary from case to case and will, of course, depend on the extent of the overjet. No more than the width of a first bicuspid is generally required. It is a good plan to err on the generous side, but only to the extent of 1 or 2 mm., since once the palatal flap has been returned it is desirable that it should not be disturbed.

The bone on the palatal aspect of both sockets is first nibbled away with a Jansen-Middleton or McIndoe bone-cutting forceps. The ostectomy section is then carried medially from the sockets to follow the markings already made. The authors prefer to confirm these by perforating the cortical bone with a fine rosehead bur, or the point of a Lindeman rotating saw. These can then be joined together by a fissure bur, such as the Toller, until two parallel cuts have been made, extending through the depth of the palatal cortex. By careful instrumentation and with use of a water coolant at all times, the cuts can be deepened sufficiently to allow removal of sections of bone without perforating the antral or nasal mucosa (Fig. 20–13B). However, no untoward consequences seem to arise if this takes place, except that it is wise to be sure no residual blood clot remains in the nasal cavity or postnasal space following disintubation.

It having been determined that the ostectomy is complete, a vertical incision is now made in the upper labial frenum and deepened to expose the nasal spine. Through a submucous approach, the nasal septum is separated from the vomer by means of a fine osteotome with the corners blunted, or even a pair of heavy scissors (Fig. 20–13A). With careful dissection damage to the nasopalatine vessels or accidental penetration of the nasal cavity should be avoided.

Finally, a flat, narrow-bladed instrument may be introduced into the wound and moved from side to side in order to check visually by its appearance through the palatal ostectomy that adequate division of the septum has been achieved (Fig. 20–13B). However, if the segment is to be raised or rotated to any extent,

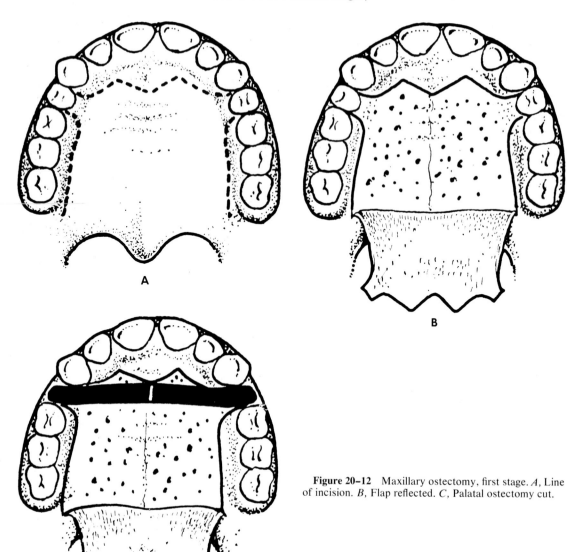

Figure 20–12 Maxillary ostectomy, first stage. *A*, Line of incision. *B*, Flap reflected. *C*, Palatal ostectomy cut.

simple division of the septum may result in its buckling, in which case a wedge resection should be carried out.

It may be noted from some of the drawings and photographs that division of the septal attachment has been done in either the first- or second-stage procedure. On reflection, the authors have concluded that it is best done at the first stage, if a two-stage procedure is proposed, but this is a matter of personal choice.

Following the ostectomy, the flap is put back into position and sutured into place with 000 braided silk sutures. The prefabricated appliance, usually one that has been used for orthodontic purposes, is positioned and any cribs for retention are adjusted. The value of a simple appliance of this nature cannot be overestimated, as it not only will minimize hematoma formation below the palatal flap but will also serve in maintaining depression of the lower six front teeth if a bite plane has been incorporated (Fig. 20–14*A*).

The interim period occupies about 15 days, during which time the patient's general condition, the integrity of the palatal flap and the fit of the splints can be determined (Fig. 20–14*B*).

On the day prior to the second operation the elected appliances for fixation are put

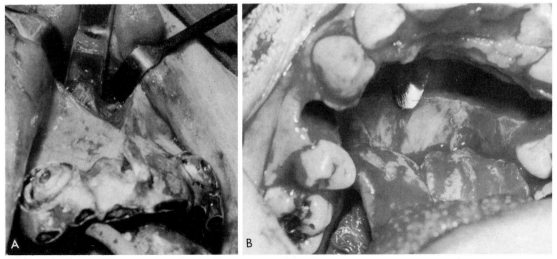

Figure 20–13 Operative procedure. *A,* Chisel dividing the nasal septum (between retractors). *B,* Retraction of the palatal flap, the palatal ostectomy cut and a Howarth's elevator passing from the divided septum into the palatal ostectomy.

onto the buccal and labial teeth. If these are cast metal cap splints, the three sections should be cemented with either crown-and-bridge or black copper cement, not mixed too thickly, so that a correct seating is obtained.

Second Stage of Operation. With the same anesthetic technique but on this occasion oral intubation, the patient is so positioned that the buccal approach can be made. A vertical incision is made in the 3/3 region, which curves mesially toward the floor of the nose. A mucoperiosteal flap is elevated and retracted distally, exposing the 4/4 socket walls. At the same time the floor and lateral walls of the nose are identified by a subperiosteal approach on both sides (Fig. 20–15).

The ostectomy cuts are now made vertically, usually the full width of the socket wall until the pyriform fossa is reached. Here they are angulated mesially above the apices of the canines and involve the lateral wall of the nose, but care should be taken not to carry out an inadvertent 3/3 apicoectomy (Fig. 20–16).

As in the first stage, it seems best to mark out the lines of the cuts in the cortical bone, using ink marks confirmed by a rosehead bur, before continuing with the second and parallel cut. It is certainly unwise to remove the full predetermined width of bone at this juncture; this should be done after mobilization of the segment has been effected.

After mobilization has been achieved, an attempt can be made to reduce the segment,

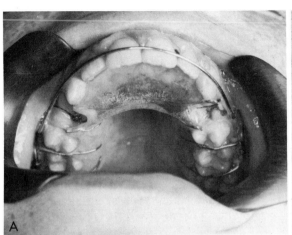
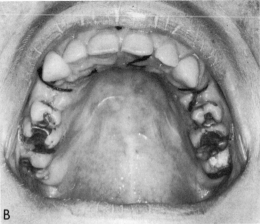

Figure 20–14 *A,* A simple orthodontic appliance retaining the palatal flap. *B,* The healed palate 14 days after the first stage and immediately prior to removal of sutures and the application of the cast cap splints.

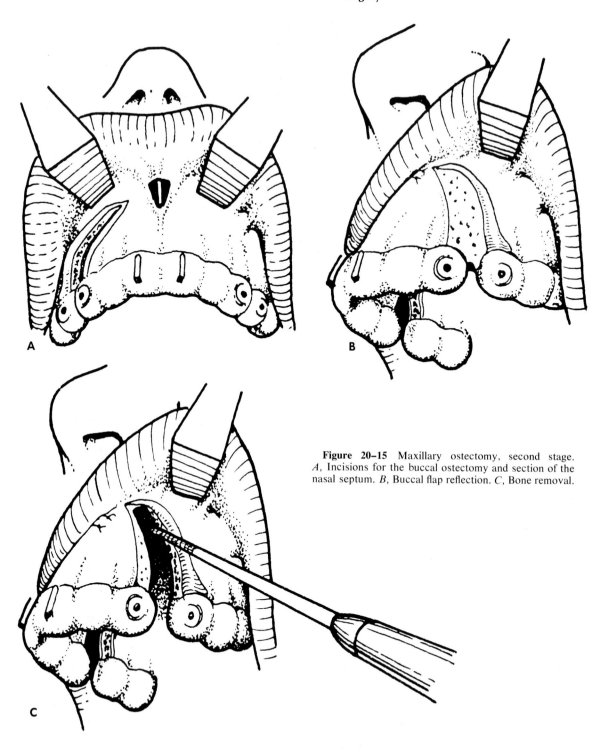

Figure 20–15 Maxillary ostectomy, second stage. *A*, Incisions for the buccal ostectomy and section of the nasal septum. *B*, Buccal flap reflection. *C*, Bone removal.

when any interference from bone spicules or inadequate resection will be immediately visible. In this way good bony contact on the interfaces should be achieved when the final reduction to the predetermined position is made. As with the palatal approach, it is almost certain that the nasal mucoperiosteum

and antral lining will be encountered, and their protection to avoid perforation adds some requirement of finesse to the procedure. Here again the curved portion of a MacDonald's dissector introduced so as to protect the lining membrane of these cavities when a bur is in use will prove invaluable. When the dis-

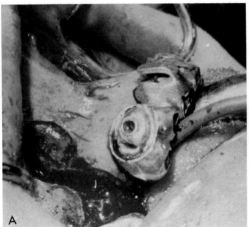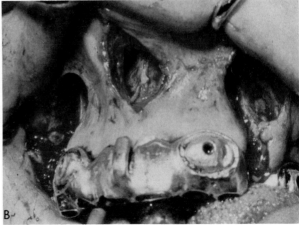

Figure 20-16   Operative procedure. *A*, Lateral ostectomy cut completed on the first side. *B*, Bony surgery completed. *Note:* We now prefer to perform septal division during the first stage of operation (see text).

sector is placed subperiosteally and held firmly in position, the bur can be used with impunity under a water jet without fear of driving it into the antral or nasal cavities.

The final reduction of the labial segment is made by a trial-and-error procedure, with removal of those fragments of bone which seem to impede the precise application of locking bars where splints have been used or where the reduction does not conform to the laboratory plan in other methods of immobilization (Fig. 20-17).

Once fixation has been achieved, the pack and endotracheal tube can be withdrawn, and, as no intermaxillary fixation is employed, an oral airway is inserted. The patient is supervised until his level of consciousness is such that a safe return to the ward can be made. When hypotension has been employed, it is advisable to nurse the patient flat for 12 hours; on the other hand, the blood pressure should not be allowed to rise too sharply in

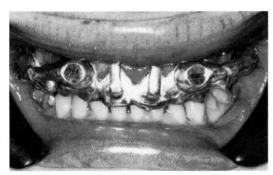

Figure 20-17   Clinical appearance 6 weeks postoperatively, showing the splint and locking bars *in situ.*

the first hour or two, in case this should encourage fresh and unwanted bleeding.

Hospitalization should not occupy more than 3 or 4 days, and, although some facial edema is encountered that can be minimized by the administration of a proteolytic enzyme, the patient should be fit enough to return to work or go on convalescence.

MANDIBULAR LABIAL SEGMENT

The indications for this form of surgery have already been given, and all that remains is to describe the surgical approach (Fig. 20-18).

Here a one-stage operation is quite acceptable, there being sufficient nourishment derived from the intact lingual pedicle to obviate the hazard of nonviability. With planning models at hand and the sectional cast metal cap splints already cemented, the surgeon may have the patient anesthetized, utilizing a nasal endotracheal tube and, if desired, a hypotensive technique.

An incision is made in the mucosa of the buccolabial fold, rather lower than the one that was first employed, which is illustrated in the diagram (Fig. 20-19). By submucosal dissection, two flaps can be raised, exposing the mentalis attachment, which should be incised horizontally, the incision being taken through the periosteum. Having encountered cortical bone, the subperiosteal elevation or division flaps or both are raised to expose both the socket walls of the teeth to be removed and the mental foramina with their nerves. These nerves, once identified, have to be closely guarded against trauma, with the minimal

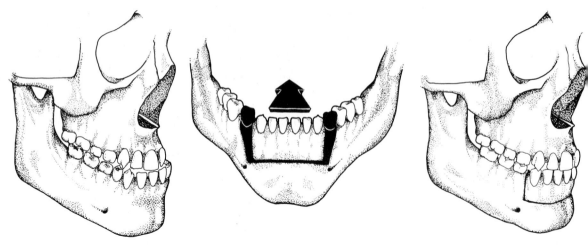

Figure 20–18 Schematic summary of the mandibular labial segment procedure.

amount of retraction. On occasions, especially when teeth $\overline{4/4}$ have previously been removed and $\overline{5/5}$ have drifted mesially, it may be necessary to exteriorize them and set them distally before the osteotomy is completed. The requisite teeth are now removed, either with forceps or by sectioning them with a dental bur, if access with forceps is restricted.

The lateral socket wall can now be nibbled away to its apex and then deepened with a bur, so that two vertical ostectomy cuts are outlined. Guidance in regard to the depth of the section can be obtained from periapical films showing the apices of $\overline{543/345}$.

In nonextraction cases, as in labial segment advancement, the vertical division can be ini-

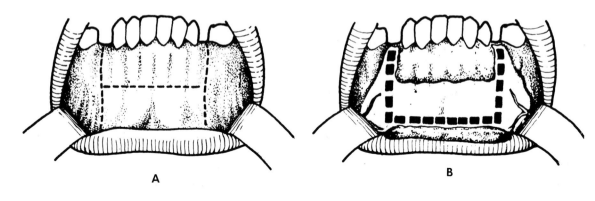

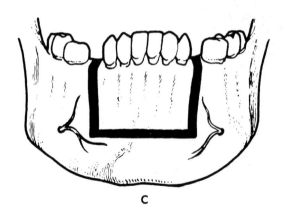

Figure 20–19 Operative stages. *A*, Incision. *B*, Flap reflected. *C*, Ostectomy cut.

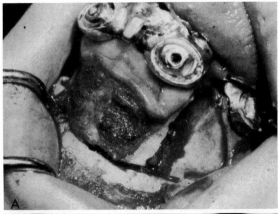
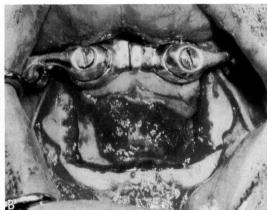
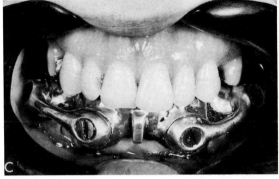

Figure 20–20 Operative procedure. *A* and *B*, The ostectomy section. *C*, After surgery and prior to splint removal.

tiated between $\overline{4-3/3-4}$ or $\overline{5-4/4-5}$ with a fine-tapered fissure bur and completed with an osteotome, modified from an enamel chisel.

The horizontal osteotomy (Fig. 20–20) is carried well below the apices of the incisors and cuspids and joins together the vertical osteotomy or ostectomy cuts. Instrumentation is a personal choice, but these authors find it again best to mark out with a rosehead bur the direction of the section and to join the markings together by a fissure bur. Still using a suitable bur, the operator deepens the osteotomy until the lingual plate is felt. Attention can now be paid to the lingual aspect of the socket walls. With the soft tissues protected by a narrow curved instrument (MacDonald's dissector), introduced subperiosteally, bur and osteotomes may be used to complete this part of the ostectomy. All that now remains for the surgeon is to in-fracture the lingual cortex in a horizontal plane, using a very thin broad-bladed osteotome, which must not be allowed to act as a wedge.

Once the labial segment is mobile, an attempt at reduction is made, and under direct vision any encroaching bone spicules or slender shelves in the socket region usually are removed. Full reduction can be judged by

the accurate location of the locking bars, and if these do click home, they can be screwed into position (Fig. 20–21*A*). As this procedure is in one stage and the entire nourishment of the segment is derived from the lingual pedicle, it will be appreciated that the soft tissues must be treated with respect. In order not to put the blood supply at risk, subperiosteal elevation and retraction on the lingual aspect should be kept to a minimum, and the bur must not be allowed to macerate the periosteum or muscle attachments on this aspect.

Should the labial segment not only have to be moved in an anterior or posterior direction but also have to be elevated, then quite a large gap will be created between the sectioned surfaces, causing a delay in union. In these cases it has been our custom to fill the space so created by osteogenic material of an autogenous nature, as this expedites new bone formation. The method employed is adequately described by Flint,[7] and entails no more than a 1-inch incision over the crest of the ilium, the cortical bone of which is hinged up as an osteoplastic flap.

The resultant scar is minimal, there is no loss of contour, and there is no inhibition in

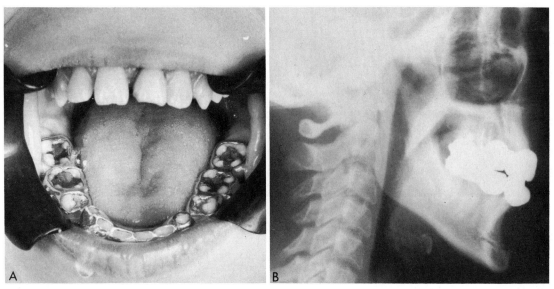

Figure 20–21   *A*, Clinical appearance of a modified cap splint, with the occlusal surfaces of the teeth left free. *B*, Lateral skull radiograph demonstrating the ostectomy cuts in maxilla and mandible.

walking. This is in contrast with the conventional bone grafts taken from the inner table, where complications and postoperative disability are far from unknown.

Finally, the soft tissues in the buccal sulcus are repaired in the normal manner, the endotracheal tube is withdrawn, and the patient is returned to the ward with an oral airway in position.

In combined procedures, when both upper and lower labial segments have to be moved, as in bimaxillary protrusion, the same type of

surgery is instituted. However, the planning may be slightly more complicated, as is shown in Figure 20–22. The models in this instance have again been reversed, with the upper model mounted on the lower arm of the articulator; in the center photograph it is apparent that the upper labial segment cannot be displaced distally until adjustment has been made in the lower arch. In the right-hand photograph, the lower labial segment has been set back and depressed, while the upper labial segment not only has been set

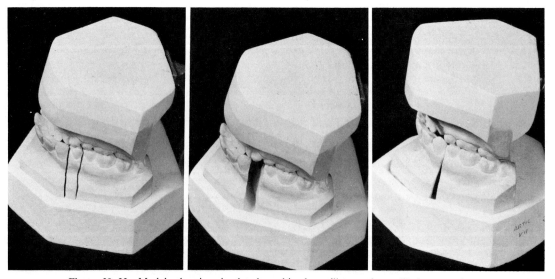

Figure 20–22   Models showing simulated combined maxillary and mandibular procedures.

back but has been given a slight element of rotation to obtain incisal contact (see Figure 20–21B).

CLINICAL APPLICATION

As segmental movement is being applied essentially for the correction of malocclusions, these cases will be considered according to Angle's classification but only in respect to incisal relationship.

CLASS II, DIVISION 1, MALOCCLUSION

The significant feature of patients in this group is the increased incisor overjet with an overbite that may be increased or decreased in extent. The overjet may be due entirely to proclination, that is, forward angulation of the upper incisors, perhaps caused by adverse lip activity or a digit-sucking habit. Alternatively, the overjet may be present with correctly angulated and upright upper and lower incisors; in this case the basic skeletal jaw relationship is at fault. It is then important to determine whether the mandible is retrusive relative to the maxilla and base of the skull, or whether the maxilla is the jaw at fault, being protrusive relative to the base of the skull. In many cases the overjet is the combination of incisor proclination and skeletal discrepancy.

The ideal case for segmental correction is the case in which the overjet is primarily maxillary in source, with minimal incisor proclination and an overjet approximately the width of a premolar. An overjet greater in extent but composed in part by incisor proclination can often be reduced to the surgical limits by initial orthodontic treatment. The amount of overjet correction obtainable by surgical movement can be increased by a combination of labial segment rotation with distal movement, but if carried out to excess this brings the upper canines above the occlusal plane to a position of infraocclusion.

Case Report No. 1

CORRECTION OF CLASS II, DIVISION 1, MALOCCLUSION IN A 12-YEAR-OLD BOY

This 12-year-old boy presented with severe Class II, Division 1, malocclusion (Fig. 20–23A) caused by a combination of maxillary protrusion, adverse soft tissues and a discontinued digit-sucking habit. The overjet was in part due to incisor proclination and the bodily forward displacement of the teeth was in part due to the skeletal discrepancy, that is, the maxillary protrusion. The mouth was sealed during swallowing by the tongue thrusting forward to contact the lip and hence the incomplete overbite. This was thought to be a secondary adaptive pattern because of the difficulty of producing the more usual lip-to-lip seal.

It was felt that the treatment time should be as short as possible on the grounds of doubtful cooperation and oral hygiene; therefore, a combined orthodontic-surgical approach was chosen. A removable orthodontic appliance with extraoral reinforcement was fitted to close the anterior spaces and retract the upper incisors to an upright position, as seen in Figures 20–23B and 20–24B. A coincident arch form was also obtained (Fig. 20–25).

At this stage, there was still a residual overjet, and, as Fig. 20–23B shows, the lower lip still lay behind the upper incisors. Feasibility analysis models, as described previously, were constructed. These showed that, although the lower incisors were relatively depressed by the tongue activity, further depression was desirable to facilitate movement of the labial segment. This depression was obtained over a further 3-month period with an appliance incorporating an anterior bite plane. The depression is demonstrated in Figure 20–24C. At this stage construction of planning models was repeated, and these demonstrated that all preparatory objectives had been achieved. Therefore, splints were constructed for movement to the desired position. Surgery was carried out, and the splints were removed 6 weeks later. The final result is shown in Figure 20–23C and 20–24D. The shortness of the upper lip is apparent, but the incisors are under lip control. Total treatment time was less than 1 year. The result 6 years later is shown in Figure 20–26.

(Text continued on page 1401)

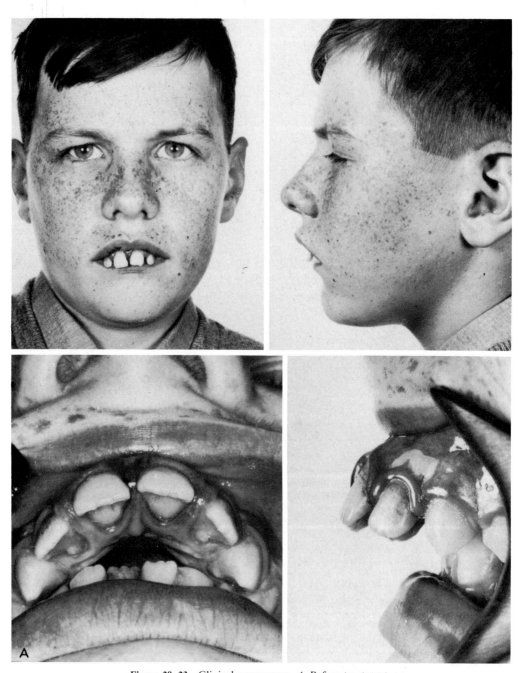

Figure 20–23   Clinical appearance. *A*, Before treatment.

(Figure 20–23 continued on opposite page)

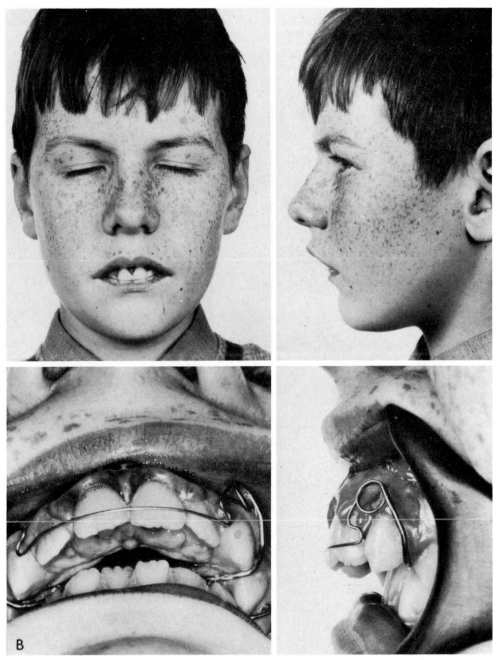

Figure 20–23   *(Continued.)*   *B*, After presurgical orthodontic treatment.

(Figure 20–23 continued on following page)

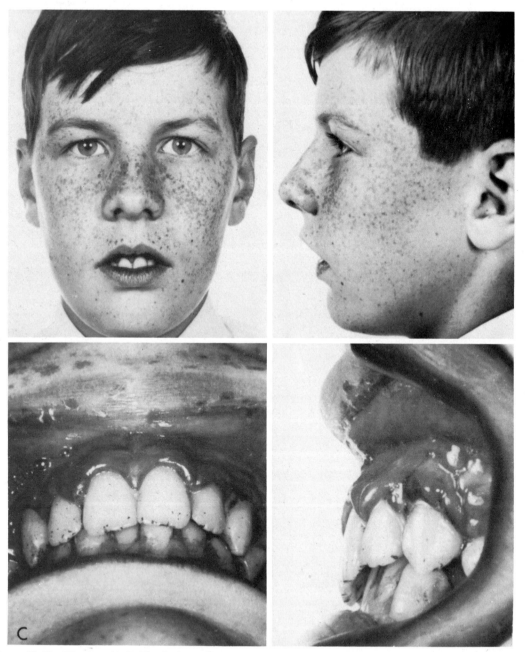

Figure 20–23 *(Continued.)* C, The final result 6 weeks after splint removal. (See Case Report No. 1 for details.)

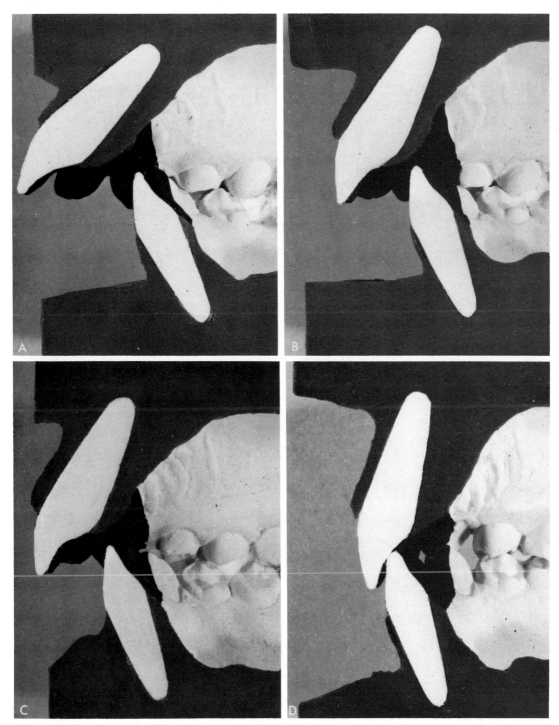

Figure 20–24 Study models (of the patient in Case Report No. 1) sectioned through 1̲/. *A*, Before treatment. *B*, After incisor space closure. *C*, The same stage after lower incisor depression. *D*, The final result. (The root outline on the models was extrapolated with a template constructed from the lateral skull radiograph.)

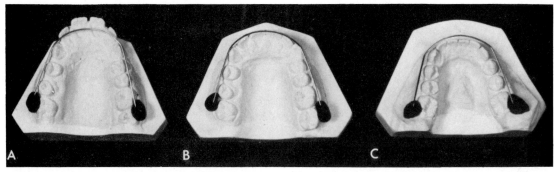

Figure 20–25 Identical arch wire superimposed over models of the patient in Case Report No. 1. *A*, Upper model before treatment. *B*, Upper model after orthodontic treatment. *C*, Lower model demonstrating the arch coincidence relative to that in *B*. The changes between *A* and *B* correspond to those between Figures 20–23*A* and *B* and 20–24*A* and *B*.

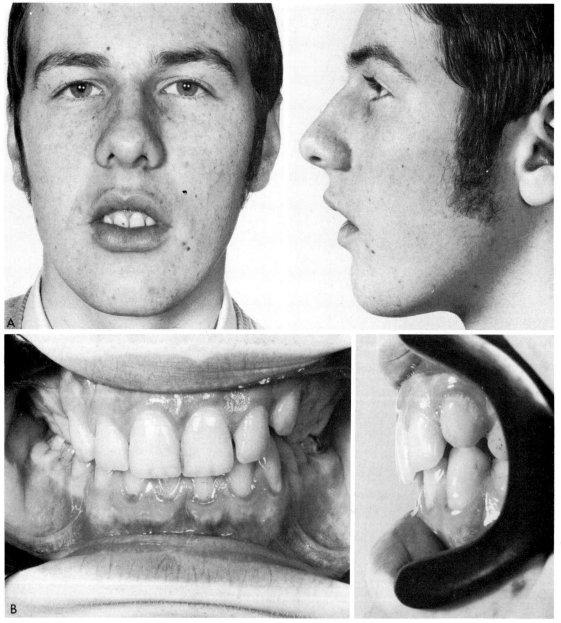

Figure 20–26 Clinical appearance of the patient in Case Report No. 1, 6 years after treatment.

CORRECTION OF CLASS II, DIVISION 1, MALOCCLUSION AND ASSOCIATED TEMPOROMANDIBULAR JOINT SYMPTOMS

This 26-year-old married patient was referred because of her temporomandibular joint symptoms. She had Class II, Division 1, malocclusion with maxillary protrusion. Observation of the patient's jaw movements and occlusal wear revealed that the forward posturing of the mandible was used to produce what to the patient was a better facial appearance (Fig. 20–27A). The lower lip contracted behind the upper incisors when the mandible was not in the forwardly postured posi-

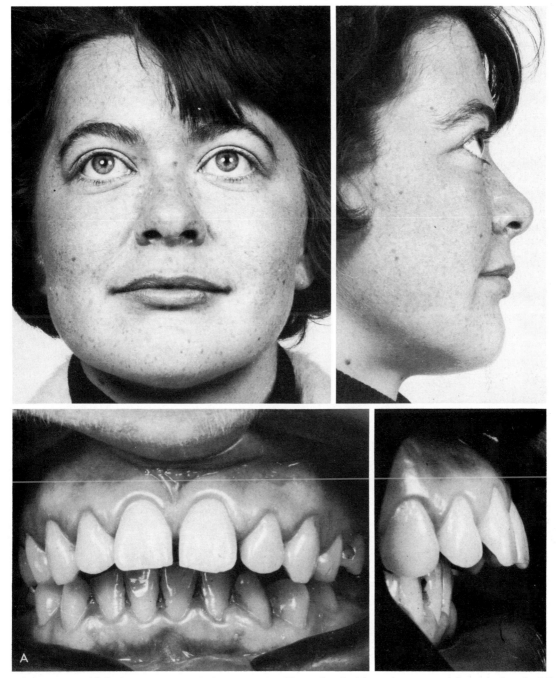

Figure 20–27 Clinical appearance. A, Before treatment. The patient had lower jaw postured forward when the full face and profile views were taken.

(Figure 20–27 continued on following page)

tion, and this accounted for the mild upper incisor proclination (Fig. 20–27*A*).

Feasibility analysis indicated that the overjet could be reduced surgically if some rotation as well as distal movement was carried out. The problem of narrowing in the intercanine area was revealed, as well as the desirability for lower incisor depression. The patient was originally completely antagonistic toward any form of therapy utilizing appliances, but when the nature of the in-conspicuous removable appliance was explained to her, this was accepted. The buccal movement of 3/3 and the depression of the lower incisors was achieved during a 4-month period. Surgery was then carried out and the overjet reduced. The changes are summarized in Figure 20–27*B*. The total treatment was accomplished within a 6-month period, and the joint symptoms have disappeared with the elimination of the forward posturing of the mandible.

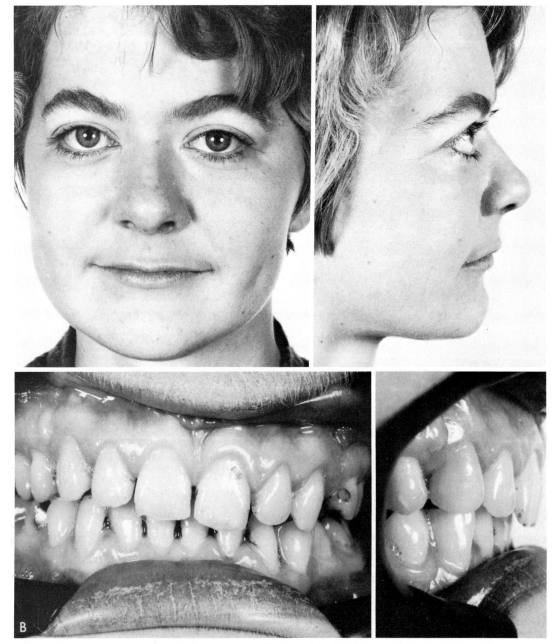

Figure 20–27 *(Continued.)* *B,* After surgical repositioning of the labial segment; the profile improvement is disguised because of the posturing in the pretreatment views, but the occlusal change is quite marked. (See Case Report No. 2 for details.)

Case Report No. 3

CORRECTION OF CLASS II, DIVISION 1, MALOCCLUSION IN A YOUNG WOMAN

This 23-year-old single nurse requested treatment to improve her "toothy appearance" (Fig. 20–28A), but with the stipulation that orthodontic appliances were not to be used and that the treatment be accomplished in 6 months, as she was emigrating! Examination showed her to have Class II, Division 1, malocclusion with bimaxillary proclination, this being illustrated well in Figure 20–

29A. To correct the malocclusion, both upper and lower labial segments needed to be rotated lingually to reduce the proclination, and additional depression of the lower incisors was also required. This was carried out by repositioning first of the lower labial segment and 2 weeks later of the upper segment. The open cap splints, as shown in Figure 20–21, are particularly useful in cases such

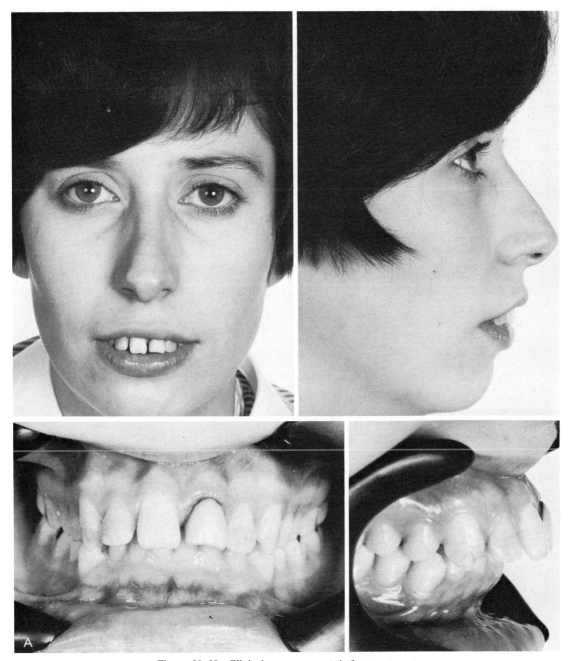

Figure 20–28 Clinical appearance. *A*, before treatment.

(Figure 20–28 continued on following page)

as this, to obtain close apposition of incisor teeth. The splints were removed 6 weeks later, and the final result is shown in Figures 20–28B and 20–29B. An effort is still required for the patient to approximate her lips, and ideally the segments could have been rotated further lingually, but this would have produced a localized open bite in the canine region. Total treatment time was less than 2 months.

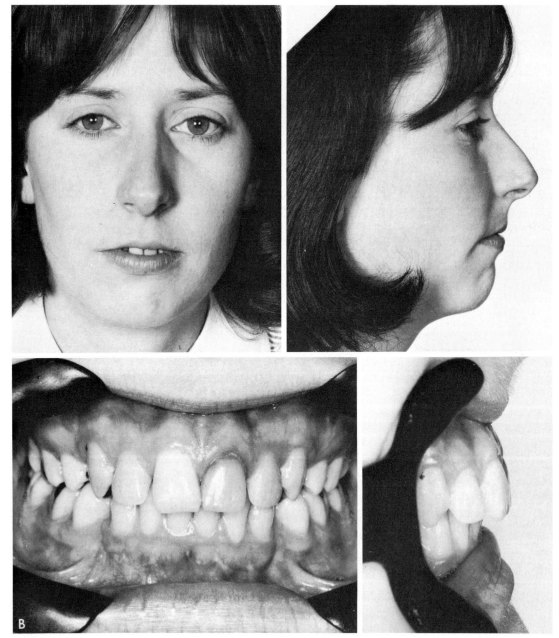

Figure 20–28 *(Continued.)* *B,* After upper and lower labial segmental surgery. (See Case Report No. 3 for details.)

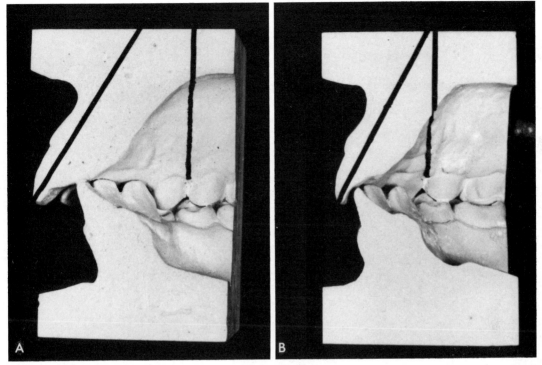

Figure 20–29   Study models (of the patient in Case Report No. 3) sectioned through 1/. *A*, Before treatment. *B*, After treatment.

Case Report No. 4

TREATMENT OF CLASS II, DIVISION 1, MALOCCLUSION IN A MENTALLY RETARDED GIRL

This 14-year-old girl was mentally retarded and was cared for at home, but her parents were disturbed by her vacant, "goofy" appearance and her constant dribbling of saliva, which caused excoriation of the skin on her chin (Fig. 20–30*A*). Cooperation was adequate to take impressions and extraoral roentgenograms, but little else. Orthodontic treatment was certainly not possible for her severe Class II, Division 1, malocclusion, which was primarily due to mandibular retrusion. Major surgery to correct the latter was certainly contraindicated, because of the necessity for intermax-illary fixation with this approach. The problem was, therefore, dealt with segmentally, by advancement of the lower labial segment and distal movement of the upper, there being a 6-month interval between operations. The result is shown in Figure 20–30*B*. Although a forward slide of the chin point would have perfected the result, the parents were happy with the improvement, and the skin problem was cured. The changes are well summarized in the serial lateral skull films (Fig. 20–31).

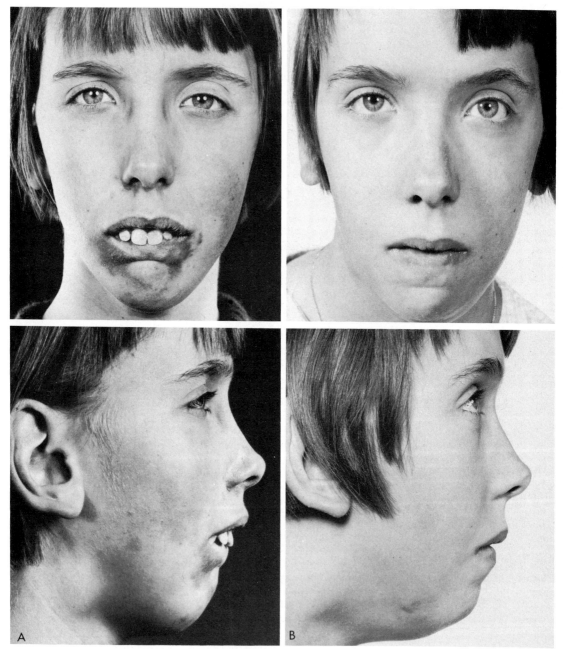

Figure 20–30 Clinical appearance. *A*, Before treatment. *B*, After surgical repositioning of upper and lower labial segments. (See Case Report No. 4 for details.)

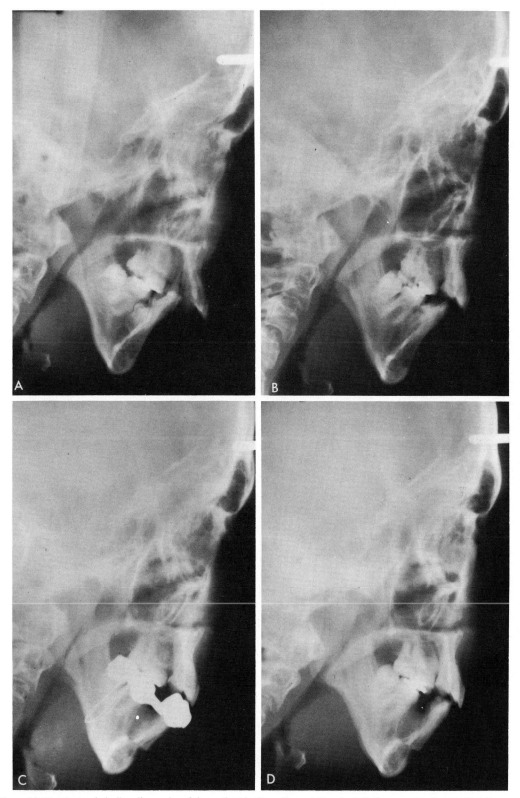

Figure 20–31   Lateral skull radiographs of the patient in Case Report No. 4. *A*, Before any treatment. *B*, After maxillary surgery. *C*, After mandibular surgery, the splint being still *in situ*. *D*, The final result.

CLASS II, DIVISION 2, MALOCCLUSION

The essential feature of patients in this group is the bimaxillary retroclination of the incisors, with the associated deep overbite. The latter may be such as to cause trauma to the lower labial or upper palatal gingiva. At rest the lower lip line is very high; that is, it may overlap most of the labial surface of the upper incisors. The object of treatment is to eliminate gingival trauma, if present, and to reduce the deep overbite. This can only be achieved by bringing both upper and lower incisors to a more normal angulation, and, as can be appreciated, the bite must be "opened" to allow this correction to be ef-fected. The stability of the result appears to relate to reducing the amount of labial upper incisor surface exposed to the influence of the lower lip, with concomitant readjustment of the axial angulation at which the upper and lower incisors meet.

The three-dimensional correction potential of segmental surgery has obvious application in the treatment of this type of malocclusion. However, since tooth irregularity within the labial segments is very common, it is rarely possible to treat a patient without orthodontic preparation, and therefore treatment times are not dramatically reduced by segmental surgery, as may be the case with other types of malocclusion.

Case Report No. 5

CORRECTION OF CLASS II, DIVISION 2, MALOCCLUSION IN A 12-YEAR-OLD GIRL

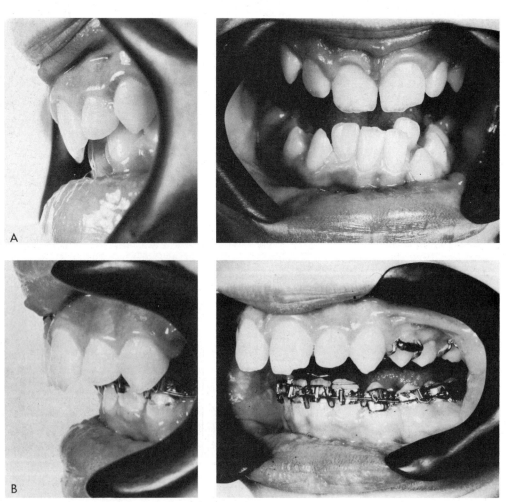

Figure 20–32 *A* to *D*, Clinical appearance. *A*, Before treatment. *B*, After proclination of the upper incisors and orthodontic alignment of the lower arch.

(Figure 20–32 continued on opposite page)

This 12-year-old girl had fairly severe Class II, Division 2, malocclusion (Fig. 20–32A), with marked crowding in the lower labial segment. The lower first bicuspids were removed, and a fixed appliance was fitted to align the lower labial segment. The residual extraction space was closed and the adjacent roots paralleled. The lower incisors were torqued to a more upright position, and during the final stages of the lower arch treatment, an upper removable appliance was inserted to procline the upper incisors to a normal angulation (Fig. 20–32B). This, in effect, converted the case into a Class II, Division 1, type with an overjet, and surgery was carried out as described previously, the object being distal movement of the upper labial segment, combined with a degree of depres-sion. In Figure 20–32C the overjet has been reduced, and the lower fixed appliance and upper splint are *in situ*. The final result is shown in Figures 20–32D and E.

DISCUSSION

The proclination of the upper incisors can often be carried out to advantage at the outset, as this provides a working clearance for the lower fixed appliance. An additional advantage is that the effect of forward posturing of the mandible can be seen, and patients with a more marked retrusive mandibular skeletal base may benefit more from a total mandibular advancement procedure than from a segmental approach.

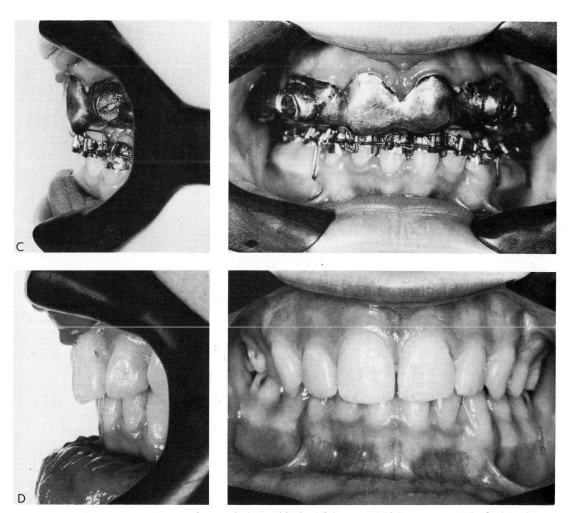

Figure 20–32 *(Continued.)* C, After surgical repositioning of the upper labial segment. D, The final result.

(Figure 20–32 continued on following page)

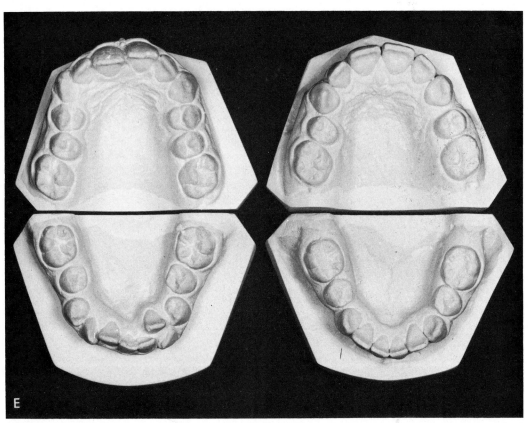

Figure 20–32 *(Continued.)* *E*, The original and final study models showing the good arch alignment. (See Case Report No. 5 for further details.)

(Our thanks are due to Dr. P. H. Ellisdon, who carried out the orthodontic treatment in this case and to whom we are grateful for the photographs.)

MILD CLASS III MALOCCLUSION

The orthodontic treatment of patients with Class III malocclusion is limited to those with a mild skeletal discrepancy, when there is an adequate degree of overbite. It consists of either proclination of the upper incisors or retroclination of the lower incisors, or a combination of the two. If there is an inadequate overbite after treatment, the teeth will relapse. The other problem is that if the lower incisors are out of muscle balance after treatment, but the overbite is adequate to maintain the new incisal relationship against this imbalance, a traumatic occlusion is then established.[9]

The surgical mobilization of the lower labial segment allows it to be moved vertically, so that an overbite can be created, and it can also be moved in a distal direction without excessive tilting. This requires qualification, since the amount of movement possible in this direction is determined by tongue size and position. This factor is now recognized in major mandibular osteotomies, in which a tongue reduction may be required for a successful result.[9]

The surgical movement of the lower labial segment, therefore, applies to cases that are skeletally just a little more severe in an anteroposterior and vertical dimension than are those treated orthodontically. It could be argued whether surgery is justified in such a mild skeletal discrepancy. The answer lies in the patient's request for facial improvement, since his or her appearance is often more prognathic than the anteroposterior skeletal discrepancy would have led one to expect. Although the height of the lower face due to a high Frankfort–mandibular plane angle may contribute something to this, the fullness and slight eversion of the lower lip seems to be the main factor.

Ricketts[12] and Williams[15] have both stated that a harmonious facial profile results if the lower incisor tips are on or close to a plane drawn from subspinale (A) to pogonion (P). (See Figure 20–35; see also Chapter 21.)

All our patients that have been treated surgically for mild Class III malocclusion have had lower incisors an average of 5 mm. or more in front of this plane before treatment. The technical aim of the treatment has been to establish a Class I incisal relationship, but this has incidentally placed the lower incisor tips close to the A–Po. plane. The postoperative result has been an improved facial profile, and this appears to support the work of Ricketts and Williams.

Case Report No. 6

CORRECTION OF MILD CLASS III MALOCCLUSION

This 15-year-old girl was originally referred for orthodontic treatment with a view to improving both function and appearance (Fig. 20–33A). She complained of her inability to incise hard foods and of her prognathic appearance.

Examination showed her to have Class III malocclusion with a mild skeletal discrepancy, the Frankfort–mandibular plane angle being high. There was an anterior open bite that was thought to be skeletal in origin. The lips were competent, and the tongue appeared to be of normal size. There was a tongue-to-lip contact during swallowing, but this was thought to be secondary to the open bite.

The prognathic appearance seemed to be due to two factors, namely, the high Frankfort–mandibular plane angle, giving an increased facial height, and the full, everted appearance of the lower lip (see Figure 20–35A). The skeletal discrepancy dictated a surgical approach confined to the movement of the lower labial segment, since the chin point seemed to be correct relative to the overall facial profile. The lower labial segment was moved superiorly and distally at the time of operation (Fig. 20–34). In this case it was only necessary to extract /4, since 4/ was already missing. The new position was maintained by a lower splint worn for 6 weeks.

The result is shown in Figures 20–33B and 20–35B, and the tracings show the improved relationship of the lower incisor tip relative to the A–Po. plane. The vertical movement obtained, as measured along the plane from the lower incisor tip to nasion, was 4 mm.

There has been a degree of relapse in the incisor relationship, but the result is now stable. A lateral

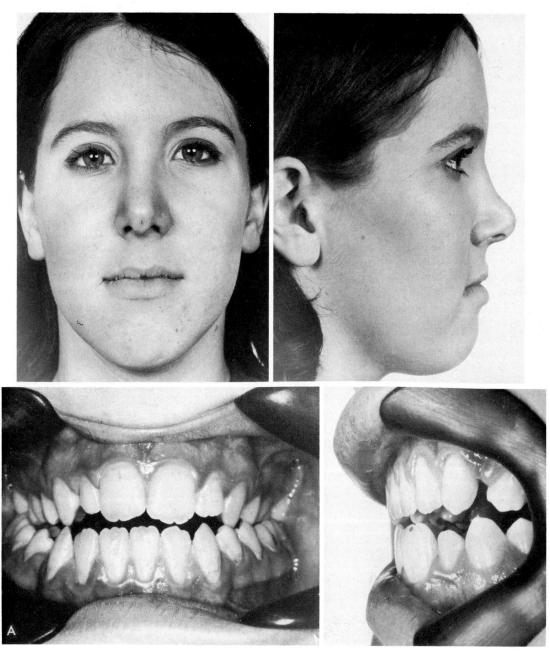

Figure 20–33   Clinical appearance. *A*, Before treatment.

(Figure 20–33 continued on opposite page)

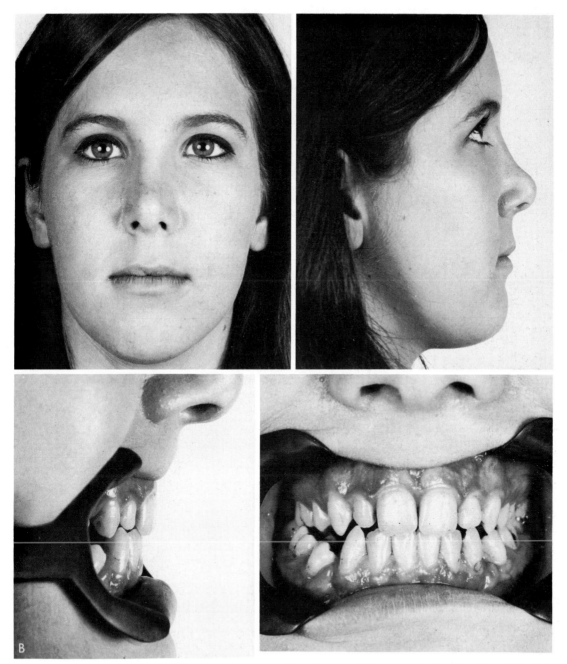

Figure 20–33   *(Continued.)*   *B,* After treatment to reposition the lower labial segment. (See Case Report No. 6 for details.)

(From Cradock Henry, T.: Localized osteotomy in cases of mild inferior protrusion, pp. 80–92. *In* Walker, R. V. (Ed.): Transactions of the Third International Conference on Oral Surgery, 1968. Edinburgh, Churchill Livingstone, 1970.)

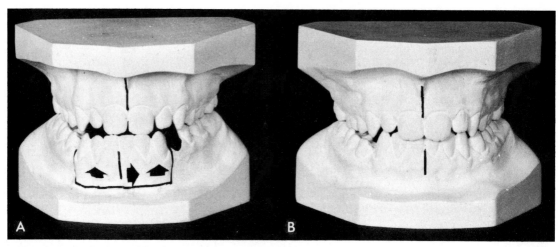

Figure 20–34   Study models of the patient in Case Report No. 6. *A*, The original occlusion. *B*, Sectioned models showing the planned repositioning of the labial segment.

skull tracing 16 months postoperatively shows the lower incisor tip to be 2.5 mm. in front of the A–Po. plane and the overbite to have decreased by 1 mm. The overall changes are shown in the lateral skull roentgenograms (Fig. 20–36). This relapse suggests that the tongue activity may have been contributing to the open bite originally, and this case illustrates the difficulty of objectively estimating tongue activity.

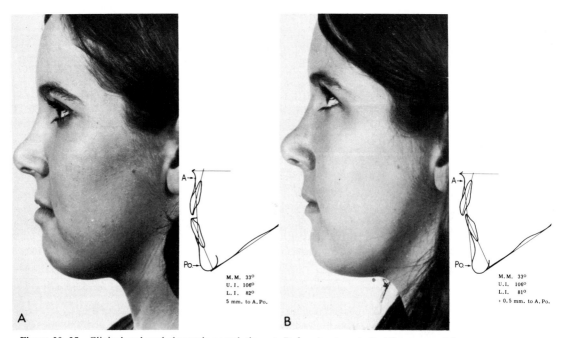

Figure 20–35   Clinical and cephalometric correlation. *A*, Before treatment. *B*, After segmental surgery.
(From Cradock Henry, T.: Localized osteotomy in cases of mild inferior protrusion, pp. 80–92. *In* Walker, R. V. (Ed.): Transactions of the Third International Conference on Oral Surgery, 1968. Edinburgh, Churchill Livingstone, 1970.)

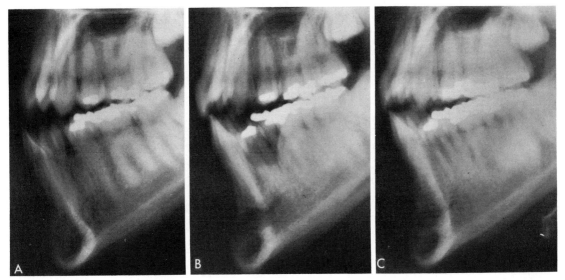

Figure 20–36   Lateral skull radiographs of the patient in Case Report No. 6. *A,* Before treatment. *B,* Immediately after splint removal. *C,* Sixteen months later.

(From Cradock Henry, T.: Localized osteotomy in cases of mild inferior protrusion, pp. 80–92. *In* Walker, R. V. (Ed.): Transactions of the Third International Conference on Oral Surgery, 1968. Edinburgh, Churchill Livingstone, 1970.)

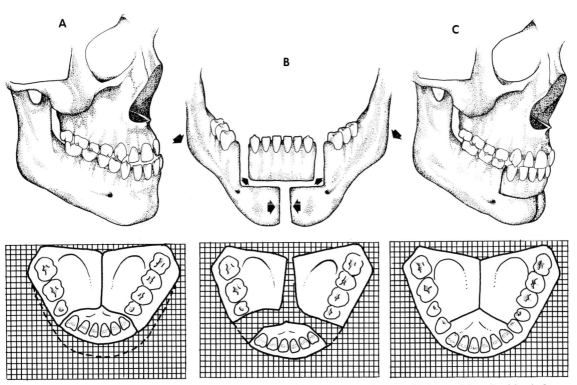

Figure 20–37   Diagrammatic representation of the skull and a corresponding mandibular model. *A,* Position before treatment. *B,* After section. *C,* The repositioning of the fragments. Note the lateral mandibular narrowing and the reduction of the chin prominence, in addition to the incisal correction.

(From Cradock Henry, T.: Localized osteotomy in cases of mild inferior protrusion, pp. 80–92. *In* Walker, R. V. (Ed.): Transactions of the Third International Conference on Oral Surgery, 1968. Edinburgh, Churchill Livingstone, 1970.)

Segmental Surgery with Associated Procedures

It is not uncommon for a Class III incisal relationship to be associated with a bilateral posterior crossbite, representing a mild but distinct discrepancy between maxillary and mandibular skeletal size. In cases such as this, the Class III incisal relationship can be corrected by the usual lower segmental movement combined with division of the symphysis in the midline with bone removed, thus allowing the horizontal rami to be moved

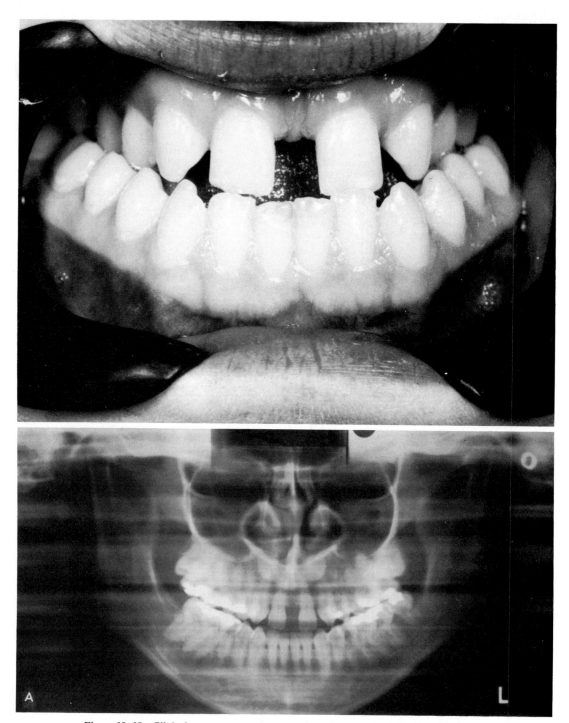

Figure 20–38   Clinical appearance and panoramic radiographs. *A*, Before treatment.

(Figure 20–38 continued on opposite page)

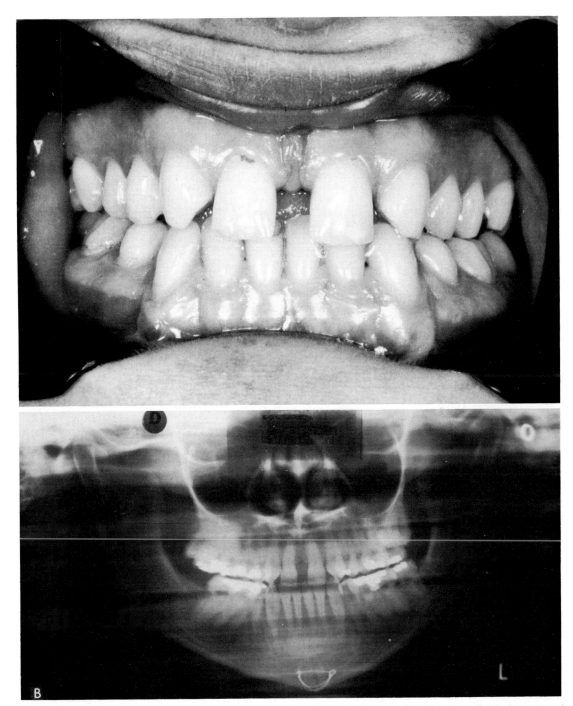

Figure 20–38 *(Continued.)* *B,* After lower segmental and symphysis surgery, which has effectively corrected both the incisal and molar occlusion. Note the good bony union and the transosseous wire still *in situ.* (See Case Report No. 7 for details.)

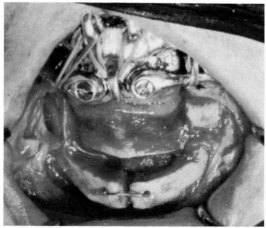

Figure 20–39 Operative view of the lower labial segment elevated into the new position and held by the locking bars. The symphysis is divided and wired into the new position, and the bony deficiency is filled with autogenous cancellous bone.

lingually and thereby correcting the crossbite (Fig. 20–37).

This technique was described both by Plumpton[11] and by Sowray and Haskell.[14]

The procedure is planned on models by sectioning of a plaster mock-up of the mandible. If the models are articulated, one should remember that rotation of the major and distal fragments will occur at the condyles and not be pivoted in the third molar region.

At surgery, first the labial segment is mobilized, and this step is followed by the vertical symphysis ostectomy, when a measured amount of bone is removed. However, as the planning is more complicated than a simple labial segment adjustment, care should be taken not to remove too much bone at the initial section. Finer adjustments are made later in the operation, until the locking bars of the three-part splint are found to fit accurately (Fig. 20–39).

Immobilization of the major fragment is effected by a single or figure-of-eight suture with 0.5 mm. stainless steel wire (Figs. 20–38 and 20–39). Access to the symphysis is easily achieved by a "degloving" procedure, and preservation of the mental nerves can be ensured by their exteriorization, if need be.

Case Report No. 7

CORRECTION OF CLASS III MALOCCLUSION WITH BILATERAL CROSSBITE

This patient was 23 years old and presented a mild Class III condition, together with a bilateral crossbite that is evident in both the clinical photograph and the radiograph. She was not a suitable candidate for any form of osteotomy of the ramus, but she did appear to be a candidate for labial segmental surgery and a symphysis ostectomy in which 1.2 cm. of bone could be excised. Six weeks after surgery, the splints were removed. It is evident from Figure 20–38B that the crossbite has been corrected, as has the Class III incisal relationship.

Case Report No. 8

CORRECTION OF CLASS III MALOCCLUSION WITH CROSSBITE AND PROTRUDING CHIN

Figure 20–40A shows a 25-year-old nurse who came to treatment primarily on account of her appearance. It was decided that an osteotomy of the ramus would be contraindicated not only because her chin would be placed in an adverse position but also because the occlusion would be traumatic and unstable. Again, distal repositioning of the lower labial segment coupled with a symphysis ostectomy satisfactorily corrected both appearance and malocclusion (Fig. 20–40B). No intermaxillary fixation was applied postoperatively, but the symphysis was wired and a bone graft inserted. The lower cap splint was retained for 6 weeks.

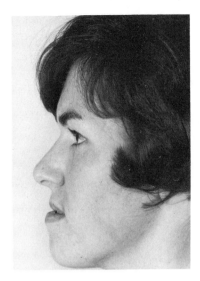
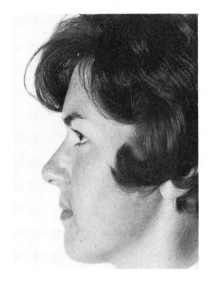

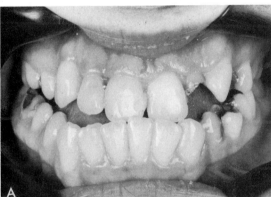
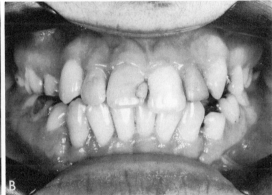

Figure 20–40   Clinical appearance. *A*, Before treatment. *B*, After segmental and symphysis surgery. Note the marked improvement of the chin position. (See Case Report No. 8 for details.)

Buccal Segmental Surgery

Adjustment of the buccal segments can also frequently be made with advantage in the maxilla, but in the mandible sectioning distal to $\overline{5/5}$ is obviously contraindicated because of the anatomic location of the neurovascular bundle.

Schuchardt described an operation for closure of an anterior open bite that involved lifting the posterior alveolar processes into the maxillary sinuses, thus in effect decreasing the height of the posterior teeth.[13] This operation was a two-stage procedure, easy to perform, but fell into disrepute mainly be-cause of the frequency with which partial relapses occurred. However, it is sometimes a very useful approach when combined with a mandibular procedure in the correction of a reverse overjet (Fig. 20–41).

Again, this surgical approach may be adapted to forms of crossbite in which no other method, surgical or orthodontic, will suffice.[4] The diagram in Figure 20–42 demonstrates a case in which the maxillary teeth from $\underline{7/}$ to $\underline{3/}$ were buccal to the lower arch.

A two-stage operation was performed, the palatal section being completed at the first operation and the buccal one 18 days later.

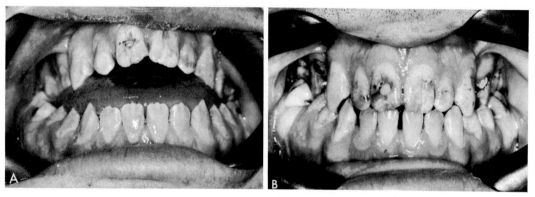

Figure 20–41 Clinical appearance. *A,* Before treatment. *B,* After performance of Schuchardt's procedure in the maxilla and a body ostectomy in the mandible. These were preceded by a tongue reduction. (See Case Report No. 9 for details.)

This allowed the right half of the maxilla to be shunted upward and inward (Fig. 20–43). The only variation from a classic Schuchardt operation was the measured ostectomy section made on the palatal aspect instead of the usual osteotomy. In a unilateral case, inter-maxillary fixation is not required, and the undisturbed contralateral side can be used as an abutment. The locking bar, if cap splints have been employed, will suffice for accurate location as well as fixation of the reduced buccal segment.

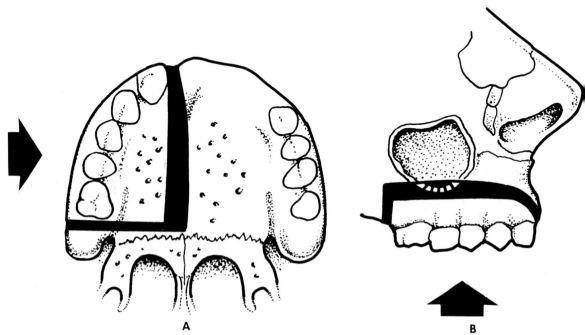

A   **B**

Figure 20–42 Ostectomy sections for a case of complete unilateral buccal crossbite. *A,* Occlusal aspect. *B,* Lateral maxillary aspect.

(From Cradock Henry, T.: Surgical correction of certain bite anomalies with particular reference to the maxillary approach. Br. Soc. Study Orthod. Tr., 80–84, 1962.)

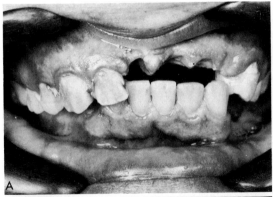

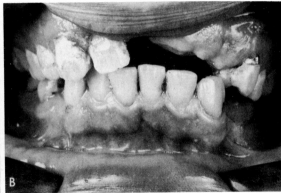

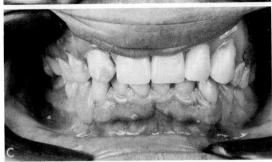

Figure 20–43 Clinical appearance (see diagrammatic representation in Figure 20–42). *A*, Complete crossbite on the right side before treatment. *B*, After surgery. *C*, Dental arch completed with a denture. (See Case Report No. 10 for details.)

(From Cradock Henry, T.: Surgical correction of certain bite anomalies with particular reference to the maxillary approach. Br. Soc. Study Orthod. Tr., 80–84, 1962.)

Case Report No. 9

CORRECTION OF CLASS III MALOCCLUSION WITH MARKED OPEN BITE

This boy of 16 years, who was mentally retarded, presented a gross anterior open bite that was combined with Class III malocclusion (Fig. 20–41*A*). This was treated by the following method: First, Schuchardt's procedure was performed, which obtained partial closure of the open bite deformity. Second, this was followed 6 months later by a tongue reduction. Third, nine months after the tongue reduction, a body ostectomy was performed. This is an example of a combined maxillary-mandibular procedure, producing the desired result in a gross case of open bite (Fig. 20–41*B*).

Case Report No. 10

CORRECTION OF UNILATERAL BUCCAL CROSSBITE

This young man had malocclusion with a crossbite (Fig. 20–43), most of the maxillary teeth on the right side being buccal to the mandibular teeth. In this instance the right buccal segment was displaced upward by 0.7 cm. and inward by 0.5 cm. to achieve normal articulation with the mandibular teeth. A prosthesis for the upper and lower jaws was then constructed, resulting in a considerable improvement in masticatory ability and appearance.

MALOCCLUSION IN CLEFT PALATE

The collapsed maxillary segment or segments in cleft palate seem, at first sight, ideally suited to the surgical procedures just described. Their practical application, however, is severely limited by the inelastic nature of the fibrous tissue of repair.

Unilateral Clefts

It is sometimes possible in this group, when a good lateral arch width exists, to lower the lesser segment and correct an infraocclusion by bringing the maxillary teeth into contact with the mandibular ones. However, this presupposes that the maxillary occlusal plane is level, which it rarely is (Fig. 20–44). Osteotomy in those cases that present a marked occlusal curvature gives a very poor result, as illustrated in the planning models (Fig. 20–45).

Bilateral Clefts

On the other hand, segmental surgery of the maxilla, in the bilateral cleft, has greater potential. One of us (T.C.H.), as a result of his experience during World War II in the secondary reduction of malunited middle third fractures by osteotomy, applied this to the cleft palate deformity[5] (Fig. 20–46). In 1947, a case with bilateral crossbite in a bilateral cleft palate was corrected by an osteotomy procedure that reproduced a Le Fort I fracture (see Chapter 18).[8] This case, and those that followed, emphasized the shortage of soft tissue that existed, together with its inability to be stretched. It was always found

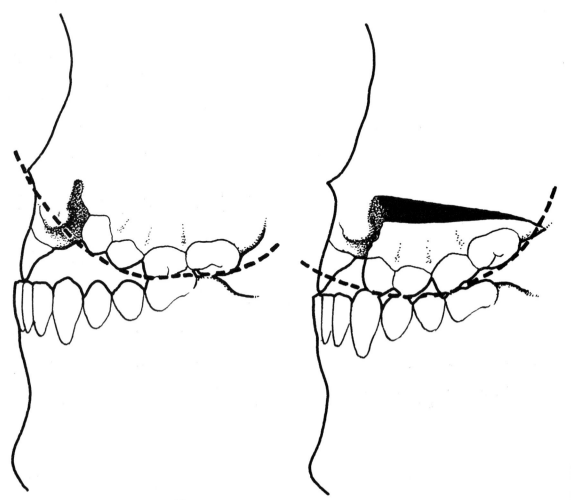

Figure 20–44 Exaggerated curve of Spee.

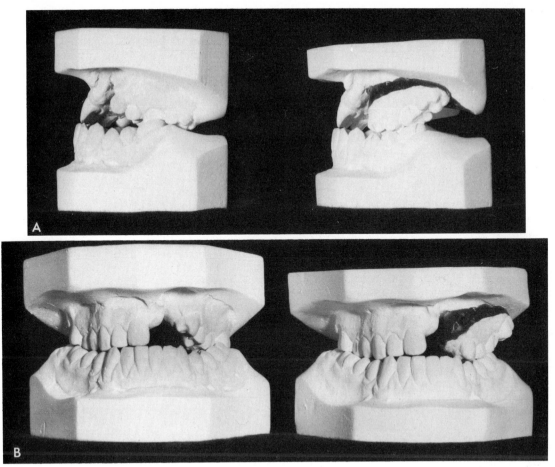

Figure 20–45 Models of a case of unilateral cleft palate. *A*, Collapse of the lesser segment and a localized anterior open bite. *B*, Surgical improvement of the lesser segment occlusion anteriorly is at the expense of the posterior occlusion. Segmental surgery is of no value in this instance.

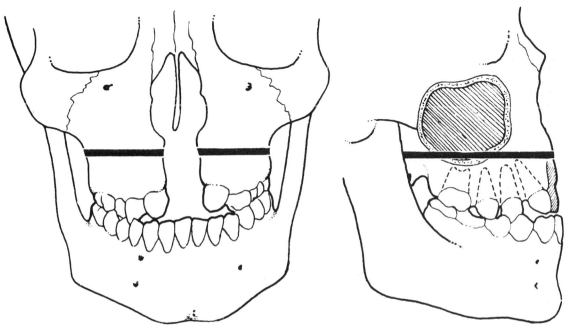

Figure 20–46 The level of the ostectomy section in a bilateral cleft case. (From Cradock Henry, T.: Surgical correction of certain bite anomalies with particular reference to the maxillary approach. Br. Soc. Study Orthod. Tr., 80–84, 1962.)

necessary, if the buccal segments were to be moved any worthwhile distance, to divide the anterior third of the repaired palate and thus re-create a fistula (Fig. 20–47C). Certainly, in the case illustrated, the occlusal improvement was marked. It helped to reduce the flattening of the middle third, and it allowed a denture of normal proportions to be fitted, but at the expense of re-creating a fistula, which is probably unjustified.

Case Report No. 11

CORRECTION OF MALOCCLUSION IN BILATERAL CLEFT PALATE

This girl of 16 years presented a severe deformity of the maxilla following surgery for the repair of a bilateral cleft lip and palate (Fig. 20–47A). The premaxilla had been partly ablated, and what remained carried a single supernumerary tooth. The two buccal segments had collapsed, with the cuspids converging toward the midline.

A bilateral osteotomy was performed. The two buccal segments were mobilized and, following division of the anterior third of the cleft, were pivoted outward. Retention involved a period of craniomandibular fixation with intermaxillary fixation. The intercanine width was increased by nearly 2 cm. and allowed the fitting of an adequate prosthesis.

One year later, the patient had a nose and lip revision performed by Sir Archibald McIndoe, and her final photographs, taken in 1970, were 18 years postsurgery (Fig. 20–47B).

This case illustrates in a practical manner both the potential and the limitations of segmental surgery in this field.

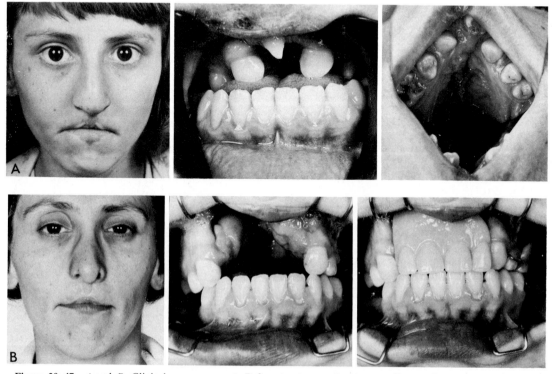

Figure 20–47 *A* and *B,* Clinical appearance. *A,* Before treatment, showing maxillary collapse and narrowing, but with an intact palate. *B,* After surgery, showing improved occlusion without and with the denture. *Note:* The correction was stable without the presence of the denture.

(Figure 20–47 continued on opposite page)

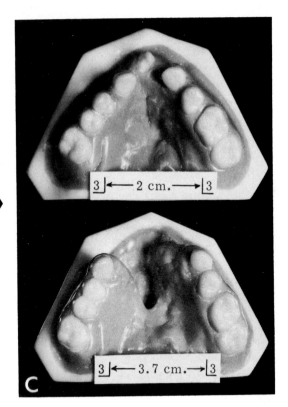

Figure 20–47 *(Continued.)* *C*, Models of the lateral arch width changes. (See Case Report No. 11 for details.)

SUMMARY

Segmental surgery is a means of moving groups of teeth and their supporting tissues in any plane of space. This provides a means of correcting malocclusion and facial disharmony in the perioral area. The method is free from complication, provided that the patient's condition is properly diagnosed and the surgery properly planned, prepared for and executed.

Cases should be jointly assessed by the oral surgeon and the orthodontist. Since this text is primarily for oral surgeons, however, the detailed orthodontic aspects have been intentionally curtailed. Segmental surgery is not a universal panacea but appears to have an important place in our treatment armamentarium, especially in the older patient, for whom expediency is important.

REFERENCES

1. Barton, P. R., and Rayne, J.: The role of alveolar surgery in the treatment of malocclusion. Br. Dent. J., *126*:11, 1969.
2. Bell, W. H., and Levy, B. M.: Healing after anterior maxillary osteotomy. J. Oral Surg., *28*:728, 1970.
3. Cohn-Stock, G.: Die chirurgische Immediatregulierung der Kieser, speziell die chirurgische Behandlung der Prognathie. Vjschr. Zahnheilk., *37*:320, 1921.
4. Cradock Henry, T.: The surgical correction of certain bite anomalies with particular reference to the maxillary approach. Br. Soc. Study Orthod. Tr., 80–84, 1962.
5. Cradock Henry, T.: Aviation injuries of the face. Hunterian Lecture at Royal College of Surgeons, England, 1945.
6. Cradock Henry, T., and Wreakes, G.: The surgical repositioning of labial segments in the treatment of malocclusion. Br. Soc. Study Orthod. Tr., *18*:329, 1968.
7. Flint, M.: Chip bone grafting of the mandible. Br. J. Plast. Surg., *17*:184, 1964.
8. Gillies, H. D., and Millard, D. R.: Principles and Art of Plastic Surgery, p. 341. London, Butterworth & Co., Ltd., 1957.
9. Hovell, J. H.: *In* Walther, D. P. (Ed.): Current Orthodontics, p. 523. Bristol, John Wright & Sons, Ltd., 1966.
10. Moore, A. W.: Cephalometrics as a diagnostic tool. J.A.D.A., *82*:775, 1971.
11. Plumpton, S.: Surgical correction of unilateral mandibular prognathism by intra-oral ostectomy of the symphysis. Br. J. Plast. Surg., *20*:70, 1967.
12. Ricketts, R. M.: Keystone triad—growth, treatment, and clinical significance. Am. J. Orthod., *50*:728, 1964.
13. Schuchardt, K.: Die Chirurgie als Helferin in der Kieferorthopadie; Fortschritte der Kieferorthopadie. Stuttgart, Georg Thieme Verlag KG, 1954.
14. Sowray, J. H., and Haskell, R.: Osteotomy at the mandibular symphysis. Br. J. Oral Surg., *6*:97, 1968.
15. Williams, R. T.: *In* Begg, P. R., and Kesling, P. C.: Begg Orthodontic Theory and Technique. 2nd ed. Philadelphia, W. B. Saunders Co., 1971.

ADDENDUM

During the 4-year interval since the writing of this chapter, wide acceptance of segmental surgery as a standard part of the treatment armamentarium of both oral surgeons and orthodontists has been seen. This is reflected by the number of new references in the literature (see list appended). Note especially those concerned with animal research into the revascularization processes of bone healing, as seen in maxillary and mandibular segmental surgery.[1,2,4] The comments that follow are included in the light of developments and experience in this period.

Class II, Division 1. With the technique described in Figure 20–13*B* and accompanying text, the anterior nasal spine was moved backward as part of the anterior tooth-bearing segment. If the patient's nose is of such a shape that a change in the nasal tip profile is undesirable, a cut *below* the nasal spine to give access to the septum keeps the nasal spine's support to the nose intact.

Class II, Division 2. The correction of this type of malocclusion by upper and lower segmental surgery is only really satisfactory with fairly normal anteroposterior jaw relationships. If there is any degree of mandibular retrognathia, a better approach is to create a Class II, Division 1, malocclusion by proclining the upper incisors and to follow this by a forward advancement of the mandible with a sagittal-split osteotomy of the ramus. (See Chapter 22.)

Class III. Experience suggests that the creation of a good positive overbite does not immediately confer stability and that the wearing of a Hawley-type orthodontic retainer for several months postoperatively is a wise precaution.

Cleft Palate. The movement of the maxillary segments is being used with increasing success in unilateral cases. However, a reasonable upper and lower arch coincidence is a prerequisite for surgery, which takes the form of a Le Fort I osteotomy (see Chapter 22), with bone grafting between the posterior maxillary surfaces and the pterygoid plates and also in the horizontal line of section.

The operation reduces the flatness of the lower part of the middle third of the face and corrects the mandibular overclosure. Extended postoperative retention is indicated.

Residual Problems. The problem of the short upper lip in patients with Class II, Division 1, malocclusion defies satisfactory resolution. However, in cases in which this is a relative situation—that is, when maxillary alveolar hyperplasia exists—the combination of a Wassmund and Schuchardt procedure to depress the whole maxillary dentoalveolar process appears to have been successful.[3,5,6] The significance of increasing the freeway space by so doing is not as yet known.

REFERENCES

1. Bell, W. H.: Revascularization and bone healing after anterior maxillary osteotomy: A study using adult Rhesus monkeys. J. Oral Surg., 27:249–255 (Apr.), 1969.
2. Bell, W. H., and Levy, B. M.: Revascularization and bone healing following total maxillary osteotomy. J. Dent. Res. (special issue), 82 (Feb.), 1973. (Abstr. No. 96.)
3. Bell, W. H., and Turvey, T. A.: Surgical correction of posterior crossbite. J. Oral Surg., 32:811 (Nov.), 1974.
4. Bell, W. H., et al.: Bone healing and revascularization after total maxillary osteotomy. J. Oral Surg., 33:253 (Apr.), 1975.
5. Hall, H. D., and Roddy, S. C.: Treatment of maxillary alveolar hyperplasia by total maxillary alveolar osteotomy. J. Oral Surg., 33:180 (Mar.), 1975.
6. West, R. A., and Epker, B. N.: Posterior maxillary surgery: Its place in the treatment of dentofacial deformities. J. Oral Surg., 30:562 (Aug.), 1972.

CHAPTER 21

DENTOFACIAL ORTHOPEDICS: A MULTIDISCIPLINARY APPROACH

VIKEN SASSOUNI, D.F.M.P., D.D.S., D.Sc.

A cardinal concern of dentistry is the understanding, recognition, prevention and treatment of malocclusion. Normal occlusion is the end result of numerous genetic and developmental factors, and the task of maintaining it by means of dentofacial diagnosis and reconstructive procedures involves all branches of dentistry (Fig. 21–1). When a patient is being treated, these divisions become artificial: all possible knowledge and skills are necessary for the ultimate benefit of the patient. This sum of services can be rendered only by a team.

A team of specialists needs a common language for communication, especially in diagnosis and treatment planning. The skills necessary to carry out treatment procedures are widely diversified, so it is at the time of diagnosis that consultations should be initiated. Knowledge of the extent and limitations of each specialty is important in order to derive the best possible treatment approach.

RECORDS

One of the bases of a common language is standardization of the records from which a diagnosis is derived. The following is a list which helps in the evaluation of a patient's condition.

1. Radiographic records
   a. Intraoral periapical films.
   b. Maxillary and mandibular occlusal films.
   c. Lateral jaw films (right and left 45°).
   d. Cephalometric films.
      1. Lateral (profile) (Fig. 21–2A).
      2. Frontal (posteroanterior) (Fig. 21–2B).
      3. Open mouth.
      4. Mandible at rest.
   e. Laminography of sections according to condition.
   f. Hand and wrist x-ray films for evaluation of skeletal age of children.
2. Dental models.
   a. Oriented according to cephalometric landmarks[8] (Fig. 21–3).
   b. Mounted on an articulator with facial transfers.
3. Photographic records.
   a. Profile and frontal facial views.
   b. Intraoral photographs.
   c. Physioprints[6] (Fig. 21–4).

These records help to answer a few fundamental questions:

1. What is the health, shape, and position of the teeth and their supporting structures? (Periapical, occlusal, lateral jaw films.)
2. Is there a healthy and efficient masticatory apparatus? (Laminography of condyles, mounted dental models on an articulator, cinefluorography.)
3. Evaluation of malocclusion. (Cephalo-

DENTAL OCCLUSION

BASIS AND RAMIFICATIONS

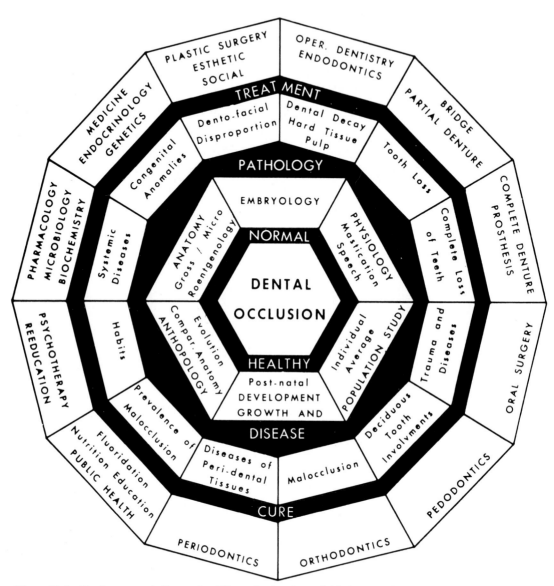

Figure 21–1 The inner area indicates the different basic science fields involved in the definition and description of occlusion. The second middle area represents the different diseases affecting dental occlusion and the outer circle indicates the branches of science involved in the cure of these diseases. (From Sassouni, V.: The Face in Five Dimensions. 3rd ed. Pittsburgh, University of Pittsburgh, Dental School Publication, 1965.)

metrically oriented dental models, cephalometric films.)

4. Evaluation of facial esthetics. (Facial photographs, physioprints, cephalometric films.)
5. Evaluation of the effects of treatment.

(All records evaluated serially by comparing before and after intervention and periodically thereafter.)

From these records, an intraoral examination and a general estimation of the patient's health, a complete diagnosis can be made.

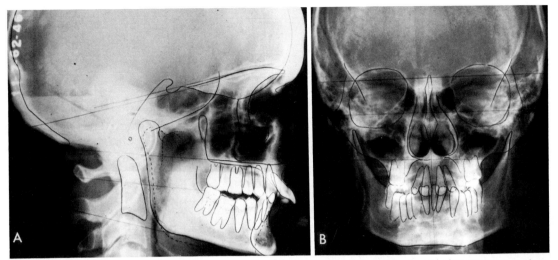

Figure 21-2 Roentgenographic cephalometry. *A*, The lateral view (profile). *B*, The frontal view (posteroanterior).

DENTOFACIAL DIAGNOSIS

In making a diagnosis, dentofacial abnormalities should be analyzed in the following sequence:
  A. Classification and description of malocclusion.
  B. Functional analysis.
  C. Assessment of facial proportions.
  D. Evaluation of growth potential.
  E. Racial and hereditary factors.
  F. Esthetic appraisal.

CLASSIFICATION AND DESCRIPTION OF MALOCCLUSION

There are three categories of malocclusion: dental, functional and skeletal. In this sec-

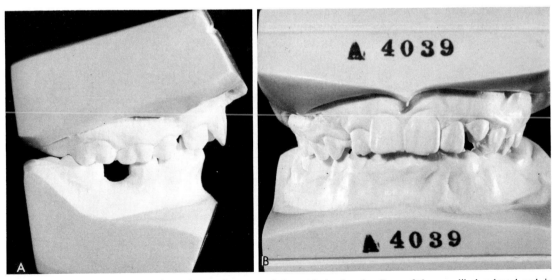

Figure 21-3 Dental models trimmed according to cephalometric landmarks. Base of the mandibular dental arch is trimmed according to the mandibular plane. The base of the maxillary dental arch is trimmed according to the palatal plane. The anterior portion of the maxillary dental casts represents the Anterior Nasal Spine. The mandibular anterior limit represents the Pogonion. The posterior borders of the casts are trimmed according to a perpendicular to the Frankfort horizontal plane. (From Sassouni, V.: The Face in Five Dimensions. 3rd ed. Pittsburgh, University of Pittsburgh, Dental School Publication, 1965.)

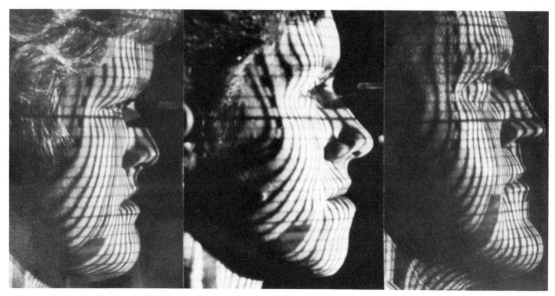

Figure 21–4 Examples of physioprints (a millimeter grid is projected on the face, and a photograph is taken at a right angle). Three types of mandibular prognathism are depicted by the physioprints. (From Sassouni, V.: The Face in Five Dimensions. 3rd ed. Pittsburgh, University of Pittsburgh, Dental School Publication, 1965.)

tion, only the dental malocclusions will be described.

The malocclusion should be evaluated by assessing the degree of the crowding and spacing in each quadrant separately. The proper midline of the dental arches should be charted, as well as any deviation in size and form.

The classification of dental malocclusion should be established in three dimensions: anteroposterior, vertical, and transverse.

1. Anteroposterior classifications: Angle's Class I (Fig. 21–5), Class II (1) (Fig. 21–6), Class II (2) (Fig. 21–7), and Class III (Fig. 21–8).
2. Vertical classification: open bite (Fig. 21–9) and deep bite (Fig. 21–7).
3. Transverse classification: crossbites (buccal or lingual) (Fig. 21–8).

FUNCTIONAL ANALYSIS

The different functions of the oral cavity—mastication, speech and breathing—are difficult to evaluate objectively in clinical practice. Most of the information is derived from the direct examination of the patient. Occasionally extensive testing is required. Certain problems are encountered frequently.

The parts of the masticatory apparatus to be evaluated are the teeth, their supporting periodontal structures, the temporomandibular joint and the facial musculature. Cusp interference during closure of the mandible may traumatize the supporting structures of the teeth or displace them or shift the mandible from its normal path of closure. It is sometimes extremely important to detect these interferences, as some Class III malocclusions are due to an anterior shift of the mandible after the incisors come to an edge-to-edge relationship. The mandible should be evaluated in its most retruded position and then in centric occlusion. Similarly, a cuspid or a bicuspid cusp may cause a lateral shift of the mandible, creating a buccal crossbite on one side, a lingual crossbite on the other and a deviation of the midline of the mandibular incisors. In the adult these interferences may cause periodontal breakdown, temporomandibular joint trauma and pain, or muscular spasm. In actively growing children a number of adjustments take place, and interferences may be temporary and self-correcting. Long observation should precede intervention.

Speech defects of peripheral origin may be associated with malocclusion (with size, position and action of soft palate and tongue). At times, it may be difficult to determine the cause, and the patient should be referred to the speech specialist. On the other hand, if an extremely large tongue is the cause, surgery can be undertaken. True macroglossia should

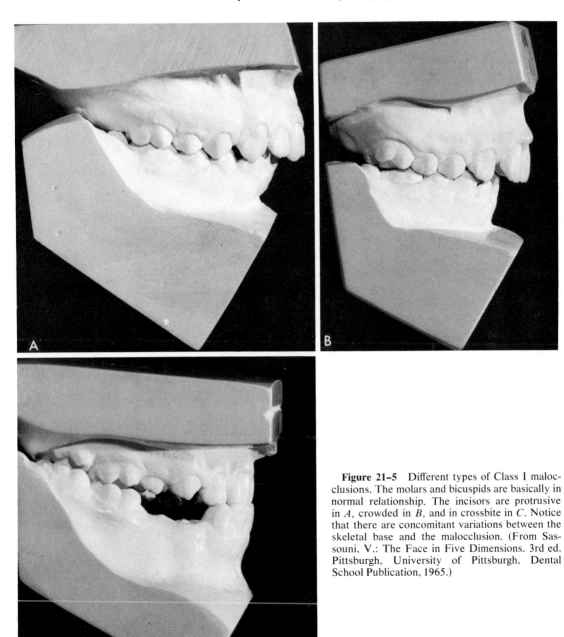

Figure 21–5 Different types of Class I malocclusions. The molars and bicuspids are basically in normal relationship. The incisors are protrusive in *A,* crowded in *B,* and in crossbite in *C.* Notice that there are concomitant variations between the skeletal base and the malocclusion. (From Sassouni, V.: The Face in Five Dimensions. 3rd ed. Pittsburgh, University of Pittsburgh, Dental School Publication, 1965.)

be differentiated, of course, from a normal tongue in a small oral cavity.

Breathing as well as speech may be affected by the tonsils and adenoid tissues. From lateral cephalometric films it is possible to recognize the tonsils and determine to what extent they constrict the pharyngeal space. Obstruction or constriction of the nasal apertures (as seen in posteroanterior films) may be of diagnostic importance in palatal expansion procedures.

SKELETAL ANALYSIS OF THE FACE

Facial proportions are evaluated by means of oriented facial photography, physioprints and cephalometric films. Because pho-

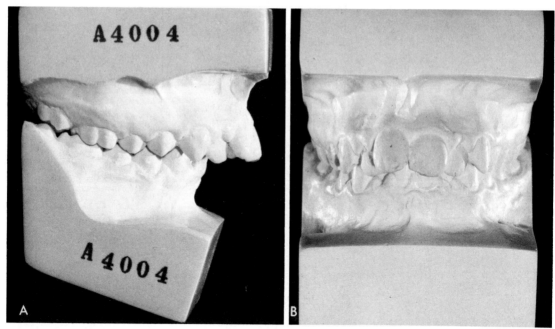

Figure 21–6 Angle's Class II, Division 1, malocclusion. The teeth are in distocclusion (the mandibular teeth distal to the corresponding maxillary ones or the maxillary teeth mesial to the corresponding mandibular ones). (From Sassouni, V.: The Face in Five Dimensions. 3rd ed. Pittsburgh, University of Pittsburgh, Dental School Publication, 1965.)

tographic records are primarily evaluated subjectively, cephalometric analysis will receive the major attention in this chapter.

Cephalometer. This instrument orients the face in a standardized position (Fig. 21–10), according to the Frankfort horizontal plane. Two x-ray sources are fixed and also oriented according to the cephalometer. The lateral x-

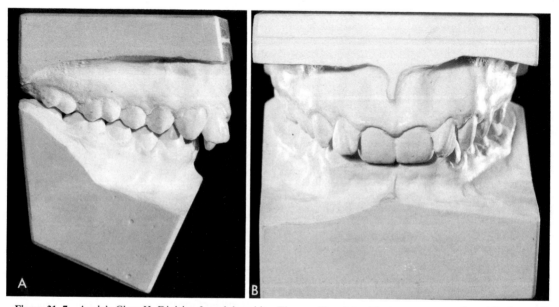

Figure 21–7 Angle's Class II, Division 2, and deep bite. The maxillary lateral incisors are protrusive while the maxillary central incisors are in lingual version. The posterior teeth are in distocclusion. (From Sassouni, V.: The Face in Five Dimensions. 3rd ed. Pittsburgh, University of Pittsburgh, Dental School Publication, 1965.)

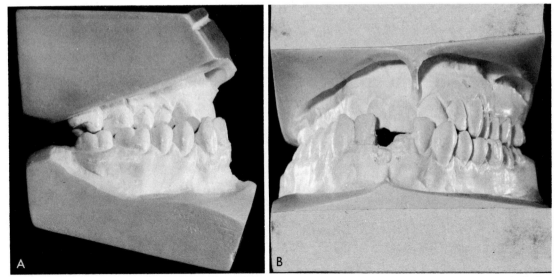

Figure 21-8 Angle's Class III malocclusion with posterior and anterior crossbite. The teeth are in mesioclusion. (From Sassouni, V.: The Face in Five Dimensions. 3rd ed. Pittsburgh, University of Pittsburgh, Dental School Publication, 1965.)

ray source is perpendicular to the median sagittal plane of the face at the level of the transmeatal axis (ear rods, external auditory meatus). The posteroanterior x-ray source passes through the intersection of the median sagittal and the Frankfort horizontal. The cassette for the lateral film is parallel to the median sagittal plane, and the cassette for the posteroanterior film is perpendicular to the median sagittal plane and the Frankfort horizontal plane. The most elaborate cephalometer was designed in 1931 by Broadbent.[1] It

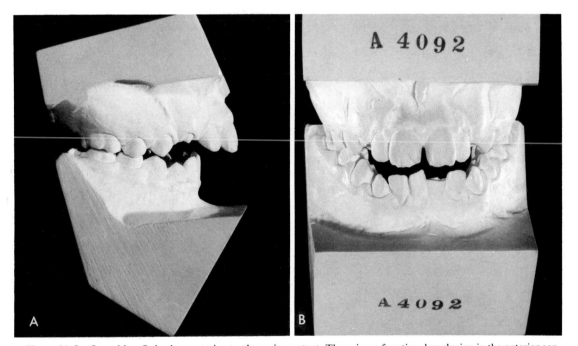

Figure 21-9 Open bite. Only the posterior teeth are in contact. There is no functional occlusion in the anterior segments. (From Sassouni, V.: The Face in Five Dimensions. 3rd ed. Pittsburgh, University of Pittsburgh, Dental School Publication, 1965.)

is still the instrument of choice. Since then a number of others have become available with some modifications.

Identification of Radiographic Anatomy and Landmarks.[4-8] THE LATERAL FILM. (Fig. 21–11. Midpoint of all bilateral landmarks is taken.)

1. Profile.

Nasion (Na): Most anterior point of the nasofrontal suture on midsagittal plane.

Anterior nasal spine (ANS): Most anterior point of the nasal floor. Tip of premaxilla on midsagittal plane.

Subspinale (A): Deepest point on the profile between ANS and Is.

Incision superius (Is): Incisal tip of the crown of the most anterior central incisor.

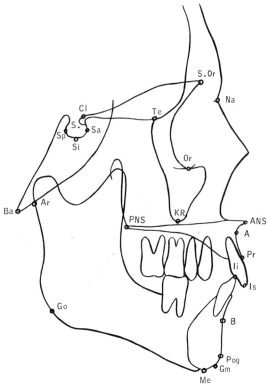

Figure 21–11 Roentgenographic cephalometric landmarks (lateral view).

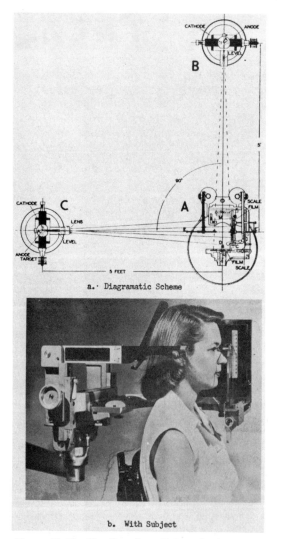

a. Diagramatic Scheme

b. With Subject

Figure 21–10 The Broadbent-Bolton Cephalometer.

Supramentale (B): Deepest point on midsagittal plane between infradentale and pogonion. Usually anterior to and slightly below the apices of the lower incisors.

Pogonion (Pog): Most anterior point on midsagittal plane of the contour of the chin.

Menton (Me): Lowermost point of the contour of the mandibular symphysis.

2. Upper face and cranial base.

Dorsum sella (Sp): Most posterior point on the internal contour of sella turcica.

Floor of sella (Si): Lowermost point on the internal contour of sella turcica.

Clinoidale (Cl): Most superior point on the contour of the anterior clinoid.

Center sella (S): Center of the contour of sella turcica, by inspection.

Roof of orbit (RO): Uppermost point on the internal wall of the roof of the orbits.

Supraorbitale (S.Or): Most anterior point of the intersection of the shadow of the roof of the orbit and its lateral contour.

Orbitale (Or): Lowermost point of the contour of the bony orbit.

Floor of orbit (FO): Lowermost point on the internal wall of the floor of the orbits.

Temporale (Te): Intersection of the shadows of the ethmoid and the anterior wall of the infratemporal fossa.

3. Mid-face and palate.

Key ridge (KR): Lowermost point on the contour of the shadow of the anterior wall of the infratemporal fossa.

Posterior nasal spine (PNS): Most posterior point on the contour of the bony palate.

4. Lower face or mandible.

Gonion (Go): Located by bisecting the posterior ramal plane and the mandibular plane angle.

5. Posterior face.

Articulare (Ar): Intersection of basioccipital and posterior border of the condyle mandibularis.

Foramen magnum:

Basion (Ba): Lowest and most anterior point.

Opisthion (Op): Lowest and most posterior point.

Bolton point (Bo): Highest point in the upward curvature of the retrocondylar fossa. In uncertain cases it may be located as the midpoint between opisthion (Op) and basion (Ba); in other words, as the center of foramen magnum.

Odontoidale (Od): Uppermost point of the tip of the odontoid process of the axis (second vertebrae).

THE POSTEROANTERIOR FILM. (Fig. 21–12.)

1. Upper face and cranial base.

Roof of orbit (RO): Uppermost point on the roof of the orbit.

Latero-orbitale (Lo): Intersection point between the external orbital contour laterally and the oblique line. (This is a roentgenographic landmark, not anatomic.)

Oblique orbital line: Projection of the greater wing of sphenoid.

Crista galli (N.C): Neck of crista galli, most constricted point of the projection of the perpendicular lamina of the ethmoid (almost at the level of planum).

2. Mid-face.

Maxillare (Mx): Maximum concavity on the contour of the maxilla between malar (Ma) and the first molar (6). Corresponds closely to the key ridge.

Zygoma (Zyg): Most lateral point of the shadow of the zygomatic arch.

3. Lower face.

Mastoidale (Ms): Lowest point on the contour of the mastoid process.

Gonion (Go): Horizontal projection of gonion from the lateral film.

Incision superius (Is): Lowermost point of the incisal edge of the maxillary central incisors.

Menton (Me): Lowermost point of the contour of the chin.

Cephalometric Analysis. Numerous cephalometric analyses have been proposed.[4] Most frequently a statistical definition of average facial proportions and the extent of "normal" variations are given. Their "standards" are dependent on the sample selected: on the basis of normal occlusion or on the basis of facial esthetics. These standards vary according to age, sex and race. One method of analysis is described here in order to permit the evaluation of individual deviations from a set of norms: the archial analysis, which is a roentgenographic cephalometric analysis of cephalo-facial-dental relationships.[5]

The basis of the construction of the archial analysis is an anterior arc that represents the line of reference which permits the evaluation of the maxillary and mandibular relationships. The anterior arc is drawn from a center ("O") unique for each face. This center is located at the point of intersection (or nearest convergence) of the four planes of

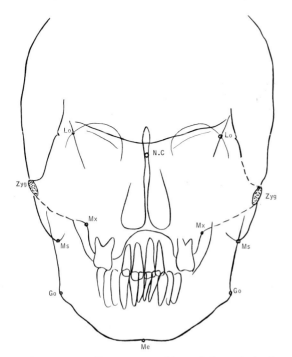

Figure 21–12 Roentgenographic cephalometric landmarks (posteroanterior view).

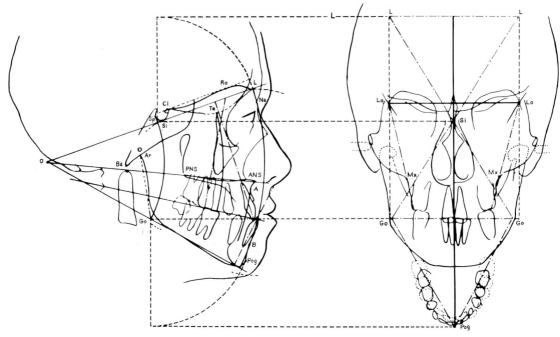

Figure 21–13   The archial analysis in three dimensions. (From Sassouni, V.: Diagnosis and treatment plan via roentgenographic cephalometry. Am. J. Orthod., *44*:433–463, 1958.)

the face: the supraorbital, the palatal, the occlusal and the mandibular planes (Fig. 21–13). With O−Nasion as the radius an arc is drawn. Normally the anterior nasal spine (ANS), the tip of the upper incisor (Is), and pogonion (Pog) should be situated on this arc. If ANS and pogonion are anterior or posterior to the arc this is interpreted as a maxillary or mandibular protrusion or retrusion, respectively. A posterior arc is drawn from the same center with O−posterior sella (Sp) as the radius; this arc normally passes through gonion.

VERTICAL EVALUATION. Normally the upper and lower face heights are equal.

Upper face height is measured from ANS to supraorbitale (S.Or) and lower face height from ANS to menton (Me).

Facial Types.[7, 9]   Based on these norms a certain number of "deviant" or "abnormal" or "extreme" dentofacial types can be defined. Each of these types represents a combination of multiple deviations frequently found present simultaneously. The four basic facial types are described in Table 21–1 and illustrated in Fig. 21–14. This classification defines only four basic types, but combinations of types (vertical and anteroposterior) are often seen.

Each facial type requires a different

Table 21–1   *Facial Types*

SKELETAL TYPES	OPEN BITE	DEEP BITE	CLASS II	CLASS III
Center O	Close to profile	Far from profile	Low	High
Planes	Steep	Horizontal and parallel	Variable	Variable
Palate inclination	Down at back	Horizontal	Down at back	Up at back
Gonial angle	Large	Small	Small	Large
Cranial base angle	Large	Small	Large	Small
Ramus length	Short	Long	Short	Variable
Corpus length	Short	Normal	Short	Long
Anterior vertical balance; lower to upper face height	Large lower face height	Small lower face height	Variable	Variable

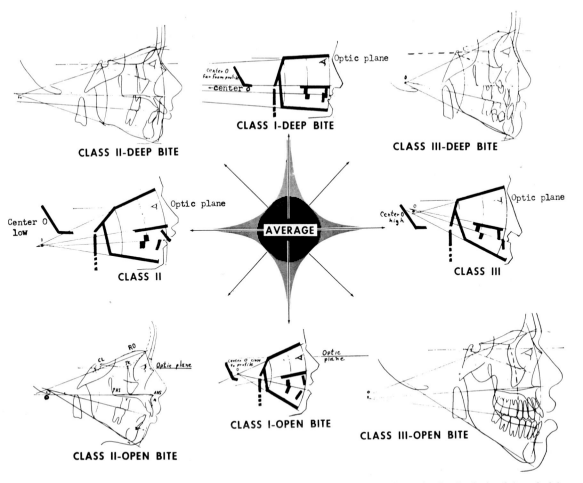

Figure 21–14 The facial types (refer to Table 21–1). (From Sassouni, V., and Nanda, S.: Analysis of dentofacial vertical proportions. Am. J. Orthod., *50*:801–823, 1964.)

method of treatment. From an orthodontic point of view the poorest prognosis is present for the "Class II deep bite" and the "Class II open bite" types.[9] It is in these two types that facial surgery may be the most clearly indicated.

EVALUATION OF THE GROWTH POTENTIAL OF THE FACE

The analysis of the facial pattern should be supplemented by information obtained about the growth potential of the patient. Different bones of the face do not grow at the same rate and do not stop growing at the same time.

The *anterior cranial base* (sphenoid, ethmoid and internal surface of frontal bone) do not grow in size or change in shape after about the seventh year of life. The *posterior cranial base* continues to grow until the individual's

early adulthood, primarily at the spheno-occipital synchondrosis.

The *palate* grows primarily downward and forward because of the growth of the nasal septum.[10] The sutures of the upper face are areas of adjustment rather than prime movers with respect to the changes of the position of the palate. The increase in size of the dental arch is brought about largely by periosteal bone apposition on the posterior border of the maxillary tuberosity. By about 14 to 15 years of age the maxilla stops growing.

The *mandible* is made up of a central core extending from the condyles to the symphysis (Fig. 21–15), with three types of processes: the alveolar process, containing the teeth; the two gonial processes, where the masseter and the internal pterygoid muscles are inserted; and the two coronoid processes where the temporal muscles are inserted.[11] The centers of endochondral growth in the mandible are

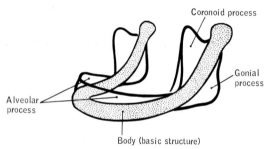

Figure 21–15 Diagrammatic representation of the central core of the mandible and its processes. (Courtesy of Arthur Symons.)

at the symphysis and at the condyles. By about 18 months of age the symphysial growth stops, but the condylar growth continues until adulthood. This is why there is little change in the shape and size of dental arches but a major change in their position during growth.

Timing of Growth. During the progress to adulthood the different structures of the face are not growing evenly; spurts alternate with plateaus. At about the time of puberty there is a general spurt of growth activity followed by a relative deceleration. Growth is difficult to predict because puberty may occur at various ages.

In females, menarche (earliest occurrence of periods) indicates a definite level of physiologic and hormonal maturation. Menarche may occur as early as 9 years of age and as late as 17. Chronological age, therefore, is not a good indicator of the biologic maturation of an individual. Because changes in the rate of growth accompany menarche, prediction of menarche will permit a more accurate prediction of growth timing. About a year prior to menarche there is a spurt of somatic and facial growth; after menarche, there is a rapid deceleration of growth until adulthood, approximately two or three years after menarche. One of the best ways to evaluate the "maturational age" of an individual is by means of an assessment of the formation and growth of the bones of the hand and wrist. An atlas is available that permits thorough comparison of the radiographs of the hands of an individual with standards for each age and sex.[3] It is interesting to note that while menarche occurs at any time from age 9 to age 17, it always occurs around 13 years skeletal age. Therefore, by evaluating the skeletal maturation serially a relatively accurate prediction (plus or minus six

months) of the time of menarche can be established.

In some surgical treatments it is critical to know whether the face (especially the mandible) will continue to grow, because growth could lead to a recurrence of the abnormal condition. In boys, the mandible continues to grow until adulthood (after age 20). It is obvious that a differential diagnosis and treatment plan based on age and sex is necessary when contemplating orthodontic and surgical procedures.

In the instance of mandibular prognathism, there is on the one hand a desire to correct the facial deformity as early as possible. This is important not only from the standpoint of functional adaptation but also because of esthetic, psychological and social demands. On the other hand, a major concern is to achieve a permanent correction of the deformity. In some cases, growth continues after resection, and mandibular prognathism reappears, necessitating a second operation.[2] The evaluation of the skeletal age of the patient in such a case may avoid premature and unnecessary intervention.

In the evaluation of the growth trends of an individual it is necessary to eliminate the possibility of pathologic conditions of congenital or systemic nature that could be responsible for the facial deformity. In addition, a critical evaluation of hereditary background of the individual may permit a more accurate and intelligent prediction.

RACE AND HEREDITY

The previous remarks bring us to the more critical evaluation of the hereditary and racial factors associated with an individual. When facial patterns were described, no distinction was made as to the predominance of any facial type in particular races. Primitive people, for example, because of their race as well as the special masticatory function required by their diet, develop a greater tendency toward mandibular prognathism and Class III malocclusion. Extreme development of the ramus and the gonial processes makes the appearance of an open bite extremely rare. On the other hand, the fact that their incisor occlusion is in an edge-to-edge relationship permits the forces of mastication to be distributed over the total dental arch, which makes unlikely the appearance of deep bite.

There are other differences between Cau-

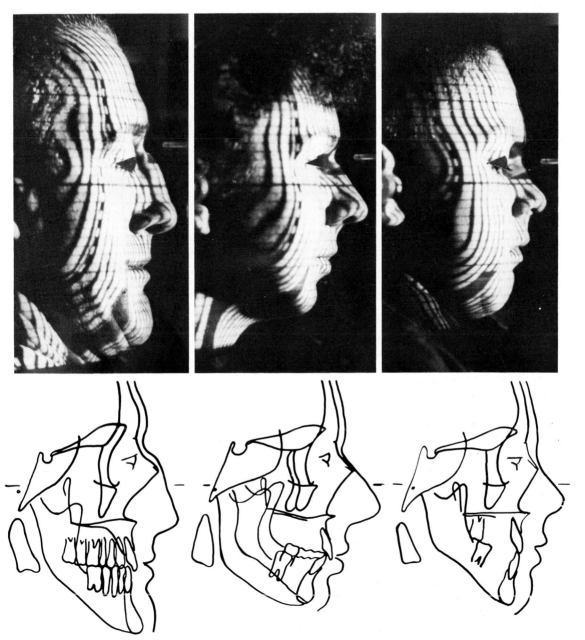

Figure 21–16 Physioprints and tracings of the cephalometric film of a family (see text). (From Sassouni, V., and Nanda, S.: Analysis of dentofacial vertical proportions. Am. J. Orthod., *50*:801–823, 1964.)

casian, Negro, and Mongolian people.[8] Probably because of the particular musculature and tooth size, there is a greater bidental protrusion in the Negro. Furthermore, the Negro has a relatively large palatomandibular plane angle, reflecting a larger lower facial height than upper facial height. From this we recognize the characteristics of the open bite skeletal pattern. These general racial character-istics provide us with a certain framework of reference but are not precise enough when treating an individual.

The immediate family background of a patient gives us a better source of information for the evaluation of his skeletal pattern. Often it is important not only to observe his parents but also to analyze them radiographically.[5, 9] Figure 21–16 shows a child and his parents. From the physioprints we can see the child's resemblance to the mother; the tracing of the child, however, shows that while the upper face (cranial base and palate) resembles that of the mother, the mandible in shape and proportion is closer to that of the father. A recent investigation of the hereditary implications of facial pattern has revealed that when the father and mother have open bite characteristics the child tends to resemble them. The same is true for the deep bite skeletal pattern, the skeltal Class II and the skeletal Class III. However, when the parents have opposite facial types the child may resemble either one of them or may seem to be a combination of both. Here again, knowledge of the hereditary background may permit us to establish a more intelligent, etiologic, systematic diagnosis leading to a differential treatment plan.

ESTHETIC AND SOCIAL CONSIDERATIONS

In addition to functional requirements, an important consideration in treating malocclusion is the esthetic balance of the face. An esthetic appraisal depends upon social and racial standards. The illustrated press, television and movies are instrumental in promoting certain facial types as the beautiful or desirable ones. They are active in forming and crystallizing the esthetic ideals of a population.

It is interesting to note that in American society a kind of character judgment has overlapped the purely physical evaluation of characteristics of the face. A person with mandibular retrusion is sometimes associated in newspaper comic strips with feeble-mindedness and is usually the scapegoat, such as the chinless (Class II) character Zero in the Beetle Bailey series. In contrast to this type is the strong-jawed individual, who is usually the sheriff, the detective or the hero. He may have true mandibular prognathism, but at this end of the scale the social lens has made an attribute out of a deformity. A comic strip example is Dick Tracy. This prognathism is supposed to be not only a sign of strong will but also a reflection of moral rectitude.

There is some danger in this association of physical characteristics and moral values. The popularity of particular facial types is temporary. What may be considered desirable or acceptable today may become undesirable tomorrow. Furthermore, what may be acceptable in American society may not be considered desirable elsewhere. Concepts of the Greek ideal of beauty have to be replaced by ideals that are relative to particular times, places and people.

Esthetic considerations are particularly important in the diagnosis and treatment planning of facial deformities because they are at the base of the motivation of many patients. It is up to the dentist to discuss the problem on an objective basis with the patient and above all to avoid imposing artifical and temporary fashions.

In summary, the diagnosis of dentofacial abnormalities should be all-inclusive. The different aspects discussed above may not all be significant in a given case. However, the establishment of a routine step-by-step analysis insures that the diagnosis will be as complete as possible and leads to a logical treatment plan.

TREATMENT PLANNING

In order to establish a treatment plan it is necessary to formulate the objectives. Only then will it be possible to select from the means available (orthodontic, prosthetic or surgical) the best one or the best combination of different ones to achieve the objectives. All treatments have common goals: to achieve the best esthetic and functional relationship of the teeth and the jaws; and to insure the greatest stability and longevity of teeth and supporting structures with an economy of treatment, of means used and of risk involved.

Possibility and Limitations of Orthodontic Treatment. Although different methods of orthodontic treatment cannot be elaborated here, it is necessary to describe some principles. The term *orthodontics* is usually associated with the movement of teeth, while we are speaking primarily about changes in bone shape, size and position. In this context it is better to use the term *dentofacial orthopedics*.

In a summarized way, from results of recent investigations, it could be stated that in a growing child it is possible to prevent the maxilla and the mandible from growing forward. It is possible to change the size of the maxilla by splitting the palate and increasing its breadth. It is possible, moreover, to increase or restrict the amount of possible movement of the mandible. Any combination of these different changes could be achieved, and this is equivalent to changing the facial proportions.

There are two categories of facial types that cannot be treated adequately by dentofacial orthopedics: Class II deep bite with mandibular retrusion, beyond the growth period, and skeletal Class III open bite. These facial types require surgical intervention to achieve the best results.

Joint Treatment Plan with Surgical, Orthodontic, and Prosthetic Teams. Different alternate plans may be considered:

1. Orthodontics and no surgery.
2. Surgery only.
3. Prosthetics only.
4. Orthodontics or prosthetics or both, followed by surgery.
5. Surgery followed by orthodontics or prosthetics or both.
6. Orthodontics or prosthetics first, followed by surgery, followed by orthodontics or prosthetics.

Case Report No. 1

ORTHODONTIC TREATMENT

Female (G.G.), age 11 years, mixed dentition, Class III malocclusion with anterior crossbite, skeletal Class III deep bite (see Figure 21–17). At rest position the mandible was more retrusive, bringing the incisors to an edge-to-edge relationship. The potential of growth was considerable, with the skeletal age being 10 years 6 months. Skeletal evaluation by archial analysis showed an underdevelopment of the maxilla and a protrusion of the mandible. This was a combination of dental, skeletal and functional Class III deep bite. However, because of the mild deficiency and the growth potential, the orthodontic approach was selected. Treatment consisted of correcting the crossbite and rotating the mandible around the condyles in a downward and backward direction. The appliance selected was the tongue blade. The child was instructed at chairside to use the tongue blade, and in 3 months the incisor crossbite was corrected. This created a posterior open bite. Further eruption of the posterior teeth stabilized the correction. The results were obtained by the removal of the incisor interference and the rotation of the mandible downward and backward. Although the maxilla was still retrusive it was expected to grow forward because of the forces exerted by the mandible.

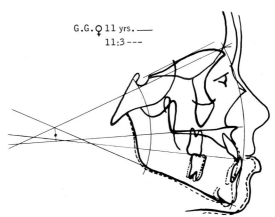

Figure 21–17 G. G., female, 11 years old. Maxillary deficiency and slight mandibular protrusion. A functional malocclusion associated with anterior crossbite. The crossbite was corrected with tongue-blade treatment, which permitted rotation of the mandible. (From Sassouni, V.: The Face in Five Dimensions. 3rd ed. Pittsburgh, University of Pittsburgh, Dental School Publication, 1965.)

Case Report No. 2

ORTHODONTIC TREATMENT

Female (S.M.), age 18 years, Class III malocclusion with anterior crossbite, skeletal Class III deep bite (see Figure 21–18). As in the previous case, the mandible assumed a more posterior posi-

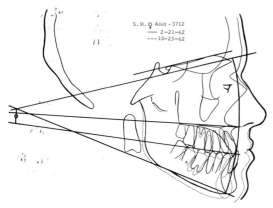

Figure 21–18 S. M., female adult. Mandibular protrusion and deep bite skeletal pattern. The mandible was rotated and the crossbite corrected by maxillary dental expansion achieved by full band appliance. (From Sassouni, V.: The Face in Five Dimensions. 3rd ed. Pittsburgh, University of Pittsburgh, Dental School Publication, 1965.)

tion when at rest. The archial analysis showed a normally positioned maxilla with a protrusive mandible. As this patient was an adult, no growth was expected. Therefore, the treatment was based purely on positional changes. In choosing between the surgical and orthodontic approaches, the orthodontic was selected primarily because of the favorable rest position of the mandible and because of irregularities of the maxillary incisors, which would necessitate correction. The treatment plan was to open the bite in order to insure the downward and backward rotation of the mandible. In addition this removed the incisor interference and permitted the anterior expansion of the maxillary incisors. The bite was opened by means of a removable acrylic plate covering the mandibular molars, and the expansion of the incisors was accomplished with a fixed appliance on the maxillary teeth. These objectives were achieved in 8 months of treatment.

Case Report No. 3

ORTHODONTIC TREATMENT

Male (R.F.), age 14 years, Class I malocclusion with anterior and posterior crossbite and maxillary incisor crowding; the canines were forced out of the dental arch to the buccal (see Figures 21–19 and 21–20). The mandibular dental arch was normal. Archial analysis showed a mandible in normal position and a retrusive maxilla. Unlike both previous cases the plan of treatment called for was expansion of the maxilla to correct the posterior and anterior crossbites. The orthopedic approach was selected because of the growth potential and the dentoskeletal nature of the maxillary deficiency. The plan of treatment required a skeletal expansion by means of an opening of the midpalatal suture. This permitted the two halves of the maxilla to be moved laterally. Space thereby created between the incisors brought the cuspids into alignment. The palatal expansion was achieved in 3 weeks, and the movement of the teeth in 1 year. The changes produced were a downward and backward rotation of the mandible (unlocked by the expansion of the maxilla) and a partial correction of the maxillary deficiency.

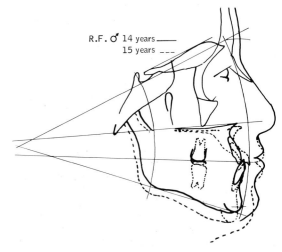

Figure 21–19 R. F., male, 14 years old. There is a maxillary retrognathism, with anterior crossbite and maxillary dental crowding. The treatment was done with a palatal splitting appliance. The crossbite is corrected, the premaxilla is growing forward, and the direction of growth of the mandible has been changed.

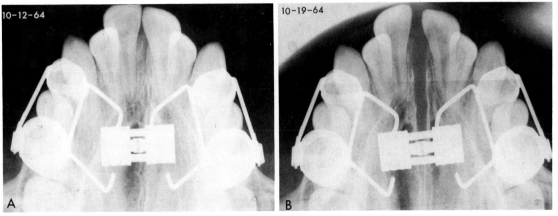

Figure 21–20   Rapid expansion of the median palatal suture of patient illustrated in Figure 21–19.

Case Report No. 4

PROSTHETIC TREATMENT

Female (D.T.), age 28 years, Class I open bite malocclusion (see Figure 21–21). The only contact between maxillary and mandibular teeth started at the second bicuspid. Skeletal evaluation by the archial analysis showed a typical skeletal open bite: short ramus, large gonial angle, steep mandibular plane, downward and backward tipped pal-ate, small total posterior height and large total anterior height. The large lower anterior facial height does not permit normal lip closure. The objective was primarily to reduce the lower facial height and establish a functional masticatory apparatus.

The orthodontic approach was unfavorable; an extrusion of the incisors to reduce the open bite

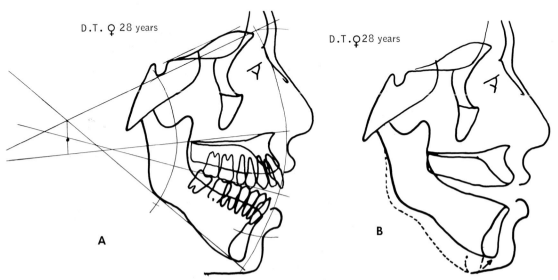

Figure 21–21   *A*, D. T., female, 28 years old. Skeletal open bite. Notice the steep planes and their convergence at center "O" close to the profile. The lower anterior facial height is 20 mm. larger than the upper. *B*, The treatment plan is to permit the mandible to rotate in a closing direction. This could be accomplished only by removing the interferences created by the presence of the posterior teeth.

would probably have relapsed. Furthermore, this would not have reduced the lower facial height. Depression of the posterior teeth may permit the closure of the mandible in a child but will not do so in an adult. A surgical approach was contemplated at two different levels: (1) A vertical osteotomy of the ramus, sliding the anterior segment downward. This would have necessitated freeing the masseter, internal pterygoid and temporal muscles, and the total possible reduction of anterior facial height would have been only about 5 mm. (until the cuspids came into contact). (2) A V cut of the body of the mandible (corpus) may have avoided interfering with the posterior musculature, but the total possible closure would have been the same (5 mm.). Furthermore, this would have required removal of the first mandibular molars

and retraction of the anterior portion of the dental arch, thus creating a Class II malocclusion. The results would not have been commensurate with the means contemplated.

The prosthetic approach was therefore indicated. It should be recognized that the jaws were kept apart by the teeth. Therefore if the teeth were removed, nothing would prevent the mandible from closing (Fig. 21–21B). Some alveolar ridge reduction was necessary. Complete dentures with very small posterior crown height permitted closure in this position.

In certain favorable instances it is possible to consider the extraction of posterior teeth only, preserving the cuspids and incisors. Then partial dentures should be adapted, again with very small crown heights.

Case Report No. 5

SURGICAL AND PROSTHETIC TREATMENT

Male (G.A.), age 37 years, Class III malocclusion (see Figure 21–22). The maxillary first and third molars were previously extracted, as well as the mandibular second bicuspids, first and second molars. The archial analysis indicated a normally positioned maxilla and a mandibular prognathism of 20 mm. The objectives were to reduce the prognathism and to reestablish a functional masticatory apparatus.

Treatment. The problem centered around which surgical approach to adopt: resection at the ramus or at the body of the mandible (corpus). If the vertical or transverse ramus resection were adopted, then in the process of moving the corpus posteriorly, the molars would have interfered and opened the bite. The alternative was to extract the molars, but the prosthodontist required the preservation of these teeth as abutments for partial den-

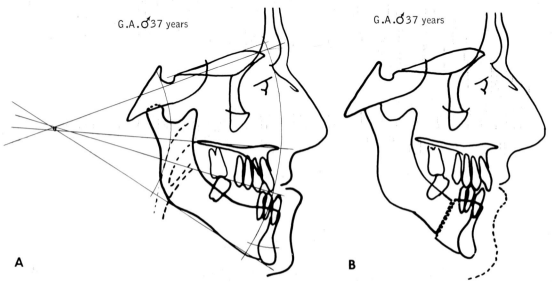

G.A.♂37 years   G.A.♂37 years

A   **B**

Figure 21–22 *A,* G. A., male, 37 years old. A mandibular prognathism due to a large gonial angle but not to a long corpus. *B,* Normally a ramus resection should have been planned here; however, because of the dental interferences and for the preservation of abutment and further because of the edentulous space, a corpus resection was performed.

tures. Furthermore, the ramus was narrow and may not have permitted enough retraction. Finally, notice the narrow pharyngeal space that might have been reduced by the retraction of the mandible. Resection of the corpus had some advantages peculiar to this patient. As there was a large edentulous space, no teeth were sacrificed; furthermore, this resection closed the edentulous space, permitting the construction of a fixed prothesis rather than a removable partial prosthesis. See Figure 21–22B.

Case Report No. 6

SURGICAL AND ORTHODONTIC TREATMENT

Female (D.C.), age 16 years, Class III malocclusion with open bite (see Figure 21–23). The archial analysis indicated a maxilla in normal position and mandibular prognathism of 18 mm. The open bite was purely dental—caused by undereruption of the maxillary incisors. There was a deep bite skeletal pattern: the lower anterior facial height was smaller than the upper. The objectives were to increase the lower facial height and close the open bite while reducing the prognathism.

The surgical treatment of choice was an oblique osteotomy of the ramus in order to retract and rotate the body of the mandible (corpus). This will temporarily increase the dental open bite, which should then be corrected by orthodontic means (Fig. 21–23B).

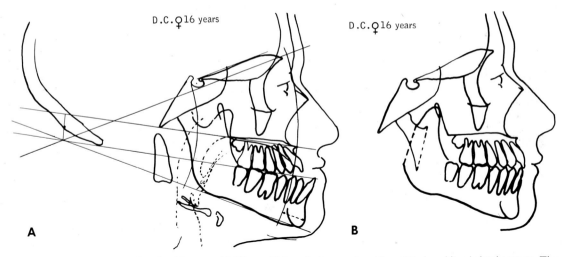

Figure 21–23 *A*, D. C., female, 16 years old. The archial analysis reveals a Class III, deep bite skeletal pattern. The severity of this case requires surgical treatment. *B*, The plan of treatment required the reduction of the mandibular prognathism and an increase of lower facial height. The oblique ramus sliding osteotomy permits these two objectives to be achieved.

Case Report No. 7

SURGICAL TREATMENT

Female (B.D.), age 20 years, Class III malocclusion with deep bite (see Figures 21–24 to 21–26). The archial analysis (Fig. 21–24) indicated a maxillary retrusion of 5 mm. and a mandibular prognathism of 18 mm. at the chin (pogonion). Gonion was only 12 mm. anterior to its normal position (in reference to the posterior arc). Therefore, this skeletal malocclusion is due partly to a

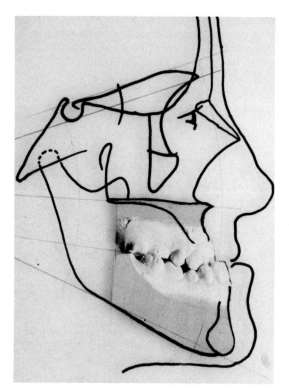

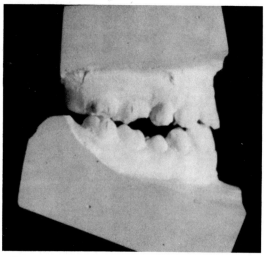

Figure 21–25   Patient B. D. When the mandible is retracted, an incisor lock can be achieved. The maxillary molars' lingual cusps interfere with complete posterior closure. They need to be reduced.

Figure 21–24   Patient B. D., female, 20 years old. Skeletal Class III deep bite. The favorable dental arch shape permits a surgical treatment only.

deficient maxilla, partly to a long corpus (long by 6 mm.) and partly to an anteriorly positioned corpus (anterior by 12 mm.). The dental evaluation indicated that if the mandible were repositioned posteriorly until the upper incisors overlapped the lowers, the posterior facial height would be increased and a buccal open bite created at the level of the first molars and second bicuspids (Fig. 21–25). Notice that in this position the lingual cusps of the maxillary molars would interfere to prevent closure. Furthermore, in this retruded position of the mandible the posterior crossbite would be corrected to a large degree, and an incisor lock could be obtained. The objectives of treatment were to retract the mandible by the amount necessary to create the incisor lock and to reduce (by grinding) the lingual cusps of the molars to close the posterior open bite.

The entire treatment was by surgical means without further orthodontic or prosthetic intervention. Because of the relatively wide ramus and the long necks of the condyles, and because the corpus was anteriorly positioned rather than large, an oblique ramus osteotomy was recommended (Fig. 21–26).

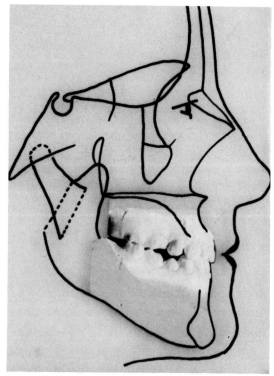

Figure 21–26   Patient B. D. Skeletal and dental reduction. The slight open bite left at the bicuspid level could be expected to correct itself.

These case reports demonstrate the necessity of close cooperation between different specialists in dentistry. They stress that no single method of treatment is sufficient to achieve the best result for each patient. When all possible avenues of treatment are contemplated, one best combination will emerge that will be best adapted to the *unique* problem presented by each *individual* patient.

REFERENCES

1. Broadbent, B. H.: A new x-ray technique and its application to orthodontia. Angle Orthod., *1*:45–66, 1931.
2. Goldstein, A.: Appraisal of results of surgical correction of class III malocclusions. Angle Orthod., *17*:59–91, 1947.
3. Greulich, W. W., and Pyle, I. S.: Radiographic Atlas of Skeletal Development of the Hand and Wrist. Stanford, Calif., Stanford University Press, 1959.
4. Krogman, W. M., and Sassouni, V.: A Syllabus in Roentgenographic Cephalometry. Philadelphia, University of Pennsylvania Growth Center, 1957.
5. Sassouni, V.: A roentgenographic cephalometric analysis of cephalo-facial-dental relationships. Am. J. Orthod., *41*:735–764, 1955.
6. Sassouni, V.: Palatoprint, physioprint, and roentgenographic cephalometry, as new methods in human identification. J. Forensic Sci., *2*:429–443, 1957.
7. Sassouni, V.: The Face in Five Dimensions. Philadelphia, University of Pennsylvania Growth Center, 1960.
8. Sassouni, V.: The Face in Five Dimensions. 2nd ed. Morgantown, W. Va., West Virginia School of Dentistry, 1962.
9. Sassouni, V., and Nanda, S.: Analysis of dentofacial vertical proportions. Am. J. Orthod., *50*:801–823, 1964.
10. Scott, J. H.: The growth of the human face. Proc. Roy. Soc. Med., *47*:91, 1954.
11. Symons, N. B. B.: Studies on growth and form of the mandible. J. Dent. Res., *71*:41, 1951.

CHAPTER 22

ORTHOGNATHIC SURGERY OF THE MANDIBLE AND MAXILLA

W. HARRY ARCHER, M.A., D.D.S.
WILLIAM H. BELL, D.D.S.
MARSH ROBINSON, D.D.S., M.D.
CONRAD J. SPILKA, D.D.S.

PROGNATHISM AND MICROGNATHISM

W. HARRY ARCHER, M.A., D.D.S.

Etiology. The overdevelopment or underdevelopment of either jaw may be due to disease, trauma or atavism. Blair said: "Once destroy that nice balance upon which the natural development depends, and the normal muscular forces will operate to exaggerate the malrelation."[20] The primary factor in some cases, according to Blair, is atavism.[18] Distinct facial types were developed and preserved in the early nations of the world. Individuals today are mostly the product of many mixtures. This mixing produces prognathism or micrognathism in some cases, while in others orthognathism is preserved.

Indications for Surgical Operation. Patients with a pronounced deformity who did not have the benefit of orthodontic treatment at the time it would have been effective, or who were beyond the treatment of the orthodontist from the start, are legitimate and proper cases for surgical intervention, provided the patient seeks relief. The author feels strongly that the patient and his family should *convince the surgeon*, by their insistence and persistence, that surgical correction of this deformity is vitally important to the patient. Surgery, particularly an elective procedure, should never be "sold" to a patient.

Deformities of this nature may be associated with psychic disturbances. The patients become introverts, acquire inferiority complexes, are morose, and suffer mental anguish. Interference with normal employment and social success may result. Functional disabilities may arise, including speech difficulties, improper mastication and inadequate nutrition.

However, as has been noted by other authors, few of these patients actually seem to be handicapped physically by malocclusion, and those who do mention this as their reason for seeking surgery are often doing so to mask their real reason: they are sensitive about their appearance. Eventually they readily admit that they actually wanted to look like "normal" people, and so sought surgical relief.

Whole-hearted confidence of the patient is a prerequisite for surgery, because during the postoperative period trying complications may arise in which both the surgeon and the patient may find their patience taxed to the limit. However, the long-term rewards must be considered.

Any oral surgeon who has corrected this condition in young people can attest to the re-

1448

markable personality changes that often occur.

Purposes of Surgery. Orthognathic surgery is performed to achieve these results: (1) improved facial appearance, (2) improved occlusion, (3) normal function of the mandible.

Blair, in an address to a dental socity group in 1907, adequately summarized the purpose of these procedures as follows: "If called upon, our endeavor should be to set the bones in the position that will ultimately give a useful occlusion, and the most symmetrical facial outline. Occlusion must be an end, not a guide, while good mechanical, and not ideal occlusion should be the object."[19]

Behrman has stated well the surgeon's responsibility in fulfillment of these goals: "The surgical correction of jaw deformities is an art as well as a science. It is not enough to have an orthodontist make a cephalometric evaluation and a study-model treatment plan. It is not sufficient to have a prosthodontist indicate the desired freeway space and design a splint. It is not enough to be slick with a scalpel, saw, and suture. The surgeon must complement this surgical skill with knowledge of facial growth and development, an understanding of orofacial musculature, speech and swallowing patterns, and a thorough comprehension of occlusion. With these, along with empathy and understanding, he will be able to fulfill the patient's desires concerning appearance and still provide a comfortable, fully functioning organ of speech, deglutition, and mastication."[9]

ORTHOGNATHIC TECHNIQUES AND ASSOCIATED COMPLICATIONS

A number of techniques have been devised to correct prognathism and micrognathism in the mandible and maxilla, as is indicated in Figure 22–1, and of these, four are discussed in detail in this chapter: vertical ostectomy, or ostectomy of the body of the mandible; subcondylar osteotomy; oblique (vertical) osteotomy of the ramus; and total maxillary osteotomy.

Behrman has studied in detail the complications associated with certain of the more common orthognathic techniques that are used in the mandible.[9] In weighing the relative merits and disadvantages of the various techniques, the surgeon should bear in mind that this is *elective surgery*.

Subcondylar Osteotomy. Behrman has noted the following complications in cases treated by subcondylar osteotomy: (*a*) hemorrhage, (*b*) facial nerve injury, (*c*) nonunion and open bite and (*d*) gustatory hyperhidrosis.[9]

Oblique (Vertical) Osteotomy of the Ramus. Complications found by Behrman in osteotomies of the vertical rami included: (*a*) hemorrhage, (*b*) facial nerve damage, (*c*) mandibular nerve damage, (*d*) inadvertent horizontal osteotomy, (*e*) inability to obtain desired repositioning, (*f*) nonunion and open bite, (*g*) extrusion of teeth, (*h*) infection, (*i*) skin scars and keloids and (*j*) condylar displacement.[9]

Sagittal-Split Osteotomy. This technique, which is an intraoral osteotomy of the ascending mandibular ramus and posterior body of the mandible in the sagittal plane, according to Behrman carries with it the following potential life-threatening complications: (*a*) hemorrhage,* and (*b*) airway obstruction and edema.

Additional complications include the following disfiguring or potentially disfiguring complications: (*c*) substantial loss of bone under aseptic conditions, (*d*) substantial loss of bone due to sepsis, (*e*) infection, (*f*) displacement of bone segments, (*g*) dislocation of the condyle, (*h*) impairment of function of the facial nerve, (*i*) impairment of function of the mandibular nerve, (*j*) impairment of function of the lingual nerve, (*k*) regression and relapse, (*l*) nonunion, (*m*) fracture and fragmentation and (*n*) limited opening of the mouth.[9]

In substantiation of Behrman's findings, Biermann, Schettler and Koberg, in their analysis of 78 cases of prognathism surgically corrected by various techniques, found that the highest rate of infection (23 per cent) was associated with the Obwegeser (sagittal-split) technique, as was the highest rate of alveolar nerve involvement (67 per cent).[17] Guernsey and DeChamplain have reported that following sagittal osteotomy "19 of 22 patients had bilateral neuropathy" of the inferior alveolar nerve, "ranging from hypesthesia to frank anesthesia. One had unilateral hypesthesia and one had no neuropathy." In the 15 cases they were able to follow of the total 22, this lack of sensation persisted from 1 to 18 months.[39] In Koblin and Reil's follow-

---

*AUTHOR'S NOTE: Two known deaths have resulted from hemorrhage.

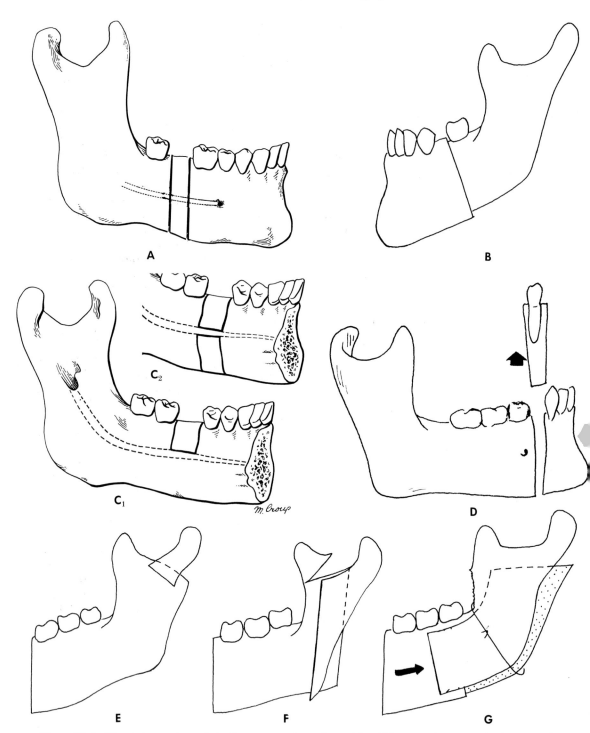

Figure 22–1 The various cuts made in the osseous tissue favored by different oral surgeons in the correction of prognathia or micrognathia of the mandible.

A, Vertical osteotomy or osteoectomy of the body of the mandible after the extraction of a first molar. *B*, Sections of the mandible fixed in their new relationship after the section of bone shown in *A* is removed.

C, Vertical sectional ostectomy of the body of the mandible to preserve the continuity of the inferior neurovascular bundle. *C₁*, First stage, cuts are made intraorally. *C₂*, Second stage, cuts are made extraorally. (See text.)

D, Ostectomy of a section of the mandible anterior to the mental foramen.

E, Subcondylar osteotomy.

F, Oblique (vertical) osteotomy of the ramus and horizontal osteotomy of the coronoid process.

G, Sagittal-split osteotomy for prognathism of the mandible.

(Figure 22–1 continued on opposite page)

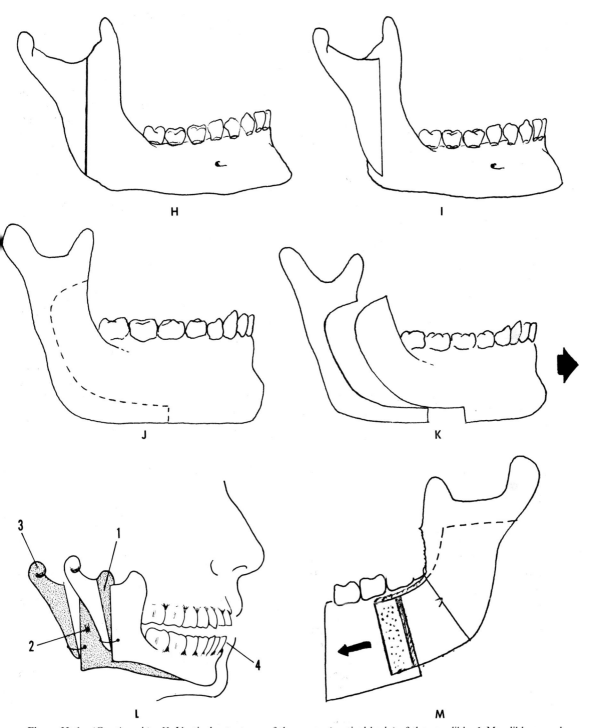

Figure 22–1   *(Continued.)*   *H*, Vertical osteotomy of the ramus (vertical body) of the mandible. *I*, Mandible moved posteriorly with the posterior cut lapping the anterior portion of the ramus.

J, Curved line of osteotomy of the ramus. *K*, Mandible moved forward to correct micrognathia.

L, Oblique osteotomy of the ramus for correction of micrognathia.

M, Sagittal-split osteotomy of the mandible for correction of micrognathia.

(*B* and *D* to *K*, Adapted from Waite, D. E.: Textbook of Practical Oral Surgery. Philadelphia, Lea & Febiger, 1972.)

up examination of 75 patients after surgical correction of prognathism by three different methods, these researchers found 5 per cent incidence of alveolar nerve injury following the Babcock-Lindemann technique in the ramus, 14 per cent in those cases of ostectomies of the body of the mandible in which the mandibular nerve (neurovascular bundle) was preserved, and 20 per cent when the Obwegeser–Dal Pont sagittal-split operation was performed.[56]

While acknowledging that "unfortunately the versatility and broad applicability of this technique is matched by an extraordinary variety of potential complications," Behrman states that the sagittal-split osteotomy is "our procedure of choice for the correction of apertognathia and retrognathia as well as for the correction of prognathism for patients who develop keloids or who have severe acne." He goes on to say, "This is not a procedure for neophytes or novices; it is not meant for the solo surgeon nor for anyone not thoroughly trained, fully knowledgeable, and totally at ease doing extensive procedures intraorally. Even the most skillful of surgeons will not be at his best if he performs this procedure only occasionally. On the other hand, like open-heart surgery and kidney transplants, when the sagittal-split osteotomy is done regularly by a well-trained, well-equipped team the results are excellent and complications are rare."[9]

Vertical Osteotomy or Ostectomy of the Body of the Mandible. Behrman found the following complications in cases treated by ostectomy of the body of the mandible: (a) nonunion and (b) fifth nerve damage.[9] I have found that nonunion will occur if immobilization is inadequate or for too short a time. It is a rare complication if immobilization is maintained a minimum of 8 weeks. Fifth nerve damage cannot be considered a complication if the technique used includes sectioning a block of bone with the inferior alveolar canal and its contents. The resulting anesthesia, deliberately produced, does not last over a year in the great majority of cases.

Note that 14 kinds of serious complications, including death, have occurred in significant percentages of patients treated by sagittal-split osteotomies, while Behrman found only two kinds of complications in vertical osteotomy procedures. I suggest that it would be logical for more cases of prognathism of the mandible to be treated by bilateral vertical ostectomy of the body of the mandible, in the best interests of patients.

OSTEOECTOMY IN THE HORIZONTAL RAMUS (BODY OF THE MANDIBLE)

W. HARRY ARCHER, B.S., M.A., D.D.S.

A preoperative appraisal is made of the patient that includes: (a) classification and description of malocclusion, (b) functional analysis, (c) assessment of facial proportions, (d) evaluation of growth potential, (e) racial and hereditary factors, and (f) esthetic appraisal. All these are discussed in Chapter 21 and will not be repeated here.

Bilateral sections of proper size are removed from the body of the mandible, usually in the second bicuspid or first molar area, creating a double mandibular fracture. The cut ends are brought together by moving the anterior segment posteriorly, and immobilizing the segments in their new position until union is complete. This procedure may be performed entirely from an intraoral or an extraoral approach. This is the author's preferred technique. The Dingman technique is a modification of this procedure. It is a combination of intraoral and extraoral approaches that may be performed at the same time or in separate stages. This technique maintains the continuity of the neurovascular bundle. (See Two-stage Osteoectomy of the Horizontal Ramus, later in this chapter.)

Osteoectomy of the horizontal rami has been the procedure of choice for many surgeons in this country. It has been criticized because of the sacrifice of teeth at the surgical site. When the freedom from the numerous potential complications that have been seen in other techniques is taken into consideration, this is an insignificant loss. Some surgeons have also objected to severing the inferior alveolar nerve and the resultant transitory anesthesia. However, this nerve may be preserved by one technique, or, if severed deliberately (as in the technique described in the following section), it regenerates readily. Oral contamination is present in this procedure, and the objection raised is the possibility of infection and nonunion. One must consider, however, that nearly all fractures of the mandible are compounded into the oral cavity, and that these fractures heal as quickly as closed fractures. We do not prophylactically administer antibiotics. The fear of respiratory embarrassment by pushing the tongue into the pharynx has been raised. This rather remote possibility is present in all the techniques for correction of a prognathic mandible. It has been observed that the tongue has a tendency to adapt itself to its new environment.

From a technical standpoint the difficulty of making four straight cuts through the body of the mandible with a Gigli saw after the continuity of the mandible has once been severed has presented a severe problem. The technique described here makes this operation easier and more accurate.

OSTEOECTOMY WITH SEVERANCE OF THE NEUROVASCULAR BUNDLE

The author prefers, in the great majority of cases, bilateral osteoectomy of the body of the mandible (horizontal rami) by removing a bilateral segment from the first molar area. If a second molar is missing, this area is selected for the removal of the segment of bone.

To simplify the removal of bilateral sections from the horizontal rami, the author now places extraoral appliances on each side of the mandible. This obviates one of the most trying and difficult procedures, the stabilization of the mandible during cutting and immobilization during healing.

In the author's opinion, this technique of removing bilateral sections of the horizontal rami with the preoperative placing of extraoral skeletal fixation devices such as the biphase pin fixation, Stader or Roger Anderson devices (see Chapter 18 for the application techniques) has these advantages: (1) The site of operation is easily accessible. (2) The operation may be performed under direct vision, so that the predetermined set-back of the procedure may be obtained. (3) There is little or no interference with anatomic structure. The muscles of mastication are not tampered with; trismus is not encountered. The mandibular sheath with the inferior alveolar nerve and blood vessels is severed, but it regenerates easily and rapidly. Facial paralysis and extraoral salivary fistulas are not seen as postoperative complications. (4) Open bite is not seen postoperatively. If present preoperatively, it may be corrected by this technique. (5) Control of the fragments both during the operation and postoperatively is facilitated by the extraoral appliance. After making the original cut, the surgeon no longer encounters the problem of controlling two and then three fragments during the succeeding cutting operations. One can readily visualize the difficulties to be encountered during osteoec-

tomy or osteotomy with freely movable fragments. (6) After the osteoectomy the mandibular fragments are easily aligned to their new relationship. Any adjustment needed in a posterior or lateral direction can be easily accomplished by the use of the lock nuts and connecting bars of the appliances. (7) By the use of the extraoral appliance, immobilization is accomplished without the patient's being subjected to keeping the teeth wired together for 8 to 12 weeks. Note that the maxillary and mandibular arch bars with intermaxillary elastic bands fixation are removed after the first 2 weeks' fixation. The details of the author's modification of the osteoectomy of the horizontal rami (body of the mandible) follow:

First Stage. The patient should have a careful physical examination before operation is decided upon. Adequate nutrition and rest should be stressed, and instituted. The surgeon should check carefully to determine whether or not the patient has bruxism. This is a contraindication.

Next, the surgeon should procure good full face and profile photographs, and close-ups of the occlusion of the teeth. Cephalograms should be made and analyzed by an authority, but the surgeon must compare the measurements obtained from his study casts with the cephalometric tracing data. The author saw one case in which cephalometric measurements alone were used and a prognathic patient became micrognathic. (Study Chapter 21.)

A complete 16-film intraoral radiographic examination and a panoramic radiograph are made, as well as posteroanterior and right and left lateral jaw radiographs of the mandible. Carious teeth should be restored, the teeth should be scaled and polished, and the patient should institute rigorous daily oral hygiene.

Two sets of good models in stone of the maxillary and mandibular teeth and arches with bite recordings are made. One set in the present occlusion is mounted on an articulator for a permanent record and for preoperative study. On the second set the surgeon should place the models in their present occlusion, and draw a vertical line through the upper right and left first molars, or right and left second bicuspids, down through the tooth on the mandible that occludes with this particular maxillary tooth. He should then move the mandibular model to the desired posterior or retruded position.

The original lines on the maxillary model

should be retraced, carrying the line down on the mandibular teeth (or edentulous ridge) now in occlusion with the maxillary teeth.

With slight adjustment to allow for the mandibular tooth, the segment of the mandibular model between the two lines represents the segment of bone to be removed from both sides of the body of the mandible. This section should be cut out of the lower model; this will indicate the amount of bone, and which teeth, if any, are to be removed. Many patients have lost their posterior mandibular teeth. The lines are drawn on the edentulous areas of the mandible. (See Case Report Nos. 1 and 2 for examples.) Occlusal adjustments are made by spot grinding where they are now indicated on the occlusal surfaces of the teeth in what will be their new relationship after surgery.

At this point the surgeon should have the patient come in, and the teeth are extracted from the section of the mandible to be removed. Wide flaring buccal and lingual flaps are reflected, and after the surgeon carefully marks with a sharp instrument in the buccal cortical bone the width of the bony segments to be removed, a series of holes are drilled through the cortical plate with medium-sized Feldman spear-pointed burs, and these are then connected by means of crosscut burs. This cut is carried down to the apices of the tooth socket. The soft tissue flaps are now replaced and sutured. This procedure definitely establishes accurate starting grooves for the Gigli saw at the time of the resection. In addition, the demineralization of the cut bone ends plus the increase in circulation that takes place after this procedure, and before the second stage, materially aids in rapid union of the fragments after the bilateral resection of the bone segments. This procedure is, of course, carried out on both sides of the mandible. The mouth wound is allowed to heal for 3 or 4 weeks. In the laboratory the cut sections are again brought together and embedded in soft plaster. Now the surgeon mounts the models on an articulator, studies the new occlusion, and marks the teeth with articulating paper. The occlusion is adjusted by spot grinding, and the surgeon marks carefully with India ink the areas that were adjusted. Wire splints are adjusted to the gingival surfaces of both maxillary and mandibular teeth on the model.

Second Stage. The patient is admitted to the hospital 24 hours before the operation. A careful preoperative physical examination of the patient is made by the patient's physician.

Laboratory studies ordered should include bleeding and coagulation time, blood count and differential, blood typing and urinalysis.

The surgeon should write preanesthetic and preoperative orders, and, in consultation with the hospital anesthesiologist, decide upon the anesthetic technique to be used. We also use mandibular local block anesthesia. The local anesthesia materially reduces the amount of supplemental anesthesia required, and the vasoconstriction helps control hemorrhage. In addition, the block anesthesia protects the brain from the bombardment of painful afferent impulses incidental to the operation.

Strict asepsis is observed throughout the operation.

The lips are coated with petrolatum, and the Molt mouth prop is inserted. The surgeon grasps the tongue with the fingers, which have been covered with gauze, and brings it forward out of the mouth. The dorsal and ventral surfaces of the tongue are scrubbed with germicidal solution, and a suture is passed through the midline $1/2$ inch from the tip.

The surgeon attaches a hemostat to the suture through the tongue and secures it to the drapes by a towel clip. This prevents the tongue from slipping back into the pharynx, where it would cause mechanical respiratory embarrassment in those cases in which nasoendotracheal intubation was impossible, or it affords control of the tongue after the endotracheal tube has been removed.

Biphase pin fixation, or Stader or Roger Anderson extraoral skeletal appliances (see Chapter 18) are applied on the right and left body of the mandible, spanning the areas from which the osseous sections are to be removed. The extraoral skeletal fixation has the great advantage that the mandible is held rigidly as a single unit throughout the operation. This is advantageous when cutting through the bone with the Gigli saw, particularly when a bilateral section of the body of the mandible is being removed. It is next to impossible to control the segments of the mandible once its continuity has been severed.

Even though extraoral skeletal fixation is to be used, Jelenko or Erich fracture splints are wired carefully to the necks of the maxillary and mandibular teeth. This will permit additional support of the mandible when two wires are passed right and left under both maxillary and mandibular splints. These wires can be twisted together during the ac-

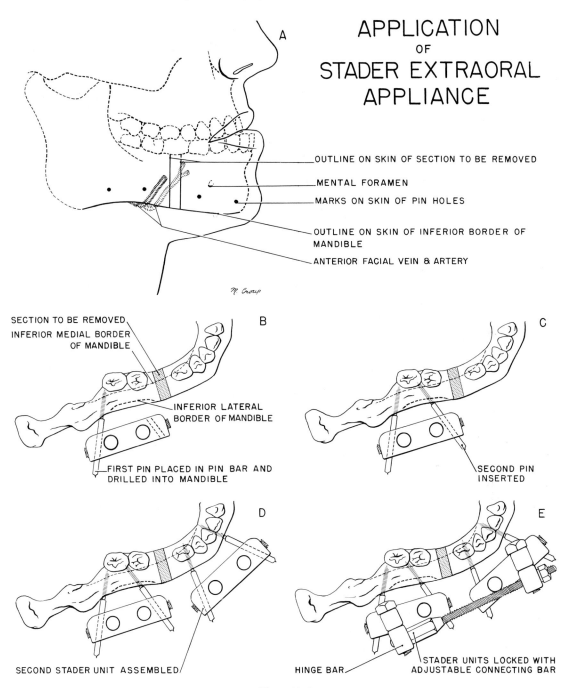

APPLICATION
OF
STADER EXTRAORAL
APPLIANCE

A

OUTLINE ON SKIN OF SECTION TO BE REMOVED

MENTAL FORAMEN

MARKS ON SKIN OF PIN HOLES

OUTLINE ON SKIN OF INFERIOR BORDER OF
MANDIBLE

ANTERIOR FACIAL VEIN & ARTERY

M. Croup

B

SECTION TO BE REMOVED
INFERIOR MEDIAL BORDER
OF MANDIBLE

INFERIOR LATERAL
BORDER OF MANDIBLE

FIRST PIN PLACED IN PIN BAR AND
DRILLED INTO MANDIBLE

C

SECOND PIN
INSERTED

D

SECOND STADER UNIT ASSEMBLED

E

HINGE BAR

STADER UNITS LOCKED WITH
ADJUSTABLE CONNECTING BAR

Figure 22-2

tual cutting of the bone. When changing the saw, the wires must be cut quickly, and when immobilization is desired new wires should be used. The splints also will permit fixation of the mandible in the new position while the extraoral appliances are being readjusted to the new desired relationship of the mandibular segments. These intraoral splints and in-termaxillary elastics are kept in position for at least 2 weeks to take the initial heavy strain off the extraoral skeletal fixation appliance. We use intermaxillary elastics rather than wiring for two reasons: (1) In case of emergencies in which it is necessary to open the mouth quickly, elastic bands may be cut or removed much more easily than wires can

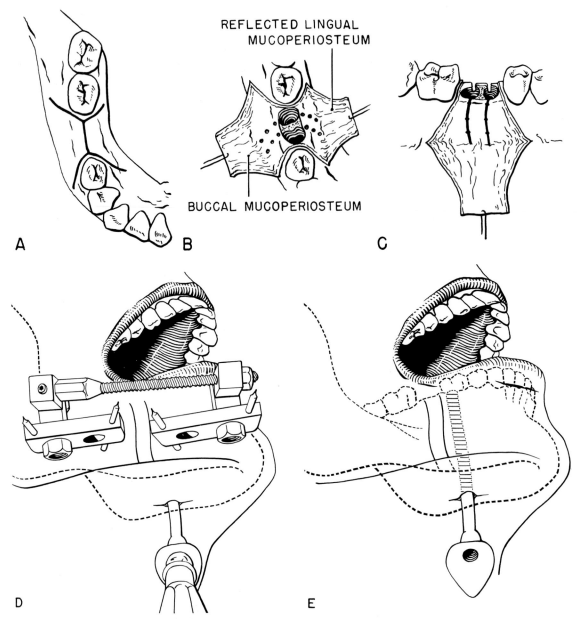

Figure 22–3 Surgical treatment for mandibular prognathism: osteoectomy of the body of the mandible.

A, The incision is made in the mucoperiosteum.

B, Holes are drilled through the cortical plate on the crest of the ridge and down on the buccal and lingual plates.

C, The holes are connected with a crosscut bur. The distal cut is made first.

D, A trocar and cannula is passed through the ½-inch incision in the skin beneath the body of the mandible along the distal cut in contact with the lingual cortical plate.

E, The trocar is removed, leaving the cannula in place. The Stader splint has been eliminated in this drawing to show the position of the cannula clearly.

(Figure 22–3 continued on opposite page)

be cut. (2) Wires stretch and then permit jaw movement, which may contribute to nonunion.

TECHNIQUE FOR PLACING STADER EXTRAORAL SKELETAL APPLIANCES. (See Chapter 18 for placement techniques for Roger Anderson and biphase extraoral skeletal pin fixation units.) The skin overlying the mandible should be scrubbed with tincture of green soap, wiped clean and painted with a germicidal solution such as tincture of Merthiolate, Metaphen or Zephiran.

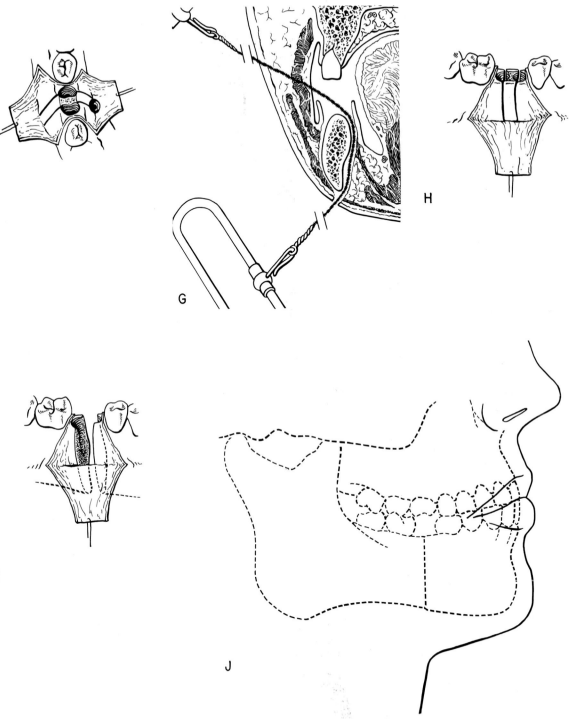

Figure 22–3 *(Continued.)* F, The cannula is in place along the distal cut, appearing in the oral cavity. The Gigli saw is now passed through the cannula and the cannula is then removed.

G, Cross section of face showing the relationship of the Gigli saw with surrounding tissues.

H, The distal cut is made first with the Gigli saw; then the mesial cut is made. When the Stader connecting bar is tightened, the segment of bone is now held firmly in place. (See text.)

I, The same procedure from step A to step H is now followed on the left side of the mandible. When all four cuts have been made, the segments of bone are removed and the fragments are brought together by adjusting the Stader splint. I shows the right side of the mandible after the segment of bone is removed.

J, Correct alignment of the mandible and improved occlusion and profile are obtained.

The surgeon should carefully outline the inferior border of the mandible with a thin line of gentian violet or an indelible pencil and make vertical lines on the skin indicating the section of bone to be removed.

Pin holes are marked with a dot of gentian violet. These pins should be located on either side as far from the cuts in the mandible as possible. They should be $1/4$ inch above the lower border of the mandible. When positioning the pin holes in the region of the angle of the jaw, the surgeon should locate the facial artery, where it passes up over the mandible, with the fingertip. This area must be avoided when marking pin locations.

The surgeon now inserts the pin in the drill chuck and puts a plastic pin bar over the pin. The pin bar is kept parallel to the body of the mandible or the symphysis. A daub of sterile petrolatum jelly is placed on the tip of the pin to prevent the tissues from winding around the pin.

In passing the sharp pin through the skin, particularly in the region of the angle of the jaw, the surgeon moves the pin laterally to permit any large vessels, such as the facial artery or vein, to be moved to one side of the pin. The pin is pushed slowly through the tissues overlying the bone until the cortical plate of bone is contacted by the pin. Although the inferior border of the mandible is marked on the skin with an indelible pencil, it must be recognized that the skin is freely movable over the body of the mandible, and the guide line can be easily moved out of position. When the pins penetrate the skin and buccinator, or masseter muscle, there may be slight bleeding. This can be controlled by pressure on the skin around the pin.

After the cortical plate is contacted, the pin is positioned so that its horizontal plane is at right angles to the body of the mandible, and its anteroposterior angle is such that the plastic bar will be parallel to the cortical plate.

Both pins are drilled through the buccal plate, the cancellous tissue, and just into the lingual plate. (Study Chapter 18 for detailed information on the technique for the insertion of pins.) The set screws in the pin bars are tightened against the pins. The surgeon should now apply the other three pin bar units as already described. The Stader unit is assembled on the pin bars, and all nuts and lock screws are tightened. The surgeon should allow 2 to 3 days for edema to subside before carrying out the third stage.

Third Stage. The next step is in the mouth. The mucoperiosteal tissue overlying the length of segment of bone to be removed on the right side along the crest of the ridge is incised. The incision is carried at either end down to the mucobuccal fold at a 45-degree angle. The same steps are taken on the lingual. (Study Figure 18–3.)

The mucoperiosteal tissue is reflected buccally and lingually, and held back by retractors. Now the surgeon passes a trocar and cannula beneath the body of the mandible through a short skin incision until it contacts the lingual mandibular surface, keeping the trocar in contact with the lingual cortical plate until the point appears in the oral cavity beneath the mucoperiosteal flap. The trocar is then removed.

One end of the Gigli wire saw is passed through the cannula, and the cannula is removed. Handles are attached, and the cheek is reflected with a metal retractor.

The jaws may be wired together right and left if additional support is needed. This is seldom necessary with the extraoral splints in position.

Next the surgeon cuts through the mandible, making the distal cut first. The cuts must be made at a right angle to the long axis of the mandible.

The surgeon must be sure that skin or lip will not be lacerated by the Gigli saw.

The surgeon moves the saw back through the cut, and along the lingual cortical plate until the point for the mesial cut is reached. As soon as the Gigli wire saw is passed back through the cut, the connecting bar is tightened so that the cut ends are held firmly in apposition. This will immediately control the hemorrhage from the inferior alveolar artery, and in addition makes the mandible a solid unit again.

The same steps are repeated for the mesial cut. The surgeon removes the Gigli wire saw from the mouth and tightens the Stader connecting bar so as to hold the cut section in place.

The procedures for the distal and mesial cut are now repeated on the left side. Both Stader adjustable connecting bars are loosened, and both segments of bone are removed.

Now the surgeon turns the adjustable connecting bar, bringing the fragments together. He must be certain that no portion of the buccal or lingual mucoperiosteal membranes is caught between the bone segments.

The new occlusion of the teeth is carefully

checked. If satisfactory, the hinge bolts are tightened on the adjustable connecting bars.

The anesthetic may now be discontinued, and the patient removed to the recovery room. When the patient has regained consciousness, intermaxillary elastics may be applied.

Regeneration of the Mandibular Nerve. In all the author's cases treated with the technique just described, there was regeneration of the inferior alveolar (mandibular) nerve, within a year on the average. This was proved not only by a return of normal sensation to the lip but also by normal response of the lower anterior teeth to the electric vitality test.

Case Report No. 1

BILATERAL OSTEOECTOMY FOR MANDIBULAR PROGNATHISM

W. H. Archer, D.D.S.

A male patient, aged 26, had difficulty in mastication, and a protruding lower jaw. He was admitted to the Eye and Ear Hospital for a bilateral osteoectomy to correct a mandibular prognathism. This condition had necessitated the preparation of a special soft diet. However, he was well nourished and finally admitted that the primary reason for seeking surgical correction of his abnormal mandible was esthetic. In fact he was so self-conscious that he worked in a coal mine and seldom went out nights. Two months prior to admission the lower right and left first molars and horizontally impacted lower right second bicuspid were extracted. Six weeks ago, preliminary vertical intraoral cuts had been made bilaterally in the body of the mandible.

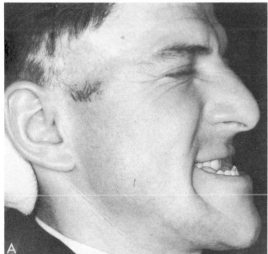

Figure 22-4 *A*, Mandibular prognathism with Class III malocclusion. (See Case Report No. 1.) *B* and *C*, Right and left views of study models.

(*Figure 22-4 continued on following page*)

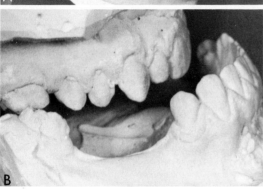

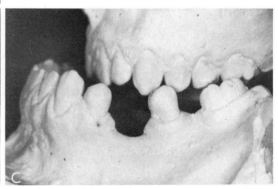

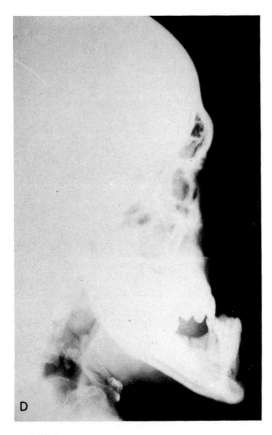

Figure 22–4 *(Continued.) D,* Lateral head radiograph showing marked mandibular protrusion.

E and *F,* Mandibular prognathism with Class III malocclusion.

G, Preoperative application of Stader connecting bar. A similar unit was placed on the opposite jaw.

(Figure 22–4 continued on opposite page)

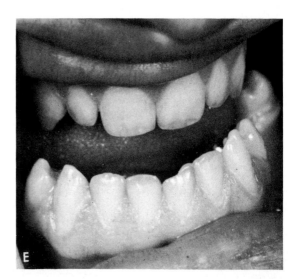

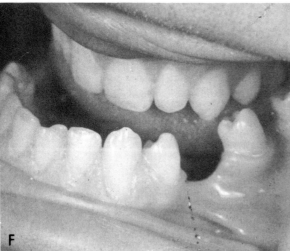

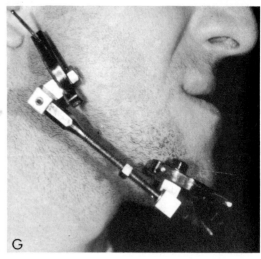

Examination. The results of a general physical examination were essentially negative. The mouth was in a good state of oral hygiene; the gingivae and oral mucosa were normal. The tongue was greatly enlarged, probably because of its use as an aid in mastication. The teeth were in a good state of repair. There was a marked prognathism of the mandible (Fig. 22–4A to F), with accompanying Class II malocclusion. When the patient attempted to bring his teeth into normal occlusion, the only teeth that occluded were the first upper molars with the lower second molars. A profile radiograph revealed the marked mandibular protrusion and poor dental function (Fig. 22–4D).

Operation: Application of Erich and Stader Splints. The Stader splints were attached bilaterally to the mandible, using the technique described in Case Report No. 3. At the same time

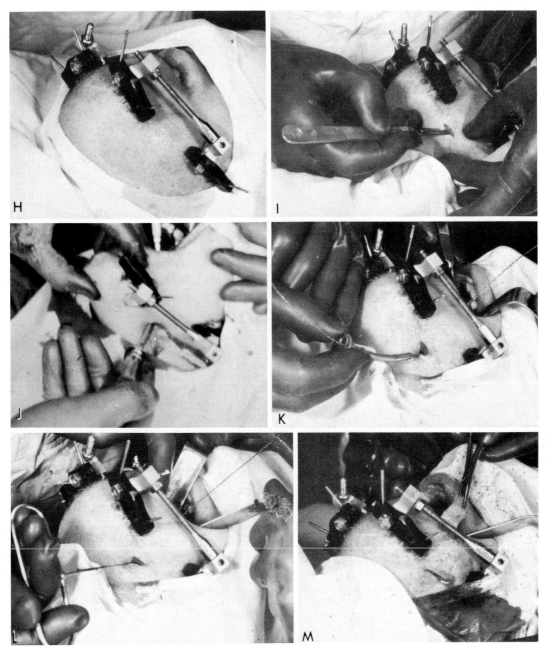

Figure 22-4 *(Continued.)* *H*, Adjustable threaded connecting bar locked in place. *I*, Short incision through the skin below the inferior border of the mandible.

J, Trocar and cannula passed through incision and up the lingual surface of the cortical bone of the mandible. *K*, Gigli saw passed through cannula, which is then removed.

L, Handles are attached to the wire saw, and distal and then mesial cuts are made through the body of the mandible from the lingual side to the buccal side. *M*, Cut section of the mandible is removed. This process is repeated on the opposite side, and bone segments are removed. The segments are approximated by rotating the threaded connecting bars and are then tightened. (See text.)

(Figure 22-4 continued on following page)

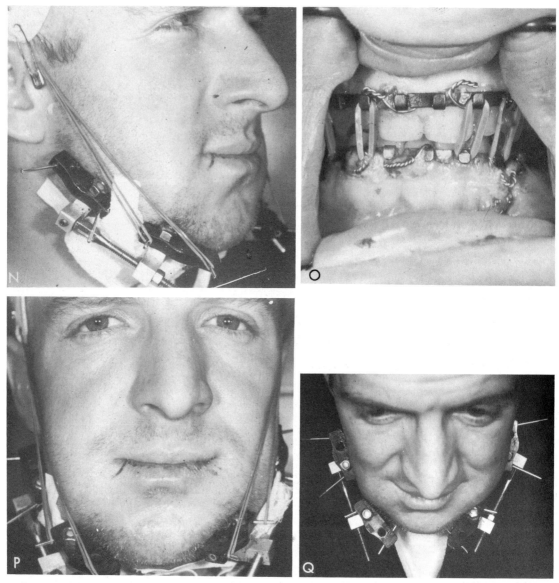

Figure 22–4 *(Continued.)* N to P, Extraoral and intraoral views taken the day following operation. *Q,* Superior view of the bilateral application of the Stader splints 3 weeks after surgery. At this time the intermaxillary fixation was removed, and the patient was permitted a soft diet and had the use of his jaws in talking and drinking for the next 6 weeks, the time required before removal of these splints. This freedom of movement is greatly appreciated by these patients. Total time of immobilization was 9 weeks. (Relapses occur when immobilization is terminated too soon.)

(Figure 22–4 continued on opposite page)

Jelenko splints were wired to the necks of the maxillary and mandibular teeth.

Postoperative Course. A few days were allowed for the patient to accommodate himself to the Stader appliance, and for slight edema of the adjacent fascial spaces to subside. The patient was then scheduled for bilateral osteoectomy.

Operation: Bilateral Osteoectomy of the Horizontal Ramus of the Mandible. Using the same technique already described, a 1.7-cm. bony seg-

ment was removed from the right side of the mandible and 1.4 cm. of bone from the left side. (See Figure 22–4G to M.)

Postoperative Course. For added support, a head cap was applied, and traction was instituted with elastics from the Stader appliance. (See Figure 22–4N to P.) The occlusion was normal (Fig. 22–4O). Radiographs taken on the seventh postoperative day revealed the fragments to be in good alignment (Fig. 22–4R to T). The patient was

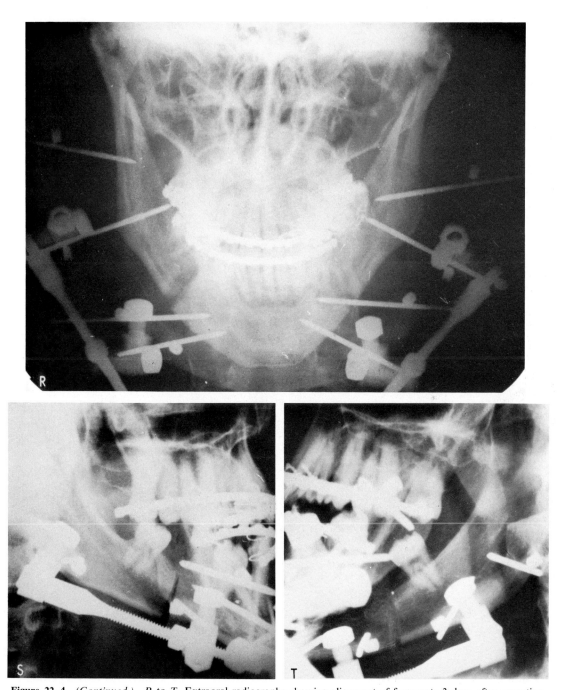

Figure 22–4 *(Continued.)* *R* to *T*, Extraoral radiographs showing alignment of fragments 3 days after operation.

(Figure 22–4 continued on following page)

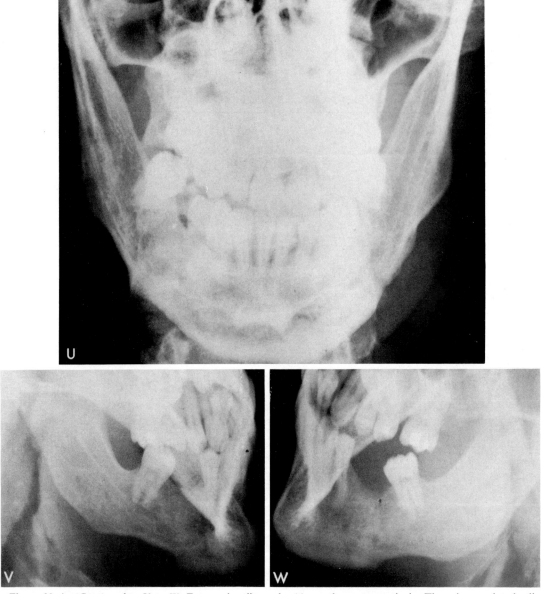

Figure 22–4 *(Continued.)*   *U* to *W*, Extraoral radiographs 11 months postoperatively. There is complete healing and return of normal sensation in the lip and teeth.

(Figure 22–4 continued on opposite page)

discharged on the sixth postoperative day, to be followed up with visits at the office.

Intermaxillary fixation was discontinued after 3 weeks. The patient's occlusion was satisfactory. The patient could open and close his mouth, eat a soft diet, and drink and talk normally for the balance of the healing period, which was 7 weeks.

Radiographs taken at this time gave evidence of satisfactory alignment of the bone segments (Fig. 22–4*R* to *T*). The Stader appliance was removed 10 weeks postoperatively. Radiographs taken 11 months after the operation are shown in Figure 22–4*U* to *W*. The patient's appearance and occlusion 1 year later are shown in Figure 22–4*X* to *Z*.

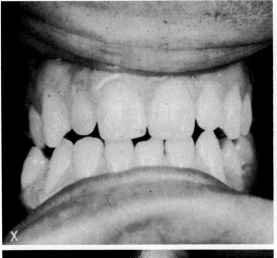

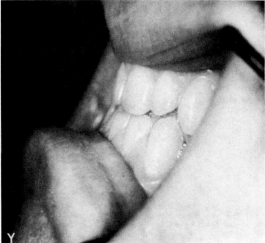

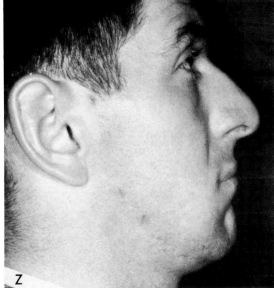

Figure 22-4 *(Continued.)* *X* to *Z*, Occlusion after removal of intermaxillary fixation. Appearance after operation.

Case Report No. 2

BILATERAL OSTEOECTOMY FOR MANDIBULAR PROGNATHISM

W. H. ARCHER, D.D.S.

A male patient, aged 23, had an unsightly appearance because of a protruding lower jaw. He was admitted to the hospital for a bilateral osteoectomy to correct the mandibular protrusion. The patient was a morose, depressed person who was self-conscious of his "chisel-chin." He exhibited the symptoms of an introvert with neurotic tendencies.

Examination. The general physical examination was essentially negative. The mouth was in a good state of oral hygiene, though the mandibular molar teeth were missing; the gingivae, oral mucosa, and tongue were normal. The patient had a marked protrusion of the lower jaw and a Class III malocclusion (Fig. 22-5A and B).

Operation No. 1. Under local anesthesia Stader splints were applied bilaterally. Intraorally, splints were wired to the maxillary and mandibular teeth. (See Figure 22-5C.) The patient left the operating room in good condition.

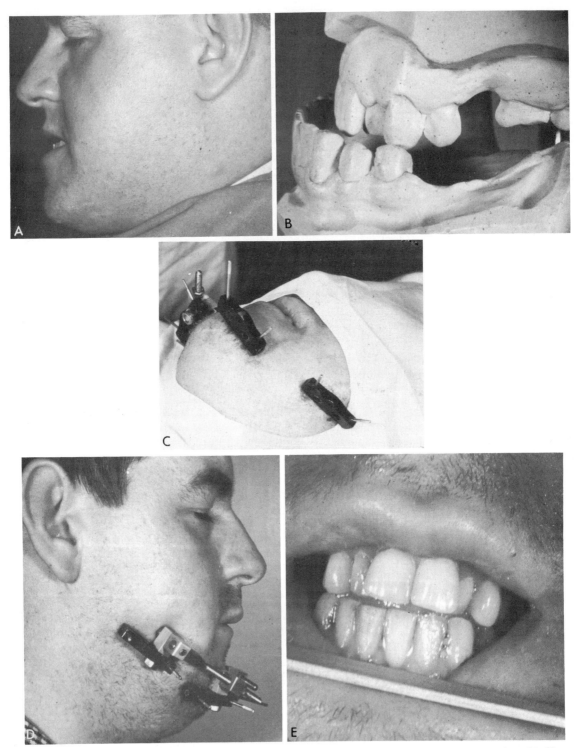

Figure 22–5   *A*, Patient with protrusion of lower jaw. (See Case Report No. 2.) *B*, Mandibular protrusion with Class III malocclusion. *C*, Pin bar in place. *D*, Postoperative view. *E*, Alignment of teeth after removal of intermaxillary elastics. *F*, Final profile. *G*, Teeth in occlusion before orthodontic adjustment.

(Figure 22–5 continued on opposite page)

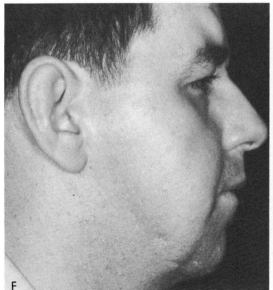

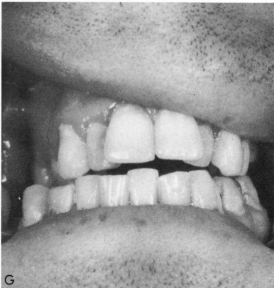

Figure 22–5   *(Continued.)*

A few days were allowed for subsidence of slight tissue reaction to the pins of the appliance, and then the patient was scheduled for the next operative procedure.

Operation No. 2.   Bilateral osteoectomy of the body of the mandible was performed with the same technique used in Case Report No. 3. (See Figure 22–5D and E.)

After the operation it was discovered that the patient had bruxism, and this grinding of his teeth while sleeping repeatedly broke apart even direct intermaxillary–mandibular wiring. Eventually the pins were also loosened and normal osseous healing was prevented.

The extraoral appliances were removed 10 weeks postoperatively. The cosmetic effect was excellent, and the normal occlusion was restored (Fig. 22–5F and G). Eventually the patient had osseous union.

Case Report No. 3

SURGICAL TREATMENT OF MANDIBULAR PROGNATHISM

W. H. Archer, D.D.S.

A woman aged 21 had a "protruding lower jaw" and poor dental function. However, her real complaint was about her facial appearance, which troubled her greatly. She was admitted to the Eye and Ear Hospital for bilateral osteoectomy to correct mandibular prognathism. She had a congenital protrusion with malocclusion (see Figure 25–6A to D). Eight weeks prior to admission, the lower right and left first molars were extracted. Fracture arch bars were contoured and wired to the necks of the maxillary and mandibular teeth.

Examination.   The results of a general physical examination were essentially negative. The mouth was in a good state of oral hygiene; the gingivae, oral mucosa and tongue appeared normal; the teeth were in a good state of repair. The throat was normal, and there were no masses or ten-

derness in the neck. There was marked prognathism of the mandible, including a Class III malocclusion.

Operation: Application of Stader Splints. Under general anesthesia,* the face and mucous membrane were prepared with green soap and tincture of Merthiolate, and the lips were coated with petrolatum. A Molt mouth prop was inserted in the mouth, and the jaws were separated. The tongue was grasped by gauze held between the fingers and brought forward, exposing the tip, which was scrubbed dorsally and ventrally with tincture of Merthiolate. A curved needle threaded with 00

---

*Today all operations are done under endotracheal and local anesthesia.

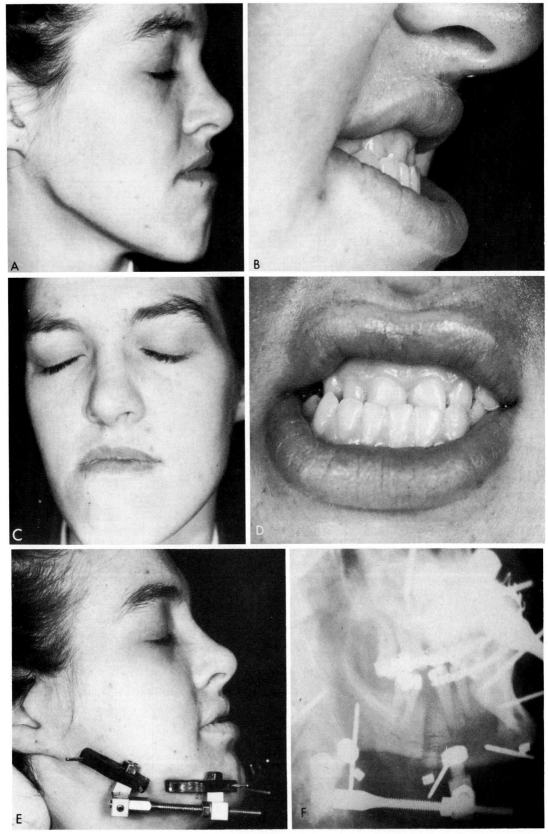

Figure 22-6   (Figure 22-6 continued on opposite page.)

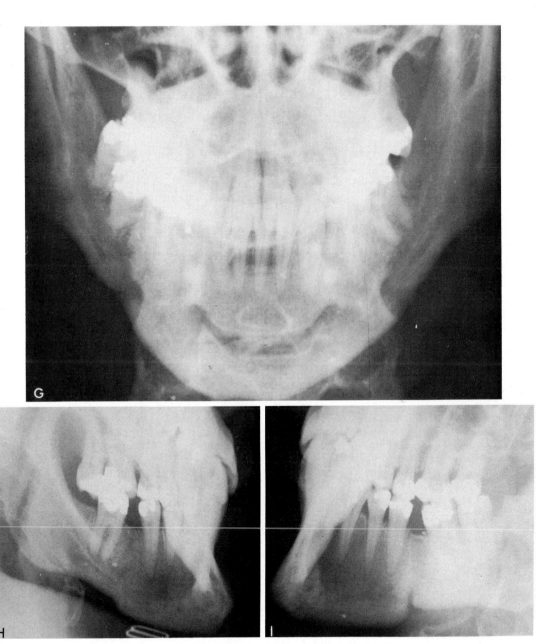

Figure 22–6 *A* to *D*, Mandibular prognathism with malocclusion. (See Case Report No. 3.)
  E, Reduction of prognathism. Mandibular segments held in correct alignment and firm apposition of the cut ends by the extraoral splint on each side of the mandible. (Right side shown here.) *F*, Lateral oblique radiograph of the mandible showing alignment and apposition of fragments. Note the approximation of the inferior alveolar canals in each segment. Completely normal sensation returned to the lip and anterior teeth in approximately 10 months.
  G to *I*, Radiographs taken 15 months after operation.

(Figure 22–6 continued on following page)

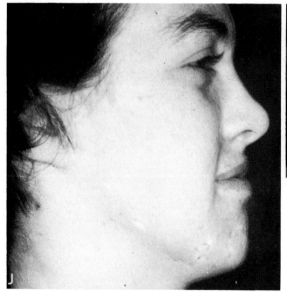

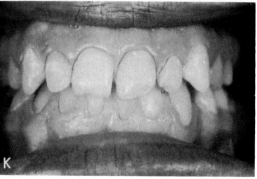

Figure 22–6 *(Continued.)* *J*, Postoperative relationship of maxillary and mandibular teeth. *K*, Patient 6 weeks after operation.

plain catgut 18 inches in length was passed through the midline of the tongue ½ inch from the tip, and brought forward for a distance of 6 inches. The needle was cut from the suture, a knot was tied in the ends of the four strands, and a hemostat was clamped on this knot and held to the cover sheet by a towel clip. The oropharyngeal partition was then placed.

The right and left inferior alveolar nerves were blocked and mandibular soft tissues were injected with local anesthetic solution. The inferior border of the mandible was outlined with gentian violet, as were the two lines outlining the section to be removed. The facial artery and vein were located by palpation as they ascended over the lower border of the mandible.

Points of entrance of the pins were determined and marked posterior to the distal cuts to be made. A pin was placed in the pin bar, the tip coated with petrolatum, and the electric drill attached. The skin was penetrated, and the pin was driven through the outer cortical plate through the medullary bone until the lingual plate was penetrated. The pin bar was then made parallel to the inferior border of the mandible, and the second pin was then drilled through the mandible in the same manner as was the first. A second set of pins and bar was applied anterior to the segment outlined. The set screws on the side of the pin bar were tightened. A hinge bar was then placed and locked in each pin bar, so that they were on the same side of the pin bars. The adjustable connecting bar was then placed between the hinge bars and adjusted so that there was no tension on the pins. All nuts and lock screws were then tightened. The same procedure was followed in placing the splint on the opposite side of the mandible. (See the drawings in Figure 22–2 illustrating the foregoing technique.)

The patient left the operating room in good condition.

Postoperative Course. Because the patient exhibited a postoperative toxic labyrinthitis, the second surgical procedure was delayed for 2 weeks.

Second Operation: Bilateral Osteoectomy of the Horizontal Ramus (Body) of the Mandible. Under general anesthesia the face and mucous membrane were prepared and a tongue suture was inserted as previously described. The patient was intubated with a nasotracheal catheter, and anesthesia was maintained.

The right and left inferior alveolar nerves and mandibular soft tissues were anesthetized. The inferior border of the mandible was outlined, as was the section to be removed.

An incision was made with a Bard-Parker blade in the molar area on the right side of the mandible on the crest of the ridge (Figure 22–3*A*, *B* and *C*). This incision was extended to the buccal and distal extremities of the original incision. The tissue was reflected with a periosteal elevator both buccally and lingually. A 13-inch directing needle was passed parallel to the lingual cortical plate through the floor of the mouth extraorally. This was used to determine the location of the extraoral incisions. The extraoral incision was then carried out parallel to the lower border of the mandible for a distance of 2 cm. distal to the point of exit of the directing needle. A trocar and cannula were then passed through this incision, emerging intraorally between the flap and the lingual cortical plate (Fig. 22–3*D* and *E*). The trocar was removed, leaving the cannula in place. The Gigli saw was then passed up through the cannula, and handles attached. A cheek retractor was then inserted to protect the lip and adjacent tissues from the Gigli wire saw. This saw was then drawn back and forth until it passed through the mandible (Fig. 22–3*G*, *H* and *I*). The saw was passed back through the cut to the lingual, and moved forward for the mesial cut. The Stader connecting bar was tightened. This immediately controlled hemorrhage from the inferior alveolar artery.

The same technique was followed in making the mesial cut, which resulted in a segment of 0.9 cm. After this cut was completed the segment was held in position by again tightening the Stader connecting bar. (This is to hold the cut segment firmly in place, thereby preventing hemorrhage while the vessels are retracting and the clot forming. In addition, the right mandible is held firmly as a solid unit during the cutting on the opposite side. Following the second cut on the left side, the connecting bar is tightened so as to hold the segment for 5 minutes to control hemorrhage from the left inferior alveolar artery and vein.)

The same technique was followed on the left side of the mandible, and the segment was cut 0.6 cm. The two segments were then removed (Fig. 22–6*E* and *F*), and the adjustable connecting bar was tightened so that the two cut ends came together. Final adjustments on the connecting bar were made to assure proper alignment of the mandible on each side, and proper occlusion. The reflected tissues were then coapted, and sutured with 000 silk. The extraoral incisions were sutured with interrupted 5–0 sutures.

The patient was removed from the operating room in good condition.

To prevent the possibility of aspiration of vomitus postoperatively, application of the intermaxillary elastics was delayed until the patient had completely recovered from the anesthetic. These were applied between the arch bars wired to the maxillary and mandibular arches.

Postoperative Course. The patient had a normal postoperative course. Immediately after the operation the patient was given 1000 cc. of glucose in normal saline solution with 3 cc. of vitamin B complex and 300 mg. of cevitamic acid intravenously. Ice packs were applied to the jaws. Penicillin, 400,000 units every eight hours, was ordered. (*Note:* Today we do not routinely order postoperative antibiotics.) The patient was given a Hyclorite mouthwash four times a day. An infrared lamp was used for a half hour four times a day. The patient was given a high-calorie liquid diet.

During the first few days postoperatively the patient exhibited moderate edema, and ecchymosis of the buccal and submaxillary fascial spaces. Slight drainage continued intermittently from the extraoral incisions.

On the third postoperative day hot, wet dressings were applied every 3 hours, and the patient had a hot saline mouthwash every 2 hours. Betalin complex, 1 cc. intramuscularly, was prescribed daily. This was increased to 2 cc. on the fifth postoperative day, at which time the penicillin was discontinued.

The edema continued to subside, and the patient was discharged on the seventh postoperative day, to be followed up at the office.

The sutures had been removed on the third postoperative day. Radiographs taken at this time revealed good alignment of the fragments (Fig. 22–6*F*) and satisfactory bony alignment. The teeth were in good alignment. Intermaxillary fixation was discontinued after 3 weeks. The extraoral Stader splint was removed 6 weeks later. Total time of immobilization of jaw segments was 9 weeks. Note, however, that the patient could open and close his mouth for 6 of the 9 weeks. The radiographs taken 15 months after the operation are shown in Figure 22–6*H* and *I*. Final appearance and occlusion are shown in Figure 22–6*J* and *K*. Normal sensation in the lip and lower teeth returned in 13 months.

Case Report No. 4

BILATERAL OSTEOECTOMY OF THE BODY OF THE MANDIBLE

W. H. ARCHER, D.D.S.

A woman, aged 23, had an unsightly appearance because of protrusion of the mandible.

History. The patient had been referred for treatment by a psychiatrist. She had been morose, depressed and an introvert. She was self-conscious because she felt that people stared at her "big jaw," and as a result she avoided going out with people as much as possible.

Medical Report. The examination results were essentially negative, except for a systolic murmur over the apex of the heart.

Oral Examination. The mouth was in a good state of oral hygiene. The gingivae, oral mucosa and tongue appeared normal. The teeth were in a good state of repair. There was marked prognathism of the lower jaw (Fig. 22–7*A* and *B*), including Class III malocclusion.

Jelenko splints had been contoured, and applied to the maxillary and mandibular arches. This was done before the patient was admitted. The first hospital operative procedure was the application of the Stader splints. This was to be carried out under general anesthesia.

Preoperative Orders. The patient was given

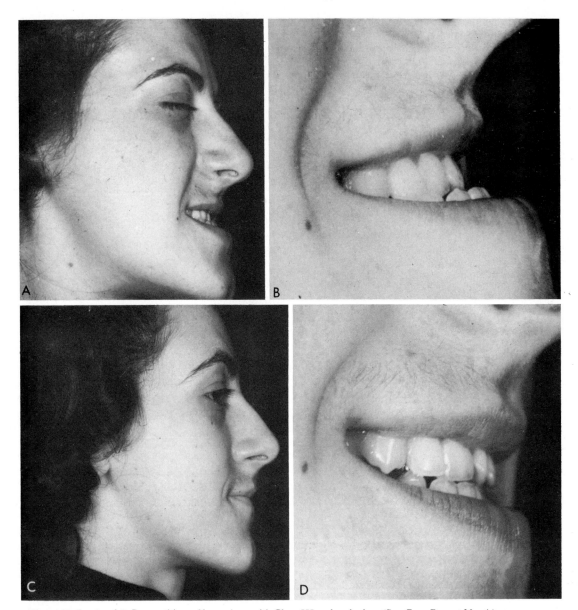

Figure 22–7   *A* and *B*, Prognathism of lower jaw, with Class III malocclusion. (See Case Report No. 4.)
C and *D*, Final result. Bilateral segments of bone were excised as necessary from the right and left bodies (horizontal rami) of the mandible, after both sides were first supported with extraoral skeletal fixation with Stader splints.

penicillin, 400,000 units (*Note:* today we do not order antibiotics routinely) and ascorbic acid, 100 mg three times a day, on the day before operation.

Operation: Application of Stader Splints. Under general anesthesia, the face and mucous membrane were prepared with tincture of Merthiolate, and the lips coated with petrolatum. A Molt mouth prop was inserted in the mouth, and the jaws were separated. A tongue suture was inserted, as previously described. An oropharyngeal partition was then placed.

The Stader splints were applied as described in Case Report No. 3.

Postoperative Course.   An ice pack was applied to the jaw for the first 24 hours. Ascorbic acid 100 mg. three times a day, and penicillin, 400,000 units every eight hours, were ordered (not now done routinely). An infrared lamp was used for 15 minutes four times a day. Fluids were forced to 3000 cc. daily.

The left side of the jaw appeared normal. The right side was swollen because of bleeding into the submaxillary region. The patient tolerated the appliance well.

The second stage of the procedure was postponed until the swelling had subsided.

Operation: Bilateral Osteoectomy of the Horizontal Ramus (Body) of the Mandible. The technique used in this case was the same as that described in the operative notes for Case Report No. 3.

Postoperative Course. Medication was the same as before, 1000 cc. of 5 per cent glucose solution was given intravenously, and 75 mg. of meperidine hydrochloride (Demerol) was prescribed every 3 hours as needed for the relief of pain.

Postoperatively, the patient exhibited moderate edema, and ecchymosis of the submaxillary spaces. After subsidence of the edema the patient had a normal postoperative course, and was discharged on the tenth postoperative day, to be followed up at the office. The sutures were removed on the tenth postoperative day. Radiographs revealed good apposition of the fragments and beginning union. The pins were overextended through the lingual cortical plate, but did not cause any discomfort. Intermaxillary fixation was discontinued after 4 weeks. The Stader appliance was removed after 10 weeks (Fig. 22-7C and D). The cosmetic effect was excellent. Normal occlusion was restored. The patient also exhibited a remarkable personality change and became much more extroverted.

TWO-STAGE OSTEOECTOMY TO PRESERVE THE NEUROVASCULAR BUNDLE

A two-stage method of osteoectomy can be used to maintain the continuity of the neurovascular bundle. The technique is described in detail in Case Report No. 5

First Stage. After the preliminary studies are completed and the sizes of the segments to be removed are determined (as described later), the teeth in the segments, if any, are extracted and intraoral cuts are made in exactly the same manner as shown in Figure 22-3A to C. These cuts must not be deeper than the depth of the alveolus, in order to avoid cutting into the inferior alveolar canal and injuring the neurovascular bundle. (See Figure 22-1C.)

Second Stage. When oral healing of the soft tissues is completed, the inferior border and buccal surface of the mandible is exposed by an extraoral incision made parallel to and about an inch below the site of the osteoectomy. If the external maxillary vessels are exposed and obstruct the operative field, they should be ligated and cut.

The original cuts in the bone are located, and with burs they are continued through the buccal cortical plate to the inferior border of the mandible. The surgeon should take care not to cut any deeper than the thickness of the cortical bone because the neurovascular bundle may be inadvertently severed with the bur. Midway along the buccal surface and along the inferior border the vertical cuts are connected by horizontal cuts. The superior and inferior buccal segments are removed, exposing the neurovascular bundle. A space is hollowed out in the exposed cancellous bone around the neurovascular bundle as it leaves the inferior alveolar canal in the proximal segment of the mandible and enters the same canal on the distal segment. This is to accommodate this bundle when the space is closed.

Two holes, one above the inferior alveolar canal and the other below it, are drilled through the body of the mandible on either side of the cut. These are for subsequent use in direct wiring of the mandibular segments. The bundle is retracted and the remaining portion of the lingual cortical plate is removed. One suture is inserted to close the soft tissue over this operative site temporarily while the same procedure is carried out on the opposite side.

The teeth are now brought into their new relationship and held there by intermaxillary elastics over splints previously wired to the maxillary and mandibular teeth. Next the mandible is wired together extraorally, and finally the soft tissues are closed.

Postoperative Anesthesia of the Mandibular Nerve. It has been the author's experience that even though every precaution has been taken *not to pinch* the neurovascular bundle between the bony ends when wiring the fragments together, these patients still have a transitory numbness lasting from several weeks to months and years. One of our patients has permanent unilateral anesthesia, the postoperative complication this technique is supposed to prevent.

Koblin and Reil[56] report that their survey of postoperative results in patients treated for prognathism by this technique revealed a 14 per cent rate of various degrees of anesthesia, lasting from 4 to 10 years. The only explanation is inadvertent trauma to the nerve during the exposure of the neurovascular bundle or during the preparation of the recesses in the cut ends around the inferior alveolar canal in which the neurovascular bundle is placed when the anterior segment of the mandible is moved posteriorly and is fixed to the body of the mandible. Also, if these recesses are too small to accommodate the inferior alveolar neurovascular bundle, unilaterally or bilaterally, it will be compressed by the apposition of the segments of the mandible and temporary or permanent anesthesia results. When one considers the fact that the great majority of prognathic patients who have had vertical bone sections containing a part of the neurovascular bundle (including inferior alveolar nerve, artery and vein) removed from their mandibles experienced complete return of normal sensation to their anterior teeth and lower lips within a year, the question arises, Why select this more difficult procedure? The answer is that the great majority of these cases do have normal sensation, either immediately or shortly after surgery.

Case Report No. 5

TWO-STAGE OSTEOECTOMY FOR A PROGNATHIC MANDIBLE
W. H. ARCHER, D.D.S.

History. The patient, a 23-year-old white female, was admitted to the Eye and Ear Hospital with a diagnosis of "prognathism—malocclusion." The patient's major complaint was a cosmetic one stemming from a prognathic mandible. The malocclusion and related problems were secondary (see Figure 22–8*A*, *B*, *C* and *D*).

Clinical Examination. *Extraoral:* The patient had a prognathic mandible. The head and neck were normal, with no other external evidence of pathology or lymphadenopathy.

Intraoral: The intraoral examination revealed two healing mandibular first molar tooth sockets. Otherwise, the oral tissues were healthy and normal in appearance.

Physical Examination and Laboratory Findings. All findings were in the normal range.

Operative Procedure. *First Stage:* One month prior to admission, the patient's mandibular first molar teeth had been extracted under local anesthesia. Using small spear-point drills a series of vertical holes were drilled in the buccal and lingual cortical plate to the depth of the sockets. These holes were then connected with a crosscut fissure bur. The distance between the two rows of bur holes was previously determined from plaster models, which were first occluded in the present occlusion (see Figure 22–8*E* and *F*); both models were marked with a straight line, and then the lower model was moved posteriorly until the mandibular anterior teeth were just lingual to the maxillary anterior teeth. The distance now between the pencil markings (see Figure 22–8*E* and *F*) represents the amount of bone which will have to be resected to correct the prognathic condition.

Second Stage: The day following admission, intraoral Stout wiring was placed on both the maxilla and mandible to provide for intermaxillary stabilization of the dental arches during and after the operation for the reduction of the prognathic mandible.

Third Stage: The following day, under endotracheal anesthesia, the following procedure was carried out: With the chin straight forward, the skin of the patient's face was prepared with aqueous Zephiran and draped in the usual manner with the head turned to the right side to expose the entire mandible. A 2½-inch linear incision was made through the skin and the subcutaneous tissues on the left side in the first molar area 1 inch below the inferior border of the mandible. Bleeders were tied off. The external maxillary artery and vein were retracted with the soft tissues. The platysma muscle was sharply and bluntly divided and the lower border of the mandible was exposed. The marginal mandibular branch of the facial nerve was avoided. The periosteum along the inferior border of the mandible was divided and reflected from the lateral and medial border of the body, exposing the previous intraoral cuts. Bur cuts were extended from these cuts to the inferior border of the mandible (see Figure 22–8*G*) avoiding the mandibular artery, vein and nerve. This 7-mm. section of bone between the cuts was divided into two parts, one superior and one inferior, and removed. Then drill holes were placed through the segments on each side of the cuts to facilitate the wiring (see Figure 22–8*H*; note the neurovascular bundle). The wound was packed with moist sponges covered with a sterile towel.

The head was turned to the left, and the same procedure was performed on the right side. The anterior portion of the mandible was mobilized, the mouth was entered by an assistant and the anterior portion was moved posteriorly into normal occlusion. At the same time the neurovascular bundle, with its mandibular artery, vein and nerve on both sides, was placed in previously made

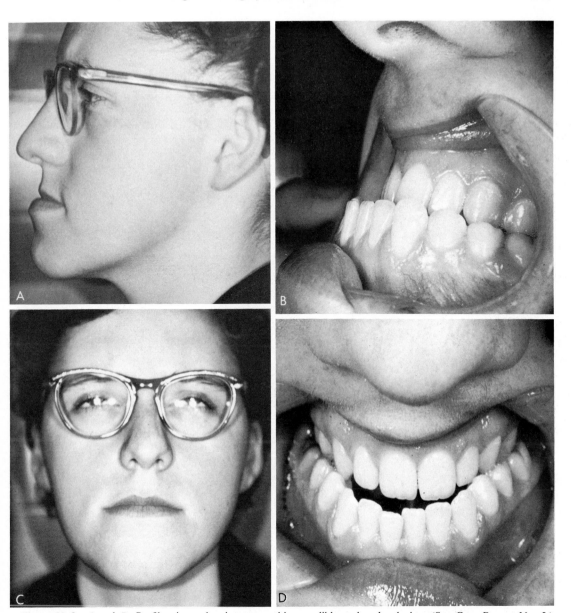

Figure 22–8 *A* and *B*, Profile views showing prognathic mandible and malocclusion. (See Case Report No. 5.) *C,* Full face view showing prognathic mandible. *D,* Prognathic mandible and malocclusion.

(Figure 22–8 continued on following page)

recesses in both fragments in an attempt to avoid pinching. Intermaxillary elastics were then applied to the intermaxillary multiloop wiring previously placed (see Figure 22–8*J* and *K*). Upon re-entering the extraoral field of operation the proximal and distal segments were found to be in apposition. Stainless steel wire, .018 gauge, was then threaded through the drill holes in each segment, twisted, cut and turned on itself, thus fixing the segments in apposition (see Figure 22–8*I*). The

same procedure was done on the other side. The tissues were closed in layers. Petrolatum gauze dressings were placed over the incisions.

Roentgenologic Report. Both horizontal rami of the mandible have been sectioned. The fragments on both sides are maintained in position by wires at the fracture sites. Arch splints are attached to both maxillary and mandibular teeth. (*Note:* Intermaxillary elastics maintained the occlusal relationship.) The fragments of the left horizontal ramus

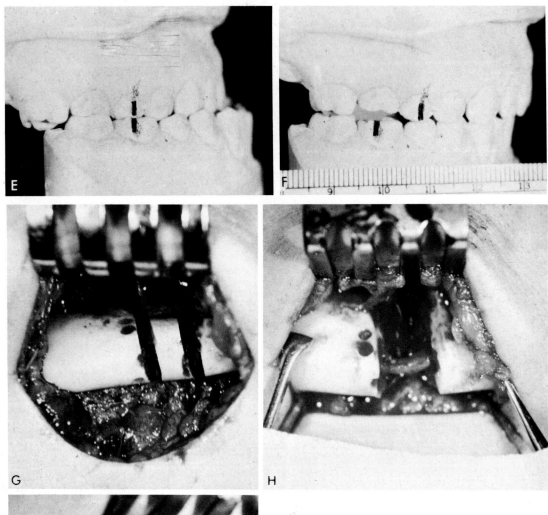

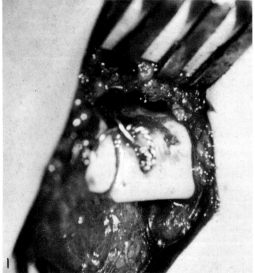

Figure 22–8 *(Continued.)* *E,* Plaster models showing existing occlusion. *F,* Distance between pencil markings represents amount of bone to be resected to correct prognathic condition. *G,* Bur cuts were extended to the inferior border of the mandible, avoiding the mandibular artery and nerve.

H, Area shows where the 7 mm. of bone was removed; note neurovascular bundle.

I, Stainless steel wire (0.018 gauge) was threaded through the drill holes in each segment, twisted, cut and turned on itself, thus fixing the segments in apposition.

(Figure 22–8 continued on opposite page)

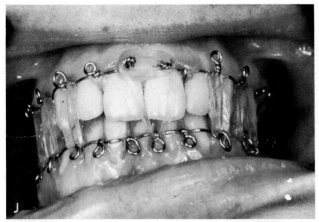

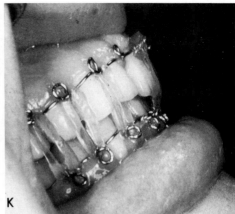

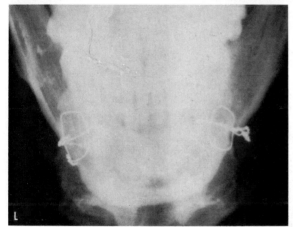

Figure 22–8 *(Continued.)* *J* and *K*, Intermaxillary elastics were applied to the intermaxillary multiloop wiring previously placed; note new relationship. *L* to *N*, One year after operation, radiographs show healed mandible.

(Figure 22–8 continued on following page)

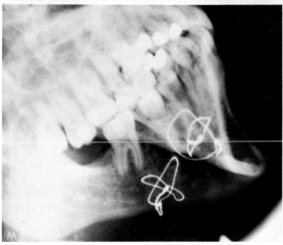

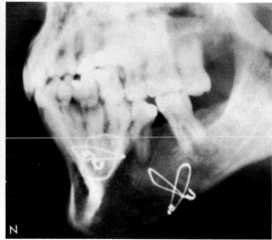

are in direct alignment. The anterior fragment on the right side is a few millimeters inferior to the posterior fragment, but the alignment appears satisfactory for union to take place.

Follow-up. The patient's hospital recovery was uneventful and she was discharged for office follow-up on the sixth postoperative day. The intermaxillary elastics were maintained for 8 weeks before removal. Radiographs and photographs

taken one year later (Figure 22–8*L, M, N, O, P, Q* and *R*) show the healed mandible and the improved profile. It is of interest to note that in spite of the extreme care taken to not traumatize either inferior alveolar neurovascular bundle or to pinch them when approximating the bone segments, this patient had numbness of the lower left lip for the following 2 years.

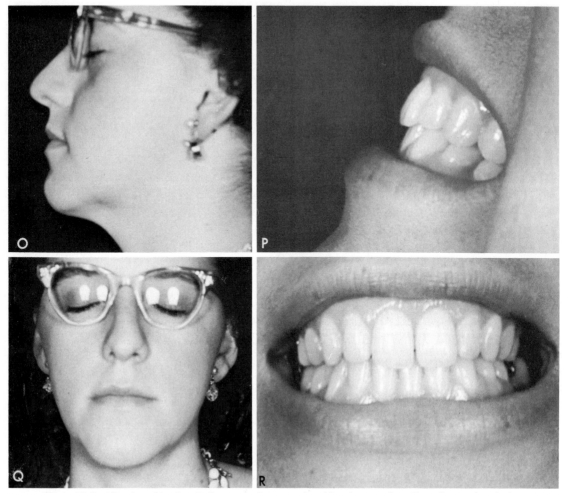

Figure 22–8 *(Continued.)*   *O* to *R,* One year after operation. Note improved profile and normal occlusion.

CLOSED SUBCONDYLAR OSTEOTOMY

CONRAD J. SPILKA, D.D.S.

Our aim in correcting the prognathic mandible, in addition to that of achieving a good functional and esthetic result, has been to reposition the lower jaw without relapse or nerve injury. There are many methods of mandibular ramus surgery, and it would appear that surgical intervention in the region offers many advantages—regardless of the procedure used. We have preferred the closed subcondylar osteotomy in selected instances, because of the simplicity of the operation and the satisfactory results.

This technique permits all the teeth to be placed into occlusion. The patient is given a good, functional jaw as well as an improved appearance. This has been successfully accomplished by cutting through the neck of the mandible at a point above where the inferior alveolar vessels enter the mandibular canal. Not only have the results been uniformly good, but the simplicity, short operative time (30 to 45 minutes) and absence of facial scars are more than enough to recommend this technique highly.

The preoperative planning should include radiographic studies and cephalometric measurements, as well as models of the dental arches, mounted on an articulator with bite recordings. By matching the upper with the lower cast we can determine what the occlusal relationship will be after the mandible has been repositioned. We can also decide whether or not orthodontic treatment is indicated before or after surgery. After all preliminary arrangements, such as the grinding of teeth, the wiring of splints to the teeth or the cementing of orthodontic bands, have been completed, the patient is scheduled for surgery.

Technique. The operation is performed bilaterally on the mandibular rami using an oblique osteotomy.[102] The line of the incision in the bone extends from the sigmoid notch to a point above the angle on the posterior border of the ramus. The skin incision, approximately 1 cm. long, is made through the skin and subcutaneous tissue. A mosquito hemostat is used to separate the tissues until the posterior border of the ramus is identified. A large aneurysm needle is inserted through the incision; it contacts the bone and remains in close proximity with the medial surface. It is advanced toward and through the sigmoid notch, where it is brought on to the face through a second incision, also 1 cm. long (Fig. 22–9A and B).

A Gigli saw is attached to the aneurysm needle and withdrawn through the first incision. Handles are attached to each end of the saw and the bone is sectioned, after which the saw is withdrawn (Fig. 22–9C). The incision is closed with 5–0 nylon sutures. The opposite side of the mandible is operated on in a similar manner. The mandible is then placed in normal occlusion and held with intermaxillary fixation for 8 weeks on prefixed fracture bars or orthodontic appliances. The orthodontic appliances are retained so that the orthodontist can correct any abnormality in the occlusion.

Relapses and Complications. In those patients in whom the mandibular body is neither disproportionately long nor abnormally wide, the closed subcondylar osteotomy has been the procedure of choice. Patients whose posterior mandibular displacement was 6 mm. or less were considered the best candidates for the operation. Relapses were noticeable when posterior displacement exceeded 6 mm. The greater the displacement the greater the risk of relapse.

The recurrence of malocclusion can be attributed to a disturbance of the pterygomasseteric sling, which will not tolerate more than a 5 to 10 per cent distortion of its muscular arrangement. Any surgical procedure that alters these muscular attachments beyond this limit inevitably will result in a relapse unless the pterygomasseteric sling is repositioned.

Relapses, complications and disappointments may occur when any operative technique is used. This has been demonstrated by Nordenram and Waller[73] in their recent investigation of the surgical techniques most commonly used.

With the subcondylar approach, the greatest concern has been the possibility of severing the internal maxillary artery and the facial nerve, or cutting through the parotid gland, which results in a parotid fistula.

Complications that have been reported can be attributed to allowing the aneurysm needle to move medially away from the bone. Damage to the facial nerve or parotid gland results when it is not recognized that the bone sectioning has been completed and the osteotomy is continued with resultant nerve and soft-tissue damage.[52]

Results of Series. In our series of 140 operations none of these complications has developed, as the point of the aneurysm needle was kept close to the bone and the osteotomy was discontinued immediately after sectioning was completed.

To evaluate the 140 operations performed over a 25-year period in which the closed subcondylar osteotomy was used, we recalled all of our patients for a clinical and radiographic examination. Those who were not available because of location were asked to answer a questionnaire. Sixty-five patients responded to the questions, either in person or by mail. The results of this investigation are shown in Tables 22–1 and 22–2.

In one patient there was a minimal unilateral gustatory hyperhidrosis. Relapses were seen when the preoperative posterior displacement exceeded 6 mm.; these relapses varied from 1 mm. to 3.2 mm. In one patient, an open bite developed that we attributed to having placed elastics on teeth loosened from protracted orthodontic treatment.

Six transient complications occurred; each of these consisted of an involvement of some terminal branches of the seventh nerve. In all instances complete recovery of function occurred in less than 4 months. Apart from the complications already mentioned, the results generally have been good. Radiographs were

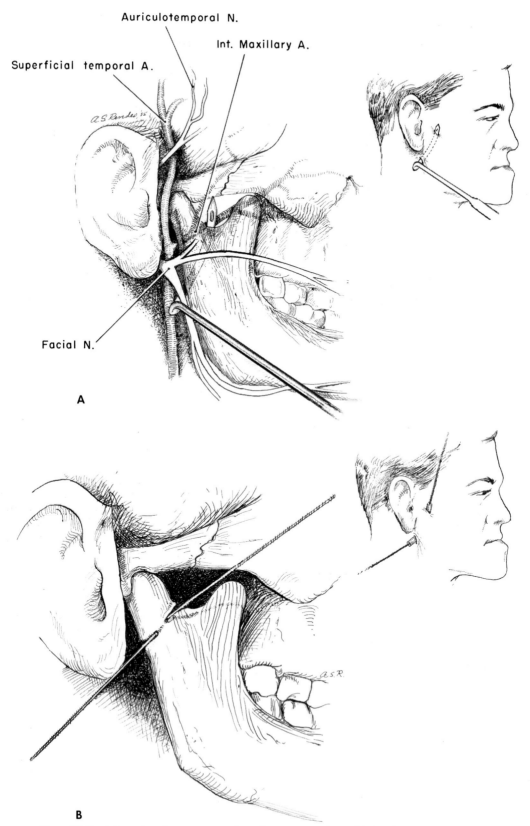

Figure 22–9   *A*, Insertion of aneurysm needle and structures to be avoided. *B*, Position of Gigli saw.

(Figure 22–9 continued on opposite page)

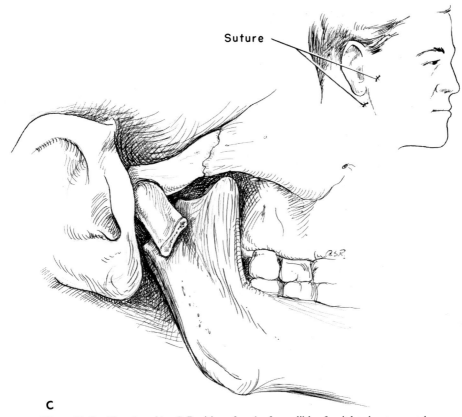

C

Figure 22-9 *(Continued.)*   C, Position of neck of mandible after it has been severed.

taken of the operative site whenever possible to determine the extent of ossification. In all of the patients for whom radiographic examinations were made, there was good bone apposition and normal bone healing. The radiographs included different views so that the bony sites could be seen from all aspects.

Summary. One hundred forty cases of mandibular prognathism have been surgically corrected with closed subcondylar osteotomy. The results have been generally good, with a minimum of complications. The results of a follow-up study with an observation time extending over a period of 25 years give convincing assurance of the merits of this procedure in selected cases.

Table 22-1   *Distribution of Cases*

YEARS	NUMBER OF PATIENTS OPERATED ON	SEX		AVERAGE AGE (YEARS)	POSTERIOR DISPLACEMENT OVER 6 mm.	RELAPSE (mm.)
		F	M			
1945–1950	10	6	4	24.2	0 cases	0
1951–1955	21	13	8	23.1	(2 cases)	
					8	1.5
					9	1.9
1956–1960	36	21	15	22.4	(3 cases)	
					12	2.7
					9	1.8
					11	2.4
1961–1965	39	26	13	23.3	(4 cases)	
					9	1.9
					12	3.0
					13	3.2
					7	1.1
1966–1970	34	20	14	21.5	(2 cases)	
					12	3.0
					7	1.1

Table 22–2 *Investigation*

QUESTION	YES	NO	QUESTION	YES	NO
1. Have you noticed since your operation that the skin above or in front of your ear sweats when you are eating?	1	64	5. Do you or did you have a paralysis of the face?	0	65
2. Have your teeth moved since the time of your operation?	11	54	6. Are you satisfied with the results of your operation?	65	0
3. Has your bite opened?	1	64	7. Is your lower lip numb or are your lower teeth numb?	0	65
4. Do you, or did you have any numbness of the face or forehead?	6	59	8. Do you or did you have a salivary fistula (that is, saliva escaping through a small opening in the face)?	0	65

Case Report No. 6

BILATERAL SUBCONDYLAR OSTEOTOMY FOR MANDIBULAR PROGNATHISM

CONRAD J. SPILKA, D.D.S.

A 23-year-old man requested an operation for improvement of his facial appearance before re-enlisting in the Army. He complained of being unable to masticate his food properly. He could not eat hard or tough food. The jaws tired easily and attempts at mastication were very wearisome. He complained of frequent episodes of indigestion.

An oral examination revealed that the only occluding teeth were the upper second molars with the lower third molars.

The operation aided the patient in mastication as well as in making a complete social readjustment. The patient returned at the end of 1 year for follow-up examination. He displayed a good, functional jaw. (See Figure 22–10A to F). Roentgenograms taken at this time showed a good bony union at the neck of the mandible. (See Figure 22–10G and H.)

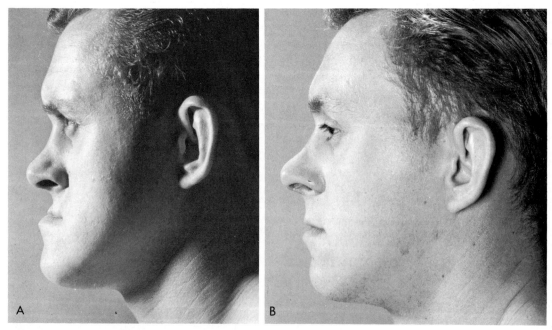

Figure 22–10 *A, C* and *E*, Preoperative photographs. *B, D* and *F*, Postoperative photographs showing improved cosmetic and occlusal result. (See Case Report No. 6 for further details.) Laminogram (*G*) and roentgenogram (*H*) taken 1 year postoperatively, showing good bony union.

(*Figure 22–10 continued on opposite page*)

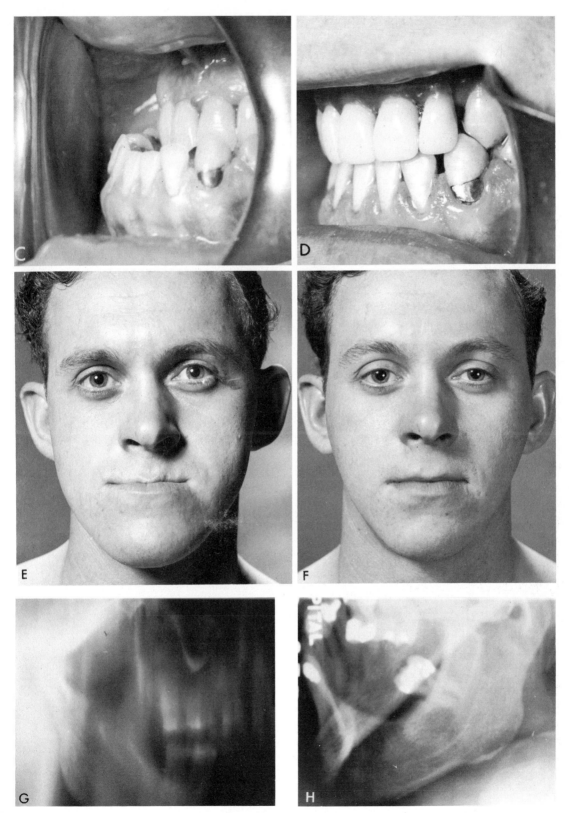

Figure 22–10 *(Continued.)*

Case Report No. 7

BILATERAL SUBCONDYLAR OSTEOTOMY FOR MANDIBULAR PROGNATHISM

Conrad J. Spilka, D.D.S.

A 27-year-old paraplegic complained of inarticulate speech and difficulty with mastication. Inspection showed a very prominent chin with overdevelopment of the symphysis menti. There were no occluding teeth. The maxillary anterior teeth were missing. Preoperative radiographs were taken to rule out any pathologic condition, as well as to demonstrate the prominence of the lower jaw. Immediately after the operation the patient displayed a new personality, and he was more than gratified with the results. Three months postoperatively an upper partial denture was constructed. This enabled the patient to chew better and to speak more distinctly.

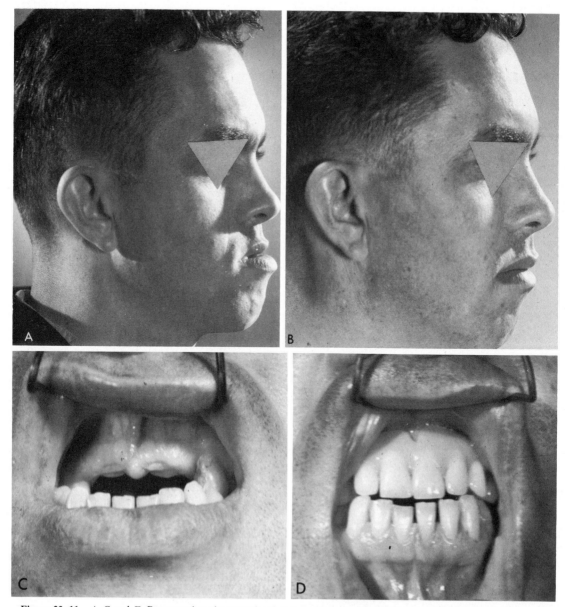

Figure 22–11 *A, C* and *E,* Preoperative photographs showing elongated prognathic face. *B, D* and *F,* Postoperative photographs showing well-proportioned face and normal jaw relationship. (See Case Report No. 7 for further details.)

(Figure 22–11 continued on opposite page)

The patient was contacted 8 years later for follow-up radiographs. Because of his paraplegic condition, he was advised to report to the nearest hospital. The radiographs were taken at the Co-shocton County Memorial Hospital in Coshocton, Ohio. These revealed a complete bony union with no evidence of fracture line (Fig. 22–11*G* and *H*).

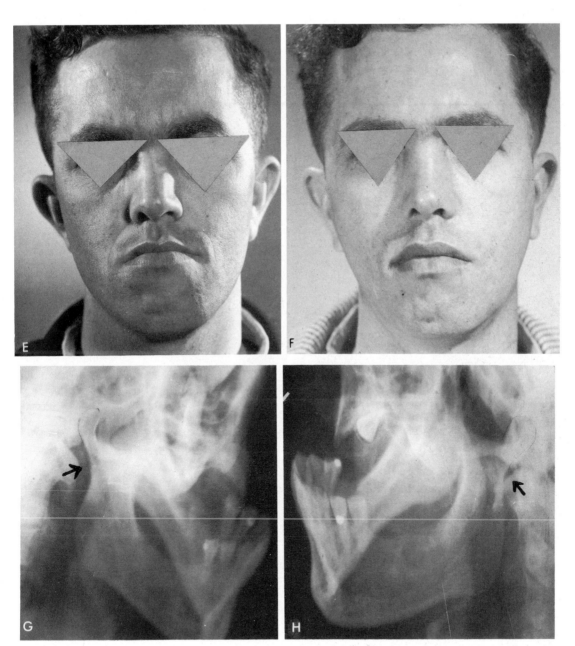

Figure 22–11   *(Continued.)*   *G* and *H*, Postoperative radiographs show complete bony union bilaterally.

BILATERAL SUBCONDYLAR OSTEOTOMY FOR MANDIBULAR PROGNATHISM

Conrad J. Spilka, D.D.S.

A 21-year-old factory worker wanted his facial appearance corrected before getting married. He had developed an inferiority complex and was embarrassed when appearing before groups of people.

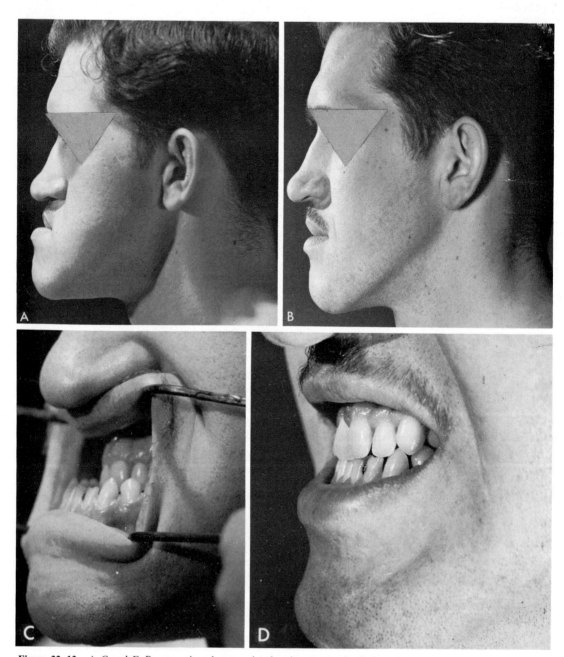

Figure 22–12 *A, C* and *E*, Preoperative photographs showing extremely elongated face; the mandible is usually long from angle to symphysis. *B, D* and *F*, Fourteen-month postoperative photographs showing well-proportioned face, normal profile, normal occlusion and absence of facial scars. (See Case Report No. 8 for further details.)

(*Figure 22–12 continued on opposite page*)

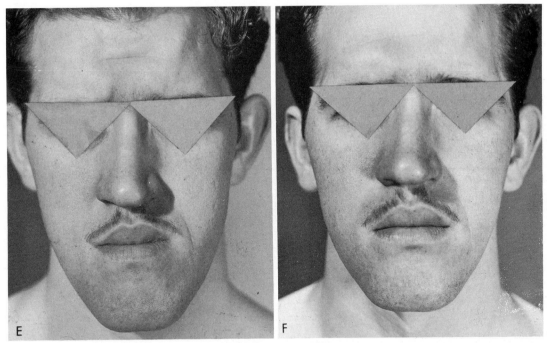

Figure 22–12   *(Continued.)*

Oral examination revealed two occluding molars. Because of the relationship of the remaining teeth, there was considerable difficulty in mastication. Postoperative results have completely changed this man's mental attitude. Now, also, he is the proud possessor of a good, functional jaw. The patient was seen 14 months later, at which time he proudly displayed a new personality and an excellent functioning jaw.

Case Report No. 9

BILATERAL SUBCONDYLAR OSTEOTOMY FOR MANDIBULAR PROGNATHISM

CONRAD J. SPILKA, D.D.S.

A 21-year-old undernourished student stated that he was not doing too well in school because of his loss of weight. He was constantly tired and attributed his undernourishment to his inability to masticate his food properly. He had developed an unpleasant attitude toward life. He was interested in getting his facial appearance changed, as well as acquiring an occlusion for proper mastication.

Examination revealed an overdevelopment of the lower jaw, with protrusion and malocclusion. There was no occlusion on the left side. On the right side, the only point of contact was the upper first molar with the lower third molar and two upper premolar pontics with the lower second molar.

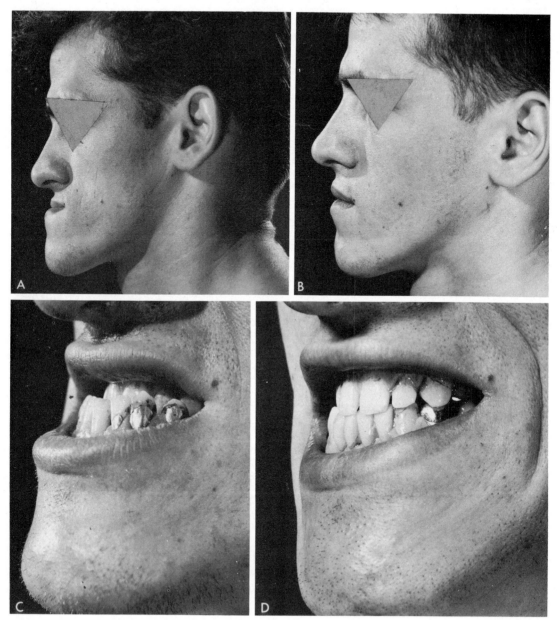

Figure 22-13 *A, C* and *E,* Preoperative photographs showing elongated face. *B, D* and *F,* Seven-week postoperative photographs showing facial symmetry and normal occlusion. (See Case Report No. 9 for further details.) *G* and *H,* Lateral views, 18 years postoperatively, showing complete bony union bilaterally.

(Figure 22–13 continued on opposite page)

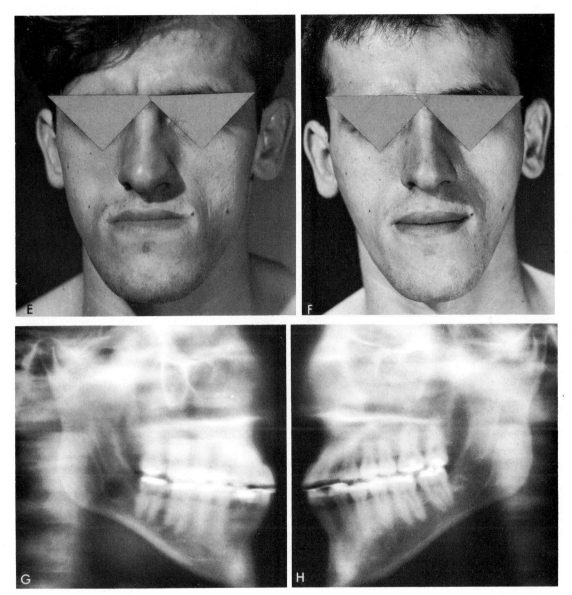

Figure 22–13 *(Continued.)*

OPEN OBLIQUE OSTEOTOMIES OF THE RAMI

Marsh Robinson, D.D.S., M.D.

In this article, some of the aspects of a new surgical procedure for the repositioning of the mandible will be presented. Since 1848, when Hullihen performed the first operation for surgical correction of mandibular prognathism,[47] many methods have been advocated. The very number of procedures shows that there are inherent difficulties in all of them. Since 1954 I have had experience with over 500 surgical corrections of mandibular prognathism and 50 surgical corrections of mandibular micrognathism. The open oblique osteotomy of the rami is presented as one method of correcting both of these deformities. Most severe deformities require the utmost in co-operation between the surgeon and the orthodontist, prosthodontist or general practitioner if the desired result is to be achieved. The surgical correction by means of the oblique osteotomy in the rami should be reserved for those cases in which there is no discrepancy in the size of the arches. It is often found, however, that even though there is no discrepancy in the sizes of the arches, the teeth either need some regulation in the postsurgical position or, more commonly, selective spot grinding must be done.

METHOD FOR CORRECTING MANDIBULAR PROGNATHISM

Accurate dental models are mounted in an arbitrary postsurgical position. They are then remounted with an overcorrection of 1.5 mm. of the prognathism and incorporating a 1-mm. opening in the second molar area. An acrylic occlusal splint covering all occlusal and incisal edges is then made. On the day before surgery, arch bars are placed on the maxillary and mandibular arches.

Surgery. An incision approximately 3 cm. in length is made about 1 cm. below the angle of the mandible in a skin line. The incision is carried down to the lower border of the ramus, with the surgeon taking care not to injure the mandibular branch of the facial nerve. The lateral surface of the ramus is then exposed by elevation of the periosteum. When the mandibular notch has been identified, a vertical osteotomy is made with a nasal saw from the anterior portion of the notch to an arbitrary point approximately 2 cm. above the angle of the mandible on the posterior border of the ramus, making as long a cut as possible and still avoiding the inferior alveolar neurovascular bundle (Figure 22–14). This cut with the saw is not carried completely through the ramus, but at the last moment an instrument can be wedged into the cut to effect final separation and thus protect the medial structures. The mandible is then moved posteriorly, with the condylar

fragment kept lateral. A similar procedure is carried out on the opposite side. These wounds are temporarily closed, the previously prepared intraoral overcorrected acrylic splint is placed between the dental arches, and intermaxillary wires are placed. The wounds are then re-entered and inspected for good bone apposition. After the surgeon has ascertained that the condylar fragments are overlapping in a lateral position and there is no soft tissue between the bones (Figure 22–14), the wounds are closed. The intermaxillary wires are removed 7 weeks later.

Comment. Many of the past difficulties associated with the surgical correction of the prognathic mandible can be avoided. With the technique of horizontal osteotomy of the rami there is the possibility of an increased anterior vertical dimension. The possibility of hemorrhage and the tragic sequela of medial displacement of the proximal fragment can be avoided by using the open approach to the vertical subcondylotomy. The postoperative jaw position in future orthodontic or prosthodontic patients should be determined by the orthodontist or prosthodontist. He can mount the casts arbitrarily in a postoperative position, regardless of the intercuspation of teeth, taking into consideration only the arch relationship in which he wishes to start his treatment. In some cases it may be advisable to complete a portion of the orthodontic treatment before the operation. In other cases the orthodontist may wish to overcorrect the mandibular prognathism in a Class II relationship of the dentition as a future starting point. In all cases of open bite as illustrated in Case Report No. 10, interosseous wires should be used. If it is a problem of pure prognathism, interosseous wires are not necessary. The reason for using an occlusal splint has been

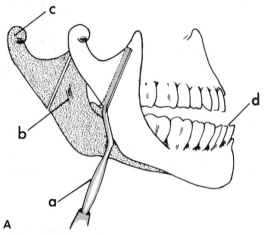

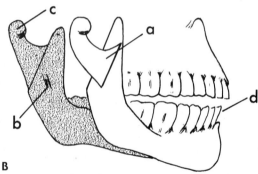

A   B

Figure 22–14 *A,* A prognathic mandible. *a,* The saw in position for osteotomy of the ramus; *b,* mandibular foramen; *c,* condyle; *d,* malocclusion of the lower teeth.

B, The same mandible after surgery. *a,* The condylar fragment is lateral to the ramus; *b,* mandibular foramen; *c,* condyle; *d,* the malocclusion is corrected.

presented previously. One female patient underwent correction twice, at the ages of 18 and 21, because of failure of intervening orthodontic treatment and possible additional growth to the jaw. The second procedure did not differ materially from the first, except that the bone in the osteotomy site was slightly thicker. This girl's second operation was performed on February 6, 1958. Since that time we have not refused any young patient who required a surgical procedure. The youngest patient treated was 8 years of age. When these young patients are treated before growth and development of the mandible have stopped, there must be a definite understanding with the parents that a second operation at some later date may be necessary.

Case Report No. 10

OPEN OBLIQUE OSTEOTOMY OF THE MANDIBULAR RAMI FOR PROGNATHISM

MARSH ROBINSON, D.D.S., M.D.

An 18-year-old white schoolboy was first seen on June 8 because of masticatory dysfunction due to mandibular prognathism and open-bite deformities. On July 5 at Santa Monica Hospital, his man-

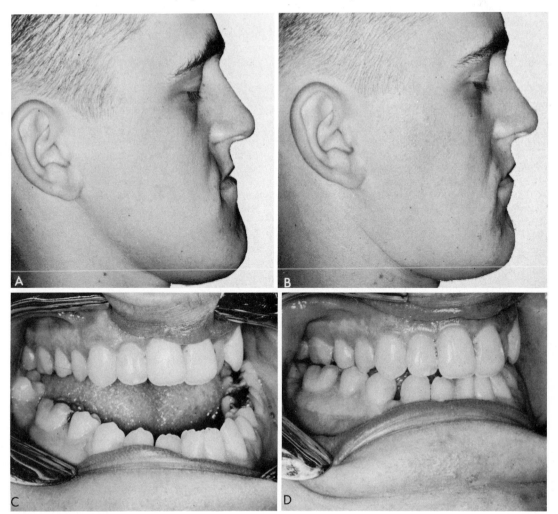

Figure 22–15 *A* and *C*, Preoperative views. Note 19-mm. deformity in occlusion. *B* and *D*, Profile and occlusion following surgery. (See Case Report No. 10 for further details.)

dibular prognathism and open bite were surgically corrected in the manner just described except that bilateral interosseous wires were placed (Figure 22–15). The patient left the hospital on the fourth postoperative day and returned to school in 2 weeks. The intermaxillary wires were removed 7 weeks after the operation. A slight amount of selective spot-grinding was done after the inter-maxillary wires and arch bars were removed.

Case Report No. 11

PROGNATHISM CORRECTED BY OPEN OBLIQUE SLIDING OSTEOTOMY OF THE MANDIBULAR RAMI*

Marsh Robinson, D.D.S., M.D.

Note.: A 14½-year follow-up is presented of the first reported case in which prognathism was corrected by open oblique osteotomy of the rami.

A 30-year-old white woman was first seen on July 24, 1954, for correction of mandibular prognathism (Fig. 22–16*A*). She complained of difficulty in mastication; biting through food was especially troublesome. There was no family history of prognathism, and the patient's medical history disclosed no trauma or surgical procedures.

Physical examination revealed that the patient could open the mouth adequately in the midline. There was a 7-mm. mandibular prognathism (Fig. 22–16*B*). There was no tenderness or crepitus in the temporomandibular joint regions.

Study models revealed no arch discrepancy, and an almost normal occlusion was produced when the mandible was moved back 7 mm. (Fig. 22–16*C* and *D*). An intraoral acrylic bite splint was made to produce the proper relationship.

On August 22, 1954, arch bars were placed. The patient was admitted to the hospital for completion of the procedure. On August 23 the patient was placed under general anesthesia and a 4.5 cm. incision was made in a skin line about 1 cm. below the right angle of the mandible. The marginal branch of the facial nerve was identified and retracted superiorly. The periosteum and all tissues were elevated from the lateral surface of the ramus. An instrument was placed on the medial surface as a guard.

Under direct vision, the osteotomy incision was made with a nasal saw from the deep portion of the notch to an arbitrary point on the posterior border about 1 cm. above the angle. This wound was closed temporarily. A similar procedure was performed on the left side. The intraoral acrylic splint was placed between the arches of the teeth, and five intermaxillary wires were placed between the arch bars. The wounds were closed.

The patient's recovery was uneventful. The fixation was removed after 7 weeks, and 1 mm. of correction was lost. Selective spot grinding produced a good occlusion. Postoperative radiographs were reported as showing bilateral oblique fractures of the rami with the condylar fragments in good position; however, the distal fragment was displaced posteriorly 1 cm.

Follow-up. The patient was last seen on February 1, 1969, 14½ years postoperatively (Fig. 22–16*E* and *F*). She had no complaints. She admitted that before the surgical procedure she had disliked her appearance, which had caused her to seek treatment.

She has never had any deficiency in function of the motor or sensory nerves of the face or mandible. After the surgical procedure she had experienced some swelling but no pain. She has had no

---

*Reproduced with permission from Robinson, M.: Prognathism corrected by open oblique sliding osteotomy of the mandibular rami. Forteen-year follow-up of a case. Oral Surg., *29*:323–327 (Mar.), 1970; copyright by The C. V. Mosby Co., St. Louis.

Figure 22–16 *A* and *B*, Preoperative profile and occlusion of patient.

C, Model showing oblique osteotomy in a prognathic mandible in an area not involved with large blood vessels, nerves, or teeth. *D*, Model showing postoperative position. Note overlapping of condylar and mandibular fragments which cannot be palpated through the large masseter muscle, the intraoral surgical occlusal splint in position which overcorrects the mandible in both the prognathic and open-bite positions, and the arch bars and intermaxillary wires used for immobilization.

E and *F*, Profile and occlusion of patient 14½ years after surgical correction (no change in occlusion had occurred in that time). (See Case Report No. 11 for further details.)

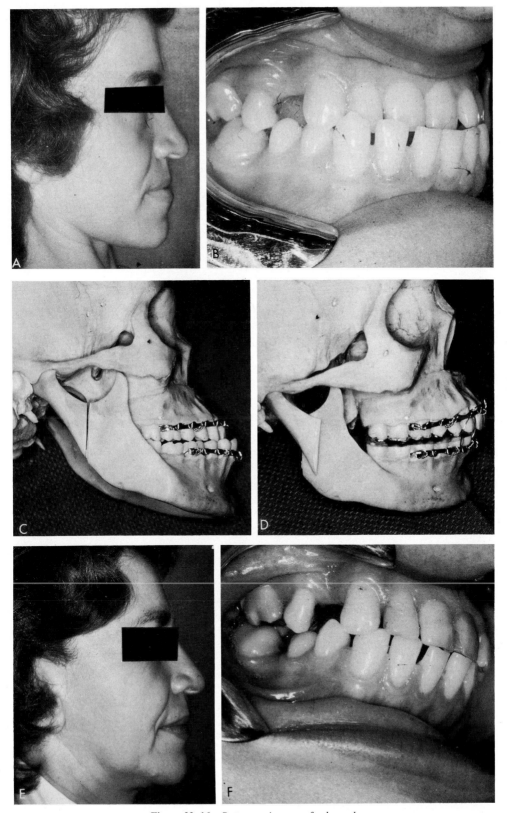

Figure 22–16 *See opposite page for legend.*

clicking or popping noise in her joints and no episodes of inadequate opening. She does not grind or clench her teeth.

Follow-up examination revealed an end-to-end bite with no change in occlusion since the operation 14½ years previously. The patient had a 37-mm. jaw opening in the midline, with no deviation. There was no tenderness or crepitus in the temporomandibular joint regions or in the muscles of mastication. There were no habit pattern facets on the teeth. There was no centric interference. The operative scars were inconspicuous and white and appeared as wrinkles.

Radiographic examination showed the overlapping osteotomies of the rami to be well healed, with evidence of the previous surgical procedure visible only to the trained observer.

COMMENT

In the years since it was introduced, the open procedure has had only a few minor changes. The skin incision is still made about 1 cm. below the angle of the jaw, but now it is extended about 3 cm. instead of 4.5 cm. The angle of the saw handle has been altered for better access to the surgical site. It has been found that no guard instrument need be used on the medial surface. The inferior alveolar neurovascular bundle can be protected by not completing the saw cut and fracturing the last bit of medial plate. The occlusal splint is overcorrected in the postoperative position to compensate for the slight loss of correction described. Patients still are hospitalized for 4 days, and the intermaxillary fixation is kept in place for 7 weeks.

METHOD FOR CORRECTING MANDIBULAR MICROGNATHISM

This is similar to the procedure for correction of mandibular prognathism. The exceptions are that the saw cut is made from the deepest portion of the notch to just anterior to the angle of the jaw (Figure 22–17). When the body of the mandible has been moved forward and intermaxillary wires have fixed it

in position, the long condylar fragment is rotated until it approximates the distal fragment. An interosseous wire is then placed to stabilize the lower end of this long condylar fragment (Figure 22–17). The postoperative care of the patient is the same as that which follows correction of mandibular prognathism, except that the intermaxillary fixation is allowed to remain for 12 weeks.

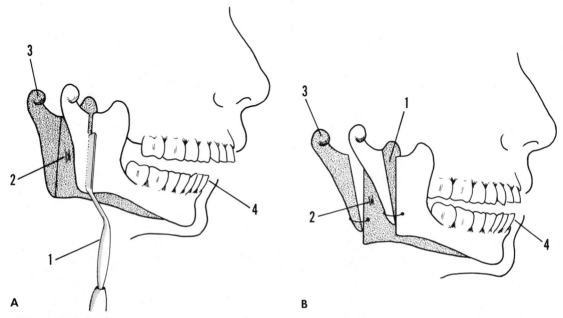

Figure 22–17 *A*, Drawing of retruded mandible. *1*, Saw in position for vertical osteotomy; *2*, mandibular foramen; *3*, condyle; *4*, malocclusion due to micrognathia.

B, Drawing of mandible after surgery. *1*, Defect which fills in with new bone; *2*, mandibular foramen; *3*, condyle; *4*, corrected occlusion.

Case Report No. 12

OPEN OBLIQUE OSTEOTOMY OF THE MANDIBULAR RAMI FOR MICROGNATHISM

Marsh Robinson, D.D.S., M.D.

An 18-year-old white schoolgirl was first seen at the Orthopedic Hospital in May because of masticatory dysfunction due to mandibular micrognathism (Fig. 22–18). The patient had sustained bilaterally fractured, displaced mandibular condyles in an automobile accident 5 years previously. She stated that since that time her jaw had been in a retruded position. On June 24, the girl's micrognathism was corrected in the manner just described (Figs. 22–18C and D and 22–19). She left the hospital at the end of one week and returned to school in 2½ weeks. The intermaxillary wires were removed 12 weeks after the operation.

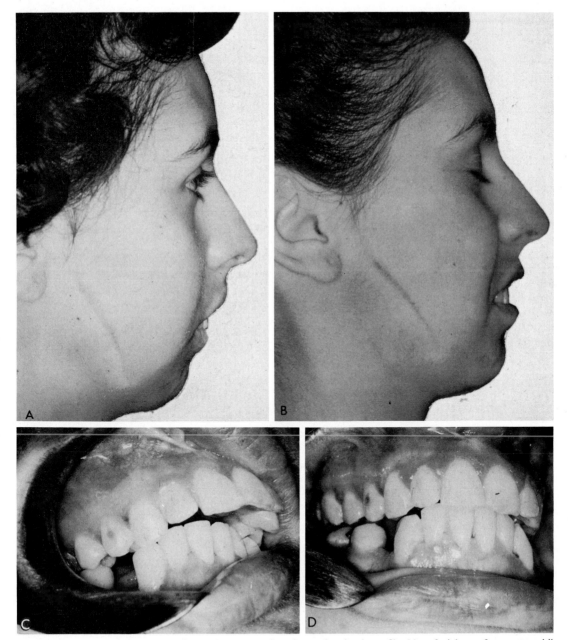

Figure 22–18 *A* and *B*, Preoperative and postoperative views of patient's profile. Note facial scar from automobile accident.

C and *D*, Preoperative and postoperative photographs of patient's occlusion. (See Case Report No. 12 for further details.)

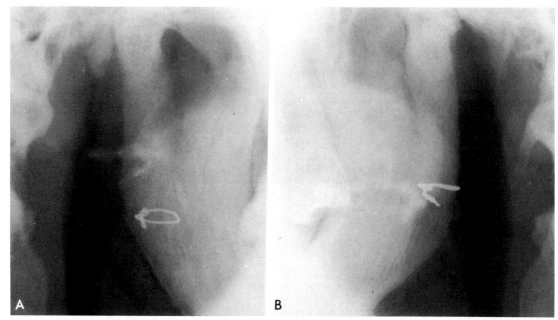

Figure 22–19   Roentgenograms taken 1½ years after surgery. Note healing of osteotomy site.

Comment. This method of lengthening the mandible is a modification of the procedure originally described in 1954 for prognathism. The only muscle pull to be overcome is that of the external pterygoid, and this can be done adequately with a small interosseous wire. In cases previously reported, iliac bone graft in the form of either a block graft or bone chips has been utilized to fill the void in the ramus area. It is thought that these pa-tients healed in spite of the bone grafts, not because of them. Recently, coronoidectomies have been done with mallet and chisel before the osteotomy is complete. It is believed that this improves the direction of the temporalis muscle postoperatively.

SUMMARY AND CONCLUSIONS

In many cases of mandibular deformity (prognathism, micrognathism, or open bite) it

Figure 22–20   *Mandibular micrognathia,* or retrusion, is correctible by elongation of the mandible following bilateral osteotomy. The elongation is maintained by either interposition of a bone graft or sliding step osteotomies of the ramus or body of the mandible. The ramus is the preferred site for the osteotomy since it spares the already deficient anterior mandible and teeth. However, the advancement is partly restricted by the muscles of mastication and the temporo-mandibular joint. Shown here is an *elongation osteotomy* of the ramus of the mandible that does not involve the coronoid or condyloid processes and permits interposition of an autogenous iliac bone graft.

Critical elements in this procedure are as follows:

1. Immobilization of the jaws in occlusion by intermaxillary fixation is essential to overcome the pull of the elevator muscles and to prevent nonunion and open bite, or apertognathia.
2. The osteotomy must be bilateral, even in unilateral micrognathia, in order to avoid malrotation of the condyle on the normal side.

Procedure: A, The orthodontic bands, arch bar and locks are in place on the maxillary and mandibular teeth. A reverse L osteotomy is outlined on the ramus of the mandible. A transverse incision beneath the angle of the mandible is indicated. *A₁,* The medial aspect of the mandible is viewed. The osteotomy is so designed as to avoid the neurovascular bundle entering the lingula. The coronoid and condyloid processes remain in their usual position and under the normal control of the temporalis (coronoid) and lateral pterygoid (condyloid) muscles. *B,* The selected correction of the micrognathia is illustrated with the teeth in occlusion and the jaws and facial profile in satisfactory relationship. A bone graft has been inserted between the distracted ramus fragments. Subplatysmal flaps are developed and forcefully retracted. The lateral edge of the masseter muscle is divided and reflected anteriorly. *C,* The osteotomy has been completed and the divided ramus is distracted. Holes are drilled in these fragments. The neurovascular bundle is illustrated at a safe distance from the nearest hole. *D* and *D₁,* A predetermined rectangular section of the iliac crest is obtained for division into two L-shaped segments. Each of these will be carved to fit the distracted spaces in the right and left rami following advance-ment of the body of the mandible into a more normal occlusion and facial contour. *E,* The appropriate iliac bone graft segment is fixed with 25 gauge stainless steel wire to restore the continuity of the elongated ramus following the bilateral distraction and advancement.

(From Rankow, R. M.: Surgery of the Face, Mouth, and Neck. Philadelphia, W. B. Saunders Co., 1968; modified from Schuchardt, K.: Erfahrungen bei der Behandlung der Mikrogenie. Dtsch. Gesellschaft Chir., *289*:651, 1958.)

OSTEOTOMY OF THE RAMUS WITH BONE GRAFT INLAY FOR CORRECTION OF MANDIBULAR MICROGNATHIA

Robin M. Rankow, D.D.S., M.D.

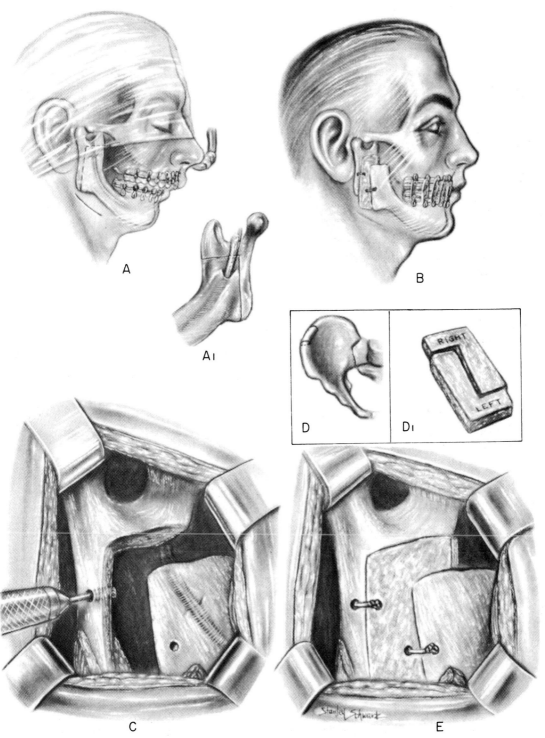

Figure 22–20 *See opposite page for legend.*

appears that a team of professionals must work together to achieve a satisfactory result. When there is either over- or underdevelopment of the mandible, it appears that the open oblique osteotomy of the rami, where indicated, is the procedure of choice, as it permits the entire basal bone of the mandible to be transferred to a new position. The great majority of results have been good, and no serious complications have developed.

TOTAL MAXILLARY OSTEOTOMY
WILLIAM H. BELL, D.D.S.

In 1927 Martin Wassmund introduced a surgical procedure for moving the entire maxilla.[106] The operation, which has since been called Le Fort I osteotomy or total maxillary osteotomy, was first used to correct an anterior open bite. The maxilla was not completely sectioned from its bony attachments, and no attempt was made to mobilize the maxilla at the time of surgery. Postoperatively, intermaxillary elastic traction was used to close the open bite and stabilize the maxilla. In view of the unsophisticated state of anesthesiology at the time, the lack of antibiotics and chemotherapeutics, and the empirical basis for maxillary surgery, this was truly a remarkable feat. Wassmund's direct approach to the maxillary deformity was clearly years ahead of its time. Total maxillary osteotomy has been used for almost 50 years with variable degrees of success.

The design of the bony and soft-tissue incisions has been continually modified to facilitate movement of the maxilla and to maintain circulation to the maxillary bone and teeth.[4, 29, 34, 45, 67, 77] Problems with mobilization and fixation have been dealt with in various fashions. Schuchardt[97] and Köle[57] devised a two-stage procedure to prevent impairment of the vascular supply to the maxilla. Postoperatively, Schuchardt used weights from an overhead traction device to reposition the maxilla forward. The second stage of his technique involved separation of the pterygoid processes from the maxillary tuberosities. Despite such measures, he became disenchanted with the procedure and concluded that the operation should not be used to treat cleft lip and palate patients. Axhausen used elastic traction after surgery to facilitate anterior movement and retention of a traumatically retrodisplaced maxilla.[5] In

an apparent attempt to circumvent these shortcomings, Gillies[38] and Converse and Shapiro[29] advocated advancing the maxilla by means of a transverse palatal cut at the junction of the palatine and maxillary bones. The success of this approach, however, was not commented upon. Bone grafting has been advocated to promote bone regeneration between the buccal bone cuts in the lateral maxillae.[31, 38] Obwegeser maintained that inserting a graft into the space between the posterior maxilla and the pterygoid plates was essential for stability.[78]

Inability to move the maxilla the desired amount and relapse of the patient's maxilla were common experiences for the innovators of this operation. The surgeon's fear that mobilization of the maxilla would devascularize and devitalize the bone and teeth was the dominant reason for such problems. Fear of traumatizing vascular structures, such as the greater palatine arteries, was also a major obstacle to success of the technique.

Gradually, as clinical experience increased, surgeons became more aggressive, and complete mobilization and adequate fixation of the maxilla were accomplished. At this stage, surgeons began to report encouraging results due to total maxillary advancement.[45, 80]

Still, the biologic basis and surgical principles for maxillary osteotomies remained obscure, and this lack of knowledge obviously contributed to postoperative devitalization

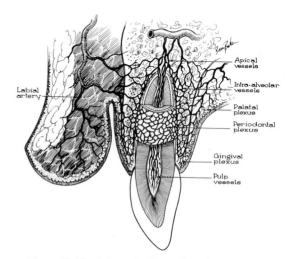

Figure 22–21 Schematic illustration of vascular architecture of anterior maxillary region. Freely anastomosing gingival plexus, palatal plexus, periodontal plexus, labial artery, intra-alveolar vessels, apical vessels and pulp vessels permit maxillary osteotomies without compromising circulation to the bone or teeth.

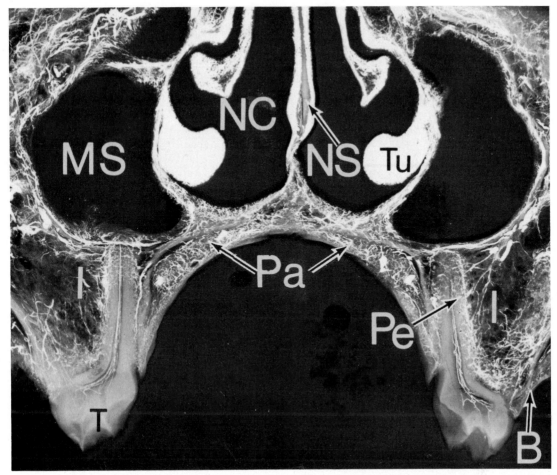

Figure 22–22 Microangiogram of 1-mm. transverse tissue slice from molar region of unoperated control animal: buccal (*B*), palatal (*Pa*), maxillary sinus (*MS*), and nasal cavity (*NC*) blood vessels penetrating bone and anastomosing with intramedullary blood vessels (*I*); periodontal vascular plexus (*Pe*); molar tooth (*T*); turbinate (*Tu*); nasal septum (*NS*).

and loss of bone and teeth. Microangiographic and histologic studies of total maxillary osteotomy performed on adult rhesus monkeys showed only transient vascular ischemia, minimal osteonecrosis and early osseous union when the maxilla was pedicled essentially only to the palatal mucosa (Figs. 22–21 to 22–24). Preservation of the integrity of the greater palatine arteries was not essential for maintaining circulation to the maxilla. The collateral circulation within the maxilla, its enveloping soft tissue and the numerous vascular anastomoses in the anterior and posterior parts of the maxilla permit many technical variations of the total maxillary osteotomy technique. Intraosseous and intrapulpal circulation was not significantly altered by buccal subapical osteotomies when bone cuts were made away from the apexes of the teeth and when maximal attachment of the

mucoperiosteum on the palatal and buccolabial gingiva of the mobilized maxilla was preserved.[13, 14, 16] These results generated courage and clinical confidence in performing total maxillary osteotomies. The present surgical technique was modified from these analogous animal investigations and previously reported clinical techniques.[35, 78, 106]

ANESTHESIA

Total maxillary osteotomy is performed in the hospital with the patient undergoing general anesthesia delivered via the nasoendotracheal route. Successfully administered hypotensive anesthesia has reduced bleeding significantly and has greatly facilitated surgical dissection.[96] Transfusions are rarely necessary, although 2 units of packed cells are

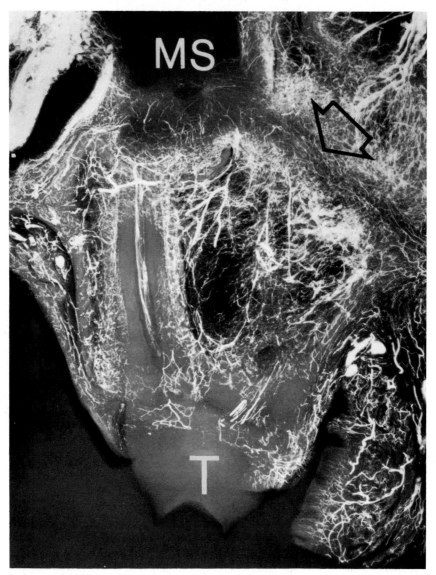

Figure 22–23   Microangiogram of molar region 4 weeks after total maxillary osteotomy shows reconstitution of circulation between osteotomized segments by proliferating vessels; maxillary sinus (*MS*); osteotomy site (*arrow*); vascularized pulp canal of molar tooth (*T*).

routinely available for use at the time of surgery if the need should arise. Reduced operative shock and decreased postoperative nausea, vomiting and edema are additional advantages. Because submucosal oozing is decreased, postoperative wound healing may also be enhanced. Despite these significant advantages, the use of hypotensive anesthesia is justified only when it enables the surgeon to carry out the operation better than he could with conventional anesthetic techniques.

With the patient in a 10- to 25-degree head-up tilt, a brachial arterial blood pressure of 60 to 70 mm. Hg is maintained with the ganglionic blocking agents pentolinium tartrate (Ansolysen) or trimethaphan camphorsulfonate (Arfonad), and halothane. A completely dry surgical field indicates excessive hypotension.

Respiratory inadequacy, bronchospasm and asthma, diabetes, cerebral and coronary vascular disease, previous steroid therapy, renal or hepatic dysfunction and Addison's disease contraindicate the use of hypotensive anesthesia. The advantages to the patient and surgeon must be weighed against the increased risks. *The technical skill and experi-*

ence of the anesthesiologist must be of a high order.[61]

SURGICAL TECHNIQUE

A horizontal incision is made through the labial-buccal mucoperiosteum above the mucogingival junction extending from one second molar region to the other (Fig. 22–24B). The incision is placed in the labial-buccal aspect of the depth of the vestibule, at about the level of the apexes of the teeth. The margins of the superior flap are raised to expose the entire lateral walls of the maxilla, zygomatic crests, infraorbital foramina and the piriform apertures. The inferior mucoperiosteal tissues are minimally elevated, so that they provide additional vascular supply to the maxillary bone and teeth. Good visualization of the posterolateral maxilla is essen-

tial and is accomplished by positioning the tip of a curved cheek retractor at the pterygomaxillary suture (Fig. 22–24B). Another cheek retractor is placed anteriorly to facilitate visualization of the anterolateral portion of the maxilla. The length of the teeth is assessed by direct visualization and palpation of the bone encasing the apexes of the teeth. These findings are correlated with measurements taken from panoramic (Panorex) or lateral cephalometric radiographs, so that a horizontal line can be etched in the bone 3 to 5 mm. above the apexes of the teeth.

Horizontal supra-apical osteotomies of the lateral maxilla are made, with a fissure bur in a straight handpiece or a high-speed reciprocating saw* under constant saline irrigation,

---

*Stryker reciprocating saw (Stryker Corporation, Kalamazoo, Michigan).

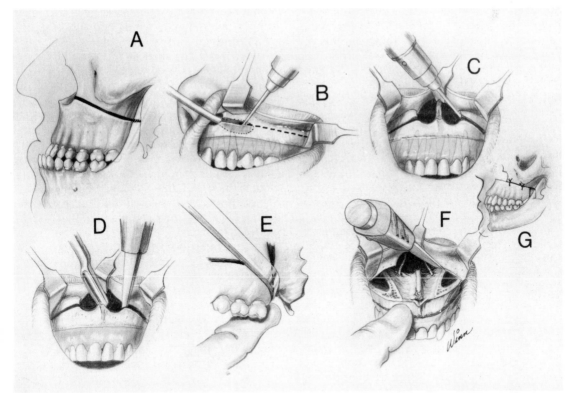

Figure 22–24 Soft-tissue and bony incisions for correction of maxillary retrusion by Le Fort I osteotomy technique. *A,* Typical dental, facial and skeletal characteristics of mandibular prognathism associated with maxillary retrusion. *B* and *C,* Horizontal incision through the mucoperiosteum in the labial-buccal aspect of the depth of the vestibule. Horizontal supra-apical osteotomy of the lateral maxilla extending from the piriform rim posteriorly to the pterygomaxillary fissure.

D, Separation of the nasal septum from the superior part of the maxilla with an osteotome; posterior lateral nasal wall sectioned with an osteotome. *E,* Separation of the maxilla from the pterygoid plate with a curved osteotome; the surgeon's finger is positioned below the palatal mucosa to feel the osteotome as it transects the bone.

F, Maxilla in "downfractured" position; mucoperiosteum has been detached and retracted away from the entire superior surface of the maxilla and horizontal plate of the palatine bone; posterior maxilla is separated from the pterygoid plates and perpendicular process of palatine bone with osteotome and burr. *G,* Repositioned maxilla fixed to the piriform rims and zygomatic buttresses with transosseous wires.

from the lateral part of the piriform rim posteriorly across the canine fossa and through the zygomatic maxillary crest to the pterygomaxillary fissure. In some cases, depending upon the existing facial deformity, by placing the anterior osteotomy more superiorly, greater augmentation of the midfacial region will result.

The mucoperiosteum is elevated from the anterior floor of the nose, nasal septum and lateral walls of the nasal cavity to facilitate separation of the maxilla from these structures. A nasoseptal osteotome is positioned above the anterior nasal spine parallel with the hard palate and is malleted to separate the nasal septum from the maxilla (Fig. 22–24D). The anterolateral nasal wall is sectioned transantrally with a fissure bur in a straight handpiece. The posterolateral nasal wall is sectioned with a sharp osteotome just above the level of the nasal floor. In many instances, however, this bone is so thin that it does not have to be osteotomized. Finally, a pterygoid osteotome is malleted into the pterygomaxillary suture to separate the maxilla from the pterygoid plates (Fig. 22–24E). By digital pressure on the palatal mucosa in the region of the hamulus, the surgeon is able to feel the osteotome as it transects the bone, while insuring that it does not traumatize the underlying mucoperiosteum. The osteotome is positioned inferiorly to minimize danger to the vascular structures in the pterygomaxillary fissure. By manipulation of the curved osteotome and manual pressure against the tuberosities, the maxilla is made partially mobile.

At this point the maxilla is downfractured. Gradually increasing inferior pressure on the anterior maxilla facilitates visualization of the superior surface of the maxilla and lateral nasal walls (Fig. 22–24F). The mucoperiosteum is elevated and retracted away from the entire superior surface of the maxilla, horizontal plate of the palatine bone and lateral nasal walls. Transection of the greater palatine vessels is of no practical consequence. Digital pressure gradually completes downfracturing of the maxilla, without the use of disimpaction forceps. The downfractured position of the maxilla provides excellent access for completely separating the maxilla from the pterygoid plates and perpendicular process of the palatine bone (Fig. 22–24F). This can be accomplished with a bur or an osteotome. By carefully levering a curved osteotome against the stable posterior bony buttress and exerting forward pressure against the tuberosities, the surgeon can completely mobilize the maxilla and move it into the desired position. The maxilla must be made mobile so that it can be moved with only light digital pressure into the desired relationship with the mandible. With a previously prepared interocclusal splint as an index, the maxilla is immobilized for 6 to 8 weeks with stainless steel wires ligated between previously placed arch bars or orthodontic arch wires Before placement of the intermaxillary fixation, a nasogastric tube is inserted in the nasal passage opposite the side of the nose that has been intubated and is usually maintained in place for 12 to 24 hours to prevent vomiting in the immediate postoperative period.

The mobilized maxilla is fixed directly to the piriform rims and zygomatic buttresses with transosseous wires whenever feasible. When the bone in these areas is too thin to support interosseous wires, however, the use of infraorbital rim or circumzygomatic suspension wires fastened to the maxillary fixation appliance is necessary. In many cases it seems preferable to use suspension wires to the mandible for optimal stabilization.

Although bone grafting has been utilized in the majority of patients, it is not routine. Indications for the use of bone grafts are determined from preoperative clinical and cephalometric studies, model analysis and clinical judgment. Substantial advancement or widening of the maxilla, augmentation of the nasolabial, malar or infraorbital areas, increase in vertical midfacial height and residual bone clefts are indications for bone grafting.

Wedge-shaped corticocancellous bone blocks are inlaid with the cancellous bone facing the antrum, so that they will not dislodge into the antrum or nasopharynx. In most cases in which the advancement is less than 6 mm., bone grafts are not used in the pterygomaxillary or lateromaxillary areas. Through the intraoral incisions, bone can be placed over the lateral and anterior maxilla, infraorbital rim and zygoma for contour restoration of these areas. The mucoperiosteal incisions are closed with interrupted horizontal mattress sutures.

If an airway problem is anticipated in the immediate postoperative period, the mobilized maxilla may be suspended by vertical lugs or eyelets previously incorporated into the acrylic wafer splint. The immediate need for intermaxillary fixation is thereby obviated. The mandible is immobilized 4 or 5 days after surgery when the nasal passages are patent.

The use of nasopharyngeal airways for 1 or 2 days may help maintain patency of the nasal passages, mold the nasal mucosa against the superior surface of the maxilla, and obliterate dead space beneath the nasal mucosa. Nasopharyngeal airways must be carefully monitored, changed and cleaned frequently so that they do not become obstructed with blood and mucus. After the airways are removed, the nasal passages are sprayed periodically with oxymetazoline hydrochloride (Afrin) nasal spray. Three or 4 days after surgery, the nasal passages are cleared of inspissated blood clots and mucus with a small aspirating tip. Patients are routinely administered antibiotics and decongestants for 7 days postoperatively or until such time as the soft-tissue incisions have healed.

After the mandible is mobilized, the splint is removed and several intermaxillary elastics are worn at night only for 2 or 3 weeks. This regimen is continued until there is synchronous jaw function, stable occlusion and clinical stability of the maxilla.

APPLICATIONS OF TECHNIQUE

With the maxilla in the "downfractured position" many technical modifications of maxillary osteotomies are feasible; the maxilla is easily sectioned sagittally, transversely or circumpalatally to facilitate simultaneous movement of the anterior and posterior maxillary dentoalveolar segments. Simultaneous anterior and posterior maxillary osteotomies, combined with the extraction of first or second premolar teeth, can frequently facilitate correction of severe occlusal problems in a single operation. The anterior and posterior maxillary dentoalveolar segments can be moved anteriorly, posteriorly, laterally, medially, superiorly or inferiorly into the desired position. Severely rotated or crowded teeth and leveling of the lower arch, however, are usually best treated by preoperative or postoperative orthodontics.

Since 1971 this technique has been used to advance, retract, raise, narrow or expand the maxilla in 20 patients. Complex dentofacial problems, such as maxillary retrusion (Figs. 22–24 to 22–27), skeletal-type anterior open bite (Fig. 22–28), bilateral buccal or palatal crossbite, maxillary dentoalveolar protrusion

and maxillary alveolar hyperplasia, have been successfully corrected.

An obtuse nasolabial angle is probably the single most important diagnostic criterion for employing total maxillary advancement. The upper-lip–nose balance can be significantly improved by reduction of such an angle. Figures 22–24 to 22–27 show how maxillary retrusion associated with mandibular prognathism in a 16-year-old boy was corrected by maxillary advancement and orthodontic treatment. Widening the alar bases of the nose and decreasing the nasolabial angle produced a marked improvement in the patient's overall facial balance.

In patients who display an excessive amount of gingiva and teeth in rest position or when smiling, owing to a short upper lip or maxillary alveolar hyperplasia, the entire maxilla or dentoalveolar portion of the maxilla can be repositioned superiorly to improve the upper-lip line–to–incisor relationship.[107] The consequent autorotation of the mandible is an effective means of increasing chin prominence. To facilitate superior movement of the maxilla, the maxillary nasal spine is reduced under direct vision. The anterior nasal floor can be grooved to accommodate the cartilaginous septum. Submucosal resection of the cartilaginous septum, turbinectomy or both may indeed be necessary when the maxilla is superiorly repositioned in excess of 10 mm.

COMPLICATIONS

Wound Healing. The incisional wounds heal without discernible vascular ischemia, infection or dehiscence. Postoperative studies have shown minimal bone loss in the interdental osteotomy sites and no periodontal problems.

Stability. Significant occlusal and skeletal relapse has been discernible in only one patient whose maxilla was advanced without bone grafting. This cleft lip and palate patient dramatically illustrated the need for bone grafting. It is beyond the scope of our discussion to focus on small positional changes of the surgically repositioned maxillae which occurred in some patients after fixation appliances were removed. Clinically, however, such changes appeared to be minimal.

Esthetics. In one patient having a previously repaired cleft lip and palate, nasal esthetics were compromised by obvious

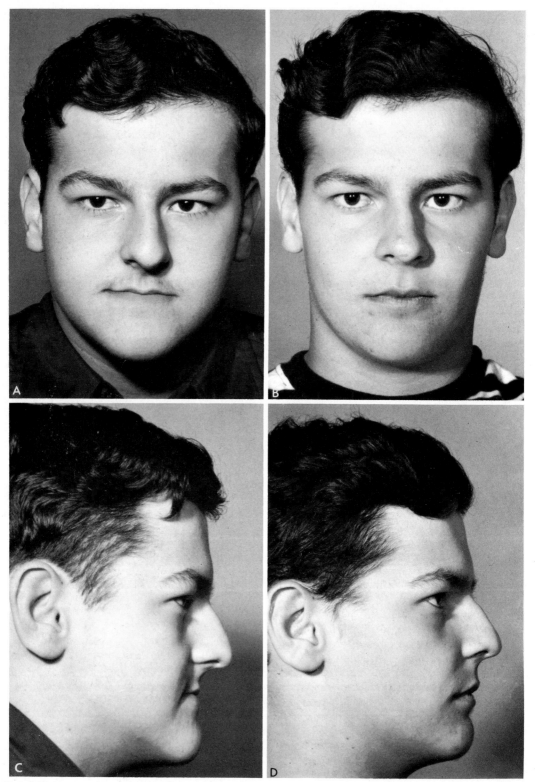

Figure 22–25 *A* and *C*, Mandibular prognathism in 16-year-old boy—poor upper lip–nose balance and narrow alar bases before treatment. *B* and *D*, Photographs after maxillary advancement, showing improved balance between the upper lip and nose, and widening of alar bases.

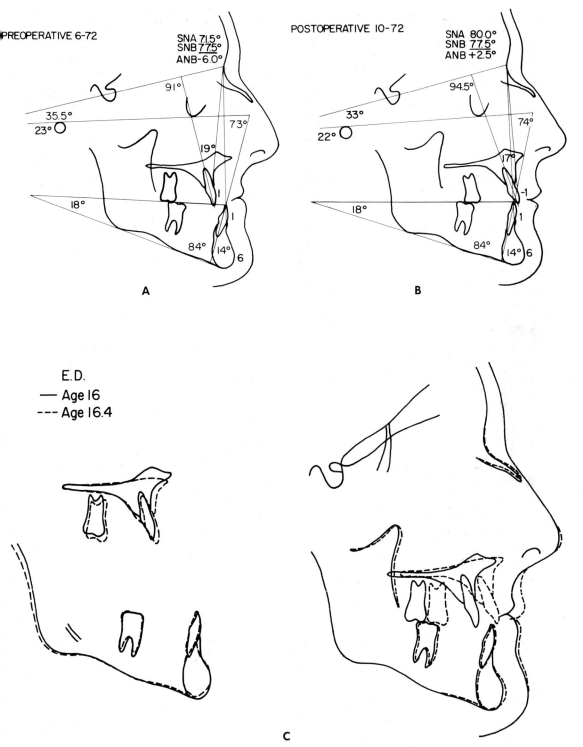

Figure 22–26 *A,* Cephalometric tracing of patient before surgery (age 16 years), showing retroinclination of maxillary and mandibular incisors, oblique nasolabial angle, maxillary retrusion, and Class III occlusal relationship. *B,* Cephalometric tracing 4 months after maxillary advancement. *C,* Composite cephalometric tracing before surgery (*solid line,* age 16 years), and 4 months after surgery (*broken line,* age 16 years, 4 months).

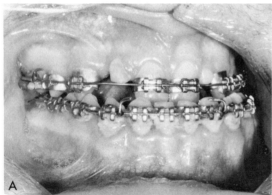

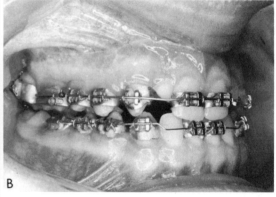

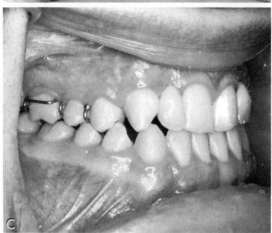

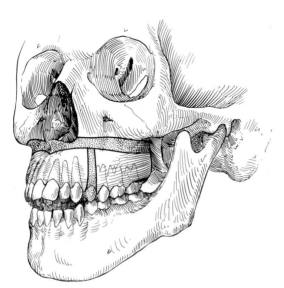

Figure 22-27 *A*, Occlusion after orthodontic alignment of teeth (age 16 years). *B*, Four months after surgery (age 16 years, 4 months). *C*, Post-treatment occlusion (age 17 years, 4 months); congenitally missing lateral incisors replaced with removable prosthetic appliance. (Orthodontic treatment was performed by Dr. James S. Cunningham, Houston, Texas.)

Figure 22-28 Modification of Le Fort I osteotomy technique—correction of skeletal-type anterior open bite and associated maxillary alveolar hyperplasia by simultaneous anterior maxillary and mandibular osteotomies and superior repositioning of the maxilla. (Stippled areas indicate horizontal and vertical ostectomy sites.)

splaying of the alar base of one side of the nose after maxillary advancement. In still another patient, there were bilateral splaying of the alar bases and fanning of the cartilaginous nasal septum after the maxilla was raised 10 mm. In both patients good facial balance was achieved after rhinoplasty. Prospective patients must be apprised of the possible need for rhinoplasty after the maxilla is advanced or raised.

SUMMARY

With proper planning and execution of surgical technique and adequate follow-up care, the maxilla can be surgically repositioned into a stable relationship with the mandible. Complete mobility, preservation of viability, by proper design of the bony and soft-tissue incisions, and adequate fixation during the healing phase are essential in obtaining this objective.

MAXILLARY OSTEOTOMY AND CLOSURE
OF DIASTEMA OF CENTRAL INCISORS
Noah R. Calhoun, D.D.S., M.S.D.

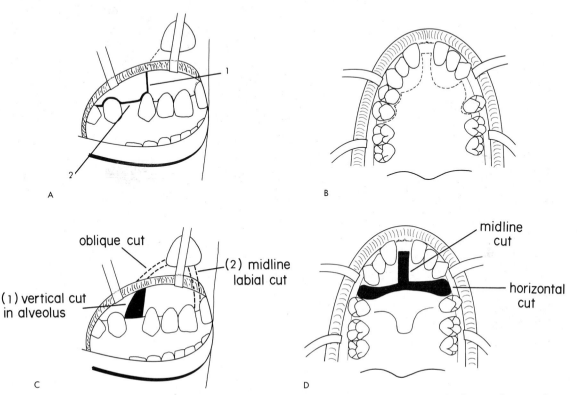

Figure 22–29   An acceptable technique for performing a maxillary osteotomy and closure of a diastema between the central incisors in which the segments are pedicled on the labial mucosa is as follows:

A, Labial mucosal incision. *1*, The vertical extension, and *2*, the horizontal extension of the incision. The vertical incision (*1*) is extended from the gingival cervix of the cuspid to the labial sulcus, and the horizontal incision (*2*) is extended from the gingival sulcus of the cuspid around the cervices of the bicuspids, if present, to the maxillary first molar area. The mucosa is elevated over the first bicuspid and cuspid area. The mucosa is tunneled from the height of the labial sulcus to the bony rim of the nasal fossa.

B, Palatal mucosal incision. This incision may extend from the first molar gingival sulcus along the sulci of the first and second bicuspids to the cuspid; a paramucosal incision may then be extended to the midline. A modification is to extend the incision in the sulci of the anterior teeth to the midline. The palatal mucosal flap is then elevated.

C, Labial bone cuts. The first bicuspid, if present, is extracted, and the vertical alveolar bone cuts (*1*) are made approximately 2 to 3 mm. superior to the apex of the cuspid. A single bone cut is then extended under the tunnel mucosa to the rim of the nasal fossa. The midline alveolar cut (*2*) is made from the palatal side.

D, Palatal bone cuts. The horizontal bone cuts are made to connect the first bicuspid bone cuts. The midline cuts are then made between the central incisors to the horizontal cut. *Note:* The horizontal cut is not completed through the nasal cortex of palatal bone until the midline cut is completed. Special care is taken not to lacerate the labial flaps and nasal mucosa. The bone cuts are completed with osteotomes and bone burs. The segments should be mobilized before they are moved into the predetermined position. The mucosal flaps are repositioned, and a watertight closure is accomplished with single interrupted sutures. The segments are kept in place with single interrupted sutures. This position is maintained with a labial arch bar and palatal acrylic stent, which were completed prior to the operation.

E, Preoperative full face photograph of a patient with a short upper lip and a diastema between maxillary central incisors.

F, Preoperative intraoral photograph showing diastema of central incisors and protrusion of the maxillary alveolar process.

G, Postoperative intraoral photograph showing correction of diastema and fixation of segments with labial arch bar.

H, Postoperative intraoral photograph showing corrected relation after removal of arch bar on first postoperative day. *Note:* Mark around labial aspect of anterior teeth is the impression of the gingiva from labial arch bar.

I, Postoperative intraoral photograph, palatal view.

J, Postoperative full face photograph. (From a film by Noah R. Calhoun: Anterior Maxillary Osteotomy and Closure of Diastema.)

(*Figure 22–29 continued on following page*)

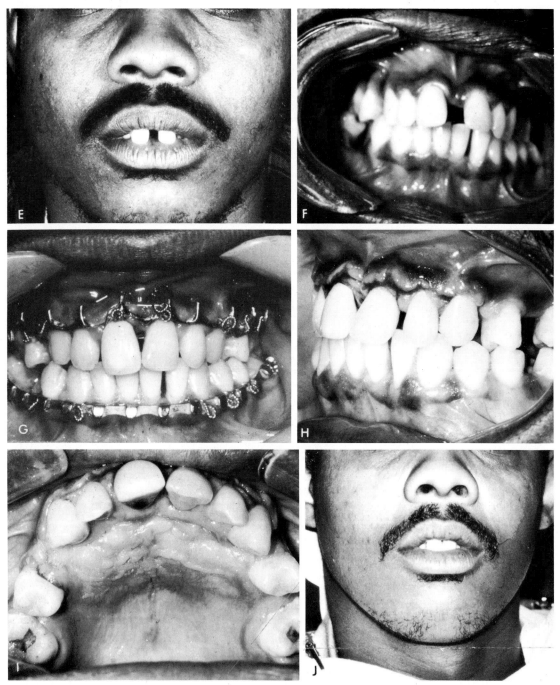

Figure 22–29   (*Continued.*)

REFERENCES

1. Aleman, O.: Ny operation for progeni. Sven. Tandlak. Tidskr., *14*:181, 1921.
2. Alfaro, R., Othon, L. G., Levine, B., *et al:* Correction of mandibular prognathism with associated apertognathia by intraoral sagittal osteotomy of rami. Oral Surg., 27:285 (Mar.), 1969.
3. Alling, C. C.: Correction of mandibular prognathism by open, oblique sliding osteotomies of the rami. J. Oral Surg., 23:199–211, 1965.
4. Antoni, A. A., Van de Mark, T. B., Weinbert, S. and Schofield, I.: Surgical treatment of long-standing malunited horizontal fracture of the maxilla. J. Can. Dent. Assoc., *31*:22, 1965.
5. Axhausen, G.: Zur Behandlung veratlteter, disloziert geheilter Oberkieferbruche. Dtsch. Zahn. Mund. Kieferheilkd., *1*:334, 1934.
6. Babcock, W. W.: The surgical treatment of certain deformities of the jaw associated with malocclusion of the teeth. J.A.M.A., 53:833–839, 1909.
7. Ballard, C. F.: Symposium on Class II, Division I, malocclusion. Part I. Morphology in relation to treatment planning. Dent. Pract., 7:269–286, 1957.
8. Ballard, C. F.: Aetiology of malocclusion—an assessment. Dent. Pract., 8:42–51, 1957.
9. Behrman, S. J.: Chapter 2. Complications associated with orthognathic surgery. *In* Irby, W. B. (Ed.): Current Advances in Oral Surgery. St. Louis, The C. V. Mosby Co., 1974.
10. Behrman, S. J.: Complications of sagittal osteotomy of the mandibular ramus. J. Oral Surg., *30*:554, 1972.
11. Behrman, S. J.: A complication of the intraoral sagittal split. Read before Consultation Clinic 51st Annual Meeting, American Society of Oral Surgeons, San Francisco, Dec. 1969.
12. Behrman, S. J.: Personal communication. New York, N.Y.
13. Bell, W. H.: Revascularization and bone healing after anterior maxillary osteotomy: a study using adult rhesus monkeys. J. Oral Surg., 27:249(Apr.), 1969.
14. Bell, W. H., and Levy, B. M.: Revascularization and bone healing following total maxillary osteotomy. J. Oral Surg., 28:196 (Mar.), 1970.
15. Bell, W. H., and Levy, B. M.: Revascularization and bone healing after anterior mandibular osteotomy. J. Oral Surg., 28:196 (Mar.), 1970.
16. Bell, W. H., Fonseca, R. J., Levy, B. M., and Kennedy, J. W.: Bone healing and revascularization associated with total maxillary osteotomy. In press.
17. Biermann, B. von, Schettler, D., and Koberg, W.: Ergebnisse der Progenieoperation in die Westdeutschen Kieferklinik (Differenential therapeutische Analyse von 98 Fällen). Paper presented at the Meeting of the Deutsche Gesellschaft fur Kiefer- und Gesichtschirurgie and the American Society of Maxillofacial Surgeons. Berlin, May 24–27, 1972.
18. Blair, V. P.: Surgery and Diseases of the Mouth and Jaws. St. Louis, The C. V. Mosby Co., 1912.
19. Blair, V. P.: Operations on the jaw bone and face. Dent. Era, 6:169, 1907.
20. Blair, V. P.: Operations on jawbones and face: Study of aetiology and pathological anatomy of developmental malrelations of maxilla and mandible to each other and to facial outline, and of operative treatment when beyond the scope of the orthodontist. Gynecol. Obstet., 4:67, 1907.
21. Boyne, P. J.: Physiology of bone and response of osseous tissue to injury and environmental changes. J. Oral Surg., 28:12, 1970.
22. Brandon, S. A.: Bilateral osteotomy of the mandible for the correction of macrognathia. Oral Surg., 2:832, 1949.
23. Caldwell, J. B.: Surgical correction of extreme mandibular prognathism. J. Oral Surg., 26:253 (Apr.), 1968.
24. Caldwell, J. B., and Letterman, G. S.: Vertical osteotomy in the mandibular rami for correction of prognathism. J. Oral Surg., 12:185, (July), 1954.
25. Caldwell, J. B., Hayward, J. R., and Lester, R. L.: Correction of retrognathia by vertical L osteotomy: A new technique. J. Oral Surg., 26:259, 1968.
26. Cameron, J. R., and Stetzer, J. J.: Bilateral resection of the mandible to correct prognathism. J. Oral Surg., 6:69, 1948.
27. Catto, M. E.: Histological study of avascular necrosis of the femoral head after transcervical fracture. J. Bone Joint Surg., 47:749 (Nov.), 1965.
28. Christenson, G. W.: Ostectomy for the correction of mandibular prognathism in cases with edentulous posterior segments. Oral Surg., *1*:535, 1948.
29. Converse, J. M., and Shapiro, H. H.: Treatment of developmental malformations of the jaws. Plast. Reconstr. Surg., *10*:473, 1952.
30. Conway, H. C., Smith, J. W., and Behrman, S. J.: Another method of bringing the midface forward. Plast. Reconstr. Surg., 46:325, 1970.
31. Cupar, I.: Die chirurgische Behandlung der Form—und Stellungsveranderung des Oberkiefers. Osterr. A. Stomatol., *51*:565, 1954.
32. Dal Pont, G.: Retromolar osteotomy for correction of prognathism. J. Oral Surg., *19*:42, (Jan.), 1961.
33. Dendy, R. A.: Facial nerve paralysis following sagittal split mandibular osteotomy. Br. J. Oral Surg., *11*:101 (Nov.), 1973.
34. Dingman, R. O.: Surgical correction of mandibular prognathism: An improved method. Am. J. Orthod., *30*:683–692 (Nov.), 1944.
35. Dingman, R. O., and Harding, R. L.: Treatment of malunion fractures of facial bones. Plast. Reconstr. Surg., 7:505, 1951.
36. Gillies, H. G.: *In* Rowe, N. L., and Killey, H. C.: Fractures of the Facial Skeleton. Edinburgh, E. & S. Livingstone, Ltd., 1955.
37. Gilles, H. G., and Millard, D. R.: The Principles and Art of Plastic Surgery. Boston, Little, Brown & Co., 1957.
38. Gillies, G. G., and Rowe, N. L.: L'osteotomie du maxillaire supérieur envisagée essentiellement dans les cas de bec-de-lièvre total. Rev. Stomatol., 55:545, 1954.
39. Guernsey, L. H., and DeChamplain, R. W.: Sequelae and complications of the intraoral sagittal osteotomy in the mandibular rami. Oral Surg., 32:176 (Aug.), 1971.
40. Harsha, W. M.: Bilateral resection of the jaw for prognathism. Surg. Gynecol. Obstet., *15*:51 (July–Aug.), 1912.
41. Hebert, J. M., Kent, J. N., and Hinds, E. C.: Correction of prognathism by an intraoral vertical subcondylar osteotomy. J. Oral Surg., 28:651, 1970.
42. Hinds, E. C.: Surgical correction of acquired man-

dibular deformities. Am. J. Orthod., *43*:161, 1957.

43. Hinds, E. C., and Kent, J. N.: Surgical Treatment of Developmental Jaw Deformities. St. Louis, The C. V. Mosby Co., 1972.

44. Hogeman, K.- E.: Surgical-orthopaedic correction of mandibular protrusion. Acta Chir. Scand., (suppl. 159):1–144, 1951.

45. Hogeman, K.- E., and Willmar, K.: Die Vorverlagerung des Oberkiefers zur Korrektur von Gebissanomalien. Fortschr. Kiefer. Gesichtschir., *12*:275, 1967.

46. Hovell, J. G.: Muscle patterning factors in the surgical correction of mandibular prognathism. J. Oral Surg., *22*:122 (Mar.), 1964.

47. Hullihen, S. P.: A case of elongation of the under jaw. Am. J. Dent. Sci., *9*:157–165, 1849.

48. Hunsuck, E. E.: Modified intraoral sagittal splitting technic for correction of mandibular prognathism. J. Oral Surg., *26*:250 (Apr.), 1968.

49. Hutton, C. E.: Patients' evaluation of surgical correction of prognathism: survey of 32 patients. J. Oral Surg., *25*:225, 1967.

50. Irby, W. B. (Ed.): Current Advances in Oral Surgery. St. Louis, The C. V. Mosby Co., 1974.

51. Johnson, W. B., and Jacobs, S.: Single-stage bilateral ostectomy of the mandible. Oral Surg., *9*:801, 1956.

52. Kaplan, H., and Spring, P. N.: Gustatory hyperhidrosis associated with subcondylar osteotomy. J. Oral Surg., *18*:50, 1960.

53. Kazanjian, V. H.: Surgical treatment of mandibular prognathism. Int. J. Orthod., *18*:1224, 1932.

54. Kemper, J. W.: Surgical correction of mandibular prognathism: Report of case. J. Oral Surg., *5*:29, 1947.

55. Kemper, J. W.: Hemiresection of the mandible for ossifying fibroma: Report of a case. J. Oral Surg., *4*:340–342, 1946.

56. Koblin, I., and Reil, B.: Die Sensibilität der Unterlippe nach Schonung bzw. Durchtrennung des Nervus alveolaris-mandibularis bei Progenieooperationen. Paper presented at the Meeting of the Deutsche Gesellschaft fur Kiefer- und Gesichtschirurgie and the American Society of Maxillofacial Surgeons. Berlin, May 24–27, 1972.

57. Köle, H.: *In* Reichenbach, Kole, and Brueckl (Eds.): Chirurgische Kieferorthopädie. Leipzig, Barth, 1965.

58. Köle, H.: Results, experience, and problems in operative treatment of anomalies with reverse overbite (mandibular protrusion). Oral Surg., *19*:427 (Apr.), 1965.

59. Köle, H.: Surgical operations on the alveolar ridge to correct occlusal abnormalities. Oral Surg., *12*:277, 1959.

60. Kostecka, F.: A contribution to the surgical treatment of open-bite. Int. J. Orthod., *20*:1082, 1934.

61. Lee, J. A., and Atkinson, R. S.: A Synopsis of Anesthesia. 6th ed. Baltimore, The Williams & Wilkins Co., 1968.

62. Lines, P. A., and Steinhauser, E. W.: Soft tissue changes in relationship to movement of hard structures in orthognathic surgery: A preliminary report. J. Oral Surg., *32*:891 (Dec.), 1974.

63. Massey, G. B., Chase, D. C., Thomas, P. M., and Kahn, M. W.: Intraoral oblique osteotomy of the mandibular ramus. J. Oral Surg., *32*:755 (Oct.), 1974.

64. McNeill, R. W., Hooley, J. R., and Sundberg, R. J.: Skeletal relapse during intermaxillary fixation. J. Oral Surg., *31*:212, 1973.

65. Merrill, R. G.: Further studies in decompression for inferior alveolar nerve injury. J. Oral Surg., *24*:233 (May), 1966.

66. Merrill, R. G.: Decompression for alveolar nerve injury. J. Oral Surg., *22*:291 (July), 1964.

67. Mohnac, A. M.: Maxillary osteotomy for the correction of malpositioned fractures: Report of case. J. Oral Surg., *25*:460, 1967.

68. Moose, S. M.: Surgical correction of mandibular prognathism by intraoral sub-condylar osteotomy. Br. J. Oral Surg., *1*:172 (Apr.), 1964.

69. Moose, S. M.: Correction of abnormal mandibular protrusion by intra-oral operation. J. Oral Surg., *3*:304, 1945.

70. Moyer, J. H., and Fuchs, M.: Edema, Mechanisms and Management: A Hahnemann Symposium on Salt Water Retention. Philadelphia, W. B. Saunders Co., 1960.

71. Murphey, P. J., and Walker, R. W.: Correction of maxillary protrusion by ostectomy and orthodontic therapy. J. Oral Surg., *21*:275 (July), 1963.

72. Nathanson, N. R., and Moynihan, F. M.: Prognathism, one-stage intraoral ostectomy. J. Oral Surg., *24*:411, 1966.

73. Nordenram, A., and Waller, A.: Oral-surgical correction of mandibular protrusion. Br. J. Oral Surg., *6*:64 (July), 1968.

74. Obwegeser, H. L.: Surgical correction of maxillary deformities. *In* Grabb, W. C., Rosenstein, S. W., and Brock, K. R.: Cleft Lip and Palate. Boston, Little, Brown & Co., 1969.

75. Obwegeser, H. L.: Comprehensive Conference on Oral Surgery. Sponsored by the American Society of Oral Surgeons, Walter Reed Army Medical Center. Washington, D. C., June, 1966.

76. Obwegeser, H. L.: Indications for surgical correction of mandibular deformity by sagittal splitting technique. Br. J. Oral Surg., *50*:157 (Apr.), 1964.

77. Obwegeser, H. L.: Eingriffe am Oberkiefer zur Korrektur des progenen Zustandsbildes. Schweiz. Monatsschr. Zahnheilkd., *75*:365, 1965.

78. Obwegeser, H. L.: Surgical correction of small or retrodisplaced maxillae. The "dish-face deformity." Plast. Reconstr. Surg., *43*:351, 1969.

79. Parnes, E. I., and Becker, M. L.: Necrosis of the anterior maxilla following osteotomy. Oral Surg., *33*:326, 1972.

80. Perko, M.: Maxillary sinus and surgical movement of maxilla. Int. J. Oral Surg., *1*:177, 1972.

81. Ragnell, A.: Den moderna plastikkirugien inclusive den kosmetiska kirugien, dess verksamhetsfalt och arbetsmetoder. Nord. Med. Tidskr., *15*:361, 1938. (Summary in English.)

82. Rankow, R. M.: An Atlas of Surgery of the Face, Mouth, and Neck. Philadephia, W. B. Saunders Co., 1968.

83. Reiter, E. R.: Surgical correction of mandibular prognathism. Alpha Omegan, *45*:104 (Sept.), 1951.

84. Ricketts, R. M.: Foundation for cephalometric communication. Am. J. Orthod., *46*:330 (May), 1960.

85. Risdon, F.: Ankylosis of the temporomaxillary joint. J. Am. Dent. Assoc., *21*:1933, 1934.

86. Robinson, M.: Micrognathism corrected by vertical osteotomy of the ascending ramus and bone chips. Arch. Otolaryngol., *69*:185–187, 1959.

87. Robinson, M.: Mandibular prognathism corrected by overlapping open vertical osteotomies of the rami: Report of 71 cases. Am. J. Surg., 98:894–897, 1959.

88. Robinson, M.: Surgical correction of mandibular prognathism in preparation for dentures. J. Prosthet. Dent., 9:340–343, 1959.

89. Robinson, M.: Prognathism corrected by open vertical subcondylotomy. J. Oral Surg., 16:215–219, 1958.

90. Robinson, M.: Micrognathism corrected by vertical osteotomy of ascending ramus and iliac bone graft. Oral Surg., 10:1125–1130, 1957.

91. Robinson, M.: Prognathism corrected by open vertical condylotomy. J. South. Calif. Dent. Assoc., 24:22–27 (Jan.), 1956.

92. Rowe, N. L., and Killey, H. C.: Fractures of the Facial Skeleton. Edinburgh, E. & S. Livingstone, Ltd., 1968.

93. Rowe, N. L.: Aetiology, clinical features, and treatment of mandibular deformity. Br. Dent. J., 108:41–64, 1960.

94. Rowe, N. L.: Secondary surgical procedures for the correction of deformities in cleft lip and palate patients. Dent. Pract., 5:112, 1954.

95. Sassouni, V.: Roentgenographic cephalometric analysis of cephalo-facio-dental relationships. Am. J. Orthod., 41:735 (Oct.), 1955.

96. Schoberg, S. J., Kelly, J. F., Terry, B. C., Posner, M. A., and Anderson, E. F.: Blood loss reduction by hypotensive anesthesia in orofacial corrective surgery. J. Oral Surg. In press.

97. Schuchardt, K.: Ein Beitrag zur chirurgischen Kieferorthopädie unter Berücksichtigung ihrer Bedeutung für die Behandlung angeborener und erworbener Kieferdeformitaten bei Soldaten. Dtsch. Zahn. Mund. Kieferheilkd., 9:73, 1942.

98. Small, I. A., and Rae, D. B.: Vertical osteotomy for retrognathia: A modified technic. J. Oral Surg., 21:505 (Nov.), 1963.

99. Small, I. A., Brown, S., and Kobernick, S. D.: Teflon and silastic for mandibular replacement: Experimental studies and reports of cases. J. Oral Surg., 22:377–390 (Sept.), 1964.

100. Smith, A. E., and Robinson, M.: Surgical correction of mandibular prognathism by subsigmoid notch ostectomy with sliding condylotomy: A new technic. J.A.D.A., 49:46 (July), 1954.

101. Spanier: Prognathie-Operationen. Zahn. Orthopadie, 1932.

102. Spilka, C. J.: Surgical correction of mandibular prognathism. Oral Surg., 9:1255 (Dec.), 1956.

103. Trauner, R., and Obwegeser, H.: Surgical correction of mandibular prognathism and retrognathia with consideration of genioplasty. 1. Surgical procedures to correct mandibular prognathism and reshaping of the chin. Oral Surg., 10:677 (July), 1957.

104. Van Zile, W. N.: Triangular ostectomy of the vertical rami: Another technique for correction of prognathism. J. Oral Surg., 21:3–10, 1963.

105. Waldron, C. W., Peterson, R. G., and Waldron, C. A.: Surgical treatment of mandibular prognathism. J. Oral Surg., 4:61, 1946.

106. Wassmund M.: Lehrbuch der Praktischen Chirurgie des Mundes und der Kiefer. Bd. I. Leipzig, Meusser, 1935.

107. West, R. A., and Epker, B. N.: Posterior maxillary surgery: Its place in the treatment of dentofacial deformities. J. Oral Surg., 30:562, 1972.

108. White, R. P., Peters, P. B., Costich, E. R., et al.: Evaluation of sagittal split–ramus osteotomy in 17 patients. J. Oral Surg., 27:851, (Nov.), 1969.

109. White, R. P., Peters, P. B., and Collins, L. R.: Surgical approach to facial deformity. Va. Dent. J., 44:8 (Oct.), 1967.

110. Wilde, N. J.: Sagittal rami section for correction of mandibular deformities. Plast. Reconstr. Surg., 43:167, 1969.

111. Winstanley, R. P.: Subcondylar osteotomy of the mandible and intraoral approach. Br. J. Oral Surg., 1:157 (Apr.), 1964.

CHAPTER 23

TRANSPLANTATION AND GRAFTING PROCEDURES IN ORAL SURGERY*

PHILIP J. BOYNE, D.M.D., M.S.

Increasingly sophisticated clinical surgical techniques, and immunologic and tissue banking research efforts have developed an environment that has made possible the evolution of a large number of new transplantation and implantation procedures in oral surgical treatment. These techniques involve the use of fresh living, banked viable and banked nonviable tissues in dental practice. New procedures of skin, bone and cartilage grafting have been developed in recent years as a direct result of the application of findings from significant research in oral surgery and allied fields.

Additionally, procedures of tooth transplantation have been revived, with new scientific approaches based on the results of laboratory research efforts. The general effect of such emphasis on regeneration of human tissues and organs by grafting and transplantation has been a marked increase in patient demand for such surgical services. Oral surgery, as a specialty, has been progressive in developing and adapting new immunologic and general surgical concepts to oral surgical care, and in offering the delivery of a health service, which gives every indication of increasing in significance in the future years.

BASIC PRINCIPLES OF TISSUE AND ORGAN GRAFTING

In the transplantation of any type of tissue, there are from a source-origin standpoint three categories of grafts:

1. *Autogenous transplants,* which represent tissues taken from the same individual receiving the graft.
2. *Homogenous transplants,* which represent tissues taken from another donor of the same species. Homografts may in turn be subdivided into:
   a. Allografts, or allogeneic homografts, which are composed of tissue taken from a donor unrelated to the recipient.
   b. Isografts, or isogenous homografts, which are composed of tissues obtained from a donor closely related to the recipient (*e.g.,* grafts between animal littermates; or, in human subjects, between siblings).
3. *Heterogenous transplants* (xenografts), which represent tissues taken for transplantation from an individual of another species (*e.g.,* an animal bone graft implanted into a human subject).

The term graft or transplant is usually applied to the transfer of *living tissues.* Nonviable tissue transfers, and tissue transplants that although living at the time of grafting later die, are termed *implants.* It is therefore not necessary for the cells of implants to survive in order for the procedure to be termed successful. The cells of a true graft, however,

---

* Portions of the text of this chapter are adapted and reproduced by permission from Boyne, P. J.: Transplantation, implantation, and grafts. Dent. Clin. North Am., *15*(2):433–453 (Apr.), 1971.

must survive and proliferate in order for the transplant to be successful.

APPLIED IMMUNOLOGIC CONCEPTS

Immune Response. When allogeneic homografts or xenografts are exchanged, a graft rejection phenomenon is frequently elicited. Such graft rejection is usually the result of a tissue reaction called the *immune response,* which is the process by which the host recipient protects its cellular integrity from the intrusion of foreign graft material that is immunologically unacceptable. Since, in clinical situations, homografts are more commonly used than are grafts from an animal or heterogenous source, the immune response usually is encountered clinically in homogenous grafting, and is called the "homograft response." This rejection of the living homogenous graft is the result of a cellular reaction of the host to transplantation antigens contained in the grafted tissue. Such reaction is usually not immediate, and a homograft transplanted to a normal subject enjoys an immunologic latent period, during which time the healing of the graft-host interface is indistinguishable from that of a fresh autograft.[11] The length of this latent period depends upon the degree of genetic disparity between the donor and the host, *i.e.,* the genetic relationship between the two.[11,17] Genetic similarity between the donor and the recipient of a transplanted tissue appears to be the major factor responsible for success of the graft. For example, a fresh isograft of skin (a homogenous transplant between closely related individuals) may remain in place for a long period of time before being rejected, whereas a fresh homograft between nonrelated individuals (*i.e.,* an allogeneic homograft) may be destroyed within a few days.

Recently, it has been found that for a given recipient, it is possible to identify nonrelated donors having genetic similarity that will permit the exchange of living transplants.[20] This work has made possible, through lymphocytic typing and other laboratory tests, the identification of kidney donors for nonrelated recipients.[19,20]

Second Set Response. The rejection and loss of a living tissue homograft leaves the recipient host in a specifically immune state of heightened resistance, which may continue for many months. During this time, if a second homograft from the same donor is transplanted to the same recipient, it will be destroyed *more* rapidly than its predecessor. This is called a "second set response." It occurs because the second graft has been made during a period of increased immunologic resistance on the part of the host.

The homograft response is thought to be due to cell-fixed antibodies and not to the circulating antibodies, which usually play a major role in the protection of the host from various diseases.

In attempting to solve the problems of tissue incompatibility in grafting from one individual to another, three approaches have been used:

1. Approaches may be used that attempt to modify the immune mechanisms of the recipient in order to block the rejection of the graft. (These have included irradiation of the recipient, and the use of various immunosuppressive drugs.)

2. Attempts at immunologic suppression may be directed at the graft itself (by means of radiation, freezing, and freeze-drying, the antigenicity of a bone graft, for example, may be attenuated).[9,14]

3. More recently, attempts have been made at attenuation of transplants by the storage of the graft tissue in an "intermediate host" prior to removal and transplantation into the final one, called the "second recipient." Such use of intermediate hosts has been applied to "storage" of primate kidneys in baboons for later transplantation to the permanent recipient.

Of these methods, the second, *i.e.,* attenuation of the antigenetic properties of the graft itself by irradiation, freezing, and freeze-drying has found more application to those grafting procedures that have been used in oral surgery. The use of immunosuppressive drugs on the donor recipient, while being used in major organ transplantation procedures, is thought to be too disruptive of normal homeostatic mechanisms to be used in the types of tissue transplantation utilized in oral surgical procedures.

HETEROGENOUS IMPLANTS (XENOGRAFTS)

The use of tissues from a heterogenous (or animal) source in oral surgical treatment, of course, does not apply to tooth transplantation, and to date heterogenous skin and fascial transplants have not been used in oral surgical procedures. (xenografts of animal skin have, however, been used clinically in the treatment of burn patients. These heterogenous skin implants have served as "temporary dressing" implants, with the surface implant serving to promote marginal healing and to decrease surface tissue fluid loss. Of course, no cell survival would be expected in this type of tissue transfer.)

However, during the past century there has been a recognized need for a readily available inexpensive source of *bone* and *cartilage* graft material that could be used in routine oral surgical procedures which attempt to restore minor as well as major facial bone defects. This need has stimulated a considerable research effort to attenuate or eliminate the antigenic factors operating in hard tissue heterografts from an animal source. Essentially, the problem has been that in order to render animal bone nonantigenic and safe for transplantation to human subjects, the organic fraction of the bone needs to be completely removed or markedly altered by very drastic chemical means.

The chemical treatment employed to accomplish this task of "despeciation" has invariably produced an inert osseous product, which, when placed in surgical defects, has not been able to stimulate, even passively, bone formation. Grafts made from such material act essentially as a *space-filling substance* and do not even passively assist the osteogenic processes of the recipient patient.

Heterogenous grafts of cartilage treated by various chemical means, however, have occasionally been used in certain facial recontouring operations in which nasal or zygomatic outlines have been restored in laboratory animals (and in a few instances in clinical patients) in areas of the face not subject to functional pressures or to the effect of muscular action. In such areas, union of the cartilagenous graft with the host bone is not of primary importance, and a heterogenous, cartilagenous implant may be completely surrounded by a connective tissue capsule and still be considered successful in satisfying the requirements for soft tissue recontouring.

HOMOGENOUS (ALLOGENEIC) IMPLANTS

In contrast to the heterografts, homogenous allogeneic tissue transplants have been used in oral surgery with considerable success. Since the genetic disparity in allografts is, of course, less than that operating in heterogenous grafting situations, and since grafts of the hard tissues of bone, cartilage and teeth contain large areas of calcified intercellular matrix, which is relatively acellular and which is not as productive of severe immunologic response as are the highly cellular soft tissue grafts, the methods used to preserve and store these tissues have not, of necessity, involved the drastic types of chemical treatment used to eliminate the allergenic factors in xenografts. Instead, storage of allogeneic homografts has tended to be of the cryobiologic type. Such cryogenic tissue storage methods have involved freezing, freeze-drying and simple cooling at "refrigerator temperatures" of +4°C.[4]

The following types of allogeneic homogenous tissues have been used in oral surgical procedures:

1. Bone.
2. Cartilage.
3. Fascia.
4. Teeth.

CRYOGENIC STORAGE OF NONVIABLE ALLOGENEIC HOMOGENOUS TISSUES FOR LATER SURGICAL USE

During the past two decades, allografts of bone, cartilage and fascia have been obtained for storage in hospital tissue banks by taking material at autopsy from human subjects or by saving tissue material taken during previous operations. Such tissue specimens are treated by various means in order to produce a satisfactory storage environment. The cryogenic methods mentioned above have been very successfully employed in this type of tissue storage. Perhaps the most sophisticated of these storage methods has been the process of freeze-drying.[4,14] Bone and cartilage grafts preserved by these cryogenic methods are more readily completely revascularized, resorbed and remodeled than are xenografts or allografts that have been treated by more drastic methods, such as boiling or deproteinization.[4,14]

Stored Nonviable Allogeneic Homogenous Skin. Cryogenically preserved allogeneic homogenous skin has been used as a graft in other types of surgery, notably as a treatment procedure in the surgical management of body burns covering large areas. (As previously mentioned, skin xenografts can also be used as temporary coverings for burned areas of the body surface.) These types of grafts (more properly called "implants"), however, do not function as viable skin transplants and serve merely as a treatment *dressing,* being rejected by the host recipient with the expected immunologic response within a few days or weeks.

Stored Nonviable Allogeneic Homogenous Bone. As previously mentioned, bone and cartilage grafts preserved cryogenically are accepted by the recipient host without rejection, primarily because, unlike many other types of soft tissues and types of organ systems having large cell populations, bone and cartilage are composed of relatively small numbers of living cells with a large quantity of calcified and noncalcified intercellular matrix that is *nonvital.* Since the survival of cells in a stored bone homograft is not necessary for the success of the implant grafting procedure, a method of storage that will bring about cell death without drastically altering the remaining osseous structure of the graft material is considered to be the best type of tissue banking techniques. Since the cells of such preserved bone and cartilage do not survive, the assistance afforded on the part of such a graft to the osteogenic process of the recipient in the regeneration of the surgical defect is purely a *passive* one. In other words, there is no active osteogenic stimulation effected by these types of grafts. Such grafts merely offer a latticework over which the bone of the host may grow to reconstruct

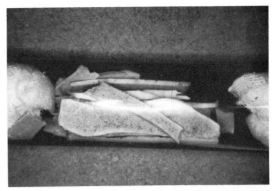

Figure 23-2 A sealed vial containing freeze-dried cancellous human bone ready for allogeneic transplantation. (In this instance the bone implant material has been cut into flat strips for later use.)

the defect (Fig. 23-1). It is obvious, therefore, that such bone transplants can be used only in smaller types of intrabone defects or in areas in which the osteogenic process of the host merely requires a small degree of assistance in order to effect good regeneration and healing. For example, freeze-dried or frozen bone homografts are partially successful in surgical treatment of large cystic defects of the jaws after the cyst lining has been removed (Figs. 23-2 and 23-3). Such grafts are of no value in attempting to lead the osteogenic regenerative processes of the host to form bone in areas in which normally such osseous growth or repair would not occur. For example, in large gap-spanning defects of the mandible, where active osteogenesis is necessary, such cryogenically preserved homogenous implants would be of little value.

Stored Nonviable Allogeneic Homogenous Cartilage. In comparison with cryogenically stored cartilage, similarly stored homogenous bone offers a larger surface area and a better latticework over which host reparative bone may grow to fill a surgical defect. Freeze-dried or frozen bone implants, therefore, tend to produce better results than do cartilagenous implants in most types of oral surgical procedures. In addition to the tendency toward fibrous tissue encapsulation, homogenous cartilage grafts tend to "warp" or revert to their previous anatomic position and form.[6] This implant property may lead to a shifting of the cartilage within its host recipient site, resulting in a nonosseous union of the cartilagenous implant with the host bone and an eventual fibrous encapsulation of the cartilage.

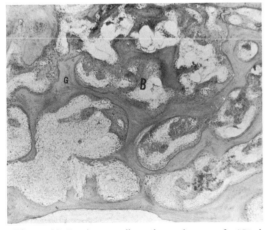

Figure 23-1 A cancellous bone homograft (*G*) is shown forming a latticework, over which new host bone (*B*) is growing to fill a mandibular cystic defect. This is an example of a graft material *passively* assisting the osteogenic processes of the host. (×125.)

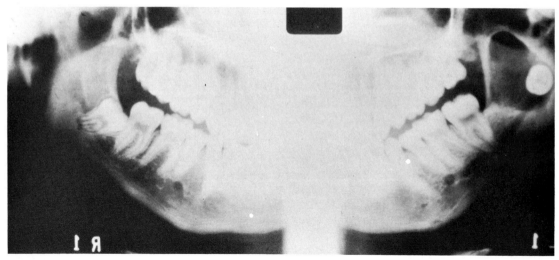

Figure 23–3 Panoramic view of a mandibular dentigerous cyst involving an impacted third molar (at far right). Such a cystic bone cavity, after enucleation of the soft-tissue cystic wall and removal of the tooth, would lend itself well to an implant of banked allogeneic bone, since only passive osteogenic assistance is necessary for host bone to regenerate in the defect.

Stored Nonviable Allogeneic Homogenous Fascia. Freeze-dried and frozen fascia has been used in oral surgical procedures involving arthroplasties and the reconstruction of the temporomandibular joint in which the fascia serves as a cushion or a "pseudodisc" for the reconstruction of the new articulating area. Such fascial implants, however, do not appear to have any marked advantage over synthetic materials such as silastic or other types of plastic implants.

Stored Allogeneic Homogenous Fully Formed Nonviable Teeth. Attempts at transplantation of fully formed teeth stored by freeze-drying and freezing have not met with routine long-term success. In cases in which *fully formed* teeth have been transplanted after having been treated in this manner, an eventual progressive root resorption tends to occur, even though the immediate clinical result is usually one of acceptance, with apparently healthy periodontal tissues surrounding the transplant. Recently investigators have attempted to reduce root resorption by treating the extracted homograft root surface with fluoride solutions and by other modalities.[18]

CRYOGENIC STORAGE OF VIABLE TISSUES FOR LATER ALLOGENEIC HOMOGENOUS TRANSPLANTATION

While the usual methods of freeze-drying, quick-freezing, and cooling to refrigerated temperatures produce death of cells and essentially nonviable grafts, there are types of freezing techniques that have been successful in the preservation of cell life for later experimental transplantation procedures.[8] Techniques of freezing in this manner have resulted in frozen blood banking, frozen sperm storage, and other types of preserved suspensions of the one-cell type. The freezing of large, complex masses of tissue and organ systems by this method, however, has not been successful to date, although a considerable research effort in this area is being made.

Cryogenic Storage of Viable Homogenous Bone and Cartilage. One of the most successful cryogenic methods of cell preservation is that of programmed freezing, in which the temperature of the graft specimens is dropped very slowly (a specified number of degrees per minute). Cryophylactic agents are used to prevent cell death, which might otherwise tend to occur in this process because of excessive concentration of tissue salts and because of the formation of intracellular and extracellular ice crystals. One such cryophylactic agent is dimethylsulfoxide. It has been shown that it is possible to preserve cell viability of osteogenic bone marrow by this method. Following a period of several days or weeks of storage at −197°C., the specimens may be thawed and transplanted back *into the same animal*, with marked osteogenic effects. Thus, *autogenous marrow* frozen in this manner has been shown to be as osteogenic as the fresh autogenous counterpart.[8]

Recent work has indicated that this preservation procedure results in the death of *all* the *differentiated cells* of the marrow, while the undifferentiated reticuloendothelial cells apparently survive the freezing process.[1] These reticuloendothelial cells, then, appear to be the essential cell types in the osteogenic grafting phenomena. However, when specimens of bone and cartilage are treated by the programmed freezing techniques that preserve the *vitality* of these reticuloendothelial cells, the grafts tend to be rejected by an *allogeneic recipient* host in a manner similar to the rejection of fresh marrow homograft. Thus, such preserved cell transplants can at present only be successfully used autogenously.

Cryogenic Storage of Viable Homogenous Tooth Buds. With these new techniques of programmed freezing, using various cryophylactic agents, it has been possible to preserve the vitality of some of the cells in certain

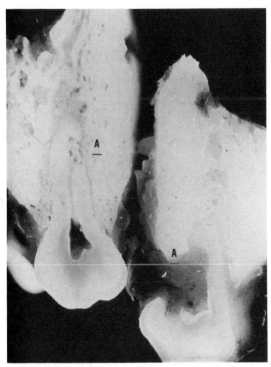

Figure 23–4   *Right,* A programmed frozen homogenous tooth transplant with marked root resorption (*A*). The pulpal tissue in this developing tooth has not survived the procedure well enough to form new normal reparative dentin.

Left, This tooth is a similarly stored homograft that had a fully formed root at the time of storage and transplantation. Some root resorption (*A*) is also evident in this tooth.

As can be seen, the cryogenic storage of these kinds of teeth was not successful in rendering the dental transplants immune to homograft rejection.

tissue systems. The use of such freezing techniques that preserve the vitality of cells, as opposed to the use of those that kill cells, has not, however, been markedly productive in the preservation and storage of tooth buds for later transplantation. While it has been possible to maintain the vitality of certain cells in the tooth germ system, it appears that the immune response causes an eventual loss of tooth bud *after homogenous transplantation.* After transplantation of a developing tooth stored in such a cryobiologic environment, there is a marked failure of the tooth bud to grow in the normal fashion necessary to produce typical dentinal and cemental tissues of the tooth organ system. Later osteoid tissue replaces the degenerating pulp as the calcified matrix of the tooth is resorbed (Fig. 23–4).

(In addition to cryogenic methods of tissue storage, attempts have been made to preserve the vitality of tooth buds by tissue culture.[10] To date, however, these methods have not been successful in preserving the normal vitality and function of a tooth organ system. These banked transplants are therefore not able to assume the role of an acceptable dental transplant postoperatively. Although these tissue culture–stored transplants may later be grafted to another recipient without immediate rejection, the tooth bud does not resume its function as a dentin- and cementum-forming organ.)

SUMMARY OF THE EFFECTS OF CRYOGENIC TREATMENT OF HOMOGENOUS TISSUES

At the present time, therefore, freezing, freeze-drying and other cryophylactic programmed freezing techniques used on homogenous bone and cartilage appear to be effective only when they produce *complete cell death,* resulting in an implant-graft material that is inert and *nonviable,* being accepted by the recipient host as a dead implant to be used only as a trellus to assist passively the normal healing processes of the host recipient.

Recent quick-freezing techniques used for the banking of small units of cancellous bone for later allogeneic transplantation into periodontal defects are thought to be banking procedures that "preserve" only a *dead graft matrix,* just as does the technique of freeze-drying, and no particular advantages are attached to the quick-freezing process.

AUTOGENOUS GRAFTS

While extensive experimental work continues on the preservation of homogenous tissues and on the development of graft material from a heterogenous source, it is clearly evident at the present time that the best type of graft material is *autogenous* in origin. The *autogenous* tissues that have been used and are presently used in oral surgery are:

1. Bone.
2. Cartilage.
3. Skin.
4. Teeth.
5. Mucosa.

AUTOGENOUS BONE GRAFTS

In the restoration of lost osseous tissue, whether it is a discontinuity defect or a recontouring procedure, viable autogenous bone remains the most effective type of graft material. There is, however, considerable disagreement as to the optimal anatomic form that this graft should take. Some surgeons have preferred to use rib grafts, fabricating transplants to the desired shape by variously notching and cutting the rib in order to facilitate bending of the graft to the desired contour. Others have preferred to take solid one-piece grafts from the iliac crest and to cut these into the desired form and shape.

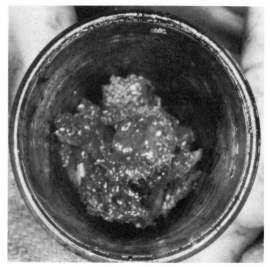

Figure 23–5 Cancellous bone and marrow taken from the ilium by an osteotomy approach just below the crest. Approximately 1 ounce of the particulate graft is shown here prior to its insertion into a metal mesh implant to restore a large mandibular discontinuity defect.

THE USE OF MARROW–CANCELLOUS BONE GRAFTS

Recent research has indicated that another type of bone transplant may be used in promoting bone repair. Specimens of hemopoietic marrow taken from the marrow–vascular spaces of the iliac crest, in combination with viable cancellous bone from the same area, are capable of inducing a strong

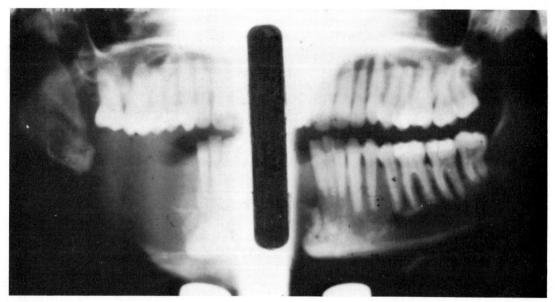

Figure 23–6 A preoperative panoramic radiograph showing a mandible resected from ramus to symphysis. The patient had had numerous operations for recurring ameloblastoma and had received three previous bone grafts that had failed.

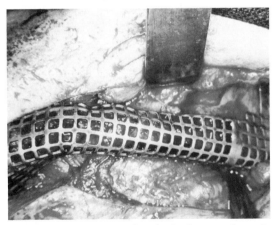

Figure 23-7 The operative site in the case shown in Figure 23-6. The metal implant mesh has been inserted and will be attached to the proximal and distal fragments by 7-mm. screws of compatible metal.

osteogenic response and of producing and stimulating the formation of bone in areas that normally would not exhibit any marked propensity toward bone regeneration. Since it has been difficult in the past to maintain a marrow–cancellous bone graft within any desired surgical site, extensive application of particulate grafts of this type has not been made. Recent studies, however, have developed a procedure whereby these marrow grafts may be applied to many areas of oral surgical treatment. The technique developed has been one in which the autogenous bone and marrow can be used feasibly in many oral surgical situations. It involves the use of a chrome-cobalt casting or a wrought titanium implant to contain the particulate marrow

graft.[2,3] Such an implant device serves to retain the graft material within the defect and to inhibit the proliferation of scar tissue into the area until adequate bony regeneration has taken place (Figs. 23-5 to 23-8).

Entire sections of the mandible may be restored by this technique.[2,3] Additionally, fracture nonunions of the body of the mandible may be treated effectively and rapidly by this procedure. The use of this type of graft material was found to have several advantages over the solid one-piece autograft in the regeneration of large discontinuity defects of the mandible:[2,3]

1. The particulate graft of marrow and cancellous bone is easily obtained with very little morbidity by making only a small opening at the iliac crest rather than taking a large portion of the ilium or a rib to effect the desired surgical result.
2. Complete healing of the grafted defects with viable bone appears to be more rapid than when the solid one-piece autograft is used.
3. Intermaxillary fixation can be greatly reduced because of the rapid spanning and osseous regeneration of the defect by new bone, and because additional support of the host bone fragments is provided by the metal implant itself.
4. Restoration of bony architecture and contour is more easily accomplished because the basic form of the regenerated bone is dictated by the metal implant itself.

In certain surgical situations, however,

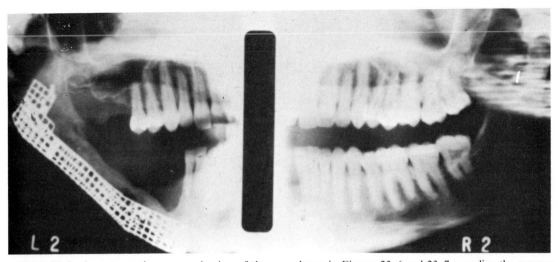

Figure 23-8 A postoperative panoramic view of the case shown in Figures 23-6 and 23-7 revealing the osseous mandibular body regenerated from angle to symphysis. The metal mesh will be allowed to remain in place and a partial denture inserted over the regenerated bone in the grafted area.

with large communications between the oral cavity and the skin areas in which intraoral dehiscence is anticipated or present at the time of surgery, it is considered more prudent not to utilize the metal-type implant but to use a solid one-piece autograft, preferably the iliac crest, to effect the restoration. Intraoral dehiscence over a metal implant may lead to total loss of the graft contained within the metal framework.

It was also found that in certain patients having large full mandibular body defects requiring complete reconstruction of the mandible, one iliac crest would not furnish sufficient cancellous bone and marrow to graft such extensive defect areas. Accordingly, a graft system has been developed involving the use of an allogeneic bone implant taken at autopsy from a donor a few hours after death. The homograft mandible is then surface-decalcified and, after having been hollowed out from the crest of the ridge inferiorly and fenestrated, the implant is then packed with fresh autogenous marrow and cancellous bone taken from the ilium of the recipient (Figs. 23–9 and 23–10).

The composite homograft-autograft was then placed in a chrome-cobalt implant which was secured to the host fragments and the soft tissues were closed.

It has been shown that surface-decalcified homografts favorably influence the osteogenic effect of autogenous marrow in labo-

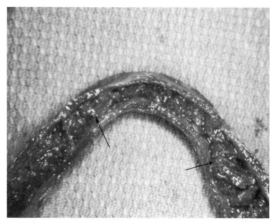

Figure 23–10 A view of the superior portion of the homograft mandible shown in Figure 23–9. The prepared homograft has been filled with autogenous marrow and cancellous bone (*arrows*).

ratory studies. The use of surface-decalcified homogenous mandibles in the manner described above materially decreases the amount of autogenous marrow and cancellous bone necessary to regenerate large mandible defects.

Marrow–Cancellous Bone Grafts in Alveolar Ridge Reconstruction. The same technique of using a particulate graft of cancellous bone and marrow and a metal implant has been effective in rebuilding deficient edentulous alveolar ridges. A considerable amount of new bone may be induced to grow on the crest of an edentulous alveolar ridge by this procedure. The metal implant is constructed to conform to the desired recontour and the optimal increase in height for the particular alveolar ridge. The implant is lined with a filter membrane* and filled with the bone graft of marrow and cancellous bone. The metal implant is allowed to remain in place for approximately 8 to 12 weeks, after which time it is removed, and a denture is prepared immediately to subject the grafted area to prosthetic function.

It is felt that the immediate use of modified prosthetic function, with the patient utilizing a soft diet, is of the utmost importance in the success of this type of bone graft application. In cases in which prosthetic function was not instituted immediately, the graft resorbed markedly over the succeeding 6 to 12 postoperative months. While the exact effect of

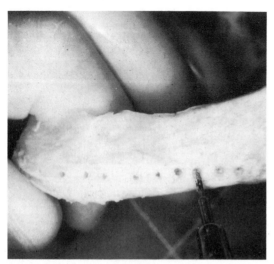

Figure 23–9 A freeze-dried, surface-decalcified allogeneic homograft for mandibular replacement. Here it is being fenestrated to provide avenues for revascularization by the autogenous marrow graft that will be placed in the "hollowed-out" central portion of the homogenous bone implant.

---

* Microweb, Millipore Filter Corporation, Bedford, Mass.

masticatory function on alveolar bone has not been carefully delineated, it is possible to say that a modified form of function appears to offer a favorable response to a bone graft in this stage of regeneration.

It has been possible to increase the height of alveolar ridges in clinical patients by as much as 1.5 cm. by this procedure. Follow-up evaluation of patients with ridges restored in this manner has indicated that approximately 30 to 40 per cent of the restored height is resorbed over a 2- to 3-year postoperative period.

Autogenous rib grafts placed in a similar manner to restore lost ridge height also undergo resorption, which in our experience is equal to or greater than that of the marrow grafts.

It therefore appears that further research is indicated in this area.

In an effort to develop a system having more favorable transmission of occlusal forces directly to bone rather than through the mandibular mucosa, and in an effort to reduce the degree of postgrafting bone resorption as well as to create an environment for a stable base upon which to construct a mandibular denture, a new approach to restoration of the deficient mandible has been evolved.[15] After a direct bone impression has been taken, a subperiosteal implant is constructed with struts raised 1 to 1.5 cm. from

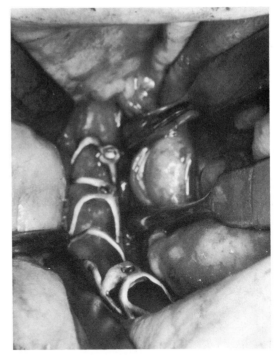

Figure 23–12 The surgical site of a subperiosteal implant–bone graft in a human patient. The space beneath the metal struts will be filled with the grafting material. The screws will be replaced with posts approximately 4 weeks after grafting.

the body of the mandible in the areas of maximum resorption. The casting is stabilized at the anterior border of the ramus and at the anterior mentum area. The space between the old deficient alveolar crest and the casting is

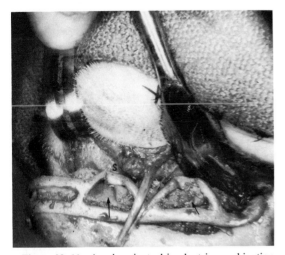

Figure 23–11 A subperiosteal implant in combination with a marrow–cancellous bone graft in a rhesus monkey. The struts of the implant have been raised 1 cm. off the old bony ridge and the space filled with the grafting material (arrows). The tissues will be closed over the combined metal implant–bone graft. At a later date, posts will be screwed into the receptor sites now occupied temporarily by screws (S).

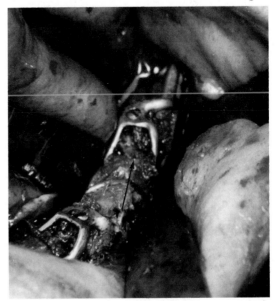

Figure 23–13 The marrow–cancellous bone graft (arrow) has been inserted beneath the metal implant in the case shown in Figure 23–12.

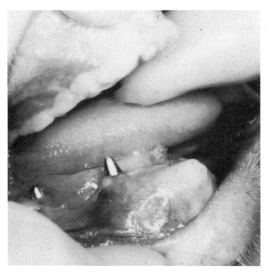

Figure 23–14 The posts have been inserted at the implant receptor sites in a rhesus monkey 5 weeks after the placement of the metal implant and the bone graft.

filled with fresh autogenous cancellous bone and marrow. Figure 23–11 shows the implant and graft in place in a rhesus monkey, and Figures 23–12 and 23–13 illustrate the procedure in a clinical human patient. The mucoperiosteum is closed over the entire graft and metal implant, which contains threaded receptor sites for later insertion of posts. These receptor sites, at the time of grafting, contain temporary screws. After complete healing of

the mucosa (5 weeks), stab incisions are made on the temporary screws and the implant posts are inserted (Fig. 23–14). The usual implant denture suprastructure is constructed. This technique has been used both experimentally in rhesus monkeys and in human patients successfully. Long-term follow-up examination is necessary, however, before a definitive prognosis may be made.[15]

The Use of Marrow–Cancellous Bone in Secondary Grafting of Alveolar and Palatal Clefts. It has been found that autogenous grafts of cancellous bone and marrow may be used with marked success in closing residual fistulas and clefts in patients from the age of 8 through adulthood.[7] Residual clefts of the soft tissue and underlying bone remaining after primary closure of the cleft palate may be effectively managed by closing the soft-tissue nasal floor, packing the defect with the autogenous bone and closing the oral flaps appropriately. *Within 8 weeks* of grafting the cuspid and lateral incisor teeth (if not lost by previous eruption into the cleft area prior to grafting) may be *orthodontically moved* into the newly grafted area (Figs. 23–15 to 23–18).

AUTOGENOUS CARTILAGE GRAFTS

While autogenous cartilagenous chips have been investigated in such a similar system as

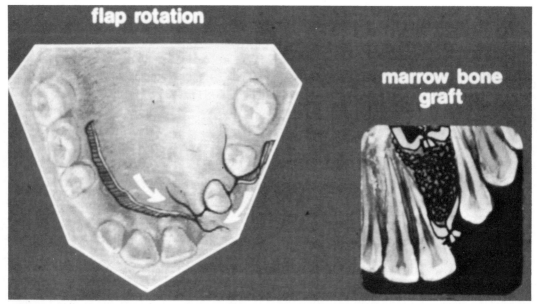

Figure 23–15 Sketch of the flap design for closure of a residual alveolar and palatal cleft in a young adult. The bone graft is placed between the soft-tissue nasal floor and the oral soft-tissue flaps (*right*).

If this procedure is accomplished prior to eruption of the cuspid, both the lateral incisor and the cuspid may be orthodontically moved into the grafted area and aligned in the dental arch.

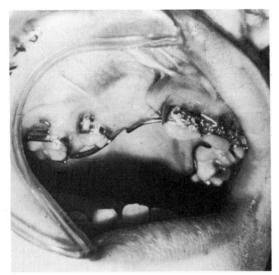

Figure 23–16 A preoperative view of a patient with a residual cleft of the alveolar ridge and palate. A patent oronasal fistula can be seen. The cuspid is unerupted but is in the process of migrating into the void of the cleft, where it would be useless.

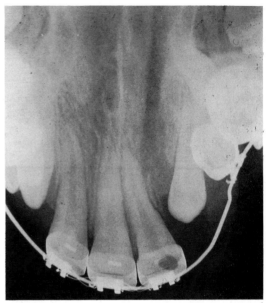

Figure 23–18 A postoperative radiograph showing the cuspid being moved into normal alignment within the grafted area in the case shown in Figures 23–16 and 23–17. The viable graft of autogenous marrow responds to the tooth movement by forming a new lamina dura as the tooth is moved into the area.

that described above, the histologic nature of cartilage is such that revascularization and remodeling by the host tissues is not as extensive as in the case of bone transplants. Cartilage does not offer the same type of grafting milieu as do cancellous autogenous bone and marrow, with their large amount of hemopoietic marrow in marrow–vascular spaces. Such hemopoietic marrow cellular elements are responsible for the osteogenic potential of the particulate cancellous bone graft. While large pieces of autogenous carti-

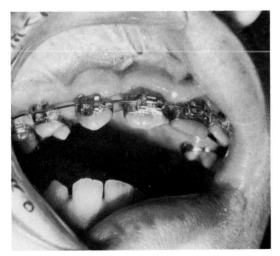

Figure 23–17 Postgrafting view of the case shown in Figure 23–16. Within 3 months of grafting, orthodontic movement was started to bring the cuspid into correct alignment, as shown here. A complete dental arch has been restored.

lage may be used in facial recontouring procedures (*i.e.,* nose, zygoma), they are not usually employed in oral surgical techniques and offer no advantages over bone grafting procedures.

AUTOGENOUS SKIN GRAFTS

Autogenous skin grafts have been used in oral surgery for some time, and more recently the use of split thickness skin in preprosthetic surgery has received additional emphasis. Skin grafts used in oral surgery may therefore be of two types:

1. Full thickness.
2. Split thickness.

Full thickness grafts are usually used in postresection surgical reconstruction in large facial defects and may be used to line the surgical cavity in such facial reconstruction procedures.

For the most part, the skin used in oral surgery is of the split thickness type, ranging from 0.015 in. to 0.025 in. The usual split-thickness graft used in oral surgery is 0.018 in. When used in the oral cavity, such a graft survives and becomes an integral part of the mucosal surface. In addition to the use of such grafts in preprosthetic vestibuloplasty, such split thickness skin transplants may be used to cover a primary stent after resection of various areas of the mandible or maxilla in eradication of tumors. The split thickness skin graft is placed over a stent, which is secured in place for approximately 7 to 10 days, at the end of which time the obturator or stent is removed and the graft is trimmed. Such a graft material serves in the latter instance as a temporary covering over the surgical site, which later may be reconstructed with a larger, thicker skin graft, if necessary, or with a composite bone and skin transplant procedure.

AUTOGENOUS TOOTH TRANSPLANTATION

As indicated previously, the allogeneic transplantation of teeth has not been productive. However, the autogenous transplantation of teeth has been employed successfully during the past few years. This success essentially has been due to the development of more refined surgical transplantation techniques.

Autogenous tooth transplantation may be undertaken under a variety of clinical conditions. The circumstances which produce the need for the surgical procedure tend to dictate the surgical method used and tend to affect markedly the final result of the operation. For example, a well-planned transplant of a lower third molar to the first molar position in the arch has a much better chance of success than the transplantation (reimplantation) of an avulsed tooth in the same relative stage of development.

The basic types of variations of autogenous tooth transplantation are as follows:

1. Surgical repositioning.
2. Reimplantation.
3. Actual transplantation.

All of the above procedures are usually carried out with use of incompletely formed teeth with open apices and vital pulpal tissue capable of forming dentin. However, at times, any of the above procedures may be undertaken on fully formed teeth, usually in conjunction with root canal treatment.

Surgical Repositioning. In surgical repositioning, the tooth is forceably torqued and moved into a new alignment after an osteotomy has first been performed to prepare space within the bony alveolus for reception of the repositioned crown. The operator attempts to keep the apex of the root in the same relative position so that revascularization of the young pulpal tissue may occur postoperatively. However, many times it is necessary to disrupt completely the relationship of the apex to the surrounding bone, thus, in effect, producing a true transplantation of the tooth.[5] Such repositioning procedures undertaken in fully formed teeth lead to nonvital transplants that are later treated with root canal fillings. At times root canal treatment in such teeth may be undertaken at the time of the forceful repositioning of the tooth.

Reimplantation. Reimplantation is a procedure undertaken to return an avulsed or extracted tooth to its original alveolus. In the case of reimplantation of avulsed or partially avulsed teeth with incompletely formed roots, it is hoped that the pulp may retain its vitality and continue to function. As a practical concept, however, this is not realistic because the patient usually presents for treatment one or more hours after the occurrence of the trauma that caused the loss of the tooth. If the reimplanted tooth is to have any degree of assurance of continuing vitality, it must be reinserted into the alveolus within several minutes of the accident at the maximum. As a consequence of delays in treatment, most reimplantations that are undertaken are *nonviable* autografts containing a considerable amount of organic material, drastically altered as a result of the length of time the tooth has been outside of the oral cavity. This drastically changed organic tissue apparently leads to ultimate rejection of the reimplanted tooth by root resorption and replacement of the normal root with new reparative bone (Fig. 23–19).

The long-term success rate of reimplanted teeth in either children or adults has not been good. However, as a temporary replacement procedure that may last for 4 to 5 years, the procedure is a sound surgical one.

Immediate endodontic therapy is necessary in reimplantation surgery involving:

1. Completely avulsed teeth with *fully formed roots.*
2. All cases of teeth with partially formed roots in which a considerable time has elapsed between the accidental avulsion of the teeth and the institution of treatment.

Tooth Transplantation. True tooth transplantation involves the complete removal of the tooth from its donor's socket and a trans-

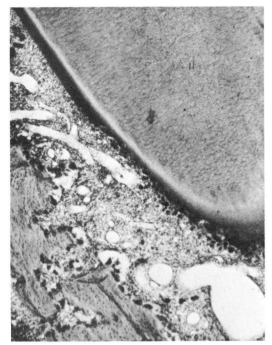

Figure 23–19 Apex of a reimplanted tooth showing osteoclastic resorption of the root. Such resorption usually progresses to eventual loss of the reimplanted tooth.

plantation to another site completely removed from its point of origin. A detailed surgical technique for the transplantation of developing teeth (usually from the third molar to the first molar position) has been well described by Hale and others.[12]

Proper case selection is most important. The optimal root development for transplantation is that exhibiting approximately 3 to 5 mm. of root apical to the crown. An acceptable technique is to prepare the recipient socket site for the transplanted tooth by enlarging the socket and removing the interseptal bone with burs. Damage to the soft tissue of the root sac through instrumentation is avoided in transplanting the tooth from the third molar site. The tooth is placed in the recipient site slightly below the level of occlusion, and it may be stabilized with an acrylic splint, or with wire ligatures crossed over the occlusal portion of the transplanted tooth (see Figure 3–83). In other techniques, no fixation device or wire or gingival packing is used.

This third molar transplant procedure enjoys a high success rate, with 5-year successes being reported in excess of 50 per cent of the cases. A common sequela, however, is failure of complete root formation following transplantation. Nevertheless, these tooth transplants are at times able to become stabilized with a healthy periodontal membrane and survive several years, even in the presence of foreshortened roots. Massive root resorption occurs at times in this technique, leading to the exfoliation of the transplant in the same manner as that occurring in the transplantation of the mature tooth with a fully formed root.

The phenomenon of root resorption in tooth transplantation in general has been thought by some investigators to be associated with degradation of organic material in the root itself during transplantation. Others have felt that the existence of a periodontal ligament on the transplanted root would preclude root resorption and "protect" the root surface from lysis. In research studies of this problem, teeth have been transplanted in conjunction with the surrounding bone in a block section.[16] These investigations have failed to show that the intact periodontal membrane or the surrounding periradicular bone confers any immunity to resorption on the transplanted tooth root.

Although the subject has been investigated extensively, it is felt that much work is still required on immune mechanisms, the physiology of bone repair, and root resorption before significant clinical advancements may be made in this important area of oral surgery.

AUTOGENOUS MUCOSAL TRANSPLANTATION

It is possible under certain conditions to graft autogenous mucosa taken from the buccal or palatal area to another recipient site in the mouth of the same individual. Such grafts usually include the full depth of the mucosa to the layers of submucosa. The transplants are sutured to the recipient site, with or without the use of a splint. A splint may be applied to produce a more optimal degree of pressure on the graft and the underlying surgical bed. The procedure of mucosal grafting in many cases has been a very successful one.[13]

Mucosal transplants have not been developed to more extensive use, primarily because of the difficulty in obtaining the relatively large amount of mucosa necessary for most soft tissue defects. Many of the defects presenting in preprosthetic surgery and maxillofacial reconstruction are of such a size that a considerable amount of soft tissue is needed for closure. Sufficiently large donor sites for such grafts are not normally available in the oral cavity. For small areas, however, mucosal grafts have been shown to be very successful.

SUMMARY

During recent years there has been a marked advancement in transplantation and grafting techniques in oral surgery. These new procedures have included those based on concepts of osteogenic marrow grafting and innovative techniques employing intraoral approaches to the graft recipient sites.

Research efforts in areas involving allied disciplines will undoubtedly produce even more optimal clinical grafting and transplantation procedures in the future, resulting in a higher level of surgical care for oral surgical patients. It is expected that autogenous bone grafting procedures used successfully now will, in the future, be extended to homogenous grafting through the use of banked viable tissues. New research in the immunologic aspects of surgical transplantation will undoubtedly make possible this further extension of the work that has been so productive during the last few years. Additionally, the use of composite bone grafts employing banked nonviable homograft matrix with autogenous marrow appears most promising.

The combination of the expertise of oral surgeons with that of other scientific specialties and disciplines will do much toward improving the delivery of oral surgical and dental health care service.

REFERENCES

1. Barkin, M., Newman, M., and Boyne, P. J.: Ultrastructure of programmed frozen hemopoietic bone marrow. Abstract No. 485, p. 169. International Association for Dental Research, 50th General Session, 1972.
2. Boyne, P. J.: Autogenous cancellous bone and marrow transplants. Clin. Orthop., 73:199–209 (Nov.), 1970.
3. Boyne, P. J.: Restoration of osseous defects in maxillofacial casualties. J.A.D.A., 78:767–776, 1969.
4. Boyne, P. J.: Review of the literature on cryopreservation of bone. Cryobiology, 4(6):341–357, 1968.
5. Boyne, P. J.: Tooth transplantation procedures utilizing bone graft materials. J. Oral Surg., 19:47, 1961.
6. Boyne, P. J., and Cooksey, D. E.: Use of cartilage and bone implants in restoration of edentulous ridges. J.A.D.A., 71:1426–1434 (Dec.), 1965.
7. Boyne, P. J., and Sands, N. R.: Secondary bone grafting of residual alveolar and palatal clefts. J. Oral Surg., 30:87–92 (Feb.), 1972.
8. Boyne, P. J., and Yeager, J. E.: An evaluation of the osteogenic potential of frozen marrow. Oral Surg., 28:764–771 (Nov.), 1969.
9. Chalmers, J.: Transplantation immunity in bone grafting. J. Bone Joint Surg., 41B:160, 1959.
10. Coburn, R. M., and Henriques, B. L.: The development of an experimental tooth bank using deep freeze and tissue culture techniques. J. Oral Ther., 2:445, 1966.
11. Guyton, A. C.: Textbook of Medical Physiology. 2nd ed., p. 174. Philadelphia, W. B. Saunders Co., 1961.
12. Hale, M. L.: Autogenous transplants. J. Oral Surg., 9:76, 1956.
13. Hall, H. D.: Vestibuloplasty mucosal grafts. J. Oral Surg., 29:786–791 (Nov.), 1971.
14. Hyatt, G. W.: The bone homograft-symposium on bone graft surgery. Am. Acad. Orthop. Surg. Instr. Course Lect., 17:133, 1960.
15. Kratochvil, F. J., and Boyne, P. J.: The combined use of subperiosteal implants and bone marrow grafts in edentulous mandible. J. Prosthet. Dent. In press.
16. Luke, A. B., and Boyne, P. J.: Histologic responses following autogenous osseous-dental transplantation. Oral Surg., 26:861–870, 1968.
17. Peer, L. A.: Transplantation of Tissue. Vol. II, p. 41. Baltimore, The Williams & Wilkins Co., 1959.
18. Shulman, L., Hovinga, J., Milstein, C., and Feingold, R.: Fluoride inhibition of tooth allograft root resorption in rhesus monkeys. Abstract No. 595, p. 201. International Association for Dental Research, 49th General Session, 1971.
19. Terasaki, P. I.: Histocompatibility Testing 1970. Copenhagen, Munksgaard, Ltd., 1970.
20. Terasaki, P. I., and Mickey, M. R.: Histocompatibility transplant correlation reproducibility and new matching methods. Transplant. Proc., 3:1057–1071, 1971.

CHAPTER 24

SURGICAL CORRECTION OF ANKYLOSIS OF THE TEMPOROMANDIBULAR JOINT*

YOSHIO WATANABE, D.D.S., M.D., D.Med.Sc.

Ankylosis of the temporomandibular joint is one of the major lesions in the field of oral surgery.[21, 30, 36, 38, 39, 43, 44] To date, its surgical treatment has been described by many surgeons, and numerous clinicostatistical observations have been made.†

INCIDENCE

According to the statistics of the Department of Oral Surgery, Okayama University Hospital,[55] during a 5-year period the total number of outpatients seen was 33,224. Of these, 33 (or 0.1 per cent) had temporomandibular joint ankylosis. Of this group, 25 were later hospitalized and treated for temporomandibular joint ankylosis. These latter patients represented 1.3 per cent of the total hospital inpatients (2028) seen during this period.

SEX AND AGE DISTRIBUTION

There was no marked difference between males and females in the incidence of temporomandibular joint ankylosis. The average

age at which it occurred was 19.4 years, with ages ranging from 2 to 63 years. The number of these patients in the upper age limit was small (only one patient, aged 63, being followed by a 39-year-old patient); therefore, if the more representative age range of 2 to 39 years is used, the average age is calculated as 18.0 years.

Approximately half of the 33 outpatients were in the 10- to 19-year age range. This is understandable, since symptoms become most apparent during this period. According to other authors the highest incidence is in the 11- to 20-year-old group, with occurrence of the condition being less frequent in patients less than age 10 and in those between ages 21 and 30.[27, 33]

In the 33 cases studied, *onset* of ankylosis usually occurred before age 10 (in 21 of 33 patients, *i.e.*, 63.6 per cent). These statistics concur with those of several other authors.[16, 27, 33, 45, 53] Onset occurred less frequently between ages 10 and 19 (10 pa-

* The cooperative assistance of Yoshiro Takanashi, D.D.S., and Kanji Kishi, D.D.S., Clinical Assistants of the Department of Oral Surgery, Okayama University Hospital, is gratefully acknowledged.

† See references 14, 16, 17, 27, 33, 34, 45, 46, 51–53 and 57.

Table 24–1 *Sex and Age Distribution*

AGE	MALE	FEMALE	TOTAL	(%)
< 10	4	2	6	(18.2)
10–19	4	12	16	(48.5)
20–29	5	2	7	(21.2)
≥ 30	3	1	4	(12.1)
Total	16	17	33	(100.0)

Table 24–2 *Locations of Ankylosis*

LOCATION	OPERATED CASES	UNOPERATED CASES	TOTAL
Bilateral	8	1	9
Unilateral			
Left	7	6	13
Right	10	1	11
Total	25*	8	33

* *Note:* 33 joints.

tients, *i.e.,* 30.3 per cent) and after age 20 (2 patients, *i.e.,* 6.1 per cent).

LOCATION AND TYPE

Operations were performed on 25 patients (a total of 33 joints); the 8 patients who did not undergo treatment were seen just for examination or were lost to follow-up.

Bony ankylosis was noted in 15 joints, fibrous ankylosis in 16 joints and indefinite union in 2 joints.

According to the results of Orlow,[33] Padgett et al.,[34] and Topazian,[45] bony ankylosis was seen in a large number of patients. In our experience, however, there was no difference in the number of cases of bony and fibrous ankylosis.

CHIEF COMPLAINT

Of the 33 patients, 24 (12 males and 12 females) complained of difficulty in opening the mouth, and 9 out of 33 (4 males and 5 females) complained of esthetic disfigurement.

CAUSATION

In the present series and those by Kazanjian,[16] Topazian,[45] and Ueno et al.,[52] traumatic injuries were the main cause of ankylosis, accounting for 10 out of 33 cases (30.3 per cent). They were followed in frequency by local infections: 5 cases of furuncle and 1 case each of osteomyelitis of the mandible, parotitis, otitis media and tonsillitis. The systemic diseases erysipelas with beriberi, measels, polyarthritis and dyspepsia each accounted for 1 case of ankylosis.

In some reports local infection is considered to be the most frequent causative factor,[27, 33] being followed in frequency by traumatic injuries, systemic diseases and congenital etiologic factors.

So-called congenital ankylosis is at present thought to evolve from a birth injury and thus to be traumatic in origin,[16, 43, 44] but no such past histories were found in the 6 congenital cases of the author's study.

It is interesting to note that of the 25 patients who were operated on, all those having had local infection or congenital factors as the cause of the joint disease had unilateral ankylosis (Table 24–4).

SYMPTOMS

Restricted mobility or immobility of the temporomandibular joint, in other words, dif-

Table 24–3 *Age Distribution and Causes of Ankylosis*

CAUSE	AGE					TOTAL
	< 1	1–5	5–10	> 10	Unknown	
Congenital	6					6
Traumatic injuries		5	1	4		10
Local infections						
Osteomyelitis				1		1
Parotitis				1		1
Otitis media	1					1
Tonsillitis				1		1
Furuncle	2	2	1			5
Systemic disease	1	1	2			4*
Unknown				1	3	4
Total	10	8	4	8	3	33

* One case each of erysipelas with beriberi, polyarthritis, measles and dyspepsia.

Table 24–4 *Location and Causes of Ankylosis*

CAUSE	BILATERAL	UNILATERAL	TOTAL
Traumatic	5	5	10
Local infections		6	6
Systemic disease	2	2	4
Congenital		2	2
Unknown	1	2	3
Total	8	17	25

ficulty in opening the mouth, or inability to do so, is always seen to a greater or lesser extent with ankylosis of this joint.

Facial asymmetry due to mandibular deformity is usually noted in cases of unilateral ankylosis and has been described by many authors. Deviation of the midline of the mandible to the affected side occurs because of less mandibular growth on that side. In the case of bilateral ankylosis, there is a symmetrical lack of growth, causing underdevelopment of the whole mandible (*i.e.,* microgenia), so that the facial contour is described by the term "bird-face."

An explanation for this hypoplasia, according to Kazanjian,[16] is that the ankylosed joint directly affects an important growth center in the condyle and thus interferes with normal growth. Lack of proper function then leads to the hypoplasia. Probably both of these factors contribute to the condition. Moreover, the effects on mandibular growth of misplaced and unused teeth in the young may be another factor.

Therefore, mandibular deformity is marked when the patient has a causative disease while the mandible is developing; it is not so marked, however, when onset of ankylosis occurs after complete development of the mandible. The earlier ankylosis occurs, the more severely the mandible is deformed, the condition sometimes being complicated by maxillary deformity, which results in asymmetry. This was confirmed by Kubota in animal experiments.[22] The effects of interference with the temporomandibular joint on the growth of facial bones was investigated in premature dogs. Underdevelopment of the mandible on the side of the affected joint was shown, particularly in the case of condylectomy of the temporomandibular joint.

Another symptom of ankylosis is the presence of many carious teeth, associated with gingivitis due to poor oral hygiene. This problem stems from difficulty in opening the mouth.

DIAGNOSIS

Ankylosis of the temporomandibular joint is easily diagnosed. Restricted mobility or immobility of the joint is readily noticed by palpating the condylar movement. Placing his fingertips in the external auditory canals or in the preauricular areas, the examiner instructs the patient to open and close his mouth. In addition, facial deformity enables one to differentiate which side is affected, since the midline of the mandible is deviated toward the affected side in the case of unilateral ankylosis. With bilateral ankylosis, "bird-face" is usually marked. Radiograms are also helpful in diagnosis.[42]

Case Report No. 1

UNILATERAL TEMPOROMANDIBULAR JOINT ANKYLOSIS WITH MICROGENIA

Patient. A 19-year-old female had had a swelling at the left preauricular area and a pus-containing discharge from her ear 20 days after birth. When she was 6 years old, her family noted that her mandible deviated to the left side. She experienced trismus at age 12, but this symptom disappeared after a period of about 1 month, during which time she had a bandage over her mandible.

The patient consulted us complaining of facial asymmetry and difficulty in opening her mouth.

Examination. The mandible deviated 15 mm. to the left, and the facial contour was typically "bird-face" (Fig. 24–1). The upper and lower incisal distance was 18 mm. (Fig. 24–2*A*). The right lower bicuspids and molars showed linguoversion.

Radiograms indicated a deviation of the maxilla and mandible to the left, with particularly marked atrophy of the body and ascending ramus of the mandible. The left condyle was flat and united with the articular fossa, and the sigmoid notch and coronoid process were difficult to see (Fig.

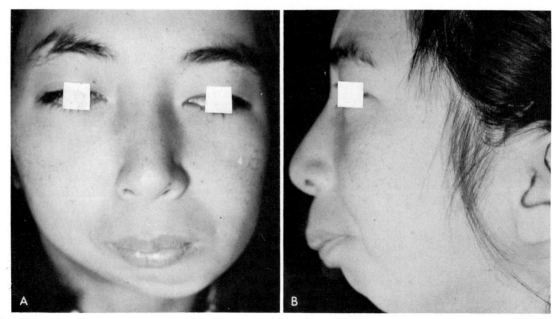

Figure 24–1 "Bird-face" appearance due to ankylosis of the left temporomandibular joint and resultant microgenia. (See Case Report No. 1 for further details.)

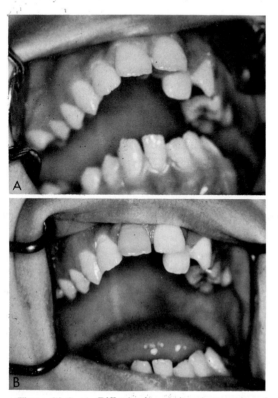

Figure 24–2 *A,* Difficulty in opening the mouth and linguoversion of teeth before operation. *B,* Wider opening after surgical correction of joint ankylosis.

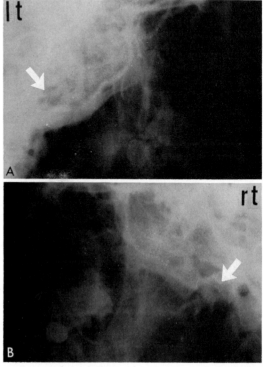

Figure 24–3 *A,* Left (*lt.*), and *B,* right (*rt.*), temporomandibular joints before operation.

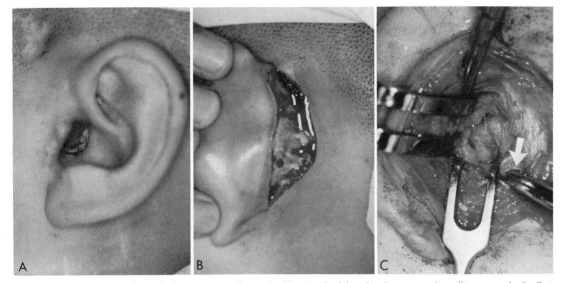

Figure 24–4 Bockenheimer-Axhausen procedure. *A*, Circular incision in the external auditory canal. *B*, Retroauricular incision. *C*, Exposure of the temporomandibular joint. The arrow points to the left external auditory canal.

24–3*A*). The right condyle was normal (Fig. 24–3*B*).

Diagnosis. Examination of the patient confirmed ankylosis of the left temporomandibular joint associated with microgenia.

Operative Notes. A circular incision in the external auditory canal (Fig. 24–4*A*) and a retroauricular incision (Fig. 24–4*B*) were made according to the Bockenheimer-Axhausen procedure. The ear lobe was retracted forward and the joint was reached from the retroauricular area beyond the external auditory canal (Fig. 24–4*C*).

In order to prevent reunion of the surfaces of the joint, a folded and sutured spindle-shaped skin flap, taken from the abdominal area (Fig. 24–5), was interposed in the joint space (Fig. 24–6*A*). The auricle was replaced and sutured (Fig. 24–6*B*) without noticeable scarring.

After the use of a mouth exerciser the patient was able to open her mouth 38 mm. (Figs. 24–2*B* and 24–7). One year later bilateral osteotomy of both ascending rami was performed with a Kärger needle (Kostečka procedure) to move the mandible forward and to the right after roentgen cephalometric measurement. Supplementary orthodontic treatment was used to correct occlusion. One

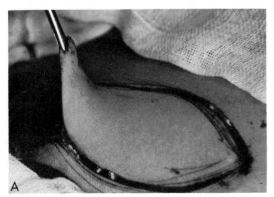
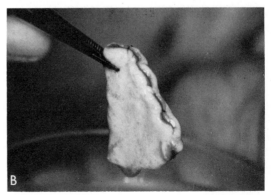

Figure 24–5 Interposition. *A*, Spindle-shaped skin flap removed from abdomen. *B*, Flap folded and sutured to interpose in the joint and prevent bony reunion.

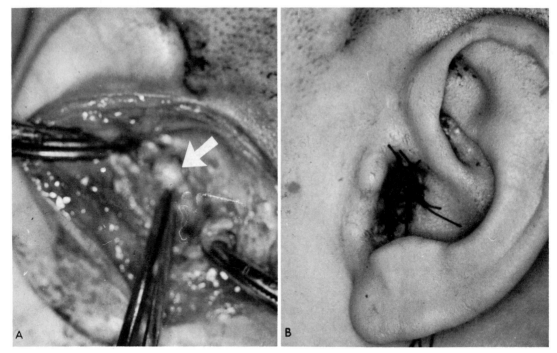

Figure 24–6 *A,* Interposing skin flap (*arrow*) inserted into joint. *B,* Suturing of external auditory canal after replacement of ear (auricle).

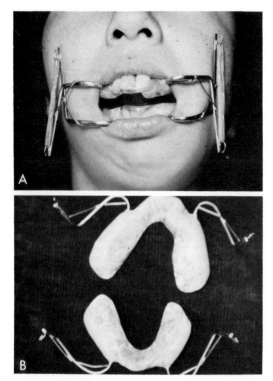

Figure 24–7 Mouth exerciser used after surgery. Note that patient is able to open mouth more widely.

month later a piece of autogenous bone taken from the right spina iliaca anterior was transplanted to the mandible, and was secondarily associated with tantalum gauze implantation[55] performed 6 months later (Fig. 24–8).

Two years later satisfactory results were obtained (Fig. 24–9).

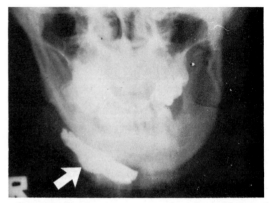

Figure 24–8 Autogenous transplant from ilium and tantalum gauze implant to correct asymmetry of the mandible.

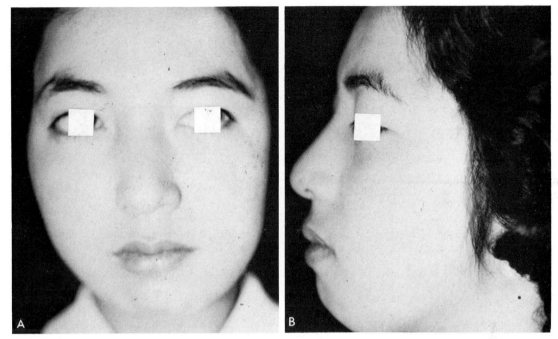

Figure 24–9 Postoperative appearance.

OPERATIVE PROCEDURE

Approach to the Joint. Several approaches to the temporomandibular joint and a variety of incisions have been used and are being employed at present. The joints are approached roughly in two ways: (1) retroauricularly[2, 3, 29, 47] or (2) preauricularly.[30, 37, 48]

When operating on the temporomandibular joint it is most important to expose the joint adequately without injuring the branches of the facial nerve and the parotid gland, which are positioned close to the joint. In this respect, the retroauricular approach is better than the preauricular, but one disadvantage of the former technique is that it takes about twice as long as the latter one to perform.

The Bockenheimer-Axhausen procedure was first performed in Japan by Nakamura in 1934.[29, 32] This procedure was utilized in operations for nine of the joints in this series. After Ueno described his preauricular incision in 1961,[48] however, the Bockenheimer-Axhausen procedure was replaced by the Ueno technique in the remaining 24 joints in this series.

Interposition. Folded skin flaps were used in all cases in this series as interposing material in the joint for the purpose of preventing bony or fibrous union or recurrence of ankylosis. Some surgeons, however, have omitted the interposition when a 2-cm. separation was made between the cut margin of the mandible and the temporal bone.[5, 12, 35, 44] Padgett and colleagues used fascia or a tantalum cup in some instances but used nothing in most cases.[34]

Topazian employed dermis or muscle in interposition arthroplasty; however, some of his patients were treated by gap arthroplasty.[45, 46] Through a comparative investigation of gap and interposition arthroplasty in the treatment of temporomandibular joint ankylosis, he showed that recurrence of ankylosis is less likely when autogenous tissue is interposed to fill the defect between the bone ends.[46]

The following interposing substances have been utilized to prevent reunion of the temporomandibular joint:

1. Vital material: temporal fascia,[16] free skin flap,[9, 24, 29, 47, 48, 53] connective tissue,[35] fat,[23] muscle,[40] cartilage,[13, 25, 41] chromic autofascia,[15] OMS membrane,[31] and JK membrane.[30]*

---

* The OMS membrane, named after Drs. Okuda, Matsuno and Satsuma, who first produced it, is chromicized small intestine from the horse. (It is now available commercially.) The JK membrane, named after Drs. Jinnaka and Kono, is chromicized autofascia.

2. Nonvital material: acrylic resin,[30] oxidized cellulose (Oxycel),[18] tantalum,[6, 10, 11, 34, 44, 51] zirconium,[50] cobalt-chromium alloy (Vitallium),[50] and Akiyama's (polyvinyl alcohol plus dimethyl polysiloxan [PVA + DMPS]) membrane.[1, 8]

The author prefers to use an autogenous skin flap taken from the abdominal area (*i.e.*, Lindemann's abdominal free skin flap) because it causes no foreign body reaction, and because it is comparatively easy to acquire at any time or in any size.

Case Report No. 2

UNILATERAL TEMPOROMANDIBULAR JOINT ANKYLOSIS

Patient. This 16-year-old female had been operated on during her childhood for congenital dislocation of the hip joint. She had suffered from measles about 13 years previously and had had a high fever which continued for about 1 month. Her mother explained that the patient had been found in bed pushing her left cheek against a pillow. Thereafter, right deviation of the mandible had progressed gradually. The patient was admitted complaining of difficulty in opening her mouth.

Examination. The midline of the mandible deviated to the right, with an apparent depressed flatness of the left mandibular body and marked facial asymmetry (Fig. 24–10). The patient could open her mouth only 7 mm. (Fig. 24–11*A*). Plani-

graphic radiograms revealed extensive radiolucency at the right temporomandibular joint and no abnormality at the left joint (Fig. 24–12).

Diagnosis. Examination of the patient confirmed ankylosis of the right temporomandibular joint.

Operative Notes. Preauricular incision according to the Ueno procedure was performed so that the affected joint could be exposed (Fig. 24–13). Fibrous union was noticed between the articular fossa and condyle; it was excised, and parts of the bone were chiseled off.

Favorable results were achieved (Fig. 24–11*B*), and the patient was discharged 16 days after her operation. She was able to open her mouth 26 mm.

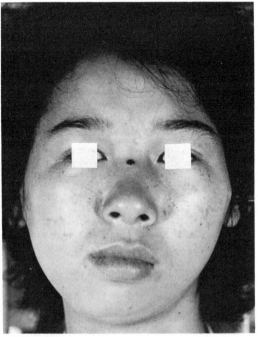

Figure 24–10 Facial asymmetry due to temporomandibular joint ankylosis caused by childhood measles. (See Case Report No. 2 for further details.)

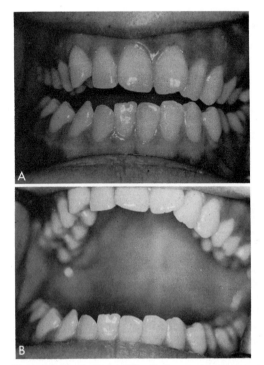

Figure 24–11 *A*, Great difficulty in opening the mouth before surgery. *B*, Greater ease postoperatively.

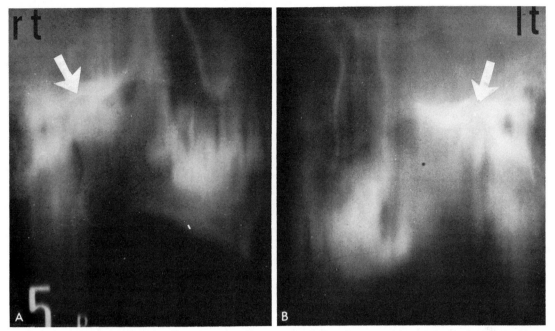

Figure 24-12 *A,* Right *(rt.),* and *B,* left *(lt.),* temporomandibular joints before surgery.

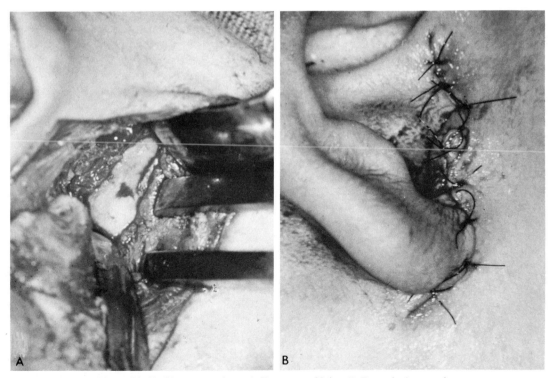

Figure 24-13 Ueno procedure. *A,* Exposure of joint. *B,* Preauricular suturing.

POSTOPERATIVE CARE

After the operation a cork stopper is always used as a wedge between the upper and lower posterior teeth. This is then replaced by an exerciser, a mouth-opening appliance (see Figure 24–7). After postoperative pain is gone the patient is encouraged to chew gum or *surume* (*i.e.,* Japanese dried squid) as an exercise at frequent intervals.

Broglia recommended the immediate initiation of orthodontic and prosthodontic procedures to obtain balanced occlusion.[4]

Following postoperative care, the correction of mandibular deformities due to ankylosis of the temporomandibular joint, such as facial asymmetry and microgenia, which were previously discussed, should be considered, since these deformities still remain after mobilization of the ankylosed joint. Treatment of these deformities is discussed in Chapter 22.

Case Report No. 3

BILATERAL TEMPOROMANDIBULAR JOINT ANKYLOSIS

Patient. This 20-year-old male was a farmer who apparently had no hereditary factors bearing on his condition. At age 10 he had fallen from a 4-m. height and suffered a contusion from the lower lip to the mental region. Owing to this injury, he had undergone surgery and subsequent immobilization of the mandible for 2 months. Since then, he had suffered from trismus.

At age 13 he had consulted a general surgeon and later an orthopedic surgeon but received no treatment. He had developed tinnitus at age 17, and since then trismus had gradually increased.

Finally he was referred to us because of inability to open his mouth (Fig. 24–15*A*).

Examination. Facial asymmetry with microgenia was marked (Fig. 24–14*A*). The digastric and sternohyoid muscles were clearly noticeable (Fig. 24–14*A*) when the patient tried to open his mouth, which he succeeded in doing by only 1 mm. (Fig. 24–15*A*). There was a scar on his lower lip, and the midline of the mandible deviated to the right.

Radiograms revealed a wide radiolucency in the area of the right temporomandibular joint and

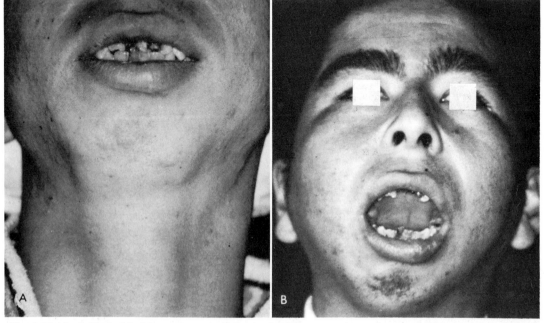

Figure 24–14 *A*, Marked facial asymmetry and microgenia with severe trismus due to ankylosis of the temporomandibular joints. *B*, After bilateral surgery, the patient was able to open his mouth. (See Case Report No. 3 for further details.)

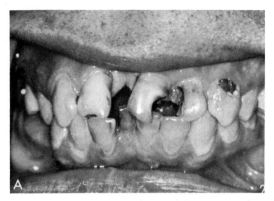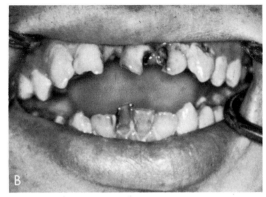

Figure 24-15 *A*, Preoperative, and *B*, postoperative, ability to open the mouth. Note also extensive caries and gingivitis due to poor oral hygiene during inability to open the mouth.

showed no condyle (Fig. 24-16); the condyle at the left joint appeared normal. Palpation revealed no movement of either condyle when he tried to open his mouth.

Diagnosis. Ankylosis of the bilateral temporomandibular joints with facial asymmetry was confirmed by examination of the patient.

Operative Notes. A preauricular incision at the right joint, made according to the Ueno procedure, showed a complete bony union in the area of the condyle. The zygomatic arch and condyle were partly excised, and a skin flap was removed, in the manner previously discussed, and was interposed between the newly formed joint surfaces.

After this surgery the patient could open his mouth only 7 mm. A week later, however, the same operation was performed on the left joint, which showed fibrous union, and then he was able to open his mouth 20 mm. (Figs. 24-14*B* and 24-15*B*).

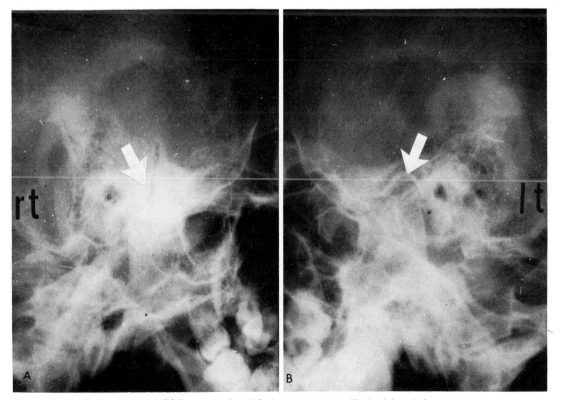

Figure 24-16 *A*, Right (*rt.*), and *B*, left (*lt.*), temporomandibular joints before surgery.

Table 24–5 *Prognosis of Temporomandibular Joint Ankylosis*

Favorable	11
Moderate	1*
Unfavorable	2*
Indefinite	11
Total	25

* Bilateral ankylosis.

PROGNOSIS

As shown in Table 24–5, the prognosis of ankylosis was not always favorable, although 14 patients experienced no recurrence of the condition. The progress of 11 patients in this series could not be determined since they were lost to follow-up.

Eschler's studies on the action of the masseter muscle following surgery for ankylosis proved that late recurrence was usually due to insufficient muscular strength.[7] This was confirmed by histologic examination of atrophy of the mandibular body and periodontium.

REFERENCES

1. Akiyama, T.: Medical application of dimethyl polysiloxan. Jap. J. Plast. Reconstr. Surg., *1:*244, 1958.
2. Axhausen, G.: Die operative Freilegung des Kiefergelenks. Chirurg, *3:*713, 1931.
3. Axhausen, G.: Beiträge zur Mund- und Kieferchirurgie. Dtsch. Zahnheilkd., *82:*103, 1932.
4. Broglia, M. L.: Anchilosi temporo-mandibolare monolaterale in bambino di 5 anni. Minerva Stomatol., *11:*26, 1961.
5. Dingman, R. O.: Ankylosis of the temporomandibular joint. Am. J. Orthod., *32:*120, 1946.
6. Eggers, G. W. N.: Arthroplasty of temporomandibular joint in children with interposition of tantalum foil: A preliminary report. J. Bone Joint Surg., *28:*603, 1946.
7. Eschler, J.: Die Muskelfunktion bei Kiefergelenkankylose und ihre Auswirkung auf Kiefer und Paradentien. Dtsch. Zahn. Mund. Kieferheilkd., *17:*400, 1953.
8. Fujino, H., Tashiro, H., Kurata, K., *et al.*: The use of (PVA + DMPS) membrane as interposition in mobilizing temporomandibular joint ankylosis. Jap. J. Plast. Reconstr. Surg., *9:*183, 1966.
9. Georgiade, N., Altany, F., Pickrell, K., *et al.*: An experimental and clinical evaluation of autogenous dermal grafts used in the treatment of temporomandibular joint ankylosis. Plast. Reconstr. Surg., *19:*321, 1957.
10. Goodsell, J. O.: Tantalum in temporomandibular arthroplasty. J. Oral Surg., *5:*41, 1947.
11. Goodsell, J. O.: Tantalum in temporomandibular arthroplasty after twelfth postoperative year: Report of case. J. Oral Surg., *16:*517, 1958.
12. Górski, M.: Zur Behandlung der Kiefergelenkankylose. Dtsch. Zahn. Mund. Kieferheilkd., *40:*97, 1963.
13. Hinds, E. C., and Pleasants, J. E.: Reconstruction of the temporomandibular joint. Am. J. Surg., *90:*931, 1955.
14. Horikoshi, T.: Clinico-statistical observation of temporomandibular ankylosis operation. J. Jap. Stomatol. Soc., *1:*275, 1952.
15. Jinnaka, S., and Kono, S.: Arthroplasty. Nippon Rinsho (Japan), *6:*323, 1948.
16. Kazanjian, V. H.: Ankylosis of the temporomandibular joint. Surg. Gynecol. Obstet., *67:*333, 1938.
17. Kazanjian, V. H.: Mandibular retrusion with ankylosis of the temporomandibular joint. Plast. Reconstr. Surg., *17:*91, 1956.
18. Kelikian, H.: A method of mobilizing the temporomandibular joint. J. Bone Joint Surg., *32:*113, 1950.
19. Kostečka, F.: Chirurgická terapie anomalií Angleovy III. třídy čili t. zv. progenie. Zubní, lék, *25:*65, 1925. (Cited by Nakamura.)
20. Kostečka, F.: Die chirurgische Therapie der Progenie. Zahnaerztl. Rundsch., *40:*669, 1931.
21. Kruger, G. O.: Textbook of Oral Surgery. 2nd ed., p. 447. St. Louis, C. V. Mosby Co., 1964.
22. Kubota, Y.: An experimental study on the influence of interference of the temporomandibular joint upon the growth of facial bones. J. Jap. Stomatol. Soc., *27:*368, 1960.
23. Limberg, A. A.: Die chirurgische Frühbehandlung der erworbenen einseitigen Mikrogenie mit oder ohne Kieferankylose. Dtsch. Zahn. Mund. Kieferheilkd., *31:*143, 1959. (Abstr.)
24. Lindemann, A.: Die chirurgische Behandlung der Erkrankungen des Kiefergelenkes. Z. Stomatol., *XXIII:*395, 1925.
25. Longacre, J. J., and Gilby, R. F.: The use of autogenous cartilage graft in arthroplasty for true ankylosis of temporomandibular joint. Plast. Reconstr. Surg., *7:*271, 1951.
26. Masuda, T., and Ishida, K.: The use of Co-Cr alloy as interposition in case of mobilization of temporomandibular ankylosis. J. Jap. Stomatol. Soc., *6:*451, 1957.
27. Miyakawa, Y., and Kawakami, H.: Clinico-statistical observation of ankylosis of the temporomandibular joint. J. Jap. Stomatol. Soc., *6:*331, 1957. (Abstr.)
28. Nakamura, H.: Surgical correction of progenia and prognathia. Nihon-no-Shikai (Japan), No. 138, 1932.
29. Nakamura, H.: Contribution to mobilization of the temporomandibular ankylosis. J. Jap. Stomatol. Soc., *10:*559, 1936. (Abstr.)
30. Oka, T.: Diseases of the temporomandibular joint (4). Dent. Outlook (Japan), *16:*164, 1959.
31. Okuda, Y., and Matsuno, M.: Arthroplasty by interposition of the OMS membrane. Surg. Ther., *12:*390, 1950.
32. Oral Surgery Department, Tokyo Medical and Dental University: Publication in honor of the tenth anniversary of Professor Tadashi Ueno, p. 143, 1961.
33. Orlow, L. W.: Ankylosis Mandibulae Vera. Dtsch. Z. Chirurg., *66:*399, 1903.

34. Padgett, E. C., *et al.*: Ankylosis of the temporomandibular joint. Surgery, *24:*426, 1948.
35. Parker, D. B.: Ankylosis of the temporomandibular joint. J. Oral Surg., *6:*42, 1948.
36. Perthes, G., and Borchers, E.: Verletzungen und Krankheiten der Kiefer. Vol. II, p. 186. Stuttgart, Ferdinand Enke Verlag, 1932.
37. Ritter, R.: Chirurgisch-orthopädische Therapie der Kiefergelenkerkrankungen. Kirschners allg. u. spez. chirurg. Operationslehre, *IV:*131. Berlin, Springer-Verlag, 1956.
38. Sarnat, B. G., and Laskin, D. M.: Diagnosis and Surgical Management of Diseases of the Temporomandibular Joint, p. 61. Springfield, Ill., Charles C Thomas, 1962.
39. Schwartz, L.: Disorders of the Temporomandibular Joint, pp. 266, 389, 394. Philadelphia, W. B. Saunders Co., 1959.
40. Smith, J. B.: Temporomandibular ankylosis. J. Oral Surg., *8:*297, 1950.
41. Snijman, P. C.: Ankylosis of the temporomandibular joint treated by osteoarthrotomy: Report of a case. Oral Surg., *15:*389, 1962.
42. Steinhardt, G.: Pathologische Veränderungen der Kiefergelenke. Handbuch d. medizinischen Radiologie, p. 877. Berlin, Springer-Verlag, 1963.
43. Thoma, K. H., and Goldman, H. M.: Oral Pathology, 5th ed., p. 858. St. Louis, C. V. Mosby Co., 1960.
44. Thoma, K. H.: Oral Surgery. 4th ed., Vol. 2, p. 605. St. Louis, C. V. Mosby Co., 1963.
45. Topazian, R. G.: Etiology of ankylosis of temporomandibular joint: Analysis of 44 cases. J. Oral Surg., *22:*227, 1964.
46. Topazian, R. G.: Comparison of gap and interposition arthroplasty in the treatment of temporomandibular joint ankylosis. J. Oral Surg., *24:*405, 1966.
47. Ueno, T.: Mobilization of the temporomandibular joint. Shujutsu (Japan), *10:*464, 1956.
48. Ueno, T.: Preauricular approach in case of mobilization of the temporomandibular joint. Jap. J. Oral Surg., *6:*206, 1960.
49. Ueno, T.: Operative technic of prognathism. Jap. J. Plast. Reconstr. Surg., *4:*123, 1961.
50. Ueno, T., *et al.*: The use of zirconium metal plate in arthroplasty of temporomandibular ankylosis. Bull. Tokyo Med. Dent. Univ., *2:*137, 1955.
51. Ueno, T., *et al.*: Temporomandibular joint ankylosis followed by microgenia: Analysis of 104 cases. Jap. J. Plast. Reconstr. Surg., *4:*73, 1961. (Abstr.)
52. Ueno, T., *et al.*: Studies on treatment and results of temporomandibular ankylosis. I. Clinico-statistical observation. J. Jap. Stomatol. Soc., *18:*246, 1969. (Abstr.)
53. Watanabe, Y.: Temporomandibular ankylosis and its surgical correction. Nihon-Iji-Shimpo (Japan), *3:*1001, 1941.
54. Watanabe, Y.: Surgical correction of mandibular deformity by autogenous bone grafting. Jap. J. Plast. Reconstr. Surg., *1:*259, 1958.
55. Watanabe, Y.: Surgical correction of ankylosis of the temporomandibular joint. Oral Surgery Lectures, Surgical Demonstrations and Dedication Program of the W. H. Archer Oral Surgery Clinic, Pittsburgh, Oct. 15, 1968.
56. Watanabe, Y., *et al.*: Tantalum gauze implantation in case of mandibular deformity. Jap. J. Plast. Reconstr. Surg., *4:*288, 1961.
57. Watanabe, Y., *et al.*: Clinico-statistical summary of 27 cases of temporomandibular joint ankylosis experienced at our department during the past ten years. J. Jap. Stomatol. Soc., *16:*1, 1967.

CHAPTER 25

COMPLICATIONS ASSOCIATED WITH ORAL SURGERY

Operations in the oral cavity may be followed by either immediate or delayed complications. These complications may be either systemic (caused by altered physiology) or local (related to surgical or anesthetic injection techniques).

Immediate Complications. Complications that may occur during an operation include syncope, cardiac arrest, myocardial infarction, acute allergic reactions to antibiotics or anesthetic solutions, angioedema and shock. Surgical and local anesthetic techniques may result in such complications as hematoma, emphysema, broken dental needles, broken roots, roots in the maxillary sinus, hemorrhage, fracture of the maxillary tuberosity and of the floor of the antrum, fracture of a large segment of the labial or buccal alveolar bone with attached mucoperiosteal tissue, inadvertent extraction of adjacent teeth, fracture or dislodgment of an adjacent tooth or filling, nerve injury, dislocation of the mandible, fracture of the maxilla or mandible, perforation of the palate, laceration of the surrounding tissues, maxillary antro-oral fistula or naso-oral fistula.

Delayed Complications. Later sequelae or oral operations include postoperative pain, secondary hemorrhage, soft-tissue infection, bone infection, pathologic fractures, systemic infection, trismus, subacute bacterial endocarditis, allergic reactions to antibiotics, epulis granulomatosa, herniation of the maxillary sinus epithelial lining through the alveolus, acute nephritis, thyroid crisis and rarely carcinoma.

SYNCOPE

Vasodepressor syncope (acute cerebral anemia or common faint) is the earliest form of shock, and it is generally transient. The signs of syncope are an ashy gray color of the skin, cold perspiration, small pulse pressure, and a feeling of dizziness, lightheadedness or nausea.

When a patient presents signs of "fainting," the back of the dental chair should be immediately lowered so that the head is lower than the feet; tight clothing should be loosened; and reflex stimulation should be secured by applying cold water to the face and by cautious inhalation of the vapors of aromatic spirits of ammonia. In a standard dental chair, lowering the head below the level of the feet is difficult, so it may be necessary for the surgeon to lift the feet manually once the patient is recumbent. Elevation of the feet straight up from a supine position will redistribute at least 1000 cc. of blood to the circulating volume in the area above the waist and rapidly help to restore adequate cerebral circulation and oxygenation.

If the surgeon has failed to note the objective symptoms of impending syncope, and is suddenly aware that his patient is unconscious, that his pupils are widely dilated, and that he is manifesting convulsive movements of the extremities as a result of the cerebral hypoxia, he should immediately carry out the steps already outlined, being careful that the unconscious patient does not slide out of the back of the chair. In addition, he should administer 100 per cent oxygen if air hunger is apparent. Persistent hypotension may require use of phenylephrine, ephedrine, Methedrine, methoxamine hydrochloride or epinephrine.

Keep the patient warm and in a supine position until he has fully recovered. Check the patient's pulse and respiratory rate, and take the blood pressure periodically.

Silent or overt regurgitation of stomach contents commonly occurs with vasodepressor syncope. Aspiration of this material could precipitate a life-threatening emergency,[1] and the surgeon or auxiliary is advised to check the airway for patency immediately after placing the patient in the supine position.

The best way to treat syncope is by prevention. Adequate premedication when indicated is helpful, but when a patient presents with a history of syncope, especially following the injection of a local anesthetic solution, it is probably advisable to put the patient in the typical recumbent "shock" position prior to the injection.

SHOCK

Shock is a circulatory deficiency that is either cardiac or vasomotor in origin and characterized by decreased cardiac output and hemoconcentration.

While psychogenic syncope is the most frequent immediate postinjection and surgical complication, the oral surgeon must not forget the possibility of hypovolemic shock, that caused by peripheral pooling of blood and cardiogenic shock (the three hemodynamic kinds of shock) during or immediately after a prolonged surgical procedure in the oral cavity.

Shock passes through several stages. The first is *primary shock* that results from reflex and emotional causes and is essentially syncope. If the primary shock is not immediately fatal, the body's defense mechanism takes over, and the patient returns to normal, or *secondary shock* appears. The skin is pale, cold, and clammy from sweat; the mucous membranes are pale; the lips, nails, tips of fingers and toes, and the lobes of the ears are grayish blue; the face appears pinched and expressionless; the eyes are sunken and fixed with a purposeless stare; the pupils are dilated and react but feebly; the pulse is weak, usually rapid, and often intermittent; the res-

pirations are rapid, shallow and irregular, and there is an occasional sigh; and the temperature is below normal. Consciousness usually is maintained, though the mind is apathetic. All these signs are evidence of decreased circulatory volume that is becoming progressively irreversible unless aggressive measures are instituted. Unlike primary shock or syncope, secondary shock does not usually undergo spontaneous remission.

Treatment. Shock can be more easily prevented than treated.

The very first step in the treatment of shock is to determine the clinical cause for this cardiovascular collapse. Is it due to hypovolemic circulation, painful stimuli or emotional upset?

Absolute rest and relief from pain or distress, if present, may be gained by administering an analgesic or narcotic. Narcotics and analgesics must be used in small amounts intravenously, as excessive narcotics tend to depress the vascular responses to oligemia. Morphine, 0.05 to 0.1 mg. per kg. of body weight, may be given intravenously, provided there are no cerebral injuries. If veins are inaccessible, the sublingual route is usually a safe alternate route, but usually a vein is available either directly or through a "cut-down" procedure.

Body heat should be maintained by keeping the normal room temperature and placing a light sheet, drape, or blanket over the patient. The patient should not be "bundled" with blankets, hot water bottles or the like.

The patient in oligemic shock should have his legs elevated 20 degrees to perfuse the vital centers properly, while the head and thorax should be elevated 5 degrees, thus lowering the diaphragm to provide better ventilation.

Lost body fluid must be restored. In all cases of shock, the pulse and blood pressure should be taken at frequent intervals, since these are one of the most reliable indicators of the severity of the shock. If considerable blood has been lost, blood transfusion is the supreme and perhaps the lifesaving remedy. A complete blood count and hematocrit at this time may indicate a hemoconcentration or higher values for hemoglobin, erythrocytes and volume of packed erythrocytes than were present preoperatively. This is a serious sign and requires energetic countermeasures. The blood count as measured by usual laboratory determinations is not immediately reduced, even by severe loss of blood. Total blood volume determinations (difficult and time consuming to perform with present methods) are necessary to thoroughly evaluate the quantitative degree of blood loss.

A previously healthy patient in shock from blood loss can be assumed to have lost at least 1000 to 1500 ml. of blood. This amount may be replaced with an equal amount of 5 per cent dextrose in a saline solution or Ringer's. A deficit greater than this should be replaced with *compatible* whole blood. Regular 10 per cent dextran is also a temporary substitute until whole blood is available. As soon as improvement has been noted, the solution should be stopped, because giving too much solution or giving it too rapidly may seriously embarrass the heart.

Adequate oxygenation of body tissues must be maintained at all times. To combat hypoxemia oxygen should be administered at 5 liters per minute through a plastic nasal catheter so that even though the blood volume and cardiac output are lowered, the blood that does circulate is carrying a full capacity of oxyhemoglobin, which then liberates oxygen to maintain the cells of the vital centers. Adequate oxygen also helps maintain body metabolism and hence body heat. Oxygen is essential in the treatment of shock.

CARDIAC COMPLICATIONS

MYOCARDIAL INFARCTION AND CORONARY INSUFFICIENCY

Although dentists seldom see myocardial infarction in their offices, a coronary occlusion may occur after surgical shock. Stress, either surgical or emotional, may induce an attack of angina pectoris if the patient has coronary artery disease and coronary insufficiency.

It is important for the dentist to recognize immediately the subjective and objective symptoms of myocardial infarctions, which are as follows: (1) midsternal or substernal pain, sometimes radiating down the left shoulder and arm, occasionally to the neck, jaws and right arm; (2) feeling of impending suffocation and death; (3) shortness of breath; (4) sudden and profuse perspiration; (5) vomiting; (6) hypotension; and (7) tachycardia.

When cardiac symptoms first appear, 1 or 2 sublingual nitroglycerin tablets ($1/200$ grain) may be given. Oxygen (with full face mask) is also indicated. If the attack is angina pectoris, dramatic relief will be noted in less than 3 minutes. Sometimes an ampule of amyl nitrite applied under the nose will relieve an anginal episode. These drugs are essentially innocuous and should be used when cardiogenic pain is suspected. Since they are vasodilators the patient may have a transient headache or possibly syncope. If the pain persists for more than 15 minutes, a myocardial infarction should be suspected. Then the following steps should be taken immediately. The assistant should call the nearest hospital and ambulance. While awaiting the ambulance's arrival, the dentist should: (1) administer oxygen; (2) alleviate pain with morphine sulfate ($1/6$ grain) or Demerol (50 mg.) either intramuscularly or intravenously; (3) if the heart rate is slow, use atropine sulfate, $1/150$ grain intramuscularly or intravenously, to prevent vagal vasoconstriction of the coronary arteries; and (4) start intravenous fluids (5 per cent dextrose in saline) slowly in case shock develops. Vasoconstrictor drugs may have to be given intravenously. The patient should be given oxygen by face mask as well as intravenous support while being transferred to hospital. The dentist should be with the patient in the ambulance; his assistant should notify the hospital cardiac care unit that the patient is on the way so that proper medical attention will be available upon the patient's arrival.

Dentists can make themselves helpful by following these essential principles and by immediately recognizing myocardial infarction during or after anesthesia or surgery.

It is the dentist's moral and legal responsibility to have emergency drugs available and be competent in using them, since the health of the dental patient is the dentist's responsibility while he is in his office. The dentist can help in managing the patient in such a manner that the condition will be alleviated rather than intensified.

CARDIAC ARREST

This is a rare complication of oral surgery, per se, but may follow the administration of any anesthetic, local or general, or it may be entirely associated with emotional stress. All dentists must be fully conversant with and capable of executing the technique of cardiopulmonary resuscitation as an emergency procedure.

CLOSED-CHEST CARDIAC MASSAGE*

W. B. KOUWENHOVEN, M.D., J. R. JUDE, M.D., AND G. G. KNICKERBOCKER, M.D.

When cardiac arrest occurs, either as standstill or as ventricular fibrillation, the circulation must be restored promptly; otherwise anoxia will result in irreversible damage. There are two techniques that may be used to meet the emergency; one is to open the chest and massage the heart directly and the other is to accomplish the same end by a new method of closed-chest cardiac massage. The latter method is described in this section. The closed-chest alternating current defibrillator[42] that was developed in our laboratories has proved to be an effective and reliable means of arresting ventricular fibrillation. Its counter-shock must be sent through the chest promptly, or else cardiac anoxia will have developed to such a degree that the heart will no longer be able to resume forcible contractions without assistance. Our experience has indicated that external defibrillation is not likely to be followed by the return of spontaneous heart action, unless the counter-shock is applied within less than 3 minutes after the onset of ventricular fibrillation.

A study was undertaken of means of extending this time limitation without opening the chest. A method was sought that would provide adequate circulation to maintain the tone of the heart and the nourishment of the central nervous system. This method was to be at once readily applicable, safe to use, and requiring a minimum of gadgets.

Method. The method of closed-chest cardiac massage developed during . . . animal studies is simple to apply; it is one that needs no complex equipment. Only the human hand is required. The principle of the method as applied to man is readily seen by consideration of the anatomy of the bony thorax and its contained organs. The heart is limited anteriorly by the sternum and posteriorly by the

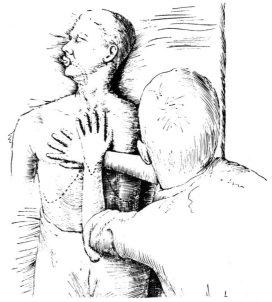

Figure 25–1 Position of hands during cardiac massage of adult. (From Kouwenhoven, W. B., Jude, J. R., and Knickerbocker, G. G.: Closed-chest cardiac massage. J.A.M.A., *173*:1064–1067 [July], 1960.)

vertebral bodies. Its lateral movement is restricted by the pericardium. Pressure on the sternum compresses the heart between it and the spine, forcing out blood. Relaxation of the pressure allows the heart to fill. The thoracic cage in unconscious and anesthetized adults is surprisingly mobile. The method of application is shown in Figure 25–1. With the patient in a supine position, preferably on a rigid support, the heel of one hand with the other on top of it is placed on the sternum just cephalad to the xiphoid. Firm pressure is applied vertically downward about 60 times per minute. At the end of each pressure stroke the hands are lifted slightly to permit full expansion of the chest. The operator should be so positioned that he can use his body weight in applying the pressure. Sufficient pressure should be used to move the sternum 3 or 4 cm. toward the vertebral column. Artificial respiration with oxygen

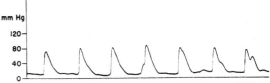

Figure 25–2 Blood pressure produced in an adult by closed-chest massage. (From Kouwenhoven, W. B., Jude, J. R., and Knickerbocker, G. G.: Closed-chest cardiac massage. J.A.M.A., *173*:1064–1067 [July], 1960.)

* Extracted from Kouwenhoven, W. B., Jude, J. R., and Knickerbocker, G. G.: Closed-chest cardiac massage, J.A.M.A., *173*:1064–1067 (July 9), 1960. Personal communication from W. B. Kouwenhoven, May 7, 1965, updating this material.

should be administered to the patient at the same time. If oxygen is not available, a second person should give mouth to mouth insufflation.

If you are alone when cardiac arrest occurs, the patient should be placed in a supine position on a rigid surface such as the floor. Apply 3 to 5 quick deep inflations of the lungs with mouth-to-mouth insufflation. Check for pulse—if absent, begin heart compressions at the rate of 1 per second. After 15 compressions stop and inflate the lungs quickly twice. Continue heart compressions and repeat the cycle until help arrives. After the helper has telephoned for an ambulance, he should take over the artificial respiration, giving a breath (mouth-to-mouth) at every fifth compression, while you continue external heart massage. He should inflate the lungs as you are raising your hands from the patient's chest.

Clinical Application.   During the past 5 years 77 patients in the Operating Rooms and Recovery Rooms at Johns Hopkins Hospital have suffered 85 cardiac arrests. Of these, 72 were resuscitated by the prompt application of cardiopulmonary resuscitation and 38 were alive when discharged from the hospital.[42]

Prompt diagnosis and treatment are mandatory, since cerebral anoxia can result in irreversible damage *within 3 minutes*.[49]

WHEN YOUR OFFICE PATIENT DIES

FRANK M. MCCARTHY, M.D., D.D.S.

Approximately half of all deaths that occur annually in the United States are a result of heart or cerebrovascular disease. The majority of these one million deaths are sudden and occur with little or no warning; 10 per cent of them are also totally unexpected, without prior diagnosis of disease.

From the standpoint of probability alone, without regard to therapy modes or to therapy stresses, the death of an office patient from natural causes is almost certain to occur at least once during the surgeon's practice lifetime.

For purposes of the following discussion, it is assumed that the patient's death has already occurred, that all proper precautions were taken, including the establishment of relative risk via physical evaluation, that informed consent was obtained, and that medi-

cal assistance was speedily summoned after the emergency developed.

When death occurs, it is a shattering experience to the deceased's relatives, to you, and to your office staff. It can be damaging to your professional reputation, and it can result in a wrongful death suit. In recent years, criminal negligence charges are becoming more common, and there have been convictions. Conviction of criminal negligence usually absolves your professional liability insurance carrier of any financial obligation resulting from subsequent malpractice action.

HUMANE AND PRACTICAL CONSIDERATIONS

There are five basic rules to follow when dealing with the office death.[1] First, preplan your resuscitative procedures with your office staff. Practice simulated emergencies several times. Do not just discuss the plan with your staff—*do it* in as rapid and as efficient a way as possible. If your procedures are not preplanned and rehearsed, you and your staff will perhaps treat a life-threatening emergency in a less than adequate manner. Keep your resuscitative kit ready for instant use. Drill your staff and retrain them periodically. Have your staff attend refresher courses. If your patient does not survive, despite your prompt and definitive treatment, you will be able to demonstrate that you did everything that could reasonably be expected of you.

Second, take extreme care when informing the next-of-kin of a death. Tell the relative in the privacy of your office that the patient collapsed, that everything possible was done, but to no avail. It is virtually impossible to extend too much grief and sympathy, *without admitting liability*. If no relative is in the office, call the most responsible next-of-kin and state that the patient has suffered a serious collapse and that everything possible is being done to revive him. Ask the relative to come quickly. Try to avoid stating positively on the phone that the patient is dead. However, do not lie. Avoid any statement about the cause of death until you have had time to review and complete your records. Just say *sudden collapse*.

Third, have the patients in your reception room excused. Have your aide say, "A serious emergency has come up and the doctor must cancel all appointments." The aide should offer new appointments, giving *no details* about what has happened.

Fourth, compile a complete record—the patient's appearance, the probable cause of death, and the resuscitative efforts. It is mandatory in most states to report a death to the coroner's office if the mechanism of death is not known, if death occurs during or following a surgical procedure, if there is a question of litigation (accident case), or if the patient has not been under his attending physician's care within a short period of time (4 days in many states). Considering the various ramifications, it is advised that any death in the oral surgery office, whether related to therapy or not, be reported to the coroner, who will then advise the surgeon whether such a death falls within the coroner's jurisdiction. Keep a record of the time of the call, the name of the coroner's deputy, and the advice if the deceased is released to you and the attending physician for certification of death. You may be glad to have an official record of the circumstances under which death occurred and your actions if questions should arise later. Also, certain insurance carriers require that they be notified immediately of any event that could result in a claim. Sudden death in the office is a leading cause of big-dollar malpractice action.

Fifth, guard your reputation. You will have to fend off pointed questions by the deceased's relatives and lay friends. The less said the better, but do not remain silent. Silence on your part will intrigue the relatives and fortify suspicions about your possible responsibility. Repeat your shock and grief, offer sincerest sympathy, but simply say that the deceased *suddenly collapsed.*

LEGAL CONSIDERATIONS

The preceding 5 humane and practical points far outweigh any legal issues at the time, but several should be mentioned.[59]

1. Do not volunteer to take care of the remains. If your directions are not followed and the next-of-kin suffers shock, you are liable. You may discuss details regarding removal of the deceased with the mortuary, but only under the specific instructions and with the express consent of the next-of-kin. You may not direct or contract for services.

2. Only the next-of-kin has the right to bury or preserve the remains.
3. The surviving spouse has the right of disposition over all relatives.
4. If you authorize an autopsy without consent, you are liable.
5. Only the next-of-kin may authorize retention of body organs.
6. The next-of-kin may not give directions contrary to the deceased's will. The Anatomical Gift Act allows the deceased to dispose of the whole or any part of his body, subject of course to the degree of the coroner's involvement.

The catastrophic experience of a death in the office must be anticipated in order to be handled in a proper, humane and practical manner. Preparation before the fact is the key.

ANGIOEDEMA

Angioedema is a symptom complex frequently recognized as having a varied mechanism of underlying hereditary, allergic and psychophysiologic factors. Many authors have discussed angioedema and urticaria jointly because of their essential similarity. However, the distinction should be made that angioedema involves the deeper tissues, while urticaria is limited to the cutis. While chronic forms of angioedema can continue for months or years and are etiologically difficult to diagnose, acute attacks of brief duration are common and frequently are self-diagnosed. Patients with a history of angioedema should not be operated on until consultation and preoperative preparations are carried out. While the primary lesion of angioedema may be innocuous by virtue of location, such as localized swelling of the lip or eyelid, edema of the glottis may follow with complete obstruction of the airway.[17] Aspirin should be considered as a possible causative agent.

Scher[56] reports a case of migratory angioedema and notes a case reported by Richards and Crombie[53] in which a 28-year-old man, who suffered from angioedema for several years, died after the extraction of a tooth under local anesthesia. Autopsy showed complete mechanical respiratory stoppage as the result of edema of the vocal cords. Patients with a personal or family history of angioedema should be treated with antihistamines before and after oral surgery.

ANGIOEDEMA OF THE LIP

A woman aged 25 came to the clinic complaining of recurrent painless swelling of the upper lip. This transient edema was confined solely to the upper lip and generally lasted from 24 to 36 hours. She could not relate the swelling to any particular foods. She stated, however, that when she was "nervous or upset" she frequently had this swelling (see Figure 25–3).

Examination of the lip revealed a markedly thickened and lengthened upper lip that was tense and elastic but normal in color both in the skin and the mucous membrane. Oral hygiene was good; the teeth were in a good state of repair; the oral tissues were normal.

Findings in oral radiographs and electric vitality tests of the maxillary anterior teeth were negative.

A diagnosis of angioedema was made. The patient was referred to the allergy clinic. Here the diagnosis was confirmed. Findings in sensitivity tests were essentially normal.

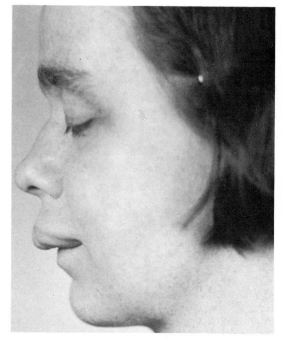

Figure 25–3 Angioedema of the lip. (See Case Report No. 1.)

TREATMENT OF ACUTE ANGIOEDEMA

According to Goltz, intubation or even tracheostomy may be needed to maintain the airway during an attack of acute angioedema.[28] Measures to combat shock should be used. Epinephrine, 3 cc. of 1:100,000 solution, may be injected intravenously or intramuscularly. Corticosteroid preparations — for example, Solu-Medrol — may be given intravenously. Intravenous or intramuscular antihistaminics (Histadyl, 15 to 20 mg.) may also be helpful. Fortunately most emergencies are of short duration, lasting at most 30 minutes.

SWALLOWED FOREIGN OBJECTS

It is surprising that foreign objects are not swallowed more often during dental and surgical procedures. In oral surgery the most frequently swallowed object is a tooth, although instruments and dental appliances have been swallowed. Johnson and Parker reported a case in which a thermometer was

swallowed. There was doubt expressed that this smooth object would pass through the gastrointestinal tract. A low roughage diet was started with unsatisfactory results 5 days

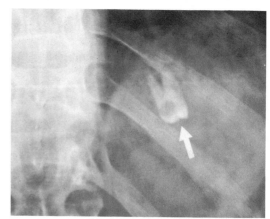

Figure 25–4 Abdominal radiograph showing the presence of a molar tooth in the stomach of a patient who had swallowed it following routine extraction. The tooth was subsequently passed without complications. (Courtesy of the Canandaigua V. A. Hospital, Canandaigua, New York. Radiographs and caption material prepared by Dr. Edward Zegarelli, Division of Stomatology, School of Dental and Oral Surgery, Columbia University, New York, New York.)

later. The surgical service proposed abdominal surgery. However, on this day the patient's diet was changed to solid food. The intact thermometer was passed 3 days later.[39] (See also Figures 25-4, 25-5 and 25-6.) The author has always prescribed a regular or a high roughage diet for patients who have inadvertently swallowed foreign objects. Radiographs should be taken to observe the passage of the object through the gastrointestinal tract. Stools must be carefully examined to recover the foreign object.

ASPIRATION OF FOREIGN OBJECTS

During operations in the oral cavity there is an ever-present danger of the patient's aspirating some object, such as a tooth, a small gauze sponge, dental prosthesis, small dental instruments or impression material, that may produce partial or complete obstruction of the airway or, if small enough, might pass through the larynx and trachea and lodge in a bronchial tube. (See Figure 25-7.) To prevent this possibility, whether the opera-

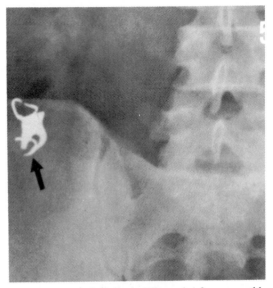

Figure 25-6 Abdominal radiograph of a removable bridge which was swallowed and eventually lodged in the ileum. This, too, was surgically removed and followed by uneventful recovery. (Courtesy of St. Francis Hospital, New York City. Radiographs and caption material prepared by Dr. Edward Zegarelli, Division of Stomatology, School of Dental and Oral Surgery, Columbia University, New York, New York.)

tion is performed under local or general anesthesia, a gauze oropharyngeal partition should be placed across the posterior area of the oral cavity.

Case reports of lives saved in dental offices and hospitals by performing an emergency tracheostomy have been published. Unfortunately, fatalities have occurred as the direct result of not performing an emergency tracheostomy.

One may be called upon to perform an emergency tracheostomy at the site of an accident, or on the floor in the home where a patient has aspirated a large piece of food or other object, using a penknife or whatever sharp instrument happens to be at hand, and without regard to asepsis. This emergency operation consists essentially in cutting down on the trachea without regard to hemorrhage, incising the trachea, introducing some makeshift tube or inserting the handle of the penknife and turning it sideways to hold the tissues apart, and then arresting the hemorrhage with pressure along the edges of the wound around the opening into the trachea. Following are the details of such an operation carried out in the more ideal environment of the dental office or hospital.

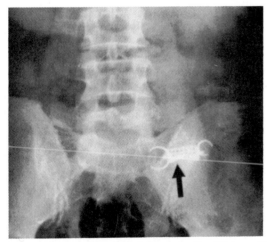

Figure 25-5 Abdominal radiograph of a 59-year-old man who unknowingly swallowed a removable bridge during sleep. Increasingly severe abdominal cramps during the subsequent 24 hours necessitated hospitalization and investigation. During surgical removal of the appliance it was found that the ileum was perforated with an associated peritonitis. Aside from a bout of postsurgical abscess, which was controlled with antibiotics, the postoperative course was uneventful. (Courtesy of Department of Radiology, Columbia Presbyterian Medical Center, New York City. Radiographs and caption material prepared by Dr. Edward Zegarelli, Division of Stomatology, School of Dental and Oral Surgery, Columbia University, New York, New York.)

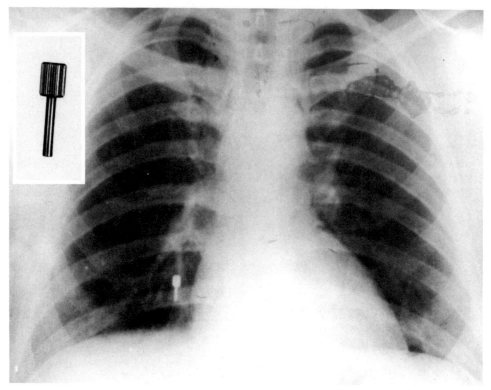

Figure 25–7   Small pin wrench aspirated during operative procedures on an upper molar.

EMERGENCY TREATMENT OF ACUTE RESPIRATORY BLOCKAGE

Surgically creating an opening into the respiratory tree is the only means of circumventing a complete blockage of the respiratory passage, thus permitting oxygen to reach the lungs to maintain life.

A *tracheostomy* is the "surgical creation of an opening into the trachea through the neck, for the insertion of a tube to facilitate the passage of air to the lungs, or the evacuation of secretions." A *tracheotomy* is the "incision of the trachea through the skin and muscles of the neck, for exploration, removal of a foreign body, or for obtaining a biopsy specimen or removal of a local lesion."[19]

An emergency *cricothyrotomy* is the surgical creation of an opening into the larynx between the anterior inferior border of the thyroid cartilage and the anterior superior border of the cricoid cartilage (see Figures 25–8 and 25–9). This is known as the cricothyroid space and is recommended as the ideal area for an emergency opening into the respiratory tree, as it is the most accessible point inferior to the glottis.[11]

Indications.   The presence of an irrevers-ible or progressive obstruction that completely prevents air flow to the lungs for a life-threatening period is an indication for surgically opening the airway below the obstruction.

The following is a sequence of events that indicates the need for emergency treatment to create an airway. A normally breathing patient suddenly manifests respiratory difficulty, with little or no exchange of gases, in spite of labored excursions of the chest wall and diaphragm. This is followed by asphyxial convulsions, rapidly increasing cyanosis, and respiratory failure. The patient does not respond to the usual treatment of asphyxia—namely, the removal of any visible source of mechanical respiratory embarrassment, such as a downward flexion of the head and neck, tongue displaced posteriorly into the pharynx, sponges or blood clots—nor does he respond to the administration of 100 per cent oxygen under pressure with a face mask, with the exhaling valve closed. The decision for surgical intervention is confirmed by observation that the patient's chest wall fails to expand when oxygen is administered under pressure.

Even if inflation of the lungs by forcing the object deeper is successful, there is still

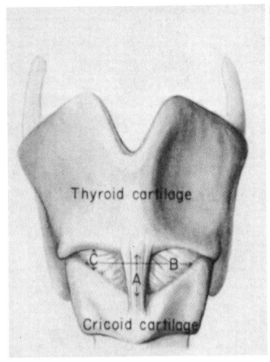

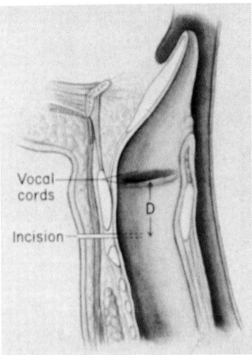

Figure 25–8   Figure 25–9

Figure 25–8 The cricothyroid space, indicated by *A*, is located between the inferior border of the thyroid cartilage and the superior border of the cricoid cartilage. *C–B* indicates the line of incision. (From Archer, W. H.: Dental Anesthesia. 2nd ed. Philadelphia, W. B. Saunders Co., 1958.)

Figure 25–9 The line of incision shown here between the thyroid and cricoid cartilages is well below the vocal cords. (From Archer, W. H.: Dental Anesthesia. 2nd ed. Philadelphia, W. B. Saunders Co., 1958.)

danger. As the patient regains consciousness the cough reflex returns, and the possibility of this foreign object's becoming impacted in the larynx on the reverse journey when the patient coughs it up must be anticipated.

There are two approaches to surgical opening of the airway: the tracheostomy and the cricothyrotomy. The former is done through the tracheal rings, the latter through the cricothyroid membrane.

For additional information on tracheostomy in patients with multiple facial injuries and jaw fractures, see pages 1549–1554.

EMERGENCY CRICOTHYROTOMY

RALPH J. CAPAROSA, M.D.

Cricothyrotomy is indicated in real emergent laryngeal obstruction if endotracheal intubation is not available or is impossible to perform. In the hands of an experienced operator or anesthetist, intubation is usually possible; however, in those rare situations in which difficulty is encountered, the attendant should not sacrifice precious time for repeated attempts at intubation that may not succeed.

Original objections to cricothyrotomy were based upon the fear of postoperative laryngeal stenosis. This will not occur if the cricoid cartilage itself is not damaged. Antibiotics should also be administered postoperatively to help prevent perichondritis, which is usually the underlying cause of stenosis.

Figure 25–10 shows the front of the neck and its underlying topography. In hyposthenic people, these areas are readily visualized. In even the most obese, there is usually a slight palpable depression between the thyroid and cricoid.

Surgical Anatomy. Externally, the cricothyroid space is usually readily identifiable. It is the concavity between the convex borders of the inferior portion of the thyroid cartilage and the superior border of the cricoid cartilage (see Figure 25–10). In searching for this area in the neck, the palpating finger should

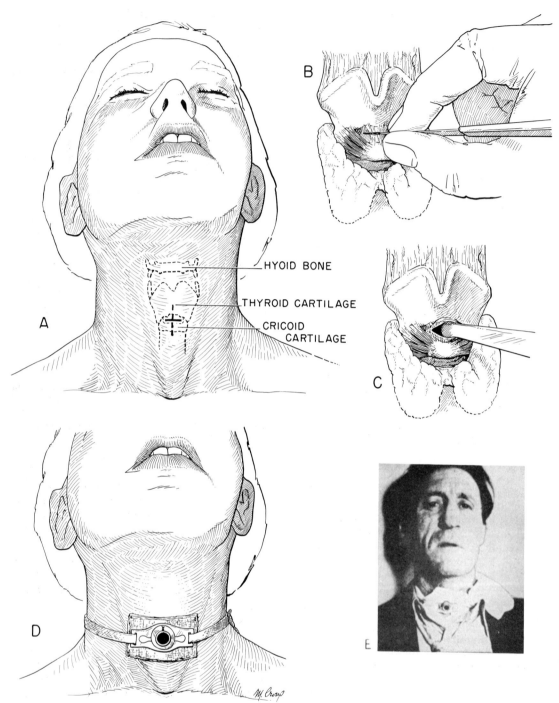

Figure 25–10 Technique for an emergency cricothyrotomy. *A,* Place patient's head in a flexed position. The anterior portion of the thyroid cartilage (Adam's apple) is palpated and its anterior border is traced inferiorly until the first depression in the midline is encountered; this depression, just superior to the cricoid cartilage, is the cricothyroid space. The dotted vertical line in *A* shows the line of incision through the skin. The horizontal black line on this drawing is in the middle of the cricoid space and indicates the line of incision to open into the airway. *B,* Grasp the knife (this is an emergency, so a penknife or any knife will do)½ to ¾ inch from the tip and *cut horizontally for one inch through the skin and underlying tissues into the airway. C,* Turn the knife and insert the handle into the trachea; then turn the handle to hold the tissues apart, creating an emergency air bypass to the lungs. If respiratory attempts by the patient have ceased, start artificial resuscitation immediately. *D,* When a tracheostomy tube is obtained, it is inserted. Oxygen can be administered through this tube. (From Archer, W. H.: Dental Anesthesia. 2nd ed. Philadelphia, W. B. Saunders Co., 1958.)

initially identify the thyroid prominence (Adam's apple). Then proceeding caudad in the midline of the neck, the first depression encountered is the cricothyroid space. This is the area through which intercricothyrotomy is performed.

Although the larynx usually lies in the midline, one must be cautioned that occasionally this structure may be deviated. In patients who are obese or who have large neck tumefactions in this area, the skin and subcutaneous tissue may have to be incised before this space can be accurately identified. In any event, it is imperative that this region be identified prior to any surgical manipulation.

The cricothyroid space is roughly a trapezoid with a cross-sectional area of approximately 2.9 square cm., and is adequate for performing an intercricothyrotomy. In order to further delineate this area, 51 adult larynges were examined, and the following measurements, as specified, were recorded (see Figures 25–8 and 25–9):

1. The contiguous distance between the anterior inferior border of the thyroid cartilage and the anterior superior border of the cricoid cartilage, represented as "A," ranged from 0.5 cm. to 1.2 cm., with the average being 0.9 cm.
2. The workable width of the cricothyroid space, represented by "B," varied from 2.7 cm. to 3.2 cm., with the mean being 3 cm.
3. The minimal workable vertical distance measured at the lateral aspects of the cricothyroid space, represented by "C," varied from 0.2 cm. to 0.6 cm., with the average being 0.3 cm.
4. The distance between the true cords and the mid-horizontal plane of the cricothyroid space, represented by "D," averaged 1.3 cm.
5. The vertical distance of the cricoid arch was 0.7 cm., while the posterior plate measured 2.5 cm. vertically.

Indications. Cricothyrotomy is indicated only in those instances of laryngeal obstruction in which an absolute emergency exists, such as the presence of a foreign body in the larynx, or when a delay would result in a fatality.

Classical tracheostomy, when performed under the proper circumstances, may be a safe procedure; but when faced with the urgency of impending asphyxia, the relative inaccessibility of the lower tracheal rings, and the anatomical vascular barriers of the region, a genuine surgical challenge is presented.

Technique. This is a second-by-second life emergency procedure. There is no time for asepsis, anesthesia or hemostasis, which can be taken care of after the airway is established.

In performing a cricothyrotomy, the structures encountered from without inward are: the skin, subcutaneous tissue, cervical fascia, medial aspects of the cricothyroid muscles, median cricothyroid ligament, medial portion of the lateral cricothyroid ligaments, and the endolaryngeal mucosa. The only major blood vessel is the cricothyroid artery. The veins are usually small, and there are no nerves of importance in this vicinity.

Figures 25–8 and 25–9 show in detail the cricothyroid areas as measured by Caparosa and Zavatsky.[11] They show that there is an adequate area through which the operative procedure can be performed safely.

A midline incision approximately 2 cm. in length should be made through the skin and immediate subcutaneous tissue over the area of the cricothyroid membrane (see A in Figure 25–10). The neck should be extended if possible. One must keep in mind, however, that hyperextension increases laryngeal obstruction and forcibly placing the patient in this position may precipitate a real crisis. However, inasmuch as the entire procedure should take no more than 30 seconds, the risk of further obstruction can be taken if the situation warrants this extension.

The incision tends to widen as the head is extended. If there is not enough widening, the tissue can then be spread apart with the index fingers and the thumb of the left hand. A transverse incision (line C–B in Figure 25–8) is then made directly through the cricothyroid membrane. (See B in Figure 25–10.) Care must be taken to avoid penetrating the mediastinum posteriorly. The broad, flat surface of the posterior cricoid serves as an excellent "back-stop" to prevent penetration into the mediastinum.

The handle of the scalpel or any other flat instrument can be inserted, turned and used to keep the airway open. (See C in Figure 25–10.) If a tracheostomy tube is available, and one should be in every oral surgeon's office (see D in Figure 25–10), it is inserted. Coughing generally follows the introduction of the tube into the trachea. To prevent its dislodgment, the anchorage tapes on the

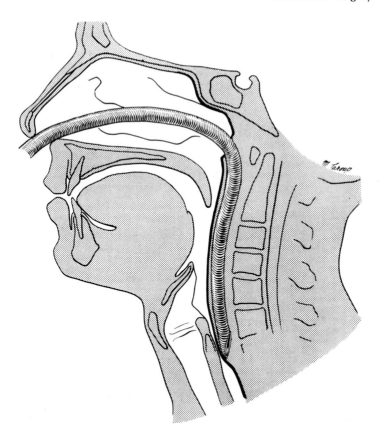

Figure 25–11 Complication with endotracheal anesthesia. Endotracheal tube advanced submucosally. (From Gaisford, J. C., Hanna, D. C., and Monheim, L. M.: Endotracheal anesthesia complications associated with head and neck surgery. Plast. Reconstr. Surg., *24*[5]:463–471 [Jul.-Dec.], 1959.)

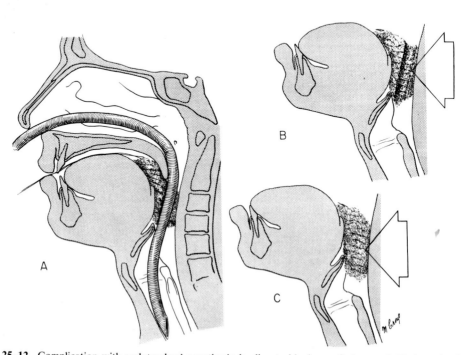

Figure 25–12 Complication with endotracheal anesthesia leading to blockage of airway. *A*, Endotracheal tube and pharyngeal packing in place. *B*, Endotracheal tube removed, packing not removed. *C*, Packing closing off airway. (From Gaisford, J. C., Hanna, D. C., and Monheim, L. M.: Endotracheal anesthesia complications associated with head and neck surgery. Plast. Reconstr. Surg., *24*[5]:463–471 [Jul.-Dec.], 1959.)

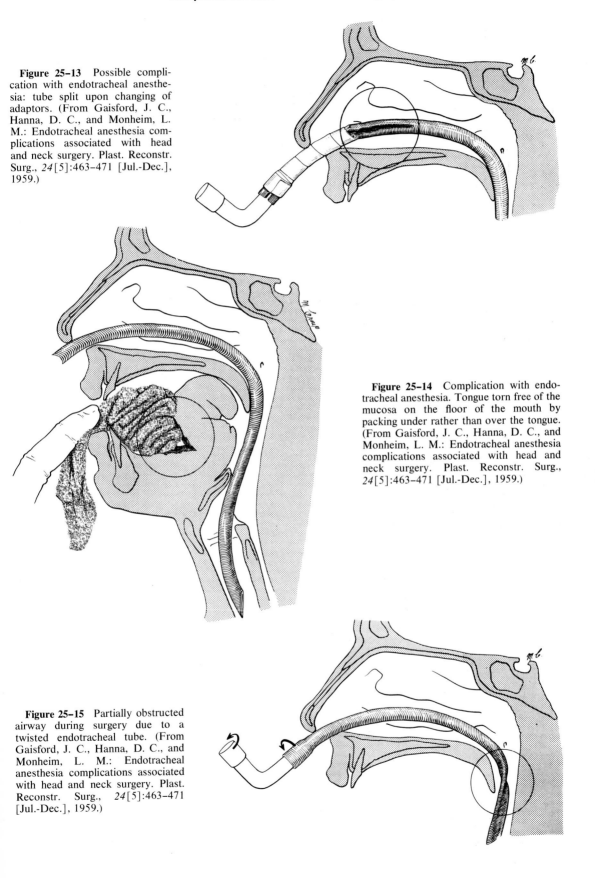

Figure 25–13 Possible complication with endotracheal anesthesia: tube split upon changing of adaptors. (From Gaisford, J. C., Hanna, D. C., and Monheim, L. M.: Endotracheal anesthesia complications associated with head and neck surgery. Plast. Reconstr. Surg., *24*[5]:463–471 [Jul.-Dec.], 1959.)

Figure 25–14 Complication with endotracheal anesthesia. Tongue torn free of the mucosa on the floor of the mouth by packing under rather than over the tongue. (From Gaisford, J. C., Hanna, D. C., and Monheim, L. M.: Endotracheal anesthesia complications associated with head and neck surgery. Plast. Reconstr. Surg., *24*[5]:463–471 [Jul.-Dec.], 1959.)

Figure 25–15 Partially obstructed airway during surgery due to a twisted endotracheal tube. (From Gaisford, J. C., Hanna, D. C., and Monheim, L. M.: Endotracheal anesthesia complications associated with head and neck surgery. Plast. Reconstr. Surg., *24*[5]:463–471 [Jul.-Dec.], 1959.)

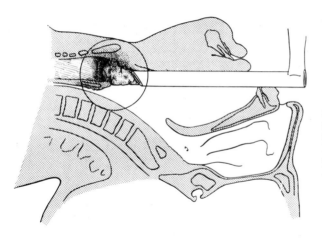

Figure 25–16 An emergency tracheostomy was required during induction of anesthetic because of severe edema from trauma caused by the laryngoscope. (From Gaisford, J. C., Hanna, D. C., and Monheim, L. M.: Endotracheal anesthesia complications associated with head and neck surgery. Plast. Reconstr. Surg., *24*[5]:463–471 [Jul.-Dec.], 1959.)

flange of the tube should be tied around the neck. Oxygen is administered through the tube. A classical tracheostomy should then be done as early as possible. It can be done as an elective rather than an emergency procedure.

A similar airway can be established by using a very large bore needle (13 gauge). Care must be taken that the needle does not slip out of position during the manipulation and attachment of oxygen inlets. It also may become clogged readily. One such needle will not permit adequate air exchange except for a short time. Two or three needles are helpful but the rapid accumulation of secretions in these needles reduces their efficiency. Thus arrangements should be made to have a classical tracheostomy done as soon as possible. At this time the foreign object is removed from the trachea. In a real emergency, however, the needle or any cutting instrument can be used.

It is suggested that every dentist or oral surgeon acquaint himself with one or more of the available techniques for establishing an emergency airway. The emergency cricothyrotomy technique can usually be mastered after several trials on a cadaver.

HEMATOMA

A hematoma is an effusion of blood into the tissues that results in a tumor-like mass. It is most frequently the result of blood vessels being pierced by the needle of the anesthetic syringe when making an injection.

The most dramatic hematoma is the rapidly developing one that within minutes produces marked swelling in the cheek (see Figure 25–18). This is the result of the needle piercing the superior posterior alveolar artery or its external, gingival branch during an injection to anesthetize the posterior superior alveolar nerve (see Figure 25–18).

The slowly developing hematoma results from a needle penetrating the pterygoid plexus of veins located just behind the

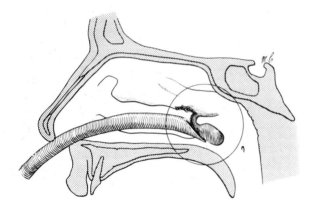

Figure 25–17 Complication of endotracheal anesthesia. Amputation of a nasal polyp during nasal intubation. (From Gaisford, J. C., Hanna, D. C., and Monheim, L. M.: Endotracheal anesthesia complications associated with head and neck surgery. Plast. Reconstr. Surg., *24*[5]:463–471 [Jul.-Dec.], 1959.)

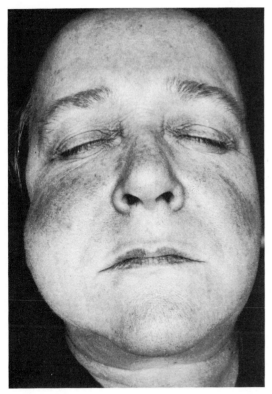

Figure 25-18 A large hematoma of the right cheek that occurred as the direct result of piercing the gingival branch of the posterior superior alveolar artery during a so-called tuberosity or zygomatic injection for the anesthetization of the posterior superior alveolar nerve. Blood rapidly poured into the buccinator space where it produced a large swelling, as shown here, within minutes.

convex posterior surface of the maxilla. (See Figure 25-19.) Also illustrated in this drawing is the recommended angle of the needle that is least likely to result in a hematoma from this venous plexus, and is mostly likely to avoid penetrating one of the branches of the posterior superior alveolar artery that enters the convex posterior bony wall of the maxillary sinus. To avoid penetrating the inferior alveolar artery when anesthetizing the inferior alveolar nerve, study Figure 25-20. The hematoma from the inferior alveolar artery into the parapharyngeal space can seriously embarrass respiration.

The artery or vein bleeds into the loose fatty connective tissue, rapidly fills the spaces between the masticatory muscles and the skeleton, and finally reaches the subcutaneous tissue of the cheek just in front of the masseter muscle. The only possible way to restrict this hematoma, according to Sicher and DuBrul[63] is digital pressure exerted upward, inward and slightly forward against the bone below the zygomatic arch and in front of the masseter muscles. During a tuberosity injection the possibility of a fast-spreading arterial hematoma must be kept in mind so that at the first sign of this accident the operator is fully prepared to take action.

Hematomas in hemophiliacs are of course serious matters and can be fatal. See Case Report Nos. 4, 5 and 6 and Figures 25-21 and 25-34.

The patient is usually quite alarmed by this unexpected large swelling in his cheek, both internally and externally, or in his throat (from an inferior alveolar nerve injection). He also must be told about the extensive blue-black discoloration (ecchymosis) of the oral, facial and neck tissues that will develop.

However, hematomas may, and do, follow operations in the oral cavity. The collection of blood in the tissue planes is gradually absorbed by normal body processes, but there is a possibility of suppuration if infected material is introduced into this area.

Some authors advocate attempting to aspirate the blood by introducing a large needle, attached to a syringe, into this area. Personally, I have never carried out this procedure, but prefer to treat the patient by having him rest and apply cold applications to the part for the first 24 hours. After that, heat should be applied to facilitate absorption of the blood.

If the hematoma is the result of arterial bleeding beneath the mucoperiosteal flap, it will be necessary to locate the artery and tie it off; if it is in the alveolar process, the bone can be compressed into the lumen of the vessel or bone wax can be rubbed into it.

Diffuse bleeding from a wound, such as that created by removal of a lower third molar, may not result in a localized collection of blood giving rise to a tumor-like mass, but rather may result in extensive edema of all the tissues of the face on the side involved as the blood is forced between and through the fascial planes. Marked ecchymosis of the buccal mucosa results and is present also in the corner of the mouth and infraorbital areas.

With the use of sutures after minor or extensive oral surgery, bleeding does not usually occur, but there may be ecchymosis, a less serious result (see section below).

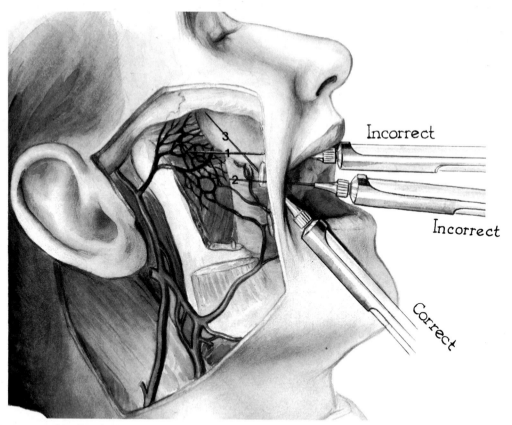

Figure 25–19 Needle *1* is shown penetrating the pterygoid plexus of veins because it is incorrectly inserted. Needle *2*, also incorrectly inserted, is penetrating. Needle *3* is the needle correctly inserted for the anesthetization of the posterior superior alveolar nerve. This technique has the least possibility of penetrating arteries or veins. (From Archer, W. H.: A Manual of Dental Anesthesia. 2nd ed. Philadelphia, W. B. Saunders Co., 1958.)

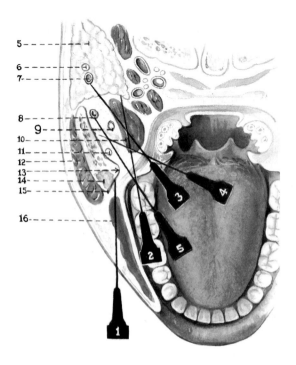

Figure 25–20 Errors in needle insertion and direction for an inferior alveolar nerve block injection. *1*, Needle inserted too far laterally contacting the internal oblique ridge. *2*, Needle inserted too far medially from the internal oblique ridge and directed medially away from the inferior alveolar nerve and through the structures seen in the drawing. *3*, The needle is inserted into the soft tissue at a grossly excessive lateral position from the internal oblique ridge and the inferior alveolar nerve. This insertion and *4* are the ones in which breakage of needles, as well as hematomas, are most frequently seen. Needle *5* shows the correct insertion and direction of the needle to anesthetize the inferior alveolar nerve, but if inserted too deeply, as shown here, there is a danger of penetrating the inferior alveolar artery, resulting in an arterial hematoma. *Anatomy: 5*, Parotid gland. *6*, Facial nerve. *7*, Posterior facial vein. *8*, Inferior alveolar artery. *9*, Inferior alveolar nerve. *10*, Internal pterygoid muscle. *11*, Lingual nerve. *12*, Masseter muscle. *13*, Internal oblique ridge. *14*, Ascending ramus. *15*, External oblique ridge. *16*, Buccinator muscle. (From Archer, W. H.: A Manual of Dental Anesthesia, 2nd ed. Philadelphia, W. B. Saunders Co., 1958.)

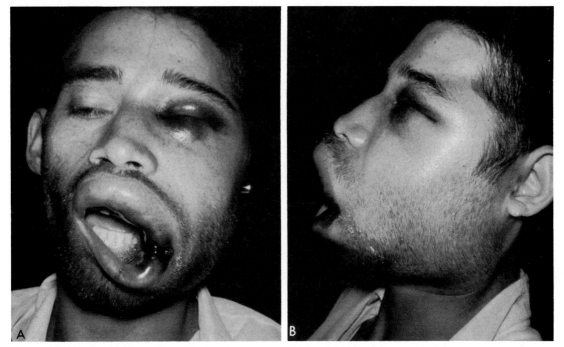

Figure 25–21 Traumatic capillary bleeding in a 24-year-old hemophiliac produced this large hematoma within 24 hours following maxillary infiltration of a local anesthetic solution for operative dentistry. Two previous prolonged episodes of bleeding had followed the extraction of teeth. The patient also experienced internal bleeding and hemarthrosis. He was treated with transfusions of fresh blood. (Courtesy of Dr. H. Serrano Roa.)

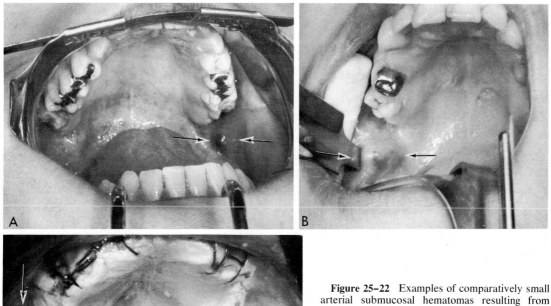

Figure 25–22 Examples of comparatively small arterial submucosal hematomas resulting from needle penetration of the buccal artery during an injection to anesthetize the long buccal nerve. *A,* Small well-circumscribed hematoma. *B,* Larger and more diffuse hematoma. *C,* A very large and diffuse hematoma (*1*) and a smaller but still diffuse hematoma (*2*). The caliber of the artery obviously plays a role in the size of the hematoma as well as in the clotting time.

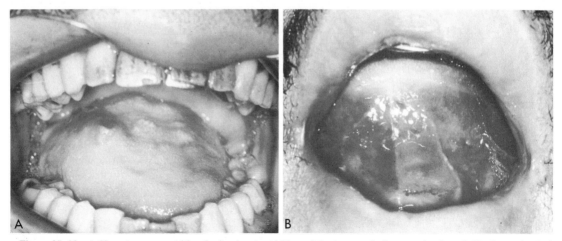

Figure 25–23 *A*, Hematoma caused by the inadvertent biting of the tongue during mastication. *B*, Ecchymosis readily apparent on the ventral surface of the tongue.

ECCHYMOSIS

Facial discoloration ranging from light red to a deep bluish purple may follow oral surgical procedures. The degree of discoloration is often related to the extent of the surgical procedure. The greater the surgical area, the more extensive flap reflection, bone trimming, and so on, the more likely postoperative ecchymosis will develop. The bleeding tendency of the patient is another important factor. Hemophiliacs, of course, will continue to bleed, but many other patients, particularly women, have a distressing tendency to bleed excessively into the mouth and soft tissues from comparatively minor trauma. These patients will always give a history of "easy bruising."

Comparatively minor surgical procedures may be followed by widespread ecchymotic areas. In the case illustrated in Figure 25–36 only the maxillary third molar was extracted, but the patient was a hemophiliac and so following closure of the soft tissues there was slow continuous bleeding out into the subcutaneous tissue and down along the sternocleidomastoid muscle, reaching the suprasternal notch and thorax. In Figure 25–25 the bleeding was confined to the submucosal area of the lip, while in Figure 25–26 follow-

Figure 25–24 Hematoma and ecchymosis following an infraorbital injection to anesthetize the anterior superior alveolar nerve for the extraction of anterior teeth. This is a rare hematoma.

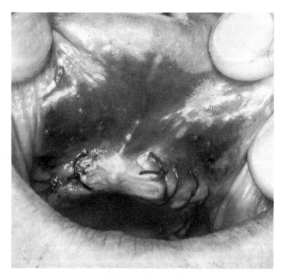

Figure 25–25 Submucosal ecchymosis from immediate postoperative continued bleeding.

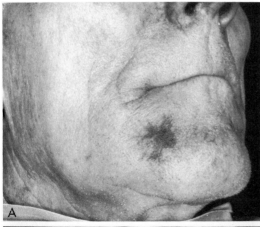

Figure 25-26   The areas of postoperative ecchymosis in these illustrations indicate slow postoperative bleeding from the mental artery, either unilaterally as in *A* and *C* or bilaterally as shown in *B*.

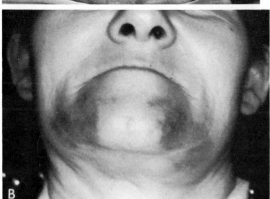

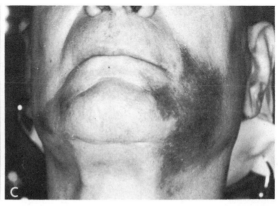

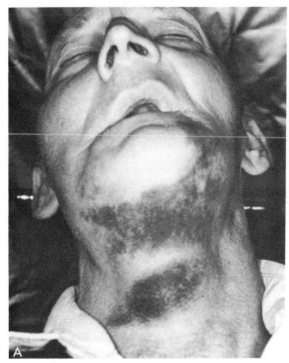

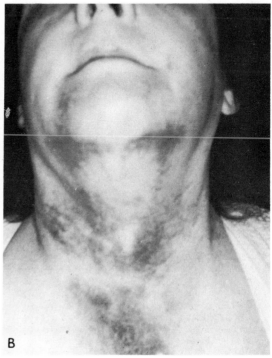

Figure 25-27   Persistent postoperative bleeding produced these large areas of ecchymosis.

ing a single extraction it was confined to the area of a single muscle insertion.

The site at which the ecchymosis appears at the surface is determined by the course the extravasated blood takes through the muscle and fascial planes and will at times be somewhat remote from the site of surgery. A knowledge of the muscles and fascia of the perioral region will help explain these apparently paradoxical ecchymotic areas. Study Figures 25–22 to 25–24 and 25–29 to 25–30.

Treatment. Heat (in any form) and massage are indicated once ecchymosis has appeared at the surface and the active bleeding or oozing has ceased. (Cold is indicated immediately postoperatively.) The discoloration is caused by the gradual breakdown of the complex organic compound hemoglobin. Treatment is aimed at stimulating the formation of new lymph channels and increasing lymphatic drainage. The deep purple fades into a lighter purple, then to greenish yellow and then back to normal. Some patients think

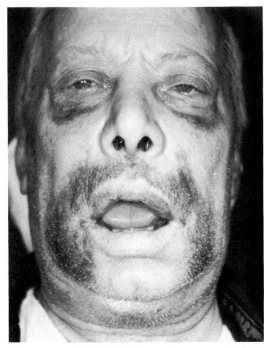

Figure 25–29 Facial view of areas of ecchymosis 1 week after maxillary and mandibular odontectomy and alveolectomy.

they are developing gangrene and need to be reassured by a detailed explanation.

HEMORRHAGE

In all surgery, hemostasis is a necessary corollary of a successful result. Probably in no other surgical area, however, does the surgeon face the vexing problems of dealing with a region subjected to constantly repeated trauma (during talking and swallowing) that cannot be put at rest, in which standard techniques of ligation of vessels are rarely applicable, and in which the final closure is not really a true surgical closure in layers in good apposition but a semi-open closure over sockets that are oozing blood through open vessels in their recently traumatized walls. Despite all these handicaps, inherent mechanisms for control of hemorrhage are present in the oral tissues much the same as a high resistance to oral flora is inherent in the tissues. However, if these mechanisms are abused or in poor working order because of systemic disease, the end result will be hemorrhage instead of hemostasis.

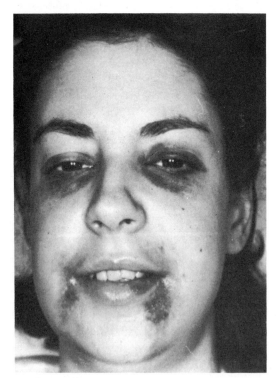

Figure 25–28 Following the excision of four impacted unerupted mandibular third molars, this patient experienced extensive edema caused not only by trauma to the operative site but also by the traction of the cheeks to expose the areas of surgery. This photograph of the ecchymotic areas taken 1 week postoperatively shows the distance the blood traveled from the operative site through the tissue planes.

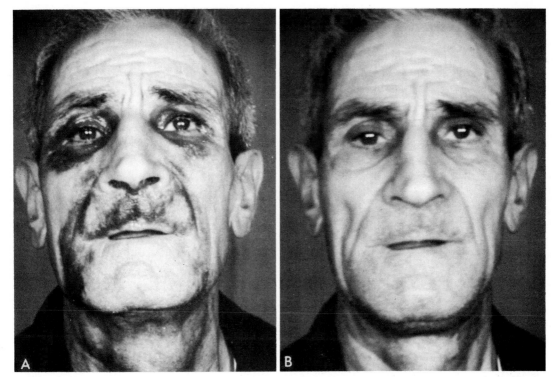

Figure 25–30 *A*, One week postoperative facial view of a patient who had undergone maxillary and mandibular odontectomy and alveolectomy. *B*, Four weeks postoperative view.

THE PHYSIOLOGY OF HEMOSTASIS*

T. C. BITHELL, M.D., AND
M. M. WINTROBE, M.D.

Hemostasis is the process which stops the flow of blood from injured vessels. Completely efficient hemostasis requires normal blood vessels and extravascular tissue, numerically and functionally normal platelets, and a normal coagulation mechanism.

The Vascular Phase. The most immediate consequence of injury to small vessels is a reduction of blood flow as a result of vasoconstriction and extravasation of blood. Vasoconstriction tends to markedly reduce blood flow through an injured area. The escape of blood into normal tissue is limited by the extravascular supporting tissue, and the increased tissue pressure which results tends to collapse venules and capillaries which may then rapidly cohere and even become obliterated. These virtually instantaneous phe-

nomena are quickly supplemented by the events of both the platelet and coagulation phases, which are initiated by the process of contact activation, and by various substances released from injured tissues, the most important being tissue *thromboplastins*, and *adenosine diphosphate* (ADP).

The Platelet Phase. Within seconds after injury, the platelets begin to adhere to the surface of the injured vessel (adhesion) and to one another (aggregation). These processes are greatly facilitated by the retarded blood flow which results from the events of the vascular phase, and rapidly produce a small platelet "plug" or thrombus. The processes of *platelet adhesion and aggregation* are complex and poorly understood, and numerous substances appear to be involved. These include a poorly defined plasma factor (the anti-VW factor) which is lacking in von Willebrand's disease and ADP derived from injured tissues, including erythrocytes, and the platelets themselves.

Like the vessels, the platelets play both a mechanical and a biochemical role in hemostasis. This involves the release of various substances which are involved in the coagula-

* Reprinted with permission from Wintrobe, M. M., *et al.*: Harrison's Principles of Medicine. 6th ed., pp. 317–319. Copyright © 1970 by McGraw-Hill, Inc., New York. Used by permission of McGraw-Hill Book Company.

tion phase. In this regard, the platelet has been likened to a sponge, since despite its small size, it contains a remarkable variety of hemostatically important ingredients. These include, in addition to ADP and ATP, various coagulation factors and the substance which is uniquely responsible for the phenomenon of clot retraction. Most important are various *phospholipids* (generically termed *platelet factor 3*) which become active in coagulation before the platelet membrane is visibly altered. It is probable that such phospholipids become activated *in situ,* the platelet membrane serving as a catalytic surface; some may also be released into the plasma in the form of lipid micelles.

In small injuries, the formation of a platelet thrombus alone may suffice to arrest bleeding, and in larger injuries, it may provide "temporary" hemostasis. However, it is generally agreed that "permanent" hemostasis depends on the formation of a firm, impermeable fibrin thrombus as a result of the process of blood coagulation.

The Coagulation Phase. Blood coagulation is the process by which fluid blood is converted into a coagulum or a clot. This process involves the interaction of various poorly defined trace plasma proteins, the "coagulation factors." The *nomenclature* of the coagulation factors has now been standardized by designating each with a Roman numeral (Table 25–1). Factor III originally referred to tissue thromboplastin, factor IV to calcium, and factor VI to the activated form of factor V. These terms are seldom used. The descriptive terms *fibrinogen* and *prothrombin* are generally preferred to the Roman numerals.

The mechanism by which the coagulation factors interact is still uncertain. Evidence suggests that they are proenzymes which are normally inert, but which are transformed into proteolytic enzymes when activated, each sequentially activating the proenzyme next in line (*the "cascade," or "waterfall," hypothesis*). *Calcium* is essential for most steps in the coagulation process, but remarkably little is known concerning its mechanism of action. Several of the coagulation factors are utilized or consumed during in vitro coagulation (factors V, VIII, XIII, fibrinogen and prothrombin), whereas the remainder are found in the serum.

The coagulation phase begins with the phenomenon of *contact activation*. Indirect evi-

Table 25–1 *Synonyms for Various Coagulation Factors*

INTERNATIONAL NOMENCLATURE	COMMON SYNONYMS
Factor I	Fibrinogen
Factor II	Prothrombin
Factor V	Proaccelerin, labile factor, accelerator globulin (AcG), thrombogen
Factor VII	Proconvertin, stable factor, serum prothrombin conversion accelerator (SPCA), autoprothrombin I
Factor VIII	Antihemophilic factor (AHF), antihemophilic globulin (AHG), thromboplastinogen, platelet cofactor I, plasma thromboplastic factor A, *facteur antihémophilique* A
Factor IX	Christmas factor, plasma thromoboplastin component (PTC), platelet cofactor II, autoprothrombin II, plasma thromboplastic factor B, *facteur antihémophilique* B
Factor X	Stuart factor, Prower factor
Factor XI	PTA (plasma thromboplastin antecedent), antihemophilic factor C
Factor XII	Hageman factor
Factor XIII	Fibrin stabilizing factor, Laki-Lorand factor, fibrinase

dence suggests that this involves a molecular rearrangement of factor XII, which as a result acquires enzymatic properties and converts factor XI into its enzymatic form. In the test tube, contact activation occurs when shed blood is exposed to electronegative surfaces, such as glass. *In vivo,* a similar effect may be produced by skin, collagen and other "foreign" extravascular surfaces.

The activated form of factor XI (factor XIa) initiates the next two steps involving factors IX and VIII, which lead to the conversion of factor X into its enzymatic form. Activated factor X forms a particulate complex (prothrombinase) with factor V and phospholipid from the platelets, which then initiates the conversion of prothrombin into thrombin.

Prothrombinase can be produced by the aforementioned sequence of reactions beginning with contact activation and involving factors XII, XI, IX and VIII. This is termed the *intrinsic pathway.* The production of prothrombinase by means of this pathway is relatively slow but requires neither tissue thromboplastin nor factor VII. A functionally identical prothrombinase can be produced in a matter of seconds by tissue thromboplastins. This involves a sequence of reactions termed the *extrinsic pathway* which, in addition to factors X and V, requires only factor VII. Consequently this pathway bypasses the steps initiated by contact activation involving factors XII, XI, IX and VIII. Thus, blood coagulation is initiated by only two processes, *i.e.,* contact activation and tissue thromboplastin; it proceeds initially via two separate pathways, *i.e.,* the tissue-activated extrinsic pathway and the contact-activated intrinsic pathway; later steps leading to the formation of fibrin proceed via a *common pathway,* requiring factors X, V, phospholipid, prothrombin and fibrinogen.

The final step in the coagulation phase, the *thrombin-fibrinogen reaction,* involves the transformation of fibrinogen into fibrin, which is the physical basis of all blood clots. This occurs in three separate steps; *viz.,* the enzymatic proteolysis of fibrinogen by thrombin which removes four peptides (fibrinopeptides), the formation of a visible but unstable fibrin polymer (soluble fibrin), and finally the formation of a stable fibrin polymer (insoluble fibrin) as the result of the action of factor XIII (fibrin-stabilizing factor). Structurally, fibrin resembles the proteins of muscle and skin and provides an extremely strong and stable framework for the "permanent" hemostatic plug.

Clot Retraction. This is the result of the mechanical shrinkage of fibrin strands within a clot. The platelets supply both the energy (ATP) and the contractile apparatus required for this process (thrombasthenin, a protein which functions like actomyosin of muscle). Despite the teleologic view that clot retraction may constitute a "physiologic" ligature which pulls the edge of a wound together, the hemostatic significance of the process remains uncertain.

CAUSES OF BLEEDING

Several factors can prevent the proper functioning of hemostatic mechanisms, resulting in abnormal bleeding. The cause of abnormal bleeding may be either mechanical or biochemical. Mechanical bleeding results from severed vessels of any size and will not stop because a clot cannot form, or because the clot breaks down or is removed from the opened end. This may be caused, for example, by the size of the vessel and the blood velocity (vein and artery), or by the numbers of small vessels or the postoperative trauma

they receive (capillary), or by other factors. Biochemical bleeding is an abnormality of the blood elements or vascular system that prevents normal clot formation and organization. This is typical in hemophilia, hepatic disorders, blood dyscrasias and other disorders (see Case Report No. 2).

In treating hemorrhage, the surgeon is faced with one of two situations: he may have seen the patient preoperatively or he sees the patient after someone else has done the surgery and the patient is in trouble.

Preoperatively all patients should be evaluated for bleeding tendencies. A history of excessive bleeding from previous extractions should alert the surgeon, but not necessarily label the patient as a "bleeder." Patients with hereditary hemorrhagic telangiectasia are not common. They frequently report nontraumatic hemorrhage from the mouth. This condition is characterized clinically by numerous small (pinpoint or slightly larger) localized bright red, purple or violet dilatations of capillaries, small arterioles, and small venules on the skin and mucous membrane and in other areas. These lesions will blanch when a glass microscope slide is pressed against them. There is no specific treatment for telangiectases. Topical hemostatic agents and electrocoagulation have been effective in the control of accessible hemorrhages.

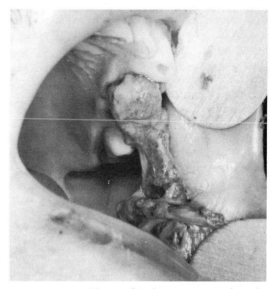

Figure 25–31 Twenty-four-hour postextraction clot that has extended from the maxilla downward, flowing over the occlusal surfaces of the maxillary teeth. This is a case of normal clotting time but prolonged bleeding. Treatment is to remove the clot and control the bleeding in the maxillary alveolus.

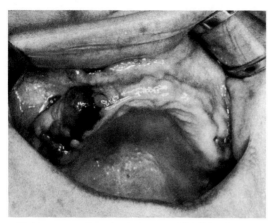

Figure 25–32 Organized postextraction blood clot exuding from the alveolus. This is found in patients with a normal clotting time and abnormal bleeding time.

The hemophiliac gives a typical familial and past medical history of bleeding. The familial history reveals abnormal bleeding associated with males only, with death of these males usually caused by massive hemorrhage. Laboratory tests will reveal a prolonged coagulation time. However, the idiopathic bleeder does not have a familial history of prolonged bleeding, nor is a lengthened coagulation time usually present. It can, therefore, be seen how easily normal familial histories and coagulation time may be misleading.

A patient with a history of bleeding should have the following laboratory tests performed: complete blood count (differential and hemoglobin); Lee-White coagulation time; clot retraction; platelet count; plasma prothrombin time and prothrombin concentration; blood type and cross matching; capillary fragility; and bleeding time.

Liver dysfunction is, in many cases, responsible for bleeding tendencies. An excellent test, therefore, is the plasma prothrombin time and prothrombin consumption. Postoperative bleeding occurs if the prothrombin concentration is less than 20 per cent of normal. Other liver function tests are indicated if the possibility of hepatic disease appears in the history. In other words, the patient requires a more thorough evaluation.

However, in many patients all presently available diagnostic tests may give negative results and clinically the patient is still a "bleeder." These patients (usually females) will develop massive ecchymotic areas and edema due to constant oozing; if the wounds are not tightly sutured they will ooze intraorally for many days. The cause of this bleeding is not known and may be a vascular (capillary) defect.

The patient who presents with active hemorrhage is a completely different problem. The first thing the surgeon should do is estimate the volume of blood that is left in the vascular system. After the application of a pressure pack over the bleeding area to control the hemorrhage by pressure, a quick evaluation of the patient's color, skin (dry or clammy), pulse and blood pressure, and duration of bleeding will reveal the possibility of impending shock. The urgency for transfusion of whole blood can thus be evaluated. The surgeon's attention can then be transferred back to the bleeding site. The first determination to be made is whether the bleeding is from the bone or from soft tissue. A good light and strong suction are essential. Mechanical compression with the finger is often an excellent diagnostic aid. If the bleeding is from the soft tissue, the severed vessel is ligated if possible or sutures are placed in such a manner as to tie off the feeder vessels. If the bleeding is from bone, the bone is crushed into the vessel if possible or pressure with gauze or surgical cement is used to control bleeding.

If bleeding persists—especially severe capillary oozing—the possibility must then be considered that the bleeding is of a biochemical origin and further studies must be instituted. Fresh whole blood should be ordered for immediate replacement as necessary until etiology is determined and specific therapy can be instituted. The use of packed cells in conjunction with high-molecular-weight intravenous fluids is a rapid method of correcting hypovolemia due to gross blood loss, and the necessary materials are readily available in most hospitals.

MECHANICAL HEMORRHAGE

Mechanical hemorrhage can roughly be divided into primary, intermediate and secondary hemorrhage. While hemorrhage from biochemical causes may follow the same pattern, it is easier to consider this in its totality.

Primary Hemorrhage

After surgical procedure in the oral cavity and closure of the wound, bleeding usually ceases spontaneously in normal patients. If this primary hemorrhage has not ceased after 4 or 5 minutes following the completion of the operation, it should be controlled before dismissing the patient. In the oral cavity, bleeding is either from bone or soft tissue.

Local Treatment of Primary Hemorrhage. If, during operations involving the bony processes, a "spurter" (artery) is severed, the bleeding can be controlled by taking a blunt instrument and crushing the surrounding bone into the point of bleeding, or bone wax can be smeared over the bleeding bony orifice. Capillary oozing from the bone either stops spontaneously or is usually controlled when the mucoperiosteal flaps are reapproximated and sutured back over the alveolar ridges. If bleeding is profuse, tightly pack the sockets with iodoform 1/4 gauze for 5 to 10 minutes under pressure, remove the gauze and then place pieces of absorbable hemostatic gauze in each socket before suturing the soft tissues into place. If local anesthesia with a vasoconstrictor is being used it must be remembered that "spurters" are not as easy to recognize and the sockets should be carefully examined to prevent these vessels from erupting when the vasoconstrictor has worn off. Where bone has been cracked, as often occurs in the buccal plate when upper molars are extracted, manual compression will reduce this greenstick type of fracture and is often all that is necessary to prevent hemorrhage if it is done at the time of the extraction.

Capillary bleeding from *soft tissues* at the time of operation is best controlled by suturing. If, for example, after an alveolectomy there is still bleeding following the insertion of the usual number of sutures, additional sutures should be inserted in that area in which bleeding occurs.

If bleeding persists, gauze pressure pads are placed over the area and firmly held in place for 5 to 10 minutes. Then, when the bleeding is controlled, additional pressure pads should be placed over this area, and the jaws held firmly together by applying an elastic bandage over the head and under the mandible for several hours.

Capillary bleeding from "raw" surfaces, such as those left after the excision of inflammatory papillary hyperplasia, hyperplastic tissue on the crest of the alveolar ridge, or epulis fissuratum, can be stopped by the careful use of the electrocoagulation instrument.

Ligation of Blood Vessels. In the event of arterial bleeding from the soft tissues, the vessel should be grasped with a hemostat and ligated by tying it directly or indirectly by the use of a circumferential suture around the soft tissue. Palatal vessels are the most commonly severed arteries in the mouth. Less frequently traumatized or severed are the inferior alveolar artery, the sublingual artery or the external maxillary artery.

If the greater palatine artery is cut, it is practically impossible to grasp and clamp it with a hemostat. Palatal pressure, great enough to stop the bleeding, should first be applied along the course of the vessel posterior to the point of bleeding and held firmly for at least 5 to 10 minutes. This gives the body's defense mechanism an opportunity to attempt to seal off the cut vessel.

A defense mechanism against bleeding, locally, is brought about by the contraction and retraction of the vessels at the site of rupture, producing a mechanical barrier to the escape of blood. Also, thromboplastic substances released from platelets and tissue juices facilitate clotting of blood, which tends to arrest the bleeding. Further, upon coagulation of the blood, a vasoconstrictor substance (serotonin) probably is liberated from the platelets, which contributes to the vascular contraction.

The author has twice stopped a major vessel hemorrhage by pressure. One case involved a severed sublingual artery and the second resulted when the external maxillary artery was pierced by an incorrectly placed pin being inserted through the skin into the mandible for extraoral skeletal pin fixation of a fractured mandible.

If bleeding resumes on release of pressure, the palatal mucoperiosteal tissue is reflected, including the point of bleeding. The anterior palatine vessels are then ligated posterior to the bleeding point by a "stick tie" (circumferential) suture through the entire thickness of the mucoperiosteum around the anterior (greater) palatine artery. The flap is then replaced and sutured to position (see Figure 25–33).

As a result of trauma (either external or from the operator's instrument), the sublingual artery in the floor of the mouth may be severed. This vessel is extremely difficult, if not impossible, to ligate when severed by a puncture wound, and the consequences can be fatal if the wound remains untreated. Bimanual pressure (one hand inside and one

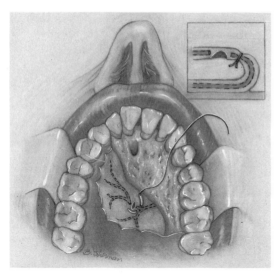

Figure 25-33 Control of hemorrhage from a severed anterior palatine artery with a "stick tie" suture passed through the mucoperiosteum medial to the cut. (Modified from Royer, R. Q. *In* Kruger, G. O.: Textbook of Oral Surgery. 2nd ed. St. Louis, The C. V. Mosby Co., 1964.)

hand outside the mouth) will usually control this bleeding until an appropriate ligation can be performed in the neck. Sometimes compression of the vessel in this manner for a minimum of 5 to 10 minutes will in itself stop the hemorrhage. Attempts to locate and clamp this artery with a hemostat are generally unsuccessful. If these attempts fail, then the lingual artery must be ligated.

The three most common sites for ligation are the lingual artery in Lesser's triangle, the external carotid artery in the neck between the superior thyroid and lingual arteries, and the external carotid in the retromandibular area lateral to the stylomandibular ligament. The reader is referred to Sicher and DuBrul's excellent text on head and neck anatomy for a detailed description of the anatomy and techniques involved.[63]

Intermediate or Recurrent Hemorrhage

This is hemorrhage that occurs within 24 hours after the operation. During the operation the patient's blood pressure may have fallen because of semi-shock, and then when the blood pressure returns to normal, as the patient recovers, there is recurrent hemorrhage. Ligatures may become untied, or, when the patient goes to bed, he removes the pressure pads, and the blood pressure "blows out" the clot, which no longer has the back pressure of the gauze sponges to support it.

Secondary Hemorrhage

Secondary hemorrhage may occur more than 24 hours following surgery; it is generally the result of the clot breaking down as the result of infection.

Local Treatment of Intermediate or Recurrent Hemorrhage and Secondary Hemorrhage. One or a combination of the following methods may be used:

1. If the sutures have become loose, the area should be anesthetized and a mat suture inserted firmly over the bleeding area.
2. Direct pressure may be applied over the bleeding area. This is accomplished by having the patient bite firmly on gauze pressure pads over the bleeding area, or by molding soft compound blocks over the bleeding area and having the patient bite into the soft compound. The surgeon should allow the compound to harden, remove and chill, trim with a knife, smooth with the torch, rechill, place it back into the mouth over the bleeding area, and have the patient bite firmly on the compound bite block. He should be certain that the compound also covers the buccal and lingual cortical plates.
3. A vasoconstrictor, such as epinephrine poured on a sponge, can be applied directly to the bleeding area; this results in a constriction of the lumen of the vessel until a new clot can form.
4. The surgeon can also apply a local agent to speed up blood coagulation. Local agents are thrombin, fibrinogen local, and thromboplastin local. All these agents are placed on gauze sponges and held over the bleeding areas, or placed into the sockets with pressure.

BIOCHEMICAL HEMORRHAGE

As previously mentioned, this type of bleeding is due to the absence of one or more of the factors necessary for a normal coagulation mechanism. It may be a genetically conditioned disorder or it may be acquired as a result of illness or through drugs that depress the formation of the necessary elements for coagulation.

CLINICAL MANIFESTATIONS OF DISORDERED HEMOSTASIS*

T. C. BITHELL, M.D., AND M. M. WINTROBE, M.D.

Certain *bleeding manifestations* are more or less *characteristic of the disorders of hemostasis.* For example, bleeding into the synovial joints (hemarthrosis) in the absence of obvious trauma and spontaneous bleeding into the skin are rarely encountered in patients with normal hemostatic function. Moreover, such signs and symptoms fall into two relatively distinct patterns, *i.e.,* those which are most common in disorders of vessels and platelets, and those which are more frequently seen in disorders of coagulation (Table 25-2). *Hemarthrosis* and its sequelae, for example, are almost diagnostic of a severe hereditary coagulation disorder, *e.g.,* hemophilia, and are exceedingly rare in vascular and platelet disorders. Recurrent crops of *petechiae,* on the other hand, are strongly suggestive of an abnormality of the vessels or platelets, *e.g.,* thrombocytopenia, and are rare in the coagulation disorders. Ecchymoses may occur in any disorder of hemostasis, but if they are the result of abnormal blood coagulation, they are large, characteristically dissect deeper structures, and may spread to involve an entire limb.

Profuse and often life-threatening hemorrhage following trivial trauma or surgical procedures is a hallmark of the coagulation disorders, and the onset of bleeding is often delayed for several hours. This phenomenon of *delayed bleeding* is rare in disorders of

---

* Reprinted with permission from Wintrobe, M. M., *et al.*: Harrison's Principles of Medicine. 6th ed., pp. 321–322. Copyright © 1970 by McGraw-Hill, Inc., New York. Used by permission of McGraw-Hill Book Company.

Table 25-2 *The Clinical Distinction between Disorders of Vessels and Platelets and Disorders of Blood Coagulation*

FINDINGS	DISORDERS OF COAGULATION	DISORDERS OF PLATELETS AND VESSELS ("PURPURIC" DISORDERS)
Hemarthroses	Characteristic	Rare
Petechiae	Rare	Characteristic
Positive family history	Common	Rare
Sex	95 per cent of hereditary forms occur only in males	Relatively more common in females
Traumatic bleeding	Onset often delayed; rapid and voluminous	Onset immediate; slow and persistent oozing

vessels or platelets, where slow but persistent oozing begins immediately following trauma.

The *sex* of the patient, the *age* when abnormal bleeding was first noted, and the *family history* are of particular importance in evaluating the disorders of hemostasis, since most disorders of vessels and platelets are acquired, whereas most serious coagulation disorders are hereditary, and among these, over 90 per cent occur only in males. The absence of a family history of bleeding, however, does not exclude the presence of a hereditary coagulation disorder.

The history remains the best single "screening" test for the presence of a hemorrhagic disorder, and the corollary to this statement is no less true. A history of surgery, major injury, or even multiple tooth extractions without abnormal bleeding is good evidence against the presence of a hereditary coagulation disorder.

Case Report No. 2

POSTEXTRACTION HEMORRHAGE IN A PATIENT WITH CHRONIC MYELOGENOUS LEUKEMIA*

Patient. A 56-year-old white man, an employee of a trade school, was admitted to the Oral Surgery and Hematology† Sections of South Side Hospital on July 9 with the chief complaint of profuse bleeding from the left mandibular molar region following four recent extractions.

---

† Jay H. Silverberg, M.D., Chief of Hematology Section.

---

* Case report prepared by William Petitto, D.D.S., Oral Surgery Resident, South Side Hospital, Pittsburgh, Pa.

History of Present Illness. On Saturday, July 6, the teeth in question had been extracted by the patient's dentist. The tissues had been approximated and sutured and the patient discharged from the office. On Sunday night, July 7, the patient's gums had started to bleed, and hemorrhage had become uncontrollable. On Monday morning at 2:00 A.M. the patient had gone to the dentist's office. Alveolar sockets had been packed and the wound resutured. Bleeding had subsided until later Monday morning, at which time hemorrhaging had recurred; at 2:00 P.M. the same day, the patient had revisited the dental office and the wound had been resutured. Bleeding had been controlled until 8:00 P.M. that same day, at which time the patient had again returned to the dentist's office. On Tuesday morning at 2:00 A.M. bleeding had resumed and the patient had called the dentist, who had referred him to South Side Hospital, to the service of Dr. W. H. Archer. The patient had been admitted at 11:20 A.M. and seen at 12:45 P.M., at which time bleeding was still present. The patient stated that he had never had bleeding difficulties prior to this time.

Past History. Findings were essentially negative, with the exception of a weight loss of 15 pounds in the past 6 months.

Oral Examination. The intraoral examination revealed bleeding from the lower left molar area and packs were in place over area of bleeding. The remaining lower teeth showed deposits of calculus, staining and apparent alveolar resorption and gingival recession. The maxilla was edentulous, and the patient was wearing a full upper plate.

Physical Examination. The patient's blood pressure was 160/88; pulse, 94; and respiration, 22. Findings were otherwise essentially negative, except for palpable axillary nodes and possible splenomegaly.

Impressions.   1. Splenomegaly? (Leukemic origin.)
2. Rule out thrombocytopenia.

DAY-BY-DAY TREATMENT AND SUBSEQUENT LABORATORY REPORTS

July 9. Admission day.

Laboratory Work Ordered: Type and cross match −1000 cc. whole blood, stat. Urinalysis: Findings essentially negative. Dr. Silverberg ordered Myleran, 4 mg. (2 tablets A.M. and P.M.), ¾ hour before meals.

Laboratory Findings: Prothrombin time, 17.0 sec.; control, 15 sec. RBC, 3,250,000. WBC, 263,000. Hemoglobin, 9.5 gm.; 61.6 per cent; color index, 0.96. Bleeding time, 2 min. Coagulation time, 2 min., 30 sec. Clotting time: clot commenced in 1 hour, clot complete in 18 hours; clot firm, difficult to break or flatten; normal retraction

of clot. Blood smear loaded with myelocytes and metamyelocytes and many myeloblasts; smear revealed findings typical of chronic granulocytic leukemia. Blood chemistry: glucose, 110; urea, 28.3; creatine, 2.1.

With these laboratory findings, consistent with myeloid leukemia, the patient was transferred to the care of the hematologist (Dr. Silverberg).

July 10. The patient was still bleeding in the A.M.; 500 cc. of blood was administered. The patient, seen by Dr. Archer at 3:30 P.M., was still bleeding profusely, with blood apparently coming from the mental foramen region.

The patient was taken to the operating room. Atropine sulfate, 1/100 grain, was administered ½ hour prior to surgery. Previously placed sutures had been torn loose by the bleeding below the soft-tissue flaps. A gap over a width of 2 to 3 cm. intervened. These sutures and old clots were removed and new, deeply placed mat sutures were inserted and tied by Dr. Archer. It was impossible to approximate tissue flaps because of the partially formed blood clot beneath the flaps. However, all bleeding was controlled when patient was removed from the operating room.

July 11. The patient was still bleeding intermittently. Large clots were present over the area and extended out of the sockets. Periodically, the patient expectorated huge clots of blood. 500 cc. blood was administered.

Laboratory Findings: RBC, 3,260,000. WBC, 256,000. Hemoglobin, 8 gm.; 56.8 per cent; color index, 0.81. Platelet count, 311,000. The majority of cells are of the primitive myeloid series.

July 12. The patient was still bleeding at 10:15 P.M.; bleeding became profuse. Ordered for cross match and holding was 500 cc. blood (500 cc. blood given). Medication: Adrenosem salicylate, 3 doses, 1 ampule every 3 hours (no effect). Blood pressure and pulse to be taken every 3 hours. Mephyton, 50 mg. in 200 cc. normal saline following the blood. 20 mg. Premarin to be administered intravenously during the night if the above failed. Nembutal, 1½ grains at bedtime.

Laboratory Findings: WBC, 190,000. Hemoglobin, 7.25 gm.; 45 per cent.

July 13. 500 cc. of blood with 20 mg. Premarin added, given during the night. In A.M., the patient was still bleeding; he was to return to operating room at noon. 500 cc. of blood was again administered before operating room. At noon the patient was taken to the operating room and resutured. Bleeding was controlled, and he was taken from the operating room with bleeding under control.

Laboratory Findings: Hemoglobin, 7.5 gm.; 48.6 per cent. Hematocrit, 30 per cent. Hemorrhage was under control during the day.

July 14. Bleeding was under control following the operating room procedure. 500 cc. of fresh whole blood was administered.

July 15. Bleeding was still under control; however, the patient was beginning to expectorate small clots of blood.

July 16. Bleeding started again during the night. *Laboratory Report:* Prothrombin time, 14.0 sec.; control, 13 sec. RBC, 3,280,000. WBC, 368,000. Hemoglobin, 8.5 gm.; 55.1 per cent; color index, 0.86. Hematocrit, 37 per cent.

500 cc. of fresh whole blood was administered.

July 17. Bleeding seemed to be under control. However, there was slight oozing. *Laboratory Findings:* WBC, 231,500. Hemoglobin, 7 gm.; 45.5 per cent.

July 18. Bleeding was still present but slight.

July 19. The patient was still bleeding slightly in A.M. 500 cc. of blood was administered. P.M., bleeding was controlled and the spleen smaller.

July 20. Bleeding commenced again. 500 cc. blood was administered.

July 21. Bleeding was still present. The patient was visited by Dr. Archer; he was returned to the operating room, and the oral tissues were resutured for control of hemorrhage. Bleeding was controlled, and the patient was taken from the operating room in good condition. 500 cc. blood was administered.

July 22. Bleeding was well under control. *Laboratory Report* (sample of blood taken on July 21, report returned July 22): RBC, 2,140,000. WBC, 209,000. Hemoglobin, 6.8 gm.; 43.8 per cent. Platelet count, 184,000.

Subsequent Blood Report: RBC, 2,800,000. WBC, 173,000. Hemoglobin, 45.5 per cent; color index, 0.81. Neutrophils, 99; lymphocytes, 1.

July 23. 500 cc. fresh whole blood was ordered and administered. Bleeding was still controlled.

July 24. 500 cc. blood was given and 500 cc. ordered for the 25th. No bleeding.

July 25. 500 cc. blood was administered. No bleeding.

July 26. No bleeding was present; tissues were healing normally and sutures still in place. *Laboratory Report* (from 7/24): RBC, 3,200,000. WBC, 100,000. Hemoglobin, 8 gm.; 51.8 per cent. Platelet count, 180,000.

July 27. No bleeding was seen, and tissues were healing very satisfactorily. *Blood Report:* RBC, 3,470,000. WBC, 144,000. Hemoglobin, 9.5 gm.; 61.6 per cent; color index, 0.90. Neutrophils, 86; lymphocytes, 14.

July 28. No bleeding was evident, and a blood report was ordered.

July 29. No bleeding was present. *Laboratory Report:* WBC, 51,250. Hemoglobin, 9.5 gm.; 61.6 per cent.

July 30. Tissues were healing normally. 500 cc. blood was administered.

July 31. The patient was comfortable, without bleeding, and tissues were healing normally. *Laboratory Report:* RBC, 2,940,000. WBC, 19,600. Hemoglobin, 9.5 gm.; 61.6 per cent; color index, 1.06. Neutrophils, 87; lymphocytes, 8; monocytes, 3; eosinophils, 2; platelets, 600,000.

August 1. The patient was discharged.

Comment. Note how, despite the many efforts at local control of hemorrhage, remission did not occur until there was a depression of the leukemic condition.

Case Report No. 3

HEMORRHAGE FOLLOWING ODONTECTOMY AND ALVEOLECTOMY*

A 51-year-old male patient was admitted September 10, for complete maxillary and mandibular odontectomy and alveolectomy.

Chief Complaint. "Big cavities and rotten looking teeth."

History of Chief Complaint. Reluctance to visit dentist due to a bleeding tendency has resulted in poor oral hygiene, extensive caries and periodontoclasia.

Past Medical History. The patient claimed that he and all male members of his family were true hemophiliacs. However, extensive surgery performed on one male member of the family, with a minimum of preoperative precaution, had resulted in no untoward postoperative bleeding. The patient stated that he himself had suffered severe cuts with no protracted bleeding; also, that small cuts clotted immediately. The only history of prolonged bleeding was from a single extraction that bled for 1 week—the patient being able to work during this time.

Note: In a subsequent discussion with the patient's brother, approximately 1 week following surgery, it was found that the patient had completely minimized his previous bleeding history. At this time it was discovered that he, as a child, had had periodic bouts of epistaxis, which though now much diminished, still occurred; that he had bled profusely when cut, and bruised easily. The brother stated that he himself had left his job as a driver for a window glass company because he had feared cutting himself.

---

* Case report prepared by Oral Surgery Resident, Eye and Ear Hospital, Pittsburgh, Pa.

Family History. No familial deaths were attributed to hemophilia.

Physical Examination. Examination revealed no abnormalities. Blood pressure was 160/95. Oral examination revealed very poor oral hygiene, periodontoclasia and extensive caries.

Preoperative Orders.

    C.B.C. and hemoglobin
    Urinalysis
    Lee-White coagulation time
    Platelet count
    Prothrombin time and concentration
    Bleeding and coagulation times
    Blood type

Nembutal, $1\frac{1}{2}$ grains at bedtime
Ascorbic acid, 400 mg. at bedtime
    For oral surgery 11:00 A.M. Pentothal
Nembutal, $1\frac{1}{2}$ grains
Morphine sulfate, $\frac{1}{6}$ grain $\Big\}$ 10:15 A.M.
Atropine sulfate, $\frac{1}{100}$ grain

Laboratory Record. Urine was clear, straw-colored, acid in reaction, with a specific gravity of 1.028; findings of albumin and sugar were negative. The blood count was essentially normal. Lee-White coagulation time was 5 minutes, 35 seconds, the platelet count, 300,000; prothrombin time: control 12 seconds, patient 17 seconds; prothrombin concentration, 40 per cent of normal; bleeding time was 2 minutes, 10 seconds; coagulation time was 2 minutes, 50 seconds.

Discussion of Laboratory Findings. Probably the one great diagnostic aid in a differential diagnosis of hemophilia (aside from familial history) is a prolonged coagulation time. This was at no time evident in the patient's preoperative laboratory work. According to Beeson and McDermott,[6] atypical cases of hemophilia are not to be suspected until some operation takes place with a hemophiliac type of bleeding following. However, postoperative bleeding was to be expected because of the low prothrombin concentration. According to Best and Taylor,[7] and Quick,[52] a bleeding tendency is not to be expected until the prothrombin concentration falls to about 20 per cent of normal (100 per cent). Although Cecil agrees with this, he also considers a 50 per cent level potentially dangerous preoperatively.

Accordingly a medical consultation was obtained, with the planned operation being approved. However, it was deemed prudent to decrease the amount of surgery; therefore, only a partial maxillary odontectomy and alveolectomy was scheduled, with 500 cc. whole blood available for transfusion.

Operation (September 12). Following the routine preparation of the face and administration of general anesthesia, local nerve block injections were made to: (1) eliminate pain stimuli to the brain, (2) reduce the amount of general anesthetic needed, and (3) provide hemostasis.

A partial maxillary and mandibular odontectomy and alveolectomy was performed, with the following teeth being extracted:

$$R \frac{\quad 5 \quad 4 \quad 3 \quad 2 \quad 1 \quad \Big|\quad 1 \quad 2 \quad 3 \quad}{\quad 8 \quad 7 \quad 6 \quad \Big|\quad 4 \quad 5 \quad 6 \quad 8 \quad} L$$

Throughout the operation it was noted that rather than the excessive bleeding anticipated, the bleeding was even less than that normally encountered. It was because of this that the surgery was extended to include a partial mandibular odontectomy and alveolectomy. A transfusion was not deemed necessary at this time; the patient was removed from the operating room in good condition.

Postoperative Orders.

    Ice bags administered to face
    Biolite beginning tomorrow morning 4 times a day
    Ascorbic acid, 200 mg. twice a day
    Zonite mouthwash beginning tomorrow morning 4 times a day
    Multiple vitamin capsules, 2 per meal
    Codeine sulfate, $\frac{1}{2}$ grain $\Big\}$ every 3 hours as
    Aspirin, 10 grains $\quad\quad$ required
    Vitamin K, 20 mg. twice a day

Postoperative Progress. The evening of September 12, the patient began to bleed profusely from all operative sites. A series of deep sutures and pressure packs seemed to control bleeding at this time. The next day there was marked edema of both cheeks, and swelling involving the posterior regions of right and left mandible. This latter swelling was due to subperiosteal hemorrhage. The patient stated that he had usually bled 4 to 5 days following previous extractions. Throughout the patient's postoperative course a very strong psychosomatic factor seemed to be associated with the duration and intensity of his bleeding. This was manifested in the seeming ability of the patient to predict when bleeding would start or stop, and the intensity of the hemorrhage. It was his belief throughout his hospital stay (although at all times he was extremely cooperative and cheerful) that his bleeding would have been of much shorter duration if he had been allowed to go home and not receive medication, for it was with the medication and transfusions that he could "feel the pressure building up" with subsequent hemorrhage.

The evening of September 13 bleeding again commenced, and although pressure packs and sutures were again inserted, bleeding was minimized but not completely controlled. The patient was placed on complete bed rest, with sedation and 250 cc. whole blood transfusion. As he had predicted, he bled profusely immediately following the transfusion, but by the following day bleeding had stopped, with the formation of small clots.

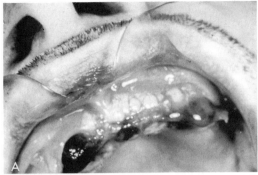
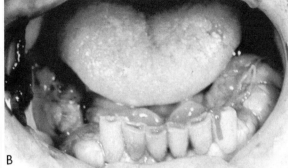
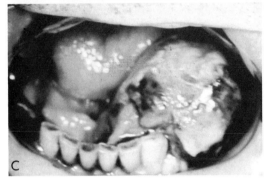

Figure 25–34 Postoperative submucoperiosteal mandibular hemorrhage. *A*, Fifth day of postoperative bleeding. *B*, Note that the sutured mucoperiosteal membrane has been stripped and lifted from the left mandibular alveolar ridge. The sutures have not broken as yet on this side, but have broken on the right side, and a mass of oozing, partially organized blood clots is visible. *C*, Thirteenth day of postoperative bleeding. On the left is an enormous partially organized blood clot which has broken through the flaps and is bleeding around the periphery. Note the pool of blood in the right ridge area. The clots in this area have broken down. (See Case Report No. 3.)

The medical consultant* advised discontinuance of transfusions until results from liver function tests were obtained. Hepatic insufficiency of undetermined origin was suspected (the patient had given no history of excessive alcoholic intake), especially in view of continued low prothrombin concentrations following administration of large quantities of vitamin K. The laboratory reports when obtained substantiated this belief. In addition to low prothrombin concentrations, the following results were reported: cephalin flocculation (24 hrs.), +4; Bromsulphalein, 10 per cent retention.

Six days postoperatively the patient had a blood pressure of 100/80, an RBC of 2,320,000 and a hemoglobin concentration of 50 per cent. Transfusions of whole blood no more than 24 hours old were instituted, 100 cc. being administered September 18. AB-negative (the patient's type) donors being difficult to obtain, the hematologist† suggested the use of O-negative fresh blood. This was done, with no reactions being encountered. Two days following the administration of 500 cc. of fresh blood per day, the patient felt and looked much better, with red count, hemoglobin and prothrombin counts increased. September 22 the transfusions were discontinued, with a recom-

mencing of oozing that afternoon; 500 cc. transfusions were reinstituted the following day.

From September 12 to 23 the hematomas present in both right and left posterior mandibular regions had continued to grow. By the latter date they had reached gigantic proportions, extending above the incisal surface of the lower anterior teeth approximately 2 cm. They extended from the first bicuspid regions to the third molar regions, and buccolingually measured 4 cm. (see Figure 25–34*C*). There was no external oozing associated with the hematomas, just a continuous oozing into the circumscribed areas. By September 24 some organization of the hematomas was noticed.

On September 27 transfusions were again discontinued. The maxillary alveolar mucosa was of good consistency and color, devoid of clots, and healing well. There was some oozing from mandibular hematomas, but this was very slight and periodic in nature. The organization of the hematomas was nearing completion, no growth being noted since September 25.

By October 1 the following blood picture was noted: red blood cells, 3,860,000 per cu. mm.; white blood cells, 7050 per cu. mm.; hemoglobin, 81 per cent; prothrombin concentration, 56 per cent; prothrombin time: control, 12 seconds; patient, 13.5 seconds.

Both hematomas had diminished in size and were beginning to slough. The patient was discharged October 2, with a final medical diagnosis of hepatic insufficiency.

THE HEMOPHILIAC: PREOPERATIVE AND POSTOPERATIVE TREATMENT

Surgical procedures of any kind constitute a definite problem in the hemophiliac patient. Case Report No. 4 illustrates the use of anti-hemophilic globulin (Fraction I) in the control of hemorrhage associated with oral surgery.

Hemophilia is a congenital entity with the following characteristics: (a) it occurs only in males; (b) family history shows a characteristic type of inheritance; (c) coagulation time of the drawn blood, but not the bleeding time, is usually prolonged; (d) there is no reduction in the number of platelets.

Use of Blood and Blood Fractions. The beneficial effects of whole blood transfusion in hemophilia have been recognized for over 30 years. The marked fall in the coagulation time following the transfusion of normal blood was attributed to the platelets by Minot and Lee in 1910, as discussed by Minot and Taylor.[47]

Patek and Stetson in 1936[51] found that the platelet-free plasma had the same beneficial effect as whole blood. Work in recent years has shown that the antihemophilic property of platelet-free plasma is closely associated with the globulin fraction of the plasma proteins. Globulin fractions free of prothrombin and thrombin have an optimal effect in bringing about a normal coagulation time in the hemophiliac patient.

Cohn's fractionation of human blood yields six major fractions. The first of these contains most of the fibrinogen and antihemophilic globulin. This fraction can be injected intravenously into human beings with safety,

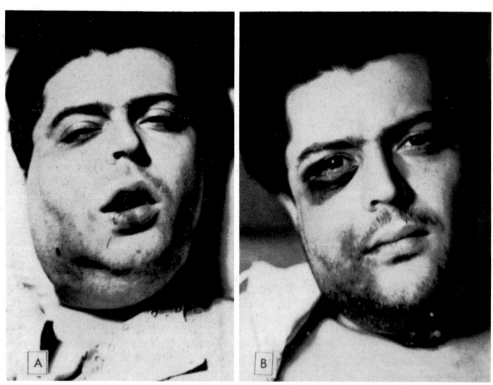

Figure 25–35 *A,* Appearance of a hemophiliac, aged 29, 4 to 5 hours after insertion of a needle posterior to the last lower right molar tooth for a regional nerve block preliminary to removal of a premolar. The anesthetic was not injected and the tooth was not removed. Immediate severe pain was experienced after the needle was inserted, and within a few minutes after the needle was withdrawn a large hematoma (arterial) formed, involving the posterior portion of the tongue, right pharynx, and right cheek. Because of impending asphyxia, a tracheotomy was done soon after this photograph was taken. *B,* Appearance 5 days later. The tracheotomy tube is in position. Daily blood transfusions were given until the wound healed completely, approximately 6 weeks afterwards. (From Jackson, C., and Jackson, C. L.: Diseases of the Nose, Throat and Ear. 2nd ed. Philadelphia, W. B. Saunders Co., 1959.)

and the coagulant effect is similar to that of whole blood. Fractions of increased purity sometimes have less antihemophilic effect than crude preparations. This may indicate that more than one factor may be defective in the clotting mechanism of hemophiliacs.

Archer and Zubrow[3] reported a case of hemophilia in which the antihemophilic globulin (Fraction I) was used to control hemorrhage from the alveolus after the extraction of a maxillary central incisor. This case is adapted in Case Report No. 4.

Case Report No. 4

TOOTH EXTRACTION FOR A HEMOPHILIAC*

W. H. ARCHER, D.D.S., AND H. J. ZUBROW, D.D.S.

History. This patient, a 25-year-old white man, had become aware that he was a hemophiliac at the age of 10, at which time he had cut his tongue during a football game. Severe hemorrhage had resulted, and he was hospitalized for 14 days. (Hospital records were not available.) At that time he had experienced his first hemorrhage in the knee joints. This had resulted in a partial loss of function, which has persisted until this time.

On February 24, the patient was admitted to a local hospital for treatment of excessive bleeding resulting from the extraction of three teeth.

The laboratory findings upon admission at that time were: red blood cells, 2,700,000 per cu. mm.; white blood cells, 4700; hemoglobin, 7.5 gm.; platelets, 240,000; coagulation time, 2 hours, 30 minutes; urinalysis: specific gravity, 1.029; 2 plus sugar; a trace of albumin; occasional leukocytes.

The notable facts about that admission were: (a) profuse bleeding from the sockets and surrounding gingival tissues, in spite of local attempts, such as pressure and epinephrine packs, to control the hemorrhage prior to admission. (b) On February 26, bleeding from the mouth continued. The patient was given a transfusion with 500 cc. of whole blood. Bleeding stopped temporarily. (c) The patient received 250 cc. of whole blood daily from March 4 to March 7 to control the bleeding. (d) Intermittent bleeding from the sockets persisted until March 18. The sockets were packed with cotton saturated with thromboplastin.

The patient was discharged 8 days after admission.

Family History. The patient was one of six children. Two of the patient's younger brothers died of uncontrollable hemorrhage at the ages of 2 years and 11 months, respectively. One brother cut his lip during a fall, and the ensuing massive hemorrhage proved fatal. The other child died of hemorrhage sustained from a blow to the mouth. The elder brother and his sister were apparently normal. Information concerning the preceding generation was vague. The patient's father had died of

a malignant disease, and the mother was still living.

Hospital Admission Notes. Three years after the first admission, the patient was admitted to the Eye and Ear Hospital, Pittsburgh, on September 28, for extraction of the upper right central incisor, which was extensively carious, with pulp necrosis and periapical infection.

The condition of the patient's mouth showed evidence of prolonged neglect. All the remaining teeth were carious, and many of the crowns were completely destroyed. It was decided to extract but one tooth at this time, evaluate the results, and plan future extractions accordingly.

The patient was seen at the office for several weeks prior to admission. During this period small rubber elastics were placed about the neck of the tooth in an attempt to produce some exfoliation, thus permitting a less traumatic extraction.

A full palatal acrylic splint with an extension over the socket was made by cutting the tooth off the stone model before processing the splint. This was examined to make certain that there would be no pressure points or undercuts that might create trauma around the socket.

Physical Examination. Significant positive findings were extensive dental caries, cervical and submaxillary adenopathy, slight enlargement of the liver, and limited function of both elbows and knees due to fibrosis.

Significant negative findings were fundi normal; no hemorrhage; heart and lungs normal.

Laboratory Findings. The urine had a specific gravity of 1.020. A complete blood count showed the following: red blood cells, 4,200,000 per cu. mm.; white blood cells, 7000; hemoglobin, 84 per cent; polymorphonuclear leukocytes, 71 per cent;

---

* Adapted from Archer, W. H., and Zubrow, H. J.: Hemophiliac: the pre- and postoperative treatment. Oral Surg., *3*:1377, 1950.

lymphocytes, 25 per cent; monocytes, 2 per cent; eosinophils, 1 per cent. The blood was typed as II "A." The venous clotting time was 35 minutes. The coagulation time was 11 minutes; bleeding time, 1 minute, 16 seconds.

Operative Procedure. Fraction I, 400 mg. dissolved in 20 cc. of normal saline solution, was given intravenously 30 minutes preoperatively. This reduced the venous clotting time (Lee-White method) to 5 minutes, 30 seconds.

Under general anesthesia the patient was draped and prepared in the routine manner. The upper right central incisor was atraumatically extracted with a No. 286 forceps. The socket was then packed with Gelfoam saturated with thrombin. An acrylic template, with an extension covering the socket, was then placed in position.

Postoperative Course. On the first postoperative day the patient bled freely. His mouth was aspirated and the template removed and cleaned. At 7 P.M. thrombin was applied to the bleeding areas with temporary effect. The patient was very apprehensive. Seconal, 1½ grains, was given immediately. The template was replaced, and a gauze dressing was placed over the template to help hold it in position. When the patient bit on the gauze, this in turn forced the template against the socket.

The thrombin was applied to the bleeding area as follows: A cotton applicator was moistened with normal saline solution, and then placed in a vial of powdered thrombin. This was introduced directly to the bleeding area, and the thrombin held in place by pressure packs or the template for 30 minutes.

The dressings were changed at 9 P.M., when there was moderate bleeding, and again at 10 P.M.

The patient suffered moderate bleeding at 1 A.M. At 6:30 A.M., early on the second postoperative day, thrombin was applied on gauze packs and placed at the lingual surface of the socket, from which most of the bleeding was coming. The template was then inserted over the small gauze dressings.

By noon the bleeding had increased, so 400 mg. of Fraction I was given intravenously, whereupon the bleeding stopped. By 2:30 P.M. dark viscous blood clots were evident under the template. The template was removed and cleaned at 8 P.M. Since there was still moderate bleeding, Gelfoam and thrombin packs were replaced, and the bleeding stopped.

At 9:45 A.M. on the third postoperative day there was still slight oozing from the lingual area of the gingiva surrounding the socket. The blood did not appear to be coming from the socket itself. Approximately one drop of blood every 10 seconds was noted at this time.

At noon, clot formation seemed firmer, but there was increased bleeding around the periphery of the clot. At this time 400 mg. of Fraction I was administered intravenously. By 1 P.M. the bleeding

had practically stopped, with just slight oozing. At 7:15 P.M. the patient was bleeding rather freely, however, and 400 mg. of Fraction I was given intravenously. The bleeding lessened.

On the fourth postoperative day a heavy clot had formed, with some retraction evident. There was no bleeding.

On the fifth postoperative day there was a large clinging clot about 1 cm. in diameter hanging from the upper incisor area. There was little oozing. The template was removed.

On the sixth postoperative day there was no bleeding. A small, well-attached clot was present.

On the seventh postoperative day there was still no bleeding, and the patient was discharged on the eighth postoperative day.

Summary of Postoperative Course. Fraction I, 400 mg., was given intravenously approximately every 18 hours, and would in each case reduce the coagulation time to between 4 minutes 45 seconds and 5 minutes 40 seconds within 30 minutes. From this time until 6 hours after injection there was only a slight increase in the coagulation time; the time remained well within normal limits. The increase in the next 6-hour period was also slight, and at the end of 18 hours the coagulation time was still below the time recorded before the administration of Fraction I.

There was no appreciable variation in blood pressure during the admission. Blood pressure upon admission was 114/91, and upon discharge was 124/78.

A fluid intake of 3000 cc. per 24 hours was maintained.

The blood picture varied little throughout. The hemoglobin remained between 80 and 84 per cent; the red blood cells, between 3,980,000 and 4,200,000 per cu. mm.; and the white blood cells, between 7000 and 7700.

The patient was extremely apprehensive during his hospital stay, and entered into a state of moderate mental depression. This necessitated frequent sedation. Phenobarbital was used for this purpose.

Summary.

1. The use of Plasma Fraction I quickly reduced the venous clotting time to within normal limits.
2. The maximal effect of the plasma fraction was observed for approximately 12 hours after injection.
3. The bleeding was often spontaneous, and it appeared to be from the gingival margins rather than from the socket itself, probably because of the gingival inflammation resulting from the use of a rubber band.
4. The bleeding could be controlled for short periods by topical application of thrombin.
5. Large clots, showing no tendency to retract, would form and interfere with the stability of the template.

6. The template, we feel, created additional trauma, thereby increasing the tendency to bleed by interfering with clot formation.
7. The rubber band around the neck of the tooth was of little help in loosening the tooth. On the contrary, because of the mechanical irritation of the rubber band, the gingival tissues were greatly inflamed, and the bleeding thereby increased when the tooth was extracted. White and Mallett reported that they observed troublesome bleeding from this procedure.[69]

Case Report No. 5

FATAL HEMORRHAGE FOLLOWING REGIONAL ANESTHESIA FOR OPERATIVE DENTISTRY IN A HEMOPHILIAC*

W. H. ARCHER, D.D.S., AND H. J. ZUBROW, D.D.S.

This case report is presented as a sequel to the preceding case report. The patient involved in both case reports is the same person, the elapsed time interval being approximately 5 years.

The following pertinent facts, made available to us, were obtained from the patient's dentist, the patient's hospital record, and the patient's family, and serve to illustrate graphically the chain of events leading to the termination of this case.

On July 13, the family dentist gave the patient described in Case Report No. 4 two left inferior alveolar nerve block injections to prevent pain in cavity preparation. However, in spite of the fact that the patient admitted numbness of the lip, he still complained of pain when cavity preparation was attempted. The appointment was terminated, as the dentist did not want to give a third injection.

A gradually increasing swelling of the oral tissues during the next 4 hours prompted the patient to call his dentist, who advised him to apply ice to his swollen face. The next day the swelling continued to increase and the patient could not swallow, so he was referred by the dentist to the family physician, who gave him a prescription (contents unknown). The patient's condition became steadily worse, and on July 15, his physician sent him to the hospital.

Extracts from hospital record were as follows:

Patient. A 30-year-old white man was admitted to a local hospital on July 15, with a provisional diagnosis of hemophilia, ecchymosis of pharynx, mouth, gingiva, face and neck (left side).

Chief Complaint. Swelling of the jaw, mouth and neck since July 13.

History of Chief Complaint. The patient was in usual health until July 13, when he received two injections of procaine (in lower jaw) for dental work. No extractions were performed. The swelling began on the same day, a few hours after the procaine injection. Patient is unable to swallow saliva—nothing by mouth since July 13—has applied ice locally since the onset.

The physical examination revealed a marked diffuse swelling of the left side of the face and neck, due to a hematoma, with ecchymosis of skin.

Throat—pharyngeal swelling.

Mouth—opening of mouth limited because of swelling; left side gingival swelling.

Chest—respiration labored because of swelling of mouth and pharynx.

Extremities—marked limitations of movement in both knees and elbows (hemarthroses).

July 15: 5 P.M. 500 cc. of whole blood was given at once with 1000 cc. of 5 per cent glucose in normal saline solution.

5:10 P.M. The physician was called to evaluate respiratory difficulty; nasal catheter and oxygen were at bedside.

6:00 P.M. The physician was called to the patient in acute respiratory distress. He attempted to open the airway and administered artificial respiration. The patient was cyanotic and had ceased to breathe; the pulse was weak and faint, rapid, of low volume. He attempted intratracheal intubation. The patient did not respond.

6:14 P.M. Circulatory failure with cessation of heart beat. The patient was pronounced dead.

Discussion. The patient discussed in this case was a true hemophiliac. This was verified by his clinical and family history.

Briefly, in 1932, he spent 14 days in a hospital for the treatment of hemorrhage from a cut in his tongue (hospital records not available). In 1944, 34 days of hospitalization and repeated blood transfusions were required to control hemorrhage following the extraction of three teeth. At this time, his coagulation time was 2 hours and 30 minutes.

In 1947 he was treated by us, at which time the extraction of an abscessed tooth was performed. Plasma Fraction I was used to reduce the clotting time to within normal limits, and to provide for clot retraction.

---

*Adapted from Archer, W. H., and Zubrow, H. J.: Fatal hemorrhage following regional anesthesia for operative dentistry in a hemophiliac. Oral Surg., 7:464–470 (May), 1954.

At this time his venous coagulation time was 35 minutes, and the bleeding time was 1 minute and 16 seconds. However, it required 8 days of local and systemic treatment, including seven intravenous injections, each containing 400 mg. Fraction I in 20 cc. normal saline the first 6 days before bleeding stopped.

At the hospital admission described in this report, the coagulation time was reported as 3 minutes and 30 seconds, and the bleeding time 2 minutes and 30 seconds. It is recognized that the coagulation time in hemophiliacs can fall within normal limits, but it is not reasonable to believe that such was the case in this patient at this time. Death occurred before a recheck of these findings, but it seems obvious that they were incorrect.

The patient had received two mandibular injections of procaine hydrochloride (2 per cent), with epinephrine, to provide anesthesia for cavity preparation. The ensuing respiratory embarrassment caused by a constantly enlarging hematoma of the superficial and deep structures pierced by the injection needle ably proves the fact that even the most innocuous procedure is formidable when performed on the hemophiliac.

When hemorrhage does occur, local attempts at hemostasis are usually unsuccessful and waste valuable time. The general hematologic picture must be corrected by injections of whole blood, plasma, or fractions containing the antihemophilic globulins.

The question of tracheostomy becomes a highly complex one in the hemophiliac. When absolutely necessary to prevent death from asphyxia, the tracheostomy may be performed, and the subsequent bleeding controlled by the infusions mentioned in the preceding paragraph. Other methods of maintaining an airway are preferable only if they assure a patent airway beyond doubt.

The patient suffering from a prolonged, gradually progressive hypoxia may reach a respiratory and circulatory crisis quickly and without warning. This is demonstrated in this case report.

To circumvent the respiratory obstruction (hematoma) present in this case perhaps the use of an emergency unit known as the "cricothyrotomy trocar tube," which is much less traumatic than Jackson's emergency tracheotomy, thereby opening a small vascular field, might have been of value. (Study Emergency Treatment of Acute Respiratory Blockage in this chapter.)

ANATOMIC DISCUSSION OF THIS HEMORRHAGE

G. E. FULLER, D.D.S.

The hemorrhage described in this case report produced a progressively enlarging hematoma. The logical site for such a hemorrhage to occur,

due to trauma of a blood vessel while making an inferior alveolar nerve injection, is in the pterygomandibular space.

The pterygomandibular space is located between the medial surface of the ramus of the mandible and the lateral surface of the internal pterygoid muscle. This space is limited superiorly by the external pterygoid muscle. Its inferior and posterior boundary is the insertion of the internal pterygoid muscle to the medial surface of the ramus. Within the pterygomandibular space lie the inferior alveolar nerve and the lingual nerve, both of which are the objectives of the inferior alveolar injection. Also traversing the pterygomandibular space are several arteries of moderate size, such as the inferior dental, mylohyoid, lingual twig, and the first division of the internal maxillary. In addition, this space contains corresponding veins that accompany the arteries just mentioned. Trauma to any one of the vessels contained within the boundaries of the pterygomandibular space could cause a hemorrhage that would flood the entire space with blood.

If such a hemorrhage and a subsequent filling of the pterygomandibular space occurred, blood would exit from this space into the following spaces: first, into the buccal space by passing between the buccinator and masseter muscles (the filling of the buccal space with blood would account for the hematoma described on the face and neck); second, by passing from the pterygomandibular space medially beneath the buccal fat pad and into the submucosa of the oral vestibule (this would explain the hematoma in the buccal mucosa); and third, the blood contained within the pterygomandibular space could enter directly into the lateral pharyngeal space. The lateral pharyngeal space is located posterior to the pterygomandibular raphe, lateral to the pharynx, and medial to the ramus of the mandible and parotid gland. The posterior limit is the alar fascial sheet. Blood entering this space may find its way into the submandibular space and to the lateral pharyngeal and submandibular spaces of the opposite side of the neck. A large quantity of blood in these spaces could cause a collapse of the pharyngeal walls. It is believed that the patient's air passage was obliterated because of such a collapse.

There are various possibilities of vessel trauma within the pterygomandibular space. The vessels most vulnerable to trauma during the course of a correct inferior alveolar injection would be the inferior dental artery and vein. These vessels traverse the pterygomandibular space from above downward. The inferior dental artery is a branch of moderate size that arises from the first part of the internal maxillary artery as the latter courses the area medial to the neck of the condyle. Its path is directed downward between the sphenomandibular ligament and the ramus of the mandible.

Early in its downward course it becomes closely associated with the inferior dental vein, a tributary of the pterygoid plexus of veins. These two vessels leave the pterygomandibular space by the mandibular canal. They are vulnerable to trauma not only at this point of exit from the pterygomandibular space, which would be the point of trauma caused during a correct needle insertion for the inferior dental nerve, but also through their course from the neck of the condyle to the mandibular foramen. This course could be reached by a needle inserted too high and too deep.

Other vulnerable vessels that arise from the inferior dental artery and vein are the lingual twigs and the mylohyoid artery and vein. The mylohyoid vessels pierce the sphenomandibular ligament just above the mandibular foramen and descend in the mylohyoid groove. These vessels exit from the space as they pass through the inferior attachment of the internal pterygoid muscle. Trauma to these vessels could be caused by a needle inserted too low and too deep.

Arteries stemming from the second part of the internal maxillary artery that are vulnerable to trauma are the buccal artery and intramuscular branches of the internal and external pterygoid artery. Veins that are tributaries of the pterygoid plexus also course in close relationship with these arteries.

The buccal vessels pass obliquely forward and downward in close relationship to the buccal nerve. These vessels are closely associated with the anterior and medial aspect of the tendon of the temporalis muscle. Here the vessels are closely related to the posterior wall of the vestibule of the mouth. As these vessels course downward in the area of the anterior border of the ramus the possibility of needle trauma, in either an inferior alveolar injection or a buccal injection, is present. Any insertion directed toward the anterior border of the ramus of the mandible may cause this trauma.

Summary. In summation, it is believed that the site of primary hemorrhage was in the pterygomandibular space, with the formation of a massive hematoma that spread to the lateral pharyngeal and submandibular spaces, and, in turn, to the corresponding spaces of the opposite side of the neck. Pressure, caused by blood filling these spaces in the neck, is thought to have collapsed the pharynx. This pharyngeal collapse caused blockage of the air passage and death ensued.

Surgical or anesthetic procedures should not be attempted in the patient with uncontrolled hemophilia. If a procedure is necessary, primary concern should be given to stimulating normal clotting activity by infusions of whole blood, plasma, or blood fractions containing the antihemophilic globulins. Local hemostatic measures will be effective only after this has been done.

Case Report No. 6

POSTEXTRACTION BLEEDING IN A HEMOPHILIAC

In this case (see Figure 25–36) whole blood was used to control bleeding, which was primarily from the pterygoid plexus of veins that had been pierced during the so-called "zygomatic injection" to anesthetize the region of the right maxillary third molar, and was secondarily from the alveolus of this tooth after its extraction.

As noted later, the right facial swelling in this patient took 5 hours to develop. Therefore, it is reasonable to assume that it was due to bleeding from the pterygoid plexus of veins following needle injury. If the posterior superior alveolar artery or its external, gingival branch had been pierced by the needle, swelling would have been present in minutes. Today this patient would be given 100 cc. of antihemophilic plasma every 12 hours until his bleeding was controlled.

Hospital Admission Notes. A 28-year-old man was admitted on April 3 to the Magee-Women's Hospital with a complaint of oral bleeding, bleeding into the tissues of the face and neck, pain in the face and neck, difficulty in swallowing and oral discoloration. The symptoms followed the extraction of the right maxillary third molar 30 hours previously. Local anesthesia had been used.

The patient was presumed to have been prepared for the tooth extraction by taking "calcium tablets." No pre-extraction coagulation time had been taken.

Five hours after the extraction, the patient had noticed swelling of the right side of the face. This swelling had continued to increase in size, causing considerable pain, so that he had been unable to sleep. There had also been moderate bleeding from the extraction wound. The next morning he had gone to the dental school, from which he was referred to the hospital.

Past History. When the patient was 5 years old he had cut his foot on a bottle. He had bled from the wound for 1 week. At that time the diagnosis of hemophilia was made. Any small cuts that he had experienced had bled profusely. Sixteen years prior to this admission he had had a tooth extracted. He had bled from the site of this extraction for 6 weeks. Bleeding had been stopped in the Homestead Hospital by means of "intramuscular

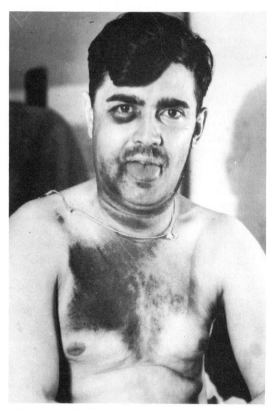

Figure 25–36 Ecchymosis following postextraction bleeding in a hemophiliac. (See Case Report No. 4.)

shots" in the arm. Thirteen years ago he had suffered a cut on the right cheek that had bled for 2 weeks, and it had been stopped by a pressure bandage. Later he had been shot through the finger, and bleeding had been severe for over a week.

The patient had had "rheumatoid pains" in the knees and elbows — sometimes in the hips, shoulders and ankles, but never the wrists. The pains had never been associated with sore throat; pains had begun about the time he started to school. Whenever a joint was involved, there was a marked limitation of motion for several days (associated with the pain), but after the pain had subsided, the motion of the joint was practically normal. This history of hemarthroses is typical in hemophiliacs.

Physical Examination. This revealed a fairly well-developed and well-nourished white man who appeared anxious about his present plight. The right side of the face was diffusely swollen because of a hematoma, and the right side of the neck seemed somewhat swollen. The larynx was on the left side of the neck, because of the extension of the hematoma into the neck and floor of the oral cavity. Examination of the mouth revealed a large, extensive extravasation of blood beneath the mucous membrane involving the right cheek, the right side of the tonsillar fossa and soft palate, the lower lip and the ventral surface of the tongue on the right

side. The floor of the mouth was elevated and with it the tongue. The cheek was moderately firm to the touch. The patient was able to talk, but with difficulty; he had some difficulty in breathing (dyspnea). There was no evidence of active bleeding into the mouth, although the patient did have blood-tinged sputum.

An emergency tracheostomy set and oxygen inhaler were placed at his bedside.

Laboratory Examination. Coagulation time was 14 minutes. A blood count showed 3,510,000 red blood cells per cu. mm.; hemoglobin was 74 per cent.

Progress Notes. On the first hospital day the patient had a transfusion of 400 cc. of fresh whole blood. By 11 P.M. the swelling was more pronounced and the right cheek was discolored extraorally.

Early on the second day the patient complained of difficulty in breathing and inability to swallow. The swelling had increased, with slight ecchymosis about the right eye. The swelling extended to the right inferior border of the mandible and anteriorly to the chin. An ice bag was intermittently applied to the face.

There was no profuse bleeding from the tooth socket. Gauze pressure pads were kept over the socket. Pressure packing in the socket had materially controlled the bleeding. The packs were carefully moistened with Monsel's solution and dried before insertion. It was apparent that bleeding into the tissues was the result of the accidental penetration of the pterygoid plexus of veins by the needle at the time the posterior alveolar nerve was anesthetized by the so-called "zygomatic injection." The blood coagulation time was 9 minutes, compared with 14 minutes on the day before.

On the third day the swelling was about the same size, but it was softer than before. The patient continued to complain of a sensation of choking. He was quite apprehensive about the bleeding. There was very little oral bleeding.

On the fourth day the patient reported that the pressure symptoms in his face and head were somewhat less. There was an extensive ecchymosis spreading downward over the neck and the anterior chest wall (see Figure 25–36); also, slight seepage around the socket packing. Ecchymosis was spreading in the buccal mucosa, and also extraorally around the eye and face. At this time 400 cc. of whole blood was given intravenously.

On the fifth day the ecchymosis of the chest wall was very pronounced. The swelling in the neck and mouth had definitely subsided. The larynx, which had been displaced to the left at the time of admission, was now almost back to normal position in the midline. The patient was able to swallow with less difficulty and asked for food. However, bleeding was markedly increased from the tooth socket.

The packing was removed and the socket repacked with iodoform gauze saturated with a paste made from 1:1000 epinephrine and tannic acid crystals. Then a large packing was placed over the socket. To help the patient keep pressure on the socket, a modified Barton bandage with elastics on the sides was placed around the mandible and over the head. The patient was given 400 cc. of blood.

On the sixth day there was no bleeding from the tooth socket. Ecchymosis was more marked, and the swelling in the neck was less than the day before. The patient felt much better and was encouraged. The blood coagulation time was 10½ minutes.

On the seventh day minor bleeding from the mouth started again. The sputum was blood-tinged. Oral examination revealed slight oozing from around the periphery of the socket; the buccal mucosa was very edematous. The socket was repacked as described before.

On the eighth day the patient was expectorating considerable blood. The socket of the extracted tooth was not bleeding. Blood was running down the buccal mucosa. The buccal tissues of the upper jaw were too edematous for accurate observation of the origin of hemorrhage, but it was probably coming from the site of the original injection. Another 400 cc. of whole blood was given, and the bleeding stopped shortly afterward. The patient felt better that evening.

On the ninth day there was no oral bleeding. The cheek was still very swollen and tense. The skin of the face, neck and chest to the nipple line was markedly ecchymotic. (See Figure 25–36.)

On the tenth day there was no bleeding; and the right cheek was not quite as swollen. The patient

felt better and wanted to get out of bed. The blood coagulation time was 7½ minutes.

On the eleventh day the patient was much less apprehensive; his mouth felt better. The socket dressing was not disturbed. He expectorated some blood in the evening.

On the twelfth day there was expectoration of blood, and the patient had no complaints.

By the thirteenth day the mucous membrane of the right cheek opposite the maxillary tuberosity was devoid of epithelium. Undoubtedly this had been the source of the acute bleeding on the eighth day.

I have observed before in cases of hematomas of the cheek following posterior-superior alveolar nerve injection (the so-called "zygomatic injection") that frequently there is a loss of epithelium of the buccal mucosa, exposing a raw bleeding surface, which is ulcerated in appearance. This is probably the result of interference with the normal circulation of the epithelium because of the intense subepithelial pressure produced by the hematoma.

From the fourteenth to the sixteenth day there was no bleeding. The swelling was gradually disappearing.

By the seventeenth day the joint pains were subsiding and the ecchymosis was disappearing.

On the eighteenth day the packing in the socket was loose and was removed with no bleeding.

The patient continued to improve, with no further complaints and no bleeding. He was discharged on the twenty-second day. He was advised not to have teeth extracted except in a hospital.

TEETH, CROWNS AND ROOTS FRACTURED DURING EXODONTIA

This subject is discussed in detail in Chapter 2 and Chapter 4. Discussion of roots in the maxillary sinus and their treatment starts on page 1623 of this chapter. Also consult pages 228 to 244 in Chapter 4.

TRAUMA FROM INSTRUMENTATION

If the operator catches the lip between the handles of the forceps and teeth (see Figure 25–37), or catches the mucosa of the floor of the mouth between the lingual beaks of the forceps and the tooth, very painful wounds are produced. Elevators may slip and plunge into deep structures, creating serious injury or hemorrhage. (See Figure 25–38.) The

author knows of one fatality from such an accident. Finger guards, which are described in

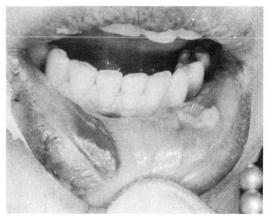

Figure 25–37 A lacerated and pinched lip that occurred when the surgeon compressed the lip between the handles of the forceps and the lower teeth during the extraction of lower molars. Note the slough on the right side and the lone bruise and puncture wound on the left.

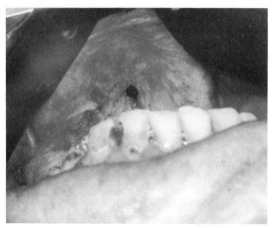

Figure 25–38 Patient stated that when the maxillary teeth were extracted 3 years ago, the dentist had had "a lot of trouble digging out the teeth and roots and his instrument slipped and tore a hole in the roof of my mouth." He refused surgery to close the fistula. He said he had "had enough."

the chapter on elevators, should always be used. (See Figures 4–7 to 4–14.)

ACCIDENTS TO TEETH

These include the extraction of the wrong tooth or teeth; loosening of adjacent teeth; fracture of a portion of the crown of the adjacent tooth; dislodgment or fracture of a filling in an adjacent tooth; loss of an adjacent tooth or teeth weeks or even months later because of extensive loss of supporting alveolar bone that was excised to permit the removal of an impacted tooth. Or this supporting bone may be thrown off as a result of the overuse of an electrocoagulating tip to destroy the base of a peripheral soft tissue tumor involving the gingival tissues.

More lawsuits result from the extraction of the wrong tooth or teeth than from any other dental procedure. If the dentist recognizes his error before discharging the patient, he should replant the tooth and wire it in position. If possible, he should fill the root canal before replantation. Obviously the way to prevent this most unfortunate occurrence is to *check* and *double check* to make certain that this is the tooth or teeth to be extracted and that the *diagnosis* justifies *the extraction.*

Before the extraction of a tooth, to avoid fracturing its crown, dislodging a filling or loosening adjacent teeth, the dentist should carefully examine the relationship of the crown of the tooth he is about to extract to those on either side. If this reveals overlapping of the crowns or fillings, then he should reduce the mesiodistal diameter of the tooth he is going to extract by cutting away a portion of the mesial and distal surfaces with a side cutting disk in the handpiece. Then he can luxate the tooth with safety.

To avoid the postoperative loss of an adjacent tooth or teeth because of excessive removal of bone, the impacted tooth should be sectioned with a bur or chisel, or a combination of the two, and removed in small segments through a comparatively small window in the alveolar bone, thus preserving the bone around the adjacent teeth.

DESTRUCTION OF TISSUE

Misuse of Alcohol in Injections. Excessive infiltration of anesthetic solutions with alcohol in osseous canals will destroy tissue, as shown in Figure 25–39.

Misuse of Electrosurgical Coagulation. A more common cause of tissue destruction is the electrocoagulating instrument, which has been grossly misused and probably has done as much harm as good. Extreme care must be used *not to overcoagulate* when controlling bleeding with this instrument or destroying the bed of tumors. This is particularly true when coagulating hard or soft tissues of thin or moderate thickness such as the palate, alveolar ridge, or cheek. Otherwise the necrosis which follows may produce a naso- or antro-oral fistula, erosion of a large vessel, extensive loss of bone and teeth, or perforation of the cheek or lip.

Coagulating instruments must be used with extreme care to avoid excessive destruction of bone. The extent of tissue destruction is determined by how much current is used and by how long the coagulating tip is in contact with the tissue. Minimum current should be used, and the tip should be moved over the surface. The dentist must know what he can expect from the various settings on the electrosurgical apparatus. He can get a lot of experience using various electrodes on a slab of beef, but he cannot get similar experience on nonviable bone. He should proceed cautiously, recognizing that he can always coagulate more if necessary but that there is no way to replace dead bone and lost teeth.

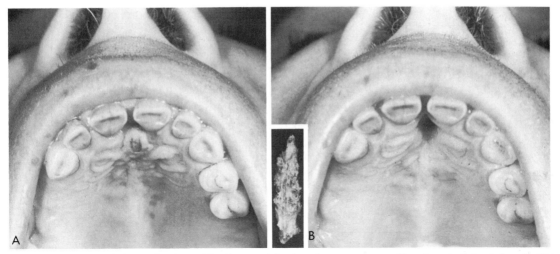

Figure 25–39 *A*, Soft tissue slough resulting from an injection of too great a quantity of an alcohol solution. *B*, Not only was there destruction of the soft tissue, but the osseous canal has also sloughed out. This can also result from overcoagulation of the contents of a neurovascular canal with an electrocoagulating needle.

FRACTURES OF THE MANDIBLE

This possibility is always present when extracting teeth and especially when removing impacted third molars or bicuspids. The incorrect use of elevators or the failure to recognize the tremendous forces that can be created by the injudicious use of these valuable but potentially dangerous instruments, has resulted in many fractures of the mandible. (See Figures 25–40 and 25–41.) While the author fortunately has not had such a complication, he has treated many fractures produced not only with elevators but also from the use of forceps. Although most fractures of this type result from overzealous application of forceps, the fact remains that well-trained and conscientious surgeons who

follow careful and accepted surgical principles will on occasion fracture a mandible. This occurrence does not necessarily imply negligence on the part of the surgeon.[61]

A basic error is the failure of the dentist to desist from applying pressures, regardless of the instrument used, that exceed those that experience should have taught him are sufficient to luxate and extract the average tooth in that particular location. As soon as he recognizes this problem, he should stop and plan another technique, such as removing surrounding bone, or sectioning the tooth if it is multirooted, in order to remove the tooth without the possibility of fracturing the mandible or, in the maxilla, fracturing the tuberosity and floor of the maxillary sinus. When a crack is heard and movement of the maxillary

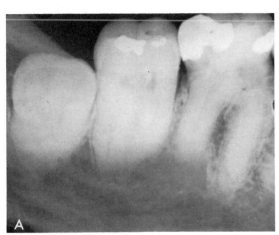
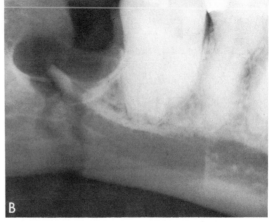

Figure 25–40 The surgeon attempted to elevate a third molar impaction (*A*) without creating a space distally by cutting off a portion of the crown or removing distal bone, resulting in a fracture of the mandible (*B*).

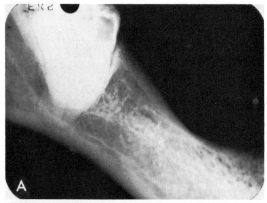

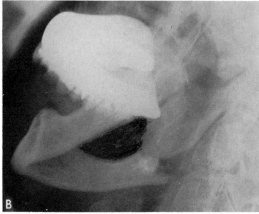

Figure 25–41 *A,* The dentist, in attempting to remove this carious impacted third molar for this 65-year-old female, cut the bone away from the distal surface, drilled a pathway along the mesial surface, inserted a 1R elevator, and applied pressure which fractured the crown of the tooth and the mandible. *B,* Note the root portion still in place and the upward and forward displacement of the vertical ramus. This was treated by reduction and stabilization with extraoral skeletal fixation with the Roger Anderson Frac-Sur units.

tooth produces simultaneous movement of the tuberosity, then further attempts to remove the tooth should cease and the patient should be treated for the segmental fracture of the maxilla (see Figure 25–42). The technique is to wire the teeth in occlusion, using the teeth on the opposite side of the jaw.

Of course when the preextraction radiographs reveal extensive destruction of bone due to a pathologic condition, the dentist should be forewarned and plan his technique to require a minimum of force to deliver the tooth.

BROKEN DENTAL NEEDLES

Since the advent of the stainless steel disposable needle, the percentage of needles broken during injections has been markedly reduced.

The great majority of needles broken during injections are those broken during a so-called mandibular injection for anesthetization of the inferior alveolar nerve. The reasons for this will be considered later. Faulty technique is more frequently the cause of broken needles than are faulty needles. To prevent, in a large measure, the breakage of needles, the following rules should be carefully observed:

1. Old or dull needles of fine gauge should not be used. Today disposable needles in sterile cases are available at relatively low cost, which makes a sharp sterile needle available at all times.

2. One-inch needles should not be used for nerve blocking; at least a 42 mm. 25 or 23 gauge needle should be used for all nerve blocking injections.

3. The dentist should thoroughly review the anatomic structures through which the needle will pass.

4. The dentist should carefully locate landmarks with the index finger and *keep this finger* in contact with the landmark throughout the injection.

5. The patient should open his mouth wide and be warned to *hold very still for just a moment.*

6. The dentist should pass the needle directly to the point of injection without stopping to inject the solution every few millimeters. A sharp needle passed swiftly but surely through tensed tissues produces much less pain (in fact, in practically 100 per cent of the cases it causes no pain) than a needle advanced a few millimeters followed by injection of a drop of solution, then advanced, followed by injection of another drop of solution, and so on. This latter procedure involves plowing the needle slowly through the tissues which ball up in front of the point, and it is not only very painful, but also conducive to needle breakage.

7. Lateral pressure should never be applied on the shaft of the needle in order to change the direction. The dentist should always remove the needle, relocate the landmarks, mentally review the technique and the anatomy in-

volved, and then reinsert the needle in the correct direction.

8. The needle should never be forced through dense tissue that is not normally found in the pathway of the needle. This generally indicates that passage is being made through a muscle. The dentist should remove the needle and follow direction "6."

9. In all injections the dentist must *make certain* that the needle is not inserted in the tissues up to the hub. In all the so-called "deep injections" for nerve blocking, there should always be 1 cm. of needle projecting from the tissue. In the infiltration injections at least 2 cm. should project from the tissues.

10. During all injections the patient should be properly positioned in the chair, so that the injection area is well illuminated and clearly seen.

Even when all these precautions have been taken, a needle may still break. After the needle has been broken and has disappeared in the soft tissues, the question arises: Should the patient be told? The answer is, yes. An attempt to remove the needle secretly, or having an oral surgeon remove it under the guise of another operation, proves to the patient, when he discovers what is being done, that his dentist has been guilty of neglect or carelessness. Either or both might be true, but the patient should not be given grounds for believing this. The proper attitude to take is that this is an unfortunate occurrence that sometimes happens no matter how much care has been exercised, one that happens to the most skilled and conscientious surgeons (which is perfectly true), and that the needle should be removed.

It is agreed that needles do not migrate through the tissues to any great extent, in spite of occasional newspaper reports of the migration of broken sewing needles from such locations as the "finger to the big toe," nor are there any authentic records of the migration of a needle into vital structures, thereby causing death. Why, then, should the broken needles be removed? Simply because the general public believes that a sharp needle may at some time cause grave injury; therefore, for the patient's peace of mind, consideration should be given to the early removal of all broken needles. However, good judgment must be used, because considerable dysfunction can result from scarring

attendant to prolonged and extreme surgery. Surgical exploration for a broken needle should be abandoned if the attempt is not successful within 30 to 45 minutes. Shira[61] states that if the needle is broken in deep tissues, or if it is difficult to localize, consideration should be given to allowing the needle to remain with no attempt at removal. I agree. This must be done with the patient's full understanding of the reasons and his consent should be obtained in writing.

Robinson's[54] conclusions are, "If the broken needle and other metallic foreign bodies could be handled within the dental profession in the same way that a piece of amalgam within the tissues is handled, life would be safer and easier. The fantasy of the broken needle in the minds of the patient and the profession has woven a web, with the help of our lawyers and our courts, which has created unnecessary surgery, disability, and death."

LOCATION OF BROKEN NEEDLE

The needle broken in the region of the mandibular sulcus should be located using the steps below. First, another injection should be made with a Luer-type syringe, being careful in the location of landmarks and the depth and direction of the needle. If anesthesia is not present, or is poor, the dentist should inject a suitable local anesthetic with this injection. The procedure should be performed where posteroanterior and lateral jaw and true lateral head roentgenograms can be made, and films and roentgen-ray equipment should be in readiness before making the injection.

The needle should be left in position but the dentist should disconnect the syringe. The Luer syringe with a Luer-lok, or a friction-type needle, is preferred, because of the ease with which the needle can be disengaged from the syringe after the solution has been deposited.

To maintain the needle in position it is necessary to suture the hub to the cheek with silk suture, otherwise the diagnostic or guide needle will be dislodged during surgery. A better guide is illustrated in Figures 25–45 to 25–47 and described in Case Report No. 7.

The dentist should position the patient's head for posteroanterior views of the mandible and make exposures, *making certain that the patient's mouth is open wide during*

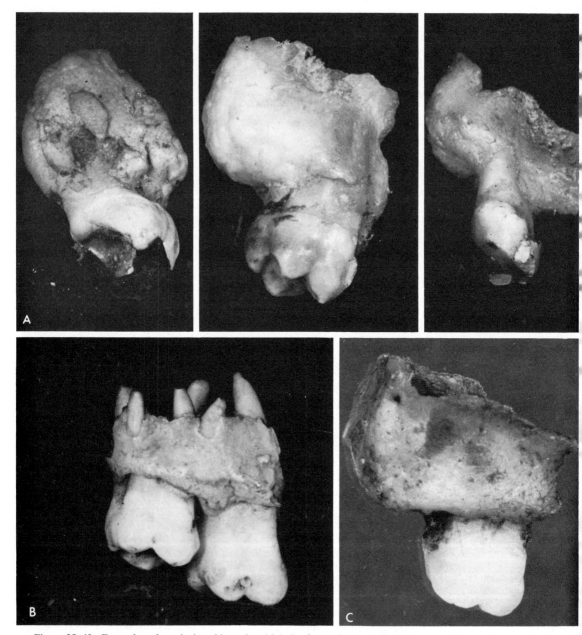

Figure 25–42 Examples of surgical accidents in which the floor of the maxillary sinus and tuberosity were fractured and torn out, thus creating very large antro-oral fistulas which are extremely difficult to close. Pre-extraction radiographs, followed by sectioning of the teeth, as described in Chapter 2, would have prevented these accidents. Or when it was seen that a large segment of bone was fractured with the teeth, then extraction attempts should have ceased and the fractured segment should have been treated as a maxillary fracture, as described in Chapter 18.

exposure. The lateral jaw plates are now exposed and followed by the true lateral head films.

The posteroanterior roentgenograms should be exposed with the mandible at a right angle to the film and the central ray passing through the vertical ramus. This film will show the position of the broken needle relative to the inner (medial) border of the ramus, provided, of course, that the injection was made on this side of the ramus. Needles that are searched for fruitlessly on the lingual surface of the ramus have occasionally eventually been found between the lateral surface of the ramus and the masseter muscle, the oral surgeon taking it for granted that the

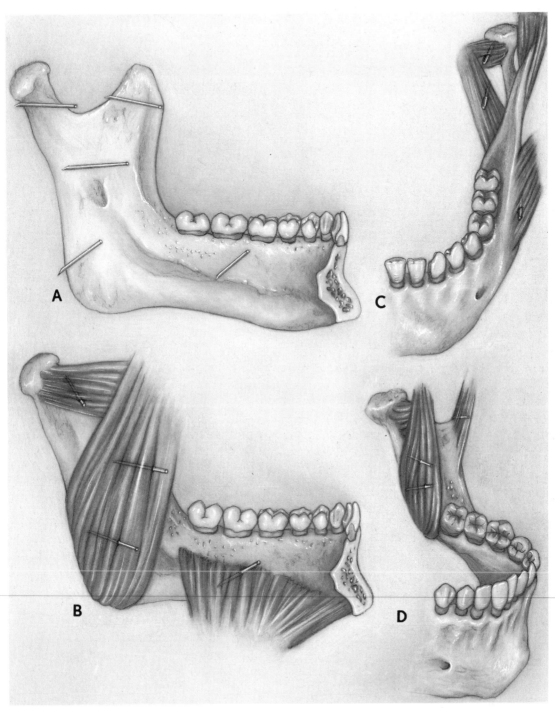

Figure 25–43 The most common locations for broken needles. *A,* The broken segments of needles represent locations in which needles have been broken during the so-called mandibular, lingual and long buccal injections of local anesthetics. *B,* Medial view showing the location of broken needles in the medial (internal) pterygoid, the lateral (external) pterygoid and mylohyoid muscles. *C,* Anterior view which shows a broken needle in the insertion of the buccinator muscle as well as in the pterygoids. *D,* Semilingual view showing a needle segment in the insertion of the temporalis muscle. (From Archer, W. H.: Manual of Dental Anesthesia. 2nd ed. Philadelphia, W. B. Saunders Co., 1958.)

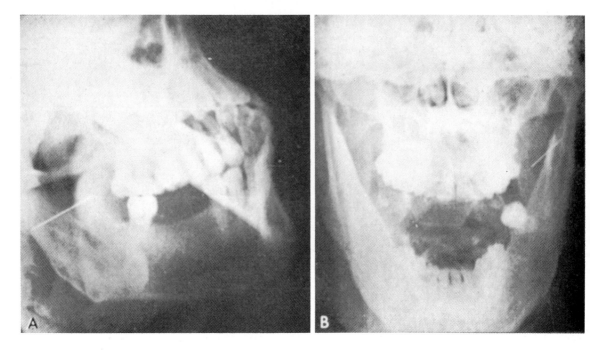

Figure 25–44 *A,* Broken mandibular needle in an adult. This is the incorrect way to visualize the needle; *the mouth should be open.* Furthermore it should be remembered that, regardless of whether the mouth is open or closed, in this view there is a foreshortening that will make the needle appear higher in relationship to the sigmoid notch and mandibular sulcus than it really is, unless it is actually in contact with bone. *B,* Posteroanterior view with the mouth open, giving the lateral relationship of the needle to the ramus. (From Archer, W. H.: Manual of Dental Anesthesia. 2nd ed. Philadelphia, W. B. Saunders Co., 1958.)

needle was on the lingual (medial) surface. The position of the needle should never be taken for granted. The position of the broken needle relative to that of the injection needle is also shown in the film.

The lateral jaw roentgenogram will show fairly accurately how far anteriorly the broken end is in relationship to the second needle and how high or low it is in relationship to the second needle. It must be thoroughly understood that the lateral jaw film exposed without the second needle in place is of little value, except to demonstrate whether or not the needle is present.

To obtain accurate information as to the exact relationship of the broken needle to the anterior and posterior borders of the vertical ramus and to the inferior border of the mandible, and to the sigmoid notch, it is necessary to expose a true lateral head roentgenogram in which the ramus involved is placed parallel to the film, with the mouth opened wide, and the central roentgen ray passing through and at right angles to the middle of the ramus. This, of course, necessitates the superimposition of the opposite ramus over the one concerned. While this does block out

the finer detail, one is able to see clearly the borders just mentioned, and the two needles.

If the roentgenographic examination does not show the guide needle close to the broken needle, the diagnostic needle should be removed, reinserted and repeat roentgenograms taken until it does approximate the broken needle. It is now locked or fixed in position so it will not be displaced during the surgical procedure of locating and removing the broken needle.

TECHNIQUE FOR REMOVAL OF MANDIBULAR NEEDLE

The patient must be positioned so that a clear view of the *anterior pillars of the pharynx* is possible. The surgeon should use a good headlight and have an assistant aid in retraction, one who can also keep the field dry with a suction tip. These are essentials.

In addition to the mandibular (inferior alveolar) injection, it is necessary to anesthetize the middle and posterior palatine nerves at the greater palatine foramen. It may be necessary to remove the needle under general anesthesia if there is considerable trismus, or

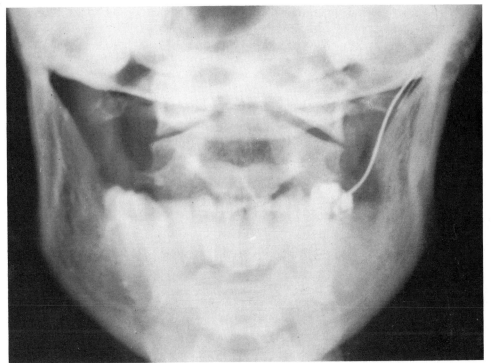

Figure 25–45

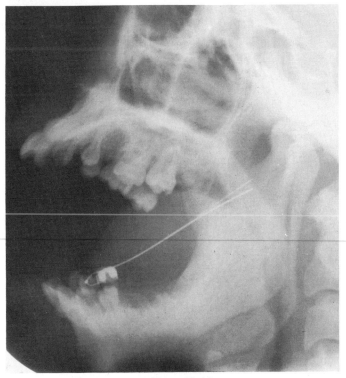

Figure 25–46

Figures 25–45 and 25–46 Anteroposterior and lateral views of a broken needle medial to the coronoid process with a sharpened 23 gauge stainless steel diagnostic wire alongside. Once the radiographs reveal the diagnostic wire in close approximation to the broken needle in both the anteroposterior and lateral views, then it is locked to an orthodontic band on the nearest tooth, in this case a mandibular second bicuspid (see Figure 25–47). (From Archer, W. H.: Manual of Dental Anesthesia. 2nd ed. Philadelphia, W. B. Saunders Co., 1958.)

if the patient is nervous or uncooperative and insists on a general anesthetic. Nasoendotracheal anesthesia with induction by an intravenous barbiturate, nitrous oxide and oxygen, fortified by one of the new halogenated agents, is the author's choice in these cases. Many of these patients, however, can be satisfactorily operated on under local anesthesia by administering $1\frac{1}{2}$ to 3 grains of pentobarbital sodium 45 minutes before operating.

The surgeon should not palpate the tissues in the region of the needle in the hope of locating it digitally. This is impossible and may force the needle deeper into the tissues.

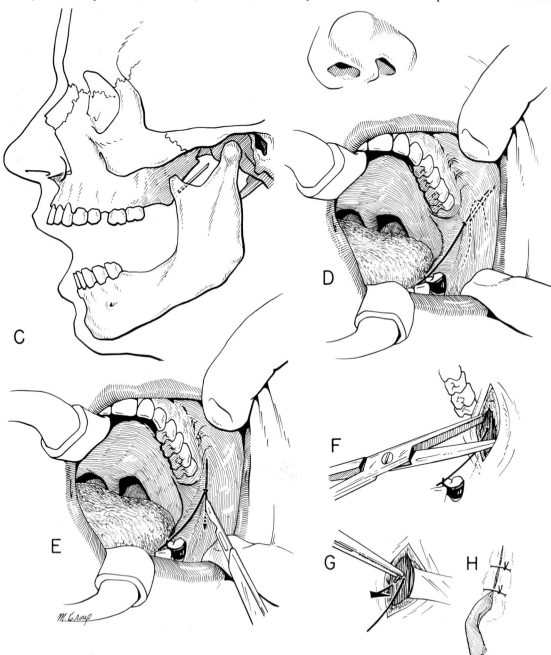

Figure 25–47 Study the text for a description of the technique illustrated here. *C,* Broken piece of needle medial to the coronoid process. *D,* Diagnostic (guide) needle inserted alongside broken needle and locked on an orthodontic band on the bicuspid. *E,* Incision through the mucosa using a No. 15 blade. *F,* Deeper tissues separated. *G,* Broken needle located, grasped with a hemostat and removed. *H,* Rubber tissue drain inserted and tissues sutured with 000 black silk. (From Archer, W. H.: Manual of Dental Anesthesia. 2nd ed. Philadelphia, W. B. Saunders Co., 1958.)

With a mental picture of the location of the needle gained from a study of the roentgenograms, and with the guide needle still in place, the surgeon incises through the mucous membrane about 1 inch above the guide needle and carries the incision down to and below the guide needle for another inch. The incision must not be carried too deeply, because the lingual nerve may be severed. The edges of the incision are separated with retractors, and deeper structures are dissected with blunt instruments. The lingual nerve may be seen and, if so, is held to one side. The surgeon dissects the overlying tissues alongside the shaft of the diagnostic or guide needle until the broken needle is contacted. The broken needle is grasped with a hemostat and removed either by working the broken end back out of the tissues into the oral cavity, or by creating traction on the needle, causing it to bend at the middle, and removing it through the pathway that the surgeon has created. A rubber tissue drain is then inserted.

The mucous membrane is sutured with two 000 black silk sutures, depending on the length of the incision. (Study Figure 25–47.)

Hot salt-water gargles and chewing gum may be prescribed postoperatively.

If there is sustained elevation of temperature (over 24 hours), the patient should be hospitalized if he was operated on as an office patient, and antibiotic therapy instituted.

It might appear from the brief foregoing description that the removal of broken mandibular needles is a simple matter. This is most definitely not so. On the contrary, it is generally a difficult, tedious and trying procedure, initial attempts frequently proving unsuccessful. I cannot stress too emphatically the absolute necessity of having excellent roentgenograms of the broken needle, plus the guide needle, and the need for the surgeon to carefully study these films, keeping in mind the distortions that may be produced when roentgenograms are made.

An example of distortion is seen in the lateral jaw roentgenogram in which the ramus is foreshortened and the needle appears higher on the ramus than it is actually. It is because of this distortion that the true lateral jaw film should be the guiding film in locating the height or depth of the needle in relationship to the long and short axes of the vertical ramus.

The foregoing statements apply to the removal of broken needles in any part of the oral cavity.

Case Report No. 7

REMOVAL OF A BROKEN MANDIBULAR NEEDLE USING A MODIFIED KAZANJIAN GUIDE*

Patient.　A girl, aged 6, was admitted to the Eye and Ear Hospital to the service of an otolaryngologist for the removal of a foreign body (hypodermic needle) from the lingual surface of the left ramus of the mandible.

Medical History.　There was no history of illness, with the exception of the usual childhood diseases.

Dental History.　The patient had gone to a school dentist for removal of a tooth. When the mandibular injection had been made, she had jerked her head. The hypodermic needle had broken and been lost in the left pterygomandibular space. The school dentist had been unsuccessful in removing the needle through minor procedures (see Figures 25–48 and 25–49).

Operative Notes.　An operation was performed on June 1 by the otolaryngologist. Under ether anesthesia an incision was made over the left pos-

terior molar up toward the ramus of the mandible, but the needle was not located. Several attempts were made, but all were unsuccessful. The operation lasted 2 hours. Additional roentgenograms were advised and further exploration advocated at a later date. The patient was removed from the operating room in good condition.

Progress Notes.　*June 1.* Routine care and antibiotic therapy, and 1 ounce of elixir of phenobarbital when the patient showed signs of restlessness, were ordered.

June 2. Consultation with an oral surgeon (W.H.A.) was ordered. His report read as follows: "There is extensive submandibular edema but as

---

* Prepared by A. S. Mangie, D.D.S., Oral Surgery Resident, Eye and Ear Hospital, Pittsburgh, Pa.

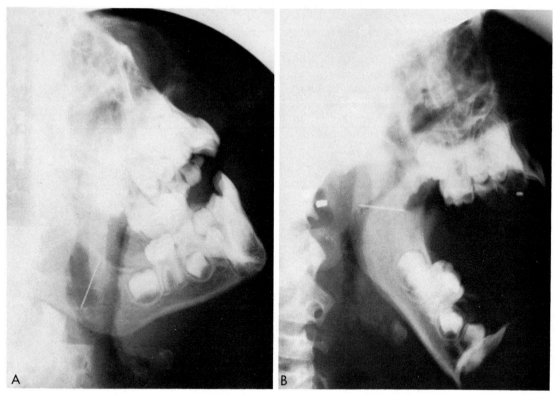

Figure 25–48 *A*, Oblique lateral jaw roentgenogram showing the foreign body. Mouth in open position. *B*, True lateral jaw roentgenogram with mouth in open position. The relative position of foreign body does not seem to change. (From Archer, W. H.: Manual of Dental Anesthesia. 2nd ed. Philadelphia, W. B. Saunders Co., 1958.)

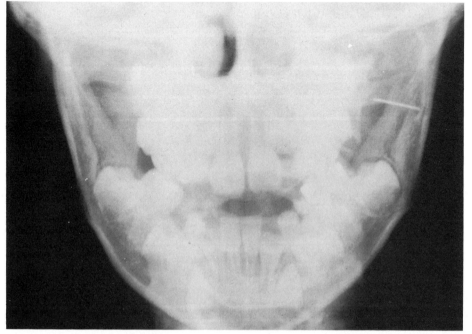

Figure 25–49 Anteroposterior view showing the buccolingual position of the broken needle. (From Archer, W. H.: Manual of Dental Anesthesia. 2nd ed. Philadelphia, W. B. Saunders Co., 1958.)

yet no induration. The patient has difficulty in swallowing. Marked trismus makes examination of the lingual area of the ramus very difficult. Temperature is 101° F."

June 3. The case was transferred to the oral surgery service of W.H.A. The edema was slightly reduced, but trismus was still marked at this time. Postponement of a further attempt to remove the foreign body until edema and trismus had completely subsided was advised. Since it was considered possible that the needle had been moved by the tissue dissection, another roentgen-ray examination after edema and trismus had subsided was advised.

June 4. Trismus was 90 per cent relieved, and submandibular edema was reduced. Considerable edema was still present in the peritonsillar area and in the region of the anterior pillars. The temperature was normal.

June 5. The trismus was practically gone, but the middle and posterior submaxillary lymph nodes were still indurated. The patient had no complaints in regard to swallowing. It was decided that she could be handled as an outpatient until the edema and induration had completely subsided, at which time the needle could be visualized roentgenographically and the patient readmitted for its removal.

June 6. The patient was discharged.

Second Admission. On October 24, the patient was readmitted to the Eye and Ear Hospital for the removal of a foreign body (needle) in the pterygomandibular space.

Physical Examination. No abnormalities were noted.

Laboratory Examination. Findings were within normal limits.

Roentgenographic Examination. The needle appeared to be in the same position as it was before the first attempt to remove it (see Figures 25–48 and 25–49).

Discussion. It was evident, because of the prolonged and extensive previous dissection of the tissues performed in an attempt to locate this needle, that the aid of a fixed guide needle in locating the foreign body was a necessity. A modified Kazanjian technique was employed, as is shown in Figure 25–50. In Kazanjian's technique a sharpened wire is passed through a tube soldered to an orthodontic band that is attached to a molar tooth and into the tissues lingual to the ramus. Study Figure 25–50 and its legend for a description of this guide needle and band.

However, this method does not permit any changes in the location of the guide or diagnostic needle. In our technique the guide needle is placed in a syringe, passed into the tissues and locked into place, and roentgenograms made. If the guide needle does not approximate the broken needle, it is unlocked, withdrawn from the tissues, reinserted into the syringe and again placed into the tissues,

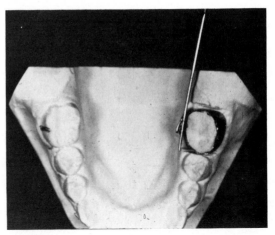

Figure 25–50   View of the orthodontic band and special guide needle made of stainless steel wire, with lug and lock wire on a stone model. The appliance is a modification of the Kazanjian technique. The band is cemented to the molar tooth. On the lug end the directional guide needle is constructed so that this end can fit into a dental syringe. This facilitates placing the needle into the tissues. The idea of the modification was that the directional guide could be inserted several times if necessary and then locked into position by bending the guide if required. See text for additional information on this technique. (From Archer, W. H.: Manual of Dental Anesthesia. 2nd ed. Philadelphia, W. B. Saunders Co., 1958.)

and roentgenograms are made. This is repeated until the guide needle approximates the broken needle. The operation itself is thereby simplified.

Preoperative Orders. (See Chapter 9.)

Operation. The operation for the removal of a foreign body (broken needle) from the pterygomandibular space was performed on October 26 by the oral surgeon (W.H.A.) and two assistants (A.S.M. and W.B.I.).*

Under Avertin anesthesia a guide needle was inserted into the tissues as though an inferior alveolar nerve injection were being made, and the needle was attached to an orthodontic band that had been placed previously. The patient was taken to the x-ray department for roentgenograms and returned to the operating room while under the anesthesia.

From the roentgenograms (see Figure 25–51) it was apparent that the guide needle crossed the long axis of the broken needle and was nearly in contact with it.

A nasoendotracheal tube was now placed, and the anesthesia carried on with nitrous oxide and oxygen mixture, supplemented by ether. An incision was made, following the guide needle posteriorly. Tissue was dissected with a periosteal ele-

* Oral surgeon, W. Harry Archer. Oral surgery residents, A. S. Mangie and W. B. Irby.

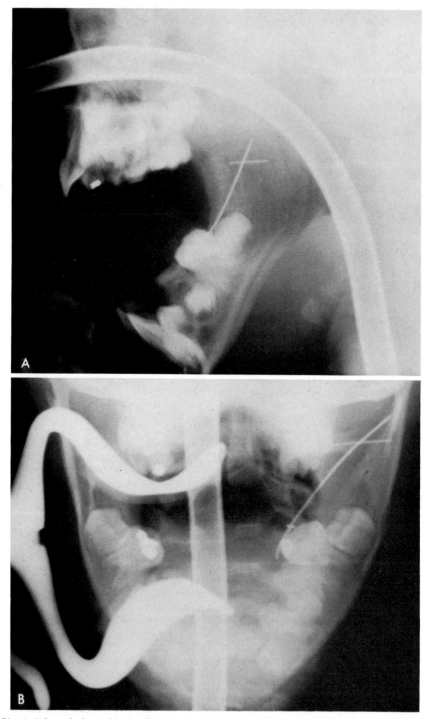

Figure 25–51 *A,* A lateral view with the directional guide in place. The long white tube is a nasoendotracheal tube. *B,* An anteroposterior view of the guide in position, and mouth held open with a Molt mouth prop. The guide seems to bisect the foreign body in both views. When this is true, an operation should be performed. The nasoendotracheal tube can also be seen in this view. (From Archer, W. H.: Manual of Dental Anesthesia. 2nd ed. Philadelphia, W. B. Saunders Co., 1958.)

vator, hemostats and scissors. About 3 cm. along the guide needle the broken needle was encountered. It was grasped with a hemostat and removed. An iodoform gauze drain was inserted, and two sutures were placed. The patient left the operating room in good condition.

Postoperative Orders. *October 26.* The following were prescribed: ½ ounce of elixir of phenobarbital four times a day as required; antibiotic therapy (see Chapter 8); Hyclorite mouthwash three times a day; application of an ice bag to left jaw for the first 24 hours following operation.

October 27. Orders included discontinuance of the ice bag and application of a hot-water bottle to the left jaw. A warm, normal saline solution was ordered to be used as a mouthwash and gargle every 3 hours.

Postoperative Notes. *October 27.* There was a moderate amount of lingual swelling, no trismus and no pain.

October 28. The iodoform gauze drain was removed. The patient's progress was very satisfactory.

October 30. The patient was discharged.

OTHER FOREIGN BODIES

During time of war, surgeons are often confronted with the problem of removal of pieces of shrapnel and other foreign bodies located in various parts of the body. Frequently the physical condition of the patient, plus the hazard of the surgical procedure, induces the decision to postpone removal of the foreign object until a later date. On other occasions, attempts to locate these objects result in a failure and the patient lives with the foreign body. No undue harm is produced by the presence of an unnatural material in the tissues of the body in many instances; on other occasions, its presence results in chronic infection with local inflammatory reaction that may persist over a long period of time, with intermittent periods of acute infection characterized by localized swelling and discomfort accompanied by the possibility of a generalized systemic effect. (See Case Report No. 8.)

Case Report No. 8

REMOVAL OF FOREIGN BODY FROM LATERAL PORTION OF INFRATEMPORAL FOSSA AND SIGMOID (MANDIBULAR, SEMILUNAR) NOTCH OF THE MANDIBLE BY THE ORAL APPROACH*

This case report is a typical example of a chronic inflammatory reaction, with intermittent acute phases that persisted in the lateral infratemporal fossa over a period of years, caused by the presence of a piece of shrapnel. Of interest also is the fact that this foreign body was located and removed by an intraoral approach after attempts to extract it at the time of the original debridement and later through an extraoral approach had met with failure.

Complaint and History of Present Illness. The patient complained of a persistent swelling, over the past 7 years, of the left side of his face. It fluctuated in size and intensity and was accompanied by trismus of the masseter muscle on the affected side. This condition had persisted since 1945, varying in severity from time to time.

Past History. This patient had suffered severe shrapnel wounds of the face in March, 1943,

during combat in North Africa. The wounds had involved the nose, left eye, forehead, and left maxillary and mandibular regions. After receiving emergency treatment, he had been transported to a hospital in Oran. It was during his recovery at this hospital that an unsuccessful attempt through an extraoral incision slightly below the zygomatic arch had been made in an effort to remove the piece of shrapnel lodged in the lateral portion of the infratemporal fossa (Figure 25–52*A* and *B*). Pain and severe trismus had persisted for approximately a month after this attempt. Several months later, the patient had been transferred to a general

---

* W. Harry Archer, R. J. Caparosa, and W. B. Irby (Oral Surgery Resident). From the Oral Surgery and Otolaryngology Services. Veterans Administration Hospital, Aspinwall, Pa.

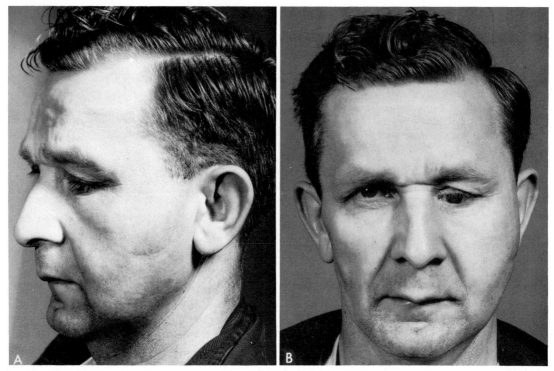

Figure 25–52 *A,* Line of incision from an unsuccessful attempt to remove a piece of shrapnel. (See Case Report No. 8 for further details.) *B,* Facial swelling during an acute exacerbation of a chronic abscess around a piece of shrapnel lodged in the sigmoid notch. The left eye was destroyed when this metallic body tore through the patient's face.

hospital in the United States. During the next 5 months of hospitalization, the surgery performed had consisted of enucleation of the left eye, plastic repair of the nose and a tendon graft from the left wrist to assist in the elevation of the left eyelid. He had returned to active duty and was discharged from the army in 1945.

Since the date of his discharge from the army, this patient has been hospitalized four times because of pain and swelling of the left side of his face. These exacerbations have occurred more frequently during the summer, seemingly because of hot weather. Upon each admission, it has been the opinion of the surgical service that surgery was not indicated, would prove unsuccessful or would result in facial paralysis.

Examination. Physical examination revealed a well-developed, well-nourished middle-aged male, wearing an artificial left eye. There were multiple scars over the nose, over the left upper eyelid and below the left zygomatic prominence. The left eyelids could be closed only with difficulty. A large, moderately tender swelling involved the left side of the face (see Figure 25–52*B*). The lungs were clear, and findings in the cardiovascular system, the abdomen and the remainder of the physical examination were essentially negative.

Oral examination revealed an edentulous maxilla and mandible. The patient was wearing dentures but could open the mouth only about 1 inch.

Radiographs of the skull and jaws disclosed a jagged, triangular radiopaque object located in the infratemporal fossa and sigmoid notch in close relationship to the coronoid process and to the anterior border of the neck of the left condyle (see Figure 25–53).

Laboratory Examination. Findings were essentially negative.

Plan of Operative Approach. A thorough study of the various possible external approaches revealed that any selected one would be complicated by the danger of injury to the parotid gland and the large nerves and vessels of the face. The sketches illustrating the anatomic layers of the face show that the foreign body lies under the main trunk of the facial nerve and also beneath the parotid gland. The masseter muscle, arising from the zygomatic arch, lies in close lateral relationship to the shrapnel, while the internal maxillary artery passes near the medial side of the object. (Study Figures 25–54 to 25–57.)

Considering the hazards of an external approach, and thoroughly aware of the difficulties in locating foreign bodies, the authors decided to attempt the removal of this shrapnel through an intraoral incision extending along the anterior border of the ramus to the tip of the coronoid process. It was believed that this approach provided a practical and less hazardous access to the foreign body.

Operation. The patient received premedication ½ hour before the operation consisting of sodium

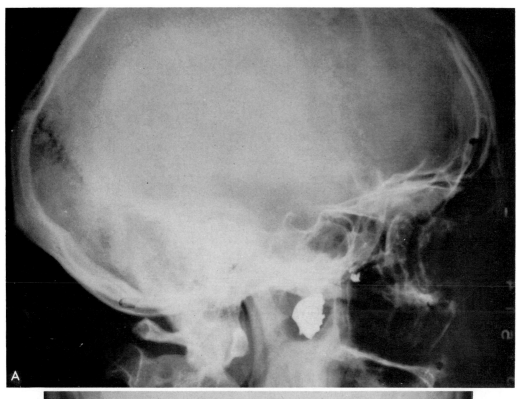

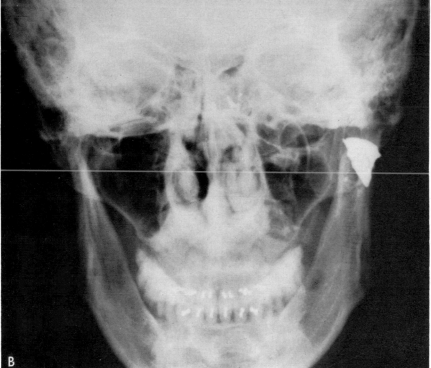

Figure 25-53   Large foreign body—shrapnel in sigmoid notch. (See Case Report No. 8.)

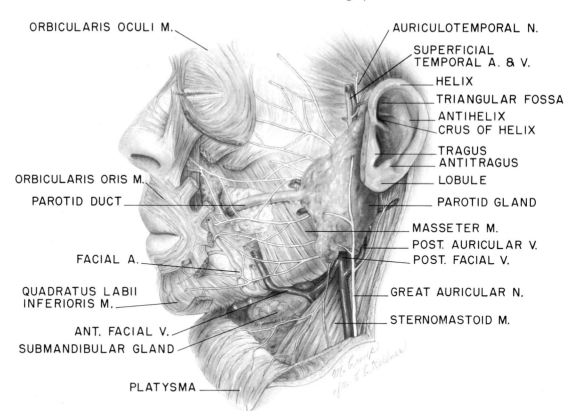

ORBICULARIS OCULI M.

AURICULOTEMPORAL N.

SUPERFICIAL TEMPORAL A. & V.

HELIX

TRIANGULAR FOSSA

ANTIHELIX
CRUS OF HELIX

TRAGUS
ANTITRAGUS

LOBULE

ORBICULARIS ORIS M.

PAROTID DUCT

PAROTID GLAND

MASSETER M.
POST. AURICULAR V.
POST. FACIAL V.

FACIAL A.

QUADRATUS LABII INFERIORIS M.

GREAT AURICULAR N.

STERNOMASTOID M.

ANT. FACIAL V.
SUBMANDIBULAR GLAND

PLATYSMA

Figure 25-54

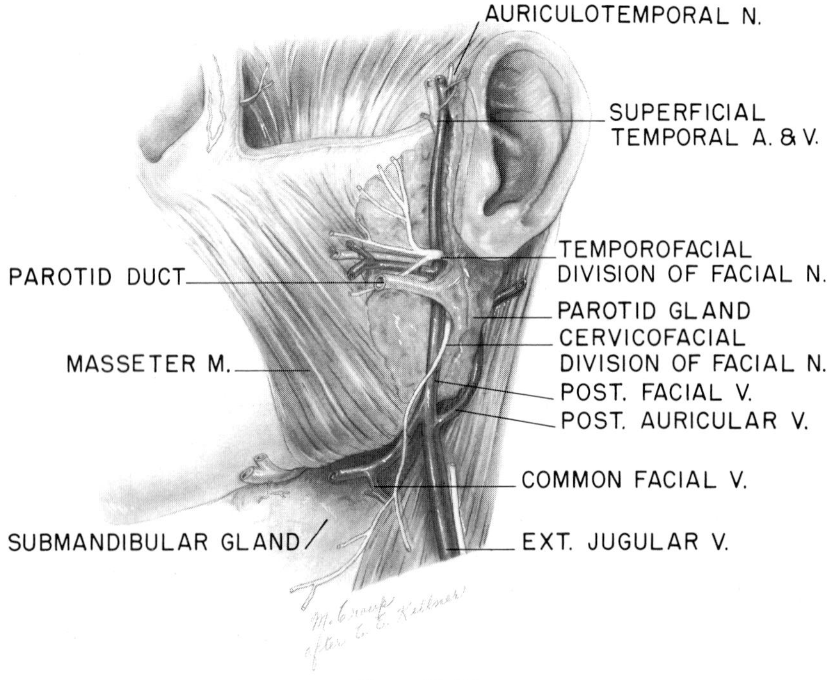

AURICULOTEMPORAL N.

SUPERFICIAL TEMPORAL A. & V.

TEMPOROFACIAL DIVISION OF FACIAL N.

PAROTID DUCT

PAROTID GLAND
CERVICOFACIAL DIVISION OF FACIAL N.
POST. FACIAL V.
POST. AURICULAR V.

MASSETER M.

COMMON FACIAL V.

SUBMANDIBULAR GLAND

EXT. JUGULAR V.

Figure 25-55

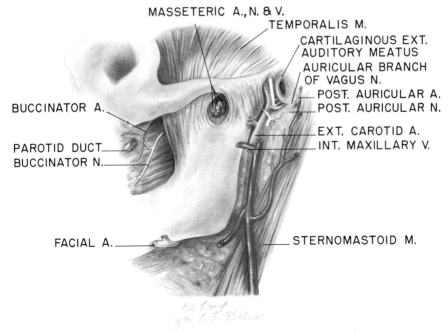

MASSETERIC A., N. & V.
TEMPORALIS M.
CARTILAGINOUS EXT. AUDITORY MEATUS
AURICULAR BRANCH OF VAGUS N.
POST. AURICULAR A.
POST. AURICULAR N.
EXT. CAROTID A.
INT. MAXILLARY V.
BUCCINATOR A.
PAROTID DUCT
BUCCINATOR N.
FACIAL A.
STERNOMASTOID M.

Figure 25–56

pentobarbital (Nembutal), 1½ grains, and atropine sulfate, 1/100 grain. Antibiotic therapy was started the day before surgery. Anesthesia was accomplished by a thiopental sodium induction, plus administration of nitrous oxide–oxygen through the nasoendotracheal route. The anesthesia produced sufficient relaxation to allow the mouth to be opened wide and stabilized with a mouth prop. The throat was carefully packed around the nasoendotracheal tube and the oral mucous membrane prepared with tincture of benzalkonium (Zephiran).

An incision was made through the mucoperiosteum opposite the anterior border of the ascending ramus, extending from slightly above the retromolar pad to the tip of the coronoid process. With a periosteal elevator, the periosteum was separated from the mesial and distal sides of the superior half of the ascending ramus, thereby exposing the tendinous insertion of the temporalis

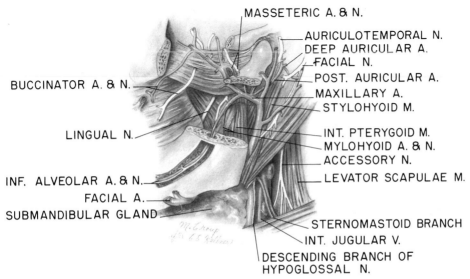

MASSETERIC A. & N.
AURICULOTEMPORAL N.
DEEP AURICULAR A.
FACIAL N.
POST. AURICULAR A.
MAXILLARY A.
STYLOHYOID M.
BUCCINATOR A. & N.
LINGUAL N.
INT. PTERYGOID M.
MYLOHYOID A. & N.
ACCESSORY N.
INF. ALVEOLAR A. & N.
LEVATOR SCAPULAE M.
FACIAL A.
SUBMANDIBULAR GLAND
STERNOMASTOID BRANCH
INT. JUGULAR V.
DESCENDING BRANCH OF HYPOGLOSSAL N.

Figure 25–57

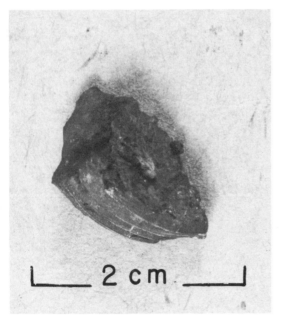

Figure 25–58   Piece of shrapnel. (See Case Report No. 8.)

sides of the coronoid process. A blunt probe was then passed along the medial side of the coronoid process toward the neck of the condyle and into the area that was assumed to be the location of the shrapnel. When a fibrous sac was punctured, considerable pus was noted, which led the operators to believe that the shrapnel was surrounded by an infected fibrous sac. An incision was carefully made in the anterior wall of this fibrous membrane, thereby exposing a portion of the foreign body. The shrapnel proved difficult to grasp and appeared to be rather securely attached by fibrous tissue. In order to dislodge it, a small periosteal elevator was passed laterally to the coronoid process and to the shrapnel, which caused the body to be moved in a mesial direction. This provided better access and allowed the object to be grasped with an Allis clamp. The shrapnel proved difficult to dislodge from its bed.

Because of the ever-present danger of rupturing the internal maxillary artery, whose wall might conceivably have been weakened by the chronic inflammation, a portion of the coronoid process was removed with bone rongeurs. This provided a much more adequate approach and allowed the shrapnel to be gently removed (see Figure 25–58). The tissues were sutured and a catheter drain inserted for irrigation. (Study Figures 25–59 and 25–60.)

Postoperative Course.   The progress of the patient was extremely satisfactory. On the day fol-

muscle into the coronoid process. Two broad and flat tissue retractors were next inserted, one on each side of the coronoid process and sigmoid notch, and the tissues were retracted. This provided access to the infratemporal fossa from both

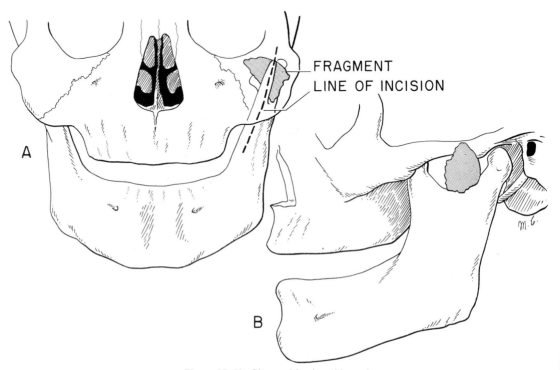

FRAGMENT
LINE OF INCISION

A

B

Figure 25–59   Shrapnel in sigmoid notch.

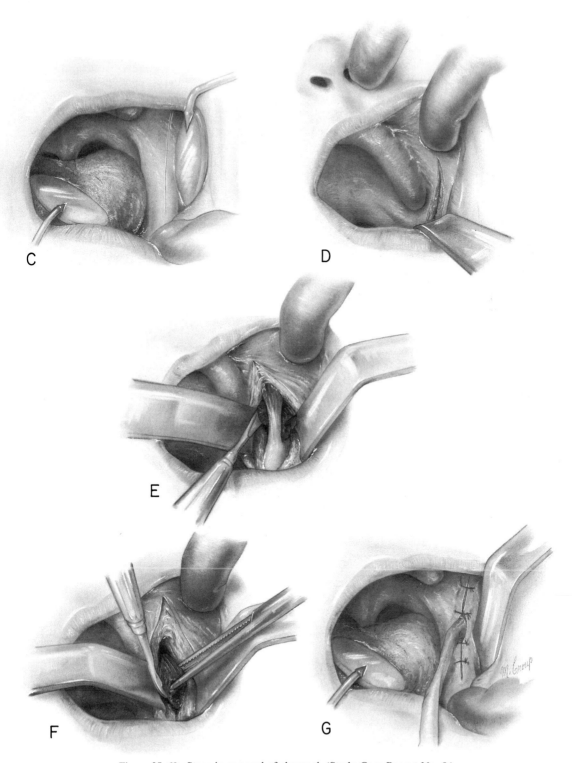

Figure 25–60   Steps in removal of shrapnel. (Study Case Report No. 8.)

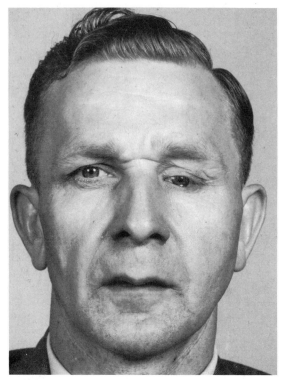

Figure 25–61 Two months after removal of shrapnel. Note reduction in facial swelling as compared with Figure 25–52. (See Case Report No. 8.)

lowing the operation, very little pain, swelling or trismus was evident. Irrigation with penicillin solu-

tion was continued through the catheter drain for 5 days, accompanied by the administration of antibiotic therapy.

The sutures and drain were removed on the fifth day. The tissue appeared healthy, and the swelling of the face had diminished considerably. On the next day, the patient was discharged to return for a 2-month check. Recheck of the patient April 14 disclosed a remarkable return of the contour of his face to normal. This represented a restoration to almost normal symmetry of a face that had remained swollen for 7 years (see Figure 25–61). The oral tissues had completely healed, and the mandibular movements were satisfactory; trismus was gone.

Comments. This case report illustrates two pertinent factors:

1. The return to normal in a 2-month interval of the contour of the face, after 7 years of deformity due to chronic inflammation, is both surprising and gratifying.

2. The familiarity of the oral surgeon with the oral cavity and surrounding structures induced the decision to attempt the removal of this foreign body from the infratemporal fossa by the intraoral route. This procedure proved to be both effective and sound, producing the desired results after attempts by the plastic and general surgeon had failed. It should be mentioned that the removal of a portion of the coronoid process was not a crippling procedure, nor is it necessary in the majority of the attempts to reach the infratemporal fossa by this approach.

(*Text continued on page 1605*)

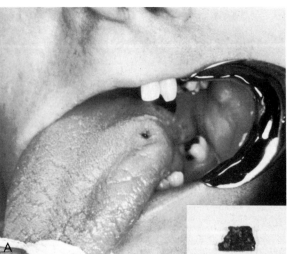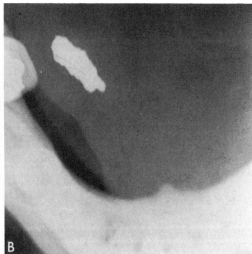

Figure 25–62 *A,* Hard black metallic object embedded in the tongue. *B,* Occlusal radiograph revealed a rough piece of metal. *Inset,* The piece of metal was removed and proved to be shrapnel.

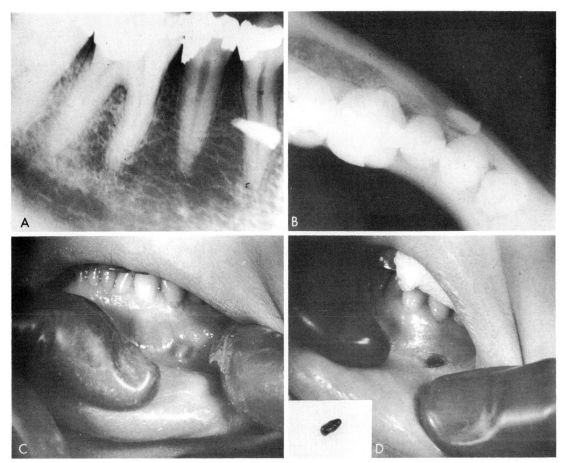

Figure 25–63 *A* and *B,* Piece of amalgam that appeared to be in bone in the periapical radiograph but was actually beneath the periosteum, as shown in the occlusal view. *C* and *D,* Amalgam just below the mucosa exposed by incision through the mucosa. *Inset,* Piece of amalgam that was removed.

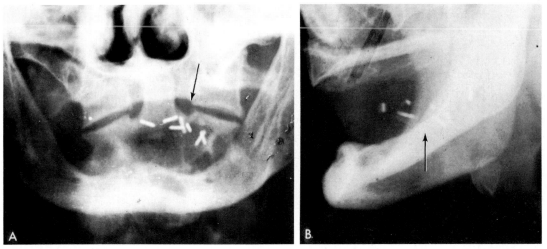

Figure 25–64 "Radium needles" in the tongue. These are not removed as long as they are asymptomatic.

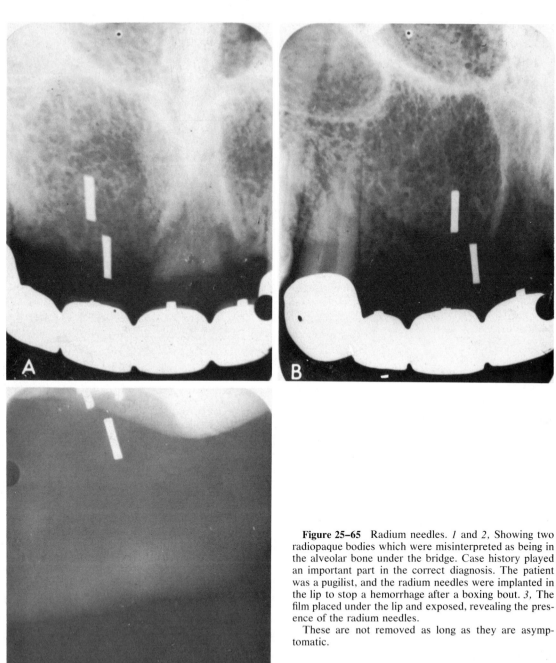

Figure 25–65 Radium needles. *1* and *2,* Showing two radiopaque bodies which were misinterpreted as being in the alveolar bone under the bridge. Case history played an important part in the correct diagnosis. The patient was a pugilist, and the radium needles were implanted in the lip to stop a hemorrhage after a boxing bout. *3,* The film placed under the lip and exposed, revealing the presence of the radium needles.

These are not removed as long as they are asymptomatic.

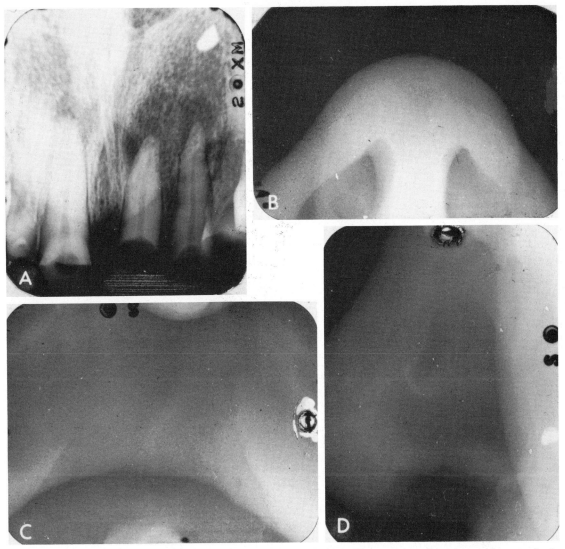

Figure 25–66 *A,* Unknown metallic object that appeared to be in bone. However, experience has taught us to check every other possible location: *B,* nose, negative; *C,* lip, negative; *D,* cheek along side of nose, positive. The high and slightly lateral direction of the x-rays threw this metallic image over the apex of the right lateral incisor.

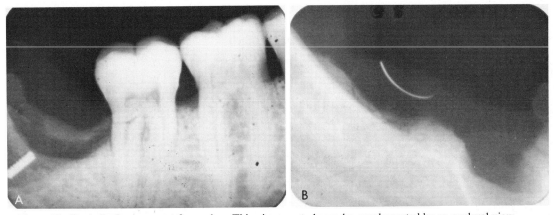

Figure 25–67 *A,* Broken crosscut fissure bur. This view must always be supplemented by an occlusal view.
B, Suture needle broken and lost in the thick, dense soft tissues in the mandibular third molar area. The absence of the eye in the needle explains the reason for the breakage. This dentist grasped the needle over the eye with the needle holder. When he exerted extra pressure to force the needle through the tissues, it broke at its weakest point, the eye. Read Rules for Suturing, in Chapter 2.

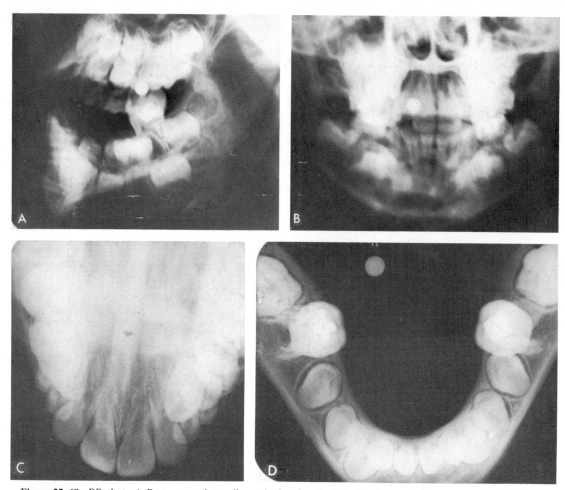

Figure 25–68 BB shot. *A,* Posteroanterior radiograph showing the BB shot between the upper centrals. *B,* Lateral jaw radiograph showing the shot at the crown of the upper right deciduous second molar. On the basis of this medical roentgenologist's report that the BB shot was in the palate, 3 operations were performed without locating the BB. *There was no intraoral radiograph taken.* When the patient was referred, the author took the occlusal view shown in *C,* proving that the BB was *not* in the palate.

Case history revealed that the gun jammed during target practice, and the boy placed the gun between his teeth and twisted the barrel, causing it to discharge. The boy insisted that he felt the BB shot strike the "roof of his mouth." A piece of broom handle was given to the patient and he was instructed to place it in his mouth as he had the gun barrel. As he did so it was observed that he raised his tongue over the end of the broom handle. An occlusal view (*D*) revealed the location of the BB shot in the base of the tongue, where it was seen in the ventral surface when the patient raised his tongue.

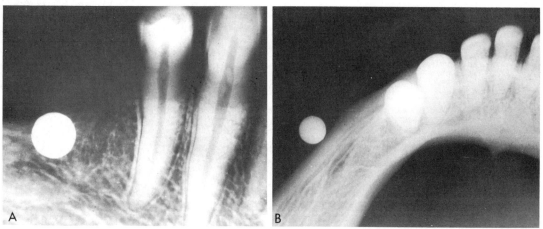

Figure 25–69 *A,* A piece of BB shot that appeared to be in the alveolar ridge was, as shown in *B,* actually below the mucosa of the cheek.

INVOLVEMENT OF MAXILLARY SINUS (ANTRUM OF HIGHMORE)

At the time of the extraction of maxillary teeth, there is always the possibility of an opening being made into the maxillary sinus. This may be the result of:

1. Removing the floor of the maxillary sinus with the tooth during the extraction of (usually) the maxillary molars.
2. Destruction of the floor of the maxillary sinus by chronic infection about the apex of a maxillary tooth. When the tooth is extracted, a pathway is established between the oral cavity and the maxillary sinus.
3. Perforating the thin epithelial lining of the maxillary sinus by incorrect use of the curette in those cases in which only this lining separates the root apex from the maxillary sinus.
4. Accidentally plunging an elevator through the bony floor of the maxillary sinus when attempting to remove a fractured or retained root.
5. Forcing a fractured or retained root into the maxillary sinus while attempting to remove it from its position in the alveolus or alveolar process.
6. Accidentally forcing an impacted maxillary third molar into the maxillary sinus while attempting to remove it.
7. Inadvertently penetrating a wall of the maxillary sinus while exposing impacted and unerupted maxillary cuspids or bicuspids. This danger is particularly great during the removal of buccally positioned unerupted maxillary cuspids.
8. Fracturing a large segment of the alveolar process containing several teeth and tearing out the floor and the lining of the antrum.
9. Enucleating a large maxillary cyst in which the bony partition has been eroded by pressure until it has disappeared and the ciliated epithelial lining

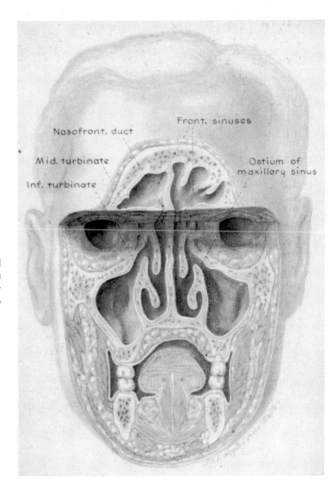

Figure 25–70 Frontal section through the head showing the relative position of the sinuses. (From Boies, L. R., Hilger, J. A., and Priest, R. E.: Fundamentals of Otolaryngology. 4th ed. Philadelphia, W. B. Saunders Co., 1964.)

of the maxillary sinus is now adherent to the cystic membrane. (The nasal cavity may also be involved. See the sections on naso-oral fistulas in this chapter, and Chapter 3.)

HERNIATION OF EPITHELIAL LINING THROUGH THE ALVEOLUS

Figure 25–71A shows the end result of the traumatic removal of the osseous floor of the maxillary sinus, lodged between the roots, when this maxillary molar was extracted but the lining mucosa of the sinus was not ruptured. The partial vacuum in the oral cavity created each time the patient swallows, plus the simultaneous increase in pressure in the maxillary sinus, has resulted in the expansion of the ciliated epithelial lining of the sinus with herniation through the alveolus into the oral cavity, as illustrated.

The case illustrated in Figure 25–71A was referred to us with a tentative diagnosis of "peripheral giant cell tumor." However, the "tumor" had been present for 6 weeks only, and its appearance followed the extraction of the maxillary second molar. The "tumor" was bluish white and was readily flattened with finger pressure. The simple test used in this case quickly differentiated an actual tumor and herniation of the lining mucosa of the maxillary sinus. The patient's nose was held, and he was instructed to attempt to inhale and exhale through his nose. When he did, the "tumor" was seen to expand slightly on exhalation, and to collapse on attempted inhalation. The "tumor" was simply a herniation of the ciliated epithelial lining of the maxillary sinus through the alveolus following a dental extraction.

The treatment is to reflect buccal and palatal flaps, carefully dissecting the mucoperiosteal membrane away from the osseous structures buccally and lingually and carefully freeing it from the hernia. These widely flared buccal and lingual flaps are then moved down and sutured over the hernia, which has been pushed back into the cavity of the maxillary sinus without tearing. It is a good practice, in these cases, after the hernia has been pushed back in the sinus, to cover the opening into the maxillary sinus with a round section of tantalum mesh gauze and then suture the mucoperiosteal membrane over the tantalum gauze.

HERNIATION OF AN ANTRAL POLYP INTO ORAL CAVITY

Figure 25–71B illustrates this postextraction sequela. This patient had a chronic maxillary sinusitis resulting from the chronically infected maxillary molar in this area. The osseous soft tissue barrier separating the apices of this tooth from the maxillary sinus was destroyed by the periapical infectious pro-

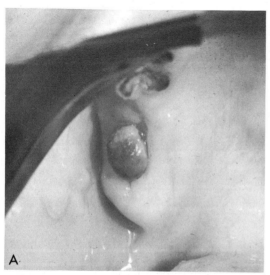 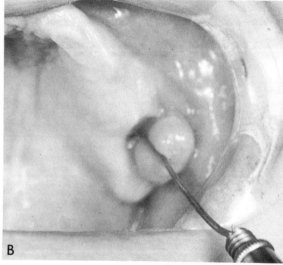

Figure 25–71 *A,* Prolapse of the antral mucosa through an antro-oral fistula. *B,* Antral polyp that has prolapsed through an antro-oral fistula.

cess, and chronic sinusitis followed with a thickened polypoid and irregular sinus mucosa. Consultation with a laryngologist is indicated in these cases. According to Jackson and Jackson, the presence of polyps does not, of itself, indicate radical removal of the sinus mucosa. As a matter of fact, the sinus membrane "may not necessarily be diseased, but with an intact epithelium and a stroma containing powerful inflammatory cells as a defense process, it is resisting disease and capable of doing so indefinitely."[37]

In the case illustrated in Figure 25–71B, the pedunculated outgrowth was cut off at its base and a circular incision was made through the mucoperiosteal membrane around the orifice of the fistula on the crest of the ridge. This collar was freed with a periosteal elevator about its circumference, inverted and sutured as shown in the drawing for the closure of a nasal-oral fistula (Fig. 25–91). Following this, the technique shown in Figure 25–75 for closing an antro-oral fistula was carried out. The cause of the chronic sinusitis, the infected molar, was removed, and the antritis subsided.

TREATMENT OF MAXILLARY SINUS– ORAL CAVITY FISTULAS

The treatment of these antro-oral openings can be divided into two phases: (a) the immediate closure of fistulas at the time the opening is made (e.g., during an extraction), and (b) the closure of long-standing fistulas.

Immediate Treatment. When the maxillary sinus floor is torn out at the time of extraction, if direct visualization of the maxillary sinus does not reveal evidence of infection, a large buccal flap is reflected and a relieving parallel incision is made in the periosteum high on the flap. This incision in the periosteum materially aids in mobilizing this flap. Next the palatal mucoperiosteum is loosened and elevated so as to expose the lingual cortical bone. Sufficient alveolar process is now removed with bone rongeurs so that the buccal and palatal soft tissues can be approximated and sutured without tension. Gauze sponges are placed over the wound; the patient is instructed to bite on these sponges. Other sponges are given to him to place over the wound when the original ones become soggy. These are removed and replaced by fresh sponges. These sponges are held in place until bedtime.

The patient should be placed on antibiotic therapy for several days, and nosedrops are prescribed that will shrink the nasal mucosa in order to keep the antral ostium open for drainage. The patient is told what has happened and is instructed not to blow his nose. If he sneezes he should open his mouth and sneeze through his mouth rather than through his nose. The use of straws for drinking is also prohibited, and in patients who smoke no excessive suction should be used when drawing in the smoke.

The patient is instructed to return in 48 hours. If inquiry does not reveal symptoms of acute maxillary sinusitis, the patient is instructed to return in 96 hours. If there are symptoms of acute sinusitis, the patient is

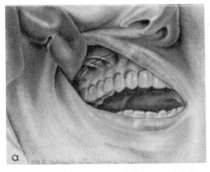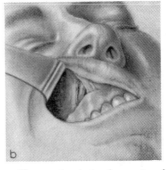

Figure 25–72 The purpose of the Caldwell-Luc ("radical antrum") operation is to clean out under direct vision the diseased tissue or foreign body in the sinus. A horizontal incision (A) is made in the canine fossa, the soft tissue is elevated, the sinus is entered through its anterior wall and enough of the wall is removed to provide adequate exposure. Then the foreign body or diseased membrane in the sinus is removed and a large window made under the inferior turbinate (B). The incision in the canine fossa is then sutured. (From Boies, L. R., Hilger, J. A., and Priest, R. E.: Fundamentals of Otolaryngology. 4th ed. Philadelphia, W. B. Saunders Co., 1964.)

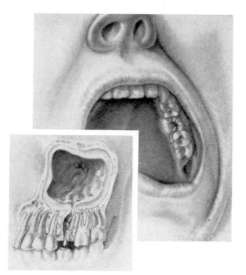

Figure 25–73 Antro-oral fistula and chronic suppurative maxillary sinusitis. Infection in the maxillary sinus must be resolved before closure of the fistula is feasible. Note the high position of the maxillary ostium. Boies *et al.* recommend: "Early care with selective (guided by sensitivity culture techniques) administration of antibiotics both systemically and locally into the sinus cavity through the fistula can control the infection and permit the normal healing process to close the fistula.

"Involvement of the sinus mucosa in the advanced chronic stage may still be amenable to similar care through the fistulous opening or intranasally through the natural ostium of the maxillary sinus.

"Where sequestration in the floor of the sinus or advanced granulomatous change in the mucosa exists, the sinus is best entered through the canine fossa and the focal areas removed under direct vision." (From Boies, L. R., Hilger, J. A., and Priest, R. E.: Fundamentals of Otolaryngology. 4th ed. Philadelphia, W. B. Saunders Co., 1964.)

referred to a rhinologist for an inferior turbinate puncture, if the rhinologist thinks it necessary, and treatment. If this is done, there is a good chance that the closure of the fistula will hold; if not, then the infection in the maxillary sinus will certainly result in a breakdown of the closure.

If, on inspecting the maxillary sinus, the second situation presents, in which the original partition between the maxillary sinus and the root apices was destroyed by infection originating in the tooth, then all infected material and polyps in the vicinity of the fistula should be removed by appropriate-sized curettes.

The buccal and lingual cortical plates are next reduced by bone rongeurs, and the soft tissues sutured firmly over the opening; sponges are placed as described. The patient is instructed as indicated earlier and is imme-

diately sent to a rhinologist so that he can make a window below the inferior turbinate into the maxillary sinus to facilitate drainage and irrigations. In many of these cases the maxillary sinus fistula will remain closed and a radical maxillary sinus operation will be avoided. In some cases a radical maxillary sinus operation will have to be performed even though a nasal window is made and the oral fistula into the maxillary sinus closes. In those cases in which the original closure breaks down, a radical maxillary sinus operation is performed by the rhinologist, and at the same operation the oral surgeon freshens the walls of the fistula, reflects the buccal flap freely, loosens the palatal tissue, and again reduces the size of the alveolar process so as to have apposition of the flaps. He then closes the fistula.

Tantalum gauze or a gold plate placed over the opening supports the soft tissue flap. See a description of this technique on page 1613.

If the fistula is on the crest of an edentulous ridge, instead of using the typical Caldwell-Luc type of incision the surgeon should make the original incision large enough so that it passes through the center of the fistula. Otherwise the Caldwell-Luc incision will cut off the circulation to the buccal flap of mucoperiosteal tissue reflected and freed by the oral surgeon in order to obtain a sliding flap of tissue to move over the fistula and suture to the palatal tissue.

If the opening into the maxillary sinus is the result of inadvertently puncturing the lining of a healthy maxillary sinus by the injudicious use of a curette or an elevator, the buccal cortical plate is reduced several millimeters, and sutures are passed from the buccal to lingual soft tissue, reducing the opening into the alveolus and protecting the blood clot.

It is not necessary to obtain absolute apposition of the buccal and lingual soft tissues in these cases of stab wounds through the epithelial lining of the maxillary sinus. It is necessary to place sponges and instruct the patient as has already been described. The placement of absorbable hemostatic gauze sponges and other foreign materials directly into the open alveolus is to be condemned. If the patient exhibits symptoms of maxillary sinusitis, he should be referred to a rhinologist. A small percentage of these cases develop symptoms of sinusitis. *Whenever you refer any of these patients to the rhinologist,*

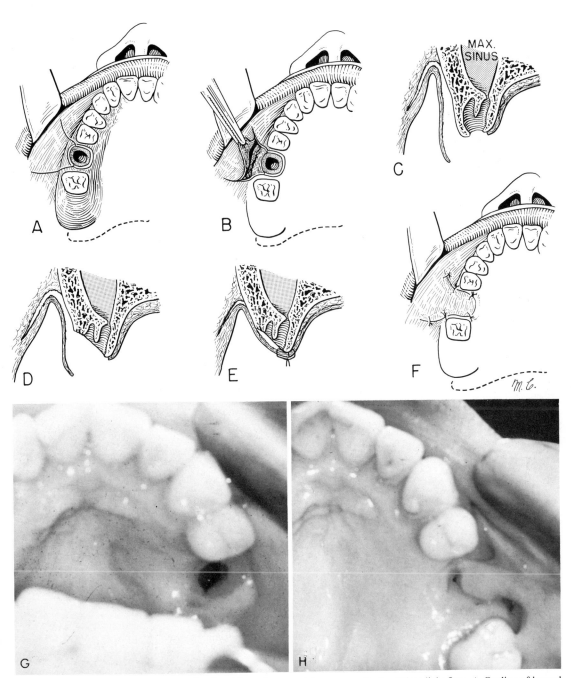

Figure 25–74 Closure of antro-oral fistula with teeth present by means of a buccal pedicle flap. *A*, Outline of buccal flap. *B*, Reflection of a large buccal flap with a relieving incision through the periosteum high in the flap and excision of antro-oral fistula. *C*, Sagittal section of *B*. *D*, Buccal and some lingual bone reduced with rongeurs. *E* and *F*, Closure of fistula with complete soft tissue apposition by sliding of buccal pedicle flap and suturing to palatal tissue. *G*, Antro-oral fistula in the second bicuspid area. *H*, Poor postoperative result because the dentist who attempted this closure violated a major rule: he did not raise a flap with a very wide base (as illustrated in *A* and *B* above) and make a relieving incision in the periosteum. Here we see the fistula is not closed and there is marked distortion of the soft tissues of the cheek and maxillary vestibule.

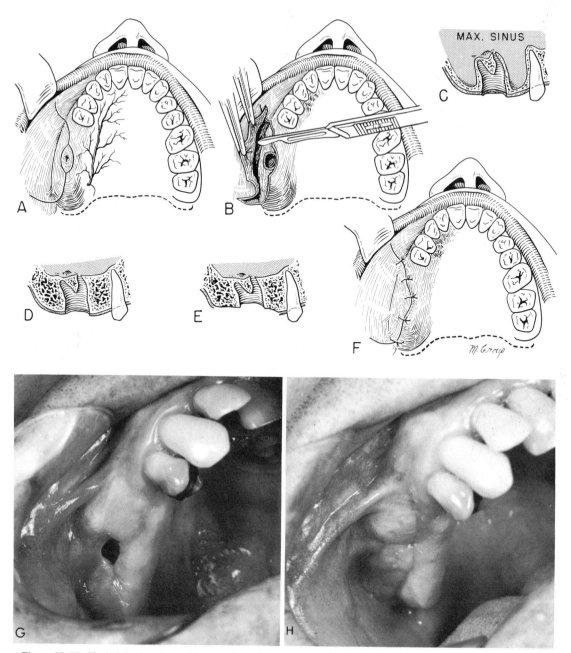

Figure 25–75 Technique for closing antro-oral fistula in an edentulous ridge.

A, Diagram of palate illustrating anterior palatine artery, antro-oral fistula, and outline of incision to be made for buccal flap.

B, Deflection of a wide buccal flap followed by a lateral incision of the periosteum as shown in Figure 25–75. The fistulous tract is excised, the edges of the mucoperiosteum surrounding the fistula are elevated and the edges of epithelium are excised. This is to prevent epithelium approximating epithelium when the flap is sutured to place. This also permits the periphery of the flap to rest on bone surrounding the opening into the sinus.

C, Lateral view of a type of maxilla with a large antrum. With this type little or no bone can be removed safely, and closure of the fistula must be done by reflecting a liberal amount of soft tissue from the alveolus and cheek, and sliding it over for closure.

D, Lateral view of another type of maxilla with a small antrum and an adequate amount of alveolar bone. This bone may be safely reduced to allow closure.

E, Following removal of bone of alveolar ridge to permit soft tissue apposition.

F, Closure complete with good soft tissue apposition.

G, Large antro-oral fistula in the posterior edentulous molar area.

H, Fistula closed by using the technique illustrated above.

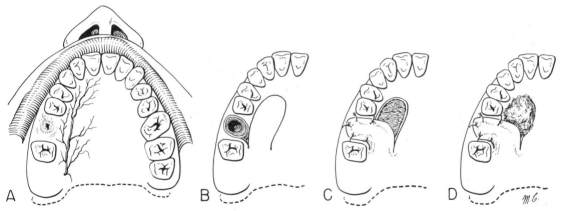

A   B   C   D   m.b.

Figure 25–76 Closure of antro-oral fistula with teeth present by means of rotated palatal pedicle flap.

A, Diagram of palate with fistula and outlining course of anterior palatine artery.

B, Incision for palatal flap. Note the small wedge of tissue removed on the distolingual side of the fistula to allow for flap rotation. Fistulous opening is freshened.

C, Flap rotated and sutured into position. There is a troublesome bulge distally.

D, Palatal defect filled with surgical cement pack to permit painless healing.

Note: A palatal incision is made so that the palatine artery will be inside the pedicle flap, thus assuring a good blood supply from the base of the flap. We are not satisfied with our results using this technique, although others are.

be sure to call him and describe what happened and what you did for the patient.

To recapitulate: when the maxillary sinus is accidentally opened during surgery, all efforts are directed toward closure of the opening. *The one thing that should never be done is to insert a gauze drain, surgical cement or any foreign body into the opening; this tends to perpetuate the opening.*

Treatment of Long-Standing Fistulas. If the fistula is of long standing the surgical treatment must be modified because an epithelized tract exists between the antrum and the oral cavity. In order to close the opening this tract must be excised, the hole covered with mucosa sutured on a firm bony surface,

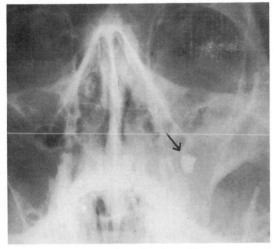

Figure 25–77 Sinusitis, chronic, with an antro-oral fistula and a foreign body in the antrum. A healthy maxillary sinus radiographically is radiolucent, while an infected one is radiopaque, as shown here. In this case an antro-oral fistula created by an extraction was incorrectly "closed" by placing a medicated cement "plug" in the fistula. Very shortly it was lost into the maxillary sinus. A "radical antrum" operation and antro-oral fistula closure using the combined skills of the otolaryngologist and the oral surgeon is now required.

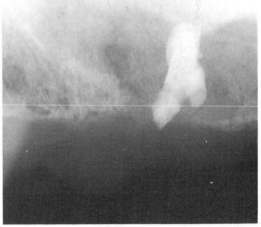

Figure 25–78 Radiograph of a medicated cement "plug" placed in an antro-oral fistula. These are contraindicated because of the possibility of the plug entering the maxillary sinus. To prevent the entrance of liquids and food until the fistula is surgically closed, a temporary base plate is made for edentulous maxillas, and "saddles" with clasps are used for dentulous patients. Both temporary devices are removed at night. (See Figure 25–79.)

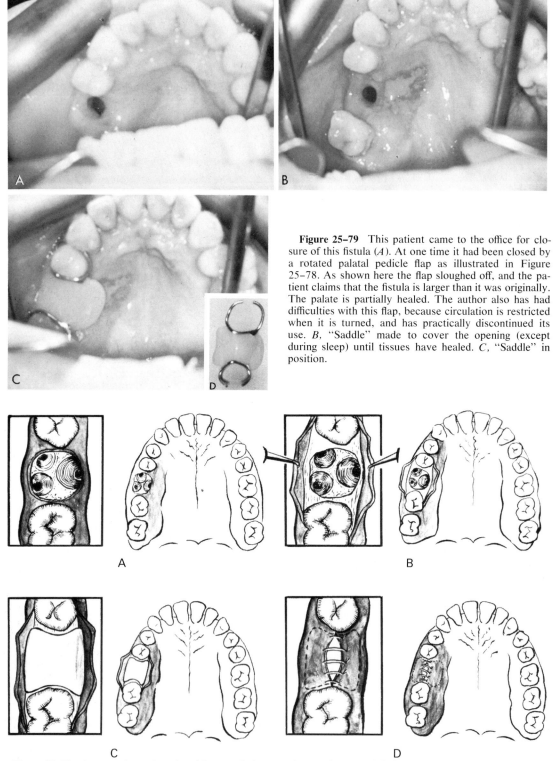

Figure 25–79 This patient came to the office for closure of this fistula (*A*). At one time it had been closed by a rotated palatal pedicle flap as illustrated in Figure 25–78. As shown here the flap sloughed off, and the patient claims that the fistula is larger than it was originally. The palate is partially healed. The author also has had difficulties with this flap, because circulation is restricted when it is turned, and has practically discontinued its use. *B*, "Saddle" made to cover the opening (except during sleep) until tissues have healed. *C*, "Saddle" in position.

Figure 25–80 Antro-oral opening closed by metal plate. *A*, Antrum is entered during extraction of maxillary tooth. *B*, Mucoperiosteum is retracted from the adjacent teeth to allow insertion of the metal plate. *C*, With the mucoperiosteum retracted, the metal plate is placed directly over the tooth socket. *D*, The mucoperiosteum is sutured back to its normal position. (From Budge, C. T.: Closure of an antro-oral opening by use of the tantalum plate. J. Oral Surg., *10*[1]:32–34 [Jan.], 1952.)

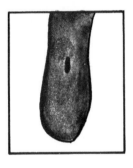
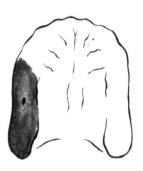
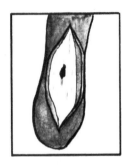
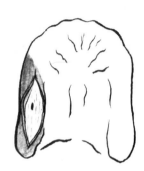

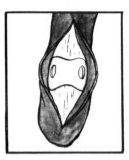
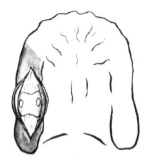
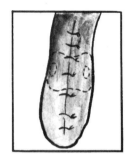
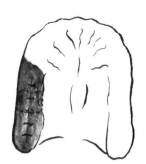

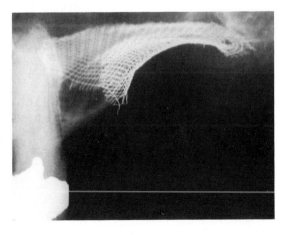

Figure 25–81 Study the text for the details of the use of tantalum or gold plates to help in the closure of antro-oral fistulas. Tantalum wire mesh gauze placed under the mucoperiosteal membrane covering an antro-oral fistula has also been successfully used. (From Budge, C. T.: Closure of an antro-oral opening by use of the tantalum plate. J. Oral Surg., *10*[1]:32–34 [Jan.], 1952.)

not over the original fistulous site (the mucosal flap must have a good blood supply), and, most important, antral secretions must be drained into the nose. Since the antro-oral fistula is below the level of the antral ostium, a window below the inferior turbinate is often necessary to divert the secretions if excessive or the ostium is not patent. The antrum must be free of infection and if not may require a curettage by the rhinologist at the time of operation. Use of antibiotics pre- and postoperatively is mandatory. The secret of suc-

cess in this operation is the judicious use of well vascularized pedicle flaps, diversion of antral secretions into the nose, and working with an antrum that is free of infection.

USE OF A METAL PLATE OR GAUZE IN CLOSING ANTRO-ORAL OPENINGS

Budge[8] describes the use of a tantalum plate for the purpose of closing antro-oral openings. A 36 gauge, 24 karat gold plate is much softer and easier to contour and adapt to the bone around the antro-oral opening. Because of this, we have taken the liberty to substitute gold into the technique used by Budge, as follows:

"On occasions during the extraction of a maxillary tooth, the antrum is entered. Immediately following removal of the tooth, the lingual and buccal mucoperiosteum is retracted from the adjacent teeth a sufficient distance to allow the insertion of the contoured U-shaped [gold] plate ([36] gauge) to cover the entire socket (see Figures 25–80 and 25–81), and to extend to the buccal and lingual aspects of the tooth socket a distance of 8 to 12 mm.

"With the mucoperiosteum retracted, the [gold] plate is placed directly over the tooth socket.

"Following insertion of the [gold] plate over the socket, the mucoperiosteum is sutured back to its normal position. The sutured mucoperiosteum will not cover the entire plate, but this is of no consequence, as the plate is to be removed after a period of from 14 to 30 days following insertion, depending on the size of the original antrum opening at the time of extraction of the tooth.

"After sufficient time has elapsed for granulation tissue to form in the tooth socket, the [gold] plate is raised from the healed tooth socket with a hooked instrument. The plate is cut in two pieces from mesial to distal and removed. Following removal of the plate, further suturing and tissue contouring is not necessary.

"To close a chronic antro-oral fistulous opening, the surgical procedures are much the same as immediate closure following tooth extraction, except the maxillary sinus should be free from infection, and the fistulous tract from the maxillary sinus to the oral cavity must be removed. . . . The [gold] plate is not removed following closure of a chronic antro-oral fistulous opening."

The use of tantalum gauze in place of metal plates is also very effective in these cases (Fig. 25–82).

ANTRO-ORAL FISTULA CLOSE TO APPROXIMATING TEETH

When the fistulous tract approximates the root of an adjacent tooth as is shown in Fig-

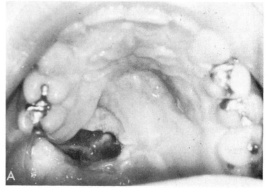

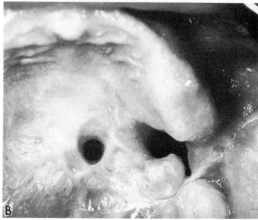

Figure 25–82 *A,* This antro-oral fistula was "closed" five times by various individuals, and this is the appearance when we saw the patient. In this case the last operation was to place a tantalum mesh over the fistula and use a palatal flap to cover the fistula. This flap, as shown here, sloughed off, exposing the mesh gauze and fistula. The mesh was removed, the exposed osseous palate was permitted to epithelialize over, and the second bicuspid was extracted. Then the fistula was closed with a large buccal flap. (See text for the indication for the extraction of an adjacent tooth.)

B, At the time this patient came to our clinic he had been operated on *nine times* for the closure of what the patient *claimed was a small opening* into the sinus. Apparently at each succeeding operation more bone was removed in an attempt to close the opening. At the last operation a palatal flap was attempted; this necrosed, and what must have been a very thin bony floor of the nasal cavity was devitalized. This exfoliated, and the patient now has a naso-oral fistula as well as an enormous antro-oral fistula. Additional surgery to attempt a closure was contraindicated. A full upper denture was constructed after the left maxillary vestibule was deepened.

ure 25–83*A,* closures frequently break down, as happened in this case. Much as we regret it, occasionally it is necessary to extract the adjacent tooth. This gives us a larger operative site, enabling us to raise a larger flap and assure that *the edges of the flap rest on bone* and not against the root, where they will never become attached. Figure 25–83*B*

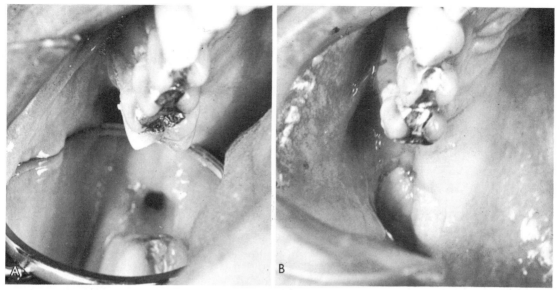

Figure 25–83 Read text under Antro-oral Fistula Close to Approximating Teeth for the technique necessary to close this antro-oral fistula.

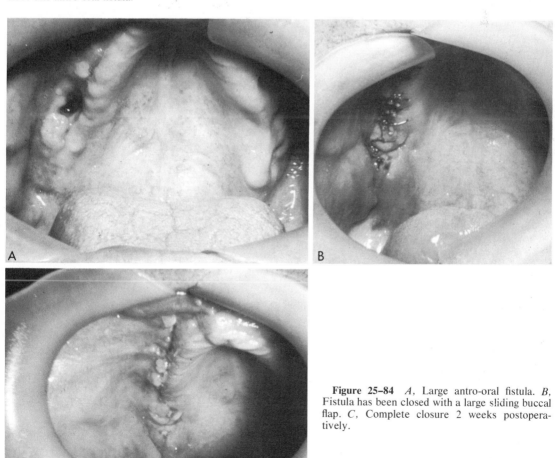

Figure 25–84 *A*, Large antro-oral fistula. *B*, Fistula has been closed with a large sliding buccal flap. *C*, Complete closure 2 weeks postoperatively.

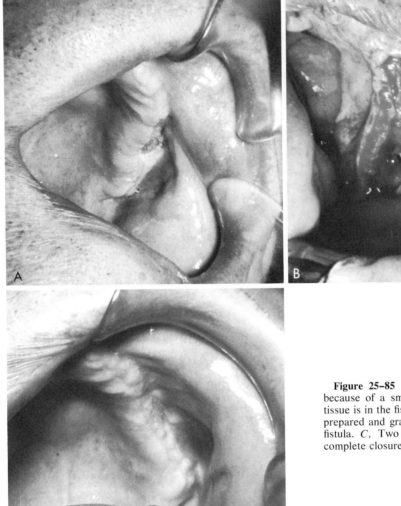

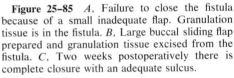

Figure 25–85 *A*, Failure to close the fistula because of a small inadequate flap. Granulation tissue is in the fistula. *B*, Large buccal sliding flap prepared and granulation tissue excised from the fistula. *C*, Two weeks postoperatively there is complete closure with an adequate sulcus.

shows the closure of a fistula after the first molar was carefully extracted so as not to enlarge the antro-oral fistula. One cannot be criticized for a first attempt to close an antro-oral fistula in these situations without first extracting the approximating tooth, but be certain to tell the patient that a second operation, with the extraction of a tooth, may be necessary to effect a closure.

NASO-ORAL FISTULA ON PALATE

These are as difficult to close as the antro-oral fistulas, if not more so. In Figure 25–90 is illustrated the technique used to close a palatal naso-oral fistula. These are seen following trauma by instruments, excision of

tumors, fractures of the maxilla which involve the palate, or, as was the case in Figure 25–90, the overzealous use of the coagulating tip.

LABIAL NASO-ORAL FISTULA

A complication of the enucleation of large anterior maxillary cysts may be the production of a naso-oral fistula where the cyst has destroyed the bony nasal floor and in which the nasal and cystic membranes are adherent. These cases should be marsupialized. In Figure 25–91 is illustrated the technique for the closure of a labial naso-oral fistula. (See Chapter 12 for technique to avoid this complication by marsupializing these cysts.)

(*Text continued on page 1620*)

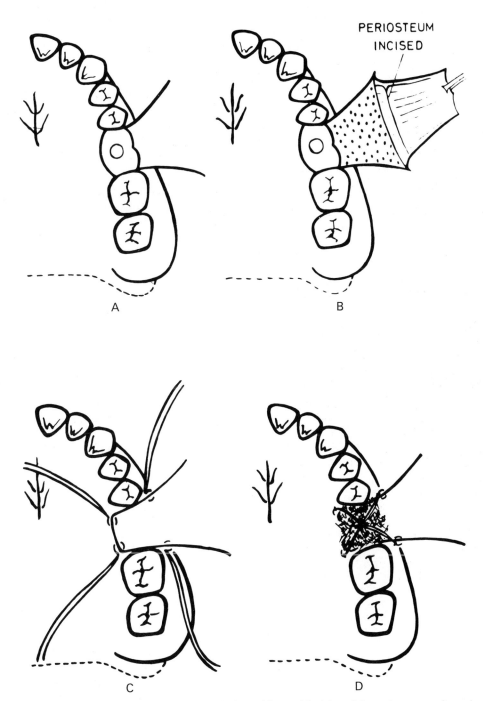

Figure 25–86 *A, B,* Diagrams showing the design of a buccal flap and incision of the periosteum on its undersurface. *C, D,* Diagrams showing buccal flap advanced following incision of its periosteum and dressing held in position with long tails of sutures. (Courtesy of F. M. S. Lee, B.D.S.)

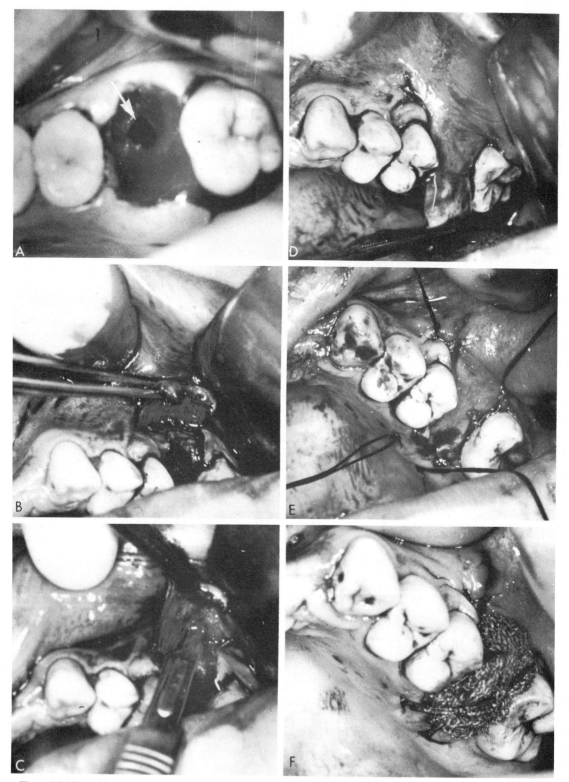

Figure 25–87 *A*, Upper left permanent first molar socket showing an obvious perforation of the maxillary antrum following a routine extraction. *B* through *F*, the essential steps in the Buccal Sliding Flap technique. See also Figure 25–88. (Courtesy of F. M. S. Lee, B.D.S.)

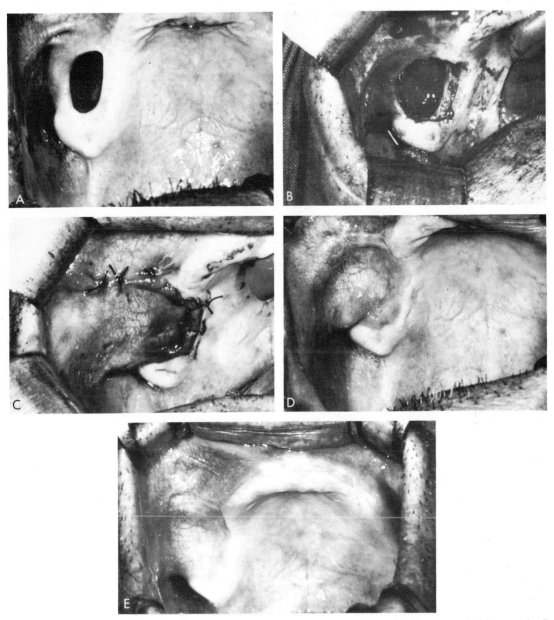

Figure 25–88 *A*, Large antro-oral fistula of several years. Several previous attempts at closure had been made. *B*, Edges of fistula were excised and a ledge of bone was prepared palatally, mesially and distally. *C*, A large buccal flap was undermined, and the periosteum was incised and sutured over the fistula as shown. *D*, One month later. *E*, One year later. (Courtesy of F. M. S. Lee, B.D.S.)

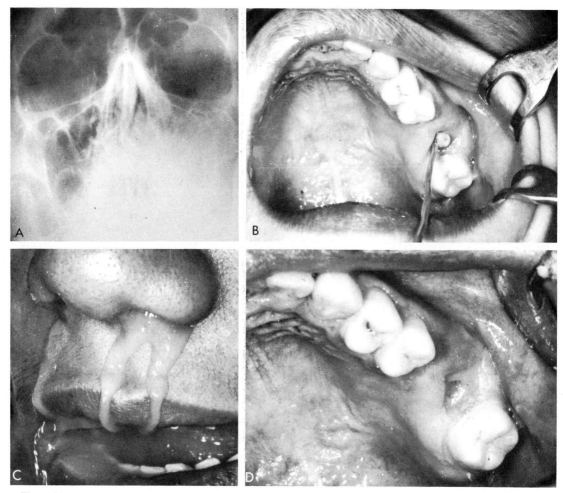

Figure 25–89 *A*, Radiograph showing a cloudy antrum on the left side. *B*, A narrow deep antro-oral fistula. *C*, Antral wash-out via oral end of fistula. *D*, Spontaneous healing of fistula occurred following resolution of antral infection. (Courtesy of F. M. S. Lee, B.D.S.)

ROOTS FORCED INTO THE MAXILLARY SINUS (MAXILLARY ANTRUM)

Some small fractured roots, inadvertently displaced into the maxillary sinus during the attempt to remove them, are occasionally "lost"; *i.e.*, they cannot be located on the radiographs. Attempts to wash them out fail. A few days later the patient may report that he was aware that something was in his nose and when he gently blew his nose, he found the root tip in his handkerchief. The root tip had been incorporated in the mucous secretion in the maxillary sinus and swept by the ciliated epithelial lining of the sinus up and out the ostium maxillary into the nasal cavity.

As one who has had personal as well as professional experience with intermittent sinusitis resulting from the unsuccessful at-tempted removal of a small root tip, I seriously question the value of or need for the removal of these roots. If the root tip is not located radiographically, the soft tissue is sutured over the alveolus and the patient is informed about the root tip and advised that it is our decision not to subject him to additional surgery unless there is postoperative sinusitis. To date I have not seen any patient who developed postoperative sinusitis under such conditions.

To avoid forcing roots into the antrum, extreme care must be exercised in the removal of the fractured roots of maxillary teeth which the radiographs reveal are in close proximity to the floor of the maxillary sinus. Apical pressure must never be applied on the end of the root fragment with an elevator. The surgeon should have *good radiographs* and good visibility at all times; he should

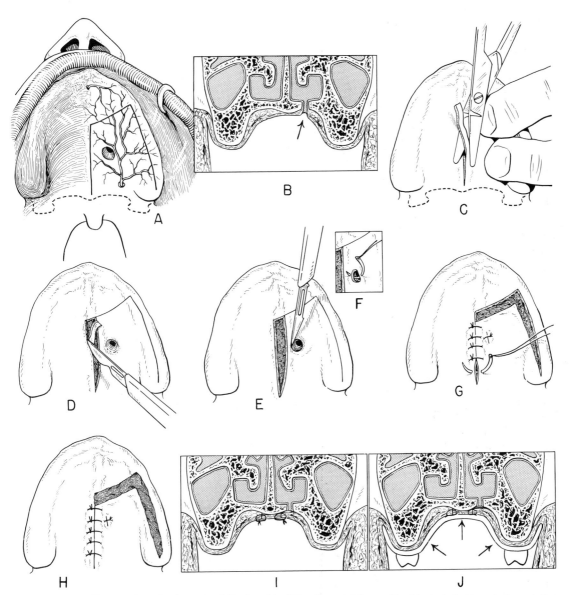

Figure 25-90 Closure of a palatal naso-oral fistula with sliding flap. *A,* Flap outlined to include the anterior palatine artery. Large sliding flap is necessary because a simple elliptical excision and undermining will produce too much tension and compromise blood supply. *B,* Cross sectional view showing fistula (arrow) and how epithelium of mouth is continuous with nasal epithelium. *C,* Flap raised and strip of tissue removed to allow room for rotation. *D,* Enough tissue is removed from the midline in order to allow the flap to be sutured to the heavier palatal tissue on the side of the midline rather than to the thin, almost avascular, tissue in the midline. *E,* Fistula is "cored"; *i.e.,* epithelium and granulations are excised from fistulous tract. *F,* Oral aspect of fistula is sutured. *G,* Flap rotated and sutured in midline. *H,* Exposed bone covered with protective pack of zinc oxide, eugenol and cotton. *I,* Cross section showing how former fistulous opening is no longer under nasal opening and where medial edge of flap is sutured to thicker palatal tissue. *J,* Denture in place (arrows), assuring good apposition of flaps and preventing submucosal hematoma.

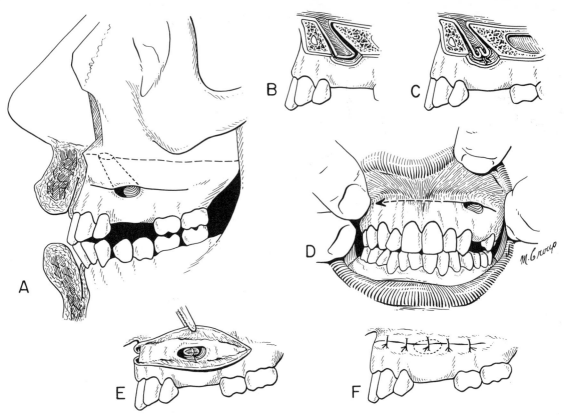

Figure 25–91 Closure of a labial naso-oral fistula. *A*, Naso-oral fistula. *B*, Cross section. *C*, Tube of tissue undermined at edges and inverted and sutured. *D*, Mucobuccal fold widely incised to allow a freely movable flap. *E*, Flap is reflected. *F*, Flap is sutured.

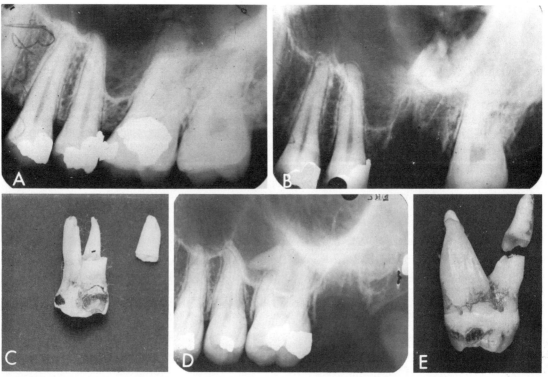

Figure 25–92 While extracting the first molar in (*A*) the lingual root was fractured and forced into the maxillary sinus when an attempt was made to remove it (*B*). It was removed (*C*), using the technique shown in Figure 25–96. *D*, Lingual root of the second molar was fractured. When removal was attempted it was forced anteriorly into the maxillary sinus between the buccal and lingual roots of the first removal. *E*, The root was removed using techniques shown in Figure 25–96.

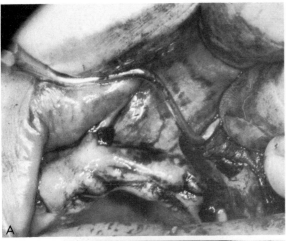
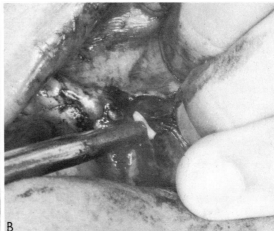
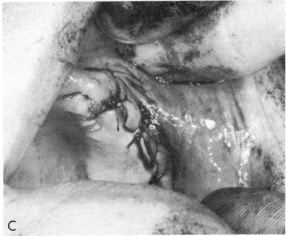

Figure 25–93 Removal of a fractured premolar root from the maxillary sinus. *A,* The mucoperiosteal flap is reflected from the gingival line and a window is cut through the buccal cortical bone into the sinus. *B,* The root is picked up by the suction tip and removed. *C,* The mucoperiosteal flap is replaced and sutured over the sockets.

never work blindly in a blood-filled socket. A small suction tip is used to keep the alveolus clear.

Radiographs of the teeth to be extracted should be studied as a valuable means of preventing the accidental forcing of tooth roots into the antrum.

The roots of the following teeth are in close relationship to the floor of the maxillary sinus in the order of their proximity: first molars; second molars; second bicuspids; third molars; first bicuspids; and rarely the cuspids.

TECHNIQUE FOR REMOVAL OF TOOTH ROOT FORCED INTO THE MAXILLARY SINUS (MAXILLARY ANTRUM)

If the root of a tooth has inadvertently been forced into the maxillary sinus, the technique described below is used for its removal.

The area is radiographed in order to locate the root. The surgeon should not attempt to remove it without a radiograph, unless he can see it clearly. Several radiographic views may be necessary in order to localize the root. It should be remembered that sometimes, even though the root has left the socket, it may not have perforated the antral membrane and may be lying under the membrane and not in the maxillary antrum itself.

If the radiograph shows the root tip in the *immediate vicinity* of the tooth socket, then the surgeon may proceed to remove it employing the technique shown in Figure 25–95.

If the root tip is shown by the radiograph to rest at a point in the sinus at a distance from the tooth socket, then the root is removed by the technique shown in Figure 25–96.

If the radiographs do not reveal the root it may possibly be washed into position by irrigation. The antrum is irrigated using an antrum-irrigating syringe. About 3 ounces of

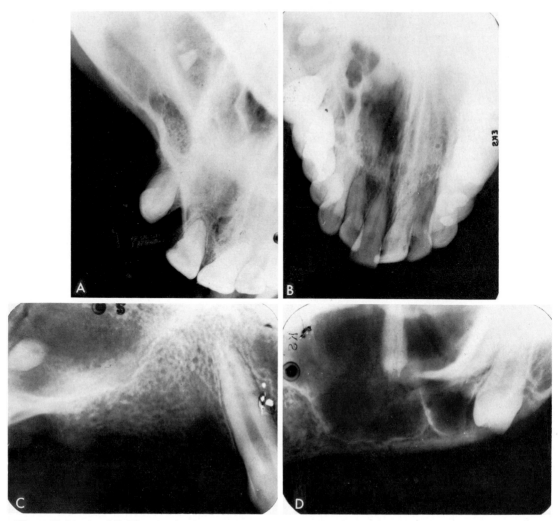

Figure 25–94 *A* and *B*. These occlusal roentgenograms are an aid in the localization of roots in the maxillary sinus and should be taken especially in those cases in which the periapical film is negative for the presence of a root. *C* and *D*. Roots in the maxillary sinus with healed ridges and no evidence of pathology in the sinuses when Waters position roentgenograms were taken of these sinuses. Therefore there is no reason to remove these roots.

normal saline solution is used at a time; a total of at least a pint should be used. Pressure should be placed on the irrigating syringe, so that the solution will be forced up against the roof of the maxillary sinus and then down around the sides and out at the opening; the idea is to have the liquid flush out the root tip.

After using each syringeful of normal saline solution, the surgeon looks up into the opening again to see whether the root tip has been carried into view at the opening. He also examines the basin into which the patient has expectorated, for the root.

If the root is not recovered, radiograph the floor of the maxillary sinus and if the root is now seen in an area removed from the alveolus, remove it as shown in Figure 25–96.

Positions of Patient and Operator. The patient must be in a *semihorizontal position*. The operator should be *sitting down* close to the patient's head, in order to have free use of his hands and to minimize stretching.

The removal of a root tip from the antrum can be a most tiresome operation. Be as comfortable as possible, and have the patient as comfortable as possible also.

COMPLETE TOOTH FORCED INTO THE MAXILLARY SINUS

The tooth most frequently forced into the maxillary sinus is the impacted maxillary third molar. Buccally impacted cuspids have also been displaced into this cavity. In this

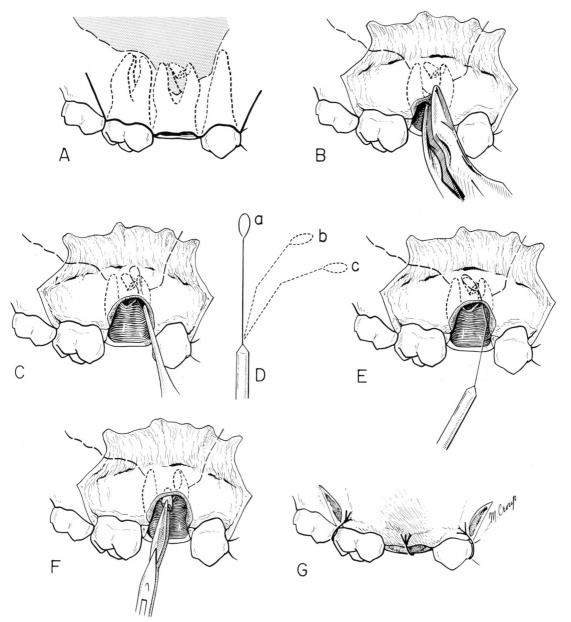

Figure 25–95 Technique for removal of a root forced into the maxillary sinus in *immediate* proximity to the periapical space. This is established by x-ray examination.

A, The apical third of the mesiobuccal root of the first right maxillary molar was fractured during the extraction of this tooth, and when its removal was attempted, it was forced into the sinus through the paper-thin bone that separated it from the maxillary sinus. It now rests in the sinus in close proximity to the original point of entry. A large buccal flap is essential for *exposure* and subsequent *closure* of this antro-oral opening. Its outline is shown by the heavy black line.

B, After the reflection of the large buccal flap, as illustrated, buccal and intraradicular bone, if any, is removed with end-cutting rongeurs for two reasons: (1) for access, and (2) to facilitate closure of the antro-oral fistula.

C, The opening into the maxillary sinus through the sinus mucosa is enlarged by a draw-cut motion with the bowl of a small straight curette. Frequently, the root apex can be trapped by the curette and removed or at least moved into position for removal by the apical fragment forceps as shown in *F.*

D, Another valuable aid in gently moving the root fragment into position for removal is to form a small loop at the end of a wire root-canal pathfinder.

E, This delicate instrument is used to snare and draw the root tip into the opening for removal.

F, The root tip is gently grasped with the fine-pointed apical fragment forceps and removed.

G, A tantalum plate is inserted as previously described. Its purpose is to help prevent pressure on the blood clot that should form in the alveolus over the antral opening. This material plus the closure of the buccal flap over the alveolus will permit the clot to organize without being subjected to pressure from the oral cavity during eating and swallowing. In order to almost completely approximate the soft tissue, buccally and lingually, a gap is left along the line of incision mesially and distally. This will heal by secondary intention. If necessary, lingual and buccal cortical bone is also removed with the end-cutting rongeurs to permit apposition of buccal and lingual soft tissues. (See text for further details.)

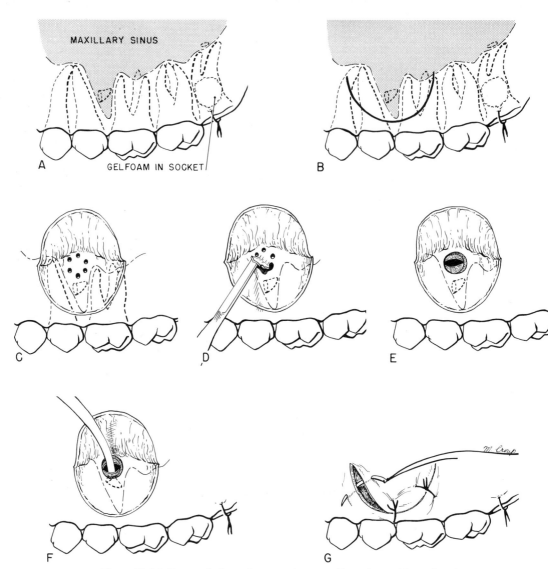

Figure 25–96 Removal of root fragment from maxillary sinus with suction tip.

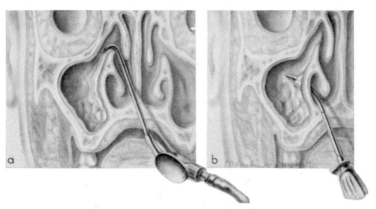

Figure 25–97 *A,* The most commonly used modern method of irrigating a maxillary sinus. *B,* A method in which a trocar is inserted through the meatal wall. (From Boies, L. R., Hilger, J. A., and Priest, R. E.: Fundamentals of Otolaryngology. 4th ed. Philadelphia, W. B. Saunders Co., 1964.)

latter situation the buccal flap made to expose the cuspid is enlarged, as is the opening made by the entrance of the cuspid into the maxillary sinus. The cuspid is located, grasped with a curved hemostat and removed. The flap is sutured back to place.

If an impacted maxillary third molar has inadvertently been pushed into the antrum, the buccal flap that had been reflected to expose the operative site is sutured back into place and then the steps below are followed. The surgeon (*a*) makes a curved incision high over the cuspid-bicuspid and molar roots; (*b*) reflects this flap; (*c*) cuts through

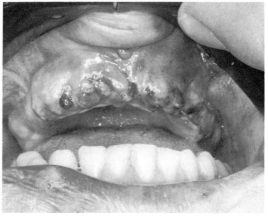

Figure 25–99 Multiple areas of postextraction pyogenic granulation tissue in the maxillary alveoli.

the thin alveolar plate, taking care not to expose the roots of any of these teeth; (*d*) enlarges the opening so that the tooth can be grasped with a curved hemostat and removed; (*e*) sutures the flap back into place.

POSTEXTRACTION PYOGENIC GRANULATION TISSUE

This postextraction complication is illustrated in Figure 25–99 and the treatment is described in Chapter 13.

ALVEOLALGIA

Dry sockets, painful sockets, sloughing sockets, alveolitis, necrotic sockets, localized osteomyelitis and postextraction osteomyelitic syndrome are all synonyms describing the same condition—faulty healing, with pain ranging from slight to excruciating in intensity, following the extraction of one or more teeth. The best term for this condition is alveolalgia, meaning pain in the alveolus.

At the Department of Oral Surgery, University of Pittsburgh School of Dental Medicine, and the outpatient department of the Magee-Women's Hospital, records of postoperative treatment for 24,575 extractions (23,886 on nonpregnant patients, 689 on pregnant patients) were tabulated for data on alveolalgia.

Some investigators have included in their studies all sockets in which there was delayed healing, regardless of whether pain was an ac-

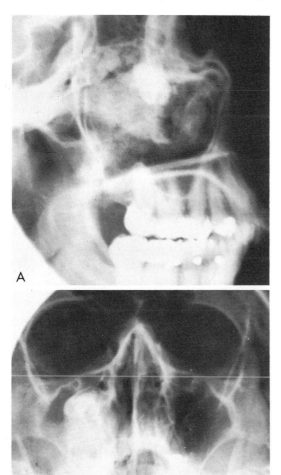

Figure 25–98 Maxillary third molar driven into the maxillary sinus by a hard, misdirected blow on the chisel during the exposure of this impacted unerupted third molar. It was removed through a window high in the cuspid-bicuspid fossa.

companying factor. This investigation considered only those sockets in which pain was actually present. The clinical picture of these two sockets is identical; why there is pain in one and not in the other, we do not know. The records in this report are of patients who returned 1 to 10 days after the extraction of teeth with a history of pain in the socket (alveolus), mandible, maxilla or ear, or radiating over the side of the face, or a combination of these.

The pain usually began the day after the extraction, or shortly after the effects of the anesthetic had worn off; this occurred in 110 cases out of 226, or about 48 per cent. As for the others, pain started in 42 patients the second day following extraction; in 31 patients the pain started the third day; in 16 patients the fourth day; in 6 patients the fifth day; in 2 patients the sixth day; and in 19 patients the pain started the *seventh day after extraction.*

Frequently a patient returns to his dentist after an extraction with a history of pain. The dentist, on examination, finds what appears to be a normal clot, and dismisses the patient with a prescription for an analgesic compound. If the dentist had taken a small curette and carefully passed it through the semitough blood clot, he would have found beneath the surface a mushy, semifluid clot in the middle and apical thirds of the socket, which would confirm the diagnosis of early alveolalgia.

Etiology. The etiology of painful sockets is believed to be varied. The following sections discuss those characteristics thought to be possible causes or predisposing factors. Infection about the apex of the tooth at the time of extraction has long been considered one of the primary causes of alveolalgia, but this hypothesis is not substantiated by actual figures. It was based on the reasoning that in cases of defensive osteitis or traumatic occlusion, there is a concentration of calcium salts about the root after the tooth is extracted; this dense bony wall prevents the ready nourishment of the clot, which collapses, exposing the cribriform walls of the socket. In those teeth that revealed radiographically diffuse or circumscribed areas of destruction in the periapical structures, or rarefying osteitis, it was reasoned that while there would be a good blood supply to the clot, the latent, low-grade organisms in the area would grow in the clot, which would provide an ideal culture medium.

However, this study does not bear out the theory. It was revealed that 82 painful sockets (38 per cent) followed the extraction of nonvital teeth, and 170 painful sockets (62 per cent) followed the extraction of vital teeth.

TRAUMA TO SOCKET AND SURROUNDING TISSUES INCIDENTAL TO THE REMOVAL OF THE TOOTH

Trauma is undoubtedly an important factor in the production of many sloughing sockets, particularly in those cases that necessitated the use of bone burs and repeated application of elevators.

Burnishing of the walls of the alveolus by the passage of a hypercementosed root will account for considerable frictional trauma. However, of the cases reported here, many resulted from the most simple extractions under ideal conditions. Neither do the figures bear out the supposition that alveolalgia is the result of faulty technique; 126 cases of alveolalgia, or 56 per cent, followed definite trauma, but 100 cases, or 44 per cent, followed simple extractions in which there was no trauma. This is not a marked difference.

INFILTRATION OF AN ISCHEMIC, TOXIC, ACID DRUG

It is the practice of some dentists to flood the labial or buccal and lingual tissues so full of the anesthetic solution that they turn white. After the tooth is extracted, the socket does not fill with blood, because of the action of the vasoconstrictor. This permits saliva, laden with bacteria, to enter and pool in the socket. This combination probably does account for some of the clotless sockets.

In the present study of 226 cases, no tabulation dealing with this etiologic factor was made, yet the observations of the author permit the general statement that it would seem that the percentage of painful sockets is greater following extractions involving local anesthesia than that after extractions in which general anesthesia was used.

EXCESSIVE USE OF MOUTHWASHES

The author's technique is to compress the expanded buccal or labial and lingual plates of the alveolar process with finger pressure, suture soft tissues, place a sponge over the wound, and instruct the patient to hold it in place for at least 1 hour and to refrain from mouthwashes for 3 hours. This is the general procedure when local anesthesia has been used. When teeth have been extracted under general anesthesia, the patient is permitted to wash the mouth immediately after recovery.

Again, no compilation in regard to this factor has been made as yet, but it does not seem that the early use of a mouthwash is an important factor.

The following case is an interesting example of sockets washed clean of blood clots. A railroader, aged 47, had 22 remaining teeth extracted under local anesthesia. He was instructed in the care of his mouth, which included the admonition to keep the ridges and mouth clean. Three days later he returned for a postoperative examination. The mouth was scrupulously clean, and every socket (alveolus) was devoid of a blood clot except in the apical third. The patient reported absolutely no pain or discomfort of any kind. He apologized for a little blood yet remaining in the sockets, and said his cotton sticks "would not go all the way up," and that he could not get them any cleaner than they were.

CURETTAGE AFTER EXTRACTION

In the past, curettage of the socket (alveolus) was a routine procedure after the extraction of all teeth. Undoubtedly, many postoperative complications resulted from this practice. Today the curette is used only to remove granulomas and small cysts from the periapical region or to remove debris that has inadvertently dropped into the socket.

ENTRANCE OF SALIVA INTO THE OPEN ALVEOLUS

This has been considered a possible cause of alveolalgia in those cases that followed the uncomplicated, not difficult extraction of vital teeth; the bacteria-laden saliva infected the otherwise sterile socket.

Claflin reported: "In all animals, these clotless sockets were produced by infecting extraction wounds with a mixed culture of streptococci from an infected human pulp; this culture was put on a cotton tampon,

placed in the socket immediately after the extraction, and then sealed with collodion. The use of collodion was necessary because it seemed that if the saliva seeped into the socket, it inhibited the bacterial growth and decreased the virulence of the bacteria."[13] Of course, since the animals used were dogs, the question that arises is whether human saliva contains the same antiseptic qualities. It is of interest to note that whereas Claflin produced sockets devoid of blood clots by infecting extraction wounds with streptococci from an infected human pulp, Grandstaff found streptococci only once in 20 cases of alveolalgia, with all the others exhibiting a mixed infection.[30]

Most writers on the subject quote Schroff and Bartels: "Fusiform bacilli and spirochetes have been found in cases of painful sockets following extraction. Upon the cessation of pain, these organisms are no longer observed in smears of exudate from the socket. Our findings, clinical and bacteriological, indicate that anaerobic organisms produce more painful sockets following extraction than do aerobes."[58]

In the author's study, smears and cultures of 40 cases of alveolalgia were obtained. The report from the bacteriologist revealed a positive growth of diplostreptococci in 80 per cent of the sockets from which cultures were taken.

PHYSICAL STATUS OF THE PATIENT

The clinical evidence on this disputed point is confusing. Gardner reported: "A few years ago a study was made to determine the possible relation of the clotless sockets to the general condition of the patient, and any such relationship was ruled out."[25]

Then, too, there are records of many patients in whom only one painful socket developed, although multiple extractions had been performed.

The investigations of Harden[35] would indicate that when pregnancy influenced the general condition, there should be a low percentage of painful sockets. He had suggested that during pregnancy there is a low protein content, but a relative increase of globulin, which is mostly fibrinogen; in the nonpregnant woman there is 0.2 per cent, which rises in the pregnant woman to 0.4 per cent. We should expect, then, a more rapid clotting of blood and a firmer, better organized clot, which would be more resistant to breakdown by infection. In a series of 294 pregnant women, 689 extractions were performed; the average pregnancy was 6½ months. In this series of extractions only 3 cases of alveolalgia were presented for treatment; this is 0.4 per cent, or 1 case of alveolalgia for every 229 extractions. Compare these figures with those obtained from the series discussed in the summary.

Additional investigation, with more careful attention given to the physical condition of the patients in whom "dry sockets" develop, will be necessary before any conclusions are reached concerning this factor in the etiology of painful sockets.

SUMMARY

Out of 23,886 extractions presented for postoperative treatment, there were 226 cases of alveolalgia (painful sockets, so-called dry sockets). This is 0.9 per cent, or 1 case of alveolalgia for every 105 extractions.

Seventy-nine per cent of the cases of alveolalgia developed in the mandible, 21 per cent in the maxilla. The low percentage in the maxilla is thought to be due to the better blood supply.

More cases of alveolalgia (62 per cent) followed the extraction of vital teeth than followed the extraction of nonvital teeth (38 per cent). No hypothesis has been proposed to explain this.

Trauma, being present in only 56 per cent of the cases, apparently does not play as important a role as previously thought. Oral hygiene has little if any influence on the development of alveolalgia.

No change from the normal blood count or hemoglobin was noted in the great majority of cases in which such counts were made.

The high percentage (80 per cent) of cases in which either diplococci or streptococci were found on making cultures seems to indicate that this organism is the most important etiologic factor in the production of alveolalgia.

TECHNIQUE OF TREATMENT

Many methods are now being used for the treatment of "dry sockets," most of which are empirical and have no sound scientific basis. The author prefers the simple but very effective method of treating alveolalgia described below.

The socket is irrigated with warm normal saline solution, dried gently and isolated with gauze sponges. A wick of iodoform gauze saturated with eugenol is then gently inserted into the socket. A doughy mixture of zinc oxide and eugenol is placed over the socket opening to act as a cover to prevent entrance of food or saliva. A moist sponge (moist to prevent the zinc oxide–eugenol paste from adhering) is placed over the socket, and the patient is instructed to bite down for 30 minutes before taking out the sponge. By this time the cover is hard enough to resist smearing through the rest of the mouth. This routine is carried out daily for 2 or 3 days.

Anesthetic Alcohol Injection. We have had a few cases of acute alveolalgia in the mandible that were so excruciatingly painful that analgesics and local treatment were ineffectual. It was necessary to anesthetize the inferior alveolar nerve to give the patient a few hours' relief from the pain. When additional nerve blocks were necessary we added 4 minims of 95 per cent alcohol to the anesthetic solution. This prolonged anesthesia from 24 to 48 hours.

Solutions containing alcohol, which is a protein precipitant, should not be injected into dense tissue such as the palatal region or into canals, unless destruction of the nerve and its immediate surrounding tissue is desired. Figure 25–39 shows the destructive effect of an anesthetic alcohol solution injected into the nasopalatine canal. The fact that too much solution was used is evident because not only was the neurovascular bundle destroyed but also the osseous canal sloughed out as a result of chemical necrosis. Fortunately, the adjacent dental alveoli were not injured.

OSTEOMYELITIS

Definition. Osteomyelitis is an inflammatory condition of bone involving primarily the soft parts. As Paget[50] pointed out, the term "osteomyelitis" is, in a sense, a misnomer: it should apply only to an inflammation of the marrow. By common usage, however, the term is generally understood to mean an inflammation of all the structures that make up

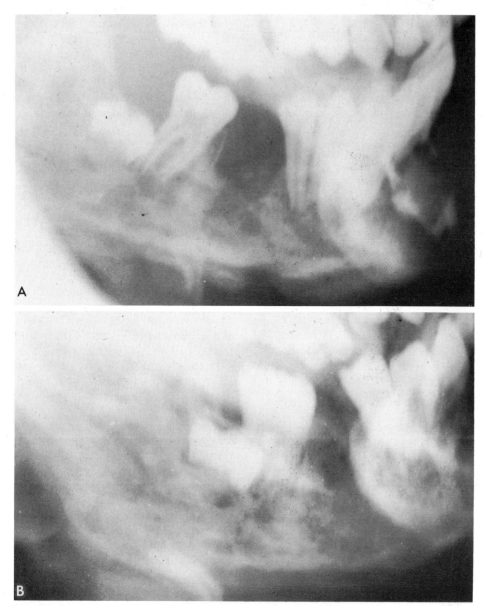

Figure 25–100 Acute osteomyelitis of the mandible in a 14-year-old girl following the extraction of a "loose" lower left first molar. This was in the preantibiotic days, and the infection spread rapidly through the left body of the mandible and symphysis to the right bicuspid area. There was a pathologic fracture of the left ramus and symphysis. The periosteum was swollen, and pus flowed freely from around the necks of the teeth. Wide intraoral drainage was established by an incision just below the gingival line from the left retromolar area to the right bicuspid area. Extraoral drainage was established in the submaxillary and submental areas. After the acute painful stage was over, drainage continued for several months, and eventually there was sequestration of this portion of the mandible and teeth. Fortunately, there was an excellent involucrum formed, and so very little facial disfigurement followed the termination of this infection.

a bone—the medulla, cortex, periosteum, blood vessels, nerves and epiphyses. The inflammation develops in the bone marrow (medulla ossium) and extends into the cancellous bony spaces (spongiosa), then spreads along the blood vessels, the fibroblastic tissues, and eventually into the periosteum. While the mineral part of the bone only modifies the inflammatory process, it is vitally affected by the inflammatory process.

Bone is living tissue; when the nutrition of the bone cells is interfered with, they die and the formation of a sequestrum results. The process by which nutrition is cut off from the

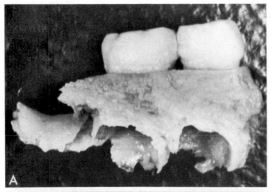

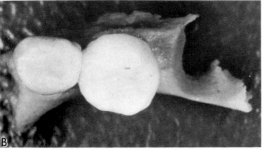

Figure 25–101 Sequestrum from the right mandible of an 8-year-old child, containing the deciduous first and second molars. This was a sequela to osteomyelitis of the mandible as a complication of chickenpox (varicella), which is a frequent predisposing factor in osteomyelitis in children. Note the portion of lingual cortical bone from around the permanent first molar. This tooth was not removed, and bone has since been replaced in part.

bony cells is quite simple. The infection travels along the course of the blood vessels and the lymphatics in the bone. The haversian vessels contain the anastomosing vessels that connect the vascular bed of the interior of the dense bony structure with the blood vessels of the periosteum. Furthermore, these canals

communicate with the canalicular structure of the calcified portions of the bone and are, therefore, essential to the nutrition of the bone cells. Inflammatory processes in the nutrient vessels mean apposition of the lumen of the vessels and thrombosis, which prevents blood from reaching bone cells. Normal metabolism in the bone cells ceases, and the bone cells die.

Bacteriology. Osteomyelitis is the result of an acute pyogenic inflammation of the bone marrow. The inflammation is due to an invasion into the bone marrow by, usually, hemolytic *Staphylococcus aureus*. In a small percentage of cases *Staphylococcus albus* is the responsible pathogenic organism. The next two organisms most commonly found are streptococci and pneumococci. Mixed cultures, which are reported, are undoubtedly due to the fact that the cultures were taken after the wound or abscess had been draining and organisms other than the primary offender had gained entrance into the wound.

Etiology. Osteomyelitis can be caused by direct extension from the source of infection, *e.g.*, teeth, sinuses, nasal cavity, sockets and soft tissues, into healthy bone. It can also be caused by hematogenous dissemination of an infection, such as chickenpox, into healthy bone.

Infection can be carried by direct extension or hematogenous dissemination into bone that has been partially or wholly devitalized by radiation necrosis, chemical necrosis, external trauma (to the bone or to the periosteum), surgical trauma (*e.g.*, overheating bone when cutting with a bur or excessive compression of bone with an elevator), or a con-

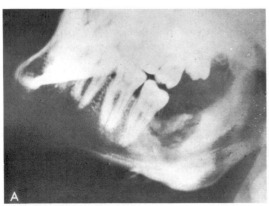

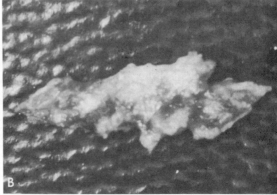

Figure 25–102 *A,* Pressure osseous necrosis as the result of excess repeated pressure on the buccal cortical bone by the shank of an elevator whose fulcrum was the buccal cortical bone. This pressure closed the nutrient canals with the inevitable nonviable bone. Twelve weeks later this large sequestrum was freely movable in a mass of pyogenic granulation tissue and was removed. There was a marked defect in the mandible at this point. *B,* Sequestrum removed.

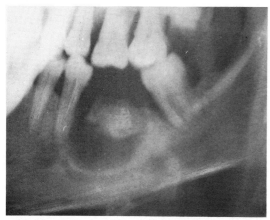

Figure 25–103 Large sequestrum that is partially exfoliated. This was a localized postextraction osteomyelitis, conservatively treated by maintenance of intraoral drainage. No antibiotics. Note clear-cut condensing osteitis about the periphery. Sequestrum was removed. No curettage.

the patient is very poor, such as occurs in metabolic diseases, vitamin deficiencies and other disorders.

Waldron reports that, unlike osteomyelitis of the long bones, which is more frequently of metastatic origin, the jaws are rarely infected by the hematogenous route.[68] It is true that primary infection, introduced by trauma — surgical or otherwise — or secondary involvement by extension of infection from dental sources or from contiguous infection, accounts for the greater percentage of cases of osteomyelitis of the mandible or maxilla.

Osteomyelitis starts as an *acute* form and unless eliminated by early massive doses of penicillin develops into a *chronic* form. There also may be periodic flare-ups of acute attacks from a chronic condition. With respect to the areas of bone involved by an osteomyelitis, there is a *localized* type, confined to a small area, and a *diffuse* type, in which the destruction spreads throughout large areas of bone. There is also a *diffuse fulminating* type that is an acute osteomyelitis of sudden, severe onset in which there is

comitant infectious process, such as tuberculosis, syphilis, or actinomycosis. Infection can also occur by means of the two routes discussed above when the general health of

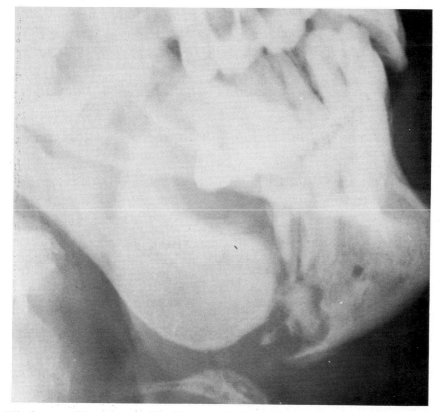

Figure 25–104 Osteomyelitis of the mandible following a fracture of the mandible by a dentist when extracting a left mandibular second molar. Sequestrum is almost free enough from the surrounding bone to permit a sequestrectomy. Unfortunately, this dentist did not fix the mandible to the maxilla in a normal occlusal relationship, which means there will be a difficult case of malocclusion to correct.

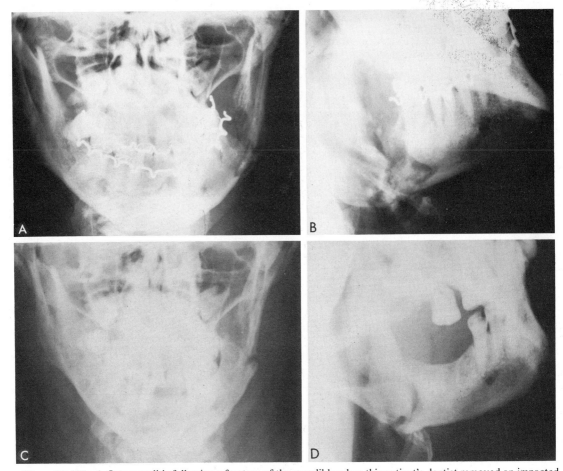

Figure 25–105 *A,* Osteomyelitis following a fracture of the mandible when this patient's dentist removed an impacted mandibular third molar. To prevent malocclusion and to maintain the normal relationship of mandible and maxilla, splints and intermaxillary elastics were applied. Massive doses of penicillin were given. Extra- and intraoral drainage was established. *B,* Large sequestra present 8 weeks later. *C* and *D,* After sequestration and extraction of teeth the vertical ramus moved anteriorly until contact with the horizontal ramus and osseous union followed. The patient now has a well-functioning mandible.

rapid destruction of large areas of bone. In the maxilla and mandible, by far the most frequent form of osteomyelitis is the subacute *localized* type. The so-called "dry socket" we term alveolalgia is, in my opinion, a localized osteomyelitis. I have seen cases in which the alveolus was thrown off in its entirety as a sequestrum. When we consider the oral flora and the ease with which this flora and odontogenic infection are introduced into the marrow during oral surgical procedures, it is truly remarkable that the incidence of osteomyelitis of the maxilla and mandible is so rare.

Symptoms. Symptoms of acute diffuse osteomyelitis in the mandible or maxilla are the usual alarming symptoms of an acute infection, such as severe pain, elevated temperature, swelling, general malaise, toxic appearance, and a high white blood cell count (8000

to 20,000). In the early stages of the disease radiographs are negative. Depending on the age and resistance of the patient and the virulence of the microorganism, it may be 2 to 3 weeks before sufficient destruction of bone has taken place to show radiographically as radiolucent areas that are larger than the surrounding spongiosa. As the disease progresses, these radiolucent areas join to give the bone a mottled or "worm-eaten" appearance.

The first symptom is pain with fever. The pain is deep-seated, and in the mandible is referred to the ear. Then the teeth become sore to percussion; eventually, as the destruction of bone increases and the infection spreads, they become loose, one after another. By this time the gingivae are dark red and edematous, as is the labial and buccal mucosa, as a result of the periostitis. Pus exudes from around the necks of the teeth when pressure is exerted on the soft tissue. By now there is usually marked swelling of the face with acute lymphadenopathy.

Treatment. In the acute stage of os-teomyelitis the patient should be immediately admitted to the hospital and given massive doses of penicillin. (See Chapter 8, "Antibiotic Therapy.") Most of these patients are severely toxic. Complete bed rest and ade-

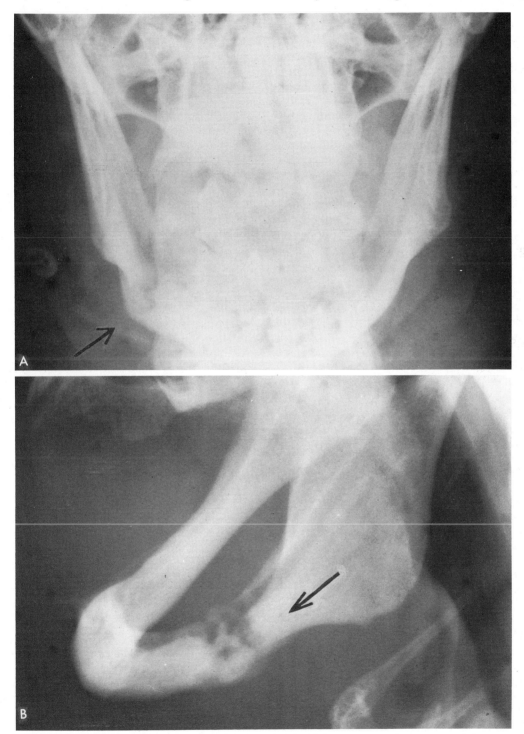

Figure 25–106 Osteomyelitis of the mandible, cause unknown. There was actually a pathologic fracture, but the involucrum (see *A*) prevented displacement. This was a low-grade chronic osteomyelitis. There were never any acute symptoms.

1636 Oral and Maxillofacial Surgery

quate fluid intake and output should be maintained. Intravenous therapy, if indicated, is given. An adequate diet that will not require excessive mastication is ordered. Polyvitamins are given with a high-protein, high-calorie diet. If antibiotic treatment is started early enough the disease may be stopped before destruction of bone and suppuration take place. If not, then surgical drainage is established as soon as pus is localized.

With good drainage, a minimum of surgery and large doses of antibiotics the acute stage subsides and the disease usually continues in a chronic form. All the acute symptoms disappear and the blood counts return to normal. In the author's experience the continuation of antibiotics does not hasten the termination of the disease.

Drainage persists and will continue until all sequestra—pieces of dead bone that have separated from the surrounding healthy bone during the process of necrosis—are removed or expelled. *At no time is vigorous curettage to be instituted in attempting to remove sequestra.* Only when the sequestrum is loose and can be *freely moved* can it be removed. Care must be taken not to disturb the granulation tissue surrounding the sequestra or to damage the involucrum. In children, extreme care should be exercised to prevent traumatizing the developing permanent teeth or their investing follicles. These tissues and teeth are extremely resistant to destruction by the osteomyelitic process.

When the amount of destruction of bone has been great, the patient must be warned about the possibility of a spontaneous fracture and is advised to take only soft foods and liquids, and to avoid yawning and any trauma to the jaw (see Case Report No. 10 and Figure 25–110). In cases of very extensive bone destruction, the mandible should be immobilized by intermaxillary ligation until sufficient new bone has been formed to prevent the possibility of a fracture.

Intraoral saucerization is indicated in localized areas of osteomyelitis. The technique involves reflecting overlying mucosa and removing peripheral sharp irregular cortical bone with a bone rongeur down to the cancellous bone.

In summary, the treatment is: (1) massive doses of penicillin in the acute stage; (2) surgical drainage when pus is localized; (3) general supportive therapy; (4) sequestrectomy *only when the sequestra are freely movable;* (5) splinting of jaw if there is a possibility of a pathologic fracture; (6) extraction of mobile teeth *only* when it is clearly evident that they have lost their bony support.

Case Report No. 9

CHRONIC OSTEOMYELITIS OF THE MANDIBLE FOLLOWING EXTRACTION OF TEETH

Patient. A 6-year-old girl was admitted to the hospital with the chief complaint of three draining sinuses of the jaw (Fig. 25–107). There was a sharp intraoral bony projection that cut her tongue.

Past History. Eight months before this admission, the patient had had two primary left mandibular molars extracted. After the extractions, an acute cellulitis of the jaw had developed; the swelling had been subsequently incised and drained extraorally. At that time a diagnosis of cellulitis had been made by her physician, and the condition had been treated with penicillin and sulfonamide drugs.

Diagnosis. The patient was admitted to the Eye and Ear Hospital for a sequestrectomy, with the diagnosis of chronic osteomyelitis of the left mandible.

Oral Examination. In the left mandibular sulcus two segments of sharp cortical plate protruded through the mucosa. These were slightly movable and were a small portion only of the two sequestra visible on radiographs (Fig. 25–108).

Laboratory Findings. The urine had a specific gravity of 1.020 and a slightly acid reaction; three white blood cells were found.

Blood coagulation time was 3 minutes and 20 seconds; bleeding time, 4 minutes and 40 seconds.

There was no growth in 72 hours from a jaw culture.

Operation. Under Avertin-ether anesthesia, after routine preparation of the face and mucous membrane, an incision was made along the mucobuccal fold from the distal aspect of the first permanent molar to the cuspid region. Tissue was reflected from the projecting bone fragment, and

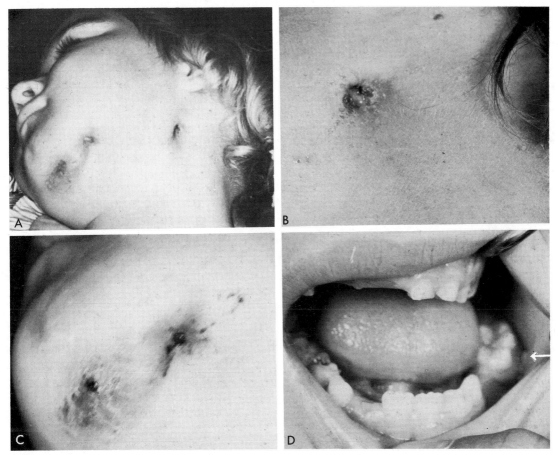

Figure 25–107 *A*, Three extraoral sinuses; chronic osteomyelitis of mandible.
B, Close-up view of sinus drainage from the angle of the ramus.
C, Close-up of double sinuses and tissue destruction in the anterior portion of the mandible.
D, Intraoral view showing one of the two bony projections through the mucosa. (See Case Report No. 9 for further details.)

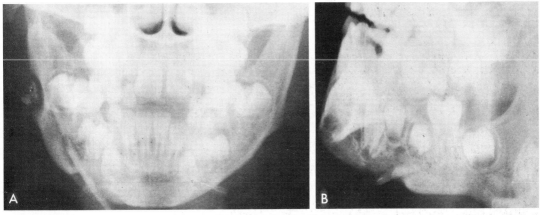

Figure 25–108 *A*, Posteroanterior radiographic view of the mandible shows the sequestra thrown off from the body of the mandible.
B, This oblique radiographic view of the mandible shows a sequestrum and what appears to be still-active osteomyelitis, judging from the "moth-eaten" appearance below the unerupted bicuspids. However, the complete cessation of drainage after the removal of the sequestra would indicate that this was a process of repair rather than destruction. It was impossible to get this patient to return for follow-up radiographs or for plastic repair of scars. The patient lived over a hundred miles away in the country. Letters from her father stated that she had no swelling or drainage.

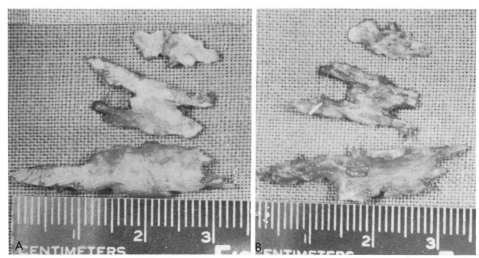

Figure 25-109 Three sequestra removed extraorally. *A,* Buccal cortical bone; *B,* cancellous side of the buccal cortical plate.

the segment was freed and removed. An iodoform gauze drain was inserted. A probe was inserted extraorally into the posterior fistula; this fistula was enlarged, and a small segment of bone was removed from it. A probe was also inserted into the anterior fistula, which was also enlarged, and a large segment of necrotic bone was removed. An iodoform gauze drain was also inserted into this fistula. The patient was removed from the operating room in good condition. A specimen of necrotic bone was sent to the laboratory for pathologic diagnosis (Fig. 25-109).

Postoperative Course. On the second postoperative day the patient was in good condition and had no complaints. She was given Crysticillin, 900,000 units daily, and penicillin, 100,000 units, was being used for intraoral and extraoral irrigation of the incision, which was still draining extraorally, but to a lesser degree.

On the third postoperative day the iodoform drains were being extruded; they were cut off, and the wound was redressed.

On the fourth postoperative day the drains were removed, and the jaw was irrigated with penicillin solution.

By the fifth postoperative day drainage had practically ceased, and the patient was discharged.

Pathology Report. The specimen consisted of two thin, bony spicules, irregular in shape, the longer 3 cm. in length and the shorter about 1.25 cm. They were only a few millimeters in thickness. Microscopically, the sections showed only necrotic bone with a small amount of surrounding chronic inflammation. A few pieces of fibrous tissue were adherent to the bone fragments. The pathologic diagnosis was necrotic bone (sequestra) from the mandible.

Case Report No. 10

ILLOGICAL, UNJUSTIFIED RESECTION OF THE RIGHT BODY OF THE MANDIBLE FOR OSTEOMYELITIS

History. Five months previously this 59-year-old male patient had had a right mandibular molar extracted. Since that time there had been moderate swelling of the cheek and oral soft tissues, with no pain but profuse intraoral drainage from the area of previous extraction.

Chief Complaint. He "couldn't stand the pus" draining into his mouth and he "wanted something done about it," in spite of a detailed description given to him about what "was wrong" with his jaw, and that nothing was surgically indicated at this

time because "the dead bone" in this area was not loose and could not be removed until it was.

He was advised about antibiotic therapy and that because of the good possibility of a pathologic fracture his jaws should be wired together. He refused this treatment and left very greatly disgruntled to "go elsewhere."

Roentgenograms taken at this time are shown in Figure 25-110*A* to *C.*

Subsequent History. Six weeks later he returned and stated that he had had his "jaw

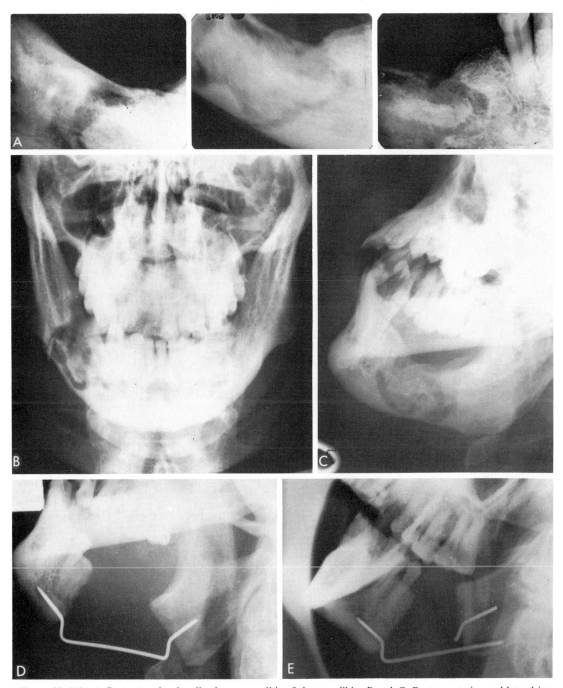

Figure 25–110 *A*, Postextraction localized osteomyelitis of the mandible. *B* and *C*, Posteroanterior and lateral jaw roentgenograms reveal the sequestrum forming, but it still was *not movable* and so surgery was not yet indicated. *D*, Postresection roentgenogram of the mandible that was performed by a surgeon in another specialty. Pathology report: "Acute and chronic suppurative osteomyelitis of the mandible." *E*, Broken Kirschner wire allows mandibular osseous fragments to collapse. *F* to *H*, Facial disfigurement and malocclusion produced by this collapse. (See Case Report No. 10 for further details.)

(*Figure 25–110 continued on following page*)

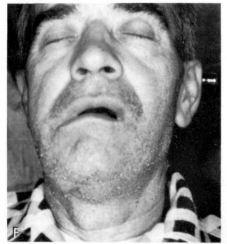

Figure 25–110   (Continued.)

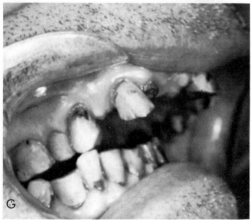

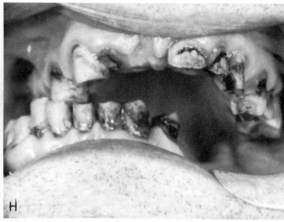

operated on" by a surgeon in another specialty and that since then he had had pain in his jaw and could not eat (see Figure 25–110D). He was sent back to the surgeon who had performed the resection of the body of the mandible and inserted the Kirschner wire in an attempt to stabilize the relationship of the mandibular fragments, pending the time when a contemplated bone graft would be inserted.

Within 2 months he again returned, this time with extreme malocclusion due to a gross displace-ment of the mandibular sections and a history of chronic pain and complete inability to eat. The roentgenogram showed that the Kirschner wire had broken (see Figure 25–110E), and the various muscular actions on the sections of the mandible had produced the facial disfigurement and malocclusion shown in Figure 25–110F to H. He was again referred to the operating surgeon. A subsequent attempt at a bone graft was a failure. Final disposition of this case is not known.

LOCALIZED OSTEOMYELITIS FOLLOWING EXTRACTION OF TEETH AND THE ENUCLEATION OF AN INFECTED RADICULAR CYST

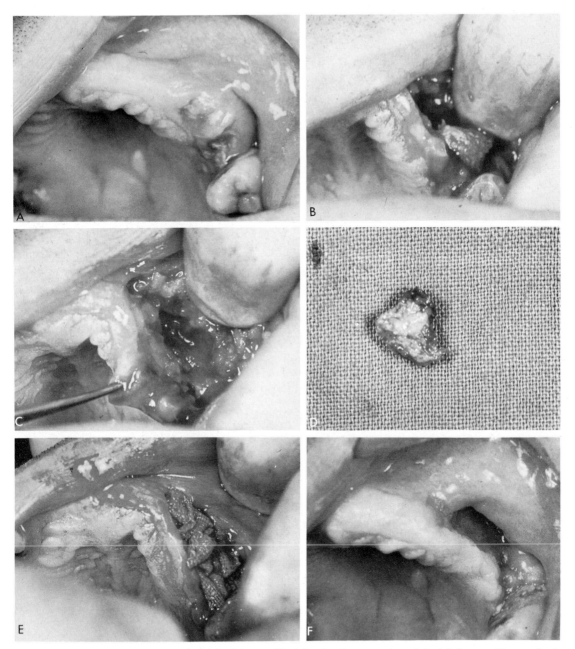

Figure 25–111 *A,* Localized osteomyelitis of the maxilla following the extraction of the left first maxillary molar in a luetic patient. Note pyogenic granulation tissue. *B,* A large semicircular incision was made, and the mucoperiosteal tissue was reflected. A large sequestrum, freely movable, was located, as seen in this view, and removed. *C,* View into the crypt in the maxilla following removal of the large sequestrum. Granulation tissue is not disturbed. Cavity is saucerized. *D,* Sequestrum with some attached granulation tissue. *E,* Cavity in the maxilla lightly filled with iodoform gauze. *F,* Epithelialized saucerized cavity. This cavity will gradually flatten out, but there will always be a depression in this area.

POSTEXTRACTION OSTEOMYELITIS OF THE MAXILLA

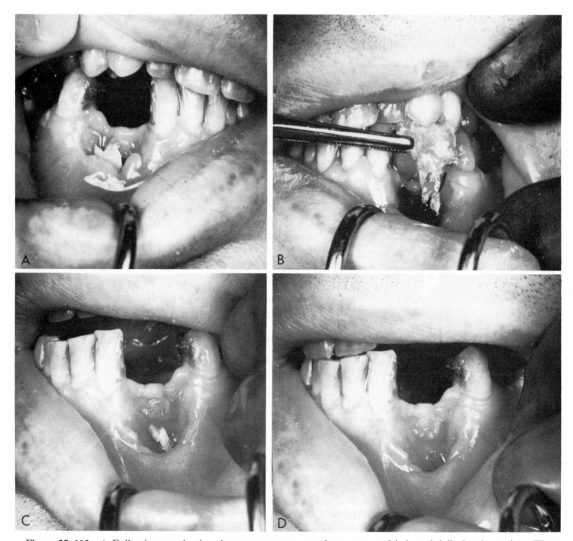

Figure 25–112 *A,* Following enucleation the osseous crypt was kept open and irrigated daily by the patient. There was no pain. In four weeks this sequestrum was freely movable. *B,* Sequestrum grasped with a hemostat and removed. Curettage is not indicated in these cases. *C,* Small sequestrum from lingual cortical plate which was freely movable and so was removed. *D,* Note final spontaneous saucerization and epithelialization.

Case Report No. 11

PATHOLOGIC FRACTURE OF MANDIBLE AS THE RESULT OF OSTEOMYELITIS, IMMOBILIZED BY EXTRAORAL SKELETAL PIN FIXATION

Patient. A 45-year-old white male steelworker was admitted to the Magee-Women's Hospital with the chief complaint of "swelling underneath the chin and pus flowing." The patient was referred from his private physician.

History. The patient stated that 2 months prior

to the time of admission he had first noticed a slight painful swelling about the size of a nickel at the inferior border of the left mandible in the mental region. The swelling had increased and become more painful, so the patient had gone to his private physician for treatment. He had been treated with three injections of penicillin per week for 2 weeks before the swelling had been incised and drained.

It had been thought that this submental abscess was the result of an acute exacerbation of chronically infected mandibular teeth. Hot, moist dressings had been used postoperatively, and the swelling did decrease somewhat. The next week the mandibular teeth had been extracted, with no postoperative complications. This had been done under local anesthesia. Three weeks later the maxillary teeth had been extracted under local anesthesia, with favorable results. Drainage of a thick yellowish pus had never stopped all during this period of weeks and treatments. The previous week the patient had noticed that the swelling in the submental region had become harder and

begun to extend almost to the midline of the mandible. He had returned to his private physician, who had admitted him to another hospital, where penicillin therapy had been instituted and radiographs taken (see Figure 25–113*A* and *B*). At this time a diagnosis of osteomyelitis of the mandible with a pathologic fracture had been made. The patient had then been referred to this hospital for treatment.

Treatment. The patient was immediately placed on large doses of penicillin. He received 400,000 units of penicillin S-R four times on the first day. The next day he received 300,000 units of aqueous penicillin every 3 hours. On the second hospital day the edema subsided and induration lessened. Pus was still draining. He was kept on the same penicillin therapy. The third day showed

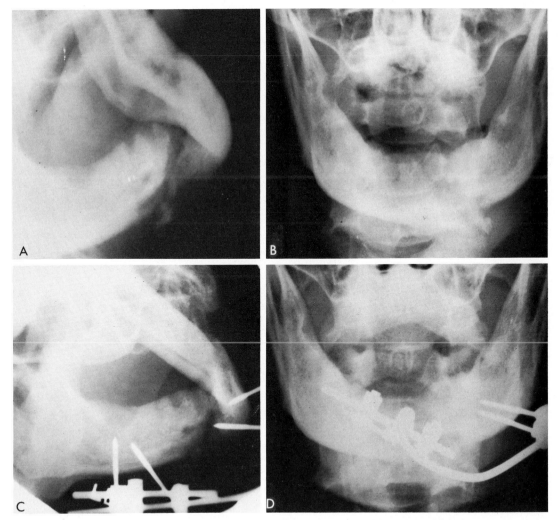

Figure 25–113 *A* and *B*, Pathologic fracture of the mandible from osteomyelitis. Note multiple free sequestra below the border of the mandible. *C* and *D*, Postoperative roentgenograms showing the immobilization of the fractured mandible with extraoral skeletal pin fixation. The pins were inserted more than 3 cm. from the fracture site. Because of foreshortening when the lateral jaw roentgenogram was taken, the one pin in the symphysis is superimposed somewhat over the fracture area. (See Case Report No. 11 for details.)

marked reduction of edema, induration and drainage. On the fifth day there was no drainage, and the induration was practically gone.

Operation. Under general anesthesia a Roger Anderson extraoral skeletal pin fixation appliance was applied, and an extraoral multiple sequestrectomy was performed. An iodoform gauze drain was placed.

Postoperative Treatment. The patient received 300,000 units of aqueous penicillin every 3 hours, received two multivitamin capsules three times a day, and was placed on a soft diet. The patient had no appreciable pain, nausea or vomiting. The induration and swelling subsided even more. The patient was up and around and complained only of numbness of the lower lip and chin on the left. Radiographs were taken (see Figure 25–113C and D).

On the second postoperative day, the dosage of penicillin was decreased to 100,000 units every 3 hours and 300,000 units of Crysticillin once a day. All drainage, induration and swelling had disappeared.

By the fifth postoperative day sensation had returned to the lip and chin, and the patient was discharged the next day.

Comment. This case shows the results that were obtained by the use of massive doses of penicillin, plus sequestrectomy in the treatment of chronic osteomyelitis of the mandible. Sequestrectomy was the most important part of the treatment.

Final Result. Six weeks later the extraoral skeletal fixation appliance was removed, as sufficient healing was present to maintain the continuity of the mandible, which had a normal contour and intermaxillary relationship. Dentures were constructed a month later.

SUBLUXATION OR DISLOCATION OF THE MANDIBLE

During surgical procedures in the oral cavity the mandible may be dislocated, either unilaterally or bilaterally, by the dentist's use of excessive pressure or by the patient's opening his mouth too wide. Dislocation also occurs under general anesthesia when the mechanical oral prop is opened so widely between the maxilla and mandible that the condyle is forcefully moved out of its fossa and over the articular eminence (eminentia articularis). The surgeon should constantly be aware of these possibilities and avoid them because treatment of this chronically annoying and painful complication is difficult and often unsatisfactory.

When a patient is under general anesthesia his normal defense mechanism against dislocation of the mandible is lost. Therefore it is very easy for the dentist who fails to recognize this fact to dislocate the patient's mandible. Many patients report the onset of hypermobility and clicking of the temporomandibular joint following an oral operation under general anesthesia. (See Figure 25–114.)

Dislocations also occur as a result of prolonged operative procedures for restorative dentistry or as a result of taking impressions for complete dentures (see Case Report No. 12 and Figures 25–115 to 25–127), or by the forceful luxation of mandibular teeth during extraction with either forceps or elevators.

Sometimes the dislocations are self-reducing and in others they must be reduced by the operator. Usually the dislocation can be immediately reduced by the patient. In other cases it is necessary for the dentist to reduce it manually by grasping each side of the jaw with his thumbs over the occlusal surfaces of the mandibular teeth and exerting pressure downward and backward. If this cannot be accomplished, then 1 cc. of local anesthetic solution may be injected into each mandibular fossa. This injection anesthetizes the external pterygoid muscle, which is holding the mandible forward, thus relaxing it and permitting the retruding portions of the mandibular musculature to retract the mandible.

The dislocation will often reduce spontaneously, sometimes with such speed as to make rapid removal of the needle imperative to prevent it from being fractured. If it does not reduce spontaneously, the mandible can be manually repositioned with little difficulty and with little risk of losing one's thumbs. An elastic Barton bandage is applied to hold the jaw in place for 48 hours. Then the patient is advised to restrict opening his mouth to the thickness of a spoon for the next two weeks while the torn or stretched capsule heals.

If the dislocation becomes chronic, the joint should be treated by the injection of sclerosing solutions to produce fibrosis. The injection of a series of small amounts of sclerosing solution mixed with local anesthetic solution (total of 6 minims) into the

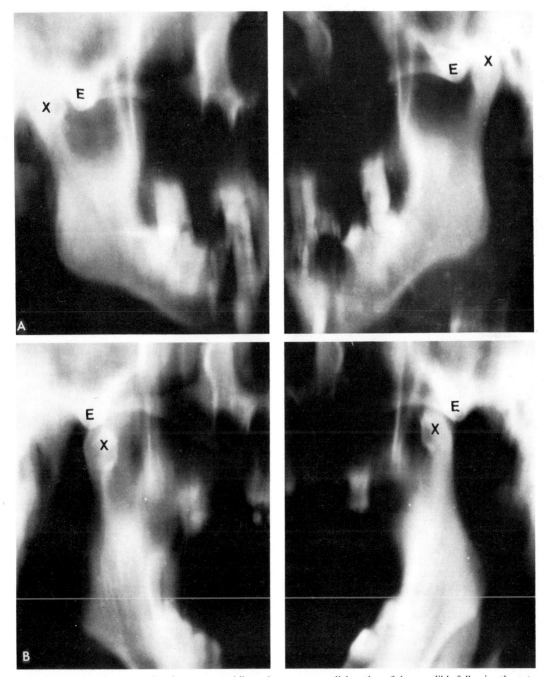

Figure 25–114 Laminograms showing recurrent bilateral spontaneous dislocation of the mandible following the extraction of teeth under general anesthesia. *A*, Condylar heads (*X*) in normal position in the articular fossa; *E* is the eminentia articularis. *B*, Condylar heads (*X*), position with the mouth open. They are now anterior and superior to the eminentia articularis (*E*).

temporomandibular joint capsule every 2 weeks for from 4 to 6 injections has been reasonably satisfactory. (See Figure 26–12.) Small amounts of sclerosing solution are used because of the acute inflammatory and painful aftermath when larger amounts of the sclerosing solutions are injected. The inflammation produced by the sclerosing solution stimulates the formation of an increased amount of fibrous tissue in the capsule, which prevents the head of the condyle from dislocating from the temporomandibular joint fossa. If this limitation of opening is found to be objectionable by the patient, the preinjection range of mandibular opening can be restored under anesthesia by separating the jaws with a mechanical mouth prop. This of course means that in all probability spontaneous subluxation or dislocation will also again be present.

Injection of sclerosing solutions in the temporomandibular joints afflicted with rheumatoid arthritis is contraindicated. More on this subject will be found in Chapter 26.

Case Report No. 12

BILATERAL DISLOCATION OF THE MANDIBLE*

Patient. A 34-year-old white woman was admitted to the Magee-Women's Hospital on September 30, with a bilateral dislocation of her mandible that had been present for 4 months (see Figure 25–115A to C).

History. In June the patient had had all her teeth extracted under intravenous anesthesia by her family dentist at another hospital. Following the operation she had been unable to close her jaws. As the result of great muscular effort during the following months, she was able to stretch her lips together over the separated jaws (see Figure 25–115B and C). For esthetic reasons she had been wearing the temporary maxillary denture shown in Figure 25–118C. (We placed the splint on this denture, as will be seen shortly.) Her dentist had unsuccessfully attempted under general anesthesia to reduce her dislocated mandible 2 weeks previously. She was referred by her dentist for reduction of this 4-month-old fixed dislocation of the mandible.

Physical Examination. This revealed a well-developed, well-nourished, edentulous white woman not acutely ill. Her mandible was solidly fixed in an anterior open position. By palpation both condyles were located anterior and superior to their respective articular eminences.

Laboratory Findings. The laboratory findings were negative.

Radiographic Examination. Radiographs of the temporomandibular joint areas revealed the crest of the left condyle 1.5 cm. anterior to and 1.15 cm. superior to the crest of the left articular eminence (see Figure 25–116A), while the crest of the right condyle was 1.5 cm. anterior to and 1.5 cm. above the crest of the right articular eminence (see Figure 25–116B).

Treatment Planning. It was obvious that this was a case of fibrous ankylosis of the bilaterally dislocated mandible. One could also speculate that in all probability the mandibular fossa was by this time also filled with fibrous tissue, so if the condyles could be brought back to the fossae, could the condyles be replaced into the fossae? Four possibilities for the reduction of the dislocation were considered:

1. To attempt again manual reduction of the dislocation under general anesthesia and muscle relaxants.
2. To construct an acrylic mandibular bite block with built-up heels, pin this and the acrylic maxillary bite block to their respective jaws and, with anterior intermaxillary elastics, the heels acting as fulcrums, move the condyles down and then with extraoral traction pull them back and up into the mandibular fossae (see Figure 25–117). The possibility of pressure necrosis of oral tissues was considered as the main objection to this plan. (The subjective symptom indicating this possibility taking place, it was thought, would be pain. One main error in this reasoning will subsequently be shown.)
3. If the second method was unsuccessful, then extraoral elastic reverse traction between pins in the zygoma and the mandible could be tried.
4. If the preceding attempts failed, then a bilateral open reduction would be attempted, and if at the time of operation this proved to be unfeasible, then a bilateral section through the necks of the condyles could be performed.

First Attempt. On October 1, under thiopental sodium and oxygen anesthesia and with muscle relaxants, the following procedure was performed: The operator's thumb was placed on the alveolar ridge of the patient's left mandibular bicuspid tooth area and his right fingers under the patient's left mandibular body; his left thumb on the alveolar ridge of the patient's right mandibular bicuspid area and his left fingers under the patient's right mandibular body. Downward, anterior and then posterior pressures applied on the patient's mandible were unsuccessful in reducing the dislocation. Next, five tongue blades were placed together and wrapped in gauze. The blades were

---

* Case report prepared by W. H. Archer, D.D.S., and A. J. Gould, D.D.S., Oral Surgery Resident, Magee-Women's Hospital, Pittsburgh, Pa.

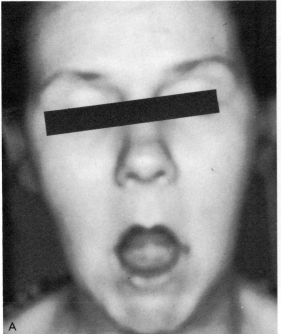

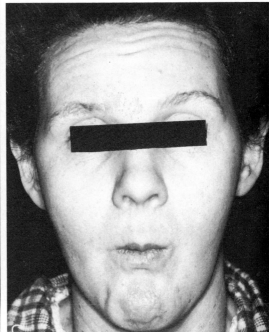

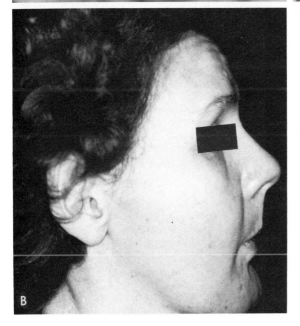

Figure 25–115 *A*, Bilateral dislocation of the mandible, which had been present for four months. Dislocation had occurred during the extraction of the patient's teeth under general anesthesia. (See Case Report No. 12 for details.)

B, Patient has to stretch her lips together over the separated jaws. Note the muscle effort necessary to close her lips.

C, Note the long lower third of the face compared with the middle and upper thirds. The muscular effort to approximate the lips is apparent.

placed between the patient's maxillary and mandibular bicuspid areas to act as a fulcrum. Then upward force was applied on the mandibular symphysis in an attempt to lever the condyles below their respective articular eminences. This attempt, too, was unsuccessful. However, the manipulations did produce 2 to 3 mm. of movement in the mandible. The patient was taken from the operating room in the same condition as she entered, with the exception that her mandible was slightly movable. This encouraged us to try the second method described earlier.

Postoperatively, the patient was dizzy and vomited excessively. On October 2 the patient was given 25 mg. of promethazine hydrochloride (Phenergan) intramuscularly to relieve the nausea. On October 3 she felt much better.

Second Attempt. Intraoral leverage was now elected in an attempt to separate the condyles from their anterior superior fibrosed location. (See Figure 25–117 for a schematic drawing of this technique.) Acrylic bite blocks were constructed, and splints were wired to each base plate (see Figures 25–117 and 25–118).

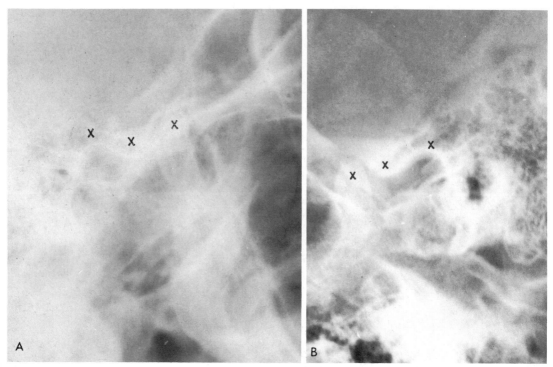

Figure 25–116 *A,* Radiograph of the temporomandibular joint area reveals the crest of the left condyle 1.5 cm. anterior to and 1.15 cm. superior to the crest of the left articular eminence. *B,* Crest of right condyle was 1.5 cm. anterior to and 1.5 cm. above the crest of the right articular eminence.

On October 4, under general anesthesia, the second operation was performed, which consisted of pinning the mandibular and maxillary bite blocks to their respective alveolar ridges with Roger Anderson pins — one into each cuspid area of the maxillary and mandibular bite blocks. The excess

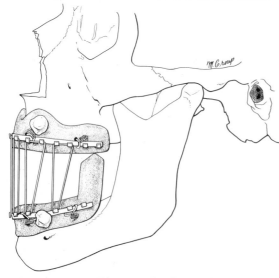

Figure 25–117 Diagrammatic sketch of the second plan to reduce the dislocation. The base plates were pinned to the maxilla and mandible, and the exposed ends of the pins were covered with compound. (See the details of this technique in Chapter 18.)

of each pin over ¼ inch was cut off, and this protruding end (left to permit subsequent removal) was covered with impression compound to protect the lips (see Figure 25–117). The pinning would prevent the dislocation of the bite blocks. The bite blocks occluded solely in the molar areas when inserted into the patient's mouth (see Figure 25–118*D*). The area of the mandibular bite block occluding against the maxillary bite block would serve as a fulcrum for two forces; the anterior force created by the intermaxillary elastics would pull the anterior mandibular bite block and mandible upward toward the maxillary bite block, and at the same time posterior force distal to the fulcrum would bring the condyles below their articular eminences (see Figure 25–117).

The patient was given intravenous glucose, 5 per cent in 1000 cc. of water. Promethazine hydrochloride (Phenergan), 25 mg. intramuscularly, was given every 3 hours, if necessary, to relieve nausea. The patient was given a liquid diet starting October 5. Three intermaxillary elastics were placed to connect the maxillary and mandibular bite blocks. The space between the edges of the bite blocks was 28 mm. On the first postoperative day, the patient reported pressure in her submandibular and sublingual areas, and she had difficulty in swallowing. On the fourth postoperative day the intermaxillary space remained at 28 mm. Until now three intermaxillary elastics had been used. At 5 P.M. this fourth day, eight intermaxillary

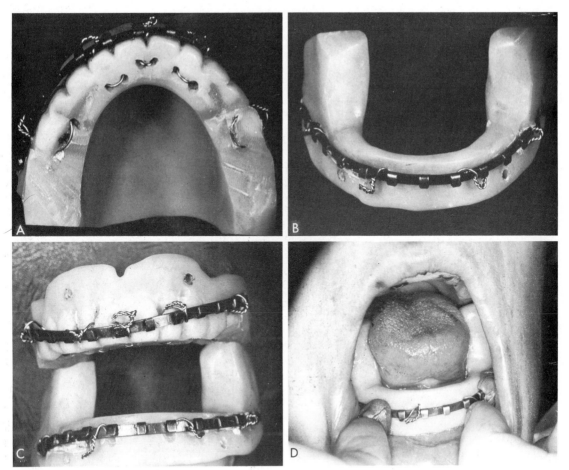

Figure 25–118 *A* and *B*, Acrylic bite blocks were constructed and splints wired to each base plate. *C*, Acrylic bite blocks with splints wired to each base plate. The upper base plate with simulated teeth was made by the patient's dentist to wear until her "permanent dentures" were made. *D*, Bite blocks occluded solely in the molar areas when inserted into the patient's mouth.

elastics were placed to connect the splints. At 9 P.M. a measurement was taken of the intermaxillary space, and a closure of 2 mm. was noted. There was slight mobility of the mandible. On the fifth postoperative day, the intermaxillary space had closed 4 mm. The patient was instructed to push up on the mandibular symphysis with her thumbs to create additional pressure on the anterior portion of her mandible. On the sixth postoperative day the intermaxillary space closed another 1 mm., total closure now being 5 mm. The mandible was slightly movable laterally right and left.

On the seventh postoperative day eight new intermaxillary elastics replaced the former ones. Total intermaxillary space decrease was measured to be 6 mm. The patient noticed that much more pressure was being exerted on her mandible. It was decided to place fresh intermaxillary elastics between the splints each day. On the eighth postoperative day the intermaxillary space was found to have a total decrease of 7 mm. The patient no-

ticed much more force being applied to her condyles. A second series of radiographs was taken and evaluated to show the amount of movement of the condyles. According to the left temporomandibular radiograph, the left condyle had moved to a position 88 mm. directly below the left articular eminence (see Figure 25–119*A*). The right temporomandibular radiograph showed the right condyle 3 mm. below the right articular eminence (see Figure 25–119*B*). This second series of temporomandibular radiographs established the fact that the mandibular condyles were moving in the desired direction. The patient was discharged October 12, the eighth postoperative day, to continue treatment at the office on an outpatient basis.

On October 16, when the patient reported to the office, the bite blocks were removed because of a strong odor of necrotic tissue. The anticipated warning signal of impending palatal soft tissue necrosis, namely pain, had not appeared. In retrospect it was obvious that the slow, gradually increasing forces produced pressure anesthesia of

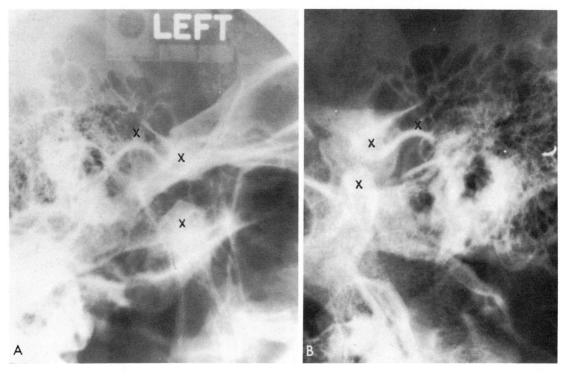

Figure 25–119 *A,* Left condyle was moved to a position 8 mm. directly below the left articular eminence. *B,* Right condyle was moved 3 mm. below the right articular eminence.

the greater palatine nerves, and therefore no pain resulted from the subsequent greater pressures. Furthermore, the increased intermaxillary pressure on the bite blocks concentrated over the posterior palatal region, including the greater palatine foramen areas, blocked the greater palatine blood supply to the mucoperiosteal membrane of the palate (see Figure 25–120*A*). The result was that large areas of this membrane sloughed off, exposing the palatal bone, which still was covered in most areas with periosteum (see Figure 25–120*B*).

There was no slough of mandibular soft tissue! Why not is a mystery to us. The same pressure was concentrated on a *smaller* area of mandibular mucoperiosteal tissue. Obviously, this method of reducing the dislocation had to be abandoned. Oral hygiene was maintained with normal saline mouthwashes, and in 3 weeks the palate was completely covered with mucoperiosteal tissue. Radiographs taken on October 23 revealed the left condyle anterior and superior to its articular eminence and the right condyle directly below its

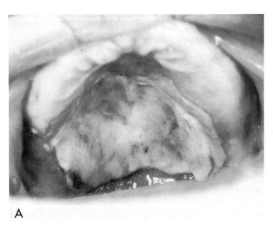
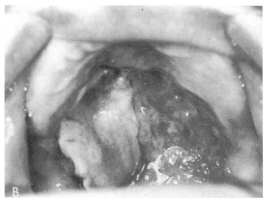

Figure 25–120 *A,* Concentrated pressure on the greater palatine foramen area blocked the greater palatine blood and nerve supply to the tissues; the area of palatal soft-tissue slough resulting from the lack of blood supply is clearly seen. *B,* Large areas sloughed off, exposing the palatal bone, which still was covered in most areas with periosteum.

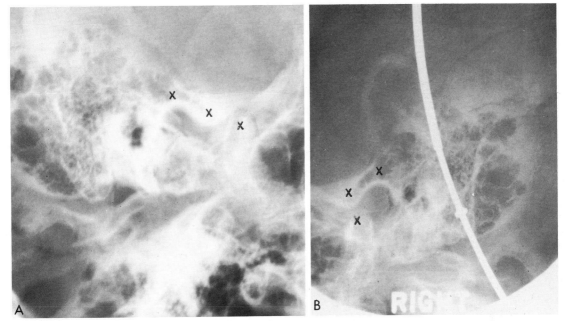

Figure 25–121 Radiographs taken October 23 revealed (*A*) the left condyle anterior and superior to its articular eminence, and (*B*) the right condyle directly below its articular eminence.

articular eminence (see Figure 25–121*A* and *B*). The patient's dislocated mandible had moved toward the right of the midline.

Third Attempt. The patient was readmitted to Magee-Women's Hospital on October 28 for the third planned phase of her treatment. Oral examination revealed that the denuded palatal process was rapidly being recovered with mucosa.

Extraoral reverse traction, as previously mentioned, was to be tried to restore normal condylar-

fossal relationships. On October 29, under local anesthesia, a Roger Anderson pin was inserted into the maxilla below the anterior nasal spine. Two pins and a connecting bar (Frac-Sur unit) were inserted into the symphysis of the mandible below the maxillary pin. A stainless steel wire was passed over the connecting bar of the Frac-Sur unit in the symphysis and through a lock nut on the maxillary pin, and the ends were twisted (see Figure 25–122). This was to stabilize the anterior

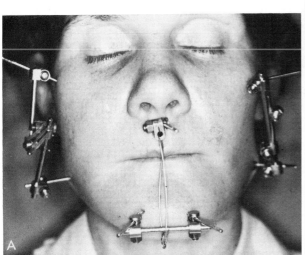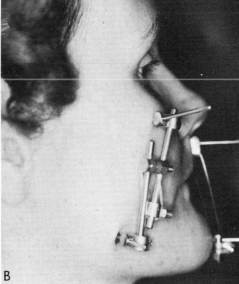

Figure 25–122 The elastic force would pull the lock nut anchors together, thereby producing inverse traction that would lower the condyles below their respective eminences.

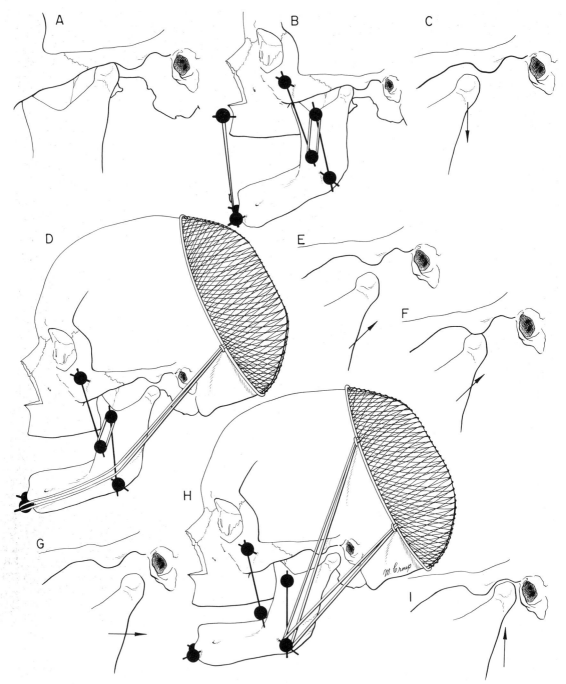

Figure 25–123   Technique for reducing a mandible that had been dislocated for 4 months.

mandible during the downward pressure on the ramus by the following technique: Roger Anderson pins were inserted into both the right and left zygomatic bones of the maxilla. Pins were inserted into the right and left body of the mandible below the zygomatic pins. To all four pins connecting bars were attached with lock nuts. The upper connecting bars extended downward, and the lower connecting bars extended upward, over-

lapping the upper bars (see Figure 25–122). A lock nut was attached to the ends of each bar. Between these lock nuts elastic bands were strung. The elastic force between these nuts transmitted to the pins would move the ramus and its condyle downward (see Figure 25–123B and C). When the condyles were radiographically shown on the second postoperative day to be below the articular eminence, backward traction was created by elastic

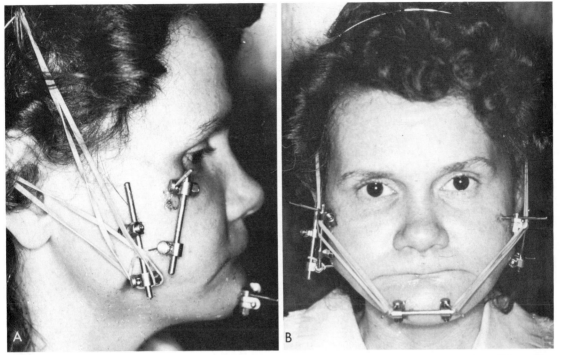

Figure 25-124 *A*, Elastic traction from a knit helmet to the Frac-Sur unit in the symphysis of the mandible, pulling the mandible posteriorly and superiorly simultaneously to move the condyles back under and up into their mandibular fossae. *B*, When the condyles were back under their mandibular fossae, posterior traction was reduced and superior traction increased to seat the condyles in the fossae.

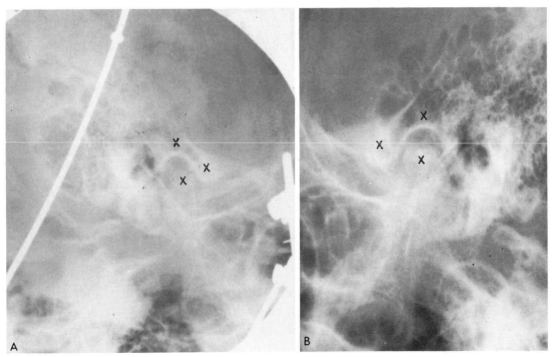

Figure 25-125 On the third postoperative day, radiographs revealed (*A*) the left condyle and (*B*) the right condyle in their respective mandibular fossae.

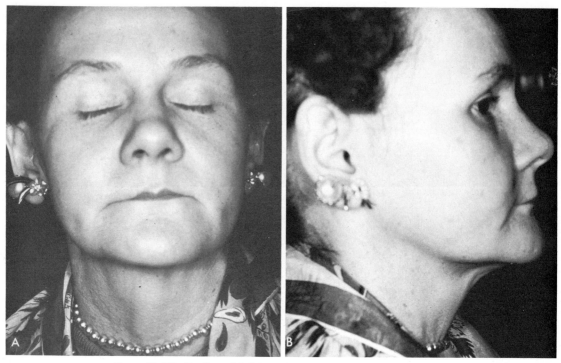

Figure 25–126   Profile and full face photographs taken on December 10.

bands strung from an orthodontic net helmet to the Frac-Sur unit in the symphysis of the mandible. The downward pressure from the posterior mandibular and zygomatic pins was continued simultaneously (see Figure 25–124). The anterior maxillary pin and intermaxillary wire were removed.

On the third day the condyles were shown radiographically to be below the mandibular fossa,

so backward and downward traction was discontinued and upward traction of the ramus and condyle instituted by elastic traction between the net helmet and posterior mandibular pins was begun, as shown in Figure 25–123D. In addition, elastic bands were now strung between the zygomatic and mandibular pins to exert upward force.

On the fourth postoperative day radiographs

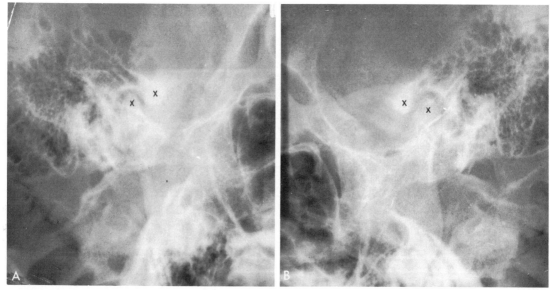

Figure 25–127   Radiographs taken 4 weeks after reduction of the dislocation. *A*, Left temporomandibular joint. *B*, Right temporomandibular joint. Note the normal position of each condyle in its fossa.

revealed the condyles in the mandibular fossae. They were maintained in this location by continued traction.

The patient was instructed to move her mandible manually up and down to stimulate circulation to the masticatory musculature, which had atrophied, to stimulate capsular circulation, and to prevent excessive fibrous tissue formation between condyles and fossae. On the fifth postoperative day the symphysis and zygomatic pins were removed. Elastics were placed between the orthodontic net helmet and the pins in the right and left body of the mandible to maintain the condyle in the mandibular fossae. The patient complained of temporomandibular joint pain and of difficulty in swallowing. The elastics were removed and the pain subsided. Apparently the elastics had exerted a force which pressed the condyles against the mesenteric and posterior auricular innervation

of the glenoid fossae, which explained the temporomandibular joint pains. The fact that this innervation anastomoses with the glossopharyngeal nerve explains the pains she experienced when swallowing. On November 17, the ninth postoperative day, all pins were removed. The patient was discharged with instructions to open and close her mandible for a distance of not more than 20 mm. To open her mandible farther would invite a second dislocation.

On December 10, the patient was found to be free from pain and able to perform all the movements necessary for mastication, deglutition and speech (see Figure 25–126). Temporomandibular joint radiographs revealed both condyles in normal position in their fossae (see Figure 25–127). The patient now has dentures that are very satisfactory. Not once has she had a dislocation since the reduction.

DYSARTHROSES FOLLOWING SUBCONDYLAR FRACTURE

Symptoms of dysarthroses caused by incorrect healing of a subcondylar fracture include: (1) pain; (2) limitation of masticatory movements; (3) annoying clicking; and (4) ankylosis.

MENISCECTOMY

In the past this procedure was used indiscriminately for pain following fracture. It is only rarely indicated. As Henny states, "Insofar as I am concerned, the operation plays no part at all in the correction of the painful temporomandibular joint. The . . . few instances [in which] a meniscectomy is indicated, in my opinion, . . . are when the patient has [suffered] whiplash, so that the meniscus is torn and crumples up to the point [that] it jams between the head of the condyle and the eminentia articularis. . . . When the patient tries to open his mouth, the jaw will not [move smoothly; it] locks in position just prior to [opening]. This can go on [until it] occurs up to 50 to 75 times a day, and in that event, serious thought has to be given to surgical intervention. I, therefore, have operated on a few of these [patients], perhaps no more than two a year." *

HIGH CONDYLECTOMY FOR PAINFUL RHEUMATOID ARTHRITIS

As Henny explains, "One major point of [high condylectomy] is to preserve the meniscus, since its preservation prevents the formation of cicatricial bands between the resected head of the condyle and the glenoid fossa and thus allows the patient to return to normal function without pain. On some occasions, the meniscus may be torn or worn through, but if that occurs, I usually repair it by closing these perforations with chromic catgut sutures. At any rate, I very carefully preserve the meniscus in every instance when I am doing a high condylectomy, which is done only for an arthritic degeneration of the temporomandibular joint. I never do one without positive radiographic evidence of osteoarthritis or rheumatoid arthritis, and then only when conservative treatment has failed." *

CONDYLECTOMY (OSTEOARTHROTOMY)

For intractable pain with ankylosis or the limitation of masticatory movements due to the malposition of the condyle, the treatment is condylectomy. (For the surgical treatment of ankylosis of the temporomandibular joint due to other factors, see Chapter 24.)

In a condylectomy, the condyle is excised

---

* Fred Henny. Personal communication, July, 1975.

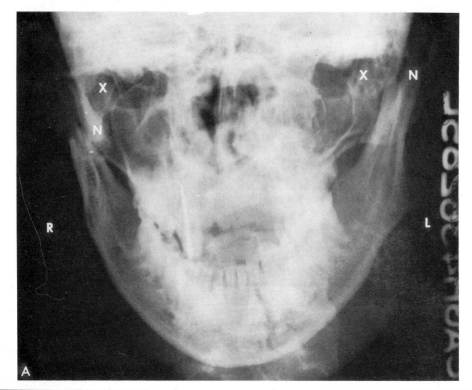

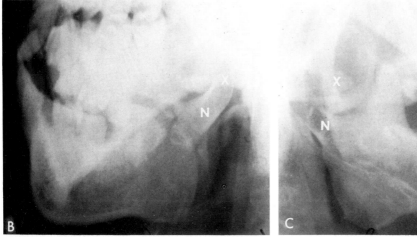

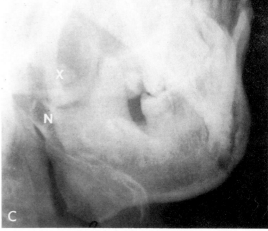

Figure 25–128 The patient had been admitted and treated at another hospital a year before for the fractures seen in *A*, *B* and *C*. *X* marks the condyles and *N* the necks of the condyles. *A*, Bilateral subcondylar fractures; a fracture through the symphysis, left zygoma and maxilla as a unit; and a fracture extending through the palate and anterior maxillary ridge. *B*, Comminuted fracture of the neck of the right condyle. *C*, Fracture of the left neck of the condyle, with the head of the condyle medially displaced from its fossa.

at the neck and freed from the joint cavity, or if it is already separated from the ramus and the joint cavity by a subcondylar fracture, and following conservative treatment in these *very rare* cases in which the patient develops chronic painful post–subcondylar fracture discomfort, the displaced condyle is located and removed. This is not an easy procedure in many cases. Fortunately *it is rarely neces-*

sary to perform a condylectomy. Condyles that are fractured and grossly displaced very seldom give rise to pain or discomfort. Unfortunately there are some who feel that the fractured condyle displaced from the mandibular fossa should be removed to prevent possible future trouble. The author has seen only one such case requiring surgery out of the hundreds of subcondylar fractures he has

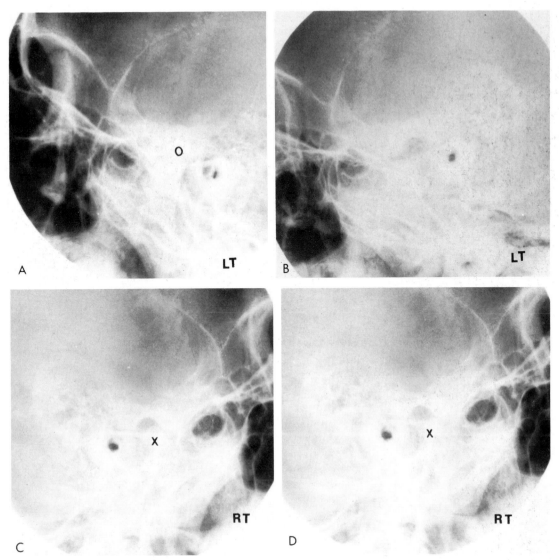

Figure 25–129 *A*, Radiograph of the left temporomandibular joint reveals calcific ankylosis of this joint. *B*, Postoperative view following removal of osseous tissue from the fossa and mandible; the jaw is in an open position. *C*, Right temporomandibular joint showing the head of the condyle in a semiluxated position but not ankylosed. *D*, Open position of right jaw with the head of the condyle on the crest of the eminentia articularis.

treated. Certainly one should at least treat these cases conservatively until it has been determined if pain and discomfort are going to develop. Partial ankylosis or blocking following subcondylar fractures is also a rare postfracture complication. If these are not amenable to physiotherapy, then a condylectomy is indicated. Pathologic changes in the joints, such as those produced by arthrosis and arthritis, with limitation of motion and pain not amenable to other treatment, may indicate the need for condylectomy.

In osteoarthrotomy for ankylosis, because the articular head of the condyle is fused to the osseous structure of the joint cavity, it is necessary not only to cut through the neck of the condyle, but also to cut through the line of fusion before the condyle can be removed.

Technique. In Figure 25–132 are shown the anatomic structures surrounding the mandibular fossa. The main difficulty is the proximity of branches of the facial nerve, which must not be injured if permanent damage is to be avoided. It must be kept in mind that dam-

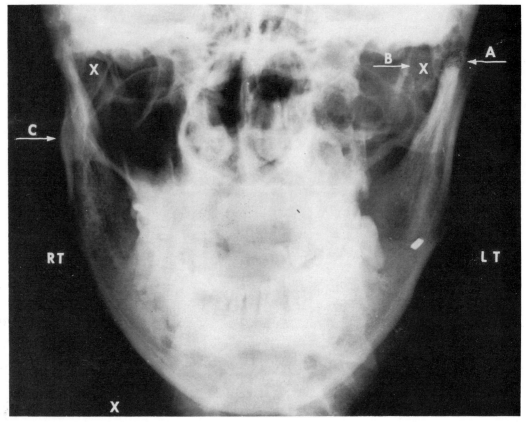

Figure 25–130 Postoperative posteroanterior radiograph of the mandible reveals: *A*, Removal of the osseous fusion between the neck of the condyle and the fossa. *B*, Isolated fractured head of the left condyle still medial to the ramus. *C*, Healed neck of the right condyle.

age to these nerves may result not only from cutting but also from trauma due to pulling or stretching the tissues in this area. The latter, however, is of temporary nature. Blood vessels such as the superficial temporal artery and vein, if encountered, are isolated, tied

and cut. If the transverse facial artery is encountered, it also is tied and divided.

Figure 25–132*B* illustrates the type of incision that should avoid, in most instances, the vicinity of the facial nerve. An incision is made through the skin and then the subcu-

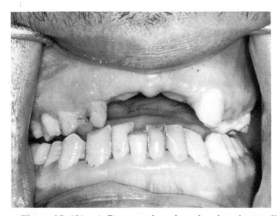
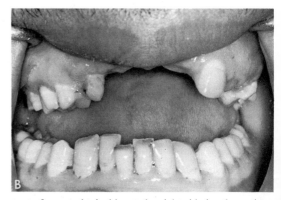

Figure 25–131 *A*, Preoperative view showing the small amount of space obtainable on the right side by the patient when he tried to open his mouth. With great effort he could "spring" the ankylosed bone on the left to permit an opening of 9 mm. for a few seconds. *B*, Postoperative view with good motion and an opening of 2½ cm.

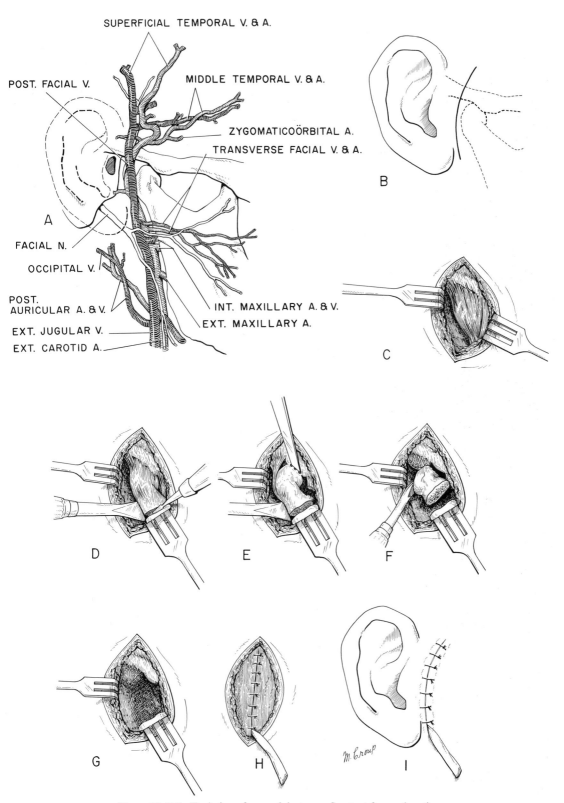

SUPERFICIAL TEMPORAL V. & A.

POST. FACIAL V.

MIDDLE TEMPORAL V. & A.

ZYGOMATICOÖRBITAL A.

TRANSVERSE FACIAL V. & A.

A

FACIAL N.

OCCIPITAL V.

POST. AURICULAR A. & V.

INT. MAXILLARY A. & V.

EXT. MAXILLARY A.

EXT. JUGULAR V.

EXT. CAROTID A.

B

C

D

E

F

G

H

I

Figure 25–132 Technique for condylectomy. See text for explanation.

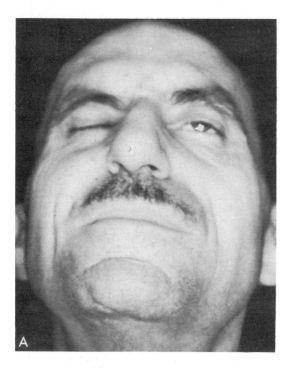

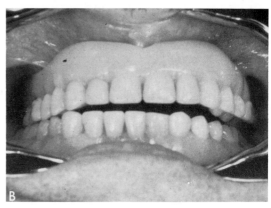

Figure 25–133 *A,* This man, aged 52, had had pain and trismus in the right temporomandibular joint, for which a right condylectomy had been performed in another city 3 years previously. After the operation the patient had noticed a right facial paralysis. He was sent to the dental clinic because he had been unable to masticate since the operation. The open bite is shown in *B.*

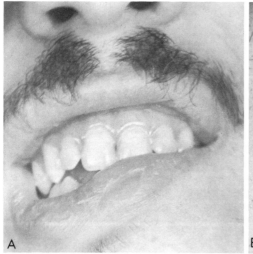

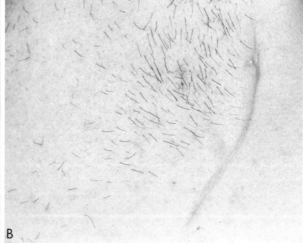

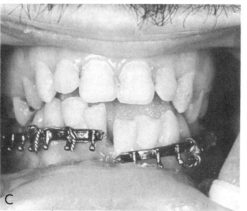

Figure 25–134 *A,* This patient is unable to move the left side of his lower lip following an open reduction for a left subcondylar fracture at another hospital. Apparently, the marginal mandibular branches of the seventh nerve were inadvertently cut. *B,* Incision used to expose the fracture area. *C,* In addition, there was nonunion of the fracture of the symphysis of the mandible. This bilateral fracture when seen by us was 8 weeks old.

taneous tissues are divided. The soft tissues at the root of the zygomatic arch are separated, and here we may encounter the superficial temporal artery and vein mentioned above. The posterior part of the masseter muscle is then detached and retracted down and forward, exposing the capsular ligaments of the joint. As the capsular ligaments are exposed, the transverse facial artery is frequently encountered; it is tied and divided. The neck of the condyle is now exposed by incising the periosteum and stripping it away by blunt dissection.

Figure 25–132*D* shows the actual cutting through the neck of the condyle with a cross-cut fissure bur. Note that a broad periosteal elevator is inserted beneath the neck of the condyle to protect the internal maxillary artery from being inadvertently severed. Figure 25–132*E* shows the chisel cutting the line of fusion between the glenoid fossa and the head of the condyle. (See Chapter 24 for the interposing of substances to prevent reunion.) In Figure 25–132*F* and *G* the condyle is removed from the cavity, the cavity is closed and sutured and a drain is inserted in the cavity, as shown in Figure 25–132*H*. The skin is next closed, as shown in Figure 25–132*I*.

Case Report No. 13

CONDYLECTOMY FOR TRUE ANKYLOSIS OF THE LEFT TEMPOROMANDIBULAR JOINT WITH TRACHEOSTOMY*

Patient. This 34-year-old man, 4 months before this admission, had sustained multiple facial injuries and fracture of the left tibia in a fall. Following discharge from the hospital, where his fractures had been treated, he had found that he could not open his mouth more than 1 cm., and this effort brought considerable pain. He was admitted for treatment of his inability to open his mouth and a right maxillary dentoalveolar abscess with facial cellulitis.

Physical Examination. Examination revealed a well-developed, undernourished Negro male who had asymmetry of the face. The right side of the face appeared elevated because the right zygoma was displaced laterally and the left zygoma medially, and the facial swelling from the dentoalveolar abscess also contributed to the asymmetry. The patient could not masticate, and his diet, semisoft and liquid, had resulted in considerable weight loss.

Complaints. (1) Inability to open his mouth more than 1 cm. accompanied by considerable pain in the left temporomandibular joint; (2) deviation of the mandible to the left; (3) pain in the right maxillary area because of an "infected tooth."

Laboratory findings were within normal limits. Findings in serology tests were negative.

Radiographic Examination. Extraoral films of the skull and mandible proved that the patient had sustained numerous fractures of the facial bones, for, as previously noted, both zygomas were displaced. The radiographs of the right and left temporomandibular joints proved the right condyle to have limited motion, and there appeared to be osseous ankylosis of the left condyle. The meniscus of the left joint could not be identified. The pos-

teroanterior view of the skull showed the head of the condyle in lateral position in relation to the mandibular fossa.

Because of the ankylosis, oral examination consisted of merely examining the buccal surfaces of the teeth with a mouth mirror. Noted were poor oral hygiene, a deformed maxilla, missing maxillary incisors, unrestorable remaining maxillary teeth, missing mandibular third molars, and most of the remaining mandibular teeth in fairly good condition.

Course. The patient was given penicillin, 300,000 units twice a day, for cellulitis of the right face; codeine, ½ grain, and aspirin compound were given for pain. Hyclorite mouthwash was ordered four times a day, and a high-calorie soft diet was prescribed. Under this treatment plus intraoral drainage, the infection subsided. A week later the patient was taken to the operating room and, under thiopental sodium anesthesia, mandibular manipulation was attempted. If movement was observed the trismus could be considered false. If movement did not occur, the patient would be judged as having true ankylosis of the left temporomandibular joint. Attempted manipulation was unsuccessful, confirming a diagnosis of true ankylosis.

Discussion. The puzzling feature of this case was the fact that the patient could *open his mouth*

---

* This patient was treated by the Oral Surgery and Otolaryngology Departments of the Veterans Administration Hospital, Pittsburgh, Pa. C. J. Novak, Oral Surgery Resident; case report prepared by A. E. Cirlone, Rotating Intern, Veterans Administration Hospital, Pittsburgh, Pa.

1 cm. In true bilateral ankylosis of the temporomandibular joint, opening of the mouth would be impossible. But, as noted previously, only the left condyle was fractured and the patient was able to open approximately 1 cm. on the right side and about ½ cm. on the left side. To verify a theory explaining this ability by the patient, the following experiment was performed, with a fresh mandible. The left condyle was locked in a bench vise and, by suspending weights up to 8 lb. on the symphysis of the mandible, it was found that the right body of the mandible could be depressed as much as 1 cm. Further experiments on six staff members as subjects proved that those muscles responsible for opening the mouth exerted a downward pull of from 30 to 50 lb. This procedure explained the patient's ability to open his mouth, through sheer muscular force springing the neck of the ankylosed condyle, despite the unilateral bony ankylosis.

Tracheostomy and Osteoarthrotomy. The patient was taken to the operating room 6 days later for left condylectomy with thiopental sodium and endotracheal anesthesia. Great difficulty was encountered in the attempt at intubation of the patient. The mandible was immobile, so the tracheolaryngoscope could not be used. Repeated attempted blind intubations were unsuccessful and produced moderate pharyngeal hemorrhage. In order to insure a patent airway, and because of the pharyngeal bleeding and probable future laryngeal edema, a tracheostomy was performed and nitrous oxide and oxygen were administered through the tracheostomy tube.

Operative Technique. An incision anterior to the external auditory meatus was made and extended from the insertion of the lobe of the ear to approximately the insertion of the superior border of the auricle, curving anteriorly to the temporal region. The subcutaneous tissue was divided and hemostasis obtained. With blunt and sharp dissection, the arch of the zygomatic process was exposed. The left condyle was in a position lateral to the zygomatic arch, ankylosed to its inferior border, and out of the mandibular fossa. A line of fusion was not evident. The fractured neck of the condyle was completely healed at an oblique angle and was incised with crosscut burs. A chisel and mallet were used to separate the head of the condyle from its ankylosed attachment on the inferior border of the zygomatic arch. The condyle was elevated out of position and the resulting rough edges of the zygomatic arch and the ramus of the mandible were smoothed with bone rongeurs and bone files. Hemostasis of the bone was secured. It was noted that the mouth was now able to open approximately 4 cm., as compared with a preoperative opening of 1 cm. 000 Catgut was used for the deep sutures and to close the layers of the fascia successively. A drain was placed into the deep cavity. 0000 Black silk interrupted sutures were used to close the skin, leaving the drain protruding from the preauricular area. A pressure dressing was placed, and the patient was taken from the operating room in good condition, having tolerated the procedure well. A mouth prop was placed between the open jaws.

Postoperative Course. The patient had no complaints during his postoperative course. He was instructed in the exercise of his mandible several times daily.

Two days after operation the tracheostomy tube, sutures and drain were removed.

Eleven days after operation a complete maxillary and a partial mandibular odontectomy and alveolectomy were performed under local anesthesia without difficulty because the patient could now open his mouth 5 cm.

Two months later, full maxillary and partial mandibular dentures were inserted. These the patient uses very satisfactorily.

EMPHYSEMA

Emphysema is swelling caused by the presence of air in the interstices of the connective tissue. On palpation a typical "crackling" or crepitant feeling is noticed that will immediately distinguish this swelling from that of edema.

While emphysema involving the face is now increasing in incidence because of the use of high-speed air rotors for ossisection and odontotomy, in past years in my experience it was seen twice. In one case it occurred after removal of a root from the antrum. The patient sneezed, and there was a large egg-shaped swelling immediately beneath the eye. The explanation is simply that air was forced from the nasal cavity into the antrum, out of the antral window made to facilitate root removal and into the soft tissues and facial musculature. Escape into the oral cavity was prevented by the sutures.

The second case followed the excision of an unerupted impacted maxillary third molar. Subsequently the patient was being treated by an otolaryngologist who, in attempting to blow a plug out of the ostium maxillare, was startled to see the soft tissues on that side of the face enlarge as he pumped air through his trocar into the antrum. It took 4 days for the

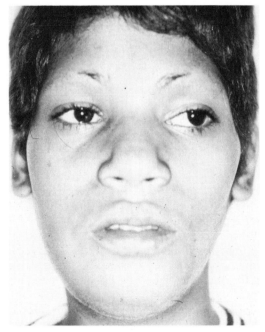

Figure 25–135 Note swelling of the right side of face and midcheek region. (From Cardo, V. A., Jr., Mooney, J. W., and Stratigos, G. T.: Iatrogenic dental-air emphysema: Report of case. J.A.D.A., *85*:144–147 [July], 1972.)

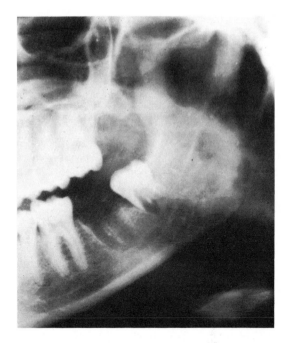

Figure 25–137 Further manipulation demonstrated further movement of air masses. (From Cardo, V. A., Jr., Mooney, J. W., and Stratigos, G. T.: Iatrogenic dental-air emphysema: Report of case. J.A.D.A., *85*:144–147 [July], 1972.)

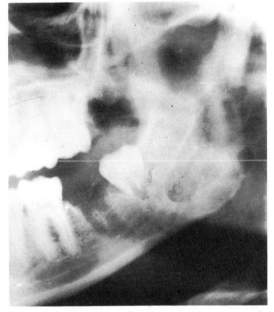

Figure 25–136 Panoramic radiograph shows two large radiolucent regions. The first of these is in the region of the sigmoid notch, and the other is in the subcondylar region. Several small loculi can be seen near the angle. (From Cardo, V. A., Jr., Mooney, J. W., and Stratigos, G. T.: Iatrogenic dental-air emphysema: Report of case. J.A.D.A., *85*:144–147 [July], 1972.)

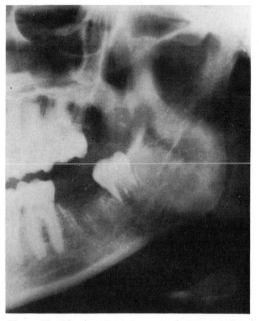

Figure 25–138 An attempt was made to move the air mass. In the second panoramic radiograph, one large radiolucent region is noted over the condylar region and the sigmoid notch. Again, several small loculi of air are at the angle. (From Cardo, V. A., Jr., Mooney, J. W., and Stratigos, G. T.: Iatrogenic dental-air emphysema: Report of case. J.A.D.A., *85*:144–147 [July], 1972.)

air to be reabsorbed. The explanation was that at the time the impaction was removed, an°opening was made through the antral mucosa. However, the mucoperiosteal membrane healed, completely closing off the antrum. When air was pumped into the sinus under pressure, the mucoperiosteal membrane was stripped off the tuberosity, and the air escaped out into the tissues of the face. The otolaryngologist was unaware of what had happened; otherwise he could have passed a large-gauge needle through the tuberosity into the mucobuccal fold and permitted the escape of the trapped air.

FACIAL NUMBNESS AND PARALYSIS CAUSED BY NERVE TRAUMA

One source of facial numbness, temporary or permanent, is trauma to a nerve. The nerve most frequently inadvertently severed, traumatized or compressed is the inferior alveolar nerve, most often during removal of impacted mandibular molars or bicuspids. Operations in the vicinity of the mental foramen may result in injury to this nerve. In both cases, anesthesia (numbness) or paresthesia (burning, tingling) of the lip on that side results. The duration of the symptom is dependent on the extent of the injury.

Regeneration of the injured inferior alveolar nerve after surgery of the mandible or after severance by a displaced fracture through the mandible takes place in a short time, provided the severed ends are in proximity to each other. Healing of the severed mental nerve at its point of exit from the mental foramen is rare, for the movement of the lip and cheek makes the approximation of the ends difficult.

When flaps are made in this area to remove impacted teeth, cysts or tumors, care should be taken to include the soft tissue overlying the foramen so that the nerves and vessels are contained within the reflected flap.

The lingual nerve is subject to injury when salivary stones are excised from the submaxillary gland by the intraoral route and, to a lesser degree, when the stone is located in the submaxillary (Wharton's) duct. A segment of the nerve might also be excised when marsupializing a ranula or enucleating a mixed tumor in the floor of the oral cavity.

The nasopalatine nerves are severed at the orifice of the nasopalatine (incisive) foramen when a palatal flap is reflected in order to enucleate a nasopalatine cyst or to remove palatally impacted teeth encroaching on this region of the palate. These nerves unite readily, however, because suturing the flap back to position brings the severed ends into reasonable approximation.

The infraorbital nerve is frequently compressed by a depressed fracture of the zygomatic bone, producing a characteristic numbness in the lip and side of the nose. This quickly disappears when the depressed zygomatic bone is moved upward and outward to its normal position.

Transverse fractures of the maxilla through the maxillary sinuses many times produce a numbness in the teeth because the branches of the maxillary nerve within the maxillary sinus, e.g., the middle superior alveolar and anterior superior alveolar nerves, are injured. These unite quickly when the fracture is reduced and immobilized.

The facial nerve may be severed by operative procedures in the region of the temporomandibular joint or invaded by tumor. This is a particularly distressing complication because of the marked facial disfigurement. In these cases the plastic surgeon offers some hope of restoration of action to the face by implanting functioning muscle from the neighboring area or by implanting fixed fascial supports in the paralyzed muscles and across the midline around the lips into the functioning muscle.

Temporary facial paralysis may result from surrounding infection, edema, toxemia, crushing or refrigeration.

BELL'S PALSY—FACIAL PARALYSIS

Bell's palsy is the name given to a peripheral facial paralysis usually involving all peripheral branches of the seventh nerve on the affected side. It is usually unilateral. Strictly speaking, it is not a complication of oral surgery, although injection of a local anesthetic beyond its usual boundaries may anesthetize one or more branches of the facial (seventh) nerve and produce a transitory paralysis which disappears when the anesthesia wears off.

Etiology and Diagnosis. A review of the muscles innervated by the seventh nerve and the course of the nerve itself will clarify the reasons for the various symptoms: inability to close the eye, wrinkle the forehead or elevate the upper or lower lip. When an attempt is made to close the eyelids, the eyeball rolls upward so that the pupil is covered and only the white of the eyeball is visible. This is known as Bell's sign.

The chorda tympani nerve, which supplies fibers of taste to the anterior two-thirds of the tongue, runs with the facial nerve for a considerable distance. For this reason, if the seventh cranial nerve is affected during its course with the chorda tympani, there will be an associated loss of taste to the anterior two-thirds of the tongue on the affected side. In the series reported here there was no apparent loss of taste except in the tumor case.

Whistling or smiling is not possible. In many cases there is pain in the area behind the ear (over the stylomastoid foramen), which may radiate to the teeth and be misinterpreted as toothache per se or as pain referred from a tooth. Since this pain will often precede the onset of neurologic symptoms, the dentist may do an extraction and in 1 or 2 days see a complete unilateral facial paralysis present for which the patient blames the dentist, quite incorrectly of course. In many cases, however, the patient has no prodromal signs, and the paralysis suddenly appears.

In true Bell's palsy there appears to be an acute localized inflammation of the facial nerve or its sheath or both, the edema of which, in the narrow confines of the facial canal, produces pressure on the nerve, resulting in paralysis. The cause of the inflammation and consequent edema is obscure. Allergic reactions, trauma, cold drafts, toxic infection and many other factors have been postulated but none have been proved conclusively.

Differential Diagnosis. Bell's palsy must be differentiated from other lesions which will produce similar facial nerve paralysis. Any central nervous system lesion (stroke, tumor, etc.) may produce a facial paralysis, but a history and careful evaluation of the patient should rule out these diagnoses. Surgical trauma that severs or compresses a branch of the facial nerve will of course also produce a paralysis distal to the traumatized area.

In Bell's palsy the onset is sudden. Some authors have reported that the paralysis is accompanied by pain that subsides in a matter of hours. In the cases reported here only 3 patients reported pain. One had acute pharyngeal and periapical infection, and 5 had exposure to cold drafts. One or the other of these is usually seen. Facial paralysis due to tumor growth involving the seventh cranial nerve is gradual in onset. Case Report Nos. 16 and 17 illustrate this etiology. Facial paralysis due to trauma—surgical or accidental—is observed after the accident or the operation. Figure 25–133 illustrates a postsurgical facial paralysis.

Treatment. Since the advent of steroids, treatment of Bell's palsy has been radically revised because steroid drugs can reduce inflammatory responses. (See Case Report Nos. 15 and 16.) Prior to their use most treatment was empirical or surgical (decompression of the facial canal), with varying results. (The cases described in Case Report Nos. 16 to 26 were all treated in the presteroid era.) Today results are much better if patients are treated early enough, although complications do result. The treatment can be divided into three phases on the basis of time.

IMMEDIATE ACUTE BELL'S PALSY. The earlier treatment is instituted, the better the prognosis. After 10 days, irreparable damage may have been done. The patient is started on steroid therapy promptly. Cortisone, 100 mg., four times daily, is used for the first 3 days. If response is prompt, dosage is reduced to 300 mg. per day (in four doses) for 3 days and then tapered off. If response is poor, dosage is increased to 500 to 600 mg. of cortisone per day for the next 3 days. These dosages will usually suffice. The dosage is gradually reduced each day and steroid therapy is concluded after 10 days. (For children dosage in proportion to weight is used.) With the advent of newer steroids with fewer side effects and higher milligram potency, an equivalent dosage must be calculated to match the potency of the above schedule. The usual precautions in the use of steroid therapy should be observed relative to ulcers, diabetes, tuberculosis, electrolyte imbalance, etc.

During the acute phase, since the eye cannot be closed, it should be protected with a covering of some sort and, if necessary, eye drops or ointment are used.

Vitamin injections, physical therapy, splints, supports, etc., do not appear to have any material effect on the course of the disease but may be used if they make the patient more comfortable. Analgesics to relieve the pain (if present) may be needed the first day or two, but this is usually the first symptom to leave when steroid therapy is instituted.

TEN DAYS TO SIX WEEKS. If paralysis persists or has not been treated, supportive measures (such as vitamins, galvanic stimulation or massage) can be tried as well as another course of steroid therapy. In some cases, remission of paralysis may be slow and 6 weeks should be allowed for "revitalization" of the facial nerve.

AFTER SIX WEEKS. If there is still a severe paralysis without evidence of recovery, surgical decompression of the facial nerve canal is a rational procedure. If evidence of recovery is present, supportive therapy, if only for the patient's psychological benefit, should be continued. After 12 months there will be little or no further improvement and, if deformity is not too severe, the patient may accept and live with it. If there is severe deformity, there are several plastic and neurosurgical procedures which may be beneficial. Anastomoses of the eleventh or twelfth nerve with the fifth nerve is sometimes successful, as is the insertion of fascial slings to relieve the drooping of the face at rest position.

Case Report No. 14

BELL'S PALSY TREATED WITH STEROIDS

DONALD DAVIDSON, D.D.S.

A 38-year-old woman had had five teeth in four quadrants extracted by her dentist 5 days prior to her first examination. She had complained of general bilateral toothaches and pain in the left ear prior to extractions. Pain in the ear had not been relieved by the extractions, and the dentist had made a diagnosis of "dry socket" and treated it the next day. Pain had been unrelieved, and the patient had developed "a funny feeling in the left eye as if it were cloudy," She had been referred to an ophthalmologist, who had found nothing pathologic in the eye or ear and referred her to the oral surgeon.

At examination a typical complete Bell's palsy of the left side of the face was present, which had apparently occurred following the visit to the ophthalmologist (3 days postextraction). She was placed on methylprednisolone (Medrol), 4 mg. four times a day, and seen 2 days later, at which time there was almost a total remission of the paralysis. The dosage was tapered off to 4 mg. three times a day for 2 days and then 2 mg. three times a day for 2 days and then 2 mg. daily for 2 days. After 4 days of therapy there was no evidence of any paralysis. The pain in the ear subsided after the first three doses of the steroid.

Case Report No. 15

BELL'S PALSY TREATED WITH STEROIDS

DONALD DAVIDSON, D.D.S.

A 16-year-old girl complained of severe pain in the left ear radiating into the teeth, head and neck. It was of 2 days' duration. The patient also complained that her face felt "numb." She was seen by the family dentist and referred for removal of impacted third molars. On examination, a very mild paralysis of the facial nerve of the left side of the face was noted; unless carefully looked for it could have easily been missed. The medical intern who examined the patient missed the correct diagnosis, calling it "facial neuralgia" on the basis of the complaints. She was started on triamcinolone (Kenacort), 4 mg. four times a day, and showed no response for 4 days except cessation of pain. The dosage was raised to 6 mg. four times a day, and in 2 days the paralysis was markedly improved, so a tapering off was started: 4 mg. three times a day for 2 days, 4 mg. twice a day for 2 days, and 4 mg. daily for 2 days. Despite the steroid therapy and mildness of the case, there was still some slight residue of lip drooping, which cleared up in about 6 weeks.

Case Report No. 16

BELL'S PALSY SECONDARY TO CARCINOMA

This case is one in which the facial paralysis was the result of involvement of the facial nerve by tumor growth. A woman, aged 52, had squamous cell carcinoma of the right external auditory canal that, in spite of surgery and radiation therapy, gradually spread into the surrounding tissues, eventually invading the seventh cranial nerve, with the typical facial paralysis shown in Figure 25–139. Here the first symptoms of seventh cranial nerve involvement were gradual in onset. There was first a mild twitching of the right eyelids, then a general weakness in the musculature of the right side of the face, gradually increasing until after several months the paralysis of the right side was complete. As the tumor spread, the fifth cranial nerve became affected, and the patient experienced trigeminal neuralgia.

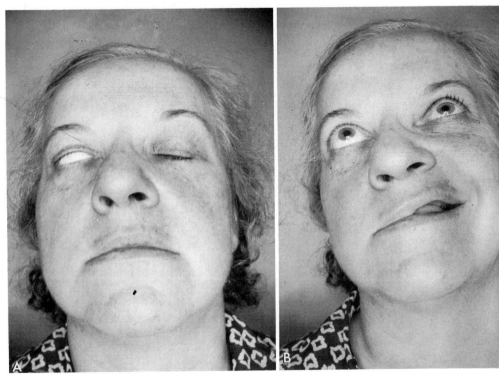

Figure 25–139 Facial nerve paralysis (Bell's palsy) due to tumor growth (carcinoma) that involved the seventh cranial nerve. *A*, Note inability to close the upper lid and turning up of the eyeball (Bell's sign). *B*, Paralysis of the right side of the lip. (See Case Report No. 16.)

Case Report No. 17

BELL'S PALSY SECONDARY TO HODGKIN'S DISEASE

This patient, a woman aged 32, had had facial paralysis for over a year, although swelling in the face had been present for only 6 weeks. The patient was referred to me for the extraction of a carious, aching mandibular molar.

According to her physician, an original diagnosis of Bell's palsy was made because she had paralysis of the seventh cranial nerve without any other symptoms.

The patient had galvanic treatment for the supposed palsy. However, when the swelling developed in the face and neck, treatment was discontinued. Subsequently a diagnosis of lymphosarcoma was made (Figure 25–140).

It was apparent that the seventh cranial nerve was involved by the extension of the malignant lymphoma.

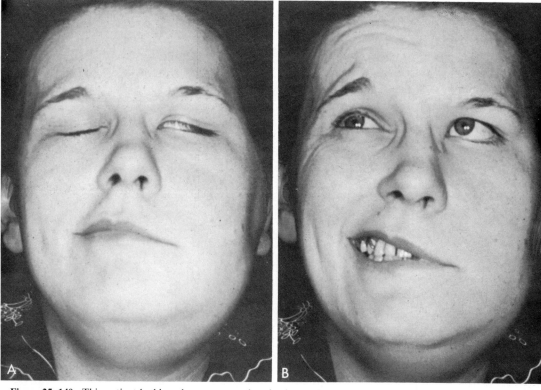

Figure 25-140 This patient had lymphosarcoma and noticed a gradually increasing paralysis of the seventh nerve as the malignant lymphoma increased in size. (See Case Report No. 17.)

Case Report No. 18

BELL'S PALSY THAT DISAPPEARED AFTER EXTRACTION

A woman, aged 28, had a typical case of Bell's palsy (Figure 25-141*A*) of 1 week's duration. Eight days previously she had had a "sore throat," and the next day she had become aware of a tender maxillary right bicuspid. On this day she had also noticed a gradually increasing paralysis on the right side of her face that, when she had awakened the next morning, was complete. She had consulted an otolaryngologist for treatment. Within 5 days her "sore throat" had been cured, but the tenderness on chewing in the right second bicuspid area had increased, and her facial paralysis was the same. The patient had become resigned to a siege of many months, when she encountered a friend who had had Bell's palsy a year previously and advised her that her paralysis had cleared up *within* a week after she had had one tooth extracted. This had prompted the patient to see her dentist, who had referred her to me. She had typical Bell's palsy of the right side of her face.

Oral and radiographic examination revealed a nonvital right lateral incisor and second bicuspid with root canal fillings. On percussion the right bicuspid was tender. Periapical radiographs showed a marked thickening of the peridental membrane. On transillumination there were marked shadows along the roots of both nonvital teeth.

The patient related the history of her friend. The author expressed skepticism, but advised the extraction of both nonvital teeth. To this the patient objected, one tooth being in the front of her mouth and not causing her any trouble, but she agreed to the extraction of the second bicuspid, which was carried out.

The next day the patient reported that her face "felt much better" and the paralysis was less. Within 1 week the paralysis had completely disappeared (Fig. 25-141*B*).

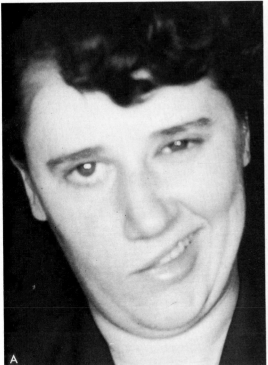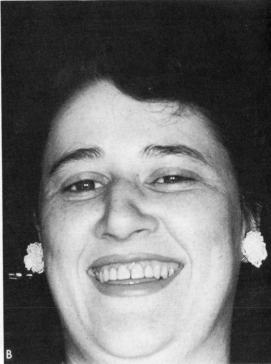

Figure 25–141 *A,* Bell's palsy of 1 week's duration. *B,* One week after extraction of a mandibular second bicuspid the paralysis of the seventh nerve disappeared. This was probably coincidental, but certainly the speedy recovery is very unusual, and the tooth had been infected. (See Case Report No. 18.)

Case Report No. 19

BELL'S PALSY DUE TO A COLD DRAFT

This patient, aged 37, was a doorman at an apartment house during the winter. One day when he opened the door, a cold draft had swept across the right side of his face. He had noticed some "stiffness" in the right side of the face as the day progressed, and the next morning he had been aware of a complete paralysis of his face (Fig. 25–142).

At examination the patient had no pain. He had extensive pericemental and periapical infection. All infected teeth were removed and physiotherapy instituted. Normal function was not restored, however, for 14 weeks.

Case Report No. 20

BELL'S PALSY OF UNKNOWN ORIGIN

This patient, aged 19, had first noticed that his face was paralyzed when he awoke one morning (Fig. 25–143). There was no history of exposure to cold or drafts.

At examination the patient had considerable oral sepsis, which was eliminated. Physiotherapy was instituted. Paralysis was present for 11 weeks.

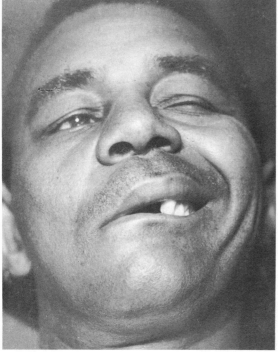

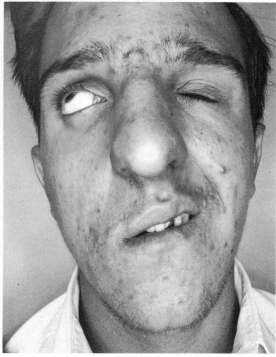

Figure 25–142 Bell's palsy due to refrigeration (cold draft). (See Case Report No. 19.)

Figure 25–143 Bell's palsy of unknown origin. (See Case Report No. 20.)

Case Report No. 21

BELL'S PALSY WITH GRADUAL IMPROVEMENT

This woman, aged 45, had been referred to our clinic for examination and an opinion. Two and a half months after the patient had had her remaining 11 maxillary teeth extracted, including the right maxillary cuspid, she suddenly had become aware of a paralysis of the right side of her face and loss of vision in her right eye, which had occurred simultaneously (Fig. 25–144). In addition, she complained of severe pain behind her ear. She had been told that a "blood clot formed on the eye tooth and struck the seventh nerve."

The ophthalmologist's report of this patient was as follows: "The right eye was slightly smaller than the left, that is, the right cornea measured 10 mm., the left measured 12 mm. Her vision was normal in either eye, with a plano in the right eye and a + 0.75 in the left. The vision in the right eye was not quite as clear as in the left."

We disagreed with the patient's reported diagnosis, but were unable to persuade her that there was no connection between the extraction and the subsequent facial paralysis and loss of vision.

She underwent medical and osteopathic treatment for over a year without any marked improvement. Gradually, in the next 4 years, mobility of the face returned. At present, 14 years later, there is still a slight drooping of the corner of the mouth.

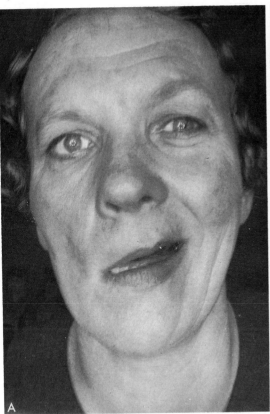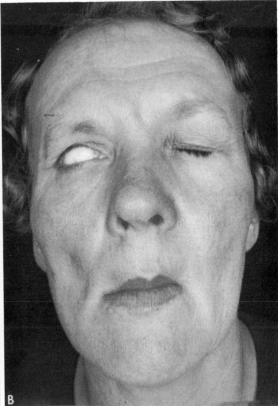

Figure 25–144 Bell's palsy 2½ months after extractions. *A*, Patient attempting to open mouth. Note paralysis of the right side of the upper lip. *B*, Patient attempting to close eye. Note the eyeball turned up in this effort (Bell's sign). (See Case Report No. 21.)

Case Report No. 22

BELL'S PALSY DUE TO COLD DRAFTS

This patient, aged 52, worked on a garbage truck as a helper. The right side of his face had been subjected to cold drafts that had swept through the cab during a cold winter day. When he had awakened to go to work the next day, his face had been paralyzed (Fig. 25–145).

Oral sepsis was eliminated, physiotherapy was instituted, and partial recovery gradually took place 6 months later.

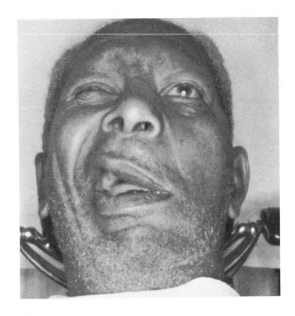

Figure 25–145 Bell's palsy following exposure to cold drafts. (See Case Report No. 22.)

Case Report No. 23

BELL'S PALSY DUE TO COLD DRAFTS

This patient, aged 63, was a doorman for a movie theater. After a cold day at work, he had noticed the next morning when he awoke that the right side of his face was paralyzed (Fig. 25–146). Occasionally that day he had had periodic pain in his left ear. He did not seek medical treatment for 2 weeks.

There was no loss of taste. However, the patient complained of blurring of vision in his left eye, but this cleared for a short period when he manually closed and opened his eyelid over the eyeball. The

blurring was undoubtedly due to the drying of the cornea.

For 2 months at a veterans hospital he underwent intensive treatment, as outlined by Alpers. At this time he showed only moderate improvement and was discharged. Extensive oral sepsis was eliminated by a complete maxillary and mandibular odontectomy and alveolectomy. Five months later there was a 75 per cent recovery. Twelve months later there was a 90 per cent recovery.

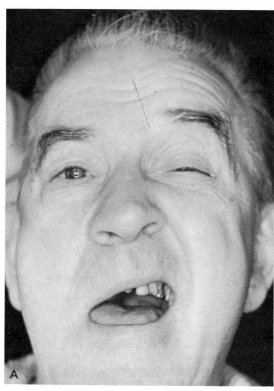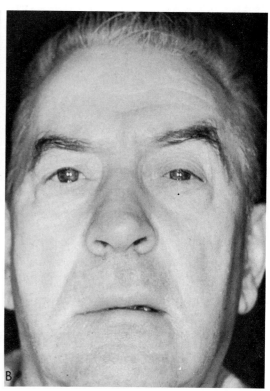

Figure 25–146 Bell's palsy following exposure to cold. *A,* Note right-sided paralysis and inability to close the right eye. *B,* Drooping of right lip. (See Case Report No. 23.)

Case Report No. 24

BELL'S PALSY DUE TO DAMPNESS AND COLD

This physician, aged 47, had been exposed to a damp cold for 4 or 5 hours during the night. The next day he had felt a sensation of numbness on the right side of the tongue. The following day the right eye had appeared irritated, as if a foreign body were present. About 7 o'clock the same evening, while shaving, the patient had noticed an

inability to raise the right side of his mouth and to close the right eye.

The following day a neurologic examination was made; with the exception of the involvement of the right facial nerve (all three branches) findings in the examination were completely negative. There was no loss of taste, nor was there a sore throat or any source of focal infection in his oral cavity.

Treatment was begun the following day. It consisted of galvanic stimulation to facial muscles three times a week. Exercise and massage were instituted. The patient received six injections of nicotinic acid intravenously, one every other day, and 100 mg. tablets of thiamine hydrochloride three times daily. Complete restoration of function occurred after 3 months' treatment.

Case Report No. 25

BELL'S PALSY DUE TO COLD DRAFTS

This patient, a nurse aged 60, had been riding on an extremely drafty bus. The next morning, June 19, she had awakened with a severe pain behind the left ear. The mouth was drawn to the left side; the left eyelid would not close; the lower lid sagged; and there was no motion in the left side of her forehead. Taste and sight were not impaired. She was forced to drink with a tube, and to push food to the right side of her face to masticate it. Severe pain continued during the first 3 weeks.

The patient visited a physician the first day. He prescribed hypodermic injections of Tetrabee, plus 100 mg. of vitamin B_6, plus galvanic current treatments after deep therapeutic treatment twice a week for 6 weeks. In addition, the patient massaged her face and did facial exercises three times a day.

At the end of 3 weeks the pain still persisted. The patient made an appointment with a neurologist, but on the day of the appointment the pain ceased. Galvanic treatment was discontinued. Tincture of nux vomica, 10 minims three times a day, and potassium iodide, 5 minims three times daily until a total of 30 minims was reached, was prescribed, but was discontinued after 20 minims because of loss of the sense of taste. Thyroid, $3\frac{1}{2}$ grains daily, was also prescribed. The patient had several chronically infected teeth removed without any appreciable benefit.

About September, the patient again started deep therapy and galvanic treatment, which were continued for 4 months. She was also taking Tetrabee, 100 mg., plus niacinamide, 100 mg., riboflavin, 0.2 mg., pyridoxine hydrochloride, 1 mg., and calcium pantothenate, 5 mg.

At this time there was slight motion in the left forehead, but the patient could not whistle, and her left eyelid closed more slowly than the right lid.

In March, 2 years later, the patient was still having facial massage and exercise. About 5 months passed before she could close the eyelid. Slight improvement appeared and continued slowly from then on. She now has 95 per cent normal muscular movement.

Case Report No. 26

BELL'S PALSY IN A YOUNG MAN

This physician, aged 25, on February 17, at approximately 6 P.M., noticed a sensation of heaviness over the right half of the face, and slight pain in the right mastoid. There was a "brassy" taste in his mouth for several hours. He was not aware of a loss of taste unless he especially tested both sides of his tongue, when it became evident that there was a loss on the right side of the tongue.

This patient had not been exposed to cold drafts, nor did he have any acute or chronic sources of infection.

Treatment consisted in infrared therapy, massage, and galvanic stimulation for 30 to 40 minutes three times a week for 3 months.

The facial paralysis was acute for approximately 3 months, when it gradually began to disappear. Fourteen months later the right side was 90 per cent normal.

GANGRENOUS STOMATITIS (NOMA, CANCRUM ORIS)

Gangrenous stomatitis is a rare disease characterized by a spreading form of gangrene which starts as a rule in the gingival tissues and spreads to and through the cheek. It is usually a terminal manifestation of a general physical debilitation caused by measles,

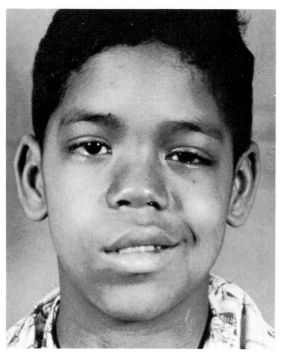

Figure 25–147 A 10-year-old male with paralysis of the seventh nerve. (Bell's palsy). No cause was determined.

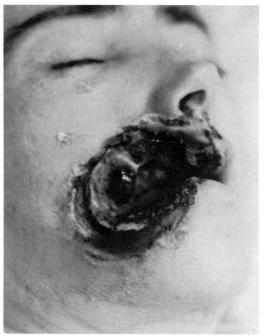

Figure 25–148 Gangrenous stomatitis (noma, cancrum oris) in a patient in terminal myelogenous leukemia. During life her white blood cell count varied from 3300 to 474,000. At the time of death it was 4900. Her maxilla was edentulous. There was no hypertrophy of the gingival tissues of the remaining lower teeth, which is frequently seen in cases of myelogenous leukemia. Note also that there is not a local defense reaction of the tissues, as shown in Figure 25–149.

leukemia, dysentery, diphtheria, typhoid fever or pneumonia.

Treatment. If the underlying cause can be quickly removed, there is hope for recovery. The two cases illustrated here were in adults with myelogenous leukemia. Local treatment consists in mild daily irrigations with weak Dakin's solution and frequent use of a warm saline mouthwash. Daily debridement should be carried out and the tissues painted with a 2 per cent solution of methylene blue.

Blood transfusions and large doses of multivitamins should be given. Penicillin in 100,000 units given intravenously every three hours will obviate the necessity of surgery.

The following case of gangrenous stomatitis (Case Report No. 27), and the one shown in Figure 25–148, were seen in the preantibiotic and prechemotherapy days.

Case Report No. 27

GANGRENOUS STOMATITIS FOLLOWING EXTRACTION OF TEETH

Patient. A white housewife, aged 40, was admitted to the hospital April 12, with a chief complaint of swelling and pain in the right cheek and neck, and difficulty in swallowing.

History. The patient stated that on awakening on the morning of April 1 her right cheek had been swollen. The swelling had been persistent, but there was no pain until 3 or 4 days later. At that time she had thought that her trouble was caused by a bad toothache, and 3 days later, or one week from the onset, she had consulted a dentist. Two teeth had been extracted from the lower right molar region. The gums were treated continuously, but the swelling and pain did not subside. For 4 days the swelling in the neck had gradually increased, and associated with this there had been pain, and difficulty in swallowing. There had been some fever associated with this condition. The pa-

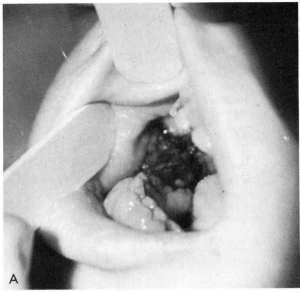 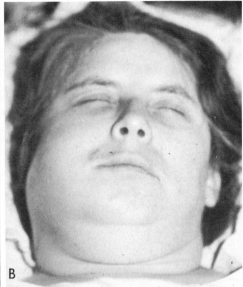

Figure 25-149 *A*, Gangrenous area in the cheek. Note the hypertrophy of the gingival tissues. *B*, Cellulitis of the right cheek and submaxillary area. (See Case Report No. 27.)

tient did not know how high her temperature was or when the fever had started. There had been no chills.

Physical Examination. This revealed an obese woman appearing to be suffering from considerable pain. There was noticeable swelling of the right cheek and right side of the neck, which was tender to the touch. The swelling was not hard, nor was there local heat or redness. Examination of the local condition revealed that the lower right second and third molars had been extracted. Gauze had been packed into the cavity in the right lower molar region. The right, mucoperiosteal membrane was edematous and slightly swollen. The gum margin was hyperemic and covered with a whitish membrane that was apparently the result of medication. (Oral hygiene was poor. Chronic gingivitis was present, but no hypertrophy.) The pharynx was slightly hyperemic. The right side of the neck was slightly enlarged, and there were palpable tender masses in the anterior margin just below the mandible. There was postcervical adenopathy of the right side.

Progress. From the day of admission the patient became steadily worse. The mucoperiosteal membrane buccal to the mandibular second and third molars became gangrenous, and this area steadily increased in size, until a large area of the buccal mucosa of the cheek was destroyed. At the same time the gingival tissues rapidly became hypertrophied until the crowns were almost covered (see Figure 25-149*A*). The facial cellulitis spread and the soft tissues became indurated (see Figure 25-149*B*). The white blood count rose from 3400 to 83,000 cells per cu. mm. the day before she died of bronchopneumonia, 27 days after admission.

Diagnosis. The diagnosis was established as (1) atypical myelogenous leukemia; (2) gangrenous stomatitis; (3) bronchopneumonia.

CARCINOMA IN A HEALING ALVEOLUS

The author had never seen or heard of carcinoma developing in a healing alveolus following a dental extraction until the case reported by Van Zile (Case Report No. 28) appeared in the literature. This is obviously a very unusual occurrence, considering the thousands of extractions done daily.

Case Report No. 28

CARCINOMA IN AN ALVEOLUS FOLLOWING DENTAL EXTRACTION*

W. N. VAN ZILE, D.D.S.

A 19-year-old white male had had a right maxillary lateral incisor, which had been fractured while eating, extracted because it was painful. There was no swelling about the tooth before the traumatic incident. Two months following the extraction, the patient noticed swelling in the extraction site. He reported back to the dispensary for examination. The oral examination revealed a granular fungating lesion of the gingival tissues of the right maxilla that appeared to be limited labially to the region of the healing alveolus where the lateral incisor had been extracted (see Figure 25–150). The lesion extended onto the palate about 1 cm. beyond the region of the alveolus. During a 6-day period of observation, before treatment, the lesion was seen to be enlarging with alarming speed. All remaining tissues were in excellent health. The pathologist's report of the biopsy specimen was squamous cell carcinoma arising from gingival mucosa involving a healing alveolus.

It was decided that treatment should consist of a surgical block resection of the right maxilla sufficiently radical to encompass the lesion with at least 1.0-cm. margins of normal tissue, to be followed with radiation at a later date in the event of recurrence. The block resection included the central incisors on the left and the cuspid and bicuspid on the right side, the labial mucoperiosteal mem-

---

* Adapted from Van Zile, W. N.: Carcinoma in a healing alveolus after a dental extraction: Report of a case. J. Oral Surg., *17*:82–85 (Jan.), 1959.

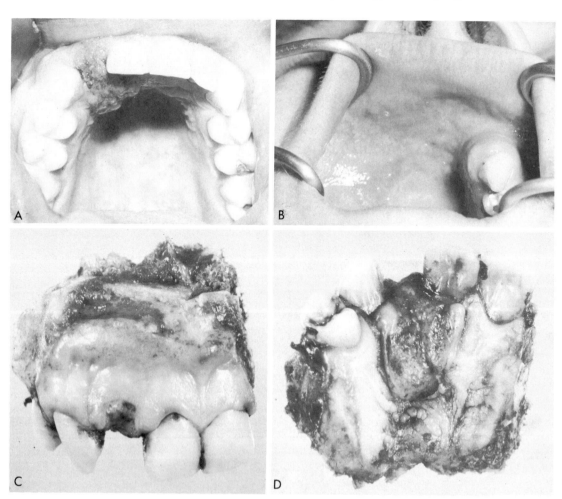

Figure 25–150 *A,* Gingival carcinoma that developed following extraction of a lateral incisor. *B,* Postoperative appearance following healing. *C,* Labial view, resected specimen. *D,* Lingual view, resected specimen. (See Case Report No. 28.) (From Van Zile, W. N.: Carcinoma in a healing alveolus after a dental extraction: Report of a case. J. Oral Surg., *17*:82–85 [Jan.], 1959.)

brane to the base of the nose and the palatal muco-periosteal membrane to the base of the nose and the nasal and antral cavity. After excision, a 1.5 cm. bony defect was seen in the antral floor. This was closed with mucosa of the lip and palate.

The patient was followed for 6 years, and there was not any indication of recurrence of the carcinoma and no metastasis developed. Normal function and cosmetic relationships were restored with a prosthesis.

VIRAL HEPATITIS AS A HAZARD TO THE SURGEON

Glazer, Spatz and Catone[27] have graphically illustrated the danger of viral hepatitis during oral surgery by presenting "cases in which oral surgeons contracted hepatitis from patients." They note that these "are distinct examples of the hazards the oral surgeon must be aware of when treating patients with hepatitis. With the increased incidence of hepatitis and drug abuse in the general population, viral hepatitis must be considered a threat to medical and dental personnel. Any penetration of tissue by contaminated materials from a chronic or active hepatitis patient can transmit the disease. This is not surprising when one considers that a plasma dilution of 1:10,000,000 can still elicit antigen in the blood. Unfortunately, the oral surgeon does not always have a choice of whether to operate, as in the first patient (Case Report No. 29), when the repair of the facial fractures was clearly an emergency. The second patient, too, needed immediate treatment to prevent the chronic dental infec-tion from progressing to acute cellulitis (Case Report No. 30).

"One partial solution is that the oral surgeon must be aware of the ease with which he can contract hepatitis from patients, and perhaps delay any dental procedure on patients who have had recent episodes of hepatitis. If it is necessary to operate, the surgical procedure must be done with infinite care."

Case Report Nos. 29 and 30 "demonstrate the highly infectious nature of hepatitis and its obvious danger to oral surgeons."

For protection of patients these authors "recommend that the physician or dentist who had had hepatitis and who is asymptomatic, but in whom a positive hepatitis-associated antigen (HAA) develops, be meticulous in sterilizing instruments, washing hands and wearing gloves, as the potential for infecting patients is apparent."*

---

* Reprinted with permission from Glazer, R. I., Spatz, S.S., and Catone, G. A.: Viral hepatitis: A hazard to oral surgeons. J. Oral Surg., *31*:504–508 (July), 1973.

Case Report No. 29

SERUM HEPATITIS ACQUIRED BY SURGEONS*

An oral surgeon and his resident were exposed in July to serum hepatitis while reducing facial fractures. Their patient was a 24-year-old man, a known heroin addict who had had a history of hepatitis for 3 months before he was injured. Results of all routine laboratory studies and liver enzymes were within normal limits. The patient was brought to the operating room, where a tracheotomy and reduction of the facial fractures were accomplished. While placing the maxillary and mandibular arch bars for intermaxillary fixation, the oral surgery resident and staff oral surgeon were known to have pricked themselves with the wires used for stabilization of the arch bars. The post-operative course of the patient was uncomplicated.

On October 13, the staff oral surgeon was admitted to the hospital because of severe polyarthralgia and malaise. During his hospital stay, dark urine, light stools, night sweats and fever developed. No icterus was present and the liver was palpable at the costal margin.

---

* Adapted from Glazer, I. G., Spatz, S. S., and Catone, G. A.: Viral hepatitis. A hazard to oral surgeons. J. Oral Surg., *31*:504–508 (July), 1973.

The patient's history was essentially noncontributory, with no history of transfusions and no other known exposure to hepatitis. The complete blood cell count showed a hemoglobin of 13.7 gm./100 ml.; hematocrit reading, 40.5 per cent; white blood cell count (WBC), 7700/cu. mm., with a differential of 63 per cent neutrophils, 31 per cent lymphocytes, 2 per cent monocytes, 3 per cent eosinophils and 1 per cent basophils. During the patient's hospitalization, the liver enzymes rose to the following levels: serum glutamic pyruvic transaminase (SGPT), 1190 (normal, 4 to 24); serum glutamic oxaloacetic transaminase (SGOT), 540 (normal, 8 to 52); lactic dehydrogenase (LDH), 571 (normal, 112 to 228); with a 3.0 mg./100 ml. for the serum bilirubin (normal, 0 to 1.5 mg./100 ml.). The alkaline phosphatase was elevated at 110. The heterophile antibody test for infectious mononucleosis was negative. At that time, the Australian antigen diagnostic test for hepatitis was not generally in use, and it was not performed.

On the basis of the incubation period, clinical and laboratory values, a diagnosis of serum hepatitis was made. A high-protein, high-calorie diet and rest in bed were ordered. The patient's condition improved, and he was discharged on November 2. He resumed normal activities after a 3-month recovery period.

On November 2, the oral surgery resident was admitted to the hospital with a chief complaint of malaise, polyarthralgia, and backache of 10 days' duration. One week before, he had experienced anorexia, a distaste for cigarettes and nausea. He had also experienced tenderness and discomfort of the right quadrant and had noticed dark urine. The complete blood cell count and differential were normal; SGOT, 1450; LDH, 620; alkaline phosphatase, 6.2; and SGPT, 1220. The heterophile antibody test was negative. The patient did not experience icterus, fever or chills. His medical history was noncontributory; he had had no transfusions and no other known exposure to hepatitis.

A diagnosis of serum hepatitis was made on the basis of the long incubation period, in addition to other appropriate tests. A high-carbohydrate diet, prednisone and rest in bed were ordered. His condition improved, and he was discharged on November 15. He was able to return to work in 2 months.

Case No. 30
SERUM HEPATITIS CONTRACTED DURING SURGERY*

On November 16, a 24-year-old white man was admitted to the hospital with a chief complaint of "bad teeth." Clinical and radiographic examination of the oral cavity disclosed severely carious and abscessed maxillary teeth and impacted mandibular right and left third molars.

Physical examination showed the patient to be moderately jaundiced, with icteric sclera and a palpable liver 6 cm. below the right costal margin. The patient also complained of dark urine, light stools, malaise and night sweats.

The patient was a heroin addict and had had hepatitis in July and February of 1970. Liver enzyme levels were also elevated; this supported the diagnosis of hepatitis. The patient was transferred to the medical service, where a biopsy of the liver disclosed chronic active hepatitis, with the normal architecture of the liver parenchyma distorted as a result of frequent collapse, loss of uniformity of cell plates and inflammatory cell and intralobular infiltrates. Occasional Councilman-like bodies were seen. Focal feathery degeneration of hepatocytes and inflammatory reaction in the portal connective stroma were evident.

The patient's condition improved, and he was medically able to tolerate the extraction of the abscessed and impacted teeth. On December 7, a maxillary odontectomy and alveolectomy and surgical removal of the impacted teeth were performed.

At the end of the procedure, it was noticed that one of the residents working on the case had a tear in his glove, probably from a suture needle, and that his finger had been punctured. The patient's postoperative recovery was uncomplicated, and he was discharged on December 8. The Australian antigen test was negative.

Approximately 5 weeks after the operation, the resident began to experience a distaste for cigarettes; he had malaise, dark urine, fever and night sweats. He was admitted to the hospital for medical evaluation on February 7. Liver enzymes were SGPT, 615; SGOT, 76; alkaline phosphatase, 120; with a bilirubin of 0.6 mg./100 ml. No icterus was experienced, and the heterophile and the Australian antigen tests were negative.

The patient's medical history was noncontributory, with no history of transfusion or other known exposure to the hepatitis virus. A diagnosis of infectious hepatitis was made on the basis of clinical and laboratory findings, and of the short incubation period. Five weeks had elapsed between the onset of symptoms and the resident's return to work.

---

* Adapted from Glazer, I. G., Spatz, S. S., and Catone, G. A.: Viral hepatitis: A hazard to oral surgeons. J. Oral Surg., *31*:504–508 (July), 1973.

REFERENCES

1. Aarons, E. F.: What if a patient dies in your office? Med. Econ., *195:* (Jan. 19), 1970.

2. Anderson, W. A. D.: Pathology. St. Louis, the C. V. Mosby Co., 1961.

3. Archer, W. H.: Manual of Dental Anesthesia, 2nd ed. Philadelphia, W. B. Saunders Co., 1958.

4. Archer, W. H., and Zubrow, H. J.: Fatal hemorrhage following regional anesthesia for operative dentistry in a hemophiliac. Oral Surg., *7:*464–470 (May), 1954.

5. Archer, W. H., and Zubrow, H. J.: Hemophiliac: the pre- and postoperative treatment. Oral Surg., *3:*1377, 1950.

6. Beeson, P. B., and McDermott, W. (Eds.): Cecil-Loeb Textbook of Medicine. 11th ed. Philadelphia, W. B. Saunders Co., 1963.

7. Best, C. H., and Taylor, N. B.: Physiological Basis of Medical Practice. 8th ed. Baltimore, The Williams & Wilkins Co., 1966.

8. Budge, C. T.: Closure of an antraoral opening by use of the tantalum plate. J. Oral Surg., *10*(1):32–34 (Jan.), 1952.

9. Burch, R. J., and Funk, E. C.: Treatment of oroantral fistula: report of a case. J. Oral Surg., *17:*58 (Nov.), 1959.

10. Burket, L. W.: Oral Medicine. 3rd ed. Philadelphia, J. B. Lippincott Co., 1957.

11. Caparosa, R. J., and Zavatsky, A. R.: Practical aspects of the cricothyroid space. Laryngoscope, *47:*577 (June), 1957.

12. Chalmers, T. C., and Alter, H. J.: Management of the asymptomatic carrier of the hepatitis-associated (Australia) antigen. N. Engl. J. Med., *285:*613–617 (Sept. 9), 1971.

13. Claflin, R. S.: The healing of undisturbed and infected extraction wounds: Abstract of thesis. The Bur, *35:*85 (July), 1935.

14. Conn, H. F. (Ed.): Current Therapy 1975. Philadelphia, W. B. Saunders Co., 1975.

15. Cook, T. J.: Osteomyelitis and osteoradionecrosis, report of two cases. Oral Surg., *16:*257 (Mar.), 1963.

16. Davis, D. G.: Malignant hyperthermia and plastic surgery. Plast. Reconstr. Surg., *44:*495 (Nov.), 1969.

17. Davis, W. H.: Emergency drugs and allergy, pp. 235–236. In McCarthy, F. M. (Ed.): Emergencies in Dental Practice. Philadelphia, W. B. Saunders Co., 1972.

18. Delaney, A. J.: A new instrument for cricothyroid tracheotomy. Trans. Am. Acad. Ophthalmol. Otolaryngol., *57:*912, 1953.

19. Dorland's Illustrated Medical Dictionary. 24th ed. Philadelphia, W. B. Saunders Co., 1965.

20. Durocher, R. T., Morris, A. L., and Burket, L. W.: Oral manifestations of hereditary hemorrhagic telangiectasia. Oral Surg., *14:*550 (May), 1961.

21. Egyedi, P.: Postoperative disturbance of the inferior alveolar nerve after removal of an impacted mandibular third molar. Schweiz. Monatsschr. Zahnheilkd., *80:*109 (Oct.), 1970. In English: Adv. Oral Surg., *2:*18, 1972.

22. Evans, R. E., and Leake, D.: Bleeding in a hemophiliac after inferior alveolar nerve block. J.A.D.A., *69:*350 (Sept.), 1964.

23. Frank, V. H.: Paresthesia: evaluation of 16 cases. J. Oral Surg., *17:*27–33 (Nov.), 1959.

24. Gardner, B. S.: Postoperative considerations regarding extraction of teeth. J.A.D.A., *16:*237 (Feb.), 1929.

25. Gaum, L. I.: Use of aminocaproic acid in oral surgery for hemophiliacs. J. Can. Dent. Assoc., *35:*599 (Nov.), 1969.

26. Georgiade, N., Mitchell, T., Lemler, J., and Heid, J.: Use of a new improved hemostatic sponge in oral surgery. J. Oral Surg., *19:*215–219 (May), 1961.

27. Glazer, I. G., Spatz, S. S., and Catone, G. A.: Viral hepatitis: a hazard to oral surgeons. J. Oral. Surg., *31:*504–508 (July), 1973.

28. Goltz, R. W.: Urticaria. In Conn. H. F. (Ed.): Current Therapy 1965, p. 507. Philadelphia, W. B. Saunders Co., 1965.

29. Gores, R. J.: The ineffectiveness of carbazochrome salicylate (Adrenosem) in the reduction of surgical bleeding. Oral Surg., *12:*814–819 (July), 1959.

30. Grandstaff, C. H.: The influence of the oral bacteria on the healing of exodontia wounds: Abstract of thesis. The Bur, *35:*95 (July), 1935.

31. Gustafson, G., and Kjell, W.: Effect of local application of trypsin on postextraction alveolar osteitis. Oral Surg., *14:*280–286 (Mar.), 1961.

32. Hale, D. H.: Treatment of recurrent dislocation of the mandible: review of the literature and report of cases. J. Oral Surg., *30:*527–530 (July), 1972.

33. Halhuber, M. J., and Kirchmair, H.: [Emergencies in internal medicine. XIX, Myocardial infarct.] Med. Klin., *52:*341–344 (Mar. 1), 1957.

34. Hall, H. D., Talley, A. W., and McCallum, C. A.: Evaluation of estrogens in extraction-induced hemorrhage. J. Oral Surg., *18:*162 (Aug.), 1964.

35. Harden, B.: Unpublished investigations at the Elizabeth Steele Magee Hospital, Pittsburgh, Pa., 1936.

36. Huebsch, R. F.: Bell's palsy: current theories of treatment. J. Oral Surg., *22:*138 (Mar.), 1964.

37. Jackson, C., and Jackson, C. L.: Diseases of the Nose, Throat, and Ear. 2nd ed. Philadelphia, W. B. Saunders Co., 1959.

38. Jacoby, J. J., Hamelberg, W., Zeigler, C. H., Flory, F. A., and Jones, J. R.: Transtracheal resuscitation. J.A.M.A., *162:*625–628 (Oct. 13), 1956.

39. Johnson, E. W., and Parker, W.: Letter to editor: Passage of thermometer through the gastrointestinal tract. J.A.M.A., *221*(3):303, 1972.

40. Killey, H. C.: The problem of the tooth or root in the maxillary antrum. J. Oral Surg., *22:*391 (Sept.), 1964.

41. Kouwenhoven, W. B., Jude, J. R., and Knickerbocker, G. G.: Closed-chest cardiac massage. J.A.M.A., *173:*1064–1067 (July), 1960.

42. Kouwenhoven, W. B., Milnor, W. R., Knickerbocker, G. G., and Chestnut, W. R.: Closed chest defibrillation of heart. Surgery, *42:*550–561 (Sept.), 1957.

43. Lee, F. M.: The displaced root in the maxillary sinus. J. Oral Surg., *29:*491 (Apr.), 1970.

44. McCarthy, F. M.: Emergencies in Dental Practice, p. 260. Philadelphia, W. B. Saunders Co., 1972.

45. McKenna, H., and MacGee, M. A.: Bleeding states in dental surgery. Aust. Dent. J., *13:*257 (Aug.), 1968.

46. Mills, L. C., Voudoukis, I. J., Moyer, J. H., and Heider, C.: Treatment of shock with sympathicomimetic drugs: use of metaraminol and comparison with other vasopressor agents. Arch. Intern. Med., *106:*816–823 (Dec.), 1960.

47. Minot, G. R., and Taylor, S. H. L.: Hemophilia, the clinical use of anti-hemophilic globulin. Ann. Intern. Med., *26:*363, 1947.

48. Nicholas, T. H., and Rumer, G. F.: Emergency airway: four basic steps required to restore ventilation. J.A.M.A., *174:*1930–1935 (Dec.), 1960.

49. O'Day, R. A., and Driggs, R. L.: Cardiopulmonary resuscitation in dental practice. *In* Quinn, T. W. (Ed.): Anesthesia and Analgesia. Dent. Clin. North Am., *17:*330, 1973.

50. Paget, J.: On a form of chronic inflammation of bone (osteitis deformans). Med. Chir. Trans. (Lond.), *60:*37–63, 1877.

51. Patek, A. J., Jr., and Stetson, R. P.: Hemophilia: Abnormal coagulation of blood and its relation to blood platelets. J. Clin. Invest., *15:*531, 1936.

52. Quick, A. J.: Hemorrhagic Diseases and Thromboses. 2nd ed. Philadelphia, Lea & Febiger, 1966.

53. Richards, R., and Crombie, H. M.: Familial angioneurotic oedema: two fatal cases after dental extractions Br. Med. J., *5215*(2):1787 (Dec. 17), 1960.

54. Robinson, M., and Lytle, J.: The broken dental needle and other metallic foreign bodies. *In* McCarthy, F. M. (Ed.): Emergencies in Dental Practice. Philadelphia, W. B. Saunders Co., 1967.

55. Safar, P.: Resuscitation in the Dental Office. J. Am. Dent. Soc. Anesth., *7:*4–8 (May), 1960.

56. Scher, I.: Angioneurotic edema. Oral Surg., *16:*286 (Mar.), 1963.

57. Schneider, S. S., and Stern, M.: Teeth in the line of mandibular fractures. J. Oral Surg., *29:*107 (Feb.), 1971.

58. Schroff, J., and Bartels, H.: Painful sockets after extraction. J. Dent. Res., *9:*81 (Jan.), 1929.

59. Sheppard, G. A.: Legal aspects of dental emergencies, pp. 499–500. *In* McCarthy, F. M. (Ed.): Emergencies in Dental Practice. Philadelphia, W. B. Saunders Co., 1972.

60. Sherry, S., and Fletcher, A. P.: Proteolytic enzymes: a therapeutic evaluation. Clin. Pharmacol. Ther., *1:*202, 1960.

61. Shira, R. B.: Surgical emergencies. *In* McCarthy, F. M. (Ed.): Emergencies in Dental Practice. Philadelphia, W. B. Saunders Co., 1972.

62. Shuttee, T. S.: Hyaluronidase in relief of postoperative trismus, swelling and pain. Oral Surg., *15:*114 (Jan.), 1962.

63. Sicher, H., and DuBrul, E. L.: Oral Anatomy. 5th ed. St. Louis, The C. V. Mosby Co., 1970.

64. Spatz, S.: Angioneurotic edema of the maxillofacial region. Oral Surg., *18:*256 (Aug.), 1964.

65. Spouge, J. D.: Hemostasis in dentistry with special reference to hemocoagulation. Oral Surg., *18:*583 (Nov.), 1964.

66. Sprague, C. C.: Re-evaluation of hemostatic agents. Arch. Intern. Med., *107:*72–73 (Jan.), 1961.

67. Van Zile, W. N.: Carcinoma in a healing alveolus after a dental extraction: Report of a case. J. Oral Surg., *17:*82–85 (Jan.), 1959.

68. Waldron, C. A.: Personal communication. Atlanta, Ga.

69. White, P. H., and Mallett, S. P.: Management of hemophilia in dental extractions. J. Oral Surg., *7:*237, 1949.

70. Wilson, C. P.: Diseases of the Ear, Nose and Throat. London, Butterworth, 1952.

71. Wintrobe, M. M., *et al.*: Harrison's Principles of Medicine. 6th ed. New York: McGraw-Hill Book Co., Inc., 1970.

72. Wishart, C.: Oral surgery in the hemorrhagic states. J. Oral Surg., *22:*178 (Mar.), 1964.

73. Zucker, M. B.: Platelet agglutination and vasoconstriction in hemostasis. Am. J. Physiol., *148:*275, 1947.

74. Zucker, M. B., Friedman, B. K., and Rapport, M. M.: Serotonin in blood platelets. Proc. Soc. Exp. Biol. Med., *85:*282, 1954.

CHAPTER 26

DIAGNOSIS AND TREATMENT OF PAIN IN THE ORAL CAVITY AND ADJACENT AREAS

DONALD DAVIDSON, B.S., M.S., D.D.S.

W. HARRY ARCHER, B.S., M.A., D.D.S.

GENERAL COMMENTS

Pain may be defined as an unpleasant sensation as perceived by the patient. It is necessary to define it in such general terms because the intensity of the stimulus causing the pain is often not directly related to the intensity of the reaction (physical or psychological) produced by the stimulus. While this is obvious in the light of common experience, it is often forgotten by the clinician when some particular operative procedure or trauma produces a subjective response in the patient disproportionate to that normally seen. The exaggerated complaints of an anxious neurotic following a simple extraction may provoke a long, futile search for other disease, and the failure of a phlegmatic elderly patient to complain may lull the clinician into overlooking a serious problem such as osteomyelitis. In brief, therefore, pain can be measured only in terms of the patient's verbalization of the problem. The good clinician must remain constantly aware of this and of the necessity of evaluating both the disease and the patient. It is the aim of this chapter to point out the pathologic processes; the evaluation of the patient is an art developed from experience fortified with knowledge gained over time. We do not wish to overemphasize the psychologic aspects of pain, because the lazy or inept clinician often relegates to the psychoneurotic category all patients whose problems he cannot immediately diagnose or who do not respond to the textbook therapy. However, the conscientious clinician must be aware of the tremendous effects of the psyche on the subjective responses commonly recognized as pain.

The procedure in the treatment of pain is obviously to make a diagnosis first and then institute appropriate treatment. Making a diagnosis, however, is by far the most difficult part of the problem, because many of the pain syndromes involving the face and oral cavity are not clearly defined and, even when somatic changes are visible, may be so interrelated with psychologic problems as to defy a cure. Much of the therapy in this area is empiric and in many cases produces a good percentage of excellent results, but since the underlying pathology is still obscure, therapy is often an art as well as a science. The treatment of many of these syndromes is beyond the province of the general practitioner and often beyond the province of the oral surgeon, but it behooves the dentist to be familiar with these syndromes so that he may recognize them and not attempt to treat them as if they were odontogenic.

ODONTOGENIC PAIN

Pulpitis. The first problem to be considered in a patient who complains of facial pain is whether it is odontogenic. Since all pain fibers from the teeth (with the exception of pulpal fibers) also carry proprioceptive fibers in association with them, *all facial pain without associated pain in the teeth* can be considered as not dental in origin *except* when there is a possibility of pulpal inflammation. Therefore the first task is usually to look for a pulpitis. It must be remembered that a pulpitis can cause referred pain to any other area supplied by any branch of the trigeminal nerve—the face, maxillary sinus, good teeth, etc.—without the offending tooth itself being readily apparent. The only dependable observation is that the pain *never* crosses the midline and the offending tooth is always on the same side as the pain. While occasional reports of such occurrences appear in the literature, we feel that these are probably diagnostic errors of etiology, *i.e.,* the contralateral pain had another cause.

X-rays often will give a clue, especially in the case of heavily filled teeth with recurrent decay or deep silicate fillings, as to which tooth is the cause of the pain.

Since upper teeth may cause pain in the mandibular area and vice versa, examination of both upper and lower teeth must be performed. The use of the electric pulp tester may be helpful if the teeth are not heavily filled with metal, but most often it is a filled tooth that is causing the trouble. Thermal tests, especially heat, are useful, particularly in conjunction with diagnostic blocks of local anesthetics. In cases where the pain appears to be referred to the areas not close to the teeth, *e.g.,* the eye or the temporal area, the teeth on the ipsilateral side can be anesthetized with a local anesthetic (combined with a vasoconstrictor to prevent diffusion) to see if the pain disappears. If the tooth is the source of pain, the pain will disappear. If the toothache can be provoked by heat or cold, small amounts of local anesthetic with a vasoconstrictor can be placed over the maxillary teeth starting from posterior to anterior and, with a suitable waiting period between injections, a possible maxillary pulpitis localized. Unfortunately, in the mandible such a serial technique is not feasible, except for the four incisors. At times the use of ice or hot gutta percha at each tooth may be productive, but here the dentist must usually either wait for signs of periodontal inflammation or guess which of the heavily filled teeth is involved. Analgesic therapy may help in making the patient comfortable during the waiting period until either clinical or radiographic evidence appears to indicate which is the offending tooth.

Some mention must be made at this time of the pulpitis caused by a deep periodontal pocket (retrograde pulpitis) or by the presence of accessory lateral root canals leading to a small pocket. These cannot be detected radiographically and may produce a pulpitis in a noncarious tooth. Trauma to the teeth with pulpal thrombosis may produce a similar picture of a noncarious tooth with a pulpitis, which is another reason for utilizing more than the radiograph to make the diagnosis.

Pulpal Calcifications. Pulp stones must also be considered in the diagnosis of pulpitis, although some controversy is involved here. We regard pulpal calcifications as the end results of low-grade inflammation similar to the calcifications seen elsewhere in the body. While they themselves may not cause pain, except by mechanical interference with circulation, we regard them as evidence that the pulp has been inflamed and may still be so inflamed. If diagnostic blocks indicate such a tooth as a cause of pain, we feel it should be extracted or the pulp extirpated. (See Case Report No. 1.)

Case Report No. 1

NEURALGIA DUE TO PULP STONES

A male patient aged 55 was referred by his physician because of a severe neuralgia, the cause of which was unknown. The patient had been taking large quantities of aspirin to obtain relief from the recurrent pain, which closely followed the distribution of the fifth nerve on the left side of his face, and was always accompanied by an earache. It was the earache which sent him first to his physician, because he felt that this was the cause of all the pain he experienced during his attacks. The physician reported that findings in the ear examination, physical examination, and history were negative.

Oral Examination. The patient stated that he did not have any "bad teeth," and had not had a toothache for years. In the maxilla only the six anterior incisors and the upper left second molar and right third molar remained. These were in a good state of repair with normal supporting tissues. The remaining mandibular teeth were the lower six anterior incisors, left bicuspids, right first bicuspid and second molar, all in a good state of repair and with normal supporting tissues. All teeth were vital, and transillumination was negative. The teeth were not sore to percussion. Radiographic examination of the remaining teeth and edentulous areas was negative except for large pulp stones in the left maxillary second molar.

Treatment. The patient was suffering intensely with widespread pain in the left side of his face and left ear at this time.

A posterior-superior alveolar nerve injection of procaine hydrochloride solution, plus infiltration over the mesiobuccal root of the maxillary left second molar, gave him complete relief from his neuralgic pain.

It was decided to extract this tooth and, after palatal anesthesia was obtained, the extraction was performed. The neuralgic pain did not recur.

Comment. This is one of a number of similar cases the author has treated. It has been stated that pain is due to venous stasis in the pulp produced by the mechanical obstruction of the pulp stone. However, this tooth was not affected by temperature changes, an effect one would normally expect if venous stasis were present in the pulp.

Pulp stones or nodules are not rare, and the presence of this calcific deposit certainly does not constitute an indication for removal of the tooth or teeth. However, if there is neuralgic pain that cannot be explained on any other basis, and the anesthetization of the tooth with the deposit stops the neuralgic pain, then that tooth should be extracted.

Impacted Teeth. Impacted teeth are also often cited as a cause of pain, but we do not consider them unless they (a) are causing resorption of an adjacent tooth, (b) are undergoing resorption themselves, or (c) are impinging on a blood vessel or nerve (especially under a denture). Most pains attributed to impacted teeth, particularly in young people, are due to pain in the muscles rather than in the teeth and are cured by removal of the teeth only because the extensive postoperative swelling and restriction of jaw movement immobilize the sore muscle.

Osteomyelitis. Osteomyelitis of the mandible deserves passing mention here because in the early stage of an acute osteomyelitis there is very intense pain with little or no other evidence of the disease. Radiographic evidence and loosening of the teeth do not occur until 48 to 72 hours have passed and irreversible bone damage has already occurred. True maxillary osteomyelitis is probably relatively nonexistent, except in newborn infants, severely debilitated patients and patients with certain rare medical problems, but osteomyelitis of the mandible does occur frequently enough to be mentioned and considered. Indications are severe pain and sensitivity to percussion of several teeth of the mandible, followed shortly by an elevated temperature and numbness of the lip due to

thrombosis of the mandibular artery and involvement of the nerve. Early diagnosis is important since rapid, heavy antibiotic therapy may prevent unnecessary loss of bone and teeth.

Alveolalgia. Postoperative alveolalgia (or "dry socket") is discussed more fully elsewhere in the text but is mentioned here because the oral surgeon is periodically called upon to treat a case in which pain persists despite all local treatment by the dentist. Careful examination will often reveal that the pain is not within the socket but on the buccal aspect, and may be caused by bone chips fractured at the time of extraction and left under the buccal mucoperiosteum. More often, the pain is actually in the masticatory muscles and is related to strain. The extraction causes the patient to transfer all chewing to the opposite side. This sets up two levers. one long and one short, between each condyle and the unilateral chewing site with the fulcrums at the condyles. The longer lever arm produces more strain on the masticatory muscles of that side. Since this causes pain on the same side as the extraction, the natural inclination is to think of a direct connection between extraction and pain and to treat the socket. Treatment, of course, consists in restoring bilateral chewing habits to relieve the unilateral muscle strain. (See Case Report

MYOFASCIAL PAIN SYNDROME CONFUSED WITH
ALVEOLALGIA (DRY SOCKET)

A 16-year-old white male was referred by his dentist for treatment of an intractable dry socket. Three weeks previously the lower right first molar had been extracted and 2 days after the extraction he had returned to the family dentist complaining of severe pain in the ear on the right side. The dentist thought the socket looked good but he cleaned out the clot and packed the socket with iodoform gauze saturated with zinc oxide and eugenol. The pain persisted despite the fact that the packing was changed daily. At the end of 3 weeks the patient was referred to us. Examination of the patient revealed a normally healing socket, acute masseteric spasm, and pain on palpation in the temporal area. The patient reported that the dentist had advised him to chew on the left side only so as not to injure the socket. It was obvious that this unilateral chewing was the etiologic factor and the patient was instructed to chew bilaterally and use aspirin as needed for pain. Within 72 hours the patient was comfortable.

Comment. This is such a common occurrence that it deserves special attention. The sudden onset of unilateral chewing, caused by an extraction, denture alteration, high filling, loss of a filling causing sensitivity or other factors, can often initiate an acute problem of myofascial pain on the side contralateral to the chewing site.

No. 2 and Pain in Muscles or Ligaments later in this chapter.)

When all odontogenic pain is ruled out, the next step is to try to identify the pain as being caused by one or another of the various syndromes that are well-recognized entities. With some of these syndromes the symptoms are so characteristic that odontogenic pain need not be considered, but in other cases the symptoms are less classical and a complete dental evaluation may be required.

PAIN REFERRED FROM ADJACENT ORGANS AND FROM SYSTEMIC DISEASES

Pain may be referred to the teeth and jaws from pathologic conditions present in adjacent tissues and from systemic diseases. While this is generally infrequent, it does occur often enough to require a degree of alertness on the part of the dentist.

Sinuses. Since the maxillary second bicuspid and first molar are very close to the antrum, and the first bicuspid and second molar are only slightly less proximate, inflammatory disease of the maxillary sinuses will make these teeth sensitive to percussion, since they are in direct contact with the inflamed area and their nerve supply passes through the inflamed area. The diagnosis is obvious here because *all* teeth in close approximation to the sinus are sensitive to percussion. In addition the pain is usually intensified when the patient is recumbent. Radiographs of the sinuses (not intraoral dental films) will usually establish the diagnosis. In older patients, carcinoma of the sinus may produce a dull, constant gnawing pain in the maxilla and must be considered and ruled out with x-rays.

Cervical Spine and Associated Muscles. Cervical arthritis, bone spurs, myositis and many other pathologic entities may produce referred pain in the face, but in our experience this always is secondary in intensity to pain at the site of the original disease and can hardly be confused with anything else.

Myocardial Pain. Myocardial insufficiency may produce a dull, diffuse pain that radiates into the lower jaw and teeth. While there is usually associated chest pain, dull diffuse bilateral* pain in the neck and mandible without chest pain can occur in coronary disease.

Salivary Glands. Intermittent obstruction of the salivary glands and ducts may produce pain that can be referred to the teeth. An examination will reveal the tender gland, and this cannot be confused with anything else except by the most careless examiner. The

---

* Even in the presence of demonstrable dental disease the spontaneous occurrence of pain bilaterally should be a warning sign to an alert clinician of some alteration of the systemic resistance of a patient. It is hardly chance that causes, for example, bilateral abscessed first molars at the same time. Some factor in the patient's resistance has probably changed, and while the changes may be trivial, such as the prodromata of a cold, they may portend serious events, such as a coronary occlusion. The surgeon's choice of anesthesia, time of surgery and so forth must be evaluated in the light of this knowledge.

cause of the swelling of the gland and the capsular distention (which causes the pain) may be hard to find, but the source of the pain itself is very obvious.

Muscles and Fascia. Pain in the muscles and fascia (including tendons) of the masticatory apparatus may resemble odontalgia, tic douloureux or atypical facial neuralgia. This is discussed in more detail under temporomandibular joint problems (see Case Report Nos. 28, 29, 30, 31 and 34).

Central Nervous System Neoplasms. When neoplasms encroach on nerves within the cranium or produce traction on nerve roots, pain is produced. In very rare cases the trigeminal nerve alone is affected, but most often there are other obvious neurologic deficits present. A detailed description is omitted since these can be so varied depending on the site of the tumor.

Bell's Palsy. A description of this condition appears elsewhere in the text, but of importance is the fact that in many—possibly 50 per cent—of these cases the patient experiences severe pain over the stylomastoid canal behind the ear *before* the facial paralysis occurs. This may last for 24 to 48 hours and usually disappears when the muscle weakness begins. Its significance lies in the fact that the pain may appear to be odontalgia, and when the paralysis appears after an extraction the dentist may have difficulty in convincing the patient that he did not cause the paralysis.

Herpes Zoster. This is a viral disease that causes skin and mucosal eruptions along the course of nerves, but rarely involves the maxillary or mandibular branches of the fifth nerve. However, in its prodromal stage there is often severe burning pain of the skin and mucosa which may be difficult to identify, since herpes zoster occurs so infrequently that the clinician may not think of it in his differential diagnosis. Once the vesicular lesions appear, however, it cannot be mistaken for anything else. After the skin and mucosal lesions disappear, changes in the nerve itself may cause paresthesias and toothaches that are not very responsive to therapy.

Collagen Diseases. Some collagen diseases may cause facial pain. See the discussion of temporal (cranial) arteritis (page 1699), the section on pain in the temporomandibular joint (page 1713), and Case Report Nos. 17 and 27.

Multiple Sclerosis. This is a disease of the central nervous system with multiple manifestations, one of which may be facial pain identical with that of tic douloureux. It occurs mostly in persons 20 to 40 years old, while most real tic occurs in those over 50 years old. (See the section on tic douloureux for a more detailed description of the pain it causes.) Patients suffering from multiple sclerosis usually have, in addition to the pain, a history of episodes of diplopia, nystagmus, transitory limb weakness or muscle fasciculations.

SPECIFIC PAIN SYNDROMES

TIC DOULOUREUX*†

This is a disease of middle age and later life.

Until the advent of the electron microscope the exact pathologic changes were unknown. In recent studies of the nerves and ganglia of patients with tic, however, investigators using the electron microscope have revealed marked changes in the myelin sheaths, both proliferative and degenerative, with the conductive portion of the nerve fiber eccentrically rather than centrally positioned. Under the light microscope these pathologic changes had never been seen. The cause of these pathologic changes still remains unknown.

The main characteristic of tic is that the pain is paroxysmal, *i.e.,* short, jabbing and lancinating, rather than steady. It is as if the victim were receiving a series of short electrical shocks. It may be intensely severe or, in the early stages, relatively mild, becoming severe in its later stages. The series of individual paroxysmal pains may last for seconds or minutes at first and for hours in its later

---

* We use this term synonomously with trigeminal neuralgia and trifacial neuralgia, although some clinicians use the latter terms for describing other neuralgias. We believe that this leads to some of the confusion in the literature with respect to diagnosis, cure rates, etc. The term pseudo tic douloureux is used by us to describe the tic-like pains which may be caused by factors such as nerve fiber compression or amputation neuromas (see Case Report No. 5), but idiopathic tic douloureux is a separate and distinct syndrome that, in its pure form, is different from all other neuralgias.

† Note that very recent theories on the etiology, pathophysiology, nomenclature and surgical treatment of tic are included in the article entitled "Trigeminal Neuralgia," beginning on page 1697.

stages. The disease has another characteristic that is very important in evaluation of "cures"—spontaneous remissions. It is often worse in the spring and fall. When the pain is severe the patient cannot sleep and may be driven to suicide. It always follows known nerve distributions of the trigeminal nerve and usually has a "trigger area," where stimulation will produce one or more "shocks." While there may be deep pain, there is *always* cutaneous pain sensation, but no hypoesthesia or hyperesthesia of the skin or mucous membranes affected exists after the paroxysm has subsided. There are no visible vascular changes. When a patient displays such a set of symptoms, extraction of teeth should *never* be performed, yet year after year we see patients who have had one or even all of their teeth extracted in an effort to relieve the pain.

Medical Treatment. In the past decade the use of anticonvulsant drugs, particularly diphenylhydantoin (Dilantin) and carbamazepine (Tegretol), has radically changed the treatment of tic. It is our feeling that medical treatment with efficacious drugs should be tried before surgery, and surgery reserved only for patients unresponsive to drug treatment. Diphenylhydantoin in doses of 0.1 to 0.2 gm. three times a day or carbamazepine in doses of 0.1 to 0.3 gm. twice a day are used in the acute phase and patients often show remission of pain within 24 to 48 hours. A maintenance dose can then be found on a trial-and-error basis by giving just enough medication to prevent the pain and not enough to cause side effects. This dosage is then gradually reduced on a daily basis so that when the patients are in remission they are not taking the drugs. (See Case Report No. 3.)

The side effects (urticaria, agranulocytosis, dermatitis, liver dysfunction) of these drugs are much greater with carbamazepine than with diphenylhydantoin; periodic blood counts and liver function tests are indicated, especially with carbamazepine. For this reason diphenylhydantoin is our drug of first choice. If the pain becomes unresponsive we then use carbamazepine, and if it becomes uneffective we switch back to diphenylhydantoin. If both drugs become uneffective, surgery is then considered.

Case Report No. 3

TIC DOULOUREUX TREATED WITH ANTICONVULSANT THERAPY

A 76-year-old male presented with classic tic of the left mandibular nerve with a trigger point directly over the mental foramen. There was paroxysmal pain radiating into the lip and jaw. He had all his teeth except the third molars, and while there was moderate recession of the gingivae there was no periodontal disease. The exposed cementum at the gingival line was slightly sensitive to thermal changes but did not provoke the tic-like pain. He stated that for the past 4 years he had experienced episodes of pain for 7 to 10 days in the spring and fall similar to the present episode but of much less intensity. The present pain, however, was unbearable. He was given a prescription for diphenylhydantoin (Dilantin, 0.1 gm.) and instructed to take two every 8 hours and return the next day, at which time he reported that the pain had ceased after the second dose had been taken. He was slightly dizzy (as would be expected from such a large dose) and was instructed to reduce his dosage to 0.1 gm. every 8 hours. This resulted in the loss of the dizzy feeling but a return of pain of less intensity than before. The dosage was increased therefore to 0.1 gm. every 6 hours, and at this dosage the patient experienced no side effects and was pain-free. After 1 week the dosage was decreased again to 0.1 gm. every 8 hours without return of pain. Over the next week the patient stopped taking the diphenylhydantoin and was pain-free.

Six months later the identical situation recurred, and he was treated in exactly the same way. Since then he has had four other episodes of pain, all well controlled with a similar routine. Five years have elapsed since the first visit.

Comment. If all cases of tic douloureux responded in this manner we would indeed have a medical panacea. However, judicious use of diphenylhydantoin can, in many cases, tide the patient over until the spontaneous remission occurs. Most of our experience has been in the use of diphenylhydantoin, and at times we supplement it with mephenesin (Tolseram), phenobarbital or diphenhydramine (Benadryl) in varying dosages if the patient develops side effects from the high dosages of diphenylhydantoin necessary to relieve the pain.

Case Report No. 4

PSYCHOSIS AND PSEUDO TIC DOULOUREUX

An edentulous male patient aged 60 came to the clinic with a complaint of pain in the lower left bicuspid region.

History. The patient stated that 3 years ago all his remaining maxillary and mandibular teeth had been extracted. Within a month a persistent pain began that manifested itself as a "pin-pricking" sensation in the lower left mental foramen region. The attacks of pain were limited to only half of the face and did not cross the median line. The patient noted that the pain was considerably increased upon shaving or washing his face, with a "trigger point" located at the corner of the lower left lip. The pain had been steadily increasing in intensity. Hot fluids or hot foods produce the pain, making it difficult for the patient to carry on normal masticatory functions. Since the patient had neurotic tendencies, psychiatric treatment was instituted after the first attack. However, the treatment was fruitless, since the patient claimed the pains became more intense. He returned to his dentist, who made a thorough x-ray examination of his mandible, but found nothing that could be the cause of the pain. The patient throughout this time became increasingly nervous and apprehensive, and threatened suicide as a possible "cure" for his ailment.

Diagnosis. A final diagnosis of chronic paresthesia, with neuralgic pain aggravated by a trigger zone, a pseudo tic douloureux, was made.

Treatment. The treatment methods considered were an alcohol injection in the lower left mental region or intraoral avulsion of the mental nerve, the latter giving more permanent relief. Therefore a mandibular injection of 2 per cent procaine was given to the patient to help him decide whether he preferred the anesthesia of the jaw to the continual attacks of pain. The painful symptoms disappeared as the inferior alveolar nerve became anesthetized. However, the patient complained bitterly about his "numb and swollen lip," and stated that he would just as soon have the pain as to have his lip "paralyzed." He was assured that his lip would return to normal and he could then decide whether or not he would rather have the pain or the numb lip. Evidently the patient preferred to withstand the continued attacks of pain, since he did not return.

Comment. This is the only case that I have seen in which the patient preferred pain to numbness. I am convinced that the symptoms this patient complained of were greatly magnified by the low threshold of pain he undoubtedly had.

Surgical Treatment. POSTGANGLIONIC SURGERY (PERIPHERAL NEURECTOMY). This type of surgery, which usually involves destruction or avulsion of the nerve at the mental foramen (see Figure 26–1), infraorbital foramen, nasopalatine foramen or mandibular foramen in the ramus, has the advantage of being relatively easy to do and carries practically no mortality or morbidity. The disadvantage is that the postganglionic fiber regenerates and, despite the most careful surgery, pain recurrence may be encountered. The use of bone wax or Silastic plugs where the nerve has been avulsed at a foramen (mental, mandibular, infraorbital, nasopalatine) tends to slow down nerve regeneration. In some patients, surprisingly enough, nerve regeneration with return of full sensation occurs *without* the return of the symptoms. (See Case Report Nos. 5 through 10.)

PREGANGLIONIC SURGERY (RETROGASSERIAN RHIZOTOMY). This is an intracranial procedure done by the neurosurgeon in which the sensory root of the gasserian ganglion is selectively cut. This produces permanent anesthesia of the area supplied by the cut nerves. This procedure carries with it a greater morbidity and mortality than does the peripheral neurectomy,* and occasional complications occur if there is loss of corneal sensation. It does produce good results in patients with true tic douloureux; in the atypical and other neuralgias it is useless. It often results in postoperative facial paresthesias, but in most cases these are not as severe as the original pain. Some patients, however, find them very uncomfortable.

There are other procedures also done intracranially by the neurosurgeon in which the nerve is not cut but decompressed (Taarnhøj procedure[76]) or compressed (technique of Sheldon and Pudenz[70]). The best results in these procedures are obtained when there is some postoperative sensory loss or paresthesia in the face such as may be experienced

---

* The microneurosurgery described in the article beginning on page 1697 apparently offers much more hope for the patient whose tic cannot be controlled by medical means, by chemosurgery or by peripheral neurectomy. We would therefore recommend it in preference to the rhizotomy mentioned here if intracranial procedures are to be employed.

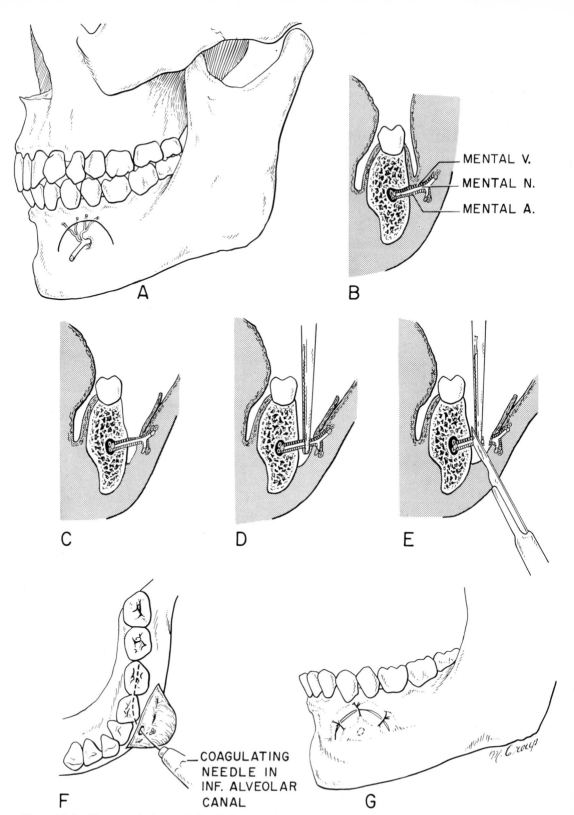

MENTAL V.

MENTAL N.

MENTAL A.

COAGULATING
NEEDLE IN
INF. ALVEOLAR
CANAL

Figure 26–1 Electrosurgical neurolysis of the mental nerve. *A,* Intraoral semicircular incision over the mental foramen. *B,* Cross-sectional view prior to incision. *C,* Same view after incision and reflection of the mucoperiosteum to expose vessels and nerve. *D,* Vessels and nerve grasped with a hemostat. *E,* With a scalpel, all grossly visible nerve is resected. *F,* Electrocoagulation of the nerve in the canal. *G,* Incision closed.

following selective section of the sensory root, and in general these procedures exhibit a greater percentage of recurrence of pain than occurs in sensory root section.

Reputable neurosurgeons still disagree as to the choice of procedure, and each weighs the greater possible complications of root section against the greater possibility of pain recurrence from compression and/or decompression and comes up with his own answer. Nevertheless, they all agree that with the proper choice of patient, *i.e.,* one with a true tic, an intracranial operative procedure gives good results in the long run. From a practical clinical standpoint, however, in cases in which more conservative management works, when the diagnosis is in doubt, and when the patient is afraid of the surgery or is a poor risk, we feel that intracranial surgery is a last resort. Attempts have also been made to section the pain fibers of the fifth nerve within the brain itself (tractotomy operation) so as to preserve sensation while abolishing pain in the face. Unfortunately, the hazards of this procedure and technical difficulties are so great that it has been virtually abandoned.

Case Report No. 5

PSEUDO TIC DOULOUREUX

A woman aged 59 had a severe lancinating pain originating in the lower jaw. She had a history of excruciating pain radiating out from the crest of the mandibular ridge in the region of the symphysis. This pain was present when her lip, or anything she placed in her mouth, touched one particular area. She had consulted several dentists and physicians, and all had agreed that she had tic douloureux.

Oral Examination. Examination of the ridges revealed both maxilla and mandible to be edentulous. All maxillary teeth had been extracted 9 months ago. The mandibular teeth had been extracted 7 months ago. The patient first noticed this pain 3 months ago. She reported back to the dental infirmary, and at that time the soft tissues were dissected back from the ridge, and a mandibular alveolectomy was performed because of sharp, irregular projections of bone on the ridge. However, the pain was not relieved by this operation.

On examining the area in which this super-sensitive spot was located, the so-called "trigger zone," I could see a grayish white line indicating the superficial location of one of the terminal branches of the mental nerve, about 0.5 mm. wide and 5 mm. long, extending from a point in the midline just labial to the crest of the ridge, and sloping distally gradually toward the mucobuccal fold in the direction of the mental foramen for a distance of 5 mm.

When all areas of the mucosa in the region of the symphysis were touched with the rounded blunt end of a cotton applicator stick, no pain was felt by the patient, except in the area just described.

When any point along this line was touched with the applicator, the patient jumped and cried out from pain. This pain, from her reaction and description, was similar to that experienced when the exposed pulp in a tooth is probed or touched. The pain quickly died down after removal of the pressure.

A test injection of 0.5 cc. of a 2 per cent procaine hydrochloride and 1:60,000 epinephrine solution was made in the region of the lower left mental foramen. After anesthesia had been established, pressure along the strip did not create any pain. The patient was asked to note when her painful symptoms returned, and was given an appointment for the following day. On her return she reported that as soon as the numbness had worn off, she had had a return of the same painful syndrome as previously.

Operation. It was decided to remove this strip of nerve tissue in an attempt to free the patient from additional attacks of pain.

Under infiltration anesthesia, with 2 per cent procaine hydrochloride, a strip of mucous membrane and nerve tissue down to the periosteum, 3 mm. wide and 15 mm. long, was removed. The surrounding mucosa was loosened, and a continuous suture introduced to approximate the edges.

After this operation the patient was free from pain, which has never returned.

Case Report No. 6

PSEUDO TIC DOULOUREUX OF THE MENTAL NERVE

A female patient aged 56, edentulous for 9 years, had been unable to wear her lower denture for the past 2 years because she was told that she had "tic douloureux" in her right jaw. She had these attacks of severe, sharp lightning-like pains radiating from her jaw into her lip only when she wore her lower denture. Repeated adjustments and remakes of her lower denture did not provide relief.

Examination revealed a thin mandible devoid of alveolar process. Digital pressure on the mandible in the region of the mental foramen quickly produced the so-called tic douloureux pain.

It was obvious that, because of the resorption of the alveolar process, the mental foramen was in the center of the mandible, and the denture compressed the mental nerve against its bony orifice, producing acute radiating pain which simulated tic douloureux.

A similar anatomic situation prevailed on the left jaw, but for unknown reasons there was no pain there.

Treatment. The mental nerve was anesthetized to determine if this was the source of pain. As long as anesthesia was present the patient could chew vigorously *without pain*. The injection also served another purpose: namely, to give the patient an opportunity to decide whether or not she preferred numbness in her lip or the pain. The patient quickly elected numbness.

She was admitted to the hospital, and under Pentothal anesthesia the mental nerve was avulsed, and the contents of the mental foramen and a portion of the inferior alveolar canal coagulated. This produced profound numbness, and for the past year the patient has worn her lower denture comfortably.

Case Report No. 7

TIC DOULOUREUX AND IMPACTED TOOTH

A 65-year-old retired coal miner was seen with a chief complaint of lancinating pain in the right lower jaw when eating, talking or swallowing. It had been present for 2 weeks and was not relieved by aspirin or narcotics. Periodontal disease was present in the lower molars, and the patient was edentulous in the upper jaw and wore a well-fitting upper denture. The attacks of pain were so severe that the patient was afraid to eat or drink. Radiographs were essentially negative except for the presence of an unerupted impacted maxillary right third molar and the periodontal disease in the remaining lower teeth. There was a trigger area just lingual to the lower right second molar. The pain radiated from the ear to the lower lip when the trigger area was touched. The teeth were not sensitive to either heat or cold.

A mandibular block of N.P.C. relieved the pain and it returned when the anesthesia wore off. Since drug therapy for tic was not satisfactory at the time this patient was seen (1959), he was admitted to the hospital for surgery. Under local anesthesia the mandibular nerve was resected for a distance of 20 to 25 mm. above the lingula at the mandibular foramen via a vertical incision along the pterygomandibular raphe followed by blunt dissection along the medial surface of the ramus of the mandible. Bone wax was packed into the mandibular foramen after removing as much of the nerve as possible with dental curettes. Postoperatively the lip was numb and the patient was free of pain. There was some postoperative trismus and

muscle spasm which disappeared totally in several months.

The patient was seen again 6½ years later with what appeared to be a classic case of tic douloureux of the second division of the right fifth nerve with a trigger point at the crest of the maxillary ridge in the third molar area. He wanted "another nerve cut" since the first operation had been such a success. The lower lip had *no anesthesia* left and he was pain-free in this area. Because the office was busy, I did not take care to carefully recheck the patient's records and, diagnosing this as a new tic, prescribed Dilantin, 100 mg. four times a day. He returned in 4 days with no relief and I then carefully checked his records and radiographs and belatedly remembered the impacted maxillary right third molar. New radiographs revealed the tooth just below the trigger area with a portion of the crown resorbed. The maxilla was blocked with a local anesthetic, the tooth was removed, and the patient was then pain-free.

The patient returned 2½ years later with a recurrence of the tic douloureux of the third division of the fifth nerve on the right side. He was placed on Dilantin, 200 mg. three times a day, and had no relief, so he was switched to Tegretal, 200 mg. three times a day. This controlled his pain and the dosage was gradually reduced to 50 mg. per day, except during occasional acute episodes of pain (every 2 or 3 months) when he had to increase the dose.

1690

Six months later he reappeared in severe pain, apparently unresponsive to both Tegretal and Dilantin. He was also in congestive heart failure. He was admitted to the hospital and after emergency treatment with diuretics, digitalis and oxygen the right mandibular nerve was blocked with 1 cc. of 95 per cent alcohol. This was done rather than nerve resection because of his limited life expectancy. This relieved his pain until he died the following year.

Comment. This case illustrates both the older and more modern approaches to tic. In 1959 surgery was the first approach, but today we would treat him with anticonvulsants first, and then, when and if the disorder became refractory to the drugs, resort to surgery or alcohol. Of interest here are two things: (*a*) how an impacted tooth undergoing resorption and producing pulpitis can mimic tic douloureux and (*b*) how some patients regain normal sensation after nerve resection without recurrence of the tic for long periods of time.

Case Report No. 8

TIC DOULOUREUX UNRESPONSIVE TO DRUG THERAPY

A 68-year-old proctologist was seen in consultation for recurrent episodes of pain in the lower left biscupid area. The pain was acute and lancinating in character and occurred about every 6 months and lasted for 2 to 3 weeks. It was provoked by eating both hot and cold foods. There was moderate gingival recession with exposure of the cementum of the roots. All teeth including the third molars were present. He had been treated by desensitization of the exposed roots without success. At first the episodes of pain were of a mild nature but gradually became more severe and he was referred for possible extractions. X-rays revealed no apical pathology and he was placed on Dilantin, 0.1 gm. three times a day. Within 48 hours he noticed some relief of pain and his dosage was increased to 0.1 gm. four times a day, which gave him total relief. After 1 week his dosage was gradually reduced until he was no longer taking the Dilantin. Six months later he had a recurrence of the pain, which was again treated with Dilantin. Four months later he had another episode of pain at which time it was necessary to use 0.1 gm. of Dilantin six times a day to achieve relief. He again gradually decreased the dose and was pain-free for a period of approximately 1 year. Over the next 5 years he had several similar episodes of pain all well controlled with varying doses of Dilantin. He then developed a recurrence of pain that was totally unresponsive to any form of drug therapy and was admitted to the hospital. A left peripheral neurectomy was performed under local anesthesia at the mandibular foramen. Postoperatively he was pain-free but developed acute urinary obstruction caused by prostatic hypertrophy that required a suprapubic cystotomy. On the fourth postoperative day he suffered a cerebrovascular accident and died within 48 hours.

Comment. This is almost a classic example of tic confused with pathologic dental processes because of the low intensity of the pain in the early stages. The pain was well controlled with drug therapy until the disorder suddenly became refractory, at which time surgery was necessary. The postoperative problems that led to the patient's death were unrelated to either the tic or his surgery.

Case Report No. 9

NASOPALATINE NERVE NEURALGIA TREATED BY AVULSION

For 3 months a 27-year-old male patient had pain in the nasopalatine region triggered by anything cold, even the oral inhalation of cold air. A nasopalatine injection of local anesthetic solution prevented the stimulation of pain even though a piece of ice was held in contact with the nasopalatine papilla. Because effective quantities of alcohol injected into the nasopalatine canal produced sloughing of the soft tissue, the author reflected a palatal flap and then avulsed the neurovascular bundles from the nasopalatine canal. Bleeding was controlled by the electrocoagulating tip and the flap replaced and sutured.

This treatment gave the patient relief. (*Note:* Occasionally nerve regeneration requires a second operation.)

Case Report No. 10

PAIN IN THE MENTAL FORAMEN REGION TREATED BY MENTAL NERVE AVULSION

A 42-year-old male patient at the time of examination had acute continuous pain in the lower left mental foramen region. This pain had been present for 8 years, ever since he had a first premolar extracted, but it was growing progressively worse; he slept fitfully at night. His physician had given him some tablets to take but they had not helped.

All lower left mandibular teeth from the central incisor to the third molar had been extracted, one at a time over the years, in the vain hope that this would relieve his pain.

A careful oral and radiographic examination was negative. An inferior alveolar nerve block injection promptly stopped the pain. The patient elected avulsion of the mental nerve rather than alcohol injections because of the more permanent relief possible with avulsion. The results of the operation were very gratifying to the patient, and at this date, 5 years later, he has not had a recurrence of pain.

Chemosurgical Treatment. The placement of drugs, such as alcohol, boiling water or phenol solutions, in direct contact with nerves is another treatment of tic. Reversible agents, such as local anesthetics, may be used for temporary relief or during diagnosis, while protein precipitants may be used for more permanent relief. Alcohol (95 per cent) is the most commonly used agent, and if injected directly around the nerve will chemically equal the effect of a neurectomy with much less trouble. (See Case Report Nos. 11 through 15.) However, for deeper injections (mandibular block, second and third division block, gasserian ganglion injection, etc.), extreme accuracy is required in the placement of the alcohol. The usual dose is 1 to 2 cc. Since the tissues adjacent to the nerve also undergo coagulation necrosis, peripheral injections may produce considerable pain and edema followed by fibrosis. If well placed, a peripheral alcohol block may last for years, but in some patients repeat injections may be required much sooner. With each succeeding injection, as a general rule, the period of relief is shorter, until so much scar tissue is built up

that no relief is obtained. In injections into the gasserian ganglion, alcohol may escape and diffuse into adjacent areas, producing severe complications. The success of this injection depends on the skill of the operator.

Some neurosurgeons, using x-ray visualization, attempt to place a special insulated electric needle into the gasserian ganglion in order to electrocoagulate the ganglion itself. Nugent, at West Virginia University, has used this technique with excellent results in drug refractory tics.[57] He inserts the needle under light analgesia. When the needle is in the ganglion (determined by stereotactic x-ray techniques), the patient is awakened and a very low current applied as the needle is moved. When the tic pain is reproduced, the operator raises the current and selectively coagulates only a portion of the ganglion, instead of electrocoagulating the entire ganglion. This appears to be less hazardous than alcohol injections, and results again vary with the surgeon's skill. Destruction of the ganglion, of course, will provide the same permanent relief as surgical intervention.

Case Report No. 11

ACUTE TIC DOULOUREUX IN THE MANDIBLE

About 2 years previously, a woman aged 67 had felt a vague pain, which came and went, in her lower jaw. In spite of her age she had all her teeth except her third molars. Her teeth were noncarious but abraded.

The pain became increasingly severe, and at the

suggestion of her physician the patient went to a dentist, who felt that a lower second molar might be causing the pain. He extracted this tooth.

After this extraction the patient had no relief, and now felt that the pain was in her upper jaw. For this reason a maxillary molar was extracted.

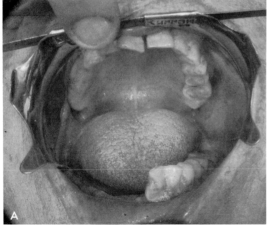

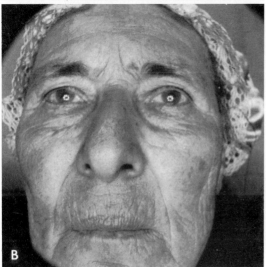

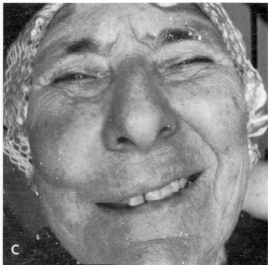

Figure 26-2 *A*, Patient's teeth were extracted one at a time to "cure" the pain. *B*, Typical frozen-face appearance in tic douloureux. *C*, Following alcohol injection, the patient is pain-free and can smile. (See Case Report No. 11.)

The pain continued, however, and increased in severity. Tooth after tooth, first from the maxilla and then from the mandible, was extracted, until all the right mandibular teeth, up to the midline, and all the maxillary teeth, up to the right cuspid, had been extracted in a vain attempt to eliminate the patient's pain (see Figure 26-2*A*).

At the time of her visit the patient had the typical fearful, frozen-face appearance of a patient with tic douloureux (see Figure 26-2*B*). If she moved her lower jaw or touched her lip, she experienced the typical sharp, knife-like pain shooting through her lip and lower jaw.

With considerable difficulty, because of the pain, an inferior alveolar nerve block was secured. This gave immediate relief. One cc. of 190 proof alcohol was mixed with 1 cc. of 2 per cent procaine hydrochloride, and the solution was slowly deposited into the mandibular sulcus. For the first time in 2 years, the patient was free of pain, and could smile (see Figure 26-2*C*).

Case Report No. 12

TIC DOULOUREUX OF THE MANDIBLE, LIP AND TONGUE

A male patient, aged 59, had a sharp stabbing pain in the tongue and lip that was started by eating or talking. The pain seemed to start in the right temporomandibular joint and end between the bicuspids. These teeth were so sore during the attack that he could not touch them with his finger. The entire lip and tongue were "painfully numb" during the acute spasm of pain. The pain lasted 10 to 15 minutes and gradually the numbness and pain tapered off for the next 20 minutes, leaving a residual soreness which lasted several hours, or until the next acute spasm of pain.

History. Five years previously he had had the apparently normal right mandibular molars extracted to relieve a neuralgic type of pain that seemed to center in those teeth; the pain was not relieved. Since then he has had periods of pain and pain-free periods, the latter sometimes lasting for months.

During the past year the painful periods had become more acute and in the past few days the severity had increased to the point where the pain was trigger-like and so intense as to be paralyzing.

Treatment. An attempt was made to determine whether the long buccal, lingual or inferior alveolar nerve was the "trigger nerve" by blocking each one individually with local anesthetic solution.

It was soon apparent that all three would have to be blocked to stop the pain completely.

Over a 15-day period 3 injections of 1 cc. of 190 proof alcohol and 1 cc. of local anesthetic solution were made so as to anesthetize the inferior alveolar, the long buccal and the lingual nerves. The pain ceased.

One year later the patient began to have a recurrence of pain. Again 1 cc. of 190 proof alcohol (without the local anesthetic solution) was injected. He has been free from pain for the past 2 years.

Case Report No. 13

TIC DOULOUREUX IN THE LOWER LIP AND MANDIBLE

A 79-year-old male patient has acute spasms of "real hot sharp pains" in the mandibular left molar region and lip. He can neither eat nor talk without stimulating the pain. Even when sleeping he will be awakened with attacks of this pain, which last several minutes, then gradually disappear. Frequently he will have another attack in 10 to 15 minutes, or he may be free of pain for an hour.

Treatment. A left inferior alveolar nerve block was accomplished with 1 cc. of 190 proof alcohol and 0.75 cc. of local anesthetic solution. The lip became numb and a recurrence of pain could not be provoked.

One year later the patient had a recurrence of the above symptoms. Numbness was no longer present in the lip. At this time the treatment was an inferior alveolar nerve block with 1.5 cc. of 190 proof alcohol and 0.5 cc. of local anesthetic solution.

One week later the patient was 90 per cent relieved, but movement of his cheek produced some pain. The pain was controlled with a long buccal nerve block with 0.5 cc. of 190 proof alcohol and 1 cc. of local anesthetic solution.

Case Report No. 14

TIC DOULOUREUX OF THE SECOND DIVISION OF THE FIFTH NERVE

For the past 2 years Mrs. R. S., aged 58, has had an increasingly severe spasmodic pain in the left maxilla, upper lip and nose. Figure 26–3 shows the patient's face during an attack of pain. Four months ago, she had all her maxillary teeth extracted because she was told they were the cause of her pain. Since then her pain has increased in severity and frequency. Movement of the upper lip triggers the pain (see Figure 26–3). A

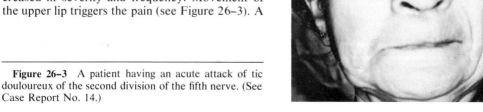

Figure 26–3 A patient having an acute attack of tic douloureux of the second division of the fifth nerve. (See Case Report No. 14.)

left infraorbital injection of local anesthetic solution stopped the pain.

The patient stated that she preferred the numbness to the pain, so on her next visit 1.5 cc.

of 190 proof alcohol and 1 cc. of local anesthetic were injected in the region of the left infraorbital canal. This has given the patient complete relief of pain.

Case Report No. 15

TIC DOULOUREUX OF THE THIRD DIVISION OF THE FIFTH NERVE

Three years ago this male patient, aged 77, who was edentulous, began to have a mild neuralgic pain in the lower jaw that gradually increased in intensity and was excited by movement of the upper right lip. Although he would sleep through the night, he always had a severe attack, which lasted from 10 to 15 minutes, on awakening in the morning. Figure 26–4 shows the patient's face during an acute attack of pain. It was with difficulty that he held reasonably still while the photograph was taken.

During the past year he has had as many as 10 to 15 attacks in 1 day, lasting from 10 to 20 minutes to over an hour. On other days he has had only the first attack in the morning and none during the rest of the day. The pain now not only involves the lower lip and jaw but extends back over the right temporal region, and within the last 10 days the right forehead has also been involved when he has the acute attacks of pain. He now has two trigger zones; the first is still the right upper lip and the second is the right forehead.

He had a series of 10 daily injections of 1000 μg. of vitamin B$_{12}$, which did not give him any relief.

A right inferior alveolar nerve block injection of 1 cc. of 190 proof alcohol and 1 cc. of local anesthetic solution gave him complete relief from pain for 4 months. He began to have pain again, so he was given another injection of 2 cc. of 190 proof

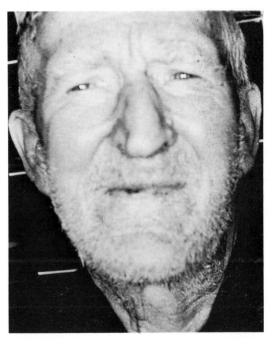

Figure 26–4 Patient with an attack of tic douloureux of the third division of the fifth nerve. (See Case Report No. 15.)

alcohol. Relief again followed, and the patient is still comfortable.

Summary of Treatment. As emphasized previously, the primary requisite in treatment is establishing the correct diagnosis. While the textbook picture is clear, any experienced clinician is aware of the fact that many cases have mixed elements that confuse the clinical picture and, as a general rule, does not like to make a firm diagnosis until he is thoroughly familiar with the patient. In some patients it may be several months before a positive diagnosis can be made. Nevertheless, the patient must be treated, so the best general philosophy to adopt is to try treatment methods at

first that, in themselves, produce as few permanent irreversible changes as possible. While at times this may be impossible, we try to avoid subjecting the patient to operative or radical chemosurgery in the early stages until we are sure of the diagnosis.

If the history the patient relates leads us to believe that tic douloureux is the correct diagnosis, we try anticonvulsant therapy first.* To confirm our diagnosis a local anes-

---

* The patient should have an adequate neurologic evaluation to rule out neoplasms, aneurysms and so forth before the start of any therapy.

thetic block is often done at the first appointment. If anticonvulsant therapy is not successful a local anesthetic block (if not done previously) is performed to make sure we have the correct nerve and to allow the patient to experience the numb sensation he will have, and this is followed by a peripheral alcohol block. For the mental nerve, nasopalatine and infraorbital nerves, if the alcohol block gives relief of pain, we repeat the blocks as necessary until they become ineffective, at which time peripheral neurectomy can be done.

One of us (D.D.) prefers not to do alcohol blocks for the mandibular and lingual nerve involvements and does an avulsion first, followed later by alcohol block if necessary, since surgery in this area is difficult after alcohol injections because of the fibrosis. The other (W.H.A.) prefers to start with and continue the use of alcohol blocks in these areas. Either technique is satisfactory and varies with the individual surgeon's choice.

Drug therapy, carefully managed, can keep many patients comfortable for their entire lives. When the disorders become resistant to drugs, peripheral neurectomy or alcohol block is our next step, and we repeat this as necessary. Only as a last resort do we feel that intracranial procedures are indicated.* It is interesting to note that in the last decade this philosophy is being adopted more and more by neurologists, and we have been seeing neurosurgeons as well as oral surgeons doing more peripheral neurectomies than ever before.

At times we are faced with a patient in whom a clear-cut diagnosis of tic douloureux cannot be made but who obtains complete relief with an injection of local anesthetic. Some of the vascular neuralgias limited to the infraorbital artery or mental artery produce such a clinical picture, and the use of alcohol blocks in these patients is worth trying if the surgeon is aware of what he is treating (see Case Report No. 16). Deeper alcohol injections for neuralgias other than true tic may only produce more pain than was originally present, and the promiscuous use of such alcohol injections must be condemned.

---

* When intracranial procedures are deemed necessary, those described in the article following would seem preferable to the rhizotomy.

Case Report No. 16

ACUTE NEURALGIC PAIN IN THE RIGHT MAXILLA

For 4 years, this female patient, aged 65, who was edentulous, had a neuralgic pain in the right maxilla that originally only bothered her at irregular intervals, and then not very severely. As time passed, the attacks became more frequent and increased in severity until they occurred daily and were acute, as shown in Figure 26–5A. (Note the frozen, agonized expression on her face.) This was not a typical tic douloureux because there was no trigger zone, and the attacks came on slowly, gradually increasing in intensity, and then slowly tapered off, with residual soreness lasting several hours.

The anterior, middle and posterior superior alveolar nerves were blocked on two occasions 10 days apart with 2 cc. 190 proof alcohol and 2 cc. local anesthetic solution each time. Figure 26–5B shows the patient's pain-free, smiling face after the second set of injections 9 days after the first ones.

The patient had complete relief for 12 weeks, at which time she began to have a recurrence. The same nerves were again blocked with the same quantity of alcohol and local anesthetic solution, which gave her complete relief for 2½ years. Again the same injections were made, and these lasted for 6 months, when the patient returned with early slight return of pain. At this and the previous time the patient and her family were advised to wait until the attacks of pain became severe, but to this neither she nor her family would agree even though it was pointed out that each series of alcohol injections theoretically gives relief of pain for a shorter duration.

The following year this patient developed a true tic douloureux, with the trigger zone in the right upper lip. She has been kept comfortable since then by extraoral infraorbital injections of 1 cc. of 190 proof alcohol with local anesthesia, averaging about one a year. The last injection was given 10 years after the first ones. This case is the longest in the author's series and provides an exception to the rule that if the patient lives long enough the nerve is no longer anesthetized by repeated injections of alcohol.

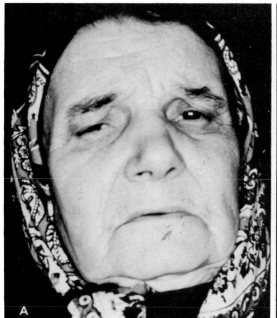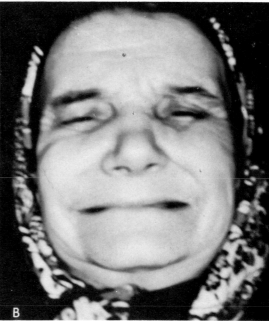

Figure 26–5 *A*, Typical facial expression of a patient with acute neuralgic pain in the right maxilla. (See Case Report No. 16.) *B*, The patient smiles with relief because she is now free from pain following an alcohol injection.

TRIGEMINAL NEURALGIA

PETER J. JANNETTA, M.D.

Trigeminal neuralgia is a symptom of hyperactive dysfunction of the trigeminal nerve, usually caused by mild compression-distortion of the trigeminal nerve at the pons by normal vascular loops.[41–47] In a review of my first 100 consecutive operative patients with trigeminal neuralgia,[47] I noted that approximately 80 per cent of these patients went to their dentists at the time of their initial attacks. Many of these patients underwent dental extractions without relief of their pain. The dentists practicing in my referral area have now become very astute in making the diagnosis of trigeminal neuralgia. Because the symptom complex is usually clear-cut and definitive microsurgical treatment is now available, it is hoped that general practitioners everywhere will come to recognize the symptoms and avoid needless extractions.

Recognition of Trigeminal Neuralgia. Trigeminal neuralgia (tic douloureux) is a symptom complex of facial pain with the following characteristics: The pain is abrupt in onset and offset and usually of brief duration. The patient almost universally can remember circumstances of the first attack in vivid detail, no matter how long ago it occurred. The pain is unilateral and is limited to the trigeminal nerve's sensory distribution. Sequential bilateral trigeminal neuralgia occurs in a small percentage of cases. Trigeminal neuralgia is about half again more common in women than in men and about twice as common on the right side of the face as on the left side. The pain is much more frequent in the lower face (third and second trigeminal divisions) than in the first division. It may occur at any time of the day, but it rarely awakens the patient from sleep. Attacks may occur spontaneously or be precipitated by moving the face, as in talking or eating, brushing the teeth, shaving, applying cold water, a cool breeze or a light touch to the face. A "trigger point," which may vary in location over a period of time, may be present. It is usually located around the nostrils in lower facial tic. The slightest stimulus to this area may precipitate an attack. The patient, therefore, will characteristically never touch the face in demonstrating the location of pain, but will carefully keep the hand off the skin. Attacks may occur irregularly and very infrequently or may occur up to 200 times per day. The patient lives in dread of the next attack. The attack is usually brief, but in long-standing cases may rarely last 30 to 60 minutes. The pain is described as lancinating, paroxysmal, "like a hot poker or electrical shock." The patient will frequently grimace remarkably during an attack.

In time, attacks usually become more prolonged and frequent, although remaining variable. As the years go by, a characteristic chronic, burning facial pain may gradually develop and become more severe. This pain may rarely supersede the tic. A certain percentage of patients (up to 33 per cent) will develop mild sensory deficit in the trigeminal distribution, as proved in careful testing.

A microsurgical operation utilizing a supracerebellar retromastoid approach to the trigeminal nerve at the brain stem has demonstrated the precise pathophysiologic changes in this clinical entity, which lends itself to definitive therapy. Abnormalities of the trigeminal nerve at the brain stem, usually vascular cross–compression-distortion, have been seen in 100 consecutive operative patients with trigeminal neuralgia.[41–47] These precise changes have not been seen in over 50 patients operated upon for problems other than trigeminal neuralgia, nor in over 250 dissections of fresh cadavers, although vessels frequently surround the trigeminal nerve. They have been noted in two brains of patients with trigeminal neuralgia who died of other problems. The following abnormalities have been noted: compression-distortion of the root entry zone of the trigeminal nerve at the pons by an arterial loop, usually of the superior cerebellar artery (in 86 patients) (Fig. 26–6), by venous compression (in 2 patients), by arteriovenous malformations (in 2 patients), and by a neoplasm that was compressing and distorting the entry zone of the nerve (in 4 patients); multiple sclerosis plaques at the entry zone of the nerve (in 4 women with multiple sclerosis); atrophy without plaque (in 2 older women with clinical evidence of old multiple sclerosis). It must be noted that an atrophic nerve surrounded by many looping arteries without clear compression-distortion was seen in one elderly woman who had undergone prior subtemporal retrogasserian rhizotomy. She was included in the first group that was operated upon in the lateral recumbent position. This finding may corroborate the positional changes in trigeminal neuralgia (i.e., tic

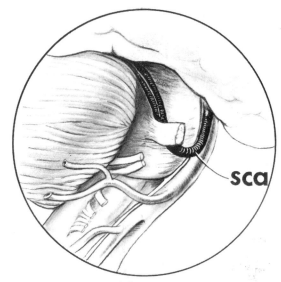

Figure 26–6 Lower facial trigeminal neuralgia. Trigeminal nerve cross-compression is caused at the brain stem by the superior cerebellar artery (*sca*).

occurs rarely in sleep because the patient is lying down rather than because he is asleep).

Operative Results. Fifty patients in this series underwent decompression of the trigeminal nerve at the brain stem *without section* of the trigeminal nerve through a supracerebellar exposure as treatment of trigeminal neuralgia. Many of these patients temporarily retained or had some episodes of trigeminal neuralgia postoperatively. This gradually faded away over a period of 2 days to 3 months. Other patients in whom more manipulation of the nerve was necessary to mobilize the vessel away from the nerve were better immediately and have remained so. The longest follow-up in the decompression group is 8½ years.

Morbidity has been mild, consisting of a prolonged headache in a number of patients. This is always self-limited. Two patients have had prolonged postoperative stance and gait ataxia. In one, an intrinsic pontine vein was coagulated and divided at the root entry zone of the trigeminal nerve. In the second patient, a second procedure was carried out because the pain was not relieved. It was found that the cerebellar hemisphere was infarcted. The lateral branch of the superior cerebellar artery was found to be occluded, while the medial branch of the artery was back on the nerve. This branch was again mobilized, and a selective section of the nerve performed. The ataxia cleared remarkably. The patient remains relieved of his pain. There has been one late recurrence due to a second artery that was cross-compressing the nerve. In three other patients mild trigeminal neuralgia has recurred early. In two patients the pain has not gone away completely, including the one mentioned above. One patient, a 79-year-old woman, suffered a postoperative cerebrovascular accident and died on the sixth postoperative day. In retrospect, I recognize that she probably should not have been operated upon. She was working full time and told us she was 59 years old. We, unfortunately, believed her.

Discussion. Trigeminal neuralgia, as noted by Gardner,[32] is a symptom rather than a disease. Dandy[16-18] noted abnormalities of the trigeminal nerve root entry zone in 60 per cent of his operative patients with trigeminal neuralgia, but he did not attempt to treat the pain by decompression of the nerve. However, he did not have the magnification and lighting of the surgical binocular microscope available to him. It is impressive to this author that Dandy was able to see as much as he did, as these vascular structures are small, and his operative approach to the nerve was from a difficult angle. Trigeminal neuralgia found to be caused by benign brain tumors and arteriovenous malformations has been termed "symptomatic trigeminal neuralgia" and placed in a separate category from the "idiopathic" common variety. This appears on the basis of these data to be an untenable subclassification. All trigeminal neuralgia is "symptomatic." The smaller causal abnormalities are just as real as the tumors, and these are now visible to us with magnification directed to the root entry zone of the nerve.

The abnormalities of compression-distortion of the root entry zone are subtle. If this were not so, the symptom complex would not be that of hyperactive dysfunction (*i.e.,* pain) but loss of function (facial numbness and temporomasseter muscle weakness and atrophy). Numbness is seen in the previously untreated patients only after prolonged symptoms. Similarly, electrical evidence of denervation of the muscles of mastication is noted, as tested by electromyography. Both these abnormalities return to normal after vascular decompression of the trigeminal nerve root entry zone, as was performed in the patients in this series.

The sequence of improvement after operation with this apparently definitive procedure differs significantly from that of any of the destructive procedures. In the former, relief of symptoms is gradual if the nerve is not touched at operation, immediate only if the nerve is manipulated or mildly traumatized. No late recurrences have been noted. In the latter form of treatment, relief is immediate but recurrences gradually supervene.

The operative procedure appears to be safe in the hands of a trained microneurosurgeon who is experienced in the surgery of the cerebellopontine angle.

Summary. Trigeminal neuralgia is a symptom of paroxysmal facial pain that has been successfully and permanently relieved in the past only by destructive operative procedures. The source of trigeminal neuralgia is compression-distortion of the nerve root entry zone, usually by a looping artery, infrequently by a bridging vein or tumor. In multiple sclerosis, trigeminal neuralgia is due to a multiple sclerosis plaque at the root entry zone. Trigeminal neuralgia can be safely relieved by a microvascular decompression procedure performed by a trained microneurosurgeon utilizing a retromastoid supracerebellar approach. The pain is relieved without concomitant numbness.

GLOSSOPHARYNGEAL NEURALGIA

In this very rare condition the patient experiences the same type of pain as in tic douloureux but in the ninth nerve with distribution to the base of the tongue, tonsils, soft palate and ear. Treatment has been intracranial section of the ninth nerve. The author is unaware whether the anticonvulsants have been tried in this disease since it is so rare. The important diagnostic feature of this entity is that the pain is stopped by anesthetizing the pharynx with a topical anesthetic where the trigger point is located.

TEMPORAL ARTERITIS

This pathologic entity is relatively rare, but its early diagnosis is important, and the patient must first consult the dentist. The essential pathology is vasculitis of the temporal artery and its branches. The etiology of the vasculitis is obscure and may be the result of a form of collagen disease, but the end result

TEMPORAL ARTERITIS

A 56-year-old female was referred by a dentist because of her inability to wear dentures. She had had, over the previous 9 months, two different sets of dentures constructed, neither of which was satisfactory, and in each case gave the dentist such a hard time that he returned her money. Intraoral examination revealed nothing dramatic, and the ridges appeared to be able to tolerate the necessary prosthesis. When asked why the dentures were unsatisfactory, she stated that they gave her a headache and she could not chew comfortably. Closer questioning revealed that the primary complaints were not in the mouth but in the temporal area and that the teeth had been reset several times in one of the dentures in an effort to find a comfortable bite.

The patient was a thin, irascible patient who appeared to be extremely difficult to please and of the type an experienced dentist recognizes as a treatment problem. When the temporal area was palpated, however, the patient nearly jumped out of the chair with pain. The temporal arteries were swollen and exquisitely tender. The patient's temperature was 100°F. and the sedimentation rate was 90 (normal 7 to 10). She was given hydrocortisone (Solu-Cortef), 500 mg. intravenously, at once plus corticotropin (ACTH Gel), 40 units intramuscularly, and placed on prednisolone tablets, 5 mg. every 6 hours. The next day she was seen by an internist and neurologist, who continued her treatment. Within a week she was a different person psychologically, and later she received a set of dentures that she wore without difficulty.

Comment. While this disease entity is relatively rare, it will probably occur in the future with increasing frequency. Prompt recognition is important, as explained in the text. In this case, the psychological changes due to the pain and severe depression might easily have led to the categorization of this patient as a psychological problem, and until she had gone blind or developed some other dramatic symptom the true nature of her disease would have been concealed.

---

is a reduction of blood flow and finally complete obliteration of the lumen of the vessel caused by inflammation and resultant thrombosis. The symptoms produced are vague unilateral pains in the head and upper jaw due to both the tenderness of the arteries themselves and the ischemia in the masticatory muscles. The pain is often intense and its distribution bizarre. In these patients, however, diagnosis is very easy because on palpation the temporal arteries are felt to be swollen and very tender, and further investigation will reveal a markedly elevated sedimentation rate and often an elevated temperature. The importance of early diagnosis in this disease is that involvement of the ophthalmic artery with a similar vasculitis is often occurring simultaneously with that in the temporal arteries, but until the patient suddenly goes blind no attention is focused on the eye. Thrombosis of the ophthalmic artery is, of course, irreversible and this catastrophe may be averted by prompt diagnosis and treatment with steroids.

PSYCHOGENIC NEURALGIAS

Into this category fall many of the pain syndromes in the literature. Their essential common denominator is that they are expressions of unconscious problems (in the psychiatric concept of the "unconscious") that take on such a variety of findings and symptomatology as to obscure their common origin. In some of these ailments their nature is obvious on the first appointment; in others their real cause is more obscure, and only after many therapeutic efforts does the truth begin to emerge.

As a broad generality one may divide these syndromes into two groups: those with and those without somatic manifestations. For those not versed in human psychodynamics, some abbreviated explanations may be in order.

Human actions are governed by thought processes and emotions that exist at four ascending levels: basic drives, unconscious, subconscious and conscious. Our basic drives (need for food, ego satisfaction, etc.) are our most primitive feelings and we learn to modify them into socially acceptable forms during our growth and development. Unfortunately this development is not smooth or equal for all people and the transition from infant to adult may be attended by much trauma to the psyche. This leaves scars in the form of unsolved problems residing in the unconscious. These bypassed problems may remain dormant until some experience in later life rouses them, or they may remain active and unsolved, like festering sores, producing constant difficulty at the conscious level. Unless a person has unusual insight, psychiatric help is needed to release these hidden unsolved problems from the unconscious. They may appear to the untrained eye as a conglomeration of peculiar unrelated symptoms. On the other hand, when the adult conscious level of the mind faces a difficult problem and represses it into the next lower level, the subconscious, this problem is usually much more superficial and much more easily recalled. Unless it has deep unconscious emotional associations, it will not produce severe manifestations. Although this description of the levels of the mind is only approximate it will be a useful frame of reference in an understanding of the psychodynamics with which we are concerned.

The other important concept to be grasped in the understanding of psychodynamics is that the concept of organic versus functional disease must be abandoned. There is no doubt that organic changes can arise as a result of psychic stimuli, especially to the vascular system (as in blushing, getting "white with anger" and so forth). Other organic changes (*e.g.*, peptic ulcer) have well-known psychogenic backgrounds and research in this field points with increasing clarity to the fact that the major factor in practically all disease is not the extrinsic causative factor but the alteration of the individual's physiology as determined by his psychologic and biochemical makeup. In essence, therefore, the presence of visible lesions (*e.g.*, vesicles, blanching, erythema and ulcers) should not blind the doctor to the fact that the initiating factor may be psychogenic. Therapy may be directed against the visible pathology with temporary relief, but the patient will never get permanent relief unless the basic problem is solved or converted to another set of symptoms.

Case Report No. 18

PSYCHOGENIC NEURALGIA AND A VERTICALLY IMPACTED LOWER THIRD MOLAR

A woman, aged 25, complained of a severe constant pain in the left side of the face and head.

History. The patient stated that this trouble had started two years ago. Whenever she became upset, the pain was so violent that she could not hold up her head. The patient would vomit and have to go to bed. After several repeated attacks, she went to her dentist, who said her teeth were all right, and referred her to a physician to treat her nerves.

The physician admitted the patient to a hospital for a general check-up, and found that her gallbladder was not normal. The patient was in the hospital for 10 days. Sedatives were administered to help her rest. She was discharged as improved.

However, the patient complained of recurrence of the symptoms at about 2-week intervals, each attack lasting about 2 days.

Eight months ago the patient again went to her dentist, who gave her sedatives, and asked her to call him if the pain persisted. She called his office 2 days later, but he was out of town, and his assistant referred her to another dentist, who also doubted that her teeth were responsible, and referred her to her family physician, who ordered sulfathiazole and salicylates. The patient did not improve, but vomited constantly for 2 days, after which she began to feel better. The patient tried self-dosing with self-prescribed proprietary remedies, but was not able to retain them.

Another physician was called, who examined the patient, and told her that she had facial neuralgia and tonsillitis. He gave her salicylates and codeine. She took 3 or 4 tablets at intervals of 3 hours, and the pain lessened. The patient continued taking codeine tablets less frequently, but was not entirely free from pain. The patient again went to her dentist about 6 months ago, and he extracted the upper left third molar in the hope that she would get some relief. This failing, he extracted the upper left second molar, which was carious, but the original complaint persisted, becoming more severe and constant. This pain was distributed over the area on the left side of the face and head supplied by the second and first divisions of the fifth cranial nerve.

About 6 weeks ago the patient had a sudden pain in the left hip. She went to her family physician, who said that the sciatic nerve was inflamed, and gave her medicine for this condition. The patient was confined to bed for 2 days. On the third night the pain "jumped from the hip into the face."

The patient was again admitted to the hospital, where she was treated for alveolalgia and for her nervous condition, and was released from the hospital after a few days of rest.

Five weeks ago the patient's mother took her to her (mother's) dentist, who examined the mouth visually and radiographically. He referred the patient to Dr. L. Friedman, who examined her and asked her to return at weekly intervals for a sinus check-up.

The patient was admitted to the Eye, Ear, Nose and Throat Hospital, after her third visit, to the services of Dr. Friedman and myself.

Examination. Findings in the physical examination were essentially negative. There was no tenderness of the face. The last two upper molars had been extracted; the other teeth were in good condition.

The diagnostic impression was trifacial neuralgia and emmetropia.

Laboratory Report. All findings were normal.

Dental Report. The patient had had a history of headaches, pain in the jaw and vague pains in the knees throughout her life. The headaches had been more severe for the past several years; they seemed to start in the left maxillary region and spread over the temple and into the patient's head. The upper left second and third molars had been removed. There was postoperative infection, with drainage from the socket, and the patient had suffered fever and chills. She was admitted to a hospital for treatment with penicillin. There was severe pain, but no swelling of the face. Since then the pain had occurred periodically, starting in the same region. The patient had had several dental examinations, none of which disclosed any source of pain.

Dental Examination. Dental x-ray examination revealed that the lower left third molar was vertically impacted, with the apex superimposed on or in the mandibular canal. The apex had a curved or grooved appearance, suggesting that it could possibly be encroaching on the inferior dental nerve. The upper left first molar showed a radiopaque substance in the pulp chamber, undoubtedly a pulp stone, and minor caries on the occlusal and distal surfaces. The pulp stones and the impacted teeth were obviously potential sources of the neuralgic pain.

Medical Report. The history was suggestive of migraine (vomiting), but was not conclusive. Although the patient might have had migraine in the past, and although there was a family history of migraine, the present pain was too constant, and suggested trigeminal disease (tic?) or perhaps toxic involvement.

Neurologic Examination. This showed no evidence of intracranial pressure or any organic involvement of the brain, spinal cord or peripheral nerves. The pain in the face was considered not to be a trifacial tic. It had none of the characteristics of a major tic, and was not limited to the anatomic distribution of the fifth nerve. It seemed rather to be a symptomatic pain incident to some local and inflammatory process in the sinuses of other neighboring tissues. In addition to the patient's background of typical migraine, with a substantiating familial history, the patient was nervous and tense and obviously had a low threshold of pain.

X-ray Examination. The accessory nasal sinuses were radiographed. The frontal sinuses showed rather poor development, but were clear, as were the ethmoid cells. There was some increase in density in both the right and left maxillary antra, which probably represented some thickening of the lining membrane. The sphenoid cells were clear.

Preoperative Orders and Course. On the patient's admission, the following had been prescribed: codeine sulfate, $\frac{1}{2}$ grain; acetylsalicylic acid, 10 grains every 4 hours as needed; Seconal, $1\frac{1}{2}$ grains at bedtime. The patient was allowed a general diet, and an ice bag as needed.

On the second hospital day the patient complained of pain during the afternoon and evening and was unable to sleep until midnight. Liver extract, 1 cc. daily, and dextrin three times a day were ordered.

The patient was ambulatory on the third hospital day. She complained of pain during the afternoon.

On the patient's fifth day of hospitalization, medication was prescribed as follows: Biolite after nasal packs, three times a day; Neo-Synephrine, 4 drops in both nostrils three times a day; 200 mg. of vitamin B$_1$ in 200 cc. of normal saline solution, intravenously, daily.

By the sixth day of hospitalization the patient was having severe pain, and it was decided to make several diagnostic block injections with a local anesthetic solution.

Operative Record. The upper left first molar was anesthetized by means of a posterior-superior alveolar nerve block, using 2 cc. of a 2 per cent N.P.C. solution and 0.25 cc. of the same solution over the mesiobuccal root, and 0.25 cc. of solution in the palate.

The patient did not have any relief from pain, so the inferior alveolar nerve was blocked with 2 cc. of the 2 per cent N.P.C. solution. Within 3 minutes the pain in the patient's upper jaw and in the head disappeared, and she was entirely free from pain for 45 minutes; the pain returned as the anesthesia wore off. Undoubtedly the pain was stimulated by the irritating influence of the lower third molar.

Under intravenous Pentothal sodium, the upper left first molar and the vertically impacted lower left third molar were removed surgically.

Postoperative Course. After the removal of these teeth the patient had freedom from pain for the first time since her admission to the hospital. She did not, however, seem to be in a hurry to be discharged. Finally, 5 days after the operation, she was told to make plans to leave the hospital. That evening she was ill again from her headache, and confided that she had "family troubles." It was now recalled, on reviewing her history, that when she was "upset," her pains were worse. It was suggested that she have a psychiatric consultation, to which she gave grudging consent.

The psychiatrist reported that, after some resistance, the patient finally described domestic difficulties involving her mother-in-law and possibly an overprotective attitude toward her own children. It was apparent that her facial and head pain might well have been a hysterical reaction to emotional conflicts arising out of this situation. Psychotherapy was recommended, on the ground that ventilation of her feelings might help her, even though the situation itself could be little relieved.

The patient was discharged on the eighth postoperative day, and given an appointment 2 weeks later. A letter from the patient, 1 week after discharge from the hospital, stated that the pain had not come back. Her jaw was still sore, her legs hurt her, and she was so shaky and tired that she often wished she were back in bed.

Five months after her discharge from the hospital the patient wrote another letter in which she said that she had not taken any of the drugs she had formerly taken and had not been to any physician, except Dr. Friedman. The domestic difficulties had been cleared up, with no more mother-in-law trouble, and the patient seemed much happier and healthier.

Comment. This is a surgeon's dilemma. This patient presented with a typical psychogenic neuralgia but was relieved by a diagnostic block of local anesthetic. Is the pain psychogenic or a real neuralgia? In retrospect, in all likelihood, the teeth were causing some pain that was greatly magnified by the patient because of her psychiatric problem. Would the patient have been cured by psychiatric therapy only? Probably not, but had such treatment not been given there is a good chance that other problems would have arisen either in the teeth or in other organ systems.

Case Report No. 19

PSYCHOGENIC NEURALGIA—PROBABLY VASOMOTOR

The following case report was written by the patient (a female, aged 57, April 12, 1955), and is printed exactly as she wrote it.

"April in 1950, had all my teeth out and dentures put right in. When I told you it was 6 months before the gum started to ache, was a mistake.

"The hurting started from the beginning, when I wore teeth, but without them it did not hurt.

"In about a year later Dr. T. cut the gum and scraped the bone, but that didn't help any. A few months later had teeth relined, as they were getting loose and he thought that might be causing it. It didn't help any.

"In winter 1952 sharp pains from lower jaw and upper gums, and in front of ear streaked up side of face. Not a continuous pain just once in awhile and at night.

"In April 1953 Dr. T. took an x-ray picture of upper gums. It showed a nerve condition.

"He sent me to Dr. R. and Dr. B. and they cut the gum and tried to separate the nerve, also scraped the bone as they said it was chipped. Next day had those pains in face and a very sore mouth.

"August I went to Dr. P. and he injected cocaine in gums, when the numbness left I had the same pains.

"From Sept., to last of Nov., I had B_{12} shots, three a week at first and then two a week. There was some relief from pain in face, but gums continued to hurt.

"March, 1954, went back to Dr. P. and he in-

jected cocaine in face and 3 of alcohol. Face was very numb, but gums still hurt, by this time pains in face was getting severe.

"I couldn't eat or touch my face or any expressing or movement of face without those pains.

"Dr. P. sent me to Dr. G., a neurosurgeon, and he operated on my head for tic, Feb. 1954 at W. Hospital. Next day had the same hurting in upper gums.

"A few days later had x-rays taken of upper and lower gums. They found the same nerve condition on right side of face, and three roots on left side.

"After the operation side of face, throat, nose and tongue, back of ear, and the whole top of head was numb. Also eye was bloodshot and I took treatments from Dr. G. until August. Also took therapy treatments for the top of head as it pained and felt like something heavy on my head. I had to quit taking them, though they did not help, because they affected the eye, and made it worse. Also was extremely nervous, and still am sometimes.

"Three weeks after the operation I went back to the hospital, and Dr. G. injected Novocain, and 2 of alcohol in face of front of ear, and that made my face more numb, and also my lips. A few days later the same pain in gums and still hurts.

"In December face started to swell, and gums where wisdom teeth were also ached, and then it would get better.

"In the past 2 months the gum has been swollen

and pains had at times, and then lets up some.

"Sometimes I can't sleep as it aches like a toothache, also sometimes the pain goes up to the face, and sometimes have an aching on top of head.

"March 28, went to Dr. W. and had an x-ray taken as I thought I may be getting another wisdom tooth.

"Gums and face were numb all evening; pain started again and when I retired it throbbed and pained worse than ever. Next morning the pain was bad and going up the side of my face in front of ear. Face was swollen more, and numbness gone."

Comment. Findings in a complete oral and radiographic examination by the author were negative.

As every neurosurgeon knows too well, cases such as described above are not a rarity and even with good early treatment are hard to cure. In this case we have the classic errors of mismanagement, misdiagnosis and repeated futile surgery that only added to the pain problem. To cure this patient would be a medical miracle at this stage.

Case Report No. 20

PAIN IN MAXILLA

This 70-year-old edentulous female patient was referred by her physician, who has been treating her for the past year for "facial neuralgia."

The patient complained bitterly about chronic neuralgic pain in the left maxilla present for the past year, gradually increasing in severity. It is not the acute spasmodic pain of tic douloureux, although the attacks come and go. The most painful area seems to be in the cuspid fossa. It is impossible for her to wear her full maxillary denture. (See Figure 26–7.)

One and one-half cc. of 190 proof alcohol and 1.75 cc. of 2 per cent local anesthetic solution were injected into the cuspid fossa. In 10 minutes the pain disappeared.

Two days later, the patient complained of pain in the region of the infraorbital foramen. It extended back into her face, which is still superficially numb. At this time 1.5 cc. of 190 proof alcohol was slowly injected into the infraorbital foramen region and massaged back into the canal. The pain stopped. The patient experienced moderate facial swelling following the injection.

One week later, the patient reported she had not had any pain since the last injection. She could wear her dentures and eat with comfort. One month after the initial visit, she was still very comfortable. She was to call if the pain returned.

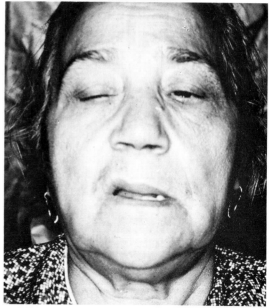

Figure 26–7 Patient suffering from continued deep neuralgic pain in the left maxilla. (See Case Report No. 20.)

Case Report No. 21

PSYCHOGENIC NEURALGIA – POSSIBLY VASOMOTOR

CARL J. BENDER, D.D.S.

According to this hospital's final narrative summary dated 8/24/61, a very alert and cooperative 71-year-old male patient had suffered from facial neuralgia since 1951. Onset was sudden and severe. The pain maintained a constant distribution. It was most severe in the left temple. From the initial site of painful stimulation, the distressing symptom radiated in the sternomastoid muscle. Occasionally, the pain spread beyond the facial midline. Daily attacks usually developed suddenly, continued for about 30 minutes and then gradually disappeared. He sometimes suffered from more than one assault in a single day.

For 3 years, the patient was treated by eight different physicians. Many types of therapy were used, but his symptoms continued. In 1954, he was admitted to a local general hospital to determine the nature of his departure from normal sensory mediation. Diagnostically, all findings were labeled as negative. It might be added that because of spinal fluid removal for analysis, he suffered a severe increase in pain.

After 8 days as a hospital patient, he returned to his home with no definite diagnosis or relief. A guarded idiopathic type of migraine syndrome of unknown origin was suggested.

Daily painful attacks continued for the ensuing 5 years, when in 1959 the patient sought the attention of a neurosurgeon. Because of his investigation, Dr. G. classified the patient's affliction as "atypical facial neuralgia." He said, "Sensory distribution had neither the characteristic nor dispersion of trigeminal neuralgia."

Upon completion of neurologic examination, Dr. G. suspected a nerve reflex disturbance of a dental origin was "the contributory cause of atypical facial neuralgia." Accordingly, the patient was referred to a dentist for purposes of adjusting his "bad bite."

After dental treatment and for about 1 year subsequently "his painful symptoms subsided dramatically." He remained asymptomatic until March 1961, when he developed an upper respiratory infection. Concurrently, painful facial symptoms again became very severe and attacks developed the same pattern as before. Except for the one year following dental treatment, the patient had had no respite from daily pain for a decade.

The patient was admitted to this Veterans Administration Hospital on June 30, 1961, for treatment of atypical facial neuralgia. His ward physician commented in the clinical record: "Please see patient regarding new dentures. This man's facial neuralgia is aggravated by poorly functioning dentures."

Dental examination disclosed a rather well-fitting upper and lower set of vulcanite dentures which the patient seemingly had tolerated for 38 years with no localized discomfort. Occlusal surfaces of all posterior teeth were flat and highly polished. From mandibular rest position to closure, his right molars occluded prematurely. With further elevator muscle pressure, either dentures, mandible, or perhaps to a greater or lesser degree both dentures and mandible shifted to the left.

This abnormal left posterior-superior movement resulted in the classical symptomatology of pain, clicking, and crepitus limited to the left side only. As far as could be determined from clinical and radiographic studies, the right articulation was normal in all respects.

Dental Treatment. It appeared very doubtful that conventional bite-registering methods would correct this unique arrangement. In fact, it was suspected that in so doing, the injury would not only be perpetuated, but also accentuated. Impinging left condylar head migration without disturbing the right counterpart was essential to restore masticatory normality—a rather difficult corrective situation because both condylar heads function as a unit.

Essig's old and almost forgotten fine technique with modification was put to use for purposes of establishing complete masticatory balance. (See also Case Report No. 29.) However, in the preparation of wax bite blocks, only left occlusal surfaces were superloaded.

After insertion of prepared bite blocks with hard, unyielding aluminum oxide plaster occlusal surfaces, the patient closed prematurely on the left side only. With the bite opened beyond normal mandibular rest position, both condylar heads were well down and forward in the glenoid fossae. Ill-defined and little understood hinge axis movements, therefore, were nullified in this open bite relationship. This being so, all parts were in an initial static stimulating phase. Occlusion, however, is not static.

The patient was then instructed to move his mandible within its full normal grinding range. During the grating process, and because both condylar heads were in a transitory functional relationship, muscles of mastication were stimulated. Upon completion of the predetermined grinding cycle, all occlusal and incisal surfaces of the bite block were contracting simultaneously.

After insertion of completed dentures, functional masticatory normality was restored. Click, edema, and pain in the left infratemporal fossa were nonexistent. Radiographic findings indicated a favorable repositioning of the left condylar head without disturbing function of the right counterpart.

The patient's new dentures, with complete functional balance including that of numerous muscles of mastication, were inserted on August 18, 1961. Since that time, he no longer suffers from "atypical facial neuralgia." In a communication dated January 13, 1965, he stated that he is still free from pain.

Comment. This is one of those cases which does not fall into a clear-cut diagnostic slot. It may be vasomotor pain, pure psychogenic pain or myofascial pain. There was undoubtedly a large psychogenic component here as well as myofascial pain. Ill-fitting dentures can aggravate both of these entities, and their correction is certainly indicated.

Vascular Neuralgias (Migraine, Horton's Cephalgia, Facial Migraine, Sluder's Syndrome and Related Entities). The essential common denominator in this group of pain syndromes that often involve the jaws is that there is usually preliminary vasoconstriction of one or more of a group of arteries and their branches followed by vasodilatation which may last from 30 minutes to many hours. The anatomic location of the arterial system affected determines the symptoms. Migraine (classic) involves the intracranial vessel producing photophobia, nausea, vomiting, and often sleep after acute vasodilatation occurs. In Horton's cephalgia, the internal maxillary artery appears to be affected, producing symptoms of deep, boring retrobulbar pain radiating to the upper jaw and sinus. (See Case Report No. 22.) The eye is congested on the affected side and the nasal cavity is blocked (due to engorgement of the nasal mucosa). Another variant involves the external maxillary artery, which produces pain that is inexplicable on an anatomical basis if one considers only nerve distribution. The pain follows the path of the external maxillary artery from the submaxillary gland into the upper and lower lip, and cuts across the distribution of V2, V3, and the cervical nerves.

The pain mechanism in these cases is easily understood. Dilated arteries are exquisitely sensitive because of nerve fibers in the walls, and the direct cause of pain is stimulation of these fibers. However, the cause of the dilatation is another matter entirely — there is no doubt of the psychic etiology. A long history of treatment including a diligent search for allergens, metabolic imbalance, nu-

---

Case Report No. 22

VASOMOTOR NEURALGIA SIMULATING TOOTHACHE

A 35-year-old white male was referred for diagnosis and treatment. He complained of severe pain of one year's duration in the right maxilla, which he described as a "deep toothache." X-rays had revealed an impacted third molar that had then been surgically removed with much trauma. This relieved the pain for about a month and then it recurred. The fillings of several teeth had been replaced by sedative cements without any relief.

At the first visit a careful history was taken, and while the pain centered in the posterior portion of the right maxilla, he also complained of pain behind the eye and deep within the head. It would often awaken him about 2 or 3 A.M. and last until 6 or 7 A.M. when he would fall asleep again. Analgesics and narcotics have provided no relief but sitting up made it less intense than it was when he was lying down. He also noticed that his eye was sore and inflamed and his nose obstructed on the right side when he had the pain. During the day he would have pain only in the late afternoon at work.

Since he was in no pain and his cardiac status was satisfactory he was given a prescription for ergotamine tartrate (Ergomar) tablets (2 mg.) for sublingual use to be taken every 30 minutes at the first sign of an attack, up to 3 every 24 hours.

He returned in one week and reported that one tablet would successfully abort the daytime attacks but that at night, since he would not awaken until the pain was intense, they did no good. He was then given a prescription for methysergide maleate (Sansert) tablets (2 mg.) with instructions to take one nightly before going to bed.

He returned the following week to report that he had had only one attack in the previous week and felt very well. He stayed on the medication for approximately 3 months using the methysergide maleate routinely before bed and the ergotamine tartrate as necessary during the day. He reported an occasional mild pain episode at night and a decreased frequency of daytime pains. After 3 months he discontinued the methysergide maleate and was relatively comfortable for almost 7 months, when the pain cycle restarted. Interestingly enough the patient commented that he thought his wife's severe illness may have precipitated the problem again. At this time it was necessary to increase the methysergide maleate (2 mg.) to one every 8 hours to control the pain. As the home situation improved, the patient's need for drugs decreased and at present he is free of pain.

Comment. This is an almost classic case of vascular (Horton's) neuralgia. Very often such excellent results are not obtainable with drug therapy, but in this case we were fortunate. At the present time, we often include a sedative or tranquilizer in our therapeutic regimen but even this does not give 100 per cent good results. The important point here is that this classic syndrome should be recognized and teeth not needlessly sacrificed.

tritional deficiencies, desensitization and other possible factors has failed to produce any consistent results. In individual cases elimination of possible allergens, histamine desensitization (the favorite for Horton's cephalgia), and other procedures have produced cures, usually temporary, with either return of symptoms or their transference to another problem. Placebo therapy would probably have given the same benefit at less risk.

There has been extensive psychological research in this field—particularly in migraine—and a characteristic personality type has emerged as that most likely to be afflicted. These patients are often compulsive, meticulous, neat, systematic people, who are very rigid in their thinking. They cannot handle the periodic neurophysiologic stresses all people experience, and instead of outward rebellion or "blowing off steam," which their personalities will not permit, they develop the migraine symptomatology. It must be understood that they cannot consciously control this—it is not a form of malingering because the mechanism is not conscious but unconscious. One of the useful analogies in the management of these patients is to compare migraine to the problem of blushing, which is due to mild surface vasodilatation and is not volitional. Migraine is comparable to an "internal blush" of greater intensity and duration.

Treatment of vascular neuralgias of the face and jaws is extremely difficult. Probably the most important factor is diagnosis so that useless therapy (extractions, etc.) is not attempted. Psychotherapy to get to the root of the problem has not given very good results, probably because this type of personality is not very receptive, and despite the apparent severity of the problem, the patient usually manages to function on symptomatic therapy. These patients, with their rigid thinking, are often hostile to psychotherapy and will not seek it unless forced to, which in itself often foredooms the effort. Consequently, the best treatment in this neuralgia (or group of neuralgias) is symptomatic and directed toward producing constriction of the dilated vessels as soon as possible. Ergot derivatives administered either sublingually, rectally, or parenterally appear to work best and a large variety are available. Sedatives and stimulants (phenobarbital and caffeine) may be added to the medication, but ergot is the prime medication. The oral administration of the drugs can be tried but their effectiveness is uncertain and the rate of absorption is too slow.

To prevent attacks of vascular neuralgias methysergide maleate (Sansert) has been used prophylactically, but the serious side effects seen with long-term use make this drug unacceptable for the purpose. The minor tranquilizers and barbiturates can be used prophylactically but their efficacy is limited.

Hysterical Neuralgia (Atypical Facial Neuralgia). * This is a psychogenic pain syndrome pure and simple. In the vascular neuralgias the psyche has used a mechanism to produce a painful dysfunction of the soma, but in this affliction there are no real somatic manifestations—just the sensation of pain. In other words, the mind manufactures the pain symptom without bothering to create somatic pathology. We have found that this is usually a much more severe psychiatric symptom than when physical findings are present, and this patient should be handled with care. A careful history and knowledge of reasonable causes of pain will usually elicit the diagnosis. The characteristic picture is of an ill-defined pain of uncertain nature and vague location, which is constant and not paroxysmal and often of long duration. The patient will rarely point to a specific site of pain but indicates a general area and will be more interested in telling how the pain is disturbing his life—his work and sleep—than in describing it. The pain has little relevance to anatomical distributions and is often bilateral. Several appointments may be necessary before this pattern is obvious and it should be a red flag of warning. This patient needs his pain syndrome in his adjustment to life and, while superficial therapy will usually not dislodge the symptom, an occasional patient under vigorous prodding by the doctor and family may abandon the pain syndrome and regress into a psychotic state. The dentist should tactfully and firmly disengage himself from this type of patient and either leave him with his pain or refer him to a psychiatrist. Under no circumstances should teeth, especially good teeth, be extracted.

---

* We prefer to reserve the term "atypical facial neuralgia" for this particular category of pain, but other authors include vasomotor neuralgias in this term. It would probably be better to abandon the term "atypical facial neuralgia" completely to eliminate confusion of the reader.

CONSTANT PAIN IN THE LEFT MAXILLA FOLLOWING MAXILLARY ODONTECTOMY AND ALVEOLECTOMY: ATYPICAL FACIAL NEURALGIA

A female patient, aged 45, stated that following the extraction of all her teeth, she had developed a constant throbbing, hammering pain that had been increasing steadily in severity. She took 12 to 16 tablets for pain daily.

A thorough oral and radiographic examination was negative, as was an examination by the otolaryngologist.

The pain was in the alveolar ridge extending from the left lateral incisor region to the third molar. She had had several "operations on the bone to remove the nerve" without relief. A left posterior superior alveolar injection of anesthetic solution did not relieve her pain, but an infraorbital injection of anesthetic solution gave her 75 per cent relief from pain. However, when the anesthetic wore off she had severe pain throughout the left side of her face (maxilla, mandible and temporal bone) and into her neck. She took ½ grain of codeine and 10 grains of aspirin every hour for 4 hours without relief. Finally she also took ½ oz. of paregoric and obtained some relief.

Because of the relief obtained from the local anesthetic solution, an infraorbital injection of 1 cc. of 190 proof alcohol and 1 cc. of anesthetic solution was made. This gave her relief for about 6 weeks.

During the next 4 months repeated injections were made to anesthetize with alcohol the terminal branches of the second division and then the second division itself. Finally alcohol did not give any relief, so the neurosurgeon resected a portion of the second division, with no relief of pain. In fact the patient claimed the pain was exactly the same as

originally, *only worse!* (See Figure 26–8.) She made trips to three major clinics outside Pittsburgh vainly seeking relief. She took psychiatric treatment without improvement.

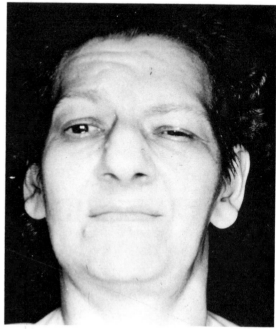

Figure 26–8 Patient with chronic continued pain of the second division of the fifth nerve *after division* of the sensory root in the skull. (See Case Report No. 23.)

DYSESTHESIAS OF THE ORAL MUCOSA AND TONGUE

Into this general grouping fall the multitude of syndromes in which patients complain either of hyperesthesia (increased sensitivity) or of hypoesthesia (decreased sensitivity) of the mucous membranes of the mouth. The complaint is usually that of hyperesthesia described as a "burning" sensation by the patient, but other patients will complain of a "scalded" sensation and a relative lack of sensation in various areas. The exact nature of these dysesthesias is obscure, and there is a complete absence of any physical or histologic findings in the affected tissues. There are two instances, however, which occur so often as to be recognizable as distinct syndromes: the burning tongue (glossopyrosis or

glossodynia) in the postmenopausal female, and the burning palate or alveolar ridge or both in the patient with new dentures. These may represent a type of pain mechanism differing from the other category of dysesthesias and are discussed below.

Most patients with dysesthesias complain of loss of taste, itching, roughness, tingling, abnormal metallic taste or tightness of a segment or all of the oral mucosa.

Psychological Dysesthesia. This often represents conversion reactions in a depression, anxiety, or other psychopathologic or neurotic state. Some of these patients are afraid of cancer and cannot verbalize their anxiety. The literature contains many cures and therapeutic measures but none of them have withstood the test of time, which is convincing evidence of their futility. Of course all possible physical causes of dysesthesia must be ruled out, such as (pernicious) anemia, severe vitamin deficiencies, compression of nerves and severe endocrinopathies. However, a cursory inspection of the mucosa and a brief history will rule out any disease severe enough to produce these symptoms. The concept of marginal vitamin or nutritional deficiencies and minor endocrine imbalance as an etiologic factor is another oft-repeated but never proved theory.

Case Report No. 24

PAIN IN THE TONGUE

Six years prior to this visit, this 50-year-old male patient had had acute pain in the right side and tip of his tongue and had insisted that his dentist extract the lower right second bicuspid and first, second and third molars. Of course, this had failed to give him any relief, so he had gone to one physician after another for the next 2 years.

He had then been referred to the Cleveland Clinic, where an extraoral alcohol block injection of the third division of the fifth nerve had been made. This had been followed by almost complete trismus for at least 3 weeks. He had had numbness in front of the right ear and in the right half of the lips and tongue.

The pain had recurred—but it was not as severe—7 months ago, and he had returned to the Cleveland Clinic, where he had been given another extraoral injection. This injection had not produced any numbness or relief of pain, so the next day the injection had been repeated. This had produced numbness and stopped the pain. In addition to the face, lip and tongue, he had had numbness around the right eye. This time the trismus and soreness had lasted almost a month.

A month before he first came to my office, the pain had started to return in his lip and had been getting worse daily. The pain was shooting and paroxysmal in the right side of his tongue. The patient could sleep at night, but when he tried to eat or talk, the pain was so intense he could do neither.

At the time of this examination, the pain was continuous in his tongue. With 2 cc. of 4 per cent procaine the inferior alveolar, lingual and long buccal nerves were anesthetized. This stopped the pain until the anesthetic wore off.

The next day the same nerves were anesthetized with 1 cc. of 190 proof alcohol and 1 cc. of 4 per cent procaine. Following this injection, the patient had a sore throat for several days, and he had 90 per cent relief from the pain in his tongue; the lip and tongue were numb.

Five weeks later, the patient reported that he had slight discomfort when he ate or talked. Numbness was not as pronounced as it had been immediately following the injection, and the patient was concerned that the pain would reach an acute stage again. The patient was advised to return only if the pain became acute.

About 10 months later, the patient reported that the pain in his tongue was returning. While not as severe as it had been when treated the previous year, it was bad enough that he wanted another injection of alcohol. One cc. of 190 proof alcohol and 1 cc. of 4 per cent procaine were injected in the area of the lingual nerve. Complete numbness of the lip and tongue followed, and the pain ceased.

Three months later, the patient reported an occasional slight pain in the tongue or jaw. He was told to return if the pain became acute.

Five months after that, the pain became increasingly severe when the patient moved his tongue, every third or fourth movement. The pain was concentrated along the side and tip of the tongue. He wanted another injection.

Injection of 1.5 cc. of 190 proof alcohol and 0.5 cc. of 2 per cent procaine was performed. This produced an intense numbness in the right lower lip and side of the tongue. The patient stated that this was a "good numbness." He had had enough injections that he could distinguish a "good" injection that would completely stop all pain.

The patient reported 1 week later that while his lip and buccal mucosa remained intensely numb, the tongue had lost most of the intense numbness and he wanted another injection. One cc. of 190 proof alcohol and 1 cc. of 2 per cent procaine were injected submucosally in the area where the lingual nerve passes forward and downward into the tongue. The side and tip of the tongue became intensely numb.

Some return of the pain occurred 20 months later. One cc. of 190 proof alcohol and 1 cc. of procaine were injected in the area of the lingual nerve. A slight return of pain was experienced 2 weeks after that, and the patient wanted another injection. The same solution was injected again.

Five months later (by now 4 years after the first visit), the patient returned with hot, needle-like, jabbing, acute pain in the right side of the tongue. He claimed that the tip of his tongue was free of pain. That morning his attack had lasted for an hour, and during the past 3 weeks he had had almost continuous pain. The patient was admitted to the Eye and Ear Hospital. The lingual nerve was exposed and 0.5 cm. of nerve excised. The patient's pain stopped.

A month later the patient complained of attacks of acute pain in the lip. The mental nerve was exposed, and a 1-cm. segment dissected out into the lip, where it was excised. The contents of the inferior alveolar canal for a distance of 1 cm. were fulgurated. The pain was relieved.

After 3 months, the pain in his tongue had returned and was controlled with 1 cc. of 190 proof alcohol and 1 cc. of local anesthetic injected into the area of the lingual nerve. The same complaint was treated with the same technique 3 months later.

Six years after the first visit, the patient was contacted; he said he had not had any pain for 2 years. The patient was still free of pain 11 years after the first visit.

Comment. This case obviously started as a psychological dysesthesia of the tongue and was converted to a traumatic (alcohol) neuritis of the lingual and mandibular nerves.

Traumatic Dysesthesia. Some dysesthesias occur in which there are both psychological and physical components. Continual mild abrasion of the skin will produce itching, burning and increased sensitivity, and the same process of irritation applied to the oral mucosa will logically produce similar symptoms.

A patient will often relieve tension by rubbing his tongue, especially the tip, on the anterior teeth or by clenching his teeth and moving his dentures back and forth in the small movements possible with all dentures. This will produce enough irritation so that, coupled with a lower pain threshold often seen in anxious patients, a burning sensation may result. A similar effect may be produced by the constant rubbing of the lateral surfaces of the tongue against the lower molars. The possibility of recurrent mild trauma, therefore, must be carefully checked in cases of dysesthesia. The tongue may show signs of inflammation and the ridges may be erythematous. (See Case Report No. 26.)

Burning Tongue Syndrome — Glossodynia or Glossopyrosis. This is one of the most frustrating syndromes to treat. It is almost completely a syndrome of women, and practically all are postmenopausal or close to menopause. They complain of burning pain along the lateral border of the tongue and the ventral edge at the posterior aspect. There is almost always a bitter, metallic, or other objectionable taste present that seems to originate under the tongue near the lingual tonsils. One would be inclined, on the basis of the peculiar complaints and the personalities of most of these patients, to attribute all the symptoms to the imagination, but it is difficult to believe that so many women in different geographical locations could have such an identical neurosis. The true nature of the problem has not been discovered.

Case Report No. 25

BURNING PAIN IN LEFT SIDE OF TONGUE

This patient, a woman aged 74, complained of a burning pain in the left side of her tongue which had been present for 10 years. She had been under medical treatment, without relief.

The patient was given a test injection. The left lingual nerve was anesthetized with 2 per cent procaine hydrochloride solution. The pain stopped immediately. The patient was discharged and told to report the results as the injection wore off.

She reported that from 1:25 to 7 P.M. she had 90 per cent relief, and from that Friday night until the following Wednesday had 30 per cent relief. Then, on Wednesday, the burning was even worse than before. The patient ate cake with lemon flavoring, which made the pain much worse. The patient much preferred a numb tongue to the burning pain she had been having.

One week following the examination, the left lingual nerve was anesthetized with 1 cc. of 190 proof alcohol mixed with 1 cc. of 4 per cent procaine hydrochloride solution.

Three days later, the patient reported that her

burning pain was practically gone. She stated that she had no numbness in the lip, though the mouth was numb. Motion of the tongue was limited. She said that she felt more relief, and felt better in general, than at any other period in the previous 10 years.

Treatment of Dysesthesias. First, a thorough examination must be made. Even though the word "cancer" has not been mentioned the patient should be firmly told that no cancer or serious disease is present. The patient may not be able to verbalize his anxieties and today, particularly, may convert cancerphobia into this symptom.

If this is not successful or does not seem indicated, the clinician should proceed cautiously because of the possibility of poor results. Except in cases of obvious neurosis, it behooves us, however, to make some effort, and cures are often possible when specific etiologic factors such as trauma can be discovered.

For trauma to oral mucosa from tension (traumatic dysesthesias) the use of tranquilizers (*e.g.*, chlordiazepoxide [Librium], 10 mg., or diazepam [Valium], 2 to 5 mg., three or four times a day) plus topical use of steroids (*e.g.*, triamcinolone [Kenalog in Orabase] every 4 hours) on the mucosa will often produce excellent results. Sometimes, just making the patient aware of the causes of the condition will effect a cure.

In nontraumatic dysesthesias in which pain or burning is confined to one peripheral nerve (*e.g.*, the nasopalatine nerve), a local block may be used, and if it produces comfort an alcohol block, surgical neurectomy or electrosurgical coagulation may be performed as indicated for the particular nerve. (See Case Report No. 25.) In these cases a careful examination for compression of the nerve by a denture, cyst, impacted tooth or other structure must be done before destruction is carried out. The use of anticonvulsants has also been tried in these cases in dosages similar to those used in tic douloureux with variable results. However, there is, as yet, no series of cases large enough to be of significance and there are many failures that may represent psychiatric problems. Empiric treatments are numerous but whether they produce better results than placebo therapy is debatable.

As of now we feel that all known medicinal treatment of nontraumatic dysesthesias represents nothing more than placebo therapy. If the doctor is aware that he is using placebo therapy this is fine, but he must understand its limitations and realize that one or more successes are not proof of its general efficacy.

Some mention must be made here of the often-diagnosed but very rare condition in which the patient is allergic to the acrylic in his dentures. If this is the case the oral mucosa will show local signs wherever the denture touches it, including the cheeks and lips, and a patch test can confirm the diagnosis. When the irritation is confined to the stress-bearing areas, trauma rather than allergy is the causative factor and unless a self-curing relining has recently been put in the denture the suspicion of allergy should be abandoned. Correction of occlusion and rough areas on the tissue side of the denture and an investigation into clenching and chewing habits are in order. (See Case Report No. 26.)

Case Report No. 26

PAIN IN AN EDENTULOUS MAXILLA DUE TO TRAUMATIC DYSESTHESIA

A 45-year-old male patient gave the following history: After extraction of the patient's teeth by another dentist, Dentist A made upper and lower dentures that from the start were unsatisfactory for several reasons. It was impossible for the patient to chew anything but the softest foods without pain in the upper jaw. The patient did not think too much about this, for he believed that it would be necessary for some time to elapse for his gums to harden. At the same time, the patient's mouth was always considerably warm, since the teeth apparently "generated heat."

After several months it became possible for the patient to eat with these teeth, but always with some difficulty and pain. The heat neither improved nor got worse. Eventually Dentist A suggested that the heat might be from a medical condition, and suggested that the patient have a complete physical check-up. The dentist implied that the pain the patient had when eating would disappear after sufficient time had elapsed.

The patient had a complete physical check-up and was told that there was nothing wrong with him. The physician suggested a consultation with another dentist.

The patient accordingly went to Dentist B, who informed the patient that poor-fitting dentures caused his touble in eating and might be a contributing cause of the heat; this dentist thought that the main cause of the heat was allergy to plastic. After some tests, which consisted in holding various compounds in the patient's mouth for varying periods of time, the dentist informed the patient that he was definitely slightly allergic to plastic, but was even more allergic to the coloring matter used in the plastic.

Dentist B made new dentures for the patient, which fitted almost perfectly. The patient had no trouble eating and no pain. He still suffered somewhat from heat, however. This effect appeared within 15 to 20 minutes after he had placed the teeth in his mouth, and was located primarily in the upper part of the mouth. It could be considerably lessened by not wearing the lower teeth, and eliminated entirely by not wearing the upper teeth. Although the patient felt that the trouble was a matter of pressure, probably due to the mechanics of the teeth, the dentist assured him that this was not so, and that his complaint was entirely caused by an allergy. The condition grew progressively worse, until after a year it was almost impossible for the patient to wear his teeth at all—even the upper plate by itself.

The patient then consulted Dentist C, who informed the patient that he had no allergy to plastic, but that all his trouble was due to poor-fitting dentures. The dentist made patch tests from scrapings, and the findings from these were negative. The dentist also made new dentures, which fitted almost perfectly, but the patient still had the heat and pain.

Two weeks after the completion of these dentures the patient had a major operation. He described his difficulties to the surgeon and asked his opinion. The surgeon thought that Dentist C's allergy tests were not conclusive, and made some himself. The results of these, too, were negative. The surgeon discounted the possibility of pressure on nerves creating heat or an effect of heat.

Six weeks after discharge from the hospital the patient went back to Dentist C. By this time innumerable small cracks had appeared in the upper plate. These, in the opinion of the dentist and of a plastic salesman or technician, could be caused only by heat in the patient's mouth (which they did not believe could be present) or by an improper amount of heat in the making of the plate. The dentist made a new denture for the upper jaw, but this did not have any effect on the heat. Within 15 to 20 minutes after placing the teeth in his mouth, the patient felt his mouth become uncomfortably warm. The warmth progressively increased until it reached a peak, in possibly an hour. It stayed the same without blistering as long as he wore the denture. The condition was helped considerably by removing the lower teeth, and could be helped completely by removing the upper plate, or both. Within 5 minutes of removing the denture, the patient's mouth returned to a normal temperature.

The patient finally consulted the author, who made some tests. Through numerous injections of an anesthetic in three different places on the roof of the mouth, the nerves were apparently blocked off. For approximately an hour the patient felt perfectly comfortable, but as the anesthesia wore off, the burning sensation returned. Later injections at only one point accomplished the same nerve block and gave the patient the same comfort, but this time for only 40 minutes.

Comment. This is one of many such cases that have come to my attention. Experience has shown that relieving the denture over the nasopalatine foramen does not give the patient relief. This patient's case occurred some years ago and at that time avulsion or electrocoagulation of the palatine nerves was the treatment of choice. Today topical steroids (*e.g.,* Kenalog in Orabase) would be used in the denture to provide symptomatic relief. The sensation the patient described as heat was really a dysesthesia, probably caused by small movements of the upper denture on sensitive mucosa. The important clue is the fact that he obtained relief when the lower denture was removed, eliminating the occlusal pressure that causes the movements when the dentures contact.

TEMPOROMANDIBULAR ARTHRITIS AND MYOFASCIAL PAIN SYNDROME

This is a pathologic entity in which pain is present either in the temporomandibular joint itself or in the masticatory muscles (or their ligaments). Because the pain may be diffuse, a very careful examination with palpation of the muscles and joint must be carried out to specifically pinpoint the area of tenderness. The patient may believe the pain is in the ear or bones of the face or even the teeth. Many patients are referred by their family dentists for removal of impacted teeth when a careful examination will reveal a tender muscle or joint. There is great controversy about the cause of these pains, and many far-fetched and anatomically and physiologically unsound theories have been advanced because one or two cures have been effected by empiric therapy of one sort or another. The research work of Laszlo Schwartz has been outstanding in this field, and the reader is referred to his book for a more detailed description of these syndromes.[69]

There appear to be two distinct conditions in these syndromes: those in which the pain is confined to the joint proper or capsule and those in which the pain is due to a sore muscle or ligament.

Pain in the Temporomandibular Joint and/or Capsule

When palpation reveals a tenderness directly over the joint itself this indicates the presence of inflammation of the joint and/or capsule, by definition an arthritis. An arthritis can be caused either by injury to the joint (osteoarthritis) or by a systemic collagen disease (rheumatoid arthritis) that produces changes within the joint. At times gout will also affect the temporomandibular joint. To rule out rheumatoid arthritis and gout, all patients who exhibit pain only over the joint and pain in the other joints should have a suitable test (latex fixation test) for rheumatoid arthritis and determination of the uric acid blood level. Since rheumatoid arthritis is a systemic disease, when this is diagnosed, the patient's physician should be informed so that he can treat any other manifestations. The temporomandibular joint should be treated by (a) the use of intra-articular steroids in acute cases to limit damage due to collagen disease; (b) the use of aspirin (10 grains, four to six times a day); and (c) relief of stress on the joint. When the patient has an elevated uric acid blood level, the gout should be treated with allopurinol and colchicine as indicated medically.

If the diagnosis of osteoarthritis can be made, treatment requires the relief of stress and strain on the joint. Intra-articular steroids are generally not helpful. Since in both rheumatoid arthritis and osteoarthritis of the joint there is often associated muscle spasm to protect the joint, the use of aspirin or other analgesics may be indicated. (See Relief of Spasm, page 1715.)

Radiographs of the temporomandibular joints in both types of arthritis may reveal anatomical changes in the condyle head and mandibular fossa. However, similar changes can be seen in x-rays of patients who have no symptoms whatsoever, so x-ray findings must be used in combination with other diagnostic measures.

Case Report No. 27

MYOFASCIAL PAIN SYNDROME SECONDARY TO COLLAGEN DISEASE

A 40-year-old white female was referred by her dentist for progressive inability to open her mouth and associated joint pain. He had constructed a splint that opened the bite posteriorly, but the patient had remained so uncomfortable that he had referred her to us for treatment. Physical examination revealed bilateral tenderness over both joints and capsules, as well as spasms of the masseter muscles. There was marked limitation of opening. The patient gave a history of migratory joint swelling and tenderness, and so she was referred for a blood uric acid test and a rheumatoid screening (latex fixation) test. Her uric acid value was in the upper levels of normal, but findings in her latex fixation test for rheumatoid arthritis were positive. It was felt that this patient had a collagen problem, and more thorough screening revealed that she was suffering from lupus erythematosus. She was placed on steroids and Indocin by the rheumatologist, with some relief of symptoms.

Comment. The symptoms of this patient should not be confused with a typical myofascial pain syndrome, because the basic pathologic process here involves a collagen disturbance of muscles and joints. Forcible trauma to these structures, such as that produced by a splint used to open the bite, will only result in further trauma to the muscles and joints.

Pain in Muscles or Ligaments

In the other 90 per cent of the cases of so-called temporomandibular joint pain, the site of the pain is in the muscles or ligaments, and these pains more properly may be classified as a "myofascial pain syndrome." Since the tissues of the head are no different from the other body tissues, the same physiologic and pathologic principles apply. Muscles are not designed to be continuously contracted (as occurs in clenching of teeth), overstretched (as occurs in opening too wide) or overused (as occurs in excessive gum chewing, unilateral chewing, etc.). All these actions produce either microtears in the muscles or ligaments, or both, or accumulation of metabolites. At a certain point, depending on the muscle tone,* the muscle will go into a protective spasm, either in its entirety or in a few of its bundles (fasciculi). This is nature's well-known effort to prevent further injury, and if the spastic muscle is used and not rested, the spasm may be extended to adjacent muscles via a reflex arc in nature's effort to protect the original site of spasm. This can produce a self-perpetuating cycle long after the original stimulus is gone, since the muscle in spasm will produce a continuous feedback into the reflex arc that continues the spasm. This was vividly described by Travell and Rinzler[77] with reference to back pain. Therapeutic measures must therefore be directed in two directions: (a) identification of the cause of the spasm and its removal if still present, and (b) use of various modalities (physical and pharmacologic) to relieve the spasm and interrupt the reflex arc.

Diagnosis of Pain in Muscles and Ligaments. In order to diagnose this syndrome, palpation of the masseter, temporalis and internal pterygoid muscles must be performed. The external pterygoid is difficult to palpate, but pain referred to the ear or head of the condyle *associated with deviation of the mandible* to the *affected side* is enough to make the diagnosis. (Remember that the external pterygoid muscle protrudes the mandible and when in painful spasm does not function well.) This is probably the second most common site of spasm, with the anterior portion of the masseter at its origin on the inferior border of the zygoma being the most common. This pain from the masseter is often described by the patient as originating from the upper molars or sinus. However, there is usually some trismus or pain on opening very wide, and if the forefinger is slipped into the mouth and the thumb placed on the cheek, the masseter may be palpated between the fingers. With the jaw relaxed, the painful, spastic muscle fibers can be easily palpated. Once felt, this can never be mistaken for anything else and the patient will identify this spot immediately as being exquisitely tender. With external palpation only, the examiner may think the zygoma is what is tender, but bimanual palpation will dispel all doubts.

Individually the internal pterygoid and the temporalis are probably affected the least, and these produce different subjective symptoms. Spasm of the internal pterygoid produces the subjective feeling of a lump in the throat or a sore throat but visual examination reveals nothing. Palpate these muscles by standing in front of the patient, crossing the hands, and using each forefinger to palpate the opposite internal pterygoid. The site to palpate is just behind the point of entrance of the needle in a mandibular block. Crossing the hands will make it easier to apply relatively equal force and the tenderness is immediately apparent. The temporalis muscle spasm most often occurs directly above and behind the eyebrow on the anterior edge of its origin in the temporal fossa and may be palpated directly. Subjectively the patient may describe this as a headache.

Thus it can be seen that the symptoms primarily depend on the site of the spasm. Very often (due to the use of the muscle in spasm) a reflex arc is set up and other muscles become secondarily involved. The spasm may spread to the sternocleidomastoid muscle (producing a stiff neck) or digastric muscle (producing pain deep in the neck or under the lobe of the ear). The trismus often seen is due merely to a quantitative increase in the number of fasciculi of the elevator muscles of the mandible involved.

Treatment of Pain and Spasm in Muscles and Ligaments. In order to intelligently and logically treat spasm a knowledge of the basic pathologic physiology is essential.

---

* Which is elevated in anxiety, meaning that spasm will occur with a much smaller stimulus.

When a muscle is subjected to trauma such as sudden stretching, small microtears occur in the muscle and/or its ligaments. This produces focal areas of derangement in the cellular metabolism with possible hematoma formation in severe cases. A similar disturbance occurs when a muscle is forced to exceed its physiologic limits in contraction either by prolonged contraction without relaxation (as in clenching of the teeth) or by overuse in which it has insufficient time for relaxation between contractions and becomes overfatigued (as in excessive gum chewing). In this case there are accumulations of metabolic wastes in the muscle (largely lactic acid) which also produce focal areas of derangement of the cellular metabolism. Regardless of the origin, therefore, both insults to the muscle produce the same result.

How does nature heal this injury? An afferent impulse is sent by receptors in the muscle to the central nervous system, which in turn relays an efferent impulse to the muscle (and if necessary to adjacent muscles) and puts it in spasm so that it cannot move and further injure itself. The degree of spasm produced depends upon how large an afferent impulse was sent to the central nervous system by the injured muscle and also upon how the central nervous system processes this impulse. In a person with marked anxiety, the efferent impulse sent back to the muscle may be much greater than that sent back in a calm individual and, as a result, a much greater spasm results.

In the extremities, muscle spasm has the effect of splinting the limb and immobilizing it against movement that aggravates the original injury. This allows the muscle to heal. In the trunk and head, however, this is virtually impossible because the normal activity of life produces movements, even in sleep. Much of the research in this problem was originally done with respect to lower back pain, but the same principles apply to the masticatory muscles. It was found that the focal areas of cellular metabolic derangement caused either by a single large trauma or by multiple small traumatic episodes might never get a chance to heal because the spastic muscle was in constant, though partially restricted, use. A muscle in spasm is obviously more vulnerable to injury when it is lengthened than when it is relaxed. Even though the original cause of the spasm had long since disappeared, therefore, the spasm was perpetuated by continual reinjury of the spastic muscle in movement when it was lengthened, and this injury produced new afferent impulses in the reflex arc. Since complete immobilization was impossible, other modalities were tried.

It was found that if the spasm could be stopped by physical or chemical modalities (heat or anesthesia) and the muscle moved passively if necessary at first and then started into gentle active movement, circulation was markedly increased in the muscle, and the removal of the metabolic wastes initiating the spasm was rapidly accentuated. This technique is the backbone of a great deal of the physical therapy used today. The sooner the muscle is put back into gentle active contraction, the faster it heals. The longer it has been in spasm, the longer the healing period, obviously, and of course if the original trauma repeats itself the cycle may be started again. Therefore, treatment involves relieving the spasm first and then, if possible, identifying the cause and eliminating it if it is still present.

RELIEF OF SPASM. In the early stages of the spasm, when relatively few fasciculi are involved, the reflex arc can often be interrupted by the use of various physical modalities applied to the skin over the sensitive area if the masseter or temporalis muscles are the prime site. These probably act much as other counterirritants, such as mustard plaster, liniments, etc., do elsewhere. The best and easiest technique is to spray ethyl chloride on the skin, being careful not to freeze it, and have the patient slowly open and close his mouth after 15 to 30 seconds. The results are often immediate, but the patient must continue to open and close his mouth for 2 to 3 minutes so that the spasm does not reappear. Use of the muscle increases circulation and removes the metabolites accumulated during the spasm. (This technique is often used on athletes.) Once the muscle functions properly, spasm will not reappear until the original etiologic factor is reintroduced. For spasm of the deeper muscles or long-standing spasm, this technique usually is not fruitful but can be tried using the spray on the area between the zygoma and neck.

Case Report No. 28

ACUTE MYOFASCIAL PAIN SYNDROME

A 23-year-old white female was referred by her physician because of her inability to open her mouth without severe pain. She had awakened the morning of the consultation without any prior history of pain or clicking in the joint or other discomfort. Her medical history was essentially normal. Physical examination revealed an acute spasm of the right masseter and temporal muscles. Ethyl chloride was sprayed topically over the right side of the face from the zygoma to the inferior border of the mandible without freezing the area. While I held my fist under the patient's jaw, the patient was asked to open her mouth slowly. Full opening was obtained against this resistance. The patient was then instructed to close slowly, and the area was resprayed. The patient was then instructed to open and close slowly and then resist this movement with her fist until the effects of the ethyl chloride on the skin were completely gone. Other than some slight muscle soreness, mobility was complete, and 10 grains of aspirin every 6 hours was prescribed. The next day full function was restored with no discomfort on opening.

Comment. If seen early, an acute myospasm of unknown cause can be treated in this manner with restoration of normal function. Sports fans (particularly baseball fans) have seen this done many times on the playing field.

If an ethyl chloride spray is ineffective, the tender points can then be infiltrated with a local anesthetic (without a vasoconstrictor) if they are accessible.* Again, the jaw must be put into function so that circulation is increased. In recalcitrant cases steroids designed for intra-articular and intramuscular use may be added to the local anesthetic injection to help reduce the inflammation reaction in the muscle which is causing the spasm.

Another technique is to open the jaw slowly against the closed fist in a direction opposite to the pull of the affected muscle. A well-known physiologic principle, reciprocal innervation, will cause a relaxation of the muscles that exert force in the direction opposite to the movement of any bone capable of moving in two directions. The more force exerted, the more the relaxation of the antagonist. This procedure, if sufficient force is applied in a direction opposite to the masticatory muscle involved and is not removed too quickly, will relax the spasm and normal function can be reestablished. Again it must be emphasized that the key ingredient in all these techniques is the restoration of muscle function so the spasm can not reestablish itself via the reflex arc.

Another technique to break the spasm, particularly in patients who grind their teeth at night, is the use of an acrylic bite plate. By opening the occlusion, the proprioceptive impulses fed back to the muscles are altered and one gets the same effect as occurs with an open bite due to inadequate posterior freeway space. Because posterior contact occurs before the muscles can develop the leverage to exert the normal chewing force, the strain on them is reduced. (Patients who have dentures with this problem complain that they cannot develop enough force to chew their food.) With the strain reduced the spasm may then be relieved.

CAUSE OF SPASM. Relieving the spasm is not enough unless the original cause was a single traumatic episode such as a wide yawn or similar accident. In most cases the cause is a combination of two factors: (*a*) increased muscular tone due to anxiety, and (*b*) muscular microtrauma due to usage in a manner that exceeds the physiologic capacity of the muscle. Sometimes the latter is the only cause but usually it is a combination of both factors. Identification of the nature of the misuse of the masticatory apparatus is the most difficult part of the therapy. This is because the abuse occurs over a period of many hours or days and ultimately requires a careful discussion and explanation to the patient so that he will observe the various habit patterns that produce trauma. He may or may not be aware, for example, of bruxism, clenching to relieve tension, unilateral chewing habits, sleeping with a hand under the jaw in far lateral positions, pipe clenching, excessive gum chewing, etc. If the patient does not have the mental capacity or interest to be an accurate reporter and observer, this stage of therapy may be extremely difficult for the doctor. Once the patient's attention is focused on the cause, however, the battle is won and the patient can literally cure himself.

---

* See pages 1725–1726 for techniques for injecting internal pterygoid.

At this point some mention must be made of malocclusion as an etiologic factor. This has been vastly overrated. All of these patients have malocclusion, but this is not the cause but the effect of the muscle spasm, which causes changes in the closure pattern of the mandible. *Under no circumstances should the occlusion be ground until all traces of spasm are removed by one or another of the modalities* for the simple reason that otherwise there is no way to determine the correct occlusion. It is highly unreasonable to ascribe this complaint to the occlusion, no matter how bad, when the occlusion may have existed for 10 years before the temporomandibular joint syndrome suddenly appeared. Except in cases where the occlusion or chewing habits have been recently al-

tered by some dental procedure (extraction, bridge, inlay, denture, etc.) that necessitates a search by the mandible for a new comfortable relationship to replace the old one (and subsequently produces muscle strain), the factor of malocclusion can be ignored. The syndrome may also be caused when a tooth has no antagonist and thus overerupts and drifts, locking the bite in an abnormal relationship in the terminal few millimeters of closure. In cases in which no dental procedure has been performed and there is no grossly visible occlusal interference and this syndrome suddenly occurs, the most logical explanation is that due to anxiety the efferent reflex arc has been greatly intensified, and therapy should be directed at that rather than at microscopic occlusal abnormalities.

Case Report No. 29

FACIAL PAIN CURED BY RESTORATION OF FUNCTIONAL NORMALITY

CARL J. BENDER, D.D.S.

Clinical findings suggest a close relationship between facial pain and dental treatment, as illustrated in this case of a 69-year-old tuberculosis patient who had successfully worn full dentures for many years.

The patient's pulmonary lesion was complicated by severe facial pains. A neurologist diagnosed his condition as a classic case of tic douloureux. His trigger zone was located near the upper right cuspid tooth. Findings in ear, nose, throat and neurologic examinations were negative, except for facial pains.

The following are observations by his ward physician, as recorded in the doctor's progress notes:

8/12/53 — "This patient has had for a long time — about 4 years — trigeminal neuralgia on the right side of his face. At times the pain is so severe the patient is forced to cry."

11/16/53 — "I believe that intramuscular injection of B_{12} is helping this patient's trigeminal neuralgia. At first, Demerol was necessary to reduce pain. Now, for the first time, he has been off Demerol and there seems to be no need of it. Members of the dental service are giving palliative help by injection of novocaine into trigger zone area."

1/20/54 — "Many types of therapy have been tried, symptomatic and temporary relief obtained, but the same symptoms have recurred ever since this patient was admitted to the hospital. The consultant in neurology recommends an alcohol block."

2/25/56 — "Weight drop noted, which may be attributed to the fact that patient has been unable or afraid to eat because of severe pain experienced with every movement of jaw."

6/12/56 — "Daily novocaine injection into trigger zone gives much relief from pain. For the past week the patient has been practically symptom-free in terms of pain. He is eating better."

7/10/56 — "The symptoms of trigeminal neuralgia are still persisting, causing severe lancinating pains, which come suddenly and end suddenly. They are brought on by movements of the face, as in talking, eating, brushing of hair, blowing of nose or touching some area of face. Medical treatment has never given relief, except temporarily."

8/15/56 — Ward physician's summary: "This patient was really in agony. The condition did not improve but progressed and became worse. At one time the patient described the pain as also affecting the ophthalmic branch and radiating to the back of the neck. Movements of the face, talking, eating or merely touching some area of the face produced severe and lancinating pain. The patient was again referred to the dental clinic, because on previous occasions he was helped a great deal by that service. He was fitted with a new set of dentures, was followed closely, and treated. For the past month, this patient has been a new man. The severe pain has not been present for many days. He is able to eat without fear, can shave without any discomfort, can blow his nose without experiencing any pain and can talk freely. One other important factor must be noted. While the patient was having these severe pains, he also complained of pain in the legs, which at times gave in, and he would fall. Since, he tells me that he has not had any pain in the legs. What was done for him should be in the dental records. All I know now is that the patient is a different man."

11/9/56—"Doing well. Symptom-free from pain for many weeks. At one time he also complained of pain in both lower extremities. These leg pains have completely subsided since the patient was fitted with a new set of dentures. I am not attributing all these changes to dental treatment, but we must admit that this has some bearing on the case."

Report from the Dental Department. Dental treatment consisted of restoring normal masticatory movements. This was achieved by constructing new dentures with complete balance of occlusion within the mandibular function range.

To register centric relationship, a simplified technique was used. The technique employed modifications advocated by Essig in 1906 for obtaining complete balanced occlusion.

The occluding surfaces of the approximately correct wax bite blocks were trimmed in the center to about a depth of 5 mm. The grooves were filled with an equal mixture of plaster, aluminum oxide, and water. To reverse the original destructive pattern of occlusion, the mixture was super-loaded in the molar area to a height of about 10 mm. After complete setting of the aluminum oxide plaster mixture and insertion of prepared bite blocks, the patient only occluded in the molar areas.

He was then instructed to move the mandible within its full normal grinding range. During the grinding process, and because the condylar heads were in a transitory functional relationship, muscles of mastication were stimulated. The grinding was continued until all occlusal and incisal surfaces of the bite block were contacting. The curvatures on the resulting dynamic occlusal plane seem to be a close approximation of the patient's inherent curve of Spee.

After completed dentures had been inserted, all parts associated with mandibular movements were in harmonious relationship with each other. The click was absent. The retromolar areas were not sensitive to digital pressure, edematous, or red.

This modification of an old, almost forgotten, fine technique established complete balanced occlusion.

Comment. This case illustrates how muscle dysfunction pain can mimic tic douloureux. True tic douloureux would not respond to this form of therapy. We feel that the original diagnosis here was in error, and had this patient been so unfortunate as to have intracranial surgery rather than good dental treatment, he would still have his pains.

Case Report No. 30

SEVERE HEADACHE CURED BY DENTAL TREATMENT

Carl J. Bender, D.D.S.

The mandible can also be forced into an abnormal protruded relationship. Such a relationship generally results from prematurely contacting occlusal surfaces of rigid, malposed posterior teeth.

The posterior teeth are the true mechanical stops of the jaws during closure. If the mandible pivots or slides forward because of extruded or malposed posterior teeth, the anterior teeth will obstruct the closing cycle. This leads to excessive wear of the anterior teeth, an abnormal forward and downward migration of the condylar head and disturbances in sensory nerve mediation.

This was illustrated in the case of a 39-year-old male being treated for pulmonary tuberculosis. According to his clinical record, the patient had had "a history of intermittent to almost constant headaches during the past few years." The following relevant observations appeared on his clinical record after diagnostic examinations had been completed:

X-ray reports of spine and skull were normal.

Examinations of spinal tap disclosed no pathologic conditions.

Neurological examination completed by the hospital's consultant reads as follows: "Has had periodic headaches of a year's duration; these have been severe and almost continuous for the past 3 weeks. Experiences stiffness and pulling in neck. May have nausea with headaches but no vomiting."

Pupils equal and react to light.

Cranial nerves normal.

Coordination good.

No muscle weakness.

Deep reflexes present and equal.

No Babinski. Sensation intact.

Tense. Long history of nervousness.

"Diagnosis: Psychophysiological autonomic reaction with headaches. Expanding intracranial lesion to be ruled out—this is very unlikely."

The ward physician's summary relative to the patient's head pains upon discharge from the hospital indicates that the patient had a long history of headaches unrelieved by medication. After dental treatment, his headaches disappeared.

Dental Examination, Treatment, Results and Comments. Except for bilaterally missing mandibular first molars, the patient had a well-designed natural dentition. Visual examination, including dental radiographic studies, disclosed no periodontal disturbances. Drifting or extrusion of all remaining teeth was minimal.

A significant abnormally developed structural pattern was detected on the maxillary bicuspids and anterior teeth. The anterodescending occlusal surfaces of the bicuspids were highly polished with very little contour loss. This was not true of the cuspids and incisors. Their lingual surfaces near the incisal angles were eroded, rough and excessively worn.

Functionally, the patient occluded prematurely on the bicuspids. With additional elevator muscle pressure, the mandible pivoted forward until the anterior teeth impeded the abnormal movement. Obviously, neither the bicuspids nor the anterior teeth in this situation served the function originally intended for each group. The patient's abnormal mandibular function resulted in crepitus, facial tiredness, and pain.

After interferences were removed by selective grinding of premature bicuspid contacting surfaces, masticatory functional normality was restored. Crepitus, tiredness, and local and central disturbances of sensory nerve mediation were eliminated. In addition, a space of about 1 mm. was created between the incisal surfaces during mandibular closure because masticatory stresses were absorbed by all posterior teeth. In effect, the patient's bite was opened in its anterior aspect by grinding down the posterior teeth. These results, seemingly impossible on a theoretical level, can actually be achieved clinically.

Case Report No. 31

MYOFASCIAL PAIN SYNDROME SIMULATING TIC

A 58-year-old white female suffering from pain in the right mandible was referred for consultation. The pain was acute and lancinating in character and was provoked when the patient ate, opened her mouth wide, or swallowed. The patient was edentulous and had a poor-fitting set of dentures. The patient first noticed the pain 2 weeks prior to consultation. Physical examination revealed a trigger point on the anterior portion of the right masseter muscle, just below the zygoma. The trigger point appeared to be in the muscle and not on the mucosa. The pain was elicited by bimanual compression of the muscle. It did not radiate into the lip, but it did radiate into the lateral aspect of the ramus and upward into the temporal area and ear. The trigger point was infiltrated with 3 per cent mepivacaine (Carbocaine), with immediate relief of pain. It was felt that this did not represent a true tic but a myofascial pain syndrome which mimicked tic. The patient was instructed not to wear her dentures, but the pain persisted. The area was infiltrated 3 days later with 1 cc. of 3 per cent Carbocaine and 40 units of Hydeltra-T.B.A. (steroid). There was marked improvement in the pain, with only some residual soreness the next day. After 3 weeks the area was no longer tender, and new dentures were constructed. The patient has remained free of pain since then.

In addition to a search for the etiologic factor in the muscle spasm, therapy can often be useful when directed toward reduction of muscle tone and decreasing the efferent response from the central nervous system in the reflex arc. Muscle relaxants (*e.g.,* meprobamate [Equanil or Miltown], 400 mg., three times a day; diazepam [Valium], 2 to 5 mg., three times a day; or chlordiazepoxide [Librium], 5 to 10 mg., three times a day) that are also tranquilizers are sometimes useful, but their side effects of drowsiness in efficacious dosages militate against their use in working patients.

For an anti-inflammatory, steroid-like effect the most useful drug is aspirin in high dosage (40 to 60 grains per day). Enteric coated aspirin is the author's choice, since little or no gastric irritation is produced, and 10 grains is prescribed four to six times a day for a period of 1 to 2 weeks. The cost is reasonable, and there are practically no side effects. Dosage can be regulated as needed after the first week or two.

For night bruxism a medium-acting barbiturate in adequate dosage or a suitable dose of any other hypnotic agent is useful. Currently we are using diazepam (Valium) in dosages of 10 to 20 mg. at bedtime.

Heat in the form of dry or wet heat is also

useful in muscle relaxation when applied to the face or neck.

SUMMARY OF TREATMENT OF SPASM. At the first appointment, a complete history should be taken and a careful examination performed. The tests necessary to rule out rheumatoid arthritis and gout should be made. If possible, attempts should be made to relieve the spasm, especially if severe and painful, with one of the above-mentioned modalities. Any necessary drugs should be prescribed and the problem explained to the patient so that the patient can find the etiologic factor. All of this requires 30 to 45 minutes, and if there is not enough time at the first appointment, the spasm may be relieved and drugs prescribed, reserving the discussion for the next appointment. If the pain and discomfort are not too severe, therapy for direct relief of the spasm may also be omitted, but the patient should be seen as soon as possible to complete the necessary explanations so the patient can check himself for etiologic factors. In some cases one visit may effect a cure. In others, especially when there is excessive nervous tension with bruxism or clenching, many visits may be required since the problem may be temporarily relieved only to recur when the muscle is traumatized again. The ultimate cure of course depends on the elimination of any recurrent traumatic factor.

SUBLUXATION, CLICKING AND DISLOCATION

Subluxation (hypermobility of the condylar head with excessive anterior movement, *i.e.*, a "loose joint"), dislocation (condylar head anterior and superior to the eminentia articularis), and clicking noises in the joint are all interrelated phenomena. In the first two a defect in the anterior restraining ligaments of the joint is probably present as a result of repeated small traumatic episodes or of one such episode, but the other factor (often overlooked) is the hyperactivity of the external pterygoid muscle. (See Figures 26–9 to 26–11.) In clicking, the problem is also due to the external pterygoid, which is attached to both the condyle and the meniscus. Normally, in a coordinated opening movement, the meniscus stays between the condyle and the anterior wall of the mandibular fossa, but if there is uncoordinated pull one or the other gets too far forward and the condyle slips off

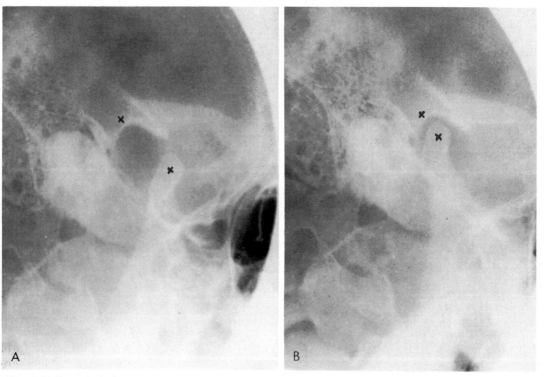

Figure 26–9 *A*, Subluxation of the left temporomandibular joint. Note that the head of the condyle is out of the glenoid fossa, anterior to the articular eminence but not superior to it. *B*, The left condyle in normal position in the glenoid fossa when the mouth is closed.

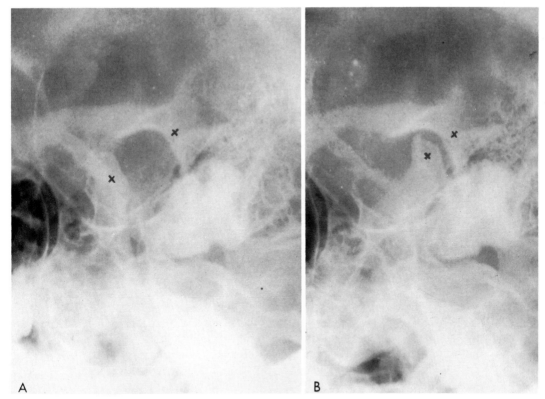

Figure 26–10 *A*, Subluxation of the right temporomandibular joint. *B*, The right condyle in normal position in the glenoid fossa when the mouth is closed.

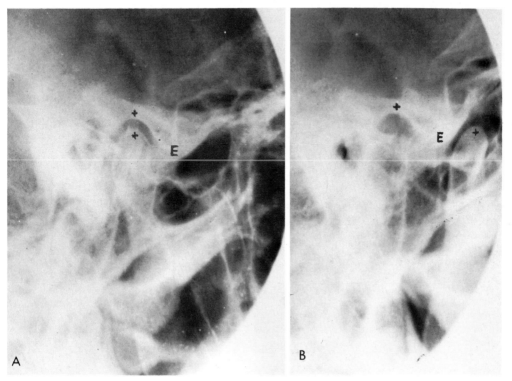

Figure 26–11 *A*, Left temporomandibular joint, mouth closed. *B*, Mouth open. Note the dislocation of the temporomandibular joint. Note also the position of the head of the condyle in relation to the eminentia articularis (*E*).

the front or back of the meniscus. This is the "clicking" noise so often heard at the opening movement.

In all these cases the common denominator is muscular incoordination. Just as in any other learned habit pattern, it may require a conscious effort to reestablish the original pattern. The normal pattern of mandibular movements starts with a rotary movement on opening followed by an anterior gliding of the condyle. If anterior movement precedes rotation, the external pterygoid has one head pulling the condyle and the other head attempting to pull the meniscus, which is still wedged tightly since there is no room for it to go forward. This is the ideal situation to provoke spasm. This internal derangement of function must be corrected by teaching the patient to consciously relearn how to open and close the jaw correctly. The correct movements—rotation first and then anterior gliding—are first explained to the patient and then demonstrated. This is done by seating the patient in the dental chair and dropping the headrest so the chin points upward in order to tense the platysma. With his finger on the patient's chin, the instructor allows the patient to slowly open his mouth but does not allow any translatory (anterior) movement to occur until adequate rotational opening is obtained. Tensing the platysma lessens the force necessary to restrain the chin. This should be done three or four times so that the patient sees that he can open and close without clicking. Sometimes placing the fingers anterior to the condyles is more helpful, for the patient can recognize when rotation ceases and anterior gliding starts. Following this, the patient should repeat the maneuver without aid. Very often he will fall back into a clicking pattern since this dysfunction has been so ingrained on the neuromuscular pattern. Several lessons may be necessary until he sees he can stop the clicking by altering his opening pattern, and then it is up to the patient to practice until he substitutes the correct habit pattern for the abnormal one. In patients who are not cooperative the injection of sclerosing solution (see below) may help break the reflex pattern. One of us (W.H.A.) prefers to sclerose the joint in all patients and the other (D.D.) prefers to try reeducation first.*

---

* Meniscectomy has proved to be ineffectual in these cases and has been generally discontinued.

Case Report No. 32

PAINFUL PROLONGED TEMPOROMANDIBULAR JOINT SUBLUXATION AND DISLOCATION TREATED WITH A SCLEROSING SOLUTION AND EUCUPINE

A 45-year-old female patient, the wife of a dentist, had trismus in the morning that took her an hour to loosen gradually.

She had continuous soreness in both temporomandibular joints and was unable to masticate anything but the softest foods. When the patient opened or closed her mouth, harsh grating sounds could be heard for a distance of 15 feet. This was extremely annoying and embarrassing to the patient.

A bilateral condylectomy had been recommended by an orthopedist.

Past History. The following history was written by the patient:

"Approximately 20 years ago, I had the first and second upper right molars extracted at both sides. These teeth had been previously treated and they were suspected of being contributing factors to an attack of rheumatic fever. I had no third molars.

At this time, no suggestion was made to me to replace these teeth with a partial plate

"About 8 months to a year later, I began to experience difficulties with my jaws locking shut. This condition seemed to be prevalent when I arose in the morning. It would be almost impossible for me to open my mouth. For a period of about a half hour, I usually had to use my hands to force my jaws open. Each time I forced the jaws apart, there was a cracking and a tearing sound in my joints and the pain was excruciating. Following this period of 'daily exercise,' I was able to open my mouth normally and I could eat a little, but not without the cracking sensation or pain. An hour or so later, my jaws seemed to be sufficiently limbered so that I could proceed through the remainder of the day with little or no trouble, except the cracking sound. Later, I partially overcame the severity of this trouble by learning to keep my jaws from completely closing at any time. However, if for any reason I happened to open my mouth too wide, I experienced practically the same trouble in reverse. The jaw would lock open.

"This condition continued for about 5 years. At this time I had a partial plate made to replace the extracted teeth, but no attempt was made to open the bite. I had very little trouble thereafter, except a continual cracking noise when I was chewing. I did experience soreness and stiffness in my jaws any time following my chewing anything hard, such as caramel or taffy. This partial plate served its purpose for nearly 13 years.

"Almost 2 years ago my jaw really slipped out of place, as shown by x-ray pictures. After the jaw was back in place and the soreness had subsided, I had a new partial plate made with the idea in mind of opening my bite. The bite actually was opened about 4 mm. This gave me considerable relief, although a grating sound was present any time I opened my jaws; there was soreness in the joints; I had to exercise care about opening my mouth too wide or eating anything which might be a little difficult to chew.

"In June of the same year,* I started to take a series of injections in my jaws. The reaction I experienced at the first injection was exceptionally severe, but each successive treatment was less bothersome. A couple of times I experienced quite a bit of pain, which lasted several hours, but for the most part, after a treatment my jaw would be a little bit stiff and sore, then by the following day it would feel normal.

"All the pain I may have suffered from the treatments, in my estimation, has been worthwhile, for it is now about 15 months since I had the last treatment and I no longer feel any pain or soreness. I have only a very slight cracking sensation in the left joint. I am able to *eat* or *chew anything.*"

---

* I gave her 4 minims of Sylnasol and 4 minims of eucupine and procaine solutions in both temporomandibular joints every 2 weeks for 4 months. Sylnasol is no longer available. Instead we use 6 minims of a 3 per cent solution of sodium tetradecyl sulfate (Sotradecol injection).

Case Report No. 33

PAIN AND CLICKING IN THE TEMPOROMANDIBULAR JOINT

About a year and a half before the present illness, the patient, a woman aged 35, began to notice pain in her right ear and jaw. The pain was aggravated when she tried to brush her teeth or to chew. The patient noticed that she sometimes had a clicking in her jaw. Occasionally, when opening her mouth, her right jaw felt as if it had "jumped out of place." On closing her mouth she had considerable pain; she also had pain when she yawned or sneezed. For the past year and a half it had been an effort to eat, especially hard rolls.

Treatment. The patient had had an injection of 0.25 cc. of 2 per cent Metycaine mixed with 0.25 cc. of a sclerosing solution* in the right temporomandibular joint cavity.

The patient reported that her symptoms were much worse in the evening and when she was in bed; if she rested on her right side, she had pain on awakening. For 3 days following the last injection she also had swelling. On closing her mouth she had the same old pain, only worse. She had no injection on this day.

The patient reported by telephone a week later that she was feeling much better. She still had a little pain when chewing.

One month later the patient stated that for 2 weeks she had felt like "a new woman." For the last 2 weeks, however, she had had a recurrence of pain in the right jaw, but not so bad as when she came in originally. She was given another injection (same as noted above) in the right temporomandibular joint.

The patient reported 10 days later that, since the last injection, she had had less swelling than after the first injection, but more pain. The pain had become constant, but she could sleep at night. The pain at present was in the temporomandibular joint. The patient preferred not to eat because of the severity of the pain, which was aggravated by talking. She had a feeling that her "teeth were too big for her mouth, also her tongue." The pain and discomfort had been made much worse after the second injection. She was now given an injection of sclerosing solution in the left temporomandibular joint.

Ten days following this injection, the patient said that, compared with her first bout, she felt better. Her ear did not bother her as much, nor was there any clicking. The pain was greater in her head than in her jaw, but was much improved. Damp weather aggravated the pain; heat and hot weather made her jaw feel better. Her nerves and "everything" felt much better now; she even chewed gum the other day, something she had not done for months. She still got a "jerky" pain in her

---

* We now use 6 minims of a 3 per cent solution of sodium tetradecyl sulfate.

jaw, but not so often and it was not so severe. She felt that she was getting better. She was given an injection of sclerosing solution in the right temporomandibular joint.

The patient reported 2 weeks later that, since the last injection, there had been only slight swelling. There was, however, marked trismus; she could open her mouth only ½ inch and could eat only soups. About 3 days later she had a terrific pain in her head from the temple region and back. This pain lasted 2 days. Every now and then she had pain in her ear, but definitely felt that there was some improvement. At present she could open her mouth satisfactorily. The patient was warned not to open her mouth too widely. She was given an injection of sclerosing solution on the left side.

Three weeks later the patient's right side felt much better than the left side. There had been no pain on the left side until after the last injection. She was given an injection of sclerosing solution in the left temporomandibular joint.

Two weeks following this treatment, the patient stated that, after the last injection, she had had

pain for about an hour, but since then she could eat without pain. She did not have the usual days of pain and discomfort that she had had following previous injections. She could now eat such things as pork chops, toasted sandwiches and other things that she had not been able to eat before the injections were started. She had pain only on yawning. She was given an injection of sclerosing solution.

At her next appointment 2 weeks later, the patient reported that, since the last injection, she had had no pain, but that her chin was "way over to the left" for 4 days. She could not eat because her teeth were not "biting right." She had no pain except when she tried to eat, and then only a little pain. In view of her report, it was decided to wait 4 weeks before considering another injection.

After this 4-week period, the patient reported no discomfort. Her jaw felt as good as it had ever felt. She had no pain in her ear or jaw, nor was there any clicking on eating. She could eat with comfort foods that required chewing, which used to produce extreme pain. The patient was discharged as cured.

Case Report No. 34

CHRONIC MYOFASCIAL PAIN SYNDROME

An 18-year-old female patient was referred complaining of pain and stiffness in the jaw, especially in the morning, inability to open her mouth wide without pain, and inability to chew hard foods without pain. Physical examination revealed a marked limitation of opening, tenderness of the right temporomandibular joint in the capsule and over the condyle, and a tender, spastic right masseter muscle. There was a long history of clicking in both temporomandibular joints for the last 4 years, but the pain had not developed until the past month. Because of the extreme discomfort, the patient was placed on aspirin, 10 grains every 4 hours, and Valium, 10 mg. before bed and 5 mg. at 8 A.M., 12 noon, and 6 P.M. She was instructed to return in 2 days. At that time she was much more comfortable, with greater mobility of the jaw, but complained about the drowsiness induced by the Valium. An examination now revealed that she initiated the opening of her mouth with a protrusive movement; *i.e.,* she started the translatory movement before the rotational movement was completed and was thus traumatizing the meniscus. She was instructed in how to open and close her jaw properly. Her daily dose of Valium was cut to 2½ mg. three times a day, but her nightly dose was kept at the same level. Within a week she had excellent movement with pain only at extreme

opening but had developed a recurrence of the clicking. She was again carefully instructed in proper methods of opening and closing, which took her approximately 1 month to master. At the end of a month she was taken off the daily Valium and aspirin and at the end of 2 months was completely asymptomatic.

Comment. This is a classic myofascial pain syndrome in which constant trauma to the joint and meniscus (as evidenced by the clicking) culminated in an acute episode of pain. This required a considerable period of time to eliminate because of the long-standing trauma to the joint. The presence of clicking noises indicates asynchronous movement of the meniscus and condylar head, and each click means that the condyle has slipped off the meniscus and forcibly hit the skull surface of the joint. This repeated trauma may not cause pain for years, depending on the patient's pain threshold and muscle irritability, but once the threshold is exceeded and acute myospasm develops, reversal is a slow process. Drug therapy will often relieve the myospasm, but the habits that produce the clicking must be corrected or the problem will recur. However, until the myospasm is corrected or at least ameliorated, accurate diagnosis of the habit pattern or occlusal imbalance cannot be made.

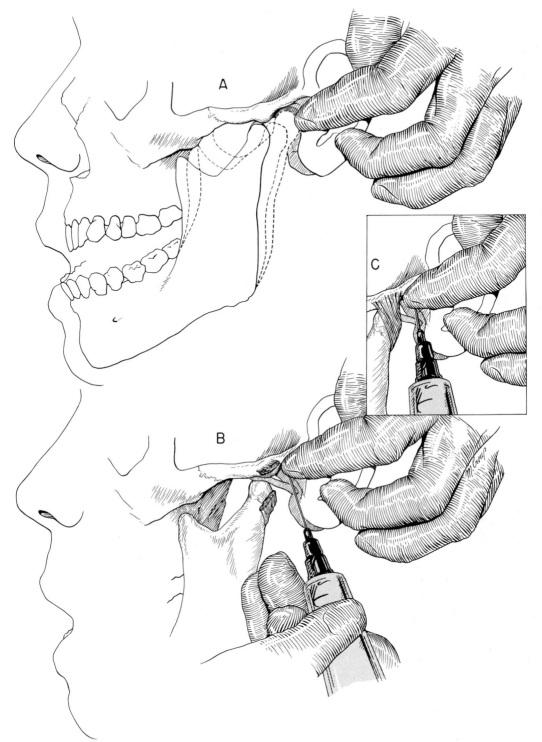

Figure 26–12 Intra-articular technique for injecting sclerosing solution or other drugs into the temporomandibular joint.

A, Palpate the area immediately anterior to the external ear with the index finger as the patient opens and closes his jaws. The excursions of the head of the condyle as it glides forward and downward on the eminentia articularis will be felt. The depression of the glenoid fossa is located as the condyle head moves out of the fossa onto the articular plane.

B, The tip of the index finger is then moved upward until the fingernail rests over the center of the glenoid fossa. The patient is instructed to hold his jaws open, or a block is placed between his teeth, and the needle is passed along the fingernail through the skin at a 45-degree angle to the facial plane, bisecting the tip of the fingernail through the skin upward and slightly anteriorly, until the articular surface is contacted.

C, The needle is then slightly withdrawn and directed upward and slightly posteriorly to the roof of the glenoid fossa. Aspirate to determine whether or not a blood vessel has been entered. If not, slowly inject the sclerosing solution or other drugs.

In subluxation the hyperactivity of the external pterygoid produces an abnormal range of movement but the pain present is due to the muscle spasm itself. In dislocation the spasm is quantitatively greater and continuous, holding the condyle forward and upward. (There are two portions of this muscle and the superior fibers extend almost vertically.) The dislocation persists not because the head is anatomically locked behind the eminentia articularis but because the muscle is holding it there. Treatment consists of either breaking the spasm forcibly by moving the mandible down and slightly posteriorly (by facing the patient and placing the thumbs on the lower posterior teeth) or injecting a local anesthetic into the joint cavity (through the skin) to anesthetize the external pterygoid insertions. The dislocation will then usually reduce spontaneously. Since the introduction of intravenous diazepam (Valium) the technique has been even easier. With regulation of the dose according to the patient's age (usually 5 to 10 mg. over 1 to 2 minutes), the drug is given intravenously and the muscle relaxation is usually so profound as to require practically no force in the reduction. The usual recovery period is 10 to 30 minutes and then the patient can safely leave.

The high frequency of recurrence of dislocations is caused by the tendency toward muscle spasm, not by ligamentous weakness. To prevent the recurrent dislocations that often occur 1 to 2 hours after the original reduction, it is advisable to place some sort of restraint (e.g., a modified Barton bandage) to prevent wide opening of the jaws for about 24 hours. If spasm is not preventable by other techniques, the use of a series of injections of sclerosing solution (4 minims of a 3 per cent buffered solution of sodium tetradecyl sulfate [sodium sutradecyl] containing 2 per cent benzyl alcohol with 4 minims of 2 per cent lidocaine hydrochloride [Xylocaine] and 1:100,000 epinephrine hydrochloride) into the joint cavity (see Figures 26–12 to 26–15) produces a high percentage of cures. (See Case Report Nos. 32 to 34.) As a last resort

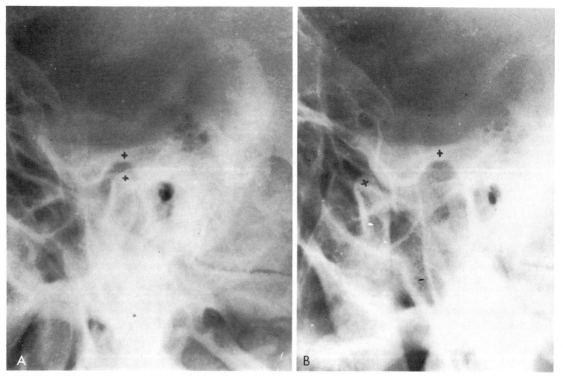

Figure 26–13 Radiographs of a case of bilateral self-reducing dislocation successfully treated with sclerosing solution. *A*, Right temporomandibular joint, mouth closed. *B*, Mouth open. Note the dislocation of the temporomandibular joint. The condyle is anterior and superior to the eminentia articularis.

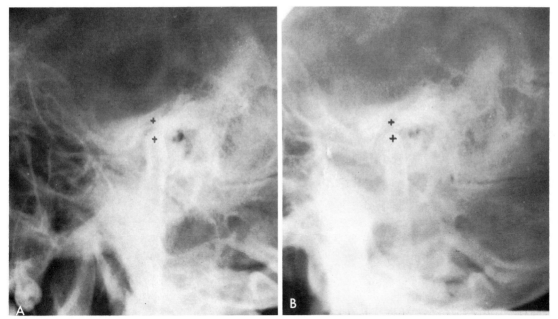

Figure 26–14 *A,* Right temporomandibular joint, mouth closed, after injection of sclerosing solution. *B,* Temporomandibular joint, mouth open, after a series of injections of a sclerosing agent. Note that the head of the condyle has not left the glenoid fossa.

a high condylectomy can be done so that no matter how much spasm occurs, the condylar level will remain below the eminentia.

DRYNESS OF THE MOUTH (XEROSTOMIA)

Dry mouth is caused by diminished secretion of saliva, a condition usually found in the aged. It may lead to redness, soreness, and painful fissuring of the mucous membranes, with eventual atrophy. Chewing and swallowing may become difficult. Inadequate amounts of saliva may result from: (*a*) a decrease in salivary gland substance (congenital hypoplasia, senile atrophy, destruction following surgical intervention, irradiation, inflammation or neoplastic infiltration); (*b*)

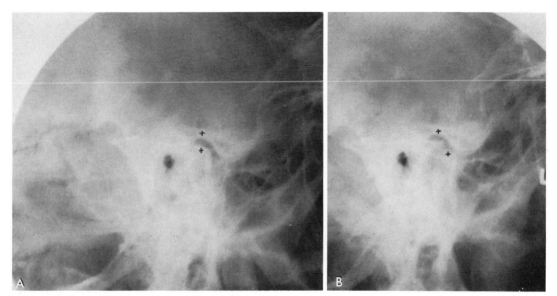

Figure 26–15 *A,* Left temporomandibular joint, mouth closed, after injection with sclerosing agent. *B,* Temporomandibular joint, mouth open, after injection of a sclerosing agent. Note that the condyle has not left the glenoid fossa.

disturbances of innervation (central or peripheral nerve lesions, emotional states, psychoses, interference with conduction of nerve impulses due to drugs, toxic agents or metabolic disturbances); (c) dehydration (patients with polyuria and dry mouth may be diabetic); (d) excessive smoking; (e) salivary calculi or stones in the salivary ducts or gland; and (f) unknown causes (Sjögren's syndrome). In Sjögren's syndrome dry mouth is associated with dryness of the eyes and mucous membranes of the nose, throat and vagina and with a deficient gastric secretion.

Treatment. Many of these symptoms suggest deficiencies of vitamin A, nicotinic acid and riboflavin and some of them are seen in pernicious anemia, iron deficiency anemia and Plummer-Vinson syndrome. There is a frequent association of the syndrome with rheumatoid arthritis and with the endocrine changes that occur in postmenopausal women.

After the preceding possibilities have been ruled out, parasympathetic stimulation to stimulate the flow of saliva should be tried. Pelner[59] recommends 7.5 mg. of neostigmine bromide three times a day after meals. Prinz[61] recommends the following "supreme sialogogue":

Pilocarpine hydrochloride	0.3 gm.
Distilled water	15.0 cc.
M.	

Sig. 5 drops three times daily in water. Slowly increase the dose by adding an extra drop every third day until 8 to 10 drops per dose are taken.

All too frequently none of these treatments is effective, and then symptomatic relief is indicated. Burket[9] recommends ordinary paraffin oil, flavored with lemon oil, to relieve many of the annoying symptoms. Denture-wearing patients with xerostomia should coat their dentures with petrolatum or one of the many lubricating jellies or a denture powder.

PAIN FROM THE STYLOID PROCESS

Kaiser-Meinhardt and Seitz[48] report five cases describing the symptoms arising from an abnormal styloid process extending downward from the lower surface of the temporal bone. The main complaints of the patients were glossopharyngeal neuralgia, dysphagia of undetermined cause, stabbing pain in the region of the ear and the mouth (otalgia dentalis), and a feeling of tightness in the neck.

In all five patients, the symptoms disappeared after surgical removal of the styloid process.

For a differential diagnosis, impacted third molars (or retarded tooth eruption), inflammatory processes in the tongue, pharynx or larynx and early carcinoma of the oral cavity, the pharynx or the hypopharynx should be considered. See Case Report Nos. 35 and 36 for further discussion of pain in the styloid process and its ligaments.

Case Report No. 35

SYMPTOMATIC CALCIFIED STYLOHYOID LIGAMENTS

K. Odenheimer, D.D.S.

A 63-year-old female patient wanted her old denture replaced. Findings in a clinical examination of her tissues were negative. However, the panoramic radiograph revealed a very large segmented, calcified stylohyoid ligament on her left side (Fig. 26–16). A more extensive search of her history revealed that she had suffered chronic pain in the region of her left ear and neck. After about 15 years of futile visits to a variety of medical spe-

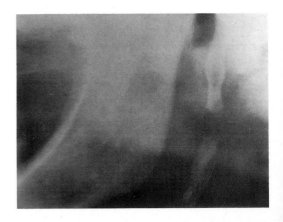

Figure 26–16 A large segmented, calcified stylohyoid ligament on the left side. (See Case Report No. 35.)

cialists, the patient had adopted the attitude that she must live with her pain. Our clinic referred her to an otolaryngologist for consultation. He concurred with our clinical diagnosis that the stylo-

hyoid was the cause of her long suffering, and he recommended surgical removal of the floating portion and a reduction of the elongated part. However, the patient refused this treatment.

Case Report No. 36

SYMPTOMATIC CALCIFIED STYLOHYOID LIGAMENTS

K. ODENHEIMER, D.D.S.

This 31-year-old male South American graduate student was unable to continue his studies because of severe paroxysmal pain in the head and neck region. After consulting several physicians, he was advised to come to the university dental clinic to rule out any dental infection. The oral examination revealed a very healthy mouth with 32 teeth and very few fillings. Findings in full-mouth periapical x-rays were negative except for the mandibular (lower) right first molar, which showed root canal treatment. Although this tooth was completely asymptomatic, it could not be ruled out at this time as a possible etiologic factor in the patient's episodes of pain, which were coincidentally on his right side. His history described the pain as neuralgic and stabbing, lasting at times for several hours. The patient could not relate it to chewing, talking, or shaving, but he sensed that turning or nodding his head often preceded his attacks. After the pain was present, it would become widespread, from the ear to the clavicle, including his throat and tonsillar region, so that localization became impossible. By the time the patient came for dental consultation, he had made his own diagnosis of cancer and only awaited our confirmation.

Experience with a few similar cases led to the suspicion that a calcified stylohyoid might be

responsible. The panoramic radiograph (Fig. 26–17) confirmed this clinical diagnosis. It was one of the largest calcified stylohyoid ligaments among hundreds of cases in our series. As in most cases, this one seemed to be jointed, and it resembled a large finger. There was also some calcification in the left neck, but much less. After the radiographic finding, we were able to produce the same excruciating pains by palpating the specific neck area and tonsillar fossa. Although we thought this would convince the patient, he refused all therapeutic recommendations, and he returned a few days later to his native land, in order to "die there," as he said.

Comments. Routine extraoral x-rays will reveal a fairly high incidence of calcified stylohyoid ligaments, some of them so large that one wonders why so few patients develop symptoms. Undoubtedly, the paucity of complaints relative to this condition catches us unaware when we do have a patient with symptoms. Variations in the size and shape of styloid processes are even seen in the same patient, as is shown in Figure 26–18.

The cases described in this and the preceding case reports should convey the extent and severity of the problem. Surgery is the only treatment and *in the hands of an expert* is a minor procedure.

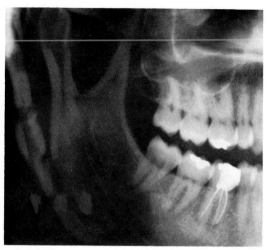

Figure 26–17 Calcified stylohyoid ligament. Note jointed appearance. (See Case Report No. 36.)

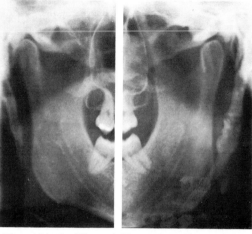

Figure 26–18 The styloid processes in one patient, showing the variation in size and shape. (See Case Report No. 36.)

REFERENCES

1. Adson, A. W.: The diagnosis and treatment of trigeminal neuralgia. Ann. Otol. Rhinol. Laryngol., 35:601–625, 1926.
2. Arai, H., and Snapper, L.: The influence of stilbamidine upon kidney function, liver function, and peripheral blood in multiple myeloma: neurologic sequelae of stilbamidine therapy. N.Y. State J. Med., 47:1867–1874, 1947.
3. Bauerle, J. E., and Archer, W. H.: Incidence of subluxation of the temporomandibular joint. J.A.D.A., 43:434, 1951.
4. Beaver, D. L., Moses, H. L., and Ganote, C. E.: Electron microscopy of the trigeminal ganglion III trigeminal neuralgia. Arch. Pathol., 17:571–582 (June), 1965.
5. Behrman, S., and Knight, G.: Decompression and compression operations for trigeminal neuralgia. Neurology, 6:363–367, 1956.
6. Bell, W. H., and Ware, W. H.: Management of temporomandibular joint pain dysfunction syndrome. Dent. Clin. North Am., 15(2):487–506 (Apr.), 1971.
7. Bender, I. B., and Seltzer, S.: The effect of periodontal disease on the pulp. Oral Surg., 33(3):458 (Mar.), 1972.
8. Blom, S.: Tic douloureux treated with new anticonvulsant. Arch. Neurol., 9:285–290, 1963.
9. Burket, L. W.: Oral Medicine. 3rd ed. Philadelphia, J. B. Lippincott Co., 1957.
10. Choukas, N. C., and Sicher, H: Structure of the temporomandibular joint. Oral Surg., 13:1203–1213 (Oct.), 1960.
11. Cleveland, D., and Kiefer, E. J.: Decompression of ganglion and posterior root of fifth nerve for trigeminal neuralgia. Arch. Otolaryngol., 59:30–35, 1954.
12. Costen, J. B.: Some features of the mandibular articulation as it pertains to medical diagnoses, especially in otolaryngology. J.A.D.A., 24:1507–1511, 1937.
13. Costen, J. B.: Correlation of x-ray findings in the mandibular joint with clinical signs, especially trismus. J.A.D.A., 26:405–407, 1939.
14. Crue, B. L., Shelden, C. H., Pudenz, R. H., and Freshwater, D. B.: Observations on the pain and trigger mechanisms in trigeminal neuralgia. Neurology, 6:196–207, 1956.
15. Cushing, H.: The major trigeminal neuralgias and their surgical treatment based on experiences with 332 gasserian operations; varieties of facial neuralgia. Am. J. Med. Sci. (new series), 160:157, 1920.
16. Dandy, W. E.: Surgery of the brain. In Lewis' Practice of Surgery. Vol. XIII, pp. 167–187. Hagerstown, Prior, 1945.
17. Dandy, W. E.: Trigeminal neuralgia. Am. J. Surg., 24:447–455, 1934.
18. Dandy, W. E.: Treatment of trigeminal neuralgia by the cerebellar route. Ann. Surg., 96:787–795, 1932.
19. Dandy, W. E.: Glossopharyngeal neuralgia (tic douloureux): its diagnosis and treatment. Arch. Surg., 15:198–214, 1927.
20. Davidoff, L. M.: The relief of tic douloureux with large doses of ferrous carbonate. Trans. Am. Neurol. Assoc., 70:176, 1944.
21. Davidoff, L. M.: Trifacial neuralgia. Oral Surg., 3:1239–1246, 1950.
22. Davidson, A. S.: Hemodynamic theory of pain production in temporomandibular joint syndrome. J. Oral Surg., 22:118 (Mar.), 1964.
23. Dott, N. M.: Discussion on facial pain. Proc. Royal Soc. Med., 44:1034–1037, 1951.
24. Ecker, A., and Perl, T.: Relief of tic douloureux by precise alcohol gasserian injection. In 2nd International Congress of Neurological Surgery of the World Federation of Neurosurgical Societies, Washington, D.C., 1961. Excerpta Medica Foundation Series No. 36, pp. E71–E72, 1961.
25. Evans, P. O.: Problems and solutions. Dent. Surv. (Apr.), 1955.
26. Fields, W. S., and Hoff, H. E.: Relief of pain in trigeminal neuralgia by crystalline vitamin B_{12}. Neurology, 2:131–139, 1952.
27. Fisher, A. A.: Allergic sensitization of the skin and oral mucosa to acrylic denture materials. J.A.M.A., 156:238 (Sept.), 1954.
28. Foster, J. M.: Facial pain. Br. Med. J., 4:667 (Dec. 13), 1969.
29. Friedman, A. P.: Facial pain. Oral Surg., 18:730 (Dec.), 1964.
30. Friedman, A. P., and Merritt, H. H.: Headache: Diagnosis and Treatment. Philadelphia, F. A. Davis Co., 1959.
31. Frazier, C. H.: A surgeon's impression of trigeminal neuralgia based on experience with three hundred and two cases. J.A.M.A., 70:1345–1350, 1918.
32. Gardner, W. J.: Concerning the mechanism of trigeminal neuralgia and hemifacial spasm. J. Neurosurg., 19:947–957, 1962.
33. Gardner, W. J., and Pinto, J. P.: Taarnhøj operation: relief of trigeminal neuralgia without numbness. Cleveland Clin. Q., 20:364–367, 1953.
34. Glaser, M. A.: Treatment of trigeminal neuralgia with tri-chlorethylene. J.A.M.A., 96:916–920, 1931.
35. Glaser, M. A.: Atypical facial neuralgia: diagnosis, cause and treatment. Arch. Intern. Med., 65:340–367, 1940.
36. Grant, F. C.: Complications accompanying surgical relief of pain in trigeminal neuralgia. Ann. Surg., 75:42–47, 1948.
37. Grantham, E. G., and Segarberg, L.: An evaluation of palliative surgical procedures in trigeminal neuralgia. J. Neurosurg., 9:390–394, 1952.
38. Hamby, W. B.: Diagnosis and management of trigeminal neuralgia. J. Am. Geriatr. Soc., 2:634–639, 1954.
39. Hassler, R., and Walker, A. E.: Trigeminal Neuralgia. Philadelphia, W. B. Saunders Co., 1970.
40. Horton, B. T., MacLean, A. R., and Craig, W. McK.: A new syndrome of fascicular headache; results of treatment with histamine: preliminary report. Proc. Staff Meet. Mayo Clin., 14:257–260, 1939.
41. Jannetta, P. J.: Microsurgical approach to posterior rhizotomy for tic douloureux. In Sweet, W. (Ed.): Progress in Neurological Surgery. In press.
42. Jannetta, P. J.: Pain problems of significance in the head and face, some of which often are misdiagnosed, pp. 47–53. In Current Problems in Surgery. Chicago, Year Book Medical Publishers, Inc., 1973.
43. Jannetta, P. J.: Trigeminal and glossopharyngeal neuralgia, pp. 849–851. In Conn, H. F., and

Conn, R. B. (Eds.): Current Diagnosis 3. Philadelphia, W. B. Saunders Co., 1971.

44. Jannetta, P. J.: The surgical binocular microscope in neurological surgery. Am. Surg. *34:*31–34, 1968.

45. Jannetta, P. J.: Arterial compression of the trigeminal nerve in patients with trigeminal neuralgia. J. Neurosurg. (Suppl.), *26:*159–162, 1967.

46. Jannetta, P. J., and Rand, R. W.: Transtentorial retrogasserian rhizotomy in trigeminal neuralgia, pp. 156–169. *In* Rand, R. W. (Ed.): Microsurgery. St. Louis, The C. V. Mosby Co., 1969.

47. Jannetta, P. J., and Rand, R. W.: Vascular compression of the trigeminal nerve at the pons in patients with trigeminal neuralgia. J. Neurosurg., *26:*150, 1967.

48. Kaiser-Meinhardt, I., and Seitz, E.: Medical and dental complications of an abnormally long styloid process. Monatsschr. Ohrenheilkd. Laryngorhinol., *93:*302–308 (Apr.), 1960.

49. Kerr, F. W. L., and Miller, R. H.: Pathology of trigeminal neuralgia. Arch. Neurol., *15:*308–319 (Sept.), 1966.

50. Logan, T. H.: Pain apparently referred across the midline from a perforated lower second molar. Oral Surg., *18:*593 (Nov.), 1964.

51. Love, J. G.: Surgical treatment of trigeminal and glossopharyngeal neuralgia: decompression of gasserian ganglion and its root for trigeminal. J. Int. Coll. Surg., *21:*1 (Jan.), 1954.

52. McKelvey, L. E.: Sclerosing solution in the treatment of chronic subluxation of the temporomandibular joint. J. Oral Surg., *8:*225 (July), 1947.

53. Markowitz, H. A., and Gerry, R. G.: Temporomandibular joint disease. Oral Surg., *3:*75 (Jan.), 1950.

54. Mason, D.: Peripheral neurectomy in the treatment of trigeminal neuralgia of the second and third divisions. J. Oral Surg., *30*(2):113 (Feb.), 1972.

55. Matson, M. S.: Pain in orofacial region associated with coronary insufficiency; report of a case. Oral Surg., *16:*284 (Mar.), 1963.

56. Moose, S. M.: Experimental injections of fibrosing solutions into the temporomandibular joints of monkeys. J.A.D.A., *28:*761 (May), 1941.

57. Nugent, R.: Personal communication, Jan., 1972.

58. Olivecrona, H.: Tractotomy for relief of trigeminal neuralgia. Arch. Neurol. Psychiatr., *47:*544–564, 1942.

59. Pelner, L.: Parotid duct obstruction without calculus: suggestion for treatment. Am. J. Dig. Dis., *9:*417 (Dec.), 1942.

60. Pelner, L., and Waldman, S.: Burning tongue. N.Y. J. Dent., *18:*218, 1948.

61. Prinz, H.: Dental Formulary. 6th ed. Philadelphia, Lea & Febiger, 1941.

62. Pudenz, R. H., and Shelden, C. H.: Experiences with foraminal decompression in the surgical treatment of tic douloureux. Presented at meeting of American Academy of Neurological Surgery, New York, October 1, 1952.

63. Rice, C. O.: Technique for the injection treatment of hernia. South. Surg., *5:*227, 1936.

64. Salman, I.: Traumatic injuries to the temporomandibular joint. J. Oral Surg., *7:*277 (Oct.), 1949.

65. Sarnat, B. G.: The Temporomandibular Joint. Springfield, Ill., Charles C Thomas, 1951.

66. Schaltenbrandt, G.: Neuralgia and other pain as observed by the neurologist. Calif. Med., *86:*362–365, 1957.

67. Schultz, L. W.: Report of ten years' experience in treating hypermobility of the temporomandibular joints. J. Oral Surg., *5:*202 (July), 1947.

68. Schultz, L. W.: A curative treatment for subluxation of the temporomandibular or any joint. J.A.D.A., *24:*1947 (Dec.), 1937.

69. Schwartz, L.: Disorders of the Temporomandibular Joint. Philadelphia, W. B. Saunders Co., 1959.

70. Shelden, C. H., Pudenz, R. H., Freshwater, D. B., and Crue, B. L.: Compression rather than decompression for trigeminal neuralgia. J. Neurosurg., *12:*123–126, 1955.

71. Silverman, S. I.: Oral Physiology. St. Louis, The C. V. Mosby Co., 1961.

72. Sluder, G.: Nasal Neurology, Headaches, and Eye Disorders. St. Louis, The C. V. Mosby Co., 1927.

73. Spiller, W. G., and Frazier, C. H.: Tic douloureux; anatomic and clinical basis for subtotal section of sensory root of trigeminal nerve. Arch. Neurol. Psychiatr., *29:*50–55, 1933.

74. Stender, A.: Discussion in Northfield, D. W. C.: Retrogasserian rhizotomy and other operations for trigeminal neuralgia: reassessment of their effectiveness and limitations. *In* Second International Congress of Neurological Surgery of the World Federation of Neurological Societies, p. E25. Excerpta Medica Foundation Series 36, 1961.

75. Svien, H. J., and Love, J. G.: Results of decompression operation for trigeminal neuralgia four years plus after operation. J. Neurosurg., *16:*653, 1959.

76. Taarnhøj, P.: Decompression of the trigeminal root. J. Neurosurg., *11:*299–305, 1954.

77. Travell, J., and Rinzler, S. H.: The myofascial genesis of pain. Postgrad. Med., *11:*425, 1952.

78. Thoma, K. H.: Oral Surgery. St. Louis, The C. V. Mosby Co., 1952.

79. White, J. C., and Sweet, W. H.: Pain. Its Mechanisms and Neurosurgical Control. Springfield, Ill., Charles C Thomas, 1955.

80. Wolff, H. G.: Headache. New York, Oxford University Press, 1963.

CHAPTER 27

THE DIAGNOSIS AND MANAGEMENT OF ORAL MALIGNANT DISEASES

MARVIN E. PIZER, D.D.S., M.S.

No one member of the health professions has a greater opportunity to recognize oral and maxillofacial cancer than does the family dentist. It is untrue to state that dentistry does not deal with "diseases of life and death."

The American Cancer Society estimated that 7600 Americans would die from oral and oropharyngeal cancer alone in 1973. An estimated 15,400 new cases were predicted to be discovered.[2] The 1974 estimate was that 24,000 new cases would be diagnosed. The dental profession, by diagnosing these lesions early, can significantly decrease the resulting deaths.

Malignant tumors that can present in the oral cavity as primary lesions are numerous, since malignant tumors can arise from epithelium or connective tissue anywhere within the mouth. The most common malignant disease is squamous cell carcinoma, of epithelial origin, which accounts for at least 90 per cent of all oral malignant neoplasms. On rare occasions there are metastases from the lungs, breasts, thyroid gland, prostate gland or gonads to the jaws or oral soft tissues.

PHYSICAL EXAMINATION

Every clinician must recognize that inspection and palpation of the head and neck, oral and pharyngeal regions are essential in order to discover and manage malignant diseases with success.

Inspection cannot be accomplished without excellent illumination. Besides the dental light, a headlight should be utilized to inspect some of the deeper recesses not seen directly. Asymmetry of the face, enlarged lymph nodes and thyroid disease can sometimes be seen before the patient is even comfortably seated in the dental chair. The lips, skin of the face, ears and salivary glands are subject to immediate inspection. Intraoral inspection should be done in an orderly fashion, the precise manner depending upon the clinician's wishes, but to include the lips, tongue, hard and soft palates, floor of the mouth, buccal mucosa, gingiva, tonsils, oropharynx, nasopharynx, hypopharynx and teeth. The clinician should determine whether flow from the major salivary glands is normal by examination of the orifices of Wharton's and Stensen's ducts. The dentist who already is skilled in the use of the dental mirror should have no difficulty in inspecting the naso-, oro- and hypopharynx. Suction may facilitate inspection of the lateral borders of the tongue and floor of the mouth near the anterior pillars of the tonsils. With gauze, the tip of the tongue should be grasped and pulled forward to better inspect and palpate the lateral borders and more posterior aspects of the dorsum of the tongue.

Digital palpation is equally, if not more,

revealing than visualization is in certain instances. Palpation of all accessible areas intra- and extraorally may reveal lesions not visible to the naked eye. Palpation supplements inspection, since the "educated" finger can appreciate the consistency and extent of a mass, its fixity and anatomic boundaries. The palpating digit can determine whether the mass is tender. An additional dimension in the physical examination is bimanual palpation when the mass is accessible, such as in the anterior portions of the tongue, lips, buccal mucosa and floor of the mouth. Much can be determined regarding a pathologic process by proper physical examination.

SYMPTOMS

The patient's inability to masticate effectively, pain, loose teeth, bad taste, spontaneous bleeding intraorally, trismus and dysphagia may all be symptoms suggestive of oral neoplastic disease. The examiner may on occasion detect foul odor from the patient, secondary to an infected or necrotic neoplasm. A persistent numbness or diminution in sensation of the face or lips, corroborated by objective examination, may be the result of local neoplastic invasion and occasionally of tumors of the central nervous system. Usually and unfortunately, however, there are no early symptoms of oral cancer.

CLINICAL APPEARANCE

Leukoplakia. *White areas* or *patches,* sometimes filmy and diffuse, that will not rub off, or *leathery white lesions,* are referred to as *leukoplakia.* These may be indicative of a completely benign condition or of varying degrees of epithelial dysplasia, carcinoma *in situ* or frank invasive carcinoma. It is important to biopsy these lesions when they do not disappear within 2 weeks to determine what they are, because clinically they are indistinguishable one from the other. Dysplastic leukoplakia has been recognized as a possible precursor to carcinoma. The overwhelming majority of leukoplakias do not show epithelial dysplasia, but when dysplasia is histologically present, the lesion must be completely excised. If diffuse, the lesion may be removed by electrosurgery. Waldron, after reviewing 1500 cases of lesions clinically diagnosed as leukoplakia or erythroplakia, has stated that about 10 per cent of these cases will show either severe epithelial dysplasia, carcinoma *in situ* or early invasive carcinoma.[26]

Erythroplakia. *Red areas* or *patches,* slightly raised and of velvety consistency, called *erythroplakia,* may or may not be well delineated. These lesions may represent early carcinoma.

Ulcers. *Ulcers* should always be examined with suspicion and, if persistent, be biopsied. Sometimes palpation will reveal underlying induration, and this is an ominous sign.

Speckled Leukoplakia. White and red areas mixed together are called *speckled leukoplakia.* These are sometimes a source of spontaneous bleeding and are usually slightly raised, with ill-defined margins. These lesions should be considered malignant until proven otherwise.

Masses. Especially when indurated and fixed, or ulcerated, *masses* may indicate malignant oral disease. If beneath normal mucosa, they may be completely asymptomatic and only detectable by palpation.

Salivary Flow. *Obstruction of salivary flow* from orifices of Wharton's or Stensen's ducts may imply invasion by a malignant neoplasm. If this has been a slow process, the patient may be asymptomatic, even though there is complete obliteration of a major salivary duct.

Pigmentation. *Brown or black pigmentation* of oral mucous membrane may represent one of the most deadly malignant neoplasms — malignant melanoma. This should be biopsied by wide excision, staying away from the tumor, if at all possible.

Certainly any unusual change in color, texture or consistency of oral mucosa *must* be investigated by biopsy if it persists longer than 2 weeks.

ETIOLOGY OF ORAL CANCER

The cause of oral cancer in man is not known; however, it is seen with such frequency in certain pre-existing conditions that a causative relationship seems likely.

Tobacco consumption, regardless of how it is used, has been incriminated in the etiology of oral cancer.

Excessive intake of alcohol added to heavy smoking provides a frequent finding in the oral cancer patient. It has been suggested that the excessive alcohol aids in absorption of tobacco carcinogens, or in production of nutritional deficiencies, setting up the squamous cells so that they become susceptible to conversion into cancer cells.

A close correlation between Plummer-Vinson syndrome and squamous cell carcinoma of the oral cavity certainly tends to implicate dietary deficiencies.

Therapeutic dosages of ionizing radiation may be a contributing factor to oral cancer.

The chronic exposure to actinic radiation, especially in the fair-complexioned patient, seems to predispose some patients to lip cancer. Blacks exhibit almost no lip cancer.

Though there is no definite evidence that chronic irritation—such as that caused by ill-fitting dentures or jagged teeth—produces malignancy, mucous membrane changes sometimes associated with chronic irritation would certainly arouse some degree of suspicion.

Wynder states that a positive correlation exists between squamous cell carcinoma of the anterior two-thirds of the tongue and syphilis.[27]

These described contributing factors may very well be cocarcinogens that trigger the carcinogen (conceivably a virus) to produce cancer. Patients who are on immunosuppressive drugs or who have been on long-term steroid therapy have a higher incidence of cancer.[7,19]

DIAGNOSIS

The diagnosis of oral cancer is established by biopsy. A negative histologic diagnosis in the presence of a clinically suspicious lesion dictates that another biopsy be performed. The clinician must satisfy himself that the clinical disease and histologic results are compatible.

Cytologic examination is of some value, but it does not replace a biopsy. It is said to have a diagnostic reliability of 86 per cent.

Toluidine blue (2 per cent), a nuclear stain, will demonstrate some dysplastic and malignant lesions. The area to be stained is gently cleansed with 1 per cent acetic acid. The dye is then placed and left on for 30 seconds. The area is then cleansed again with 1 per cent acetic acid. If the dye is retained, the lesion is blue. Nonspecific ulcers, fibrin, and inflammatory lesions may stain positively, while carcinoma covered by hyperkeratosis will not stain at all. Therefore, there is only limited value with this technique. It is probably most useful in outlining a known malignant condition, as small satellite lesions may become demonstrable.

Radiography is sometimes helpful in determining extensive neoplastic involvement of the maxilla or mandible, but it cannot be relied upon. Invasion by neoplastic cells may show a normal radiographic appearance until late in the disease. Dental periapical films give better detail than do lateral jaw films. Stereoscopic films, panoramic radiographs and laminograms are all of value, particularly when the neoplasm is of osseous origin or when bony involvement is clear-cut, and information regarding extension into the sinuses or other adjacent anatomic locations needs evaluation. Radiographs of the chest, skull and long bones may inform the clinician about whether an oral malignant tumor has metastasized. Scans of various organs and blood chemistry often assist in determining whether metastatic disease is present.

Examination of the neck, including inspection and palpation, may reveal to the surgeon whether there is clinical metastasis to lymph nodes of the neck.

Serum LDH (lactic acid dehydrogenase) has been suggested as an enzyme that is elevated in patients with head and neck cancer. Effective treatment of the malignant disease supposedly reduces the enzyme to normal levels. In our experience, LDH studies have been an unreliable index in regard to whether effective therapy has been employed.

The student or clinician interested in malignant disease of the mouth should familiarize himself with the TNM classification system of the oral cavity. (See Chapter 29, "Radiation Therapy of Lesions of the Oral Cavity.")

TREATMENT

Once the dentist sees a lesion that within 2 weeks has not responded to conservative treatment, he is obliged to establish a definite diagnosis by biopsy. If the family dentist does not wish to do the biopsy, the patient should be referred immediately to an oral surgeon or another dental colleague capable of rendering this service. (See Biopsy Technique in Chapter 13.)

When an intraoral malignant disease is

diagnosed, the best modality of therapy must be decided upon without delay. If a tumor board is available in the community, it may be used; if not, the equivalent would be to send the patient to the kinds of specialists for consultation that would normally constitute a tumor board. The reason for the team approach to intraoral malignant lesions lies in the fact that there is generally more than one acceptable form of treatment.

The ideal tumor board should include oncologists who specialize in surgery of the head and neck, a radiotherapist and a chemotherapist. The team should also include an oral surgeon, oral pathologist, otolaryngologist, prosthodontist, internist and plastic surgeon. After examination of the patient, the decision of this board regarding initial therapy must be final.

If, for example, radical excision of the jaw and tongue with combined neck dissection has been deemed best for the patient, then the services of the surgical oncologist are indicated. The prosthodontist should be informed about the nature of the surgical procedure prior to surgery so that this professional can afford the patient comfort postoperatively with a prosthesis and prepare for a definitive rehabilitation program. The oral surgeon and prosthodontist assisting the cancer surgeon at the operating room table may provide many benefits to the patient. If the tumor board decides that wide local excision is indicated, not involving a neck dissection, the services of the oral surgeon should be utilized; when irradiation or chemotherapy is indicated, then the respective specialist is needed.

The postoperative care and follow-up examination must be the responsibility of the specialist who has treated the patient. Should complications or recurrences present, then the patient should be referred again to the tumor board or its equivalent for additional evaluation and treatment.

Surgery, irradiation, or both, are the major modalities used in treating oral cancer. Chemotherapy is primarily used in palliative treatment of this disease; however, it has also been used prior to surgery and irradiation.

On occasion, multiple modalities of therapy may be necessary to provide the patient with the most favorable prognosis. Factors determining the modality of therapy depend on histopathology, location and size of the lesion, physical findings of the head and neck,

presence or absence of metastatic disease, age, and general physical and mental condition of the patient. Assessment concerning whether this is a recurrent or possibly a metastatic neoplasm must always be taken into consideration. Adequate oral and facial rehabilitation must not be denied a patient. He must be allowed to return to society with acceptable cosmetic and functional results.

Lip cancer is the exception in which a tumor board is not deemed necessary, as most lip cancers respond favorably with either irradiation or surgery when treated by competent practitioners.

The family dentist should be completely informed of his patient's progress and prognosis so that he can intelligently employ a program of practical dental care. Even in cases in which neoplastic disease does not involve the oral and maxillofacial region, the family dentist should consult with a knowledgeable physician about the patient's prognosis. The dentist must always be aware that malignant disease from other parts of the body may metastasize to the mouth, and any unusual oral changes in a cancer patient should be biopsied. The dentist who treats a terminal cancer patient would be unkind to institute extensive reconstructive dentistry when the patient's expected longevity is minimal.

CARCINOMA OF THE LIP

Carcinoma of the lip accounts for approximately 25 per cent of cancers in the oral region and 15 per cent of malignant lesions involving the head and neck. The American Cancer Society estimated, for example, that 1900 new lip cancers would be diagnosed in 1973 in the United States.[2] Careful oral examination by the dentist and physician could almost exclude the morbidity and mortality of this disease by early diagnosis.

At least 95 per cent of lip carcinomas involve the lower lip, members of the male sex constituting well over 90 per cent of the cases in the United States, with a male-to-female ratio of 14:1.[14] This disease is rare in blacks. Leffall, Professor and Chairman, Department of Surgery at Howard University College of Medicine, reports only 2 cases in black patients in the past 12 years.[17] The disease is seen primarily in patients over 40 years of age. The upper lip is seldom involved by this disease, but when a growth is present there, it has a higher incidence of metastases and consequently is a more serious lesion.

The clinical appearance may vary from chronic ulceration to a wart, fissure, thickened mass, raised crusty lesion resembling a "fever blister," and sometimes a white or red lesion that will not rub off.

The usual location on the lower lip is halfway between the commissure and the midline. The lesions at the commissure appear to have a poorer prognosis than do the other lower lip lesions. In a large study by Bernier and Clark, only 15 per cent of the cases were in the midline.[8]

There are three main macroscopic varieties seen:

1. The *verrucous variety* is the rarest and appears cauliflower-like or papillary in growth, with frequent ulceration in the deep crevices. These may be expansile lesions superficially, but there is minimal tendency toward infiltration of the underlying structures.

2. The *exophytic* lesion is the most common variety, grows slowly and appears as a warty mass with a nodular white surface that is usually ulcerated in the center when it enlarges. There may be some crusting on the surface of this lesion from the exuding serum. This growth is usually of low-grade malignancy, and consequently there is minimal invasion of underlying structures and no real propensity toward metastases.

3. The *ulcerative type* of lip carcinoma usually presents as a small ulcer on the surface of the lip; however, it is the most aggressive of the three varieties. It frequently does not start out as a premalignant lesion and evolve into a malignant one, as the others may do. It shows a higher grade of malignancy histologically than do the other two varieties and is capable of extensive infiltration. It is more likely to metastasize if allowed to persist.

In addition to squamous cell carcinoma, other histologic varieties arising from the mucosa of the lip are basal cell carcinoma, melanoma and salivary gland tumors. The latter three are extremely rare. Squamous cell carcinoma accounts for about 99 per cent of all malignant disease in the lip. These lesions are usually well differentiated and even when discovered late frequently have not metastasized. The undifferentiated, or anaplastic, lip carcinoma, though rare, will metastasize to the regional lymph nodes first, namely, the submental and submaxillary nodes, and eventually to the jugular chain.

Distant metastases to lungs, liver and so forth are extremely rare. The 5-year survival rate of patients with lip carcinoma reported by most authors ranges from 80 to 90 per cent. Even with extensive oral and regional involvement (bone, muscle, skin and lymph nodes), the 5-year survival rate is at least 60 per cent.[5]

The modalities of treatment basically include either irradiation or surgery, seldom the combination. Since surgery can frequently be done on an outpatient basis under either local or general anesthesia, with minimal loss of time to the patient, the surgical approach to most lip carcinomas is preferred.

The treatment for this disease will vary depending upon the size of the lesion, histopathologic findings and whether there are metastases to lymph nodes or distant metastases. The premalignant lesions are treated by a vermilionectomy, or *lip shave*. The very early squamous cell carcinomas are treated by lip shave and a "trough" or U excision of the muscle underlying the mucosa. This technique is especially valuable when other small suspicious lesions are noted on the lip. Carcinomas of the lip that can be removed with a margin of 1.5 cm. of healthy tissue in all directions and do not involve more than one third of the lip should be removed by a shield excision or wedge resection. The ulcerative variety, because of its greater aggressiveness and tendency toward being less differentiated histologically than the exophytic or verrucous carcinomas, should be treated by wider excision when suspected clinically. Primary closure with excellent cosmetic and functional results can be obtained when one third of the lip is resected. In the more extensive lesions in which more than one third of the lip must be excised, it is necessary to resort to plastic procedures such as the Abbé-Estlander operation, or modifications of this operation, in which a flap is rotated from the opposite lip in order to have an adequate closure. These procedures frequently leave a small oral aperture as well as a cosmetic defect at the commissure of the lip. A second operation for reconstruction of the lip is generally performed 4 to 6 weeks after the first procedure. The choice of procedures to enlarge the oral opening with satisfactory cosmetic results is multiple.

Prophylactic neck dissections have no place in the management of lip cancer; however, when a lymph node is suspected of having metastatic disease, the neck should be treated as with any other head and neck cancer.

In cases in which there are lymph node me-tastases, we prefer to perform excision of the primary carcinoma first and then a neck dis-section in 2 to 3 weeks. In some cases, inflammatory nodes in the neck will disap-pear, but if still present 3 weeks postopera-tively, they should be biopsied with the intent of doing a neck dissection if positive.

Most failures are due to recurrences of the primary lesion or those in the neck nodes or both. The rare distant metastases will fre-quently result in the demise of the patient.

Case Report No. 1

LIP SHAVE IN EARLY SQUAMOUS CELL CARCINOMA

Patient. A 55-year-old white male was referred to the office for dental extractions in April.

Chief Complaint. Loose teeth with gingival infection.

History of Present Illness. During routine oral examination, "rough" spots and crusting of the lower lip were noted. The lip was stained with 2 per cent toluidine blue, and this revealed multiple areas retaining the dye. Following the indicated extractions, the patient was told to return in 2 weeks for repeat toluidine blue staining, which again revealed the initial findings. Prominent reten-tion of the dye was noted to the right of the mid-line, with another two areas of the left lower lip, one halfway between the midline and commissure and the other near the corner (Fig. 27–1A and B).

Medical Evaluation. The patient admitted to smoking 3½ packs of cigarettes per day and exces-sive intake of alcoholic beverages. The remainder of his medical history was noncontributory.

Operative Technique. An excisional biopsy of the *two* small ulcerations of the lower left lip, seen primarily by staining with toluidine blue, was ac-complished. The lip was anesthetized with mental nerve blocks with 2 per cent mepivacaine (Car-bocaine) hydrochloride with 1:20,000 levonor-defrin (Neo-Cobefrin). The specimens were sent to the pathology department for diagnosis, after being carefully labeled.

Pathology Report. *Microscopic Diagnosis:* (1) Moderate epithelial dysplasia associated with ulceration, left corner of the lip.

(2) Early squamous cell carcinoma, oral mucosa, lower left lip (halfway between midline and corner of the lip). The specimen is adequately excised (R. P. Elzay, D.D.S., M.S.D.).

Postoperative Course. Additional examination of the neck for possible clinical evidence of metas-tasis, radiographs of the chest, skull and facial bones, complete blood count and differential count, BSP (liver function test) and a serology test were performed. Only the liver function test re-sults were not within normal limits. Because there were other areas of the lower lip that took a posi-tive stain with 2 per cent toluidine blue, a vermil-ionectomy and U resection were advised.

Operative Technique. With 2 per cent mepiva-caine (Carbocaine) hydrochloride with 1:20,000 levonordefrin (Neo-Cobefrin) injected into the mental foramen bilaterally, the lower lip was anes-thetized. The patient was given 75 mg. meperidine and 8 mg. diazepam (Valium) intravenously pre-operatively. The patient was prepared and draped in the usual fashion. Beginning with the conventional technique for a lip shave, and after removal of the vermilion mucous membrane, a U or trough-shaped wedge of muscle was excised, along with adjacent skin and mucous membrane, to insure wider margins of healthy tissue (Fig. 27–1C and D). The wound was closed by suturing of the mucous membrane to the skin with 0000 inter-rupted silk sutures (Fig. 27–1E). The entire speci-men was sent to the pathology department after being labeled properly.

Pathology Report. *Microscopic:* Specimen is adequately excised. Severe epithelial dysplasia and hyperkeratosis, oral mucosa, right lip near midline (R. P. Elzay, D.D.S., M.S.D.).

Postoperative Course. The patient was worked up medically to resolve abnormal findings in liver function studies, and he has been followed on a 3-month basis. There have been no complications, and he has had excellent cosmetic results (Fig. 27–1F and G). Local block anesthesia was used in preference to infiltration to prevent possible dis-semination of neoplastic cells and distortion of anatomic structures.

Comment. This malignant lesion was an in-cidental finding in a patient referred to the office for dental extractions. Clinically, the lower lip was not particularly suspicious except for the "rough," crusty spots, which were small and suggestive of possible minor irritation from cigarette paper or even "chapped lips." Toluidine blue was helpful in clearly demonstrating the excoriation of the lip epithelium and its persistent positive staining in the same places on two occasions, 2 weeks apart. This prompted excisional biopsy and subsequent definitive surgery. When there are small multiple lesions, either early squamous cell carcinomas or those showing varying degrees of epithelial dysplasia, lip shave (vermilionectomy) combined with U resection should result in an excellent prognosis, good function and very acceptable cosmetic results. The U resection is generally reserved for the early carcinomas.

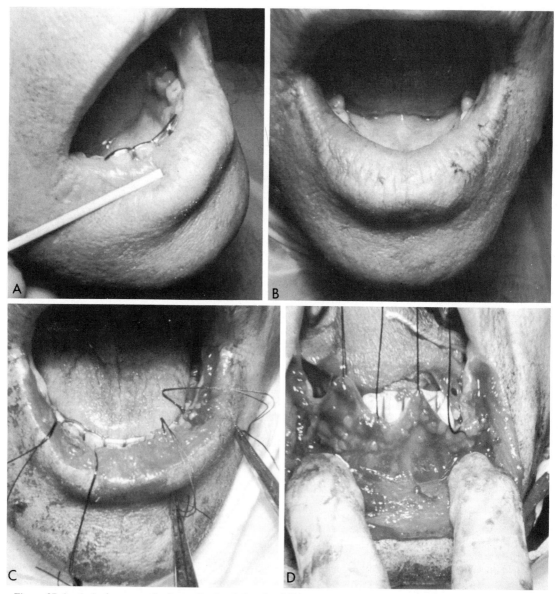

Figure 27–1 *A,* A change on the lower lip that is barely visible when viewed by the naked eye. *B,* Lip stained with 2 per cent toluidine blue, revealing multiple suspicious areas. Area near the left midline of the lip was early carcinoma not seen by the naked eye. *C,* Completed vermilionectomy of the lower lip. Silk sutures placed on the labial mucosa prior to ∪ resection. *D,* Trough or ∪ resection essentially completed.

(*Figure 27–1 continued on opposite page*)

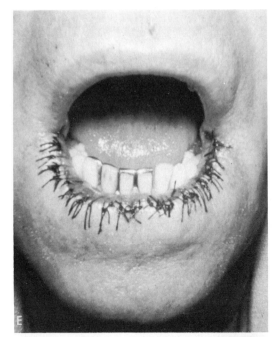

Figure 27–1 (*Continued.*) *E*, Immediate postoperative appearance. Mucous membrane sutured to the skin. *F*, Patient 6 weeks postoperatively. *G*, Six weeks postoperatively with lips closed.

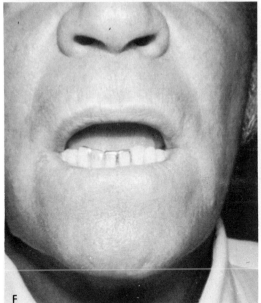

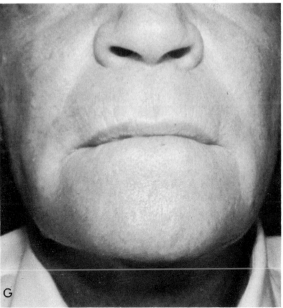

Case Report No. 2

SHIELD EXCISION FOR ULCERATIVE CARCINOMA OF THE LIP

Patient. A 68-year-old white male was referred to the office for dental extractions in June.

Chief Complaint. Mobile teeth from extensive periodontal disease.

History of Present Illness. On examination, an ulceration halfway between the midline and corner of lower right lip was noted. The lesion was found to stain positively with toluidine blue (Fig. 27–2*A*

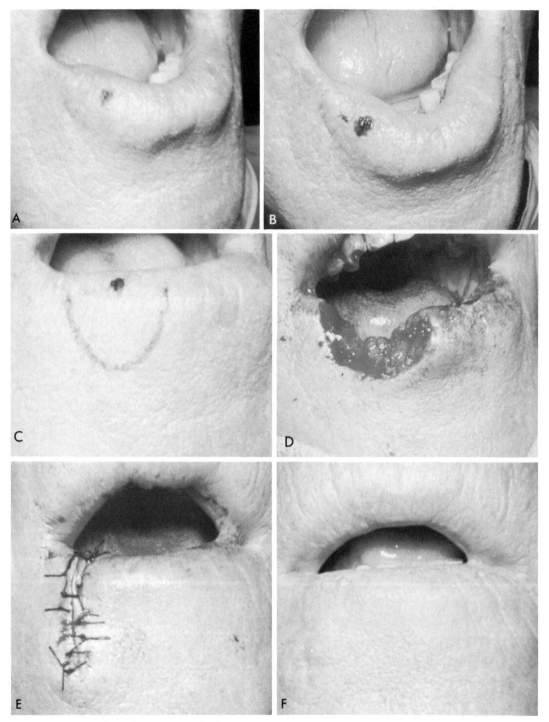

Figure 27–2 *A*, Patient with a history of skin cancer having a suspicious-looking area on the lip. The lesion is apparently of many years' duration. *B*, The lesion retained 2 per cent toluidine blue dye and showed a questionable small satellite lesion adjacent to it. *C*, Incision is outlined with methylene blue; at least 1 cm. of grossly normal tissues is necessary for safe margins. *D*, Full thickness of lip resected; bleeders have been tied off. *E*, Immediate postoperative appearance. The defect is closed in layers, the skin with 0000 and 5-0 silk in interrupted and vertical mattress sutures. *F*, Two-month postoperative appearance. Excellent cosmetic and functional results.

and *B*). Dental extraction was performed, and the patient was told to return in 2 weeks for a recheck of the lower right lip.

Medical Evaluation. Coronary artery disease with a history of myocardial infarction, hyperuricemia and glaucoma was revealed. The patient's surgical history revealed herniorrhaphy for ventral hernia and excision of basal cell carcinomas of the skin. He denied using tobacco at this time but admitted to heavy cigarette smoking for 30-plus years prior to myocardial infarction 5 years before this examination.

Course. Two weeks after the initial visit, repeat staining with toluidine blue was positive. Clinically, the lesion had not changed. Neck nodes were not palpable. The patient was admitted to the hospital for lip surgery. Chest radiographs revealed left ventricular hypertrophy. The remainder of the laboratory findings were within normal limits.

Operative Technique. The anesthetic, 2 per cent lidocaine (Xylocaine) with 1:100,000 epinephrine, was injected into the right and left mental foramen regions. An incisional biopsy of the lip lesion was taken for frozen section, and a diagnosis of squamous cell carcinoma of low-grade malignancy was made. The patient was prepared and draped. With a clean set of instruments, the lesion was totally resected by means of a shield excision. Skin, muscle and mucous membrane were resected with clinically normal tissue margins of at least 1 cm. in all directions. Bleeders were tied off with 000 chromic catgut. The wound was closed in layers, starting with mucous membrane, then muscle (both closed with 000 plain catgut interrupted sutures), and finally skin (closed with 5-0 silk interrupted and vertical mattress sutures). (See Figure 27–2*C* and *D*.) The patient left the operating room in satisfactory condition. The specimen was labeled and sent to the pathology department.

Pathology Report. *Quick Frozen Section Diagnosis:* Carcinoma of low-grade malignancy.

Microscopic Diagnosis: (1) Advanced senile keratosis (margins clear), lower lip.

(2) Fragments of mucous minor salivary gland, essentially unremarkable (Paul Snow, M.D.).

Course. The patient's course was uneventful, but because of questionable diagnosis consultation with another pathologist, Dr. Richard P. Elzay, an oral pathologist, was sought.

Pathology Consultation. The report from Dr. Elzay read in part:

. . . There is evidence of senile elastosis, and I can recognize how this could be classified as senile keratosis; however, it is my experience that a lesion such as this on a mucous membrane surface will behave as squamous cell carcinoma. I believe there is microscopic invasion of the specimen but that it is adequately excised and fortunately treated early enough that this patient should have no further problems. . . .

> Richard P. Elzay, D.D.S., M.S.D.
> Professor and Chairman
> Department of Oral Pathology
> Virginia Commonwealth University

Postoperative Course. The patient's postoperative course continued to be uneventful. There was no recurrence, but close follow-up was mandatory. Afil cream (antiactinic cream) was prescribed for the patient to use when outdoors. A good cosmetic result was obtained (Fig. 27–2*E* and *F*).

Comment. Senile keratosis on oral mucous membrane is essentially a malignant disease and behaves like squamous cell carcinoma. On skin, senile keratosis is a benign lesion that some general pathologists classify as premalignant. It is important to know that histologically identical lesions can be serious in one anatomic site and benign in another. The shield excision may be combined with a vermilionectomy (lip shave) when other premalignant lesions are suspected of involving the lip.

Case Report No. 3

WEDGE RESECTION FOR "FEVER BLISTER" CARCINOMA OF THE LIP

Patient. A 52-year-old Caucasian male was referred to the office by his internist regarding a lesion of the left lower lip in October.

Chief Complaint. Ulcerated lesion, left lip near the corner of the mouth, with a crusting surface (Fig. 27–3*A*).

History of Present Illness. The patient indicated a history of spontaneous bleeding from this lesion of 8 months' duration. He admitted to smoking one pack of cigarettes a day for approximately 20 years, but said he had quit smoking 6 years ago. He also admitted to moderate consumption of al-

cohol. The patient spends a large amount of time working outdoors.

Medical Evaluation. The lesion measured about 1 cm. in circumference, with an ulceration in the center. The periphery of the lesion was red and felt "leathery" on palpation. There were no palpable neck nodes. The patient had no other medical problems except for asthma.

Course. The lesion was stained with 2 per cent toluidine blue and retained the dye. Exfoliative cytologic findings were negative for malignant cells (Fig. 27–3*B*). A smear revealed the presence of

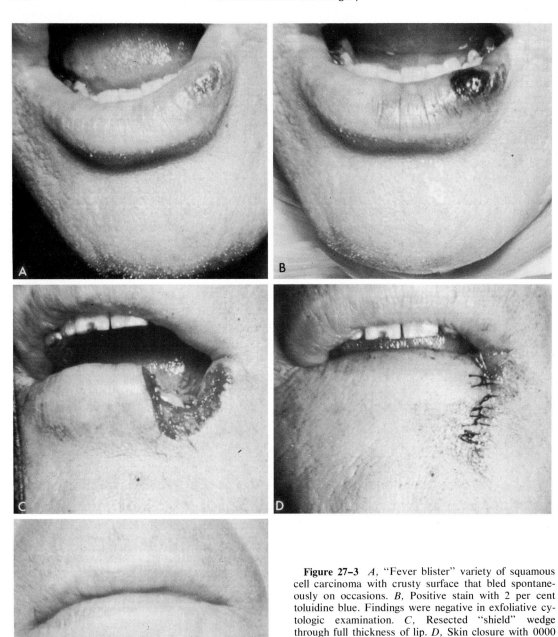

Figure 27-3 *A,* "Fever blister" variety of squamous cell carcinoma with crusty surface that bled spontaneously on occasions. *B,* Positive stain with 2 per cent toluidine blue. Findings were negative in exfoliative cytologic examination. *C,* Resected "shield" wedge through full thickness of lip. *D,* Skin closure with 0000 silk interrupted sutures. It is essential to approximate vermilion borders first before closing skin to achieve a good cosmetic result. *E,* Patient 18 months postoperatively. Minimal cosmetic and no functional loss.

Staphylococcus aureus, and antibiotic sensitivity studies showed this strain of *Staphylococcus aureus* to be sensitive to tetracycline. The patient was put on this antibiotic for 1 week. Chest radiograph, blood chemistry and serologic findings were all within normal limits. When the patient returned 1 week later, there was no improvement; hospital arrangements were made for a frozen section of the lesion and the necessary definitive surgery.

Operative Procedure. The patient was brought to surgery after premedication with 75 mg. of meperidine hydrochloride (Demerol), $1/150$ grain of atropine sulfate and 75 mg. of pentobarbital sodium (Nembutal) intramuscularly. When arriving at the operating room, the patient had some nausea and general abdominal discomfort. He was given 50 mg. of cyclizine (Marezine) intramuscularly, which relieved his symptoms.

The lower lip was blocked by injection of 2 per cent lidocaine (Xylocaine) with 1:100,000 epinephrine bilaterally into the region of the mental foramen. An infraorbital nerve block of the left maxilla was also administered in case an Abbé-Estlander flap would be needed. The patient was prepared and draped in the usual fashion. An incisional biopsy was taken for frozen section, and the first specimen was unrevealing. A second, larger specimen was removed, and this was reported by the pathologist to be carcinoma.

The patient was again prepared and draped, and a clean set of instruments was used. Under the previously administered local anesthesia, a wedge resection (or shield excision) was performed, taking no less than 1 cm. of normal margins on all sides of the lesion (Fig. 27–3C). The bleeders were tied off, and the mucous membrane was closed with 000 chromic catgut interrupted sutures. The muscle was next closed with 000 plain catgut interrupted sutures, and the skin was finally closed with 0000 silk interrupted sutures (Fig. 27–3D). The lesion was covered with Neosporin and a pressure dressing applied. The patient tolerated surgery and anesthesia and left the operating room in good condition. The specimen was labeled and sent to the pathology department.

Pathology Report. *Quick Frozen Section Diagnosis:* Carcinoma. The specimen was a wedge-shaped resection of the lower lip that had a surface diameter of up to 2.1 cm. and a depth of up to 1.9 cm. There was a central defect, in part due to the specimen excised for frozen section examination. This cavity shows hemorrhagic surfaces. The excision exhibited margins of grossly normal skin clearance varying from 0.1 to 0.2 cm. Upon section of the lesion, it was seen to extend to a depth of at least 1.2 cm. The tumor was semifirm in consistency and focally hemorrhagic. The specimen was trisected perpendicularly to the surface lip axis and totally submitted to examination.

Microscopic Diagnosis: Epidermoid carcinoma (Grade II to III) of lower lip (wedge resection); margins and depth were clear (J. H. Roe, Jr., M.D.).

Postoperative Course. The patient's subsequent course was completely uneventful. There was no recurrence, and the patient had good function and very acceptable cosmetic results (Fig. 27–3E).

Comment. In spite of the fact that a specimen with borders of at least 1 cm. of clinically healthy tissue was excised, the lesion microscopically revealed only 0.1 to 0.2 cm. of normal skin clearance. It is known that the specimen will shrink when removed and put into a fixative, but also a lesion can be microscopically present in clinically normal-looking tissue. Therefore, at least 1 cm. of normal-looking tissue should be excised with a neoplasm, and close follow-up is essential. Occasionally it may be necessary to bring a patient back to surgery to obtain better margins.

Case Report No. 4

SHIELD EXCISION AND FLAP ROTATION FOR CARCINOMA OF THE LIP*

Patient. A 67-year-old Caucasian male presented with an exophytic lesion of the left lower lip of unknown duration in August (Fig. 27–4A). A general surgeon had biopsied this growth, and it was diagnosed as granuloma pyogenicum. The patient was using an ointment prescribed by his surgeon to "dry up" the lesion. The patient was persuaded to undergo an incisional biopsy because of the suspicious appearance of the growth. The lesion measured approximately 5 by 3 cm.

Medical Evaluation. The patient's history was noncontributory. Chest radiographs indicated no metastases, and the patient had no palpable nodes in the neck.

Pathology Report. *Microscopic Diagnosis:* Squamous cell carcinoma, well differentiated (R. M. Howell, M.D.).

Operative Procedure. The patient reported to the hospital for definitive surgery in September; this was performed under local anesthesia, with 2 per cent lidocaine (Xylocaine) with 1:100,000 epinephrine. Right and left mental nerve blocks and left infraorbital nerve block were administered. The patient was prepared and draped in the conventional fashion. A shield type of incision was outlined with methylene blue with a minimum of 1 cm. of clinically normal tissue on all sides of the neoplasm. A triangular area was also outlined on

---

* Adapted from Pizer, M. E., and Kay, S.: Mouth Cancer—Concepts of treatment. Va. Med. Mon., *99:*148–166 (Feb.), 1972.

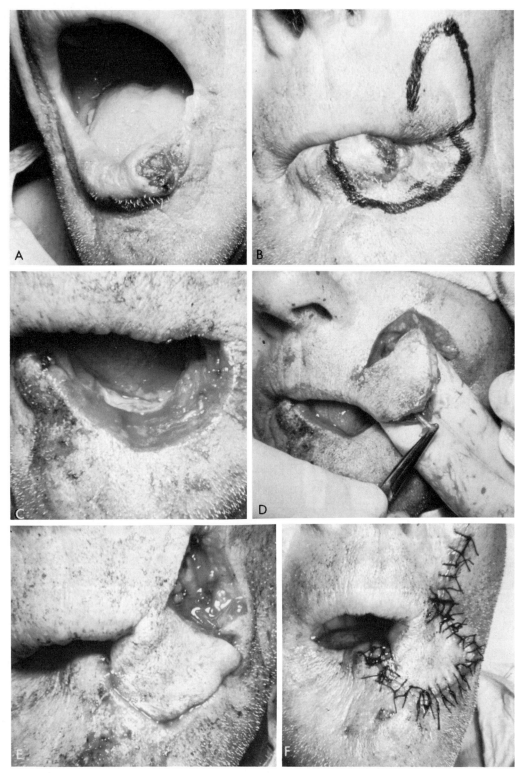

Figure 27–4 *A*, Exophytic squamous cell carcinoma involving almost one half of the lip. *B*, Methylene blue outline of incision for removal of malignant tissue and of flap to be rotated from upper lip. *C*, Malignant lesion on lower lip excised. *D*, Full thickness flap from upper lip being mobilized. Note medial pedicle which contains superior labial artery to nourish flap. *E*, Flap from upper lip rotated into defect of lower lip. *F*, Wound closed in layers. Immediate postoperative appearance.

(*Figure 27–4 continued on opposite page*)

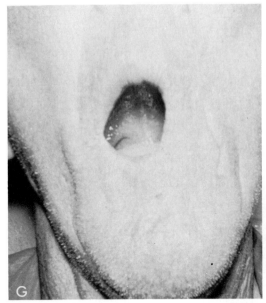

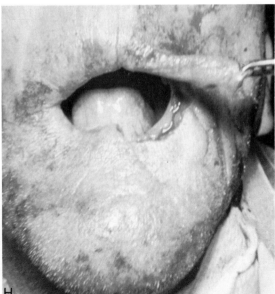

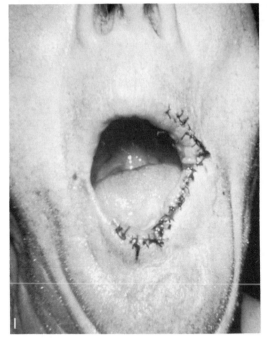

Figure 27–4 (*Continued.*) *G*, Small oral aperture requiring enlargement. Surgery should be performed about 4 to 6 weeks after the first operation. *H*, The vermilion of the upper and lower lips is mobilized for placement into the triangular muscle bed as the new upper lip. The muscle of the commissure is cut horizontally, opening the mouth. The lower lip is made by undermining labial mucous membrane and suturing it to the skin. *I*, Appearance following enlargement of oral aperture. Patient can open mouth wide and has satisfactory cosmetic and excellent functional results. (*A, B* and *F*, From Pizer, M. E., and Kay, S.: Mouth cancer – Concepts of treatment. Va. Med. Mon., *99:*148–166 [Feb.], 1972.)

the upper lip, the length slightly longer than the approximated excision and the width about one-half that of the proposed defect (Fig. 27–4*B*). A pedicle of about 7 mm. from the mucocutaneous junction was retained on the medial aspect of the upper lip flap, for this contains the superior labial artery, which must be preserved.

The malignant lesion was excised through and through, the bleeders were tied off, and a bed for the flap was prepared (Fig. 27–4*C*). Following excision of the neoplasm, clean instruments for flap mobilization and rotation were used. The upper flap was mobilized through and through and then rotated into the lower lip (Fig. 27–4*D* and *E*). A three-layer closure was performed on both upper and lower lips. The mucosa was closed with 000 plain catgut, the muscle with 0000 chromic catgut and the skin with 5-0 silk sutures, in that order, with the upper lip closed first and then the lower lip (Fig. 27–4*F*). Special care in lining up the vermilion edges is important for good cosmetic results. A pressure dressing was applied to the upper and lower lips. The patient tolerated surgery and left the operating room in good condition. The specimen was sent to the pathology department.

Pathology Report. *Microscopic Diagnosis:* Epidermoid carcinoma, moderately well differentiated, oral mucosa, lip. Specimen appears adequately excised (R. P. Elzay, D.D.S., M.S.D.).

Postoperative Course. A stitch abscess developed that was treated with penicillin and removal of the suture. All sutures were removed on the seventh postoperative day. The pedicle is usually left alone for about 6 weeks, and then a second operation is performed to enlarge the oral aperture (Fig. 27–4G). Because of the distance the patient had to travel for treatment, this second procedure was not performed for approximately 11 months postoperatively.

Operative Procedure. Under local anesthesia, the following procedure was performed: The patient was prepared and draped in the usual fashion. An incision beginning through the mucosa at the mucocutaneous junction near the corner of the left upper lip was made and carried down to encompass 1.5 cm. of the lower lip, where the incision was then brought back intraorally to near its origin in the upper lip. The width of mucous membrane necessary to make a presentable vermilion border was undermined and mobilized. This flap was freed from the underlying tissues, leaving exposed muscle in the lower lip and corner of the mouth. A triangular wedge of skin adjacent to the mucocutaneous border at the commissure was excised. The base of the triangle was adjacent to the corner of the lips. The size of the triangle depends on the amount of oral aperture desired. Following excision of this skin, a horizontal incision through the muscle and mucosa was made, thus opening the oral aperture. The mobilized mucosal flap taken from the upper lip, commissure, and lower lip was then transposed laterally to complete the new upper lip. This mucosal flap was then sutured intraorally with 000 interrupted silk sutures and to the skin with 5-0 interrupted silk sutures (Fig. 27–4H). The intraoral mucosa of the lower lip was mobilized down to the mucobuccal fold with small scissors and then brought forward and sutured with 5-0 interrupted silk sutures to the cutaneous margins of the lower lip defect (as is done in a conventional lip shave). The patient tolerated the procedure and left the operating room in good condition.

Postoperative Course. All sutures were removed on the seventh postoperative day. Excellent postoperative results were obtained. The patient was able to wear dentures and had satisfactory cosmetic results (Fig. 27–4I). There has been no evidence of recurrence or metastasis to date (4 years later).

Case Report No. 5

SHIELD EXCISION AND FLAP ROTATION FOR ULCERATIVE MIDLINE LIP CARCINOMA

Patient. A 50-year-old white male presented with an ulcerative lesion of unknown duration in the midline of his lower lip in August.

Medical Evaluation. The midline lip lesion measured about 1.5 cm. in circumference and felt indurated well below the surface ulceration (Fig. 27–5A). Clinical findings were negative in regard to palpable neck nodes upon physical examination. All other findings were within normal limits, including those from a chest radiograph. The patient admitted to heavy cigarette smoking, moderate use of alcohol and an occupation which required outside work.

Operative Procedure. Bilateral mandibular nerve blocks, a left infraorbital nerve block and infiltration of the left upper lip and cheek were accomplished with 2 per cent lidocaine (Xylocaine) with 1:100,000 epinephrine. The patient was prepared and draped in the usual fashion. With a No. 15 Bard-Parker blade, a wide shield-shaped full thickness of lip with 1.5 to 2.0 cm. of visibly healthy tissue on all sides was resected (Fig. 27–5B). Bleeders were clamped and tied with 000 chromic catgut. A second incision, with clean instruments, was made in the corner of the left lower lip, down to the depth of the excised tumor, through skin, muscle and mucous membrane. Bleeders were again tied in the usual fashion. This full thickness of lower lip was then transposed medially to close the midline defect, thus leaving a defect at the left corner of the lip (Fig. 27–5C). The midline lip defect was closed in layers, first mucous membrane with 000 chromic catgut, then muscle with 0000 chromic catgut and finally skin with 0000 silk sutures, with care to line up the mucocutaneous junctions evenly.

A triangular flap of the left upper lip was then outlined with methylene blue, the width of the flap being half the width of the lower lip defect and the length slightly more than that of the defect. A full thickness of upper lip was then mobilized, leaving a medial pedicle of about 8 mm. attached for the superior labial artery (Fig. 27–5D). All bleeders again were tied and the bleeding controlled. This flap was then rotated down into the lower lip bed and sutured in layers to close the defect, with care to approximate the vermilion borders (Fig. 27–5E). The triangular defect of the upper lip was

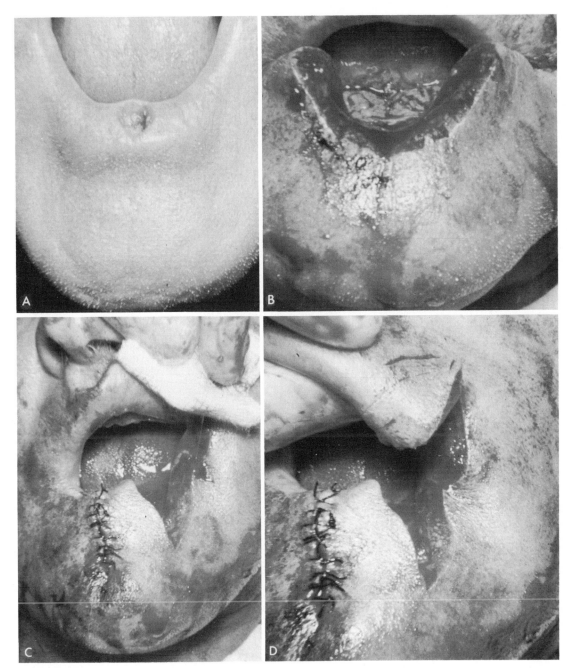

Figure 27–5 *A*, Ulcerative variety of squamous cell carcinoma. Induration palpable well below the visible lesion. *B*, Cancer excised. Satellite lesions (cancer) found histologically a distance from presenting main lesion (see Pathology Report). Wide excision is necessary for ulcerative carcinomas of the lip. *C*, Corner of the lower lip incised and a flap brought medially to close the midline defect. Wound closed in layers. Vermilion edges must be approximated accurately. *D*, Flap being mobilized from upper lip, leaving a pedicle on the medial aspect.

(*Figure 27–5 continued on following page*)

next closed in layers. The patient tolerated the procedure well and left the operating room in good condition. The specimen was properly labeled and sent to the pathology department.

Postoperative Course. No complications. Alternate skin and mucous membrane sutures were removed on the fifth postoperative day and the remaining sutures on the seventh postoperative day.

Pathology Report. The description read in part as follows: ". . . Noted at some distance from the centrally located epithelial neoplastic mass along

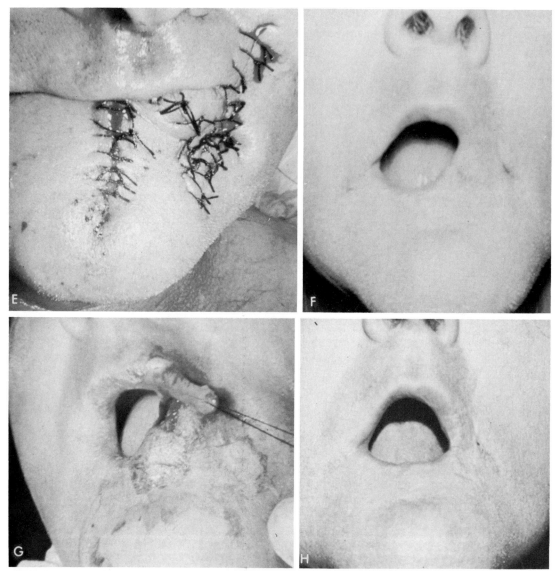

Figure 27–5 (*Continued.*) *E*, Flap is brought into defect in corner of the lip and the entire wound is closed. An additional suture was added to the skin in the midline after this photograph was taken. *F*, Patient healed postoperatively, but requiring surgery for enlargement of the oral aperture. *G*, Flap being rotated from vermilion of upper and lower lips to make new upper lip; lower lip is constructed by undermining the mucous membrane and suturing it to the skin. Aperture enlarged by horizontal incision through the skin, muscle and mucous membrane adjacent to the commissure of the lip. *H*, Patient's appearance 1 year postoperatively. Excellent cosmetic and functional results.

what chronically would be the vermilion border are a few scattered somewhat atypical to frank neoplastic epithelial foci; however, these areas are located some distance from the lateral surgical margins."

Comment: Microscopically, all surgical margins appear free of tumor.

Microscopic Diagnosis: Well differentiated squamous cell carcinoma. See Comment (R. M. Howell, M.D.).

Operative Procedure. A second procedure was performed to enlarge the oral aperture (Fig. 27–5*F*). (See Case Report No. 4.) Under local in-

filtration anesthesia with 2 per cent mepivacaine (Carbocaine) hydrochloride and 1:20,000 levonordefrin (Neo-Cobefrin), the following procedure was performed: A mucous membrane flap was developed from the left upper, lower and corner aspects of the vermilion of the lip. This flap was mobilized. Next a triangular segment of skin adjacent to the corner of the lips with the base next to the commissure was excised down to muscle. Bleeders were tied off. Then, a vertical incision through muscle and mucous membrane from the middle of the base to the apex of the triangle was made, thus opening the oral aperture and making a bed for the mobilized mucous membrane to be attached superiorly for the expanded upper lip. It is essential to have a dry field before suturing the vermilion flap to the skin and mucous membrane (Fig. 27–5G).

The denuded lower lip was treated like closing a lip shave; the labial mucosa was undermined and freed by sharp and blunt dissection down to the mucobuccal fold. The mucous membrane was then sutured to the skin of the lower lip over muscle, including that made by the triangular excision of the skin. This closure of mucous membrane to skin was done with interrupted 5-0 silk sutures for both the upper and lower lips. The mucosal aspects of the upper and lower lips were sutured with 000 interrupted chromic catgut.

Some scar tissue on the cheek resulting from the original surgery and containing an orocutaneous fistula was excised and closed in layers. All tissue excised was sent to the pathology department. The patient tolerated surgery and anesthesia and left the operating room in good condition.

Pathology Report. *Microscopic Diagnosis:* Skin, reaction to implanted hair, no evidence of neoplasia (R. P. Elzay, D.D.S., M.S.D.).

Postoperative Course. Alternate skin and mucous membrane sutures were removed on the fifth and seventh postoperative days. Functional and cosmetic results were satisfactory (Fig. 27–5H). There was no evidence of metastasis or local recurrence.

Comment. This being the ulcerative variety of lip carcinoma, wider margins than usual were excised. This was fortunate, for there were microscopically evident satellite malignant lesions at a distance from the clinically visible and palpable lesion. It is imperative to label all specimens sent to the pathology department accurately to insure that if some margin of the tumor is not clear of disease, the pathologist can tell the surgeon where malignant growth still exists anatomically. (See the initial pathology report.) Another manner of handling this large defect would have been to bring both corners of the lower lip to fill in the major midline defect and then to rotate pedicle flaps from each side of the upper lip into beds prepared at both corners of the lower lip. Upper lip carcinomas are treated in essentially the same fashion as those of the lower lip.

CARCINOMA OF THE BUCCAL MUCOSA

Approximately 10 per cent of oral cancer involves the buccal mucosa. About 90 per cent of the patients with this lesion are male. Tobacco and betel nut chewing are closely associated with squamous cell carcinoma of the buccal mucosa, and the neoplasm is frequently seen in the United States in combination with leukoplakia. Histologically, almost all malignant lesions of the buccal mucosa are squamous cell carcinoma, although occasionally adenocarcinoma from minor salivary glands is seen.

Carcinoma of the buccal mucosa tends to be well differentiated, but in contrast to lip cancer is prone to be more aggressive. Radiation and surgery are effective modalities of treatment. The surgical management may be complex, since the carcinoma may be in the retromolar region, at the occlusal plane or near the commissure of the lips. There may be involvement of the maxillary or mandibular sulcus. (See Figure 27–6.) If surgery is proposed, through and through excision is generally required, with plastic closure. The plastic reconstruction may necessitate flaps from the forehead or shoulder, or skin grafts frequently taken from the thigh. Lesions 3

cm. or less in circumference, without cervical metastasis, can be treated with wide local excision. Careful postoperative observation for neck involvement is essential. The 5-year survival rate is 60 per cent of patients without involved neck nodes, 24 per cent when palpable neck nodes are found and an overall rate of 43 per cent.[5]

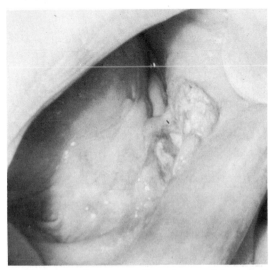

Figure 27–6 Squamous cell carcinoma of the buccal mucosa involving mandibular sulcus and alveolar process.

COMBINED TREATMENT OF BUCCAL CARCINOMA

Patient. This 69-year-old white female was referred to the office by her family dentist for a swelling of the right buccal mucosa in March (Fig. 27–7*A*).

History of Present Illness. The patient dated the onset of her present problem from the age of 12, at which time, while having a tooth restored, trauma to the right buccal mucosa about the area of the parotid orifice occurred. She stated that she had had periodic "clogging" of the right parotid gland since this experience, but admitted that there had been periods of 3 to 4 years without any symptoms.

At the time of her first visit she had a mass about 1.5 cm. in circumference protruding from beneath the mucosa. It was firm and freely movable but tender to palpation. The mass was just anterior to Stensen's orifice. Stensen's duct was explored with a lacrimal probe and found to be completely patent, with saliva flowing from it. It was noted that the maxillary right first molar was periodontally and periapically involved, and it was suggested that this tooth be removed as a potential source of her problem. This was done by her local dentist. When the patient returned to the office in 2 weeks, the mass was exactly as it had been on her first visit. Surgical exploration was advised for diagnostic and therapeutic reasons.

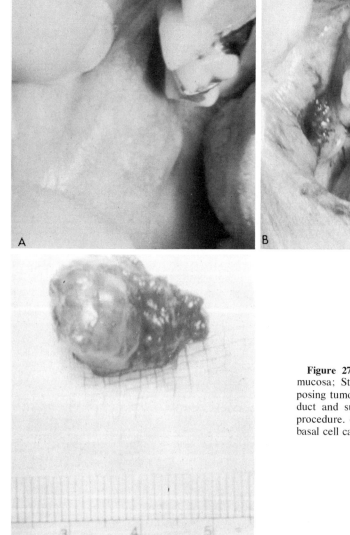

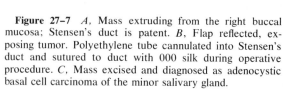

Figure 27–7 *A,* Mass extruding from the right buccal mucosa; Stensen's duct is patent. *B,* Flap reflected, exposing tumor. Polyethylene tube cannulated into Stensen's duct and sutured to duct with 000 silk during operative procedure. *C,* Mass excised and diagnosed as adenocystic basal cell carcinoma of the minor salivary gland.

Past Medical History. The patient's past history was noncontributory.

Operative Technique. The patient was prepared and draped, and she was given infraorbital and mental foramen injections extraorally as well as an inferior alveolar nerve block intraorally, with buccal nerve infiltration. The anesthetic used was 2 per cent lidocaine (Xylocaine) with 1:100,000 epinephrine. Once the oral region was anesthetized, Stensen's duct on the right side was dilated with No. 1 and No. 2 lacrimal probes and cannulated with a polyethylene tube. The polyethylene tube was sutured to the duct and left there with sutures through the adjacent buccal mucosa at the orifice (Fig. 27–7B). Following this, a horizontal incision of about 2 cm. was made in the buccal mucosa anterior to the opening of Stensen's duct. By a combination of sharp and blunt dissection, the mass was excised. The wound was closed with 000 interrupted chromic sutures through the mucosa and buccinator muscle. The patient tolerated surgery and anesthesia and left the operating room in good condition. The specimen was labeled and sent to the pathology department (Fig. 27–7C).

Pathology Report. *Microscopic Diagnosis:* Adenocystic basal cell carcinoma of minor salivary gland origin, buccal mucosa (Dee R. Parkinson, M.D.).

Postoperative Course. The patient did well postoperatively, and all sutures were removed on the fifth postoperative day. Consultation with an internist, radiotherapist, general surgeon and pathologist resulted in agreement that this patient needed additional surgery. It was decided to refer her to the National Institutes of Health, National Cancer Institute, at Bethesda, Maryland. A thorough work-up revealed no evidence of metastatic disease. Bilateral sialograms of the parotid glands revealed no evidence of a space-occupying lesion.

On June 12, the patient was brought to surgery at the National Institutes of Health. A right submandibular incision carried along the angle of the mandible to the ear and temporal hairline was made, and a flap was reflected to expose the parotid gland. Branches of the facial nerve were identified and preserved. The dissection was carried forward anteriorly to the region where the first surgery was performed. About 3 cm. of tissue around the area of the scar was resected, including buccal mucosa; this included the orifice and distal end of the parotid duct. The duct was then reimplanted. A split thickness skin graft from the thigh was placed into the resultant defect in the buccal mucosa. The skin of the face was closed in the usual fashion.

Pathology Report. The pathology report showed extensive tumor invasion of epineural lymphatic vessels. One small nest of tumors was located within a distance of 10 skeletal muscle fibers of the superficial margin. Because of the close surgical margins, the patient was referred for radiation therapy postoperatively. The histologic diagnosis again was adenocystic carcinoma of the right buccal mucosa.

Postoperative Course. The patient was asymptomatic and continued to appear free of disease. She had no resulting facial deformity.

Comment. On rare lesions, one's own tumor board or team may be hesitant about the best approach in the treatment of a neoplasm. In these situations consultation with other tumor specialists is indicated to provide the patient the best possible prognosis.

CARCINOMA OF THE HARD PALATE

Malignant disease in the hard palate is usually seen in patients over 50 years of age, with the involvement in males perhaps slightly over 50 per cent. Squamous cell carcinoma and adenocarcinomas are seen on the hard palate. The adenocarcinomas frequently occur at the junction of the hard and soft palates on either side of the midline. Adenocarcinomas metastasize late but may invade deeply into adjacent tissue.

Treatment of malignant tumors of the hard palate requires radical resection of soft tissues as well as underlying bone, thus necessitating entrance into the nasal and antral cavities. Preoperative preparation with a prosthetic appliance will make the patient more comfortable postoperatively. If the neck is clinically free of disease, an elective neck dissection is not done. Again, careful postoperative observation is essential. The 5-year survival rate is essentially the same as that for malignant diseases of the gingivae.

TREATMENT FOR CARCINOMA OF THE PALATE AND CERVICAL METASTASES*

Patient. This 56-year-old white male was referred to the office by his family physician for a lesion of the right hard and soft palates in April.

Present Illness. A right palatal lesion of 2 months' known duration, firm, painless, ulcerated in the center and having rolled edges was noted.

Findings in a cytologic examination by the physician were negative.

___

* Adapted from Pizer, M. E., and Kay, S.: Mouth cancer—Concepts of treatment. Va. Med. Mon., *99:*148–166 (Feb), 1972.

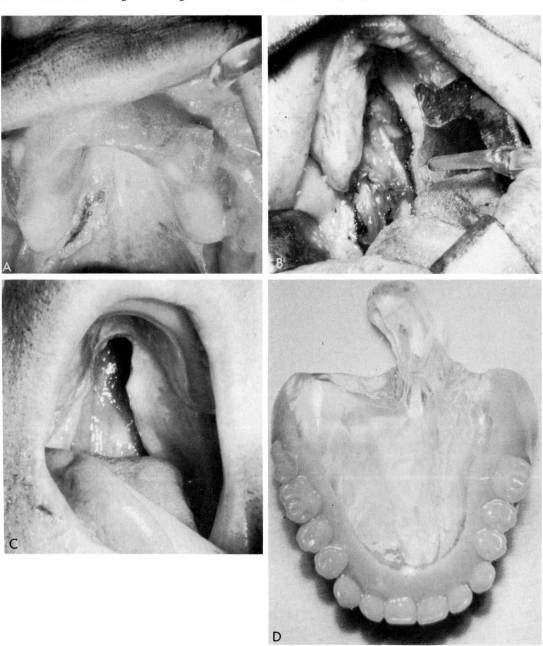

Figure 27–8 *A,* Lesion at the junction of the hard and soft palates. Findings of exfoliative cytologic examination were negative for malignant cells. Frozen section of lesion revealed squamous cell carcinoma. *B,* Appearance immediately following resection of the hard and soft palates. *C,* One-month postoperative appearance. Prosthesis prepared prior to surgery is preferred when the extent of resection is anticipated. *D,* Full maxillary denture with extension filling in surgical defect. Patient had no speech or swallowing impairment. (*A, B* and *D,* From Pizer, M. E., and Kay, S.: Mouth cancer—Concepts of treatment. Va. Med. Mon., *99:*148–166 [Feb.], 1972.)

Past Medical History. The patient admitted to heavy cigarette smoking and excessive intake of alcohol. He was admitted to the hospital in May, and the history taken at that time and the physical examination revealed no additional clinical findings. Radiographs of the facial bones, skull and chest revealed no evidence of neoplasia. There were no clinically palpable neck nodes.

Operative Technique. Under general endotracheal anesthesia, the patient was prepared and draped in the usual fashion, and a small section of tissue was taken for frozen section. The pathologist reported this to be squamous cell carcinoma of low-grade malignancy.

The malignant mass of the hard and soft palates was then defined by palpation and visualization. A wide excision of the tumor, with at least 1 cm. of normal tissue surrounding the lesion, was achieved. Some underlying bone in the region of the palatal portion of the right tuberosity was excised for pathologic examination. The uvula was also removed, since the muscular structures going to it were removed as part of the surgical procedure. The glossopalatinus muscle was left intact. The base of the defect, as well as the surrounding soft tissue walls, was electrofulgurated. Bleeding of the bone was controlled with bone wax and that of the soft tissue by electrofulguration. The patient tolerated the procedure well and left the operating room in good condition.

Pathology Report. *Microscopic Diagnosis:* Well-differentiated squamous carcinoma of hard palate, verrucoid type. *Addendum:* A small segment of bone that was placed in decalcifying fluid is free of involvement by neoplasm. A small number of mucous glands are present within one of the pieces of tissue, as seen on the slide (Michael Vassallo, M.D.).

Postoperative Course. The patient was followed closely. In July, a raised granular mass was noted in the center of the soft palate. It was excised under local anesthesia and was found upon microscopic examination to be granuloma pyogenicum. The following month, this same area in the middle of the soft palate was again suspicious-looking, and repeated biopsy revealed this also to be granuloma pyogenicum. The patient was advised to have his denture checked to rule out chronic irritation.

In October, for the first time a palpable lymph node was detected high in the anterior cervical chain. The patient was referred to a general surgeon, who biopsied this node and found it to be squamous cell carcinoma, Grade I, metastatic. A right radical neck dissection was performed by Robert L. Adeson, M.D., and no other neck nodes were found to be positive. Findings in chest radiographs and a complete work-up were all within normal limits, except for some calcification in the arch of the aorta.

In December, a white lesion on the gingival crest of the edentulous left mandible (first molar region) was noted, biopsied, and found to be a fibroma.

In May of the following year, palpable nodes became obvious in the anterior cervical chain of the left side of the neck. Frozen section revealed these to be epidermoid carcinoma, Grade II to III. A left radical neck dissection was performed by Robert L. Adeson, M.D. Metastases were found in 8 out of 13 cervical nodes.

The patient did well, and chest radiographs indicated no metastases, but in March, another year later, a hard mass was noted over the left clavicle. This supraclavicular mass was excised by the same general surgeon, and this was histologically diagnosed as myositis ossificans. The neck and palate revealed no evidence of disease.

Course. The patient was followed periodically, revealing no additional evidence of disease. He expired suddenly of a myocardial infarction, without any evidence of malignant disease, 8 years after diagnosis of palatal carcinoma. (See Figure 27–8*A* to *D*.)

Comment. Attempts to prevent this patient from consuming excessive alcohol and tobacco were to no avail. There were never any local recurrences; the primary tumor apparently was controlled. Interestingly enough, only one positive neck node was found on the ipsilateral side of the neck, but multiple positive nodes on the contralateral side. To have done an ipsilateral elective neck dissection after excision of the primary neoplasm would probably still not have prevented metastases to the contralateral side, as metastases may go to either side. The finding of myositis ossificans as a left supraclavicular mass is interesting and an unusual finding.

CARCINOMA OF THE GINGIVAE

Gingival lesions are distributed equally among both sexes, and the average age is about 60 years.[5] The mandibular gingivae are more frequently involved than are maxillary gingivae. Histologically, the tumors are usually well-differentiated carcinomas.

These malignant neoplasms are detected clinically by gingival ulceration and bleeding, and occasionally when a patient complains about an ill-fitting denture. Radiographic findings are usually negative in early gingival carcinomas. The diagnosis is made by biopsy.

The clinician should always suspect bony involvement in gingival cancer, and consequently resection of bone is indicated. The extent of resection will depend on the size of the lesion. If there is extensive mandibular gingival involvement, and submaxillary nodes or other cervical nodes are involved, then an en bloc resection (including primary tumor, mandible and the cervical metastases) should be performed. (See Figure 13–221A to C.) Bone grafting at the time of surgery is ill-ad-

vised because of the number of failures. In maxillary gingival carcinomas with neck node involvement, the patient will need two procedures: excision of the primary tumor and a neck dissection. The latter procedure may be delayed for a brief period after the primary lesion has been resected. In the clinically negative neck, we do not generally suggest an "elective" neck dissection or radiation, only close observation. The 5-year survival rate of patients with no palpable neck nodes is about 63 per cent; positive neck nodes reduce the 5-year survival rate to about 18 per cent.[5]

Case Report No. 8

TREATMENT IN GINGIVAL CARCINOMA

Patient. A 47-year-old white female was referred to the office for treatment of a diagnosed squamous cell carcinoma of the gingivae in March.

Chief Complaint. A lesion had been noted on the crest of the mandibular right lingual gingiva between the cuspid and first bicuspid by her periodontist. This lesion was biopsied, and it was reported by the pathologist to be well-differentiated squamous cell carcinoma.

Pathology Report. *Microscopic Diagnosis:* Well-differentiated squamous carcinoma, lingual gingiva opposite lower bicuspid area.

Note: The surgical line in some areas is close and passes through the neoplasm, warranting wider excision or close follow-up (Freydoon Athari, M.D.).

Medical History. Essentially, the patient was a healthy female, with a history of tuberculosis 25 years previously that had been cured.

Present Illness. The patient had histologically diagnosed squamous cell carcinoma of the gingiva. Findings in routine blood tests, urine studies and chest radiographs were all within normal limits. After consultation with the cancer team, a repeat biopsy of the gingiva at the site of the malignant growth was decided upon. The patient was admitted to the hospital for this procedure.

Operative Technique. Under local anesthesia, the lingual mandibular right gingival tissue from the mesial aspect of the first molar to that of the cuspid, from the crest of the ridge down to the floor of the mouth, was excised. Frozen sections were all negative for neoplastic disease. Vaseline gauze was inserted into the defect over the exposed cortical bone and was sutured to the soft tissues with 000 interrupted chromic sutures. The patient tolerated surgery and anesthesia and left the operating room in good condition.

Pathology Report. *Quick Frozen Section Diagnosis:* No tumor seen. Diagnosis deferred pending permanent sections.

Microscopic Diagnosis: Pseudoepitheliomatous hyperplasia, fibrosis and chronic inflammation, right lower gingiva (Dee R. Parkinson, M.D.).

Course. Many consultations were had with general pathologists in the area regarding the original diagnosis. The opinions were about equally divided. Some pathologists called the original lesion definitely malignant and others, pseudoepitheliomatous hyperplasia. The original slides were sent to Dr. Richard P. Elzay at the Virginia Commonwealth University, whose report read in part:

. . . It is my opinion that this represents a well-differentiated epidermoid carcinoma. The lesion obviously has been caught early and completely excised in the initial biopsy. . . .

Richard P. Elzay, D.D.S., M.S.D.

Further consultations with other general pathologists raised doubt, and finally the initial slides were sent to the Armed Forces Institute of Pathology in Washington, D.C. The following report was sent to our office:

. . . This letter confirms our telephone conversation of 26 April. We received 2 microscopic slides. *AFIP Diagnosis:* Squamous cell carcinoma, gingiva. This case was reviewed by several members of the staff, and there was general agreement that this lesion represents a well-differentiated squamous cell carcinoma.

R. W. Morrissey,
Colonel, U.S.A.F., M.C.
The Director

Examination and report by
Dr. John N. Trodahl

After much consideration with members of the

tumor team, it was felt that a marginal resection of the right mandible was indicated. All periapical and lateral jaw radiographs were essentially negative for suspicious changes in the bone.

Operative Technique. The patient was prepared and draped in the usual fashion. Under intravenous sedation and local block anesthesia, a marginal resection of the mandible was performed from the right lateral incisor to the first molar. An H-type of incision was made in the buccal and lingual mucoperiosteum down to the sulcus to expose the cortex of the mandible on both sides. With a dental drill, the entire block of bone was resected, leaving the inferior border of the mandible intact.

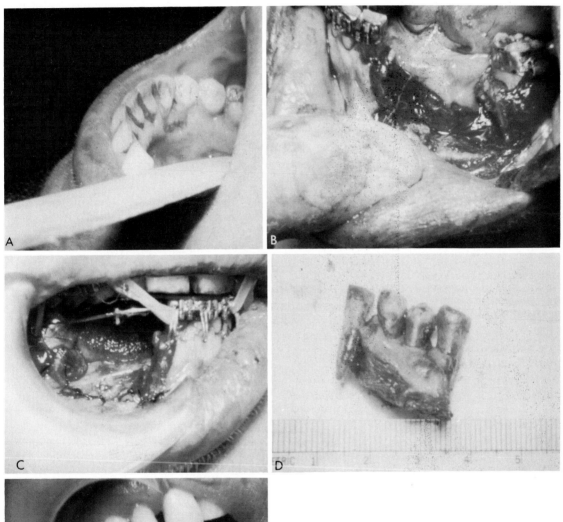

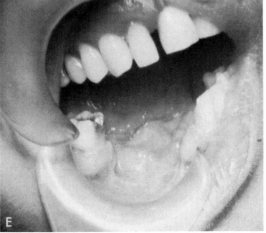

Figure 27–9 *A*, Gingival carcinoma between cuspid and first bicuspid. Note sharply defined borders of the lesion. *B*, Marginal resection of mandible down to, but not including, neurovascular bundle. *C*, Immediate postoperative appearance. Mucosa undermined on buccal and lingual sides of the mandible for primary closure. Mandible is immobilized to prevent pathologic fracture. *D*, Resected specimen containing four teeth. *E*, One-year postoperative appearance. An additional incisor was extracted for prosthetic reasons. Patient wears a partial lower denture which fills in the surgical defect.

There were no extractions of teeth, as these were included in the resected bone. Four teeth were in this bone block.

Following the resection, the soft tissues of the buccal mucosa and floor of the mouth were undermined and then brought together to cover the exposed mandible. The wound was closed with 000 interrupted silk sutures. The mandible was then immobilized against the maxilla by intermaxillary fixation to prevent pathologic fracture. The tissue was labeled and sent to the pathology department. The patient left the operating room in good condition.

Pathology Report. *Microscopic Diagnosis:* Vital teeth and associated mandibular and soft tissue—normal (R. P. Elzay, D.D.S., M.S.D.).

Postoperative Course. The patient's postoperative course was uneventful. The patient wears a prosthetic appliance that fills in the surgical defect. An additional incisor was removed for prosthetic reasons at a later date. (See Figure 27–9*A* to *E*.)

Comment. Differences of opinion by competent pathologists concerning the histologic diagnosis caused a great deal of frustration in this case. Even those pathologists agreeing with the diagnosis of malignancy differed in opinion about the treatment. Some pathologists thought that all of the lesion had been removed, while others felt that there was no malignant disease, and still another thought that the lesion had not been completely excised. It is essential to persist in obtaining professional opinions until the responsible clinician is satisfied with the tissue diagnosis. Only then can he or she decide what modality of treatment should be utilized to offer the patient the best prognosis.

CARCINOMA OF THE SOFT PALATE AND POSTERIOR ONE-THIRD OF THE TONGUE

The posterior one-third of the tongue, or base of the tongue, tonsils, lingual tonsils, pharyngeal walls and soft palate are anatomically in the oropharynx. These malignant lesions are usually (90 per cent) seen in the male over 50 years of age.[5] Lesions at the base of the tongue are seldom diagnosed early, whereas neoplasms of the soft palate are easier to detect. Clinically, the patient may have difficulty in swallowing, as the tongue may lose much of its mobility from the invading tumor. Pain may be referred to the ear. Speech and swallowing may also be altered with a malignant involvement of the soft palate.

Histologically, the lesions are usually squamous cell carcinomas and are usually much less differentiated (more anaplastic) than are the carcinomas of the more anterior portions of the mouth. Adenocarcinomas and malignant lymphomas occasionally involve the soft palate and base of the tongue.

Malignant tumors at the base of the tongue have an extremely poor prognosis. Treatment by surgery—a total glossectomy and neck dissection—or by radiotherapy produces a 20 per cent 5-year survival rate. Soft palate carcinomas in patients with clinically negative findings in the neck have a 46 per cent 5-year survival rate, but this rate is only 14 per cent when cervical metastasis has occurred.[5] Lymphomas respond more favorably to irradiation than to surgery. Early carcinomas of the soft palate, when well differentiated, may best be treated surgically, and when anaplastic, by radiotherapy.

Case Report No. 9

TREATMENT OF EPIDERMOID CARCINOMA OF THE TONSILLAR REGION

Patient. A 48-year-old white male was referred to the office with a "sore mouth" of 3½ weeks' duration.

History of Present Illness. An extensive, fungating lesion of the right retromolar region, extending into the floor of the mouth, soft palate, tonsillar pillar and fossa, was noted. There was a tender anterior cervical lymph node, not fixed or indurated, at the level of the sling between the anterior and posterior digastric muscles. The patient was a severe diabetic of 6 years' duration, with diabetic retinopathy. He admitted to heavy smoking and drinking for the past 25 years. He was admitted to the hospital for biopsy and medical evaluation in March.

Operative Technique. The patient was prepared and draped in the usual fashion, and under nasotracheal anesthesia, an incisional biopsy of the lesion was performed. Findings in an examination of the larynx and hypopharynx were negative. The patient left the operating room in good condition.

Pathology Report. *Microscopic Diagnosis:* Epidermoid carcinoma of the tonsillar area, Grade III (William F. Enos, M.D.).

Course. Chest radiographs revealed bilateral emphysematous changes. Findings in skull radiographs were negative, but those in radiographs of the mandible were reported as "probably an extension of squamous carcinoma to the bone." In the radiographs taken 3 weeks prior to these, however, this area had been reported as a normal right mandible. After consultation with a tumor team, it was decided that cobalt-60 radiation therapy should be instituted. A tumor dose of 6000 R. was delivered to the right tonsil and 6500 R. to the right cervical nodes from a cobalt-60 source, starting on March 23 and finishing on May 5.

The patient was seen in the office on May 9, with no clinical evidence of disease of either mouth or neck. In August, the patient developed an acute bifurcation infection of the mandibular right second molar. The tooth was extracted under local anesthesia; at the same time, some suspicious-looking mucosal changes in the region of the retromolar triangle were biopsied. The patient was given intramuscular penicillin at the time of extraction and kept on oral penicillin for 1 week postoperatively.

The pathology report from this biopsy revealed epidermoid carcinoma, Grade II to III, of the right retromolar region. Chest radiographs were repeated and revealed no evidence of metastatic disease; periapical radiographs of the mandible disclosed no evidence of bone disease. Consultation again resulted in a decision to proceed with additional irradiation. Radiation therapy was started on August 13 and completed on September 15. A tumor dose of 4000 R. was delivered to the lesion of the right alveolar ridge by a cobalt-60 source.

The patient did well until June of the following year, when he developed another "periodontal

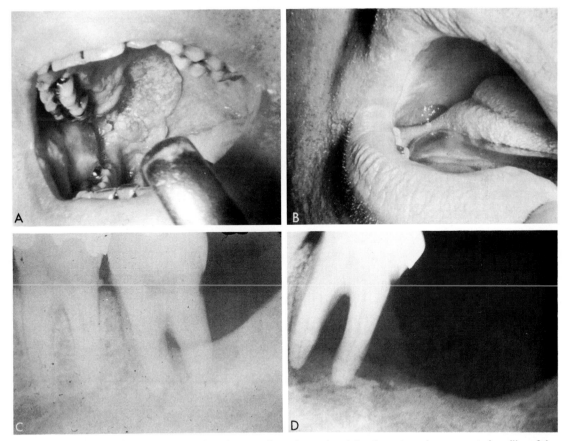

Figure 27–10 *A,* Clinical appearance of squamous cell carcinoma involving the retromolar area, anterior pillar of the tonsil and soft palate. *B,* Clinical appearance 6 weeks after completion of cobalt-60 therapy. No clinical evidence of disease. *C,* Clinical appearance 5 months after radiation treatment; the second molar must be extracted because of periodontal disease. Tissue distal to the second molar was biopsied and diagnosed as squamous cell carcinoma. Note intact bone around first molar. *D,* Destruction of bone around first molar 10 months after extraction of second molar. Biopsy of the socket revealed squamous cell carcinoma. Without the patient's history, film is suggestive of extensive periodontal disease. For patients with this kind of history, biopsy is always indicated following extraction.

abscess" of the mandibular right first molar. High dosages of penicillin were used, as in the previous extraction, and this first molar was removed without complication. Soft tissue in the first molar socket was curetted and sent to pathology for histologic examination. (See Figure 27–10*A* to *D*.)

Pathology Report. The above tissue from the first molar socket was reported to be epidermoid carcinoma, Grade II to III, retromolar region, right mandible.

Course. With this pathology report, it was felt by the tumor team that further consultation should be sought, since the patient could not tolerate additional irradiation, and he was an extremely poor surgical risk. He was referred to the National Institutes of Health, National Cancer Institute, at Bethesda, Maryland. Findings in a complete work-up for distant metastases were negative. A right radical neck dissection and hemimandibulectomy were performed. An orocutaneous fistula developed postoperatively, and a multistaged repair of the neck wound, with tubed pedicle grafts, was initiated.

The patient was admitted to the National Institutes of Health six times over a 3-year period for closure of fistulas with previously prepared pedicle tube flaps, drainage of a right preauricular abscess and other complications.

On January 4, 10 years after he was originally seen in our office, a communication was received from the National Institutes of Health, stating that "this patient has developed a new primary cancer in the left floor of the mouth near the midline." A left neck dissection in continuity with resection of the lesion in the floor of the mouth was performed. The pathologic findings were reported as squa-

mous cell carcinoma, left side of the floor of the mouth, with metastatic squamous cell carcinoma to 3 of 30 left cervical lymph nodes. The patient had slowly become totally blind and was therefore severely incapacitated.

Comment. When removing acutely infected teeth in an area which has been irradiated, consultation with the radiotherapist before an extraction is mandatory. High dosages of antibiotics are indicated in an effort to prevent osteoradionecrosis. In cases such as these, it is prudent to biopsy the soft tissue in the socket after extraction to rule out possible neoplastic invasion of the bone. In removing the mandibular right first molar, periodontal and neoplastic involvement look similar radiographically.

Tumor boards should not hesitate to consult with other institutions when the prognosis appears dismal.

Many of the postoperative complications noted in this case report were secondary to this patient's severe diabetes mellitus. Possibly some were secondary to irradiation.

The preoperative irradiation in this case was effective in eliminating the carcinoma from the tonsillar region, the soft palate and the floor of the mouth. However, it was not so with bone. Certainly irradiation in this case was completely justified as an initial modality, for it possibly made what was initially an inoperable lesion into an operable one. A second intraoral primary tumor on the opposite side developed approximately 10 years after the initial primary lesion was diagnosed, suggesting the patient's continued susceptibility to oral neoplastic disease.

Case Report No. 10

RADIATION THERAPY OF SQUAMOUS CELL CARCINOMA OF THE RETROMOLAR TRIANGLE*

Patient. A 77-year-old white male was referred to the office for a consultation regarding an intraoral lesion in February.

History of Present Illness. A tumor was found on the left retromolar triangle, involving the floor of the mouth, lateral border of the tongue and soft palate. A history was difficult to obtain because of the patient's inability to speak English. Biopsy revealed the presence of squamous cell carcinoma. Consultation was held with a general surgeon, an otolaryngologist and a radiotherapist, all of whom agreed that irradiation should be utilized as the initial modality to shrink the lesion, and then the patient could be reevaluated. A left anterior cervical node was firm and discrete, suggestive of meta-

static involvement. Radiographs of the mandible and the chest revealed no evidence of neoplastic disease.

Treatment. Cobalt-60 was administered beginning a week after extraction of the remaining teeth. The patient received 10 treatments to the left tonsillar region, soft palate and left posterior mandible, for a total dose of 3100 rads of cobalt-60. Immediately prior to each administration of cobalt-60, an intratumor injection of 11 per cent carbamide peroxide in a water-free gel base, dis-

---

* Adapted from Pizer, M. E.: A query to radiotherapists. Va. Med. Mon., *100:*222–223 (Mar.), 1973.

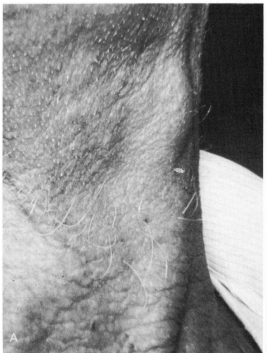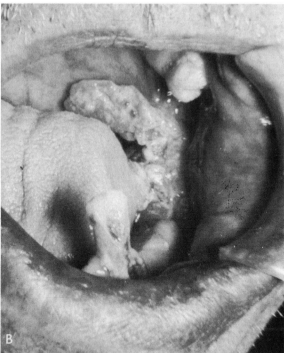

Figure 27–11 *A*, Examination of patient's neck suggests serious intraoral disease. Note the prominent cervical lymph node. *B*, Intraoral examination and biopsy of oral cavity tissue confirm squamous cell carcinoma of the retromolar region, floor of the mouth, tongue, anterior pillar, tonsil and soft palate.

solved in 2 per cent mepivacaine (Carbocaine) hydrochloride with 1:20,000 levonordefrin (Neo-Cobefrin), was administered. The lesion responded dramatically. The patient refused further radiation therapy and was last seen in June. (See Figure 27–11*A* and *B*.)

Case Report No. 11

TREATMENT OF MALIGNANT MELANOMA OF THE TONGUE*

Patient. A 35-year-old Eurasian male was seen at the office in August.

Chief Complaint. Pain in the left tonsillar region.

History of Present Illness. For 2 weeks, the patient had had tenderness of the left tongue and tonsillar region. His past medical history was essentially noncontributory; the patient admitted to smoking one pack of cigarettes a day.

Examination revealed a raised, firm red lesion that was ulcerated, extending from the foliate papillae on the left lateral border of the posterior one-third of the tongue to the anterior tonsillar pillar. It was extremely tender to palpation and bled easily upon digital pressure. There was a tender lymph node high in the anterior cervical chain, but it was neither fixed nor indurated. It felt like a "shotty" lymph node resulting from inflammatory disease. There were no other symptoms.

The patient received antibiotic therapy for 1 week, but this did not change the basic appearance of the lesion. It was felt that a wide surgical excision of this lesion was indicated, since it was pigmented and suspicious-looking. Twelve days after the initial visit, the patient underwent surgery.

Operative Technique. After being prepared and draped, the patient was premedicated with 85 mg. of meperidine hydrochloride, $\frac{1}{120}$ grain of scopolamine hydrobromide and 85 mg. of sodium pentobarbital (Nembutal) given intravenously. A left mandibular nerve block, using 2 per cent lidocaine (Xylocaine) with 1:100,000 epinephrine, was ad-

_____

* Adapted from Pizer, M. E.: A query to radiotherapists. Va. Med. Mon., *100:*222–223 (Mar.), 1973.

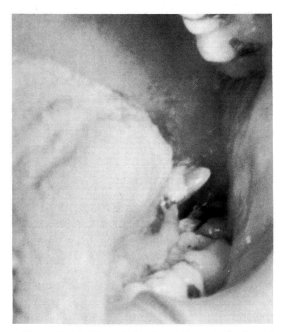

Figure 27–12 Pigmented lesion at the posterior lateral border of the tongue; the flat protruding area is part of the neoplasm. Incisional biopsy was contraindicated, and wide excisional biopsy indicated for diagnosis. Final diagnosis: malignant melanoma.

ministered. With a No. 15 Bard-Parker blade, wide excision, with good margins in all directions, was performed. Bleeders were tied off, and the wound was closed with 000 silk interrupted sutures. The patient tolerated surgery and anesthesia and left the operating room in good condition. (See Figure 27–12.)

Postoperative Course. The patient's postoperative course was uneventful. He had a sore throat and dysphagia.

Pathology Report. *Microscopic Description:* A surface layer of stratified squamous epithelium that exhibited a large mass of neoplastic epithelial cells spindling and streaming off into swirling masses and bundles of cells invading deep into the subjacent connective tissue was seen. These neoplastic epithelial cells exhibited hyperchromatism, increased nuclear cytoplasmic ratio and numerous bizarre shapes.

Diagnosis: Spindle cell carcinoma (R. M. Howell, M.D.).

Definitive Follow-up. I felt that this was a most unusual lesion, a very serious tumor, and referred this patient immediately to the National Institutes of Health, National Cancer Institute, for a consultation.

The pathologists at the National Cancer Institute requested the original slide, and it was read as

. . . undifferentiated malignant tumor, mucosa of left posterior tongue. We favor the diagnosis of malignant melanoma. Because of the histologic pattern and lack of

pigment in the neoplastic cells, the diagnosis of spindle cell carcinoma cannot be totally excluded.

L. Max Buja, M.D.

Course. An exhaustive preoperative work-up for possible metastatic disease revealed no abnormal findings. The patient underwent surgery in December. A wide local excision of the previous site on the left posterior lateral border of the tongue along with excision of the glossopalatal fold was performed with a primary closure. A left radical neck dissection was also performed at this time. All the above-mentioned surgery failed to reveal any residual tumor, and the patient was discharged from the National Institutes of Health with a diagnosis of primary malignant melanoma of the tongue.

Follow-up Communication. The following letter was received:

Dear Dr. Pizer:

I am sending this duplicate pathology report on to you in anticipation that you might care to have it for your files. How pleased we were to find no evidence of residual tumor in the specimen. I wish that more procedures could result with such a favorable prognosis. To have allowed this man to go without definitive treatment with the history with which he was referred to us would have been in poor medical judgment. While someone always asks questions concerning a negative specimen, those of us who daily deal with cancer find that these are the patients who so frequently will do much better if they are aggressively handled rather than temporizing by waiting for evidence of recurrence we know will eventually develop.

We had a slight delay in his convalescence with a wound infection. This has rapidly subsided with out-patient treatment and we expect that by now he has been seen again in your office. We look forward to a cooperative long-term follow-up between your office and ours.

Sincerely,
Alfred S. Ketcham, M.D.
Clinical Director and Chief
Surgery Branch
National Cancer Institute

Subsequent Course. The patient did well for 2 years, but in October (14 months after his initial office visit) on a postoperative visit to the National Institutes of Health, there was suspicion of a lesion of the left tonsil. He was admitted to the hospital and examined under general endotracheal anesthesia. The tonsil was found to be involved by a tumorous process. Shortly thereafter, a tracheostomy and esophagostomy with a partial left mandibulectomy and partial left neck dissection were performed.

Pathology Report. The final pathology report revealed (1) malignant tumor, consistent with malignant melanoma, of the left tonsillar area, and (2) metastatic malignant melanoma of the adjacent left hypoglossal nerve.

Comment. The following February, the patient was found to have metastases to the liver and the vertebrae. He was treated with chemotherapy and was considered to have terminal disease.

This is one of the most lethal of all malignant tumors. The tumor, which initially appeared to have been treated surgically with excellent results, still recurred 2 years later. In spite of good surgical margins, the nature of this neoplasm presents a most dismal prognosis. An initial incisional biopsy might have disseminated the tumor early, resulting in distant metastases, and possibly a very early demise of this patient. It is essential to excise pigmented lesions widely for making a pathologic diagnosis and affording the patient a "fighting chance."

MALIGNANT LESIONS OF THE ANTERIOR TWO-THIRDS OF THE TONGUE

This part of the tongue is the freely movable portion that extends from the circumvallate papillae to the root at the junction of the floor of the mouth. The American Cancer Society in 1973 estimated that 2800 new cases of cancer involving the tongue would be diagnosed that year. It is the second most common intraoral cancer. The disease is seen mostly in men over age 40.

Histologically, squamous cell carcinoma accounts for 95 per cent of the lesions involving the anterior two-thirds of the tongue. The lesions vary histologically from poorly differentiated to well differentiated. Rarely found are sarcomas, the most common of which is the rhabdomyosarcoma; less rare is the adenocarcinoma. Malignant melanoma is exceedingly rare and is probably the most lethal tumor.

Epidermoid carcinomas, which are small (3 cm. or less) and exophytic, are almost always treated surgically by wide local resection. For larger lesions in the anterior one-third of the tongue that invade adjacent soft tissue but not bone, and that are associated with nonpalpable cervical nodes, treatment may consist of irradiation followed by surgery, if necessary. When there is tongue, floor of the mouth and bone involvement, radical neck dissection, partial mandibulectomy and excision of the primary lesion (an en bloc or composite resection) are indicated, even if the cervical nodes are not palpable. It is estimated that 50 per cent of patients with the latter type of involvement have metastatic cervical nodes, even if palpation does not reveal spread of disease to the neck. In the presence of distant metastases, or a primary lesion that cannot be controlled or contained, neck dissection is usually discouraged in pref-

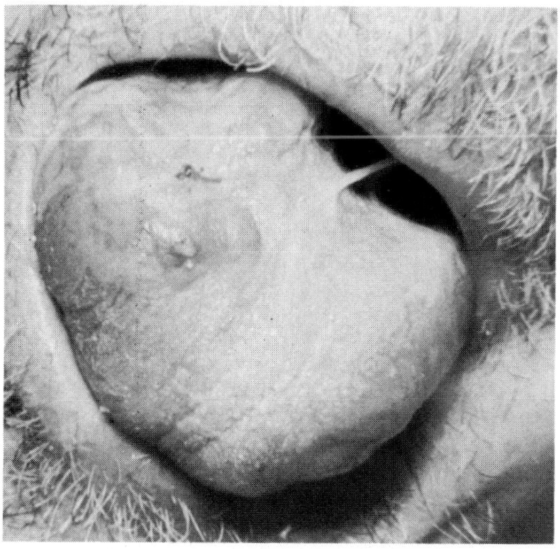

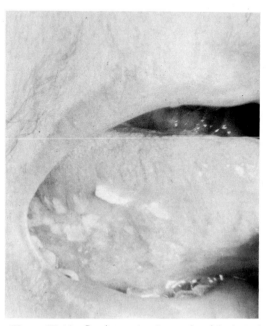

Figure 27–13 Entire dorsum of the right side of the tongue is involved by this fungating squamous cell carcinoma. The patient also had neck metastases.

Figure 27–14 Carcinoma *in situ* at the right lateral border of the tongue. The patient, receiving chemotherapy for extensive malignant disease, died of leukemia before his tongue could be treated.

erence to irradiation and chemotherapy. The 5-year survival rate is influenced primarily by whether or not there is cervical node involvement. Without neck involvement, at least 53 per cent of patients survive the 5-year postoperative period, but with neck involvement approximately 16 per cent survive 5 years.[5] (See Figures 27–13 and 27–14.)

Case Report No. 12

TREATMENT OF SQUAMOUS CELL CARCINOMA OF THE TONGUE

Patient. A 60-year-old white male was referred to the office by his family physician for a lesion on the right lateral border of the tongue in February.

History of Present Illness. The patient had noted an uncomfortable place on his tongue approximately 3 weeks before. He had visited his local physician and had received antibiotics, which the patient felt had made the lesion smaller.

Medical Evaluation. The patient had a history of benign hypertension and rheumatic fever with resultant rheumatic heart disease. These findings were verified by radiographs and electrocardiogram studies. He admitted to heavy cigarette smoking for many years but denied more than social alcohol.

Upon intra- and extraoral examination, the only positive finding was a firm, fixed, raised mass approximately 1.3 cm. in circumference on the lateral border of the right side of the tongue, about 1.5 cm. anterior to the foliate papillae or about 2 cm. from the glossopalatal fold. The lesion showed a minimal positive stain with 2 per cent toluidine blue dye. Another small nonspecific-looking ulcer, about 2 to 3 mm. in circumference, was noted on the right lower lip. The patient stated that this ulcer had just appeared. Careful examination of the neck revealed no evidence of palpable nodes. The patient underwent surgery for an excisional biopsy of the tongue in February.

Operative Technique. The patient was prepared and draped in the usual fashion. Under a right mandibular nerve block, using 2 per cent mepivacaine (Carbocaine) hydrochloride with 1:20,000 levonordefrin (Neo-Cobefrin), a wide excisional biopsy of the tongue lesion was performed. There was much bleeding that was controlled by electrocoagulation and 000 chromic ties. The wound was closed with 000 silk interrupted sutures, and the patient left the operating room in good condition.

Pathology Report. *Microscopic Diagnosis:* Squamous cell carcinoma, well differentiated. Margins free of neoplastic transformation (W. T. Sweeney, M.D.).

Course. A consultation was held with the patient's cardiologist, family physician, radiotherapist and general surgeon. After a complete medical work-up, laboratory studies and radiographs of the skull, mandible, chest and spine, no evidence of metastatic disease could be demonstrated. It was felt, however, that even though the pathologist reported clear margins around the lesion, an additional local resection was indicated. The patient was admitted to the hospital, and this procedure was performed 12 days after the orginal surgery.

Operative Technique. The patient was prepared and draped in the usual fashion, and under nasotracheal anesthesia, the following procedure was performed. The area of the original excisional biopsy was identified by the retained black silk sutures. A 000 silk suture was placed through the midline and lateral border of the tongue for retraction of the surgical site. Then, with a No. 15 Bard-Parker blade, a wide resection of the site of the previously diagnosed squamous cell carcinoma was performed.

About 1.5 cm. of clinically healthy tissue around all the previous margins was excised in all directions. Bleeders were tied off for control of major bleeding. Multiple sections from different borders were then sent to the pathology department. There was no evidence of neoplasia at the margins. The wound was then approximated and closed with a combination of vertical mattress and interrupted 000 silk sutures. The patient tolerated surgery and anesthesia and left the operating room in good condition.

Pathology Report. *Quick Frozen Section Diagnosis:* Edges and depth clear of tumor.

Microscopic Diagnosis: Segment of right side of the tongue removed because of previous diagnosis of "squamous cell carcinoma" (pathologic consultation elsewhere).

Tissue from right side of the tongue showing inflammation and granulomatous response incident to previous surgery (Dee R. Parkinson, M.D.).

Postoperative Course. There were no immediate postoperative complications. The patient was seen again in April, and at the site of the original lesion there was an area that had not healed as well as the remainder of the mucosa. It bled easily upon pressure and also retained 2 per cent toluidine blue dye. During this same visit a raised irregular area was noted on the vermilion border of the left lower lip; it too retained 2 per cent toluidine blue dye. Under local anesthesia in the office, both of these areas were excised for microscopic examination.

Pathology Report. *Microscopic Diagnosis:* (1) Acanthosis and chronic inflammation of the tongue. (2) Severe epithelial dysplasia of the lower left lip (W. T. Sweeney, M.D.; R. P. Elzay, D.D.S., M.S.D.).

Postoperative Course. The patient's condition was followed on a 3-month basis, and because of the lip finding in April, an incisional biopsy of the lower lip was done under local anesthesia in July to determine further whether a lip shave was indicated.

Pathology Report. The report read in part: "There does not seem to be evidence that would

indicate a 'lip shave' at this time; however, close clinical follow-up would seem indicated."

Diagnosis: Hyperkeratosis and actinic degeneration (W. T. Sweeney, M.D.; R. P. Elzay, D.D.S., M.S.D.).

Postoperative Course. The patient's condition has been followed closely, and presently he is free of mouth and neck disease. Because his occupation requires his being outdoors much of the time, he wears a wide-brim hat to protect his lips as well as an antiactinic lipstick. (See Figure 27–15*A* to *D*.)

Comment. Medically, each procedure required antibiotic prophylaxis because of the patient's rheumatic heart disease. The course we followed

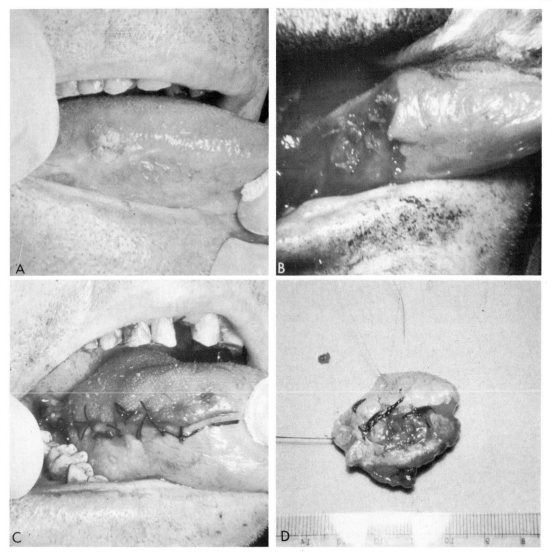

Figure 27–15 *A,* Initial appearance of the lesion at the lateral border of the tongue. Excisional biopsy confirmed well-differentiated squamous cell carcinoma. *B,* Partial glossectomy as definitive treatment for this lesion. Approximately 25 per cent (middle one-third) of the tongue was excised. *C,* Closure of the tongue with 000 silk interrupted and 000 silk vertical mattress sutures. *D,* Excised mass; note black silk sutures retained from original biopsy to identify exact location of the primary lesion. Other sutures were added to indicate to the pathologist the anterior-posterior, superior-inferior and medial borders of the specimen.

was dictated by the small size of the tongue lesion, it being histologically well differentiated and completely excised on initial biopsy. Our greatest concern was the anatomic location of this lesion. The patient's apparent susceptibility to carcinoma and epithelial dysplasia warrants close follow-up.

The 2 per cent toluidine blue dye did not significantly stain this malignant lesion owing to the hyperkeratosis overlying it. This is another reason why no other clinical test can substitute for a biopsy.

CARCINOMA OF THE FLOOR OF THE MOUTH

Anatomically, the floor of the mouth includes the space over the mylohyoid and hyoglossus muscles. It extends from the inner surface of the mandibular alveolar process to the root of the tongue and reaches posteriorly to the base of the anterior pillar of the tonsil. This is the most common site of intraoral carcinoma, and it was estimated that 6000 new cases would be diagnosed in 1974, according to the American Cancer Society and their 1973 statistics. Lesions of the floor of the mouth overwhelmingly afflict men over age 50. Histologically, nearly all lesions are squamous cell carcinomas, but on occasion, adenocarcinomas arising from the minor salivary glands are found.

Small lesions, especially exophytic carcinomas, are excised by local wide resection.

Lesions of 3 cm. or less that encroach upon the alveolar mucosa are treated by combined resection of the mandible and floor of the mouth. The extent of bone that is removed is left to the judgment of the surgeon. In these cases, when the cervical nodes are not palpable, neck dissection is not performed. When the lesion is large, is infiltrative and involves mucosa overlying an alveolar process or obviously involves the mandible, then a neck dissection in continuity with the intraoral primary tumor and mandible is indicated, irrespective of the status of the cervical lymph nodes. The 5-year survival rate when the patient has palpable nodes is only 30 per cent, compared with 60 per cent when the patient has no neck node metastases.[5] (See Figures 27–16 and 27–17.)

In general, adenocarcinomas are more sluggish in their growth and tend to remain localized longer than do squamous cell car-

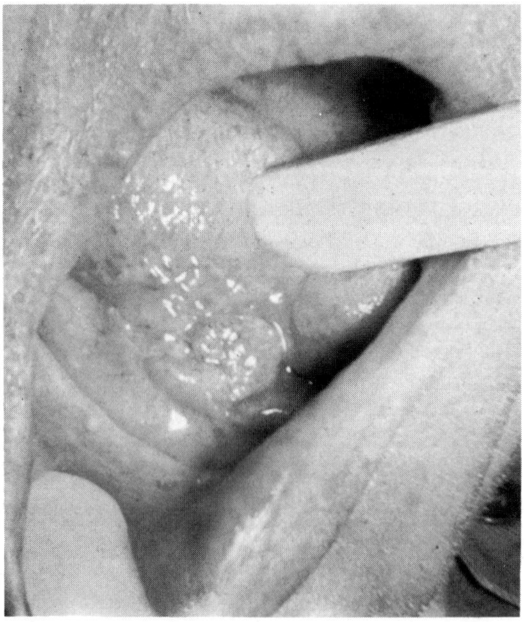

Figure 27–16 A 79-year-old man whose chief complaint was inability to wear his lower denture was found to have squamous cell carcinoma of the floor of the mouth. Cervical nodes were not palpable. Tumor was treated with interstitial radium.

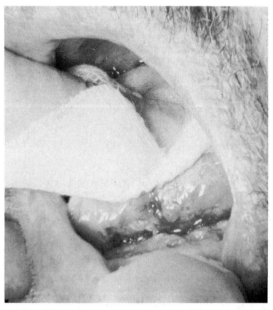

Figure 27–17 Advanced squamous cell carcinoma of the tongue and floor of the mouth with cervical node metastases.

cinomas. They are persistent and tend to recur locally. They metastasize by way of the lymphatic system and blood stream but only late in the course of the disease. The treat-

ment for adenocarcinomas arising in the salivary glands is wide excision. Sometimes radiation is administered postoperatively in an effort to prevent recurrence.

Case Report No. 13

TREATMENT OF CARCINOMA OF THE FLOOR OF THE MOUTH*

Patient. This 57-year-old white male was referred to the office in January by his internist, who detected a lesion in the floor of his mouth on a routine physical examination.

History of Present Illness. The patient presented with a raised, firm, ulcerated lesion, measuring 2 by 2 by 1 cm. in the floor of the mouth, just left of the midline and posterior to the opening of Wharton's duct. There was some clinically visible leukoplakia around the lesion. The patient admitted to use of tobacco and alcohol, and he had a history of essential hypertension and bronchiectasis. No cervical nodes were palpable on examination.

Operative Technique. An incisional biopsy of the lesion was performed at the first office visit in January.

Pathology Report. *Microscopic Diagnosis:* Infiltrating squamous cell carcinoma, predominantly Grade I (M. Freund, M.D.).

Course. The usual tumor team consultation and medical work-up were done to rule out metastatic disease. The patient was brought to surgery approximately 2½ weeks later.

Operative Technique. The patient was prepared and draped in the usual fashion, and under bilateral lingual nerve blocks the following procedure was performed. An incision was made with a No. 15 Bard-Parker blade in the floor of the mouth at the attached gingiva, from the symphysis to the region of the second bicuspid on both sides of the mandible. The incision was carried down to the bone, and with a periosteal elevator the musculature and attachments of the geniohyoid and genioglossus muscles were detached. Then, with a combination of sharp and blunt dissection, the mylohyoid muscle and the entire floor of the mouth were lifted upward and carried back to the region of the second bicuspids, where the incision was carried horizontally across the entire floor of the mouth. The resected mass was removed *in toto,* and this included the two sublingual glands and the musculature in this area. Following this, a full thickness mucous membrane graft was taken from the left buccal mucosa and brought into place in the floor of the mouth. It was sutured to the remaining mylohyoid and genioglossus muscles and adjacent mucous membrane with 000 inter-

rupted silk sutures. The graft was supported in place by a Penrose drain from the floor of the mouth to the skin of the submandibular area by 0 chromic sutures. This was done to prevent hematoma formation beneath the graft. The patient tolerated surgery and anesthesia and left the operating room in good condition. The specimen was labeled and sent to the pathology department.

Pathology Report. *Microscopic Diagnosis:* Epidermoid carcinoma, Grade I, floor of the mouth. The edge and depth appear clear (Dee R. Parkinson, M.D.).

Postoperative Course. In August a small, raised lesion was noted in the left floor of the mouth. It was excised under local anesthesia in the office, and the biopsy report revealed this to be granulation tissue.

The patient was followed periodically by examination, chest radiographs and blood count. A white lesion was noted in March 5 years later at the right corner of the lips on the mucous membrane. It was removed under local anesthesia in the office and found histologically to be "hyperparakeratosis and acanthosis."

In January the next year, exactly 6 years postoperatively, he complained of dysphagia. Both the neck and mouth appeared clinically normal. The patient was referred for a barium swallow, chest radiograph and otolaryngology consultation. The barium swallow and chest radiograph revealed no abnormality.

In spite of the negative findings with a barium swallow, the symptoms persisted, and under direct laryngoscopy that same month the patient was found to have a large ulcerative lesion of the vallecula invading the epiglottis and the base of the tongue to within 1 cm. of the circumvallate papillae. There was an isolated papillomatous mass measuring about 1 cm. in diameter located at the posterior wall of the cervical esophagus at the level of the cricoid. Biopsies were taken from all of

---

* Adapted from Pizer, M. E., and Kay, S.: Mouth cancer—Concepts of treatment. Va. Med. Mon., 99:148–166 (Feb.), 1972.

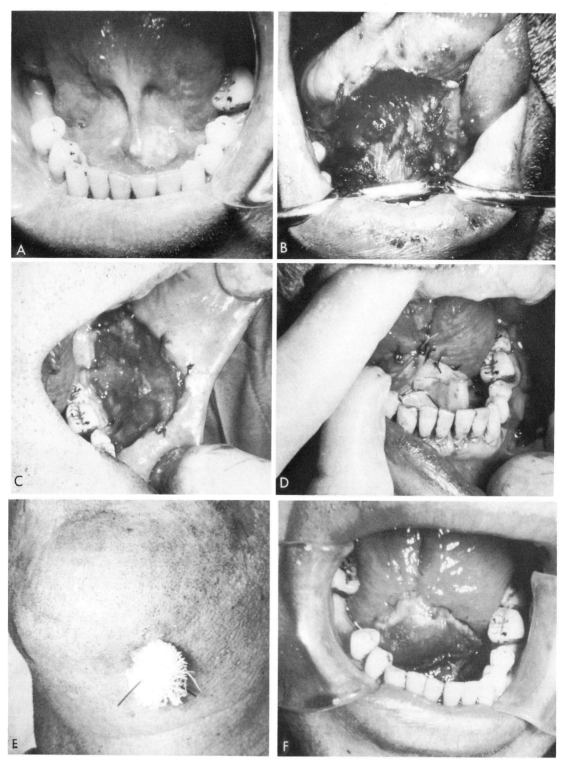

Figure 27–18 *A*, Lesion of left floor of the mouth noted by internist during routine physical examination. Clinically visible leukoplakia was noted around lesion. *B*, Immediate appearance of floor of the mouth following resection for squamous cell carcinoma. *C*, Full thickness mucous membrane graft from the buccal mucosa (donor site) to be placed in the floor of the mouth. *D*, Buccal mucosa graft sutured to the tongue and floor of the mouth; graft held in place firmly by thyroid drain to prevent hematoma formation underneath graft. *E*, Sutures from thyroid drain brought from the floor of the mouth through the skin and sutured to gauze dressing on the side of the neck. *F*, Buccal mucosa graft taking well 2 weeks postoperatively.

(*Figure 27–18 continued on opposite page*)

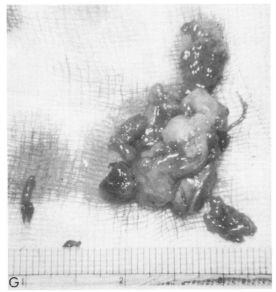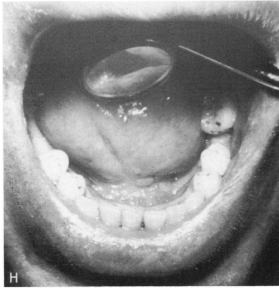

Figure 27–18 (*Continued.*) *G,* Malignant mass excised from the floor of the mouth. *H,* Floor of the mouth 1 month after surgery, with minimal scar tissue. Buccal mucosa healed by secondary intention.

these areas (by Miguel A. Acevedo, M.D.), and all were reported as epidermoid carcinoma. It was explained to the patient that surgery could be performed, but that it would be extremely extensive and would leave him with significant functional deformity. He refused surgery and was informed that the only other option was radiotherapy. From February 8 through April 4, he received deep x-ray therapy to the lingual vallecula, epiglottis and cervical areas. The tumor dose was estimated at 6300 rads at the level of the epiglottis. There was a remarkable disappearance of the disease. He has done well following radiation therapy. On an office visit 6 months after radiation, he was asymptomatic and clinically free of disease. The patient is being followed closely by the radiotherapist, otolaryngologist and our office. (See Figure 27–18*A* to *H.*)

Case Report No. 14

TREATMENT OF CARCINOMA OF THE FLOOR OF THE MOUTH*

Patient. A 71-year-old white male was referred to the office by an oral surgeon and radiotherapist for residual carcinoma of the right floor of the mouth.

History of Present Illness. In June this patient was seen in our office for a lesion in the right floor of the mouth and on the lateral border of the tongue. An incisional biopsy was done, and a microscopic diagnosis of an "infiltrating, well-differentiated epidermoid carcinoma, with tumor extending to all margins," was reported.

Because of the patient's extremely poor general health, the oral surgeon and family physician referred the patient to a radiotherapist for consultation. A cancerocidal dose of cobalt-60 was administered to the tongue and floor of the mouth. After the irradiation (in November), a letter was received from the radiologist that read in part:

Dear Dr. Pizer:

I saw the patient today. He has induration extending from the frenulum of the tongue on the right along the floor of the mouth for a distance of about 5.5 cm. In the anterior portion on the right is a small ulcer, and one is also present posterior to this that was not there the last time I saw him. I think much of the thickening is fibrosis from the radiation, but the two ulcerated areas are probably persistent disease. I feel that this can be excised widely, but I doubt if the patient will tolerate general anesthesia. . . .

Charlotte P. Donlan, M.D.

* Adapted from Pizer, M. E., and Kay, S.: Mouth cancer—Concepts of treatment. Va. Med. Mon., *99:*148–166 (Feb.), 1972.

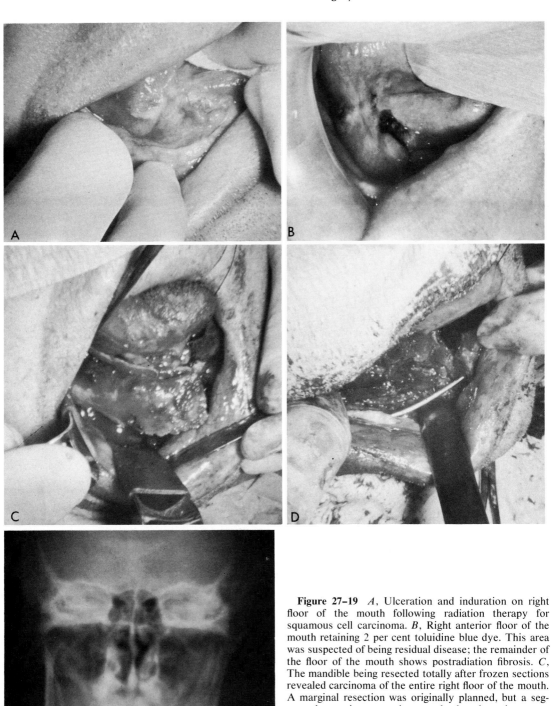

Figure 27–19 *A*, Ulceration and induration on right floor of the mouth following radiation therapy for squamous cell carcinoma. *B*, Right anterior floor of the mouth retaining 2 per cent toluidine blue dye. This area was suspected of being residual disease; the remainder of the floor of the mouth shows postradiation fibrosis. *C*, The mandible being resected totally after frozen sections revealed carcinoma of the entire right floor of the mouth. A marginal resection was originally planned, but a segmental resection was subsequently thought to be necessary. *D*, Steinmann pin inserted into holes drilled into the right ramus and left symphysis of the mandible. *E*, Radiograph of Steinmann pin in position following resection of the mandible.

(*Figure 27–19 continued on opposite page*)

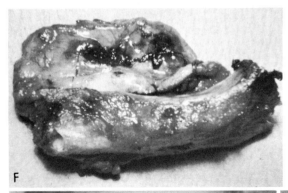

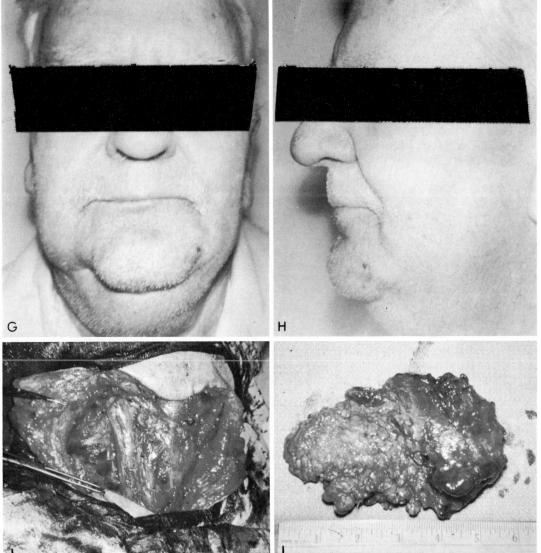

Figure 27–19 *(Continued.)* *F,* Resected mandible with floor of the mouth and marginal glossectomy. *G* and *H,* Facial appearance of patient 8 weeks postoperatively. *I,* Neck exposed for radical neck surgery. *J,* Malignant mass removed from right side of the neck during neck dissection. (*A, B, D* and *E,* From Pizer, M. E., and Kay, S.: Mouth cancer—Concepts of treatment. Va. Med. Mon., 99:148–166 [Feb.], 1972.)

Course. Further consultation was held with the internist, chemotherapist and general surgeon. It was agreed that wide local excision in the anterior floor of the mouth would be the treatment of choice.

The patient had obstructive pulmonary disease and arteriosclerotic heart disease with atrial fibrillation and a rapid ventricular response, as well as a ventral hernia.

He admitted to smoking cigars excessively until 5 months previously and to consuming alcohol moderately.

He was hospitalized and a medical work-up was carried out to rule out metastatic disease, as well as to prepare him for surgery. No evidence of cervical lymph node metastasis or other metastatic disease could be demonstrated by laboratory, radiographic or clinical examinations. Digitalization with digoxin (Lanoxin) was carried out, and it was felt that general anesthesia would be acceptable. The patient was brought to surgery on November 26.

Operative Technique. The patient was prepared and draped in the usual fashion, and under nasotracheal general anesthesia, an incisional biopsy in the anterior right floor of the mouth was taken for frozen section. This was found to be squamous cell carcinoma. Another incisional biopsy was done in the floor of the mouth at the most posterior portion, and it too revealed carcinoma. Therefore, it was decided that a segmental resection of the mandible in continuity with the lesion of the floor of the mouth and tongue was required.

A large incision was made on the crest of the ridge from the left mental foramen to the ascending ramus of the right mandible. The mucoperiosteum was reflected on the entire buccal cortex to the inferior border of the mandible, and then with surgical burs the right mandible from the region of the left symphysis to the ascending right ramus was totally resected, including the right floor of the mouth and essentially the right half of the tongue. Major bleeders were tied off, while smaller ones were electrocoagulated. The deep portions of the submaxillary gland and sublingual gland were removed in the dissection. Following this, the retained musculature was sutured together in an effort to close up the dead space created by the dissection. A Steinmann pin was measured and contoured to fit the area of the resected mandible. Holes were made in the medullary bone, and then a Steinmann pin was inserted into the holes to fill the void from the left mandible to the residual right ramus. Bone wax was placed into the mandibular canals of the left mandible and the angle of the right mandible. The remaining anterior portions

of the genioglossus muscle were sutured with silk to the Steinmann pin in the symphysis region. The entire right buccal mucosa was undermined, and the left residual tongue was sutured tightly to the buccal mucosa for a watertight closure. The patient lost approximately 1 unit of blood, and this was replaced. A nasogastric tube was inserted, and the patient left the operating room in satisfactory condition. All specimens were labeled and sent to the pathology department.

Pathology Report. *Microscopic Diagnosis:* Epidermoid carcinoma, Grade I, with central ulceration, floor of the mouth (margins and depth clear of tumor). Mandibular bone: negative for tumor metastases (Dee R. Parkinson, M.D.).

Postoperative Course. There was a stormy postoperative course, with cardiac and pulmonary complications. It was necessary to transfer the patient to the cardiac care unit. The patient was finally discharged from the hospital approximately 3 weeks after surgery.

The Steinmann pin was removed about 1 month postoperatively. The following January, a mass was noted in the right submaxillary triangle; it was extremely firm and somewhat tender. Because there was some intraoral suppuration as well as exposed bone, it was felt that this might be an inflammatory lymph node. The patient was put on antibiotics, but the mass did not respond. He was referred for tumor team consultation, and surgical exploration of the neck was decided upon. A right radical neck dissection was performed by Robert L. Adeson, M.D. This mass was found to be metastatic carcinoma, and other cervical lymph nodes were also involved by disease.

The patient was followed by both oral and general surgeons. The mouth was clean; however, neck infection with a recurrent tumor was clinically evident. The patient was referred to the chemotherapist and was put on methotrexate.

The neck lesion did not get worse, but the patient became discouraged and depressed, staying in bed most of the time. He was admitted again to the hospital in July (13 months after his original office visit) and expired 8 days later of bilateral bronchopneumonia. An autopsy was performed, and no evidence of distant metastases was found, with the exception of the muscle of the right cervical region of the neck.

Comment. Chemotherapy had contained the neck lesion, but this probably would not have continued for much longer. Additional irradiation or surgery or both might have been resorted to if the patient had survived to permit further treatment. (See Figure 27–19*A* to *J.*)

Case Report No. 15

TREATMENT OF EARLY EPIDERMOID CARCINOMA
OF THE FLOOR OF THE MOUTH

Patient. A 53-year-old white female patient was referred to the office by her family dentist in March for a lesion of the floor of the mouth.

History of Present Illness. The patient presented with a red granular lesion in the right anterior floor of the mouth near the opening of Wharton's duct. The lesion measured 1.5 by 1.5 by 0.5 cm. It felt firm when palpated and was tender. No flow of saliva could be expressed from the orifice of the right Wharton's duct, and attempts to probe the duct were unsuccessful. The lesion was of 8 months' known duration, and according to the patient, there had been no increase in size during this period. The lesion retained 2 per cent toluidine blue dye. There were no palpable nodes in the neck.

The patient admitted to smoking one pack of cigarettes per day and the social use of alcohol.

Medical Evaluation. The remainder of her history was essentially noncontributory.

Course. Exfoliative cytologic examination was performed on the lesion, and the findings were negative for malignant cells. The patient was extremely apprehensive and requested that the surgery, if necessary, be done in the office. The lesion persisted, and 8 days after the initial visit to the office, surgery was performed.

Operative Technique. The patient was premedicated intravenously with 100 mg. of meperidine hydrochloride, 1/120 grain of scopolamine hydrobromide and 100 mg. of sodium pentobarbital (Nembutal). Bilateral mandibular nerve blocks con-

taining 2 per cent lidocaine (Xylocaine) with 1:100,000 epinephrine were administered. The patient was prepared and draped. A wide excision of the lesion was performed, transecting both Wharton's ducts. The patient tolerated surgery and anesthesia. The lesion was sent to the pathology department for diagnosis. (See Figure 27–20A and B.)

Pathology Report. *Microscopic Diagnosis:* Oral mucosa, right anterior floor of the mouth, early invasive epidermoid carcinoma, moderately well differentiated. Specimen appears adequately excised (R. P. Elzay, D.D.S., M.S.D.).

Postoperative Course. The patient's postoperative recovery was completely uneventful. Chest, skull and mandible radiographs, blood chemistry and complete physical evaluation were all within normal limits. Consultation with the general surgeon and radiotherapist resulted in complete agreement to undertake no additional treatment at that time.

The left submaxillary gland was noted to be larger and more pronounced on palpation than the right. Both ducts had been transected during resection of the lesion. There were bilateral swelling and firmness of the submaxillary glands with no evidence of an intraoral orifice releasing saliva. The patient was told that there was no way of knowing whether these submaxillary glands were involved by tumor or were simply obstructed by fibrosis from the surgery. (The right submaxillary duct was involved by neoplastic disease at the time of surgery.) She was given the choice of an

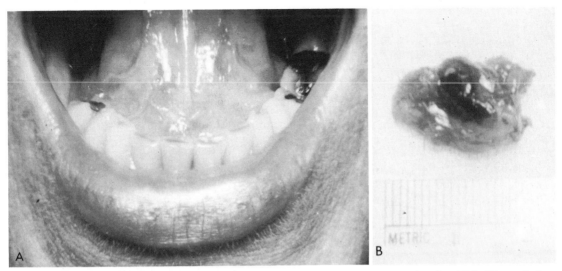

Figure 27–20 *A,* Lesion on the right anterior floor of the mouth of 8 months' known duration. Right Wharton's duct was not functioning. Findings of exfoliative cytologic examination were negative. *B,* Wide local excision of lesion diagnosed as squamous cell carcinoma. Note that tumor retains toluidine blue dye.

intraoral operation to make new ducts for the sub-maxillary glands or of having both glands re-moved. Every conceivable effort was made to encourage bilateral sialodochoplasty, but the patient refused and preferred excision of the submaxillary glands. The patient was hospitalized, and the medical work-up to rule out metastases revealed no clinical or laboratory evidence of disease. She was brought to surgery in November.

Operative Technique. The patient was prepared and draped in the usual fashion. Under naso-tracheal anesthesia, a right submandibular incision was made about 1.5 to 2 cm. beneath the inferior border of the mandible and was carried through the skin, subcutaneous tissue and superficial and deep fascia. Bleeders were tied off and the gland was identified. By a combination of sharp and blunt dissection, the gland was entirely removed from the right submaxillary triangle. The duct was doubly ligated with 000 silk sutures and cut from underneath the mylohyoid muscle. The wound was closed in layers, a drain was inserted, and the skin was closed with 0000 interrupted silk sutures. Exactly the same procedure was performed on the left side. Following this procedure, toluidine blue dye was applied to the lower right floor of the mouth where an area of approximately 2 mm. of tissue was positively stained. The tissue was excised and sent to the pathology department. The patient tolerated surgery and anesthesia and left the operating room in good condition.

Pathology Report. *Microscopic Diagnosis:* Chronic sialoadenitis, submaxillary gland, bilateral. Tissue from floor of mouth showing acanthosis and fibrosis (Dee R. Parkinson, M.D.).

Postoperative Course. The patient's postoperative recovery was completely uneventful. Her condition was followed closely on a 2-month basis. Her mouth and neck remained normal; however, at times the patient appeared extremely depressed, and psychiatric consultation was advised. On occasion, the patient presented in the office under the influence of alcohol. Our efforts to seek help for her problems were rejected. In December (21 months after her initial office visit), the patient expired from alcoholic encephalopathy. A postmortem examination was performed, and there was no evidence of any malignant disease.

Comment. This was obviously a case of early carcinoma. Clinically, the lesion appeared as an erythroplasia. The other ominous finding was a nonfunctioning right Wharton's duct. Since there was no evidence of ductal sialolithiasis, neoplastic invasion was a logical assumption. This lesion was basically a midline neoplasm, so that when there was bilateral enlargement of the submaxillary glands, one could assume possible metastases to these glands. The only reason to assume otherwise was the fact that both Wharton's ducts were nonfunctional as a result of surgery and postoperative fibrosis. Why there was no right submaxillary gland enlargement preoperatively, resulting from the occluded and diseased right Wharton's duct, is speculative. In retrospect, at the time of the surgery, identification of the transected submaxillary ducts and insertion of a polyethylene tube to maintain the patency of the left side and possibly restore function on the right side might have prevented the postoperative submaxillary gland enlargements and subsequent surgery.

MALIGNANT TUMORS OF THE MAXILLA AND MANDIBLE

Any of the malignant tumors of bone may involve the maxilla or mandible. (See Figure 27–21.) Burkitt's lymphoma, which is frequently seen in the maxilla and mandible of African children, rarely occurs in the United States.

Fibrosarcomas, chondrosarcomas and osteogenic sarcomas have the same clinical course and respond to essentially the same treatment. They may occur at any age; sometimes we get the impression that these lesions

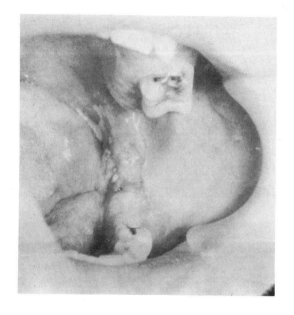

Figure 27–21 Mucosal involvement by tumor affecting the mandibular posterior ridge tissue and lingual mucosa. The maxillary molars were extruded and chronically traumatized the mandibular ridge. *Diagnosis:* Squamous cell carcinoma.

are related to trauma. The mandible appears to be affected more often than the maxilla. Clinical manifestations of these tumors are pain, edema, sometimes mobile teeth and mucosal ulceration. Radiographs may reveal spiking of the roots and in many instances may simulate osteomyelitis. Paget's disease is said to be a predisposing factor for osteogenic sarcoma. Diagnosis is made by biopsy. Osteogenic sarcoma has a better prognosis in the mandible than in other skeletal bones but still presents a poor prognosis. These malignant tumors are extremely aggressive and metastasize by way of the blood stream. Radical resection of bone offers the best modality of treatment.

Endothelioma, or Ewing's sarcoma, is a tumor that may affect the mandible or maxilla. It has an extremely poor prognosis, since it grows rapidly and metastasizes early. Diagnosis is made by biopsy. This malignancy is found primarily in young males. The treatment of choice is radiation therapy, because it is an extremely radiosensitive tumor.

Lymphosarcomas are a rare affliction of the jaw bones. A combination of surgery and radiation is used in an effort to control this neoplasm.

Secondary invasion of the jaws by adjacent malignant tumors and their treatment have been discussed. Metastases to the jaws from other parts of the body must be biopsied in an effort to determine the possible location of the primary malignant tumor. Conservative treatment to make the patient comfortable should be the objective in these cases.

Case Report No. 16

TREATMENT OF POSSIBLE MANDIBULAR MALIGNANT LYMPHOMA

Patient. This 60-year-old white female was referred to me by an oral cancer detection team of dentists in the Appalachian part of Virginia in September.

History of Present Illness. The daughter of the patient, a medical technician, related the past medical history. The patient had worked at Oak Ridge, Tennessee, during World War II years and had been associated with atomic energy research when she was told that she had abnormal blood counts. There had been some question as to whether she might have had leukemia, but the fact that the patient was still alive and basically well disproved that diagnosis. Approximately 2 years previously, a small lesion had been noted on the left alveolar ridge in the anterior mandible that was painful and prevented her from wearing her full lower denture. She had been seen by a dentist who excised this lesion, and histologic examination had revealed "lymphogranuloma with multiple giant cells." The lesion had recurred again within a month and had been excised again, only to recur.

Medical Evaluation. Upon examination, the firm mass on the left anterior alveolar ridge of the mandible was tender to palpation and was approximately 2.5 cm. in circumference. A purulent exudate was draining from the central portion of the lesion. Radiographs and frozen section of the lesion were unavailable. An incision was made into the lesion, and it was obvious that there was bone involvement. Because of the suspicion that this might be an unusual lesion, owing to its history, and because the patient was financially incapable of receiving specialized care, it was decided to do a marginal resection of the mandible. The cervical nodes were not palpable.

Operative Technique. See technique for marginal resection in Case Report No. 8. (See Figure 27–22A and B.)

Pathology Report. *Microscopic Description:* Numerous fragments of soft tissue composed of large masses of neoplastic cells, which appeared to be lymphoid in nature, with a background mixture of lymphocytes, which appeared to be streaming throughout, were noted. This lymphoid element exhibited mitotic figures, some pleomorphism and nuclear and cytoplasmic structures. The lymphoid element was noted to involve most tissue fragments submitted. A surface layer of stratified squamous epithelium overlying subjacent connective tissue that contained a large nidus of the neoplastic lymphoid tissue was noted.

Microscopic Diagnosis: Malignant lymphoma, type unknown—possibly reticulum cell sarcoma (R. M. Howell, M.D.).

Postoperative Course. Considering the preceding diagnosis, further studies and treatment were obviously necessary. Cooperation from the American Cancer Society, the State Health Department (Dental Division), and the National Institutes of Health resulted in the patient's being admitted to the National Institutes of Health, National Cancer Institute, at Bethesda, Maryland, in October.

The slides from Virginia Commonwealth University and the original excisional biopsy performed 2 years before were reviewed. Clinical and

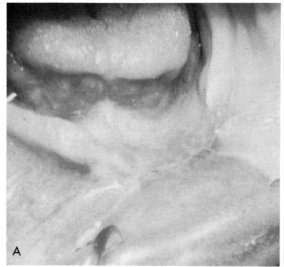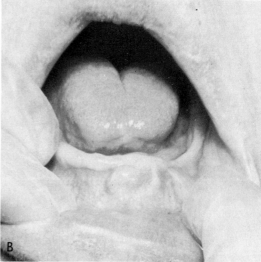

Figure 27-22 *A,* Recurrent neoplastic lesion on the left mandible, which had been excised twice previously, was removed this time by marginal resection. *Diagnosis:* Malignant lymphoma or possible reticulum cell sarcoma; final histologic diagnosis undetermined. *B,* Well-healed postoperative site, 1 month after surgery.

radiographic examination, including periapical and panoramic films of the mandible, showed no lesion of the bone. An exhaustive medical work-up revealed no evidence of neoplastic disease.

Oral and general pathologists at the National Institutes of Health, Pathology Department, reviewed all the slides and agreed that the original lesion excised 2 years before was identical histologically to the most recent lesion that was excised in September. The impression was that this lesion might represent a reactive process with extensive lymphoreticular infiltration. However, the possibility that the process represented a malignant lymphoma or even an undifferentiated carcinoma could not be excluded. Upon review of sections through the bone blocks obtained from the recent marginal mandibular resection, it was felt that the lesion could not be classified exactly but that the surgical margins were clear.

A letter from the National Institutes of Health, dated January 3, read as follows:

Dear Dr. Pizer:

We are a little bit unhappy that we could not arrive at a definitive diagnosis on Mrs. F. Having discussed this with you and considering our reluctance to call this a malignant disease, I'm sure you understand the temporizing attitude we've taken. Let's hope that the anticipated long-term cooperative follow-up between your office and ours on this patient will prove that conservatism is a wise judgment. If any problems do develop, please do not hesitate to contact us.

May I again take this opportunity to thank you for your continued interest in the Surgery Branch. We are challenged with the problems that you find through your ingenious manner of patient surveillance.

Sincerely,
Alfred S. Ketcham, M.D.
Clinical Director and Chief,
Surgery Branch
National Cancer Institute

Postoperative Course. The patient is alive and free of neoplastic disease 2 years after discharge from the National Institutes of Health.

Comment. Some lesions defy a definitive microscopic diagnosis by the many superbly competent oral and general pathologists. In these cases only careful scrutiny of the patient and time determine the seriousness of the disease.

Case Report No. 17

TREATMENT OF EPIDERMOID CARCINOMA (OF LOW-GRADE MALIGNANCY) OF THE MAXILLA*

Patient. This 57-year-old white female was referred to the office by her family physician in January regarding an area of tenderness and swelling with spontaneous bleeding on the right tuberosity of the maxilla.

History of Present Illness. A swelling of the right soft palate and tuberosity region of the right

* Adapted from Pizer, M. E., and Kay, S.: Mouth cancer—Concepts of treatment. Va. Med. Mon., 99:148–166 (Feb), 1972.

maxilla was noted. The patient had an edentulous maxilla and stated that the swollen area of the right posterior maxillary ridge bled on occasion. Her denture was not ill-fiting. Periapical radiographs of the right maxillary ridge revealed a questionable radiolucent area in the tuberosity region with some loss of trabeculae. This area was tender to palpation, and there was a break in the continuity of the mucous membrane at the crest of the ridge where blood had escaped. The initial impression was that of an inflammatory process or localized osteomyelitis. However, the patient did state that she had been operated on at this same anatomic site about 20 years ago by an oral surgeon who had told her that she had a "serious disease." She did not remember the name of the surgeon, and every effort to find information relating to this operation was to no avail. She was admitted to the hospital for a complete medical work-up and exploration of the right maxillary ridge and soft palate in January. There were no significant physical or laboratory findings, and the patient underwent surgery on the third day after hospital admission.

Operative Technique. The patient was prepared and draped in the usual fashion. Under nasotracheal anesthesia, a mucoperiosteal flap was reflected, beginning at the posterior part of the right tuberosity of the region of the canine fossa. With this flap reflected, destruction of the cortical bone was visualized in the edentulous second and third molar regions. The area was curetted. Some soft tissue and bone were removed for microscopic examination. There was more than the usual amount of bleeding. Following curettage, absorbable cellulose gauze (Surgicel) was placed in the wound, and the mucoperiosteum was returned and sutured with 000 interrupted chromic sutures. Following this, the swelling of the right soft palate was examined. Digital examination of the nasopharynx did not reveal any evidence of a tumor. Aspiration was performed with a 14 gauge needle, and no material was aspirated which might have revealed this to be a cyst. However, owing to the enlargement of this soft palatal mass, it was felt advisable to proceed with an incisional biopsy. This site was closed with interrupted 000 chromic sutures. The patient tolerated surgery and anesthesia and left the operating room in good condition.

Pathology Report. *Microscopic Diagnosis:* (1) Biopsy of soft palate with lobule of mucous glands. (2) Biopsy of hard palate with mucoepidermoid carcinoma of low-grade malignancy (Dr. Legier, Pathologist).

Postoperative Course. The patient's postoperative recovery was uneventful. The patient was discharged from the hospital on the fifth postoperative day. The tissue report was a complete surprise, and with these slides, I consulted four outstanding oral pathologists. Each agreed independently that this was a mucoepidermoid car-

cinoma of low-grade malignancy. I consulted a surgeon with both dental and medical training who strongly suggested that the right maxilla and soft palate be resected. The patient was sent to a radiologist for a consultation, and the letter that was received read in part:

Dear Dr. Pizer:
. . . Examination of the biopsy site on the right side of the soft palate revealed it to be healed as well as the tissue over the alveolar margin of the maxilla where the bone has been curetted. This mucoepidermoid carcinoma is a very low-grade type of malignancy that does not respond to irradiation. The lesion that was removed from this area some 20 years ago probably represented the same tumor. The patient may have no recurrence of this lesion for at least another 10 to 15 years. With recurrence, two things should happen: (1) bone will be destroyed, and (2) there will be a breakdown of tissue with bleeding in the area in question. To do any radical surgery or en bloc dissection at this time, I feel, would do the patient a disservice. She should be seen at regular intervals, and occlusal films of this area should be done to pick up any increase in bone destruction.

If at any time the tumor becomes more aggressive, then total extirpation of the area with all the complications that follow such surgery will have to be faced.

Thank you for the privilege of seeing this patient and please do not hesitate to call if I can be of any further assistance.

Sincerely yours,
Charlotte P. Donlan, M.D.

Course. The decision of whether to proceed with additional surgery or follow the recommendations of the radiologist was a difficult one, but considering the patient's past history of a lesion that probably resulted from the same disease in this area 20 years ago and the nature of this tumor, it was decided to institute "masterful inactivity." The patient was sent to her family dentist, and a new maxillary denture was made. Periapical and occlusal radiographs were taken every 3 months during the first postoperative year and every 4 months during the second postoperative year. In December (almost 2 years after the patient's original office visit), a suspicious-looking area of the right soft palate was biopsied and found to be "chronic sialadenitis of the soft palate." An ulcer at the surgical site overlying the right tuberosity was biopsied the following October, and the histologic findings revealed "mucosa showing ulceration, marked parakeratosis and severe inflammatory reaction."

In June (8 months later), the patient was clinically asymptomatic, the mouth looking essentially normal and the neck, as usual, with no palpable nodes. There was some clinically redundant tissue in the right tuberosity region that was suggestive of denture irritation. Periapical and occlusal films, however, *did reveal* some demineralization in the region of the floor of the antrum. It was felt that surgical exploration was indicated, and the patient was brought to surgery.

Operative Technique. Under heavy intravenous sedation and local infiltration with 2 per cent lidocaine (Xylocaine) and 1:100,000 epinephrine, an incision was made on the crest of the ridge from the posterior aspect of the tuberosity to the canine fossa. Upon reflection of the mucoperiosteum, gray tissue and spongy bone clinically similar to the findings of the first operation were noted. With an osteotome and mallet, a marginal resection of the posterior one-third of the right maxilla was performed. The antral cavity appeared free of disease. Mucous membrane was removed to the level of the resection on both the buccal and palatal sides, while leaving enough mucosa for a primary closure. The patient tolerated surgery and anesthesia and left the operating room in good condition.

Pathology Report. *Microscopic Diagnosis:* Tissue submitted for examination shows an infiltrating tumor—mucoepidermoid tumor (M. Freund, M.D.).

The following letter was also received regarding the preceding pathology report:

Dear Dr. Pizer:

In accordance with our telephone conversation, I should like to state that I found the sinus membrane present within the submitted specimen to be free of tumor infiltration.

Knowing that this patient is a telephone operator for whom intact speech is important and the tumor being of the kind for which we can presume that distant metastases are so rare and the patient being cooperative with you, I would advise that the patient be kept under observation and a more radical operation be postponed for as long as possible.

Sincerely yours,
M. Freund, M.D.
Pathologist

Course. Consultations again were held with the radiologist, general surgeon, family physician and

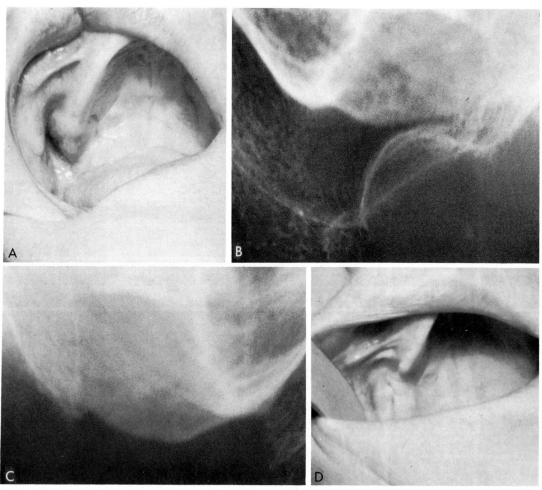

Figure 27–23 *A,* Swelling of and spontaneous bleeding from edentulous right tuberosity. Maxillary denture does not fit as it did previously. *B,* Periapical film of the right tuberosity reveals some demineralization and loss of trabeculae. *C,* Radiograph showing marginal resection of posterior right maxilla with low-grade mucoepidermoid carcinoma. *D,* Clinical appearance of resected posterior maxilla. Patient wears full maxillary denture successfully. (*A, B, C* and *D,* From Pizer, M. E., and Kay, S.: Mouth cancer—Concepts of treatment. Va. Med. Mon., *99:*148–166 [Feb.], 1972.)

pathologist, who also reviewed the original slide. It was decided to follow the patient at 3-month intervals with clinical examination and periapical and occlusal radiographs. Routine chest films and the usual complete blood count and differential count are done every 6 months, as in the past. The patient is clinically and radiographically free of disease. It is now 8 years since her first operation and 5 years since the second. (See Figure 27–23*A* to *D*.)

Comment. Recognizing this to be a slow-growing tumor of low-grade malignancy with minimal tendency to metastasize, we felt that conservatism would be the best approach for this patient.

She is a cooperative patient, who allows close observation at all times. Radical surgery would have prevented her from performing her duties as a telephone operator and thus would have crippled her financially and emotionally. However, if the decision of the tumor consultants had been different, we would not have hesitated to do a much more radical operation. The patient is now retired from her job, and should additional surgery be necessary, the prognosis would still be excellent. It would be interesting to know if the operation performed 28 years ago in this same region of the oral cavity was for removal of this same pathologic lesion.

CONCLUSION

There is much controversy with respect to treating intraoral malignant lesions. We therefore use the team approach, the nucleus of the group being an oncologic surgeon, a radiotherapist, a chemotherapist and an oral surgeon. The team also includes an internist, pathologist (oral pathologist, when possible), prosthodontist and plastic surgeon. There are no "standard operative procedures" for our patients, since we endeavor to study each patient and "tailor" the therapy based on the present available knowledge regarding oral malignant lesions.

PREVENTION

From what is presently known, eliminating tobacco and excessive alcohol consumption could conceivably make squamous cell carcinoma of the oral cavity a less common disease. The medical treatment of dietary deficiencies and anemias may also significantly reduce oral carcinomas. Fair-complexioned patients should be informed that chronic exposure to the actinic rays of the sun, in some individuals, may be carcinogenic to the lip and skin.

Dentists and physicians must examine each patient's mouth carefully and remove any and all suspicious lesions. So-called premalignant lesions must be totally removed, and the patient should be followed closely.

All patients who have been *treated* for oral malignant disease should be followed periodically by examination of the head and neck on a 3-month basis for the first 3 years, and then on a 4-month basis for the rest of their lives. Any suspicious site is quickly biopsied to determine the nature of the lesion. Chest radiographs, complete blood count and differential count are done every 6 months for the first 3 years, and then on a yearly basis. The patient is asked to do away with smoking or any etiologic factors that may contribute to the disease. Staying out of the sun (for patients with lip cancer), removing chronic oral irritations and correcting dietary deficiencies are all part of the postoperative care. Good oral hygiene and close cooperation with the family dentist and physician must be insisted upon.

An excellent study showed the high risk of the oral cancer patient for developing *multiple primary malignant lesions*. This study revealed that 34 per cent of these patients developed a second primary site of disease; the majority of these lesions (65 per cent) occurred in the oral, respiratory or upper gastrointestinal tract.[22]

Those in the dental profession are charged with the legal and moral responsibility of maintaining the patient's general health by professionally insuring good oral and maxillofacial health.

REFERENCES

1. Ackerman, L. V., and del Regato, J. A.: Cancer: Diagnosis, Treatment and Prognosis. St. Louis, The C. V. Mosby Co., 1970.
2. American Cancer Society: 1973 Oral cancer statistics. J. Oral Surg., *31*(6):495 (June), 1973.

3. Baker, H. W.: Diagnosis of oral cancer. One. CA, *22*(1):30–39 (Feb.), 1972.

4. Baker, H. W.: Benign oral tumors and tumor-like conditions. CA, *22*(2):102–109 (Mar.-Apr.), 1972.

5. Bales, H. W.: *In* Rubin, P., and Bekemeier, R. F. (Eds.): Clinical Oncology for Medical Students and Physicians. 3rd ed. New York, American Cancer Society, 1970–1971.

6. Beattie, E. J., Jr.: Therapeutic attitudes: Cooperators and competitors. *In* Rubin, P. (Ed.): Cancer of the head and neck. J.A.M.A., *215*(3):459–460 (Jan. 18), 1971.

7. Bellanti, J. A.: Immunology, p. 324. Philadelphia, W. B. Saunders Co., 1971.

8. Bernier, J. L., and Clark, M. L.: Squamous cell carcinomas of the lip. Milit. Surg., *109:*379–405, 1951.

9. Bhaskar, S. W.: Synopsis of Oral Pathology. St. Louis, The C. V. Mosby Co., 1965.

10. Conley, J.: How to examine the oro-naso-laryngopharynx for cancer. *In* Rubin, P. (Ed.): Cancer of the head and neck. J.A.M.A., *215*(3):456 (Jan. 18), 1971.

11. Dunlap, C. L., and Robinson, H. B. G.: Practical application of experimental cancer research. *In* Rubin, P. (Ed.): Cancer of the head and neck. J.A.M.A., *215*(3):457–458 (Jan. 18), 1971.

12. Elzay, R.: Personal communication. Richmond, Va., 1973.

13. Frazell, E. L.: The care of patients with oral cavity and lip cancer: Surgical principles. J.A.M.A., *215*(6):957–958 (Feb. 8), 1971.

14. Gorlin, R. J., and Goldman, H. M.: Thoma's Oral Pathology. 5th ed. St. Louis, The C. V. Mosby Co., 1970.

15. Guralnick, E.: Malignant tumors of the oral cavity.
In Guralnick, E. (Ed.): Textbook of Oral Surgery. Boston, Little, Brown & Co., 1968.

16. Jesse, R. H.: The treatment of oral cancer. CA, *22*(4):209–215 (July-Aug.), 1972.

17. Leffall, L. D.: *In* Holleb, A. I.: Editor's interview: Head and neck cancer. CA, *21*(5):288–291 (Sept.-Oct.), 1971.

18. Osterkamp, R. W., and Whitten, J. B.: The etiology and pathogenesis of oral cancer. CA, *23*(1):28–32 (Jan.-Feb.), 1973.

19. Penn, I., and Starzl, T. E.: Malignant tumors arising de novo in immunosuppressed organ transplant recipients. Transplantation, *14:*407–417, 1972.

20. Pizer, M. E.: A query to radiotherapists. Va. Med. Mon., *100:*222–223 (Mar.), 1973.

21. Pizer, M. E.: The oral cancer team. Va. Dent. J., *45*(2):5 (Apr.), 1968.

22. Pizer, M. E., and Kay, S.: Mouth cancer – Concepts of treatment. Va. Med. Mon., *99:*148–166 (Feb.), 1972.

23. Southwick, H. W.: Elective neck dissection for intraoral cancer. *In* Rubin, P. (Ed.): Cancer of the head and neck. J.A.M.A., *217:*454–455 (July 26), 1971.

24. Thoma, G. W.: Causes of death in patients with oral cancer. Oral Surg., *30:*817–823 (Dec.), 1970.

25. Totten, R. S.: Tumors of the oral cavity, pharynx and larynx: Pathologic aspects. *In* Rubin, P. (Ed.): Cancer of the head and neck. J.A.M.A., *215*(3):454–455 (Jan. 18), 1971.

26. Waldron, C. A.: Personal communication. Atlanta, 1973.

27. Wynder, E. L.: Etiological aspects of squamous cancer of the head and neck. *In* Rubin, P. (Ed.): Cancer of the head and neck. J.A.M.A., *215*(3):459–460 (Jan. 18), 1971.

CHAPTER **28**

THE SURGICAL TREATMENT OF ORAL MALIGNANT DISEASES AND THEIR CERVICAL METASTASES

JOHN C. GAISFORD, M.D.

Certainly no textbook on oral surgery is complete without a detailed discussion of the treatment of oral malignant neoplasms. Since the metastatic spread of these tumors is primarily to the neck, the dentist should be well acquainted with the accepted therapy for this problem, as well as with that for the intraoral problems.

The purpose of this chapter is to discuss the management of these tumors, not their anatomy, etiology, pathology and differential diagnosis. This is not meant to imply that the latter phases can be slighted or omitted; detailed knowledge of each subject mentioned is vitally important if one is to understand and treat cancer of the oral cavity adequately.

Many resident physicians, dentists, interns and nurses see head and neck cancer patients during their treatment. Since this disease exists where it can be observed by others, and since the breathing, eating, smelling and seeing structures may be involved, a feeling of despair often develops among these groups regarding treatment and the patient's chances for permanent cure or help. Even in this seemingly medically enlightened age, the teaching of head and neck cancer diagnosis and treatment in medical, dental and nursing schools is pitifully meager, and discussion of the moral and practical approach to the management of head and neck cancer patients is almost nonexistent. It has become quite

apparent that head and neck cancer is still—as it has always been—very inadequately managed. Because there is no "one" accepted treatment, many types of treatment approaches are used and most of them are woefully inadequate, and many are actually wrong.

The complete management of an extensive head and neck cancer is time-consuming and many times complicated and may eventually end in the distressing demise of the patient. There is no comparison between a patient dying of cancer of the intestinal tract, lung or brain and one dying of head and neck cancer. Cancer of the head and neck is exposed so that the patient and all his relatives and acquaintances can see it—dressings can never be kept clean, neat and free of odor at all times on an expanding, messy cancer of this area. And when the eyes, ears, mouth and nose are slowly encroached upon, the office visits by the patient and telephone calls by the relatives increase. In addition, this is one phase of medicine in which family physicians for some reason are reluctant to accept the major role. It is the exceptional "family doctor" who makes a real effort to become involved. He and the surgeon or radiotherapist who may have accepted the patient for definitive care, slight though the chance may have been for cure, are expected by all concerned to nurse that patient through to

1779

end, whether that ending is happy or sad.

Who then should assume complete charge of the patient with cancer of the head and neck? I think the answer to this, after the preceding dissertation, must be quite obvious. He is the one who is first of all completely honest professionally. He must permit the individual patient to be treated in the best manner available — radiation, surgery, or a combination of the two — or must make the decision, in concert with his consultants, that no treatment at all is to be instituted. Ideally, he should have excellent surgical training, a working knowledge of radiotherapy and adequate training in surgical pathology so that he knows the life history of every tumor cell type. He should have an inherent desire to work with this difficult group of disease entities and be able to adjust to family pressures and to constant dealings with the slow, miserable deaths which are such a constant accompaniment of this disease. He should be sufficiently farsighted that he plans for complete care in the rehabilitation of the individual patient. It is totally unacceptable to assume that treatment is complete after the cancer is removed. Many of these patients are free of the cancer but will be permanent surgical cripples if reconstruction or the use of prosthetic devices is not attempted.

Incidentally, age, per se, is never a contraindication to major head and neck cancer operations. Certainly, treatment should not be denied simply because a patient is considered "old." Older people withstand long, involved surgical procedures about the head and neck with surprising regularity. Advancements in anesthesiology have also increased the ability of older patients to withstand extensive surgical procedures. In addition, one reason extensive surgery about the head and neck is necessary and reasonable is that cancer frequently remains localized to the head and neck for a long period of time before metastasizing below the clavicles.

Our thinking has changed considerably in the last few years regarding primary reconstruction following the removal of primary cancers. Formerly, it was thought that reconstruction should not be undertaken until it was relatively certain that the cancer was controlled. Our approach to this problem has changed completely and we now carry out as much primary reconstruction as is consistent with safe surgery. Statistics show very clearly that when a serious cancer of the head and neck is adequately treated by surgery initially, a recurrence usually is not controllable by any means. This, then, clearly points out the fact that the patient is entitled to as much comfort as he can possibly be offered for as long as he lives. We, therefore, do not hesitate to go to extremes to reconstruct as adequately and as soon as possible any surgical defect created by the removal of a tumor.

The actual performance of these surgical procedures is really not difficult. They can all be done with a minimum of well-directed effort. This, however, is one major reason that head and neck tumors are frequently badly managed. The surgical technique may be quite acceptable but the judgment behind the decision to carry out a surgical procedure may be highly questionable. Is any one specialty group endowed with all-inclusive abilities to take care of these problems? The answer is an unqualified "no."

The professional who is most adequately equipped should be the one to do this work. It matters little to which specialty group he belongs — general surgery, otolaryngology, plastic surgery, or oral surgery — but in all fairness to his patient he must be completely trained to do this job well.

The management of oral malignant disease requires cooperation among various specialists. It is absolutely mandatory, in order for the patient to obtain maximum benefit from his treatment, that dentist, surgeon, radiotherapist and family physician work together closely and with open minds. All oral lesions must be cared for immediately. Since the dentist is frequently the first to see a patient who has an oral cancer, he is obligated to have the patient cared for properly. He should have treatment started on an emergency basis. It is unpardonable to do such things as local cauterization of an intraoral ulcer; yet this is by no means an uncommon occurrence. The oral ulcers and questionably neoplastic areas must be inspected and biopsied, and the proper treatment promptly decided upon. If this is not done, and a delay of weeks to months occurs, the lesion may metastasize to cervical lymph nodes, making the prognosis extremely poor. If delay is protracted, occasionally there may be metastases to distant sites (below the clavicle), thereby resulting in an incurable disease.

The surgeon is often far too anxious to operate on these cancers. The radiotherapist is frequently overambitious in his belief that he can cure most lesions. The surgeon and radiotherapist must therefore consult with each other regarding therapy for each controversial case. Frequently, surgery and radiotherapy in combination will produce the best result in the treatment of oral cancer.

RADICAL NECK DISSECTIONS

Radical neck dissections are common operations performed by those doing head and neck cancer surgery. They are done to control the spread of malignant cells from the primary cancer to cervical lymph nodes, because if the secondary spread of cancer is not halted, curing the primary lesion is useless. Irradiation of cervical metastases is frequently contraindicated. If one were to give a cancerocidal dose of x-rays to the lymph nodes on one side of the neck, the patient probably would not survive because the total amount of irradiation would be so great.

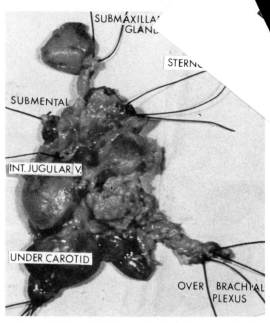

Figure 28–2 Radical neck dissection specimen—playtsma muscle not attached. Sutures mark the specimen for ease of handling by the pathologist.

However, situations do arise which might demand the use of x-ray therapy in an otherwise surgical case. If a patient is medically unable to withstand a major operation, or if he should refuse surgery, certainly x-ray treatment should be considered.

A *prophylactic* radical neck dissection is done when no clinical cervical metastases are demonstrable. This operation is indicated only for carcinoma of the tongue (bilateral dissection if the primary cancer is at or near the midline) and floor of the mouth.

A *therapeutic* radical neck dissection is the term given to the dissection performed when clinically demonstrable cervical metastases are present.

A *complete* radical neck dissection implies the removal of the following structures from the mandible above, trapezius muscle posteriorly, clavicle inferiorly, and midline of the neck anteriorly: (*a*) platysma, sternomastoid, omohyoid, digastric and stylohyoid muscles; (*b*) inferior portion of the parotid glands; (*c*) submaxillary gland; (*d*) all the lymphatic tissues of the neck; (*e*) fat and superficial vessels in the region over the brachial plexus; and (*f*) the internal jugular vein and all veins superficial to it (Fig. 28–1).

The contents of the neck are removed *en masse* without being separated into various segments. It is vitally important that the

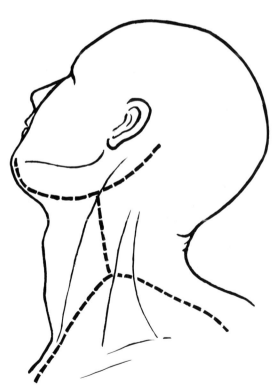

Figure 28–1 The commonly used double-Y incisions for complete radical neck dissection. The neck is widely and adequately exposed by turning back four large skin flaps. See Figures 28–54 to 28–56 for the MacFee parallel transverse incision, which gives a better cosmetic result.

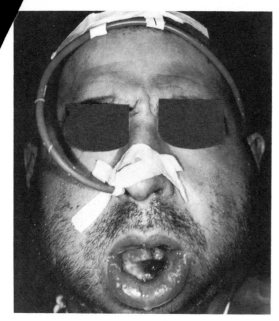

Figure 28–3 Three days following a one-stage bilateral complete radical neck dissection. The patient shows moderate facial edema.

surgical specimens from neck dissections and all malignant or suspected malignant growths be properly tagged with sutures. A rough drawing is made routinely of the specimen and it is properly labeled for identification purposes (Fig. 28–2). This specimen can be examined much easier by the surgical pathologist. The pathologist can then give the surgeon more specific information: namely, whether the tumor has been adequately removed, the degree of involvement, and the areas involved. From this information, one can often determine what the final outlook for long-term survival will be. If numerous lymph nodes contain tumor, one can assume that a certain number of these already have developed distant metastases. The prognosis is better if nodes high in the neck rather than those lower down, near and behind the clavicle, are involved.

Bilateral radical neck dissections may be done as one- or two-stage procedures. The internal jugular veins may or may not be removed in a one-stage procedure; the removal of both internal jugulars at times causes marked facial edema but may cause surprisingly little (Fig. 28–3). The decision to do a bilateral one-stage radical neck dissection is made only after very careful deliberation, since the procedure is an extremely serious undertaking. Usually the indication for this operation exists when a primary cancer within the mouth already has metastasized to both sides of the neck, and splitting the operation into two procedures would increase the chance for cutting into tumor and thereby increase the chances for local recurrences.

The author believes that the only indication for a suprahyoid or upper neck dissection is the physical inability of the patient to withstand the complete procedure. This is an inadequate cancer operation.

ANESTHESIA

Endotracheal anesthesia is the most adaptable method for surgery of the head and neck. Pentothal is still used, particularly for induction, but Fluothane is becoming more popular. This permits long procedures under the safest conditions. Minor procedures are performed under local anesthesia.

An anesthetist clearly acquainted with the problem under consideration is important to head and neck surgery. The endotracheal tube should be securely fastened at the nostril (in a nasotracheal anesthesia), with care being taken that the ala is not forced superiorly by the endotracheal tube, since this can cause necrosis of the nostril. The external endotracheal tube attachment should lie flat over the face to permit adequate and comfortable draping of the patient. The tubes leading to the anesthesia machine should be so attached

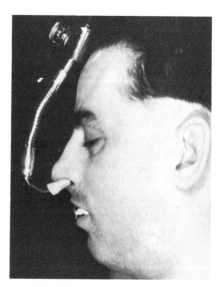

Figure 28–4 Endotracheal tube attachment which permits free motion of the head during operation. The apparatus can be firmly and easily secured to head.

to the head of the patient that the anesthetist has no reason to be near the patient's head (Fig. 28–4). There should be freedom of the patient's head and neck so that they may be turned from side to side by the surgeon as necessary during the course of the operation. A long tubing at the antecubital space allows both arms of the patient to be placed at the patient's sides and permits easy administration of the anesthetic. A cooperative anesthesiologist makes this part of the work much more satisfactory.

After major mouth and neck surgery, it is mandatory that endotracheal tubes be left securely taped in place until the patient has control of his tongue and attempts to speak. If a tracheostomy is done at the conclusion of the operation, as is routine after most jaw resections, obviously the endotracheal tube is removed as the tracheostomy tube is inserted. A tracheostomy is usually done as part of the combination jaw-neck resection, because for 24 to 72 hours postoperatively the patient may have difficulty in breathing. Since the lingual muscles attached to the mandible are sectioned, the tongue can easily fall back in the oropharynx, obstructing breathing. This, accompanied by swelling from surgical trauma, may necessitate an emergency tracheostomy if a tracheostomy has not been done.

PREMALIGNANT LESIONS

Premalignant lesions are those lesions which are thought to progress to cancer if not eradicated. See Chapter 27 for a discussion

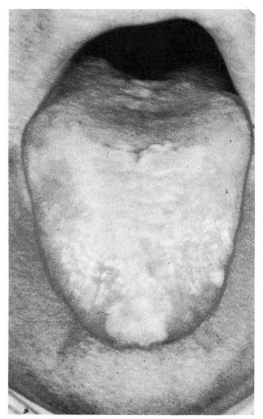

Figure 28–6 Extensive leukoplakia of dorsum of tongue.

of leukoplakia (Figs. 28–5 and 28–6) and related lesions.

MALIGNANT LESIONS

LOWER LIP

Relatively small cancers of the lower lip are treated by surgical V-wedge or shield (see Chapter 27) excision with primary closure. The line of surgical excision should be 1 to 1.5 cm. from either edge of the tumor (see Figures 28–7 to 28–10).

Large cancers that, after wide excision, make the lip short are reconstructed by the use of the switch-flap (Abbé-Estlander) from the opposite lip (Figs. 28–11 to 28–18).

Radiotherapy can give good results in many cases. Generally, surgery is a more expeditious form of therapy. The operation is done under local anesthesia and often can be performed as an outpatient procedure. Careful histologic examination of the excised specimen reveals whether the tumor has been

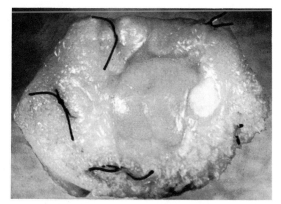

Figure 28–5 Resected specimen of the tongue. The round, white leukoplakic area was classified not malignant after the original biopsy. One year later carcinoma developed in the posterior portion.

Figure 28-7

Figure 28-8

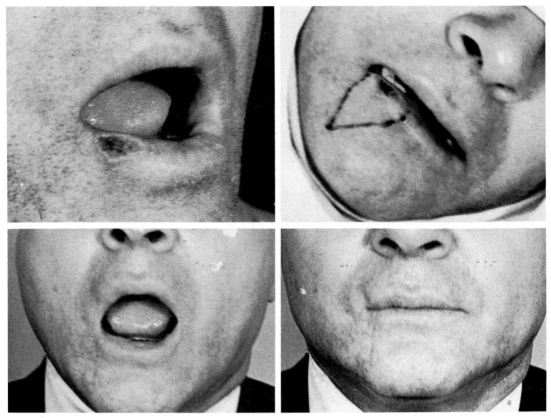

Figure 28-9

Figure 28-10

Figure 28-7 Squamous cell carcinoma of the lower lip.
Figure 28-8 Methylene blue outline of the amount of tissue to be removed.
Figure 28-9 Lip healed. Note that only a slight lip deformity results.
Figure 28-10 Resulting scar of lower lip is minimal.

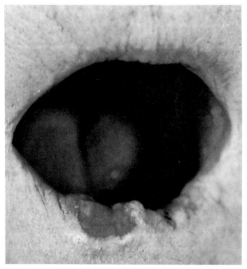

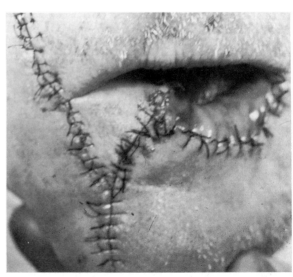

Figure 28-11 Cancer of the left lower lip and leuko-plakia of right lower lip.

Figure 28-12 Excision of cancer, stripping of leuko-plakia, Abbé flap from upper lip.

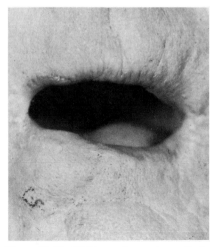

Figure 28-13 Eight months postoperatively.

removed with adequate margins of uninvolved tissue. If the pathologist feels that there is residual tumor, or that the line of surgical excision is close to the tumor, more tissue can readily be removed.

UPPER LIP

Cancer of the upper lip is unusual; probably not more than 3 per cent of all lip cancers involve the upper lip. In the author's experience, only two cancers of the upper lip have been found. One of the two was a basal cell carcinoma. (The vast majority of lip cancers are the squamous cell variety.)

The treatment is the same as for cancer of the lower lip (see Figures 28-19 to 28-22).

Figure 28-14   Figure 28-15   Figure 28-16

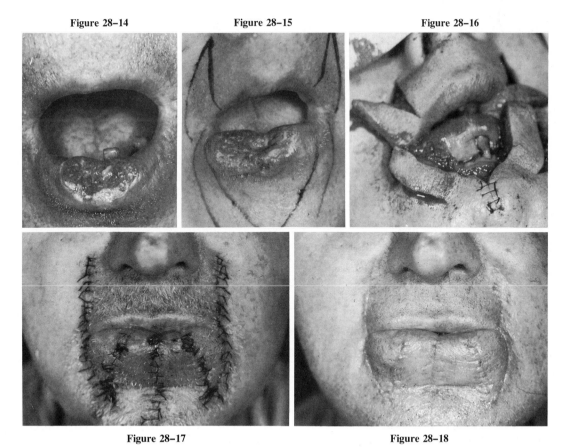

Figure 28-17   Figure 28-18

Figure 28-14 Recurrent cancer, lower lip.

Figure 28-15 Growth after 6 months while the patient is deciding about treatment; methylene blue marking of proposed incisions is shown.

Figure 28-16 Double upper lip pedicle cut after removal of cancer and advancing of two lateral flaps.

Figure 28-17 Seven days postoperatively.

Figure 28-18 Two months postoperatively.

Figure 28–19

Figure 28–20

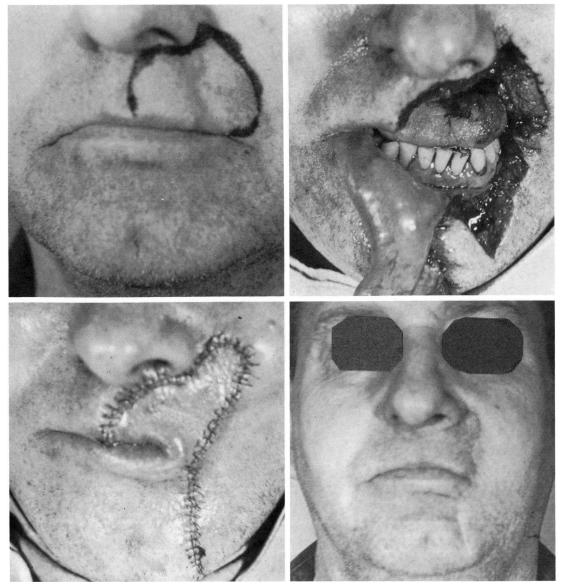

Figure 28–21

Figure 28–22

Figure 28–19   Fibrosarcoma of the left upper lip.
Figure 28–20   Lip resected, pedicle cut from the lower lip.
Figure 28–21   Lower lip pedicle rotated and sutured into upper lip, followed by closure of the lower lip.
Figure 28–22   Final result following enlargement of the angle of the mouth.

BUCCAL MUCOSA

This is a relatively common location for primary cancer. Frequently, the patient with buccal mucosal cancer also has areas of leukoplakia (see Figure 28–23).

Treatment. Surgical excision is the treatment of choice. These lesions are not particu-

larly radiosensitive and usually are relatively easy to eradicate completely. The surgical defect, even though wide, can usually be closed primarily, since wide mobilization of the cheek is always possible. When wide areas are resected, a split-thickness skin graft can be applied and does well within the mouth (see Figures 28–24 to 28–27).

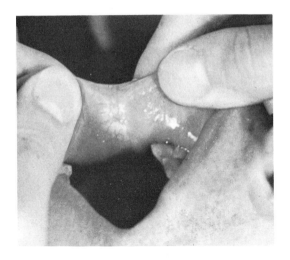

Figure 28-23 Carcinoma of buccal mucosa. Under local anesthesia, a local excision was performed as an outpatient procedure.

MUCOPERIOSTEUM (GUM) OF MANDIBLE

When the cancer primarily involves the mandibular gum, one must assume it is too close to bone to locally strip away from the bone. Not infrequently, the gum lesion will extend as far as the base of the anterior tonsillar pillar, and the entire lesion must be removed in continuity.

Treatment. Resection of the mandible with a wide margin of grossly uninvolved ad-

Figure 28-24

Figure 28-25

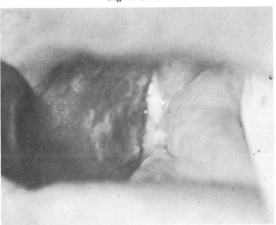

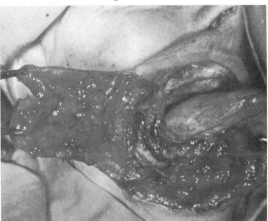

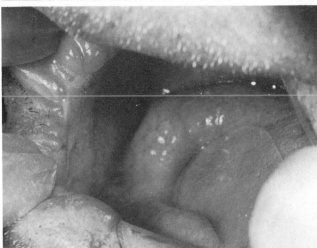

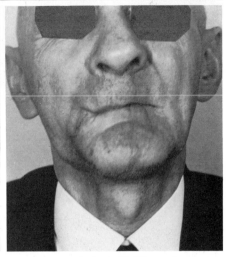

Figure 28-26

Figure 28-27

Figure 28-24 Recurrent cancer within a large area of leukoplakia in buccal mucosa.

Figure 28-25 Lip split, cheek flap laid back and cheek split with removal of the cancer.

Figure 28-26 Split skin graft has been removed from the abdomen and is growing well as the new lining for the cheek.

Figure 28-27 View of the patient 4 months postoperatively.

jacent tissue is mandatory. Tonsillar pillar lesions, as will be discussed later, are here treated surgically. These lesions are treated as extensions, not primary lesions, and are excised in continuity with the primary lesion on the mandible. Usually one must sacrifice large portions of the mandible (hemimandibulectomy is almost routine with the author) for small or large bony lesions, since cancer not infrequently travels up the mandibular canal. Cancer which has traveled along the mandibular canal usually is not demonstrable roentgenographically, so in this case one must be radical. For this reason, it is usually better to disarticulate the mandible on the involved side and section it at a considerable distance from any demonstrable bony tumor.

The oral surgeon has unlimited opportunities for working out and applying techniques for control of the remaining portion of mandible after partial resection. The functional and cosmetic result is far better if the remaining lower jaw is firmly held in proper occlusion until healing by the usual fibrosis takes place. The mandible is usually solidly fixed in four to six weeks. Permanent discontinuation of whatever type of splinting was chosen can usually be done after this period of time. Several methods may be used to maintain the remaining portion of mandible in its proper position. These are interdental wiring, extraoral skeletal fixation, various

sliding projections from a lower plate into an upper plate, and temporary or permanent splinting by insertion of a Kirschner wire between the resected ends of the mandible. Immediate or delayed bone grafts (autogenous or bank bone), and many forms of metal and plastic materials have been used. Each case must be individualized and the technique thought to be wisest in the management of that particular case followed (see Figures 28–28 to 28–31).

Many times the result is such that the patient does not wish to undergo bony reconstruction; his appearance is acceptable and he can eat, and that is all he desires.

From personal experience, the author has concluded that a prophylactic tracheostomy should always be performed at the conclusion of any operation in which the mandible has been resected. To omit this procedure is to invite obstruction of the airway, either in the immediate postoperative period before the patient has completely recovered from the anesthetic or after 24 to 48 hours, when laryngeal edema causes obstruction.

The tracheostomy tube can usually be removed safely after 72 hours, but if there is any question about residual laryngeal edema, or if there is poor support to the tongue because of radical surgery, the tube may safely be left in place indefinitely.

Temporary tracheostomy should be considered in the elderly and the debilitated, as they

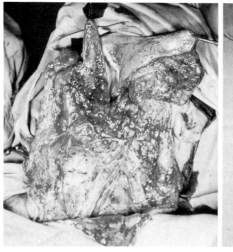
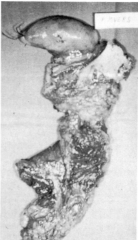
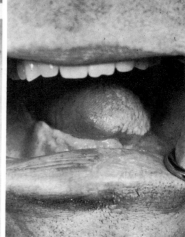

Figure 28–28   **Figure 28–29**   **Figure 28–30**

Figure 28–28   Radical neck dissection, hemimandibulectomy, and hemiglossectomy followed by insertion of a heavy Kirschner wire, for cancer of mandible and tongue.

Figure 28–29   Resected specimen—neck contents, mandible and tongue.

Figure 28–30   Intraoral view of patient 4 months postoperatively.

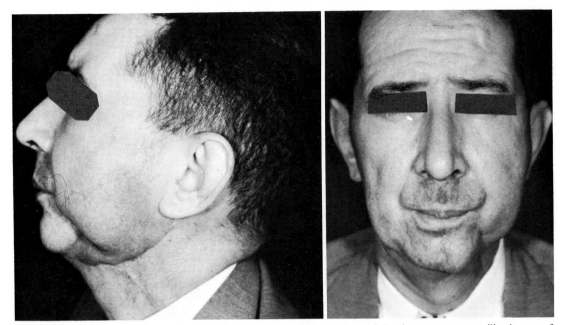

Figure 28–31   Profile and front views of patient 1 year postoperatively and following an autogenous iliac bone graft to left mandible.

are much more apt to experience respiratory embarrassment than younger, stronger people, even without having the continuity of the mandible interrupted.

MANDIBLE

Lesions of the mandible itself are treated in an identical fashion to lesions of the gum of the mandible: by radical surgical resection (see Figures 28–32 to 28–37). Usually a neck dissection is performed as part of the definitive surgery when the jaw is removed by way of an extraoral incision. The thinking here is that the ideal time to do a clean neck dissection is the first time the neck is entered, not after it becomes scarred by surgery or radiation.

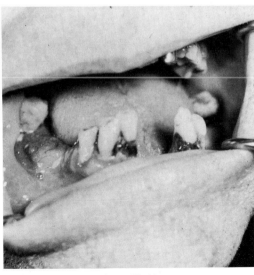
Figure 28–32

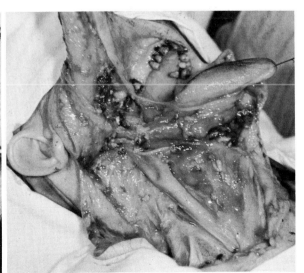
Figure 28–33

Figure 28–32   Cancer of body of the mandible with clinically evident cervical metastases.
Figure 28–33   Radical neck dissection and hemimandibulectomy.

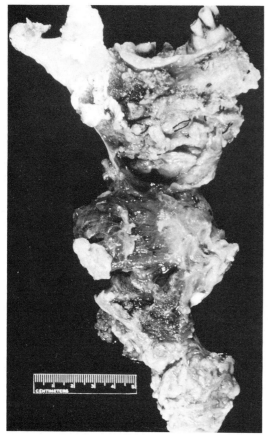

Figure 28–34   Resected specimen.

MAXILLA

Cancer of the maxilla is difficult to treat for three reasons: first, the disease is usually advanced when its presence is brought to the attention of the one who is to treat the lesion; second, cancer of the maxilla quickly extends to areas completely inaccessible to present methods of therapy (pterygoid space, sphenoid bone); third, adequate treatment for cancer of the maxilla is so devastating that it should be undertaken only when a reasonably optimistic outlook can be assured.

Treatment.   When possible, surgical extirpation of maxillary cancer is the preferred treatment. Complete disarticulation of the maxilla is rarely attempted, since the operative mortality is unreasonably high. Partial resection is justifiable and probably gives results as good as those of more extensive procedures. Usually exenteration of the orbit is performed along with removal of the maxilla. The depths of the wound and the posterior

A

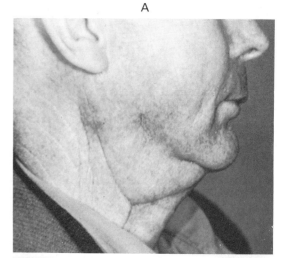

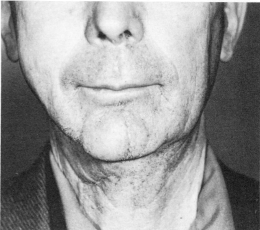

B

Figure 28–35   *A* and *B*, Four months postoperatively. No replacement of the mandible. The patient is alive and free of disease 12 years postoperatively.

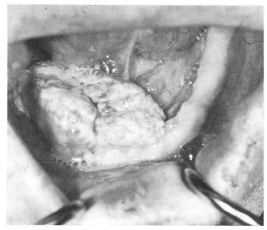

Figure 28–36   Advanced cancer of mandible and floor of mouth, with cervical metastases. Radical neck dissection, resection of jaw from angle to angle, floor of mouth and inferior surface of tongue.

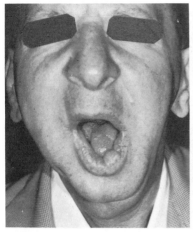
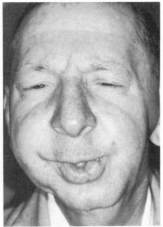
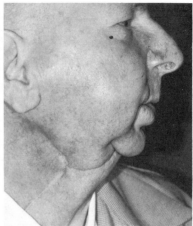

Figure 28–37 Two months postoperatively. Resected mandible was immediately freed of soft tissues, autoclaved, and reinserted at initial operation. It became exposed and had to be removed 2 weeks postoperatively, but the tissues became fixed in a very normal fashion. This patient remains free of disease 9 years postoperatively.

aspect of the cheek flap are always lined with a split-thickness skin graft to prevent unsightly puckering of the flap and to permit an intraoral prosthesis to fit adequately (see Figures 28–38 to 28–43). A temporary prosthesis may also be inserted at the time of surgery to prevent unwanted contractures in the face. An interested dentist or prosthodontist can play a major role in this type of practical rehabilitation.

Contraindications to radical maxillary surgery are distant metastases and extension locally to areas not surgically resectable.

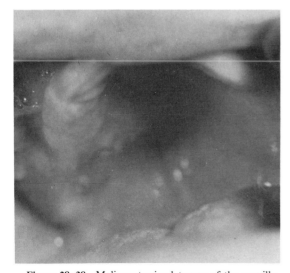

Figure 28–38 Malignant mixed tumor of the maxilla, with almost complete involvement of the floor of the orbit.

FLOOR OF THE MOUTH

Cancer of the floor of the mouth is frequently found. This lesion, if allowed to go untreated, frequently extends to the lateral aspect of the tongue and to the gum of the mandible. Next to cancer of the tongue, primary cancer of the floor of the mouth is first in metastasizing to the lymph nodes of the neck.

Treatment. Those who treat intraoral cancers disagree on how lesions in this region should be managed (see Chapter 27). It is the author's opinion that, when no clinical cervical metastases exist, lesions which have not extended as far as the mandibular gum may be treated by irradiation. In approximately six weeks, if radiation therapy is undertaken, a complete radical neck dissection should be done on the same side as the primary lesion. If the primary lesion reaches the mandibular gum and there are clinical metastases in the neck, a much more radical approach is carried out. The primary lesion and intervening mandible are widely resected in continuity with a radical neck dissection. Occasionally, when no clinical involvement of the mandible is present, the lesion of the floor of the mouth may be resected in continuity with a radical neck dissection, and the tongue and floor of the mouth dragged down beneath the mandible, preserving the entire mandible, the so-called pull-through operation (see Figures 28–44 to 28–46).

Prophylactic complete neck dissections are

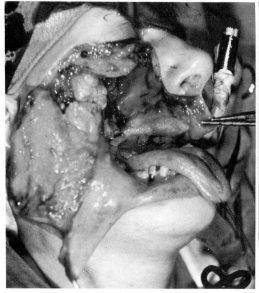

Figure 28–39

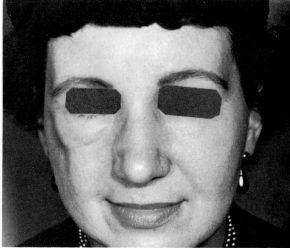

Figure 28–40

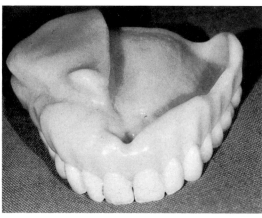

Figure 28–39 Weber-Ferguson incision. The cheek flap is laid back and the maxilla, along with the orbital floor, resected. The eye is preserved and the orbit slung on a hammock of fascia lata.

Figure 28–40 Postoperative view. Inside of the cheek and inferior aspects of the orbital contents covered with a split-thickness skin graft from the abdomen.

Figure 28–41 Oral prosthesis.

Figure 28–42 Postoperative view, oral prosthesis in place.

Figure 28–43 Postoperative view of the patient.

Figure 28–41

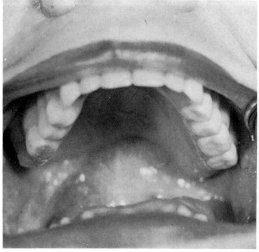

Figure 28–42

Figure 28–43

Figure 28-44

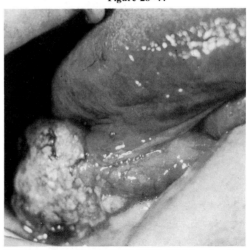

Figure 28-44 Cancer of the floor of the mouth with clinically evident cervical metastases.

Figure 28-45 Radical neck dissection, with the tongue and floor of the mouth pulled down under the mandible. The neck contents and primary lesion are amputated in continuity in full view of the surgeon.

Figure 28-46 Postoperative intraoral view. The tongue is sutured to the mucoperiosteum of the mandible. In several months, the tongue may be split and a split thickness skin graft inserted to free the tongue and permit the application of a denture.

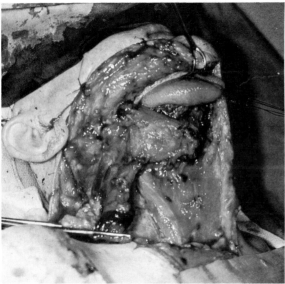

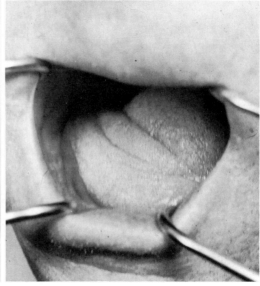

Figure 28-45

Figure 28-46

performed for only two primary lesions—those of the floor of the mouth and those of the tongue. It is thought that these two metastasize frequently enough that lives may be lengthened and more may be saved by early operation. Possibly, these two lesions metastasize more often because of the never-ending milking of the lymphatics by the muscles of the regions in which they are located.

TONGUE

The tongue is usually divided into two parts, the anterior two-thirds and the posterior third. The anterior two-thirds is anterior to the circumvallate papillae. The posterior third is actually located in the oropharynx, behind the anterior V-shaped line of the vallate papillae.

Cancers of the tongue characteristically are located on the lateral aspects of the organ and frequently extend into the floor of the mouth and onto the anterior pillar of the tonsil.

Treatment. Surgery is the preferred treatment for cancer of the tongue. This is true regardless of whether the cancer is located in the anterior or posterior portion. Formerly it was felt that posterior lesions drained to lymph nodes that could not be reached by neck dissections. Experience has proven that this is not so. A radical neck dissection is

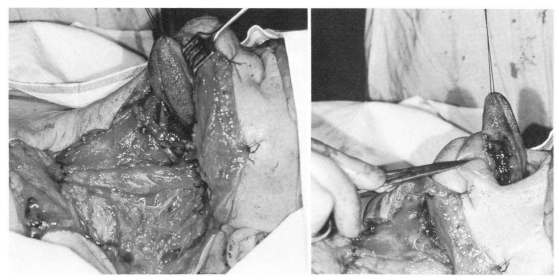

Figure 28–47   Figure 28–48

Figure 28–47   Radical neck dissection, with the tongue pulled down under the mandible into the neck.
Figure 28–48   Operation completed. The tongue is replaced after the carcinomatous area has been excised and repair of the surgical defect begun.

always performed at the same time as the glossectomy. The mandible may be resected at this time or the tongue removed in continuity with the neck specimen as the "pull-through" operation, preserving the mandible (see Figures 28–47 to 28–52).

TONSIL, PHARYNX AND SOFT PALATE

Cancer may involve the tonsil, the anterior pillar of the tonsil, the pharynx (nasopharynx, oropharynx, hypopharynx) and the soft pal-ate. Radiotherapy is preferred for treatment of cancers in the nasopharynx, tonsil, tonsillar pillar, and soft palate. Surgery may be considered for other pharyngeal lesions, particularly if cervical metastases exist, but many of these lesions also must eventually be managed by radiotherapy (Fig. 28–53).

PROSTHETICS

An additional and important member of the head and neck cancer team is the prosthetist.

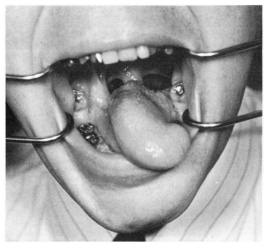

Figure 28–49   Postoperative intraoral view.

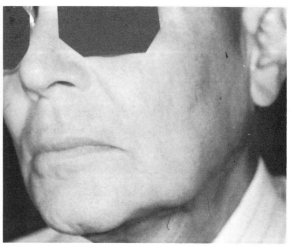

Figure 28–50   External view.

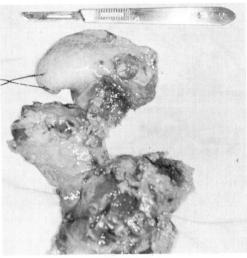 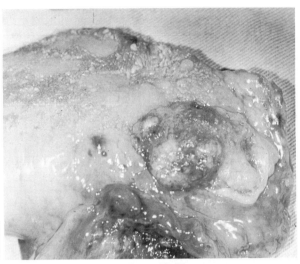

Figure 28–51   **Figure 28–52**

Figure 28–51   Resected specimen (tongue and neck contents) in continuity.
Figure 28–52   Close-up of the tongue with the carcinoma.

It is not enough to resect cancer radically—one must be prepared to reconstruct the surgical damage with the patient's own tissues or to cover the defect with artificial appliances.

Many of the patients who have an oral cancer are in the fifth, sixth or seventh decade of life. A considerable percentage of these patients will not want, nor is it advisable for them, to go through additional surgical procedures to rebuild their lost tissues. Prostheses are often the answer for them.

IMPROVEMENTS IN TECHNIQUE

It is frequently thought that surgery and surgical techniques change very little over the years. Actually, constant change is occurring. The practicing surgeon must remain aware of change and, when possible, add his innovations, when practical, acceptable and proven, to the general literature so that others may take advantage of his improvements and work them into their own surgical armamentarium. A few of these innovations are illustrated in brief photographic case reports.

(*Text continued on page 1805*)

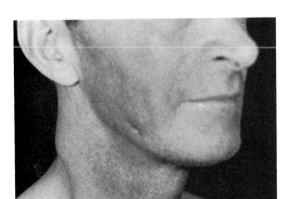

Figure 28–53 Carcinoma of the tonsil with metastasis. The cervical metastasis is located in the typical place for the tonsil. The most acceptable treatment is irradiation of the primary and secondary areas.

Photographic Case Report

THE MACFEE PARALLEL TRANSVERSE NECK INCISION

Figure 28–54

Figure 28–55

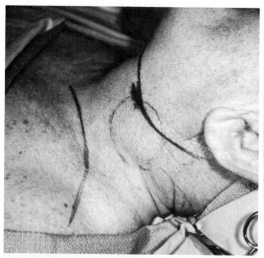

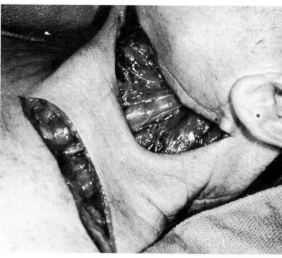

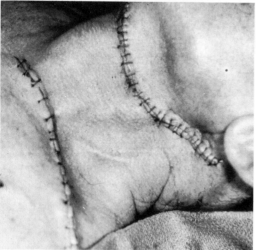

Figures 28–54 to 28–56 This case represents a man with metastatic disease in the neck, for which a radical neck dissection was performed. The MacFee parallel transverse incision technique was used to obtain a better cosmetic result. This is particularly useful in patients who are concerned not only about their tumor problem but also about the appearance of their necks after the operation has been performed. Figure 28–54 shows the metastatic node (circled) in the neck and the inked-in proposed lines of incision. Figure 28–55, a photograph taken at the completion of a neck dissection, partially shows the dissected neck, but with the neck clean. The retraction for proper exposure in this type of neck incision is more difficult and requires more assistance than that for the double-Y incision, but in some instances this particular incision still may be preferred to others. Figure 28–56 illustrates the completed operation; suction tubing is brought out through the lower flap. It is obvious that the scarring in this particular neck will be minimal following this rather extensive surgical undertaking.

Figure 28–56

A VARIETY OF FLAPS

Figure 28–57   Figure 28–58

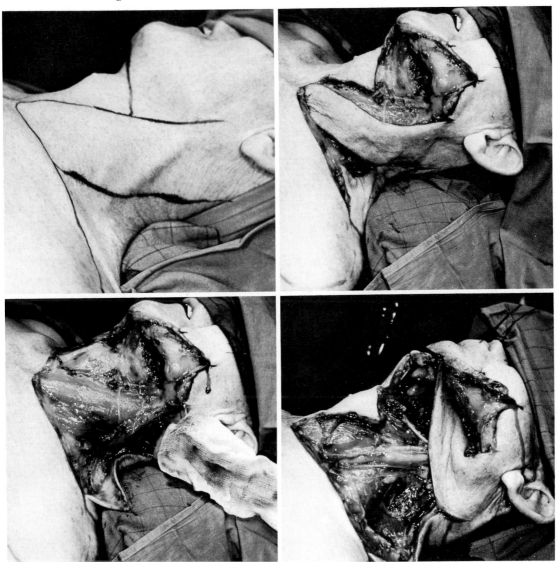

Figure 28–59   Figure 28–60

Figures 28–57 to 28–63 In the past few years a distinct change has occurred in the primary reconstruction of intraoral areas following the resection of primary intraoral tumors. A considerable amount of basic planning in these new surgical techniques can be attributed directly to Dr. Vahram Y. Bakamjian of the Roswell Park Cancer Hospital in Buffalo, New York. The Bakamjian deltopectoral flap in many respects provided the necessary background for additional thinking and planning in primary cervical and intraoral reconstruction over the past few years.

The surgery illustrated in Figure 28–57 utilized a variety of flaps, planned so that immediate reconstruction could be undertaken following a left radical neck dissection and resection of the left floor of the mouth and lateral aspect of the resected tongue for cancer. A deltopectoral flap based on the sternal area and carried over the shoulder was outlined. A second flap was based on the mastoid area and carried out inferiorly and obliquely across the neck to the superior aspect of the clavicle. Other flaps were raised superiorly, medially and posteriorly. In Figure 28–58, the neck dissection has been completely performed and the floor of the mouth and lateral tongue have been resected in continuity. The mastoid flap was elevated completely, as seen in Figure 28–59, and at this point the deltopectoral flap was cut and rotated superiorly to cover the carotid vessels while the mastoid flap was drawn into the oral cavity under the mandible to line the denuded areas of the floor of the mouth and the tongue (Fig. 28–60).

(*Legend continued on following page*)

Figure 28-61

Figure 28-62

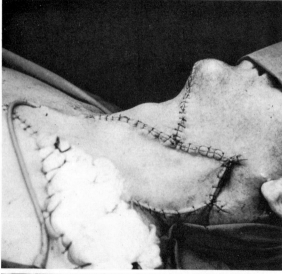

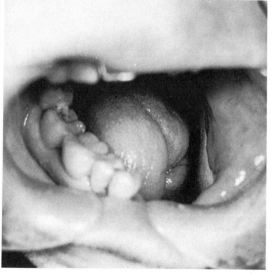

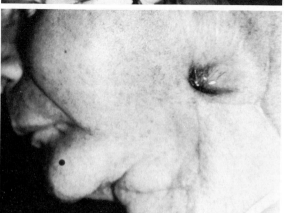

Figure 28-61 shows the completed procedure with a free split skin graft used to cover the area on the chest and shoulder, which is a denuded site after the deltopectoral flap has been raised. Placing a free graft over this rather innocuous area is simple and the flaps used to cover the important anatomic structures of the neck were sutured into position. A suction tubing was brought out through the inferior aspect of the dissected area. This obviously left an orocutaneous fistula beneath the mastoid flap, to be closed at a later date, usually in approximately 3 weeks. Figure 28-62 shows the healed intraoral area with the excellent mobile flap in its healed position, allowing free motion of the tongue and preventing pooling of saliva, a very serious problem for the patient when the floor of the mouth is filled and covered with a free split skin graft that cannot move. Figure 28-63 shows the external aspect of the neck with the orocutaneous fistula, a fistula that causes no particular discomfort for the patient because it can be covered with a small dressing and in many instances does not even drain.

Figure 28-63

Photographic Case Report

BILATERAL FOREHEAD, OR "VISOR," FLAP

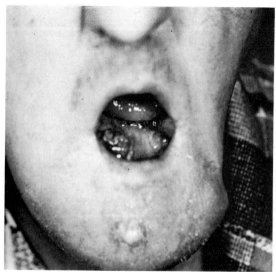

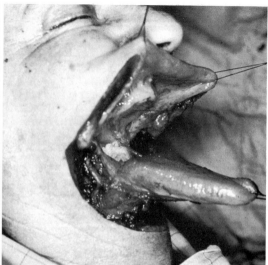

Figure 28-64

Figure 28-65

See opposite page for legend.

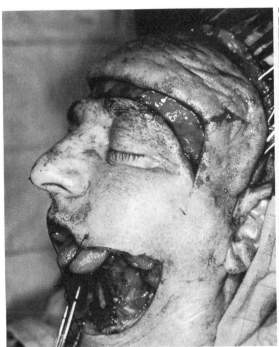

Figure 28–66

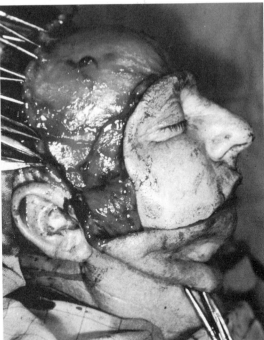

Figure 28–67

Figures 28–64 to 28–68   These figures show another type of reconstruction in an effort to benefit the patient immediately from the day of his ablative surgery. This man has a very extensive intraoral cancer directly invading the mandible and chin, making it impossible even to determine where his cancer might have started (Fig. 28–64). This is a far-advanced, neglected lesion, but this does not mean that definitive treatment may not still be in order. Surgery consisted of a very extensive removal of the involved area, with resection of the mandible from the left temporomandibular joint to the right temporomandibular joint, the entire lower lip and chin, with resection of a portion of the upper lip and the necessary overlying skin (Fig. 28–65). A bilateral forehead or visor type flap was outlined and cut (Fig. 28–66), based on both superficial temporal arteries. This visor flap was then brought down over the face (Fig. 28–67), to be placed into its new position in the raw area just created from the primary resection. A temporary tracheostomy was performed, and in approximately 3 weeks a minimal procedure was performed under local anesthesia to divide the two lateral pedicles and replace the soft tissues that were not to be used. While this initial procedure did not create a result which could be considered excellent from a cosmetic standpoint, (Fig. 28–68), it did close the mammoth surgical defect immediately and allowed this man to speak, eat and control his saliva as soon as healing was complete, in approximately 2 weeks. With removal of the entire forehead skin and its replacement by a split thickness abdominal skin graft, the forehead area was quite acceptable from a cosmetic viewpoint. The forehead skin does lend itself to immediate use in the form of pedicle tissue, with no reason for a surgical delay.

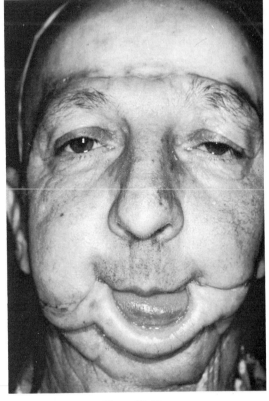

Figure 28–68

UNILATERAL FOREHEAD FLAP

Figure 28–69

Figure 28–70

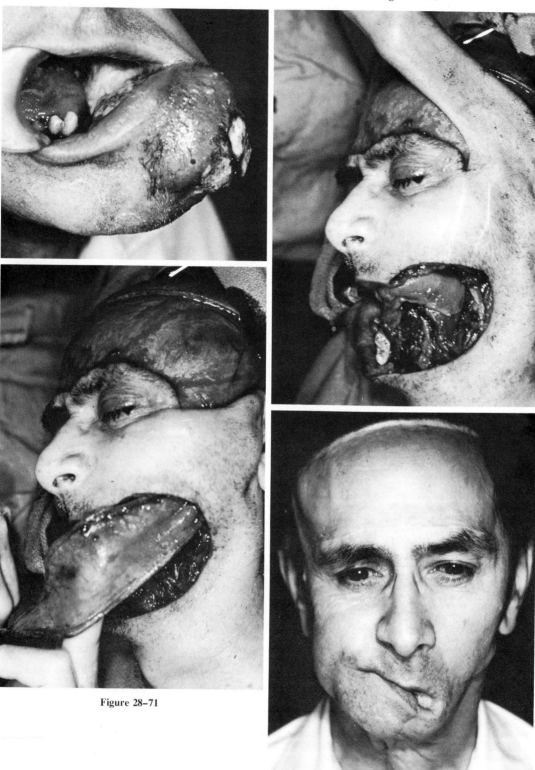

Figure 28–71

Figure 28–72

See opposite page for legend.

REPLACEMENT OF HEALTHY BONE TEMPORARILY REMOVED
TO PROVIDE ACCESS TO THE OPERATIVE SITE

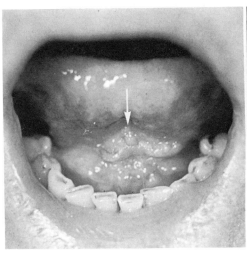

Figure 28-73

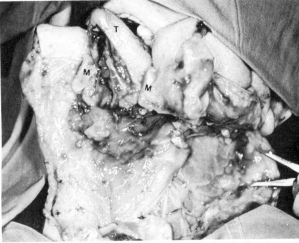

Figure 28-74

Figures 28-73 to 28-75 Of specific interest to surgeons and oral surgeons alike are the ways in which the mandible can be replaced following temporary removal of all or part of it. The mandibular problem in Figure 28-73 was created by the presence of a primary tumor in the anterior midline of the floor of the mouth. This man underwent a radical neck dissection, with removal of the anterior floor of the mouth and the inferior aspect of the tongue. A central section of the symphysis of the mandible, approximately 2 inches long, was specifically removed to allow better exposure and removal of all the cancer. In Figure 28-74, the tongue (*T*) and the cut end of the mandible (*M*) are marked, the latter showing where bone was temporarily removed. The primary cancer was well away from the bone, and the bone was removed only to provide the necessary access. Then the mandibular bone was reinserted, wired and pinned as a free autogenous graft (Fig. 28-75). The result was excellent, and the patient had no further cancer problem with his mouth or neck.

(Figure 28-75 on following page.)

Figures 28-69 to 28-72 Another type of reconstruction utilizing a forehead flap that can be used immediately following the removal of a tumor is shown here. Figure 28-69 shows very extensive and obviously neglected cancer involving the left mandible, floor of the mouth, lower lip, cheek and chin. Again, a major resection was undertaken to remove all of this area, including the mandible from the left temporomandibular joint to the midbody of the right mandible. A forehead flap was immediately outlined, cut and raised with the tip running from the right preauricular region and based on the left superior temporal and postauricular arteries (Fig. 28-70). There was never any question about the viability of this flap and no thought was given to a surgical delay in its use. The flap was brought into the mouth by turning it on itself, bringing it inferiorly and positioning it anterior to the zygomatic arch (Fig. 28-71). One can see the extreme distance this flap might be moved if necessary. In this instance it formed the entire lining for the very extensive raw intraoral area. The entire left anterior chest and remaining neck skin were then rotated as a huge flap to be brought to the midface and to cover the intraoral lining flap so that shrinkage would be at a minimum. It must be remembered that any flap used in any area must have a cover and that if any flap is left without skin coverage it will retract and contract, distorting the appearance of the area being reconstructed. The patient's appearance after this surgery (remember that this is a one-stage procedure and has not had revisions) is shown in Figure 28-72. Obviously, this man at this time can profit by fascia lata slings, local resection of paralyzed reconstructed tissue and other types of flaps and grafts, all of this to be done at a time elected by both patient and surgeon.

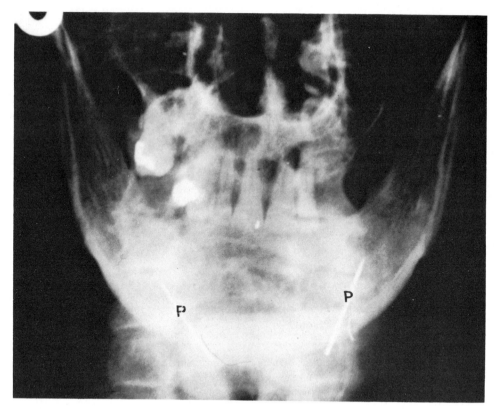

Figure 28–75

Photographic Case Report

STABILIZATION OF BONE GRAFTS

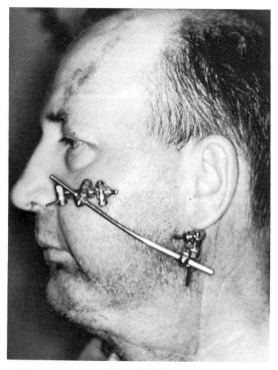

Figures 28–76 and 28–77 This report illustrates the use of an immediate iliac bone graft to replace bone removed from the left mandible following a left radical neck dissection and primary jaw resection (Fig. 28–76). The extraoral skeletal pins and bar fixation with the Roger Anderson appliance represent one method to hold a bone graft in good position. The posteroanterior radiograph of the patient (Fig. 28–77) shows that in addition to the Roger Anderson extraoral splint, interdental wiring, circumferential wiring, attachment of superior arch bars to the superior bony skeleton and primary wiring of the autogenous graft to the recipient area, have been employed to hold the maxilla and mandible together and assure solid healing of the graft. This is a complicated way to hold a bone graft so that it will heal postoperatively, but one has to choose the procedure to fit the individual patient, with some patients and fractures being considerably more cooperative than others. This means that the operating surgeon must be capable of performing a variety of procedures for the same basic problem, rather than fitting his one operation to all local situations.

(*Figure 28–77 on opposite page.*)

Figure 28–76

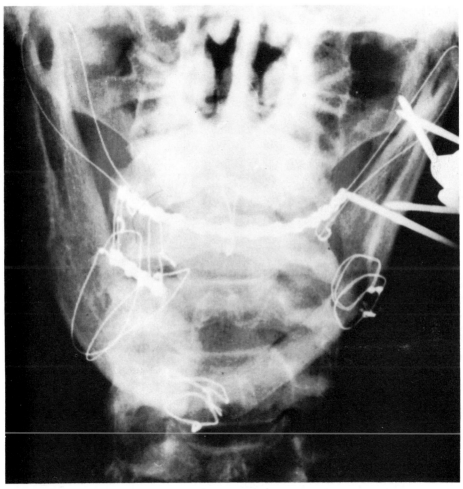

Figure 28–77

Photographic Case Report

RIB GRAFTS

Figure 28-78

Figure 28-79

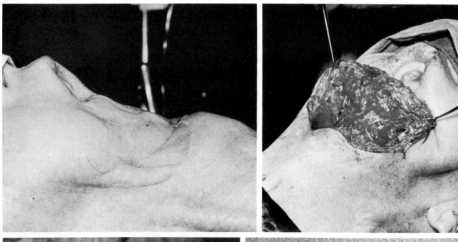

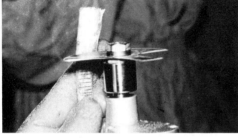

Figure 28-80

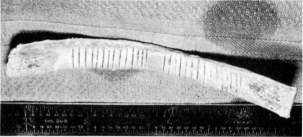

Figure 28-81

Figures 28-78 to 28-81 There has been considerable discussion regarding the relative merits of rib grafts and iliac bone grafts. Having had considerable experience with both types of grafts, we have reached the conclusion that the rib graft is useful as "filler" type material for an onlay bone graft after solidification of other types of grafts has occurred but that it is poor material for a primary graft between the two resected ends of a mandible. This case illustrates one way of using a rib graft when it is to be contoured to insert into this area. Figure 28-78 shows a patient who has lost his anterior mandible, resulting in a marked deformity and preventing him from chewing any solid food. The soft tissues are open to receive the bone graft in Figure 28-79. After the rib has been removed, a series of transverse cuts (Fig. 28-82) are made through the concave side so that the graft can be bent to fit the defect. These cuts are made with an electric saw and do tend to weaken the graft. Figure 28-81 shows the rib before it is inserted, with the cortical bone removed at both ends.

We have given up completely the use of rib grafts as the primary graft because they "melt" away.

Photographic Case Report

ILIAC BONE GRAFT

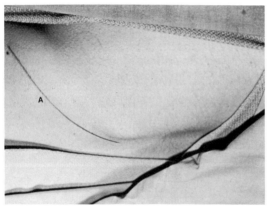

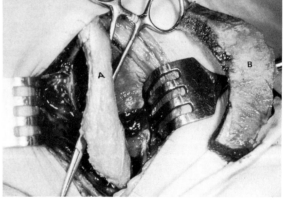

Figure 28-82

Figure 28-83

See opposite page for legend.

Figures 28–82 to 28–84 Our approach to the routine iliac bone graft is illustrated here. A generous incision is made over the iliac crest area (*A* in Figure 28–82), and the bone easily exposed. Our preference is to outline and cut a piece of ilium at a point inferior to the iliac crest, allowing the crest to remain intact and permitting the contour of the hip area to remain normal. This also gives more support to this particular area. Figure 28–83 shows the intact iliac crest (*A*); the large segment of bone (*B*) removed is resting on the retractor. One must be careful to use the correct side so that the bone will fit the defect in the jaw, as does the bone (*B*) in Figure 28–84. (This mandibular defect in a teen-age boy was caused by removal of a large benign ameloblastoma.) The graft, as can be seen in Figure 28–84, was wired inferiorly and superiorly, and no other attempts were made to secure it. Healing was prompt and complete, with no complications.

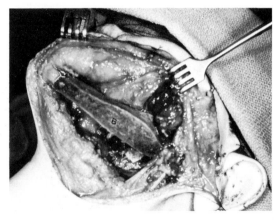

Figure 28–84

CONCLUSION

The most important points in the management of cancer of the oral cavity are: (*a*) prompt, accurate diagnosis of the lesion; (*b*) a thorough and proper understanding of what type or types of therapy should be carried out for cancer present in each part of the oral cavity and neck; (*c*) the fortitude to treat these lesions properly, in spite of the difficulties which at times arise with the patient (and often his family) after radical surgery; and (*d*) the honesty to admit when a patient is beyond medical help and not add to his misery by nonspecific or questionable forms of treatment.

CHAPTER 29

RADIATION THERAPY OF LESIONS OF THE ORAL CAVITY

CHARLOTTE P. DONLAN, M.D.

Malignant neoplasms of the oral cavity account for 5 to 8 per cent of all malignant disease and for 23,000 new cases of cancer a year and about 10,000 deaths.[9] Ninety per cent of these tumors are squamous cell carcinomas.

Oral cavity lesions include those occurring on the upper and lower lips, buccal mucosa, alveolar ridges, floor of the mouth, hard and soft palates, anterior two-thirds of the tongue and posterior one-third of the tongue (base).

BENIGN LESIONS

Surgical treatment of benign lesions found in the oral cavity is discussed in Chapter 12. Only those benign growths amenable to radiation therapy are cited here.

Cavernous hemangiomas respond well to small amounts of radiation, delivered by an intraoral cone when possible. If an external cone must be used, the teeth and gums are shielded by lead as indicated. Soft-tissue hemangiomas are treated with 200 to 800 rads, depending on the size of the growth and the age of the patient. In older patients with more resistant tumors the dosage is higher. Bone hemangiomas are treated with a dose of 1000 to 1200 rads.

An *epulis granulomatosa*, on occasion, may be treated in the same manner as a hemangioma, but a tissue dose of only 200 to 300 rads is given.

Treatment of *eosinophilic granuloma* of the mandible involves the same factors as those listed under Terminology and Techniques, No. 1; a bond dose of about 700 rads is typically administered. However, the patient should have a complete series of tests to rule out histiocytosis X. Histiocytosis X, as introduced by Lichtenstein in 1953, includes three distinct syndromes: eosinophilic granuloma, Hand-Schüller-Christian disease and Letterer-Siwe disease.

MALIGNANT LESIONS

The stage of oral cavity carcinoma may be recorded according to the guidelines set forth in the Clinical Staging System for Carcinoma of the Oral Cavity, presented by the American Joint Committee for Cancer Staging and End Results Reporting,[2] with modifications suggested by Fletcher:[36]

T – Primary Tumor

TIS: Carcinoma *in situ*.

T1: Tumor 2 cm. or less in greatest diameter.

T2: Tumor larger than 2 cm. but not larger than 4 cm. in greatest diameter, with minimal extension to adjacent structures.

T3: Tumor larger than 4 cm. in greatest diameter, with limited or moderate extension to adjacent structures.

T4: Massive primary tumor.

N — Regional Lymph Nodes

N0: No clinically palpable cervical lymph node(s); or palpable node(s) but metastasis not suspected.

N1: Clinically palpable homolateral cervical lymph node(s) that are not fixed; metastasis suspected.

N2: Clinically palpable contralateral or bilateral cervical lymph node(s) that are not fixed; metastasis suspected.

N3: Clinically palpable lymph node(s) that are fixed; metastasis suspected.

M — Distant Metastasis

M0: No distant metastasis.

M1: Clinical and/or radiographic evidence of metastasis other than to cervical lymph nodes.

The preceding TNM classification and the stage groups that follow are clinical evaluations and are not changed after the patient has been assigned to a group. If, after the histology report, it is expedient to add new information bearing on the patient's condition, the letter P should be used in place of the T (*e.g.,* P1, P2 and P3).[2] These categories cannot be compared to the TNM classification.

The following stage grouping is suggested for use at present on the basis of a retrospective field trial:[2]

Stage I:	T1	N0	M0			
Stage II:	T2	N0	M0			
Stage III:	T3	N0	M0			
	T1	N1	M0			
	T2	N1	M0			
	T3	N1	M0			
Stage IV:	T1	N2	M0	T1	N3	M0
	T2	N2	M0	T2	N3	M0
	T3	N2	M0	T3	N3	M0

Or, any T or N category with M1

After the diagnosis has been made, the pathologist, surgeon, radiotherapist and oral surgeon should jointly decide on the appropriate treatment. Radiation or surgery, in certain cases, controls the disease. A combination of both is necessary in other cases. Radiation also plays a large role in the palliative treatment of oral malignancies. Patients selected for palliative treatment, however, should be chosen with as much care as those selected for control treatment, considering that inadvised radiation can add to the discomfort of the patient rather than ameliorate it.

The amount of radiation administered for any tumor is limited by the tolerance of the normal tissue. Radiocurability is influenced by the location of the tumor, its pathologic characteristics, the amount of tumor cell infiltration and the connective tissue response. The time-dose-volume parameters influence malignant cell and normal cell recovery times. The aim is to produce tumor eradication without producing necrosis in the normal tissues.

Radioresponsiveness cannot be equated with radiocurability. A tumor may regress promptly after radiation treatments, only to reappear quickly. The radioresponsiveness is dependent to a large measure on the amount of oxygen available to the tissues, the phase of the cell cycle, temperature changes, hormones, chemicals and previous radiation.[30]

As a rule, more dissolved oxygen in the tissue increases the response to radiation, while less oxygen decreases it. Hypoxic cells are about three times more resistant to radiation than cells with more available oxygen.[31] Cells in the resting phase of the cell cycle are also less responsive. If the temperature of the body is lowered, resulting in constriction of blood vessels and consequent decreased blood flow to the tissue, response is less. With an increase in temperature the blood vessels dilate, carrying more oxygen to the tissues, and as a result the response to radiation is greater.

Previous radiation may so alter the tumor bed, through increased fibrosis and decreased blood supply, that the malignant cells become resistant to further radiation. In effect, repair, repopulation and reoxygenation determine the radioresponsiveness of the tumor once radiation has been started.

Squamous cell cancers of the oral cavity do not seem to be influenced by hormones.[31] Chemotherapy for these tumors is discussed later in this chapter.

LIP

Squamous cell carcinoma occurs on both lips but is more common on the lower lip. The incidence of squamous cell carcinoma of the upper lip is the same in men and women, but on the lower lip it occurs more frequently in men. Upper lip lesions metastasize more

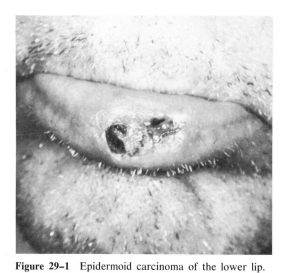

Figure 29–1 Epidermoid carcinoma of the lower lip.

readily, as do lesions at the commissure and those with buccal extensions.[1]

T1 and T2 lesions can be controlled equally well with radiation or surgery. For T3 and T4 lesions, the method that will give the best functional, as well as cosmetic, result is preferred. If the lesion is large, but little of the lip is destroyed, irradiation is the treat-

ment of choice. With large destructive lesions, mandibular involvement or metastases, surgery is the preferred treatment. Each case must be evaluated individually. It is possible to have a T2N1 lesion such that the lip might be radiated and a node dissection performed. Postsurgical recurrences would be irradiated and postradiation recurrences excised. The postsurgical site of recurrence would require a plastic repair if it were to be re-excised; therefore, radiation should be the chosen treatment. Conversely, the previously radiated tissue would not tolerate any further radiation without necrosis; however, a plastic repair would not be as extensive in this case as for a postsurgical site of recurrence.

The rare spindle cell carcinoma or salivary gland tumor of the upper lip should be excised.

Malignant lip lesions represent 25 per cent of all oral cancers.[1] Ten to 15 per cent of patients with these lesions develop metastatic nodes, which are removed surgically. No prophylactic neck dissections are performed.

The 5-year control rate if the disease does not involve the nodes is 90 per cent, and with

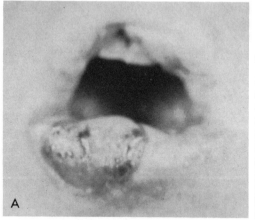

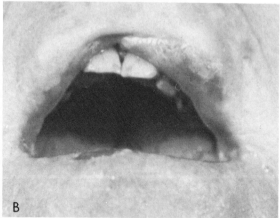

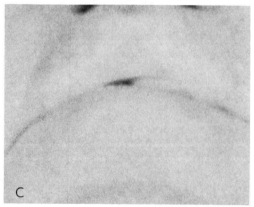

Figure 29–2 *A*, This patient had had carcinoma of the upper lip treated by surgery. He returned 4 years later with a lesion of the lower lip. *B*, Following treatment with irradiation, the lip shows a radiation reaction with moist desquamation. *C*, Healed lip.

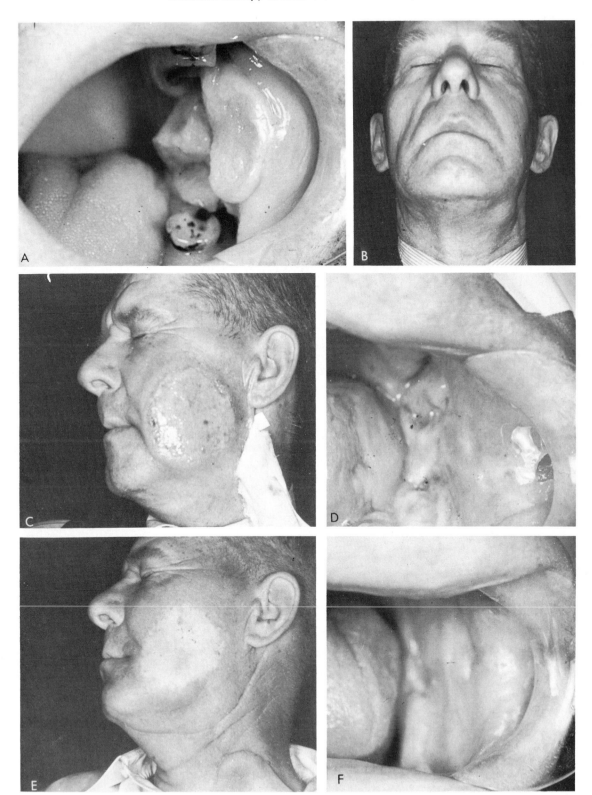

Figure 29–3 *A*, Exophytic carcinoma of the buccal mucosa before treatment. *B*, Extraoral appearance of carcinoma of the left cheek with metastasis to the left submaxillary nodes. *C*, Severe skin reaction following x-ray therapy. *D*, Appearance following neck dissection. *E*, Note flat, white scar following healing of radiation reaction. *F*, Healing of buccal mucosa following destruction of tumor. (Courtesy of W. Harry Archer, D.D.S.)

node involvement, 30 to 35 per cent, if neck dissection is done.[57]

BUCCAL MUCOSA

Squamous cell carcinoma of the buccal mucosa constitutes about 10 per cent of all oral cancers, and 8 of the 10 per cent occurs in men.[1] Lesions are often associated with leukoplakia. The verrucous type of lesion rarely metastasizes; however, 50 per cent of the others develop metastases in the course of the disease. Well-defined lesions with normal tissue around them that have not invaded bone nor metastasized respond well to radiation and surgery. I prefer to use radiation for these lesions. Lesions infiltrating the cheek are better treated surgically because recurrence after radiation is usual. Very advanced lesions can be treated better with radiation than surgery and with less discomfort to the

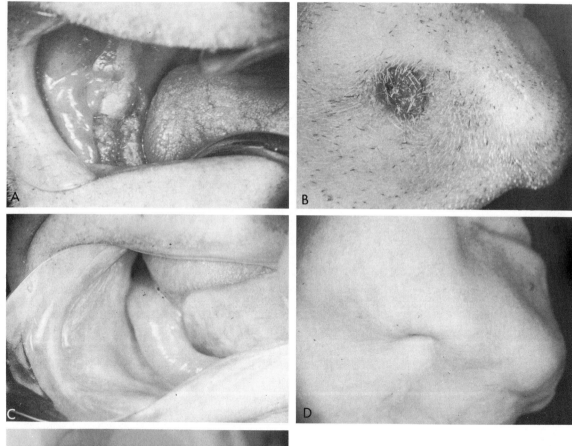

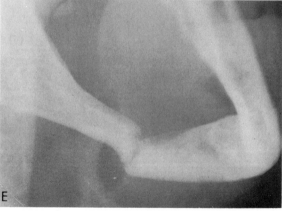

Figure 29–4 *A*, Carcinoma of the inferior alveolar ridge, with pathologic fracture of the mandible. Large fungating lesion growing between molar and cuspid areas. *B*, Following healing of radiation therapy reaction. Tumor destroyed. *C*, Draining sinus from infected pathologic fracture of the mandible. *D*, Following healing of radiation therapy reaction. Draining sinus closed and tumor clinically destroyed. *E*, Healed pathologic fracture of the mandible. (Courtesy of W. Harry Archer, D.D.S.)

patient. Eighty per cent of small uncomplicated lesions treated with radiation can be controlled for a minimum of 5 years. When there is extension of the malignant disease, the control rate is 10 per cent.[57] Ash gives an overall 5-year control rate of 35.3 per cent.[4]

ALVEOLAR RIDGE

Squamous cell carcinoma of the upper and lower alveolus accounts for about 25 per cent of all oral cancers and is eight times more common on the lower alveolus.[1] The verrucous carcinoma rarely metastasizes, but the ulcerative lesion frequently involves bone. Lesions not invading bone are radiated, but I personally have used radiation treatment for some patients with early bone involvement

(whose poor cardiac status precluded surgery) with good response. Prognosis is more favorable for lower alveolus lesions, with about a 35 per cent 5-year control rate.[39] Upper alveolus lesions respond well to radiation if they are not over 3 cm. in size. Surgery for recurrent or persistent lesions controls the disease if no metastases are present at the time of surgery.

PALATE

Malignant lesions of the palate account for 11 per cent of all oral cancers.[62] Squamous cell carcinoma occurs on both the soft palate and the hard palate, but adenocarcinoma of the cylindromatous type is more common on the hard palate. Lesions of the soft palate me-

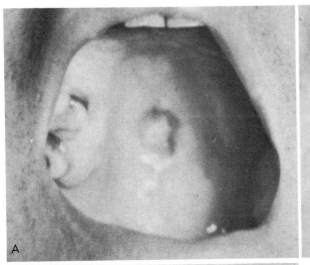
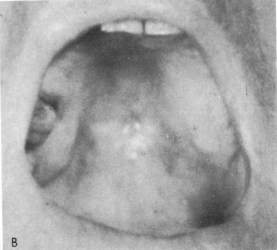
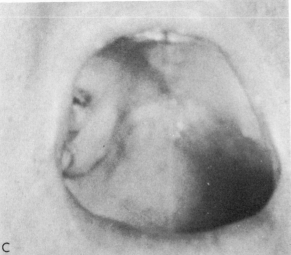

Figure 29–5 *A*, Adenocarcinoma of the palate. *B*, Treated with an intraoral cone with 6500 rads in 7 weeks. *C*, Five weeks after treatment.

tastasize twice as frequently as do those of the hard palate. Soft-palate lesions are treated with radiation, since surgery results in too much disability. Hard-palate lesions are treated by surgery, or surgery and radiation. About 50 per cent of hard-palate lesions are controlled, but fewer than 10 per cent of soft-palate lesions are checked, owing to their rate of metastasis.[1]

TONGUE

Squamous cell carcinoma of the tongue constitutes 25 per cent of all oral lesions.[1] The anterior two-thirds of the tongue is the most common site of the disease. Many lesions go unnoticed for months, often being attributed by the patient to a gastric upset or "canker sore." With lesions at the base of the tongue, metastases frequently develop before the patient has symptoms of pain, dysphagia, hoarseness or dyspnea.

The lesion may vary from a hard-edged ulcer to a warty growth or indurated plaque. Occasionally, only marked induration can be palpated. In the United States the incidence of this tumor is higher in males by a ratio of 4 to 1, in contrast to the 1 to 1 male-female ratio in Scandinavia.[1] A small lesion (1.5 to 2.0 cm.) on the tip or lateral border of the tongue can be excised very easily. Rarely, at present, is an intraoral cone used in the radiation of tongue lesions. For larger lesions on the anterior two-thirds of the tongue, with no extension to the floor of the mouth, radiation therapy is preferred for several reasons, the most important being that, from the patient's point of view, no impairment of speech occurs. From the medical standpoint, the mortality rate is much lower.

Interstitially inserted radium needles are used in many cases involving the anterior two-thirds of the tongue. Occasionally, external beam therapy is given to reduce the bulk of the lesion and infection before radium needle insertion.

Patients not suited for this therapy are treated with cobalt-60 by opposing fields with a bolus or wedge filter. Lesions at the base of the tongue are treated with cobalt-60, and the lymph nodes are often included in the fields of radiation.

Typically, 50 per cent of patients with carcinoma of the tongue have palpable lymph nodes.[1, 27] Thirty-five to 40 per cent who have no palpable nodes upon admission develop them later.[1, 27, 57] For this latter reason, in patients with involvement of the anterior two-thirds of the tongue, elective neck dissection is often performed on the side of the primary lesion several weeks after completion of treatment of the lesion.

When total surgical management of the anterior lesions has been completed, the neck nodes are dissected in continuity with the renewal of the tongue tumor.

Survival is dependent on the size and location of the primary lesion. Lesions less than 2 cm. in diameter on the mobile part of the tongue with no metastases have a 5-year control rate of 80 per cent. If metastases are present, the rate drops to 20 per cent.[1]

FLOOR OF THE MOUTH

Squamous cell carcinoma of the floor of the mouth accounts for about 16 per cent of intraoral cancer[62] and is most common in men. An adenocarcinoma arising from a salivary or mucous gland may be seen occasionally, as well as the rare endothelioma.

Irradiation is usually the chosen treatment for lesions of the anterior floor of the mouth, because of the mutilating surgery necessary for control of the tumor. If invasion of the mandible or metastatic nodes are present, surgery may be necessary. Posterior lesions are also treated by radiation if the bone is not involved. Often, the lesions are advanced and treatment is only palliative. Many surgeons elect to do a regional node dissection 3 to 6 weeks after radiation of the primary site because of the high rate of metastasis. For patients with inoperable lesions and metastatic disease, radiation is given.

RADIONECROSIS

Although bone absorption of radiation is less when cobalt-60 is used, the amount of radiation delivered to the mandible during therapy for certain intraoral lesions is sufficiently high to predispose the patient to osteonecrosis. The soft tissues of the bone, odontoblasts and rich capillary network are particularly vulnerable to irradiation damage.[70] If caries develops, or if the mucosa is traumatized, bacteria have ready access to the partially devitalized bone. The single nutrient blood vessel in each side of the mandible, because it is encased in bone, permits no dilatation in response to inflammation and edema. Consequently, the blood supply to the tissues beyond is impaired.

Rubin suggested the terms *simple radionecrosis* for bone uninvolved by cancer but heavily radiated and thus damaged, and *radionecrosis* for bone in which tumor and infection are present.[70] I recommend that the former be treated conservatively, as detailed by MacComb,[50] and the latter radically by surgery, when the patient's condition permits.

The study of experimental osteomyelitis in dogs by Ng and associates, as cited by Rubin,[70] clearly demonstrated that, in addition to a minimal dosage of radiation, trauma resulting in ulceration followed by infection is necessary for the production of osteomyelitis. The mandible of adult dogs was exposed to radiation in 1000-R. increments, with total doses ranging from 3000 to 8000 R. Ulceration occurred after exposure to 4000 R. or more. Osteomyelitis was not seen in the absence of ulceration. If the teeth were removed before radiation, osteomyelitis was reduced. The experiment demonstrated the familiar triad of radiation, trauma and infection causing necrosis of bone, which we see in the human subject.

Del Regato's classic study showed that teeth not in the field of radiation would develop caries if the salivary glands were radiated enough to decrease the flow of saliva.[26] The reduced salivary flow, increased viscosity of the saliva, decreased pH of the saliva and its increased total nitrogen content created a most favorable environment for the production of caries, which eventually led to radionecrosis.

A study was conducted at the University of Texas at Houston in which patients scheduled to receive radiation therapy were placed into one of four groups, according to dental findings at examination. These groups were: edentulous, poor, fair, and good. Patients with mouths in "poor" dental condition had all remaining teeth removed, whereas "fair" patients had extractions only in the fields of radiation, and "good" patients had no extractions. There was a control and a treatment group within each major category, the control patients receiving the formerly accepted patient care. Dentulous ("good" and "fair") "treatment" patients were given custom-made flexible mouth guards that were used to apply 1 per cent sodium fluoride gel solution directly to the tooth surfaces for 5 minutes each day. The procedure was started during the first week of irradiation and was continued indefinitely. The results showed a 21 per cent incidence of postirradiation bone necrosis in the treatment groups, compared with the 37 per cent encountered previous to the study. The incidence in patients having no extractions (those in the edentulous and "good" dental groups) was only 12 per cent, compared with that in patients having total or selected extractions ("poor" and "fair" groups), which was 32 per cent. However, the overall postirradiation rate of tooth decay decreased by 39 per cent. The sodium fluoride gel was effective, but total care seemed to be the most important factor in reducing bone necrosis and caries.[24]

If the goal of treatment is cure rather than palliation, I recommend extraction of all the teeth with alveolectomy and maintenance of the patient on antibiotics, while waiting 10 to 14 days for good healing before initiation of therapy. The patient with sound teeth and good oral hygiene (who is rare in these cases) has no teeth extracted. However, the possibility of future complications is explained to the patient in detail and the importance of good oral hygiene stressed. The edentulous patient is advised to wear dentures only at meal time and not at all during the reaction of the mucous membrane to radiation treatment. When the reaction has subsided, he may wear the dentures after they have been evaluated for proper fit.

Every effort is made to maintain good oral hygiene during and after treatment. A dilute hydrogen peroxide mouthwash is prescribed for periodic use daily. Gentle lavage with pulsative jets of a mild salt solution is recommended after meals and before retiring (a Water-pik set on low gives the right pressure). The patient is seen by the dentist every 4 to 6 weeks for 6 months and is warned that if his teeth become hypersensitive to heat or cold, or if he has a toothache, he is to see the dentist as well as the therapist promptly.

If the salivary glands are included in the treatment field, the risk of postradiation necrosis is greater. With megavoltage therapy, however, the fields can be better delineated, and dryness of the mouth occurs less than with conventional therapy.

Through education of the patient, dental prophylaxis and a coordinated program carried out by the dentist, surgeon and therapist, postradiation necrosis and bone decay are reduced. Nevertheless, the tissues of many of these patients have been compromised by years of poor nutrition, excessive use of alcohol or tobacco or a combination of all three. When subjected to a cancerocidal dose of radiation or combined therapy with drugs and radiation, some patients still develop osteonecrosis, despite all efforts at prevention. This is the calculated risk that the patient and medical team take in an attempt to cure a very malignant disease.

CHEMOTHERAPY

A number of chemotherapeutic agents have been used alone or in combination with radiation in the treatment of head and neck cancer. The amount of drug tolerated is limited not by the tumor area but by the normal tissues throughout the body. The goal of finding a drug that is specifically selective for tumor cells has not been realized. The results of combination therapy are influenced by the response of the cell population to radiation, the response to chemotherapeutic agents, and the basic immunity of the host. The combination of drugs and radiation has resulted in the control of some advanced squamous cell carcinomas of the head and neck, which might not have been controlled otherwise.

The drugs in order of established value in the treatment of squamous cell cancer of the head and neck are methotrexate, 5-fluorouracil and hydroxyurea. No drug is effective against oral adenocarcinoma.

Methotrexate is a folic acid antagonist that prevents cell replication by inhibiting DNA synthesis.[20] It has been used alone and with radiation but seems to be most effective when given before and after radiation. The drug is administered orally, by infusion or intratumorally. In cases of head and neck cancer it is given for about 7 to 14 days before irradiation is started. After irradiation is initiated, the drug may be continued until a toxic reaction occurs. The chemotherapy produces mucositis, as does radiation, which under combined therapy is more intense and lasts longer than with either treatment alone. The results of Friedman and colleagues'[37] and Kramer's[42] studies, in which combined therapy was used, were particularly good in the advanced cases. Friedman and associates obtained a 42 per cent 2-year local control rate

with combination therapy, which they had not achieved with radiation therapy alone. The few patients I have treated by this regimen have shown impressive enough improvement for me to continue its use in the patient with advanced disease.

Methotrexate is rapidly excreted in the urine within 4 to 8 hours. Its toxic effects, including stomatitis, depressed bone marrow and gastrointestinal symptoms such as nausea and diarrhea (a patient may have all or only some toxic effects), disappear from 4 to 14 days after the drug is discontinued. Impaired renal function precludes the use of the drug.

5-Fluorouracil (5-FU) is an antimetabolite that inhibits thymidylate synthetase, the enzyme necessary in the methylation of 2'-deoxyuridylic acid to form thymidylic acid, a precursor of DNA.[20, 82, 86] This inhibition results in cell injury and death. 5-Fluorouracil is also incorporated into RNA. The drug is given for 3 to 4 days before radiation is administered and then twice weekly until a toxic reaction, *i.e.*, bone marrow depression, diarrhea or nausea, occurs. The mucous membrane and skin reaction resulting from combination therapy with radiation and 5-fluorouracil is more severe than with radiation alone. The 3-year survival rate is 9 out of 13 patients, or 53 per cent, with combined 5-fluorouracil and radiation therapy, as compared with 1 out of 16 patients, or 6 per cent, with radiation alone.[86]

Hydroxyurea, an analogue of urea, is not a structural antimetabolite but is a highly selective inhibitor of DNA synthesis; it induces blocking of the formation of deoxyribonucleotides from ribonucleotides.[20, 69] The drug is excreted by the kidneys within 12 hours. It causes bone marrow depression, as do the other drugs. Hydroxyurea is given in divided doses for 7 to 10 days before radiation is started. Administration of the drug is continued for 8 to 9 months, if the bone marrow is not too depressed.

Rominger treated patients with advanced head and neck lesions with hydroxyurea and obtained his best results with previously untreated patients.[69] None of the lesions were permanently controlled, but the response was greater than that anticipated from radiation therapy alone. Tumors disappeared temporarily in some cases. In my experience with combined hydroxyurea and radiation treatment in a small number of cases, the drug has produced very prompt regression of lesions, but with recurrence in all patients.

One of the first drugs used against head and neck cancer was *menadiol sodium diphosphate* (Synka-vit), a synthetic water-soluble vitamin K analogue. A trial study of the drug was recently repeated by Krishnamurthi and associates, using Synka-Vit and radiation for the treatment of buccal mucosal cancers.[44] No significant difference between the control and other groups was found.

The alkylating agent cyclophosphamide (Cytoxan) in a number of trials has proved to be of little value alone or in combination with radiation in the treatment of head and neck cancer.

Intra-arterially administered hydrogen peroxide has been found to be a favorable potentiator of radiation effect, but the procedure does not lend itself readily to the treatment of patients undergoing a long-term course of irradiation.[82] Treatment of patients under hyperbaric oxygen tension poses many problems which preclude this method of therapy for the average patient. Those patients who have been able to breath atmospheric oxygen with 5 per cent carbon dioxide for an hour before radiation therapy seem to have better tumor response to treatment. This is a practical and feasible way to attempt to improve the oxygenation of the tumor bed. Pizer suggested injecting oxygen directly into the center of the tumor, since oxidizing agents in the circulation can extend into the tumor only as far as its vascularity will permit.[60] He proposed that Oxygel, which contains 11 per cent urea peroxide in a water-free base, be dissolved in 3 per cent mepivacaine hydrochloride (Carbocaine) solution. Four to 8 minims injected directly into the tumor and then about 10 minims held in the mouth over the tumor tissue for about 5 minutes immediately prior to irradiation might possibly increase the radioresponsiveness of the tumor.

The use of chemotherapy seems to have no place in the treatment of early lesions of the head and neck. For the patient with advanced disease, however, it is of definite value, if the patient's general condition will tolerate the treatment.

RADIATION THERAPY

DOSAGE

For years the roentgen (R.) has been used both as a unit of radiation quantity and as a unit of absorbed energy. With the advent of high energy sources, the roentgen could no longer be used in this way. With higher energy radiation, absorbed energy is largely a function of the photon energy of the incident radiation for a given material.[54] Therefore, it is more useful to define a unit that represents the quantity of radiation deposited in the absorbing material (*e.g.,* water, muscle or bone). The unit chosen was 100 ergs of energy absorbed per gram of material, the rad. This unit, which applies to any absorbing material, was introduced in 1956. The International Commission for Radiological Units in 1962 distinguished the roentgen as the unit of exposure and the rad as the unit of absorbed dose or energy absorbed in the depth of the material. One roentgen is loosely defined as the quantity of irradiation that gives one electrostatic unit of charge from all electron processes initiated by the incident radiation in 1 cc. of air under standard conditions. Since it is difficult to measure rads directly, exposure is measured in roentgens, and by means of a conversion factor the number of rads is calculated. The conversion equation follows:[54]

rads per minute (absorbed dose rate) =

$$\text{roentgens per minute (output)} \times \\ \text{depth dose in roentgens (\%dd)} \times \\ \text{conversion factor (f)}$$

The teletherapy units are in the megavoltage range, such as large sources of radioactive cobalt (^{60}Co) that give off beams of almost monoenergetic million-volt radiation equivalent to an x-ray machine operating at 3 MV., and linear accelerators in the 4- to 8-MV. range.[54] A few institutions have machines operating in the 10- to 20-MV. range. In the kilovoltage range are conventional machines operating at 250 kV., 140 kV. and 100 kV.

Cobalt-60 (^{60}Co) is a satisfactory radiation source for therapy. The radiation has a skin-sparing effect and decreased absorption in bone, in comparison with radiation from conventional units. The treatment fields can be well-defined, and scatter of rays is in a forward direction instead of laterally.

The radiation from linear accelerators up to 10 MeV. (million electron volts) has decreased absorption in bone, but above 10 MeV. absorption increases. The electron voltage (in MeV) can be selected according to the depth of the lesion, which is an advan-

Table 29–1 *Absorbed Doses (per 100 R.) in Muscle and Bone for Some Typical Radiation Beams**

| GENERATING VOLTAGE OR RADIOACTIVE SOURCE | RADS (PER 100 R.) ||
	In Muscle	In Bone
100 kV.	92.0	414.0
200 kV.	94.0	191.0
250 kV.	94.9	146.0
^{137}Cs	95.7	92.5
^{60}Co	95.7	92.0
4 mC.	95.6	92.1

* From Meredith, W. J., and Massey, J. B.: Fundamental Physics of Radiology. Baltimore, Williams & Wilkins Co., 1968.

tage in the treatment of recurrent disease, particularly of the oral cavity. Tapley and Fletcher reported in their series of head and neck cancer cases that acute skin reactions were severe and late changes pronounced if the electron beam was used alone.[83] If the electron beam was used only as "boost" therapy after other radiation, the effects were less serious.

Most radiation therapy today is teletherapy, but some plesiotherapy (short-distance radiation) is still used in the form of radium, cobalt-60 or radon implants. The method of measurement for these radioactive substances is based on the standard that the exposure rate from a point source of 1 mg. of radium with a filter of 0.5 mm. of platinum will deliver 8.26 R. (roentgens) per hour at a 1-cm. distance from the point source. If the filtration is greater, the number of roentgens is reduced. Tables for correction of filtration are available, as are tables for calculation of dosages from multiple sources. The radioactivity of cobalt-60 needles is expressed in radium-equivalent strength, so that the same tables can be used for both. Radon decays rapidly and is usually left in the body permanently but is not used as much as formerly. The radioactivity of 1 mC. of radon being expended in 133.3 hours is equivalent to the radiation of a comparable source of radium, 1 mg., left in place 133.3 hours.

The total treatment time and dose, the number of increments of therapy per week and the size of each increment are very important factors in the radiation treatment of cancer. The tolerance of normal tissue is the factor that limits the total dose delivered. Ellis, in 1965, devised the nominal standard dose (N.S.D.), which is a function of the number of treatments, their frequency of application and the dose per treatment.[31] The N.S.D. represents, as a single number or dose, the expected effect of a course of fractionated therapy.

The nominal standard dose or radiation-equivalent therapy (rets) of 2220 rads, for example, gives the same radiobiologic effect as 7200 rads given in 26 fractions over a period of 35 days.[31] With such a standard it will be possible, hopefully, to compare the results from many institutions to determine the best time-fraction method of treatment. Currently, there is much discussion about the N.S.D. and other units that have been proposed, but no particular unit has been universally adopted.

REACTIONS

Cobalt-60 therapy is associated with less skin reaction, both in degree and duration, than that seen with conventional treatment. If a bolus is used in cobalt-60 therapy, erythema and moist desquamation of the skin occur, as they do if tangential fields or wedges are used, and if the skin is within the treatment volume. With conventional therapy these skin reactions are more severe and take longer to heal. Late atrophy with telangiectases usually occurs after conventional therapy, whereas with cobalt-60 therapy it is rare. With cobalt-60 therapy a patchy mucositis develops during the third week of treatment, becomes confluent, and heals within a short time after therapy is completed. The mucosal reaction with conventional treatment lasts longer and heals more slowly. With electron beam treatment some severe skin and soft-tissue reactions may be seen. Interstitial treatment with radioactive materials produces severe mucositis, which takes a number of weeks to heal.

TERMINOLOGY AND TECHNIQUES

The International Commission on Radiological Units and Measurements recommended for quality specification of x-ray beams that the kilovoltage at which the machine is operating and the half-value layer of the beam be mentioned for radiation therapy up to 2 MV. Above 2 MV., only the kilovoltage or megavoltage is specified.[54]

Definitions of some basic terms used in radiation therapy follow:

kV.: Operating kilovoltage of the machine.

HVL: Half-value layer; the filtration needed to reduce the beam to one half of its original value (it is one way of comparing qualities of beams).

TSD: Target-to-skin distance; distance from the radiating source to the patient's skin.

SSD: Source-to-surface distance; distance from the radiating source to the patient's skin.

Wedge filter: Filter used to modify the treatment beam to produce more homogeneity, especially on curved surfaces.

STD: Source-to-tumor distance; distance from the radiating source to the tumor.

The following list specifies techniques of radiation therapy for lesions of the oral cavity:

1. 140 kV., HVL 0.1-mm. Cu filter, TSD 35 cm.; 200 rads in one treatment—tissue dose. Patient is seen weekly. Treatment is repeated if necessary in 2 to 3 weeks.

2. 200 kV., HVL 1.0-mm. Cu filter, TSD 50 cm.; 5 increments per week; 1000 to 1200 rads per week. Tumor dose is 6000 to 6500 rads.

3. a. Lesions are over 3 cm. in diameter and 1 cm. thick. 200 kV., HVL 1.0-mm. Cu filter, TSD 50 cm.; 5 increments per week. Tumor dose is 6000 to 6500 rads in 5 to 6 weeks.

Lead shield is placed behind the lip to protect intraoral structures.

b. Lesions are under 3 cm. in diameter and less than 1 cm. thick. 140 kV., HVL 0.5-mm. Cu filter, TSD 50 cm.; 5 increments per week. Dose is 6000 rads over 4 weeks.

c. Lesion is bulky, is ulcerated and involves most of the lower lip, where surgery is contraindicated. Cobalt-60, SSD 70 cm., paired wedge filters with bolus; 3 to 5 increments per week. Dose is 6000 rads over 5 to 6 weeks.

4. Buccal mucosal lesions are rarely treated with intraoral cones, but for a small lesion near the commissure a cone might be used if a good margin (1 cm.) of normal tissue is included. 140 kV., HVL 0.5-mm. Cu filter, TSD 35 cm.; 3 increments per week. Total tissue dose is 6000 rads in 5 weeks. For other lesions cobalt-60 with wedge filters at 90-degree angles is employed with SSD 70 cm.; 5 increments per week. Total tumor dose is 6500 rads in 5 weeks. (Okumura and associates used 10 to 16 MeV. with a 2-mm. lead shield against the lesion. This resulted in reactions in other parts of the oral cavity. Treatment is effective for lesions less than 5 mm. thick.[59]

5. Alveolar lesions are treated with wedge filters at 90-degree angles or with radiation by parallel oblique fields with bolus;

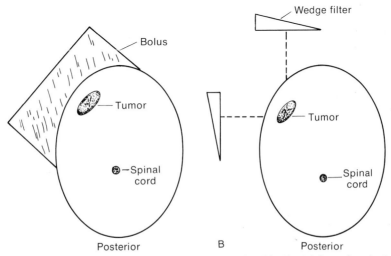

Figure 29-6 Radiation therapy of the alveolar ridge (the patient's head is viewed from above). *A*, Parallel oblique field. *B*, Wedge field.

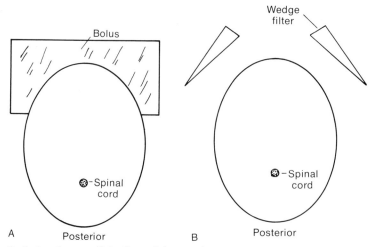

Figure 29–7 Radiation therapy of the floor of the mouth. *A*, Parallel opposing field. *B*, Wedge pair.

4 to 5 increments per week. Tumor dose is 6500 to 7000 rads in 5 to 6 weeks with cobalt-60.

6. Soft-palate lesions, if small, can be treated with an intraoral cone, as in technique 3b. Large soft-palate lesions and hard-palate growths suitable for radiation may be treated with cobalt-60 by a single field, opposing fields, or an open field on one side and a wedge on the other, depending on the volume to be treated; 4 or 5 increments per week. Tumor dose is 6500 to 7000 rads in 6 to 7 weeks.

7. Lesions of the floor of the mouth can be treated with cobalt-60 by parallel opposing fields with bolus or wedge pairs; 4 to 5 increments per week. Tumor dose is 6500 to 7000 rads in 6 to 7 weeks.

8. For lesions of the anterior two-thirds of the tongue:
   a. Interstitial radium needles may be used alone. Overall length of the needle is approximately 3 cm., with the active portion in the center. The radium is distributed so that each centimeter contains 1 mg. of radium. Tumor dose is 8000 rads.
   b. External radiation with cobalt-60 may be given by a single field for a tumor dose of 2000 rads over 2 weeks; 4 increments per week before radium is inserted. Tumor dose with radium or other radioactive source is 6000 to 6500 rads.
   c. May be treated by cobalt-60 alone, as in technique 7.

9. Lesions of the base of tongue may be

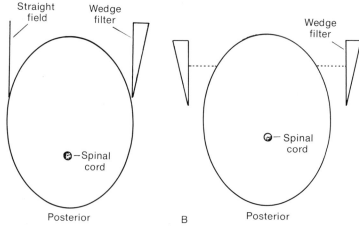

Figure 29–8 Radiation therapy of the anterior two-thirds of the tongue. *A*, Single radium needle and single wedge. *B*, Wedge pair.

Table 29–2 *Incidence of Radiation Failures and Their Surgical Management (1948–1965)* †*

ANATOMIC SITES	NUMBER OF PATIENTS TREATED BY IRRADIATION	NUMBER OF IRRADIATION FAILURES	SURGERY FOR IRRADIATION FAILURES		
			Number	*Disease above Clavicle*	*Distant Metastases*
Anterior two-thirds of tongue	225	77	35	13	4
Floor of mouth	179	40	21	5	1
Lower gum	42	19	10	3	1
Buccal mucosa	85	21	11	3	—
Hard palate	4	2	1	1 ‡	—
Upper gum	9	2	0	—	—

* From Crews, Q. E., and Fletcher, G. H.: Comparative evaluation of the sequential use of irradiation and surgery in primary tumors of the oral cavity, oropharynx, larynx and hypopharynx. Am. J. Roentgenol. Radium Ther. Nucl. Med., *111*(1):73–77 (Jan.), 1971.

† Minimum of 3-year follow-up.

‡ Postoperative death.

§ One case recurred after 34 months; patient is living with disease at 38 months.

treated with radiation by parallel opposing fields, including or excluding the cervical lymph nodes, depending on the extent of the disease. The nodes may be included for a portion of the treatment and then the field size decreased; 4 to 5 increments per week. Tumor dose is 6000 to 6500 rads in 5 to 7 weeks.

DISCUSSION

Statistics from the literature relating to oral malignant diseases indicate that patients with early lesions have a good recovery rate, whereas those with larger lesions or metastatic disease in the nodes have a low rate of recovery. In order to increase the survival rate, many treatment plans have been conceived and evaluated. Only a few have been set down, however, for most of them give comparable information.

A number of investigators have found from 39.3 to 43 per cent of lymph nodes to be microscopically positive in patients with oral cavity tumors who have had elective neck dissections with no clinical evidence of disease.[5, 43, 79] Many surgeons, for this reason, favor elective neck dissection in patients with lesions of the tongue and floor of the mouth. Before elective neck dissection, some clinics have given irradiation to the nodes in the hope of decreasing the 25 to 28 per cent recurrence rate following surgery without preoperative radiation.[5, 6, 8] Also, elective irradiation of the neck for patients with squamous cell carcinoma with a high incidence of predictable node metastasis is being advocated because of the marked decrease in new cancer of the neck when this approach has been used. Berger and associates reported that new cancer was reduced to 1.7 per cent.[8]

Table 29–2 shows the results of irradiation

Table 29–3 *Radiation Necroses Surgically Treated (1948–1965)* †*

ANATOMIC SITES	NUMBER OF PATIENTS TREATED BY IRRADIATION	NUMBER OF PATIENTS WITH NECROSIS SURGICALLY TREATED	DISEASE ABOVE CLAVICLE
Anterior two-thirds of tongue	225	15	1
Floor of mouth	179	16	2
Lower gum	42	3	1
Buccal mucosa	85	4	—
Hard palate	4	0	—
Upper gum	9	0	—

* From Crews, Q. E., and Fletcher, G. H.: Comparative evaluation of the sequential use of irradiation and surgery in primary tumors of the oral cavity, oropharynx, larynx and hypopharynx. Am. J. Roentgenol. Radium Ther. Nucl. Med., *111*(1):73–77 (Jan.), 1971.

† Minimum of 3-year follow-up.

Table 29–4 *High-Dosage Preoperative Irradiation (1948–1965)* †*

ANATOMIC SITES	NUMBER OF PATIENTS	DISEASE ABOVE CLAVICLE	DISTANT METASTASES
Anterior two-thirds of tongue	10	3	—
Floor of mouth	8	2	1
Lower gum	11	2	2
Buccal mucosa	6	1	1
Hard palate	0	—	—
Upper gum	1	—	—

* From Crews, Q. E., and Fletcher, G. H.: Comparative evaluation of the sequential use of irradiation and surgery in primary tumors of the oral cavity, oropharynx, larynx and hypopharynx. Am. J. Roentgenol. Radium Ther. Nucl. Med., *111*(1):73–77 (Jan.), 1971.

† Minimum of 3-year follow-up.

of lesions at different oral cavity sites, and Table 29–3, the number of cases of surgically treated radiation necrosis, according to the study of Crews and Fletcher.[23]

Crews and Fletcher treated patients with advanced lesions that were infiltrating or invading bone with 5000 rads over 5 weeks or 6000 rads over 6 weeks and, at times, with radiation to the neck nodes followed by a total resection. The results of this treatment are shown in Table 29–4.

Blady's figures indicate concisely the poorer prognosis of the patient with metastasis to the cervical lymph nodes (Tables 29–5 and 29–6).

The compilation of statistics from the American Cancer Society publication *Clinical Staging System for Carcinoma of the*

Table 29–5 *Incidence and 5-Year Survival Rate**

PRIMARY CANCER	INCIDENCE (PER CENT)	5-YEAR SURVIVAL (PER CENT)
Anterior two-thirds of tongue	45.0	16.2
Base of tongue	70.0	24.0
Floor of mouth	41.0	19.0
Cheek	37.0	23.0
Soft palate	47.0	17.0
Tonsil	66.0	21.0
Nasopharynx	71.0	15.0

* From Blady, J. V.: The present status of treatment of cervical metastases from cancer arising in the head and neck region. Am. J. Roentgenol. Radium Ther. Nucl. Med., *111*:56, 1971.

Oral Cavity – 1968 is a retrospective analysis of 1570 cases (Table 29–7). Unfortunately, the type of treatment used is not indicated.[2]

CONCLUSION

Malignant diseases of the oral cavity take a greater toll than seems necessary in our "enlightened" era. Many cases of cancer could be prevented by proper attention to dental hygiene and by education concerning the excessive use of tobacco and alcohol. The educational message about the relationship of cigarette smoking to lung cancer has made its impression on a certain segment of the population but has not really prevailed against the lure of cigarette smoking in the overall population. Many who were convinced of the hazard of the cigarette retired to the false security of cigars and pipes only to become victims of lip or tongue cancer.

Out of the successes and failures of individual forms of treatment have emerged cer-

Table 29–6 *5-Year Survival Rate and Cervical Metastases on Admission**

PRIMARY CANCER	5-YEAR SURVIVAL		
	Overall (per cent)	*With Metastases (per cent)*	*Without Metastases (per cent)*
Anterior two-thirds of tongue	43.0	16.2	55.0
Base of tongue	26.0	24.0	48.0
Floor of mouth	37.3	19.0	59.5
Cheek	51.0	23.0	56.0
Soft palate	41.0	17.0	68.0
Tonsil	35.0	21.0	55.5
Nasopharynx	32.5	15.0	54.0

* From Blady, J. V.: The present status of treatment of cervical metastases from cancer arising in the head and neck region. Am. J. Roentgenol. Radium Ther. Nucl. Med., *111*:56, 1971.

Table 29–7 *5-Year Survival, by Stage, of 1570 Patients with Carcinoma of the Oral Cavity**

BUCCAL MUCOSA

	N0	N1	N2	N3
T1 stage 1	72%	5/8†	—	—
T2 stage 2	61%	9/25†	—	—
T3	8/15†	5/17†	0/3	0/8
	stage 3 = 42%		stage 4 = 0%	

FLOOR OF MOUTH

	N0		N1	N2	N3
T1 stage 1	21/31†	68%	2/2†	0/1†	0/5†
T2 stage 2	21/29†	70%	12/23†	1/5†	2/8†
T3	4/9		5/12	0/4	0/10
	stage 3 = 50%			stage 4 = 9%	

ANTERIOR 2/3 TONGUE

	N0	N1	N2	N3
T1 stage 1	90%	1/4	—	—
T2 stage 2	64%	6/21	0/1	0/3
T3	8/15	1/7	0/6	1/17
	stage 3 = 34%		stage 4 = 6%	

POSTERIOR 1/3 TONGUE

	N0		N1	N2	N3
T1 stage 1	2/4		4/8	0/5	0/4
T2 stage 2	15/34	44%	7/15	3/13	1/10
T3	2/15		4/26	0/8	2/21
	stage 3 = 26%			stage 4 = 0.7%	

SOFT PALATE

	N0	N1	N2	N3
T1 stage 1	73%	2/6	0/2	1/1
T2 stage 2	48%	5/8	0/2	0/9
T3	9/27	0/9	0/4	0/9
	stage 3 = 32%		stage 4 = 5%	

HARD PALATE

	N0		N1	N2	N3
T1 stage 1	14/15	93%	—	—	—
T2 stage 2	10/25	40%	1/3	—	0/4
T3	4/22		1/12	1/3	0/5
	stage 3 = 16%			stage 4 = 8%	

LOWER ALVEOLAR RIDGE

	N0	N1	N2	N3
T1 stage 1	64%	5/7	0/1	0/3
T2 stage 2	49%	6/12	—	2/7
T3	2/18	8/18	0/6	1/13
	stage 3 = 37%		stage 4 = 10%	

UPPER ALVEOLAR RIDGE

	N0		N1	N2	N3
T1 stage 1	8/13		1/3	—	—
T2 stage 2	18/28	64%	3/6	—	—
T3	9/24		2/9	—	1/4
	stage 3 = 36%			stage 4 = 1/4	

* From American Joint Committee for Cancer Staging and End Results Reporting: Clinical Staging System for Carcinoma of the Oral Cavity. Chicago, 1968.

† <u>Number patients living 5 years</u>
  Total number patients in group

tain patterns of progress, in which we use one kind of therapy to complement another. Though hampered by lack of knowledge of the basic physiologic process by which a normal cell is transformed into a cancer cell and of the body reactions that control the transition, the improvement in the survival rate of individuals with many characteristic types of lesions testifies to the efficacy of the cooperative approach, based on the optimal combination of surgery, radiation and che-motherapy. In the next decade further progress is certainly to be expected as additional chemotherapeutic agents become available and as a wider spectrum of megavoltage radiation sources come into use—and one would like to add, as a variety of high-energy particle beams become available.[38] However, research has not advanced far enough to enable physicists to perfect these sources, much less considering, for the present, the release of these sources to radiation therapists. How far away we are from a radical advance in the treatment and cure of cancer depends on the breakthroughs yet to come in our understanding of the basic biologic, chemical and virologic processes of the body cell. Pending the attainment of that fundamental knowledge, our heuristic approach has proved valuable and successful enough that we should continue it and strive for even closer cooperation among the medical specialties that are useful in combating cancer.

HARD- AND SOFT-TISSUE RADIONECROSIS

W. HARRY ARCHER

Most authors who refer to osteoradionecrosis fail to mention soft-tissue necrosis, which also produces discomfort and disfigurement. A curative dose of radiation, of whatever type, must often be associated with unwanted destruction of normal tissue, and this risk must be accepted by the patient if his life is to be saved.

Effects of Radiation on Skin and Subcutaneous Tissue. Erythema of the skin appears briefly and reappears 3 or 4 weeks later. Extensive radiation produces edema and desquamation of epithelial cells and denudation of the surface. Alterations in the sebaceous and sweat glands result in drying and scaling of the skin, and epilation often occurs. The epithelium becomes thin and atrophic, while superficial vessels become occluded. These changes, plus thickening of the intima and thrombosis of the vascular bed, lead to necrosis of the soft tissue.

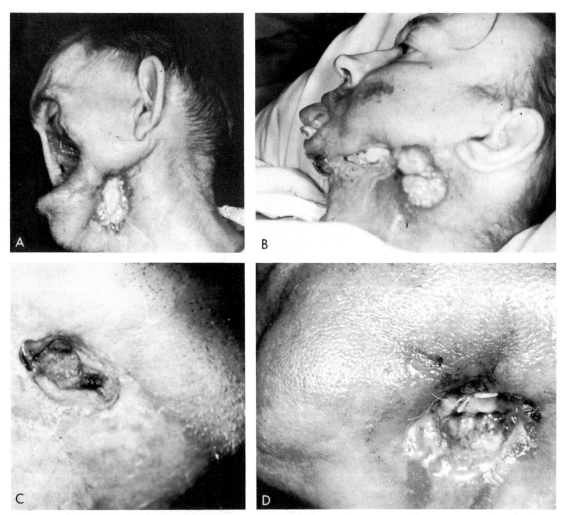

Figure 29–9 Four examples of postradiation necrosis of the skin and subcutaneous tissues with exposure of the mandible, which is nonviable in most cases. Such patients are most difficult to treat successfully. After sequestration and healing of the soft-tissue periphery, plastic surgery may be helpful in some cases. (Courtesy of W. Harry Archer, D.D.S.)

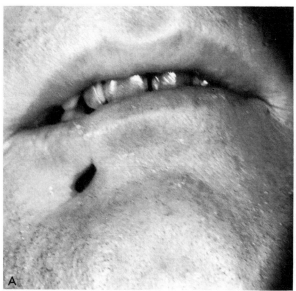 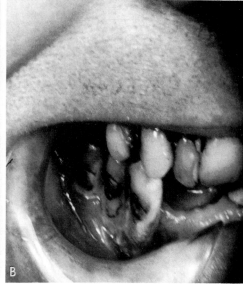

Figure 29–10 *A*, Healed postradiation soft-tissue necrosis following radiation therapy for an epidermoid carcinoma of the lip. *B*, Healed postradiation necrosis of the mucoperiosteal membrane. There was also a superficial osteoradionecrosis, and several mandibular anterior teeth and their supporting alveolar process were lost as the nonviable bone was sequestrated. The patient refused plastic surgery. (Courtesy of W. Harry Archer, D.D.S.)

TREATMENT. After the necrotic tissue sloughs out, peripheral healing of the viable tissue forms an opening into the oral cavity. Plastic surgery can be attempted, but the failure rate is high because radiated tissue notoriously fails to heal satisfactorily.

Effects of Radiation on Osseous Tissue. Bone is relatively resistant to radiation, but a heavy dosage can upset the normal balance between bone formation and resorption, and damage to the vascular bed is usually permanent. This makes radiated bone particularly susceptible to infection. Surgery, such as the extraction of teeth, results in infection because of the lack of a normal postoperative inflammatory defensive response.

Some authorities claim that the preoperative administration of antibiotics prevents infection and osteoradionecrosis; but more than a minimal disturbance of the vascular bed would not enable the antibiotic to reach the operative site. If the blood supply has been reduced, even massive doses of an antibiotic will not prevent postextraction infection and osteonecrosis.

In the author's opinion, the efficacy of antibiotics in these cases is greatly overrated. If the vascular bed can transport the antibiotic, it can also produce an inflammatory response and satisfactory healing, as we saw in some cases in the preantibiotic days. Teeth should be extracted prior to radiation and an extensive alveolectomy performed, as described in Chapter 2.

Intact oral mucoperiosteum over radiated bone frequently breaks down, and osteoradionecrosis develops without any trauma to the mucoperiosteum. The pathogenesis is not known, but all "authorities" state that three factors are involved: radiation, trauma and infection. Radiation obviously plays a part, but trauma and infection are not proven causative factors.

Pain as a sequela of osteoradionecrosis depends on the extent of osseous involvement and on whether acute infection of the investing soft tissue is present.

TREATMENT. Pain is allayed with analgesics or alcohol blocks, and infection is treated with antibiotics and establishment of drainage. Rough bone is smoothed with burs and files. Attempts to saucerize these areas and reach viable bone practically always fail. If the nonviable areas are small, sequestration and epithelialization will take place. The use of electrocoagulation on exposed bone, as advocated by some authorities, has been fruitless in the hands of the author.

For cases in which pain, trismus, recurrent infection and extensive exposure of bone indicate widespread nonviable bone, or in spontaneous fracture of the mandible (Fig. 29–11), hemiresection or block resection is

OSTEORADIONECROSIS OF THE MANDIBLE
WITH SPONTANEOUS FRACTURE

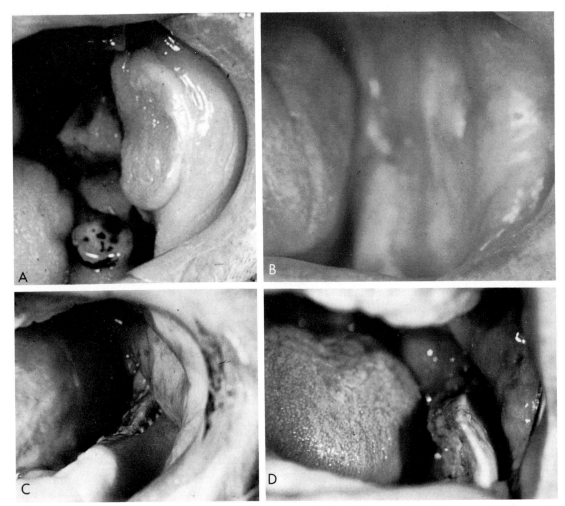

Figure 29–11 *A*, This epidermoid carcinoma of the left cheek is that of the same patient whose case is illustrated in Figure 29–3 and described on page 1809. *B*, Three months after completion of radiation therapy. *C*, Twenty months after treatment the overlying mucoperiosteum broke down as the result of osteoradionecrosis of the mandible. The patient was pain-free except during two episodes of submaxillary cellulitis. The rough surface of the disintegrating bone produced annoying irritation to his tongue, and so the exposed bone was periodically smoothed with burs. *D*, Spontaneous fracture of the horizontal ramus. A resection of a portion of the anterior segment of the mandible was performed and was followed by normal healing. The fracture line followed a rather clear-cut demarcation between viable and nonviable bone. For this reason no posterior bone was excised. (Courtesy of W. Harry Archer, D.D.S.)

indicated. The intraoral route, as described by Meyer, is preferred because incisions through radiated tissues frequently fail to heal.

MacDougall and associates stated, "Any operation which further reduces an already diminished blood supply should be avoided. An external approach to the mandible which divides the facial and labial vessels and places an incision in devitalized soft tissue,

should not be performed. . . . A 10-year experience with this operation [intraoral mandibulectomy] has proven entirely satisfactory; pain ceases to be a problem almost immediately, trismus soon disappears, fistulas heal spontaneously; in a short period, the depressed metabolic functions return to normal. Because of established fibrosis the cosmetic disability resulting from the mandibulectomy is of a minor degree."[51]

OSTEORADIONECROSIS OF THE MANDIBLE AROUND AN INFECTED THIRD MOLAR WITH SPONTANEOUS FRACTURE

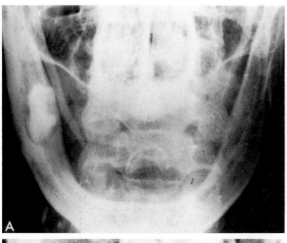
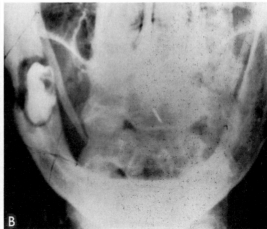
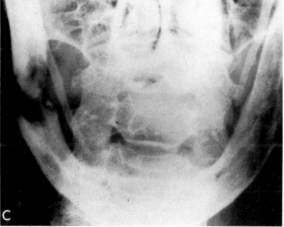

Figure 29–12 *A*, Roentgenogram of the mandible prior to radiation therapy for epidermoid carcinoma of the tonsillar area. *B*, Roentgenographic evidence of osteoradionecrosis and infection with a pathologic fracture of the mandible. *C*, The third molar has been removed, and the loss of bone as sequestra were formed and removed is evident in this roentgenogram.

Discussion: Why this carious and infected third molar was not removed before radiation therapy is a mystery. Its presence practically assured that post-radiation complications would develop. This patient was pain-free and was treated conservatively. Sequestra were removed as they formed. When drainage ceased, the patient did not return for further treatment.

It is of interest to note in the roentgenograms the exceptionally long styloid processes. We have seen one such case in which a long styloid process was fractured by the taking of impressions for a lower denture. No treatment was given for this fracture and none was needed. (Courtesy of W. Harry Archer, D.D.S.)

INTRAORAL MANDIBULECTOMY
Irving Meyer, D.M.D., M.Sc., D.Sc.

For this operative procedure general anesthesia is preferred, but local anesthesia (1 per cent lidocaine with 1:50,000 epinephrine) can be used. Local anesthesia is also administered by infiltration injections to aid hemostasis and as a supplement to general anesthesia.

The first step is intraoral incision with a No. 15 blade, starting as high as possible on the anterior border of the ramus of the mandible and continuing down to the retromolar area on the superior surface of the body of the mandible. The incision is carried anteriorly along the alveolar crest, around the exposed bone, to the midline and then dropped vertically, deep into the mucolabial vestibule. Finally, the incision is made deep through the lingual mucoperiosteum, distal to the caruncle of Wharton's duct on the involved side (Fig. 29–13*A* and *B*).

The mucoperiosteum is reflected by employing a periosteal elevator with a gauze sponge over the flat end. It is first stripped from the labiobuccal surface of the mandible, starting from the midline vertical incision and proceeding posteriorly. The mental foramen is exposed, and the exiting vessels and nerves

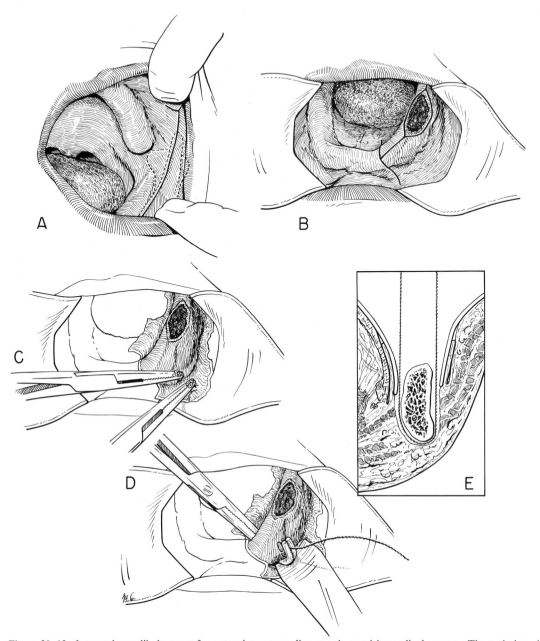

Figure 29–13 Intraoral mandibulectomy for extensive osteoradionecrosis requiring radical surgery. The technique is that of I. Meyer, with two alternate steps (G_2 and I_2) suggested by W. Harry Archer, D.D.S. Study the text for a detailed description of the technique illustrated.
(*Figure 29–13 continued on opposite page*)

are clamped with two clamps, cut and tied separately with 000 chromic catgut. The lateral surface of the mandibular mucoperiosteum is stripped straight back to the insertion of the masseter and the inferior border of the ramus. The elevator is then passed beneath the inferior border of the mandible and directed posteriorly to the angle. This will give a clean lateral and inferior border almost to the angle (Fig. 29–13C).

The lingual side of the mandible is stripped clean of the mucoperiosteum in the same manner. Starting from near the midline incision, the surgeon directs the elevator downward and backward to strip away the mucoperiosteum, the insertion of the anterior belly of the digastric muscle, the insertion of the mylohyoid muscle and the submaxillary gland.

A right-angle gallbladder clamp is intro-

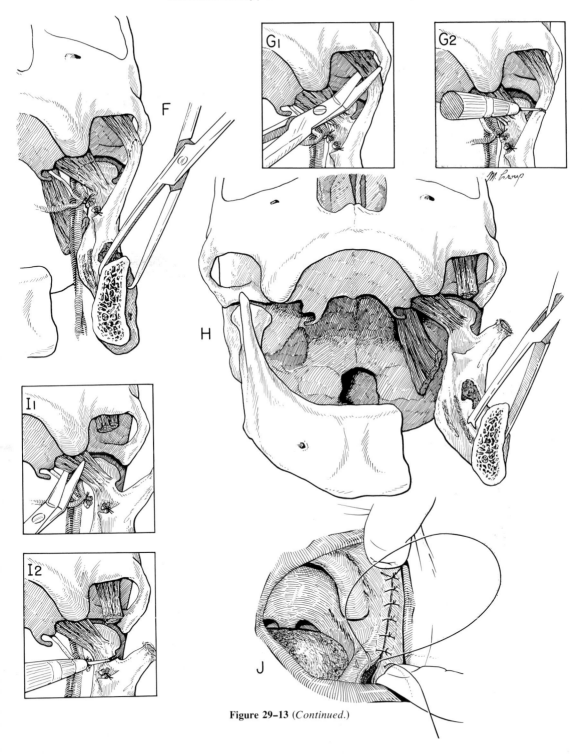

Figure 29–13 (*Continued.*)

duced on the lingual surface just in front of the mental foramen, and a Gigli saw end-loop is passed onto the buccal side of the mandible so that it can be caught with the teeth of the gallbladder clamp (Fig. 29–13D). The saw is drawn beneath the jaw with the clamp and out to the lingual side. Handles are attached to both ends of the saw, and the jaw is sectioned, with the soft tissues protected with elevators and retractors (Fig. 29–13E). As much of the anterior curve of the mandible as possible should be preserved for esthetic reasons. The cut ends of the mandible may require the application of bone wax for hemostasis.

Grasping the cut end of the jaw with bone forceps and turning the posterior portion of the mandible outward will permit easier stripping of the lingual mucoperiosteum at the middle portion of the medial aspect of the mandible. The neurovascular bundle entering the jaw bone is seized between two clamps and sectioned; a tie is placed only behind the posterior clamp, because there can be no bleeding from the jaw side (Fig. 29–13*F*).

Stripping of the lingual periosteum is continued as high as possible onto and around the neck of the condyle and the coronoid process. This will detach the insertion of the internal pterygoid, temporalis and external pterygoid muscles. The elevator must be held against the bone in order to avoid damage to the internal maxillary artery.

Stripping of the lateral aspect of the mandible should be completed so that the masseter is lifted from the bone. It is sometimes necessary to use heavy curved scissors to complete the sectioning of the tendon at the insertion of the masseter.

The coronoid process presents the most difficulty and requires the use of heavy scissors. Again, use caution in order to preserve the internal maxillary vessels (Fig. 29–13G_1). (The author of this text prefers to sever the coronoid process and its attached temporalis muscle with a crosscut bone bur – Fig. 29–13G_2.)

Bone forceps are used to twist the mandible, and the head of the condyle is rolled out of the glenoid fossa (Fig. 29–13*H*). Heavy scissors are used to cut any remaining capsular attachments (Fig. 29–13I_1). (The author of this text prefers to sever the condyle by cutting through the neck with a bur – Fig. 29–13I_2.) The jaw bone is then easily delivered.

Hemostasis is effected with 000 plain catgut. Gelfoam is sometimes placed in the glenoid fossa to control oozing from the capsule. The empty space is closed in layers with 000 chromic catgut and the mucosa is closed with 000 black silk.

Rarely is it necessary to place a drain. If infection is present, a 3-inch iodoform drain may be desirable for 24 hours.

REFERENCES

1. Ackerman, L. V., and Del Regato, J. A.: Cancer: Diagnosis, Treatment and Prognosis. St. Louis, The C. V. Mosby Co., 1970.
2. American Joint Committee for Cancer Staging and End Results Reporting: Clinical Staging System for Carcinoma of the Oral Cavity. Chicago, 1968.
3. Andrews, R. J.: Radiobiology of Human Cancer Radiotherapy. Philadelphia, W. B. Saunders Co., 1968.
4. Ash, C. L.: Oral cancer: A 25 year study. Am. J. Roentgenol. Radium Ther. Nucl. Med., *87:*417–430, 1962.
5. Barhrs, O. H., and Barber, K. W.: Value of radical dissection of structure of neck in management of carcinoma of lip, mouth and larynx. Arch. Surg., *85:*49–56, 1962.
6. Benak, S., Buschke, F., and Galante, M.: Treatment of carcinoma of the oral cavity. Radiology, *96:*137–143 (July), 1970.
7. Berger, A.: Examination of neoplastic and non-neoplastic lesions of the oral cavity. N.Y. State Dent. J., *16:*10, 1950.
8. Berger, D. S., Fletcher, G. H., Lindberg, R. D., and Jesse, R. H.: Elective irradiation of the neck lymphatics for squamous cell carcinoma of the nasopharynx and oropharynx. Am. J. Roentgenol. Radium Ther. Nucl. Med., *111*(1):66–72, 1972.
9. Bernier, J. L.: Personal communication, Washington, D.C.
10. Bernier, J. L.: The Management of Oral Disease. St. Louis, The C. V. Mosby Co., 1955.
11. Bernier, J. L.: Carcinoma of the lip. J.A.D.A., *36:*262, 1948.
12. Bernier, J. L.: Differential Diagnosis of Oral Lesions. St. Louis, The C. V. Mosby Co., 1942.
13. Berry, R. J.: Radiotherapy plus chemotherapy – Have we gained anything by combining them in the treatment of human cancer? Frontiers of Radiation Therapy and Oncology. Vol. 4. New York, S. Karger, 1969.
14. Blady, J. V.: The present status of treatment of cervical metastases from cancer arising in the head and neck region. Am. J. Roentgenol. Radium Ther. Nucl. Med., *111:*56, 1971.
15. Cahn, L., and Slaughter, D. P.: Oral Cancer: A Monograph for the Dentist. Rochester, N.Y., American Cancer Society, 1962.
16. Campos, J. L., Lampe, I., and Fayos, J. V.: Radiotherapy of carcinoma of the floor of the mouth. Radiology, *99:*677–682 (June), 1971.
17. Carlier. G., *et al.*: [Odontoradionecrosis after irradiation with cobalt bomb.] Rev. Stomatol., *65:*289–290 (June), 1964.
18. Churchill-Davidson, I.: The oxygen effect in radiotherapy – Historical review. Hyperbaric Oxygen and Radiation Therapy of Cancer. Frontiers of Radiation Therapy and Oncology. Vol. 1. New York, S. Karger, 1968.
19. Colby, R. A., Kerr, D. A., and Robinson, H. B. G.: Color Atlas of Oral Pathology. 2nd ed. Philadelphia, J. B. Lippincott Co., 1961.
20. Cole, W. H.: Chemotherapy of Cancer. Philadelphia, Lea & Febiger, 1970.
21. Coleman, C. C., and Hoopes, J. E.: The treatment of radionecrosis with persistent cancer of the head and neck. Am. J. Surg., *106:*716 (Nov.), 1963.

22. Cook, T. J.: Osteomyelitis and osteoradionecrosis: Report of two cases. Oral Surg., *16:*257–260 (Mar.), 1963.

23. Crews, Q. E., and Fletcher, G. H.: Comparative evaluation of the sequential use of irradiation and surgery in primary tumors of the oral cavity, oropharynx, larynx and hypopharynx. Am. J. Roentgenol. Radium Ther. Nucl. Med., *111* (1):73–77 (Jan.), 1971.

24. Daly, T., and Drane, J. B.: Preventive oral care for the irradiated cancer patients. Dent. Surv., *46:*36 (Nov.), 1970.

25. Dargent, M., and Bertoin, P.: [Radionecrosis of jaw bones: Indications and techniques for dental extractions.] Ann. Odontostomatol., *21:*5–12 (Jan.-Feb.), 1964.

26. Del Regato, J. A.: Dental lesions observed after roentgen therapy in cancer of the buccal cavity, pharynx and larynx. Am. J. Roentgenol. Radium Ther. Nucl. Med., *42:*404–410, 1939.

27. Donlan, C. P.: Irradiation in cancer of the tongue. Am. J. Roentgenol. Radium Ther. Nucl. Med., *60* (4):511, 1948.

28. Du Sault, L. A.: Dose-response at each fraction in a radiotherapy series. Frontiers of Radiation Therapy and Oncology. Vol. 3. New York, S. Karger, 1968.

29. Elkind, M. M.: Some principles for a rational, cell-based development of combined radiation-drug therapy. Frontiers of Radiation Therapy and Oncology. Vol. 4. New York, S. Karger, 1969.

30. Elkind, M. M., Withers, H. R., and Belli, J. A.: Intracellular repair and oxygen effect in radiobiology and radiotherapy. Frontiers of Radiation Therapy and Oncology. Vol. 3. New York, S. Karger, 1968.

31. Ellis, F.: Nominal standard dose and the ret. Br. J. Radiol., *44:*101–108 (Feb.), 1971.

32. Ellis, F.: Time, fractionation and dose rate in Radiotherapy. Frontiers of Radiation Therapy and Oncology. Vol. 3. New York, S. Karger, 1968.

33. English, J. A.: Radiation biology pertinent to dentistry. J.A.D.A., *70:*1442–1449 (June), 1965.

34. Fazekas, J. T., Green, J. P., Vaeth, J. M., and Schroeder, A. F.: Postirradiation induration as a prognosticator. Radiology, *102:*409–412 (Feb.), 1972.

35. Finney, J. M., Bolla, G. A., Collier, R. E., *et al.*: Differential localization of isotopes in tumors through use of intra-arterial hydrogen peroxide. Am. J. Roentgenol. Radium Ther. Nucl. Med., *94:*783, 1965.

36. Fletcher, G. H.: Textbook of Radiotherapy. Philadelphia, Lea & Febiger, 1966.

37. Friedman, M., DeNarvaes, F. N., and Daly, J. F.: Treatment of squamous cell carcinoma of the head and neck with combined methotrexate and irradiation. Cancer, *126:*711 (Sept.), 1970.

38. Hammond, A. L.: Cancer radiation therapy: Potential for high energy particles. Science, *175* (4027):1230–1232 (Mar.), 1972.

39. Hauser, R.: [The importance of teeth in osteoradionecrosis of the mandible (and what the radiotherapist must know).] Radiologe, *4:*339–344 (Oct.), 1964.

40. Hobaek, A.: Dental prosthesis and intraoral epidermoid carcinoma. Acta Radiol., *22:*259, 1949.

41. Kallman, R. F.: Repopulation and reoxygenation as factors contributing to the effectiveness of fractionated radiotherapy. Frontiers of Radiation

42. Kramer, S.: Use of methotrexate and radiation therapy for advanced cancer of the head and neck. Frontiers of Radiation Therapy and Oncology. Vol. 4. New York, S. Karger, 1969.

43. Kremen, A. J.: Results of surgical treatment of cancer of the tongue. Surgery, *39:*49–53, 1956.

44. Krishnamurthi, S., Shanta, V., and Sastri, D. V.: Combined therapy in buccal mucosal cancers. Radiology, *99:*409–415 (May), 1971.

45. Lambson, G. O.: Papillary epithelial hyperplasia of the palate: A clinical and histologic study of 139 cases. Thesis, University of Missouri at Kansas City (School of Dentistry), 1963.

46. Lampe, I.: Radiation therapy of cancer of the buccal mucosa and lower gingiva. Am. J. Roentgenol. Radium Ther. Nucl. Med., *73:*628, 1955.

47. Lee, R. E., White, W. L., and Totten, R. S.: Ameloblastoma with distinct metastases. Arch. Pathol., *68:*23, 1959.

48. Levitt, S. H., and Bogardus, C. R., Jr.: Advantages and disadvantages of intensive split-dose radiation therapy. Frontiers of Radiation Therapy and Oncology. Vol. 3. New York, S. Karger, 1968.

49. Lindberg, R. D., Barkley, H. T., Jr., Jesse, R. H., and Fletcher, G. H.: Evolution of the clinically negative neck in patients with squamous cell carcinoma of the facial arch. Am. J. Roentgenol. Radium Ther. Nucl. Med., *111*(1):60–65 (Jan.), 1971.

50. MacComb, W. S.: Necrosis in treatment of intraoral cancer by radiation therapy. Am. J. Roentgenol. Radium Ther. Nucl. Med., *87:*431–440, 1962.

51. MacDougall, J. A., *et al.*: Osteoradionecrosis of the mandible and its treatment. Stomatol. Ref. Curr. Med. Lit., *2:*19–20 (Summer), 1964.

52. Marchetta, F. G., Sako, K., and Badello, J.: Periosteal lymphatics of the mandible and intraoral carcinoma. Am. J. Surg., *108:*505, 1964.

53. Martin, C. L.: Long time studies of metastatic cervical lymph nodes treated with irradiation. Am. J. Roentgenol. Radium Ther. Nucl. Med., *108* (2):247–256, 1970.

54. Meredith, W. J., and Massey, J. B.: Fundamental Physics of Radiology. Baltimore, The Williams & Wilkins Co., 1968.

55. Montgomery, P. W., and von Haan, E.: A study of exfoliative cytology in patients with carcinoma of the oral mucosa. J. Dent. Res., *30:*308, 1951.

56. Moss, W. T.: Therapeutic Radiology. St. Louis, The C. V. Mosby Co., 1959.

57. Murphy, W. T.: Radiation Therapy. Philadelphia, W. B. Saunders Co., 1970.

58. O'Brien, P., Carlson, R., Steubner, E. A., and Staley, C. T.: Distant metastases in epidermoid cell carcinoma of the head and neck. Cancer, *27* (2):304–307 (Feb.), 1971.

59. Okumura, Y., Tomoyuki, M., and Kitagawa, T.: Modification of dose distribution in high-energy electron beam treatment. Radiology, *99:*683 (June), 1971.

60. Pizer, M. E.: A query to all radiotherapists. Va. Med. Mon., *100:*222–223, 1973.

61. Pizer, M. E., and Kay, S.: Mouth cancer – Concepts of treatment. Va. Med. Mon., *99:*148–166 (Feb.), 1972.

62. Robbins, S. L.: Pathology. 3rd ed. Philadelphia, W. B. Saunders Co., 1967.

63. Robinson, H. B. G. (Ed.): Tumors of the Oral

Regions. Dent. Clin. North Am., 619–758 (Nov.), 1957.

64. Robinson, H. B. G.: Diagnosis of cancer of the oral mucosa. J. Oral Surg., 4:985, 1951.

65. Robinson, H. B. G.: Medical and dental aspects of oral malignancy. Postgrad. Med., 6:355, 1949.

66. Robinson, H. B. G.: Oral malignancies: The dentist's responsibility. Dent. Radiogr. Photogr., 21:1, 1948.

67. Robinson, H. B. G.: A clinic on the differential diagnosis of oral lesions. Am. J. Orthod., 32:729, 1946.

68. Robinson, H. B. G.: Ameloblastoma: A survey of 379 cases from the literature. Arch. Pathol., 23:831, 1937.

69. Rominger, J. C.: Hydroxyurea and radiation therapy in advanced neoplasms of the head and neck. Am. J. Roentgenol. Radium Ther. Nucl. Med., 111 (1):103–108 (Jan.), 1971.

70. Rubin, P., and Casarett, G. W.: Clinical Radiation Pathology. Philadelphia, W. B. Saunders Co., 1968.

71. Sandler, H. C.: Reliability of oral exfoliative cytology for detection of oral cancer. J.A.D.A., 68:489, 1964.

72. Sarnat, B. G., and Schour, I.: Oral and Facial Cancer. Chicago, Year Book Publishers, Inc., 1950.

73. Scanlon, P. W.: Split-dose radiotherapy for head and neck cancer. Frontiers of Radiation Therapy and Oncology. Vol. 3. New York, S. Karger, 1968.

74. Schüle, H.: [Etiology and pathogenesis of osteoradionecrosis following tooth extraction in radiation-injured tissue.] Dtsch. Zahnaerztl. Z., 20:647–652 (June), 1965.

75. Shafer, W. G., Hine, M. K., and Levy, B. M.: A Textbook of Oral Pathology. 3rd ed. Philadelphia, W. B. Saunders Co., 1963.

76. Shapiro, B. L., Gorlin, R. J., and Jordan, W. A.: Role of exfoliative cytology in oral cancer detection. Oral Surg., 17:327, 1964.

77. Small, J. A.: Ameloblastoma of the jaws. Oral Surg., 8:281, 1955.

78. Smith, I. H.: Cobalt 60 Teletherapy. New York, Hoeber Medical Division, Harper & Row, 1964.

79. Southwick, H. W., Slaughter, D. P., and Trevino, E. T.: Elective neck dissection for intraoral cancer. Arch. Surg., 80:905–909, 1960.

80. Stein, J. J., et al.: The Management of the teeth, bone, and soft tissues in patients receiving treatment for oral cancer. Am. J. Roentgenol. Radium Ther. Nucl. Med., 108(2):257 (Feb.), 1970.

81. Suit, H. D.: Time factor in dose fractionation. Frontiers of Radiation Therapy and Oncology. Vol. 3. New York, S. Karger, 1968.

82. Sullivan, R. D.: Clinical Cancer Chemotherapy Including Ambulatory Infusion. Lahey Clinic Foundation, Boston, Mass. Springfield, Ill., Charles C Thomas, 1970.

83. Tapley, N. duV., and Fletcher, G. H.: Current techniques with 6-18 MeV. electron beam. Am. J. Roentgenol. Radium Ther. Nucl. Med., 105: 172–177, 1969.

84. Thoma, K. H., and Robinson, H. B. G.: Oral and Dental Diagnosis, 6th ed. Philadelphia, W. B. Saunders Co., 1960.

85. Uotila, E., et al.: Osteoradionecrosis of the jaw. Odontol. Tidskr., 73:239–249 (Apr.), 1965.

86. Vermund, H., Gollin, F. F., and Ansfield, F. J.: Clinical studies of 5-fluorouracil as adjuvant to radiotherapy. Frontiers of Radiation Therapy and Oncology. Vol. 4. New York, S. Karger, 1969.

87. Webster, J. R.: Osteoradionecrosis. Ala. J. Med. Sci., 1(2):209–210 (Apr.), 1964.

CHAPTER 30

SURGICAL REPAIR OF THE CLEFT LIP

HERBERT J. BLOOM, D.D.S.

More than 20 centuries of thought, ingenuity and skill have been brought to bear on the defects known as cleft lip and cleft palate. Therefore this chapter, understandably, covers only the general and principal aspects of this subject. The oral surgeon who must treat and help to rehabilitate the patient with a cleft lip or a cleft palate is urged to become familiar with the great volume of literature concerning these developmental defects that have been a sorrowful affliction to mankind throughout his known history.

HISTORICAL BACKGROUND

The earliest known records of surgical attempts to correct orofacial congenital clefts date back to the beginning of the Christian era. The writings of Celsus (25 B.C.–A.D. 50) allude to palatal surgery, as do the accounts of others during the succeeding 300 years, but a Chinese surgeon described cleft lip surgery in approximately A.D. 390. The Renaissance, responsible for introducing a new dimension in medicine, brought more complete reports on techniques for the correction of this deformity. Pierre Franco, Ambroise Paré and Gaspare Tagliacozzi are but a few of those identified with closure of orofacial clefts during the sixteenth century.

Although during the next three centuries the special techniques of numerous surgeons were recorded, the most significant progress in the surgical correction of the deformity was made during the nineteenth century. In 1816, Von Graefe introduced the surgical repair of the soft palate, a procedure confirmed, but modified, by Roux 3 years later. Stevens, shortly thereafter, following the technique described by Roux, is credited with the first successful operation of this type performed in the United States. Malgaigne in 1844 described his "deux lambeaux" lip repair technique, a procedure modified by Mirault the same year. The basic Mirault operation, adapted by many clinicians of the day, persisted for 100 years. The most influential refinement in Mirault's technique was made by Blair and Brown, whose report was published in 1930.

Wound dehiscence occurred almost invariably after palate closures in this period; innovations were numerous in attempts to overcome wound tension and lateral pull of muscles. Dieffenbach resorted to twisted wire sutures and lateral relaxing incisions; Mettauer tried multiple stab incisions to gain tissue relaxation; and after the classic anatomic report of Sir William Fergusson, the myotomy of palatal and pharyngeal muscles came into vogue.

Closure of the velum eventually was accomplished, but it was not until Von Langenbeck reported on the mucoperiosteal flap in 1861 that surgeons of the day progressed toward successful closure of the hard palate. Von Langenbeck's lateral relaxing incisions were made close to the alveolar ridges, extending from posterior myotomy incisions to the anterior dentition. The mucoperiosteum over the palatal shelves was elevated and displaced, altered in accordance with variations in inclination of the underlying bony plates, and the soft palate was dissected free of its attachment to bone. The bilateral bipedicle flaps were then sutured in the midline. The fundamental principles of Von Langenbeck's operation remain the basis of most modern surgical procedures for correction of the cleft palate.

The twentieth century has had its share of cleft palate surgical ingenuity. Brophy compressed the maxillary segments by force, a procedure that led to short palates and midfacial deformities. The W–V incisions to increase palatal length were suggested by Ganzer and Halle; Veau and Ruppe closed the nasal mucoperiosteum separately to decrease scarring; Dorrance further modified the push-back operation and fractured the hamular processes to relieve tension on the velum; Brown advocated freeing the palatine vessels to gain added displacement of the mucoperiosteal flaps; and Wardill changed Ganzer's W–V anterior incisions to allow for closure of the cleft of the premaxilla. Subsequent contributions enhanced surgical technique and improved the results attained. They include the classification of defects, procedures and devices for appraising the degree of velopharyngeal insufficiency, cephalometric radiography and cinefluorography.

Cheiloplastic procedures have undergone equal, if not greater, evolutionary changes during the twentieth century than in the prior centuries. Le Mesurier, utilizing a technique described by Hagedorn in 1844, devised the quadrangular flap that reconstructed the cupid's bow of the vermilion portion of the lip. This operative technique, described in 1949, provided the impetus for subsequent techniques that have accounted for remarkable improvements in cosmetic results. Tennison's single triangular flap, modified by Randall, and Skogg's double triangular flap are based on the principles established by Le Mesurier, eliminating the undesirable features of the single triangular flap while retaining the advantages responsible for its popularity for more than a decade.

The most recent advance in cleft lip surgery came in the late 1950's with Millard's rotation-advancement flap technique. Today, a popular and widely used method of cleft lip surgery, it provides for placement of the incision so as to simulate the ridge of the philtrum, accomplishes normal lip configuration and nostril symmetry, and provides possibly the most acceptable cosmetic result.

The challenge to correct one of the most personally devastating birth defects has been the focus of the valiant efforts of innumerable surgical practitioners throughout many centuries, only a few of whom have been mentioned here. We must be grateful for past accomplishments, and with these in mind, we may regard the present with compassionate respect. As the enigmatic aspects of the deformity become increasingly discernible to the concerned and dedicated specialist, we can anticipate the great accomplishments of the future.

OBJECTIVES OF CLEFT LIP SURGERY

Surgical repair of the cleft lip is an attempt to create what are regarded as normal anatomic features. The end result should be both functionally and cosmetically acceptable; our culture places a high priority on the latter effect. Ideally, the surgeon strives to achieve an intact and functioning orbicularis oris musculature, lip uniformity, a curving cupid's bow with its vermilion midline tubercle encompassed within an even white line bordering the mucocutaneous junction, and matching philtral ridges with intervening philtrum dimple. He plans his procedure anticipating a straight septum supporting an elongated columella, symmetric alar cartilages with restored nasal floors and equal nostril sills that produce equivalent nares (Fig. 30–1). The lip should be supple and the scars inconspicuous.

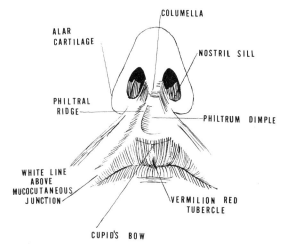

Figure 30–1 Anatomic landmarks of a normal lip and nose.

Despite the skill of the surgeon, known procedures rarely achieve the ideal result. Several surgical techniques reproduce normal appearance immediately in the postoperative patient, but the essential criterion for success is the long-term maintenance of this satisfactory cosmetic result throughout the advancing age of the patient. Too many poorly planned, unskillfully performed or overly radical operations yield distorted anatomic configurations as growth patterns progress.

TIMING THE LIP SURGERY

Each surgeon not only selects a particular operative procedure but also expresses a preference for the time the surgery is to be performed. Times of operations for lip repair in infancy will range from the first 48 hours of life to 6 months of age, depending upon the surgeon's judgment. Surgeons inclined toward earlier repair base their decisions on such matters as the psychologic influences on parents and siblings, the molding action of the united lip on the cleft maxillary arch, the greater healing potential of very young tissues, the increased resistance to surgical trauma and the avoidance of subsequent hospitalizations. They report that the closed lip prevents drying of the oral and respiratory mucosa, thereby decreasing susceptibility to upper respiratory infection.

Surgeons who favor delaying the operation believe that the larger lip resulting from natural growth processes is compatible with a greater degree of surgical apposition. The longer interim also permits comprehensive evaluation of the patient's total status, and there are those of the opinion that having parents become closely acquainted with the magnitude of the problem results in their appreciation of the several issues related to correction and rehabilitation.

Although there is no agreement as to when the surgery should be performed, most surgeons adhere to the proven "rule of 10": 10 weeks of age, 10 lb. in weight and at least 10 gm. of hemoglobin per 100 ml. of blood. With the exclusion of cases involving medical contraindication, from 2 to 3 months of age probably is the optimum time for lip closure.

Several years ago clinical investigators conceived the "lip adhesion" procedure, the goal of which is to close the lip early, but with a minimal cutaneous band across the defect, without undermining soft tissue to gain the mobilization required for a more effective and cosmetically acceptable closure. Proponents of the lip adhesion procedure suggest that it provides most of the advantages of early closure: tolerable appearance, orthopedic molding of the maxillary arch with progressive decrease in cleft width, and reduced incidence of upper respiratory disease. At the same time, it permits subsequent definitive corrective surgery without the obstacle of excessive scar tissue, which is concomitant with standard lip techniques requiring extensive undermining necessary for the advancement and repositioning of tissue. The subsequent operation is performed after the child is 1 year old, and the most undesirable feature of this sequence is that during the first year the child lives with a considerably less-than-normal-appearing lip. Nevertheless, the rationale is becoming increasingly accepted.

SURGICAL TECHNIQUES

UNILATERAL CLEFT LIP

Cleft deformities are infinitely varied in tissue inadequacies and displacements. In the unilateral cleft lip, certain normal landmarks usually are present, and the cheilorrhaphy is based on a projected visualization of the correct position of these landmarks and on shifting them to a normal relationship with the opposing segment.

Throughout the years, a myriad of techniques have been employed to accomplish effective shifting of tissue in order to use efficiently the tissue that is present, and to compensate for that which is absent and causes distortion. Today, most cleft lip operations can be classified within four broad categories: (1) linear, (2) triangular, (3) quadrangular and (4) rotation. Each category has its special usefulness under specific clinical circumstances, and the value to the surgeon of being familiar with all the techniques and their respective clinical applications cannot be overemphasized. The opportunities for preoperative planning are almost limitless, but "the die is cast" with the initial incision.

The *straight-line, or linear, closure* is the simplest and oldest technique of the modern era of cleft lip surgery. Because of consistently poor postoperative cosmetic results, its use today is confined to achieving early molding of the maxillary arch. Secondary corrective procedures must invariably be planned for and performed during the early years of the child's life.

The *triangular flap* was first developed as a lateral triangular flap by Mirault, Blair, Brown and McDowell and was widely employed between 1930 and 1950. The principle involves shifting a large triangular flap of tissue from the lateral (cleft) side to the medial segment. Although it is an improvement over the straight-line scar, it obliterates the normal landmarks of the cutaneous surface and results in a poor cupid's bow.

Tennison and Randall are given credit for the triangular flap operation as it is currently performed. Precise, reproducible stenciled markings serve to designate the opposing lip segments as components of a premeasured Z-plasty. The laterally based triangular flap is introduced into the medial segment just above the vermilion border. The cupid's bow is preserved and a pleasing lip contour is created. Disadvantages of the triangular flap are related to interference with reconstruction of a normal philtrum and tension at the inferior part of the lip.

The *quadrangular flap* technique developed by Hagedorn, but modified and popularized by Le Mesurier, involves the rotation of a quadrilateral flap from the cleft side to the intact medial segment. One of the principal advantages of the procedure is the resultant good cupid's bow, but the technique is difficult to execute. As the face develops, there is a tendency toward excessive length of lip on the cleft side, and shifting of the midline yields lip distortion.

The *rotation-advancement principle,* introduced by Millard in the late 1950's, perhaps comes closest to being the ideal repair procedure for the unilateral cleft lip. Tried and proved over a 15-year period, this technique has gained acceptance throughout the world, which justifies a review of its basic steps.

In contrast to the need for mathematic accuracy in planning Randall's triangular flap procedure, the rotation-advancement flap technique is designed to be executed by freehand incisions with allowable margins for flexibility during the operation. Unless the surgeon is experienced with this technique, however, accurately positioned preincision markings made on the cutaneous surface

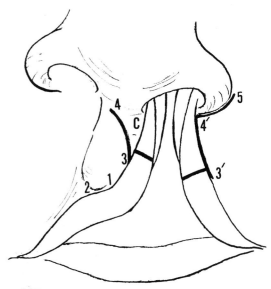

Figure 30–2 Preincision markings for rotation-advancement operation. Points 2, 1 and 3 mark cupid's bow. Incision from 3 to 4 allows for downward rotation of lip. The distance between 3 and 4 should eventually be equal to that from 3′ to 4′.

serve as valuable guidelines. Dots can be placed in the skin with a 25 gauge needle dipped in 5 per cent methylene blue solution. Incision lines may be outlined either with the needle or with a fine-tip surgical pen.

The following preliminary markings are useful in preparing for the rotation-advancement operation (Fig. 30–2):

1. Mark the cupid's bow:
   a. Point 2 is the peak on the mucocutaneous junction on the noncleft side.
   b. Point 1 is the depression at the midline—the center of the tubercle.
   c. Point 3 is the opposite peak of the cupid's bow (1 to 3 = 1 to 2).
2. Outline the rotation flap on the noncleft side:
   a. Mark point 4 below the columella at the midline. (POINT 4 MUST NOT BE POSITIONED LATERAL TO THE COLUMELLA.)
   b. With a fine-tip marking pen outline the incision as a curved sweep from point 3 and point 4.
3. Outline the advancement flap:
   a. On the mucocutaneous junction on the cleft side, mark point 3′ at the prominence of the vermilion—the lateral peak of the cupid's bow.
   b. Mark point 4′ at the nostril still on the mucocutaneous junction (3′ to 4′ = 3 to 4).

c. Mark point 5 on the alar base at its lateral extent.

The *incision* is started with the rotation flap at point 3, and with a curved sweep through the full thickness of the lip, the incision is extended in the direction of point 4. The ultimate length of this incision is determined when the cupid's bow assumes a normal horizontal position. Point 4 may be lateral to the midline but may not be lateral to the columella; extending the incision beyond the columella will result in disproportionate lengthening of the lip on the cleft side.

As the cupid's bow is rotated downward to a horizontal position, the defect created by the rotation incision widens. The gap created when the vermilion is placed in its normal position must now be filled by the advancement flap from the lateral segment (Fig. 30–3). With the lip at its future position, the distance between points 3 and 4 is measured with self-locking calipers. This distance must now be equal to that between points 3′ and 4′, and the vermilion is excised between these points. The incision is usually carried through the skin. The resultant slight concavity of the cut surface of the lateral segment can be adapted to the slight convexity of the medial segment. In order to add substance to the advancing flap, an incision from

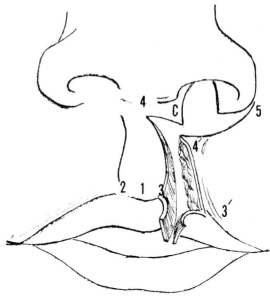

Figure 30–4 The incision between 3′ and 4′ creates the advancement flap. The incision between 4′ and 5 mobilizes the flap to allow its advancement into the rotation gap.

point 4′ is extended under the alar base to point 5 (Fig. 30–4).

An intraoral incision along the mucolabial sulcus mobilizes the lateral segment and frees it from the maxilla. Extending this incision into the nasal vestibule allows for elevation of

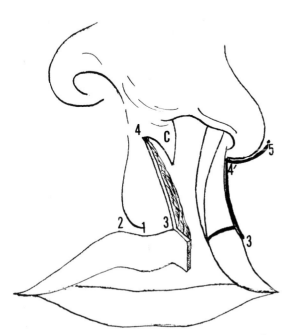

Figure 30–3 Incision from 3 to 4 develops the rotation flap; with the lip rotated downward to normal position, the distance from 3 to 4 is measured and becomes the distance from 3′ to 4′.

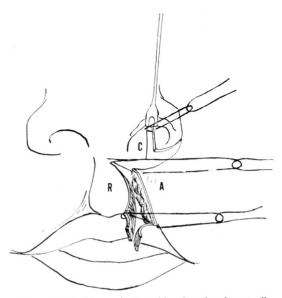

Figure 30–5 Closure is started by elevating the nostril, permitting small flap C to augment the columella. With the rotation flap (R) retracted downward, producing a gap, the advancement flap (A) is positioned into the gap. Key sutures are placed: 4 to 4′, 3 to 3′.

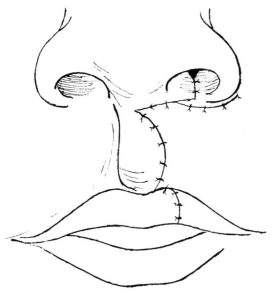

Figure 30–6 Meticulous placement of sutures provides a uniform lip, curving cupid's bow, matching philtral ridges, normal columella and symmetric alar cartilages.

the ala and its medial displacement with the lateral segment.

Closure is started by first elevating the cleft ala with a skin hook, so that small flap *C* on the medial segment advances into the columella (Fig. 30–5). It is retained in this position by interrupted 6-0 silk sutures. With flap *R* rotated downward, point 4′ is advanced to point 4, and point 3′ to point 3. The concavity of the lateral segment fits into the convexity of the medial segment (Fig. 30–5). Point 4′ of the advancing flap is accurately sutured into the crevice, point 4, of the rotation gap. The rotation-advancement flaps are now contiguous, and completion is a matter of meticulous placement of sutures. To approximate muscle 0000 chromic catgut is used, and 6-0 silk is employed to close the margins of the skin. The mucosa is usually closed last with 0000 chromic catgut (Fig. 30–6).

BILATERAL CLEFT LIP

The correction of bilateral cleft lip poses several unique problems to the surgeon, and results are usually less satisfactory than those obtained with repair of the unilateral cleft lip. Tissue deficiencies and displacements are critical; characteristic features include a protracted premaxilla, an underdeveloped prolabium with insufficient vermilion, a short columella, a flattened nose and absence of normal anatomic landmarks.

Accumulated scientific data have yet to resolve two controversies: (*a*) the matter of whether or not to produce retrodisplacement of the protruding premaxilla to facilitate closure for an immediately more satisfactory appearance; and (*b*) whether closure of the defects should be performed in one stage or in two stages. Consensus tends to favor the avoidance of positioning the premaxilla posteriorly at the time of initial surgery. The surgically closed lip in itself progressively retropositions the premaxilla without the probability of interference in midfacial growth that may follow surgical trauma to the nasal septum. Most surgeons also favor the one-stage operation, thus precluding the inherent risks of successive surgical exposures. Moreover, experience suggests that closure of the second side at a later date frequently is technically more difficult, since the premaxilla often is found to have rotated toward the previously closed side.

The number of complex geometric patterns advocated for repair of the bilateral cleft lip is no less than that suggested for the unilateral cleft lip. Each pattern has been advocated with a declaration of its being a progressive innovation, but none has demonstrated remarkable advantages over the simple closure that adheres to two fundamental standards: (*a*) preserving the prolabium, and (*b*) moving lateral lip elements into, but not beneath, the prolabium. Regardless of the technique employed, the surgical correction of bilateral cleft lip is likely to be less satisfactory than that of its unilateral counterpart, and subsequent corrective procedures must be contemplated.

The lack of normal anatomic features makes preincision markings a matter of judgment and experience. With a 25 gauge needle dipped in 5 per cent methylene blue solution, the following 4 points are marked on the sides of both clefts (Fig. 30–7):

1. On the prolabium:
   a. Point 1, at the base of the columella (skin).
   b. Point 2, at the peak of cupid's bow on the vermilion.
2. On the lateral segment:
   a. Point 1′, at the inferior edge of the ala (skin). Both 1′ points should be symmetric.

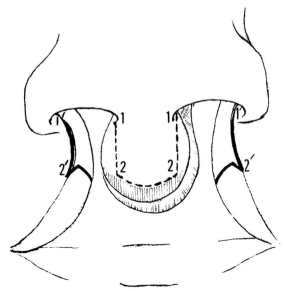

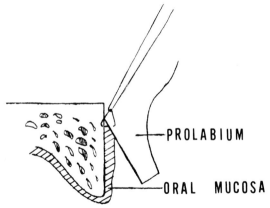

Figure 30–9 The oral (labial) mucosa is elevated to the height of the increased depth of the mucolabial sulcus and sutured to its new position. The alveolar process has a mucosal covering; the inner surface of the prolabium is raw.

Figure 30–7 Preincision markings for the correction of bilateral cleft lip. Points 1 (base of columella) and 2 (peak of cupid's bow) are marked on the prolabium. The distance from 1′ to 2′ equals that from 1 to 2.

    b. Point 2′, on the vermilion (so that 1′ to 2′ = 1 to 2).

Starting on the prolabium, a vertical incision joins point 1 with point 2. With a slightly circular incision, points 2 and 2′ are connected, care being taken to preserve the "white line" just above the vermilion border. The full-thickness prolabium is now dissected free from the maxilla to the depth of the mucolabial sulcus. The oral mucosa from the prolabium is elevated to cover the premaxillary alveolar process to its maximum depth (Figs. 30–8 and 30–9).

    The surgeon then turns his attention to the lateral aspects of the cleft and makes the incision joining point 1′ to point 2′. The vermilion-mucosal flaps of the lateral segments are unfolded, as illustrated in Figure 30–10.

These mucosal flaps (A) are then advanced toward the midline and sutured to line the cut oral surface of the prolabium (Fig. 30–11). The vermilion of the lateral segments is preserved in order to be advanced below the prolabium in the formation of the central portion of the cupid's bow.

    The segments (1′ to 1 and 2′ to 2) are brought in proximity with a skin hook; muscle is approximated with 0000 chromic catgut, and skin margins are coapted with 6-0 silk. The vermilion flaps are advanced and sutured at the midline, and to the prolabium,

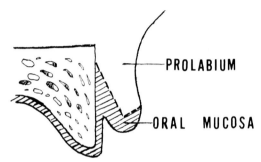

Figure 30–8 Sagittal section through prolabium demonstrating the oral (labial) mucosal surface to be dissected free of the prolabial tissue.

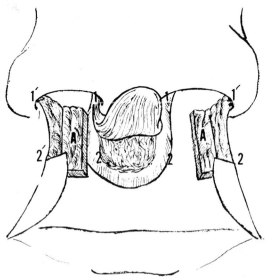

Figure 30–10 Incisions from 1′ to 2′ are of sufficient depth to allow unfolding of the vermilion-mucosal flaps (A). These flaps, when advanced medially, line the inner raw surface of the prolabium.

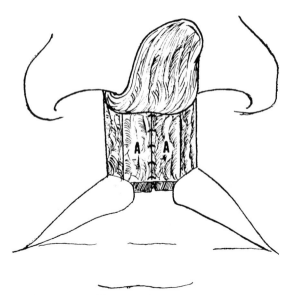

Figure 30–11 Flaps *A,* advanced toward the midline and sutured, provide the lining for the prolabium.

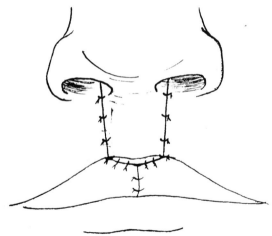

Figure 30–12 Muscle and skin are approximated at points marked. The mucocutaneous white line of the cupid's bow of the prolabium is preserved.

with maximum fullness of vermilion at the site of the lip tubercle (Fig. 30–12).

POSTOPERATIVE CARE

The particular situation dictates the need for arm restraints and the application of the Logan bow, both, if necessary, being applied in the operating room. Since closure of the wound without tension is an essential requisite to a successful outcome, use of the Logan bow should be limited to wound protection. Bacitracin or some other antibiotic ointment may be applied to the suture lines two or three times daily for the first 4 or 5 postoperative days. It depresses nasal and oral contaminants and restricts the formation of crusts.

The patient is fed through an Asepto syringe during the first week, after which a commercial cleft palate nipple may be used. Conventional soft rubber nipples with holes enlarged sufficiently to provide flow without sucking are acceptable substitutes.

Alternate skin sutures are removed on the third postoperative day; all other sutures are removed on the fifth day, when the patient may be discharged from the hospital. A narrow strip of collodion-saturated gauze is applied over the lip after all skin sutures have been removed. It should extend generously to each side, providing support to the wound and aiding in its hygiene. The gauze remains in place for at least a week or until it is spontaneously dislodged and can be lifted easily from the skin surface.

REFERENCES

(See References for Chapter 32.)

CHAPTER 31

A VARIATION OF THE ROTATION-ADVANCEMENT PRINCIPLE FOR USE IN WIDE UNILATERAL CLEFT LIPS: THE TECHNIQUE OF ASENSIO

OSCAR ASENSIO DEL VALLE, D.D.S.

RAMIRO ALFARO A., D.D.S.

The medial portion of a cleft lip presents the following characteristics: a philtrum with oblique deviation in relation to the facial midline and with vertical retraction toward the affected alar wing, and a columella deviated toward the opposite side. This deviation in relation to the vertical axes of the face is the first problem that must be corrected surgically.

The labial portion of the affected side is vertically contracted toward the affected alar wing, resulting in loss of vertical dimension. The base of the alar wing on the affected side is inserted at a lower position than that on the nonaffected side in relation to the horizontal (interpupillary) plane.

These asymmetries are present to a greater or lesser degree in all cases of cleft lip, with the exception of those in which the cleft affects only the vermilion. These abnormal relations must be corrected surgically, and facial structures should be positioned normally and in harmony with the facial planes.

This chapter describes a modification of the rotation-advancement method that we have found extremely valuable in the surgical management of wide unilateral cleft lips. This modification is simple to perform and allows one to obtain adequate vertical height on the lateral side without sacrificing lateral vermilion.

This procedure can be easily accomplished under local anesthesia by means of infraorbital blocks and local infiltration; the patient is adequately sedated prior to receiving local anesthesia.

PREOPERATIVE MARKING AND MEASUREMENTS

The following points are marked in standard fashion (see Figure 31–1): Point 1 represents the peak of the cupid's bow on the noncleft side; point 2 is the midpoint of the philtrum; and point 3 is marked on the mucocutaneous border such that the distance between 1 and 2 equals the distance between 2 and 3, and therefore point 3 designates the peak of the cupid's bow on the cleft side. Points 14 and 15 represent the labial commissures. Point 8 is the alar base on the noncleft side, and point 4 is the base of the columella on the noncleft side. The curved rotation incision from 3 to 4 is marked more or less in a standard fashion. It is not necessary to at-

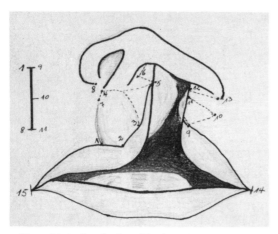

Figure 31–1 Standard marking in variation of rotation-advancement operation (Asensio technique) for wide unilateral cleft lips.

tempt to make this line straight. The rotation flap can take the form of a round flap because it will easily fit into the lateral side with the modifications to be described. In order to obtain full rotation of the flap in an inferior direction and to insure that the two peaks of the cupid's bow are positioned on a horizontal level plane parallel to the interpupillary plane, or even such that point 3 is 0.5 to 1 mm. lower than point 1 to allow for scar contracture, the back cut of the rotation flap is marked by points 4 and 7.

Points 5 and 6 are marked in such a way as to allow for a flap of tissue to be used for formation of the floor of the nose, so that a raw surface will be formed on the nasoseptum for insertion of the alar wing and so that tissue can be advanced into the columella.

LATERAL LIP ELEMENT

The following marks are made in a manner differing from the standard rotation-advancement technique: The distance from the cupid's bow peak to the commissure on the noncleft side (1 to 15) is transposed to the lateral lip element in order to arrive at point 9, and thus the distance from 1 to 15 is equal to that from 9 to 14. This is a critical measurement which insures that the cupid's bow–to–commissure distances on the noncleft and cleft sides will be equal. Extension along the vermilion border to obtain the additional length on the lateral side is not necessary. Almost always, point 9 corresponds precisely to the end of the white line, and thus we have another reliable method of obtaining the

commissure-to-philtrum distance on the cleft side.

Upon elevating the ala on the cleft side with a hook, we can locate its base and mark point 13, which corresponds to point 8. Points 11 and 12 are marked so that this flap will fill the gap created by the back cut, represented by points 4 and 7. The surgeon must be careful not to include tissue from the inside of the nose that contains vibrissae, particularly in females. A generous flap should be obtained so that it will fill the back cut gap. Excess width and size of the flap can easily be obtained and can be trimmed later to fit the gap properly. A small amount of tissue may be taken from the inside of the ala, such as in the Weir excision. The incisions from 9 to 10 and from 10 to 11 are marked such that they are equal to each other. In addition, note that the distances from 9 to 10 to 11, from 1 to 8, and from 3 to 4 are equal.

OPERATIVE PROCEDURES

INCISIONS

Medial Lip Element. The surgeon makes a full thickness incision beginning at point 3, curving upward under the columella to point 4, and then proceeding to the back cut from 4 to 7. Incisions from 4 to 5 and from 5 to 6 are then made, with the latter incision being extended internally at the base of the nasal septum to correspond to the desired insertion of the lateral nasal ala. Supraperiosteal un-

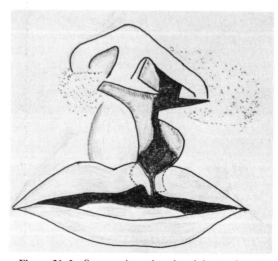

Figure 31–2 Supraperiosteal undermining to free the orbicularis oris up to the alar base.

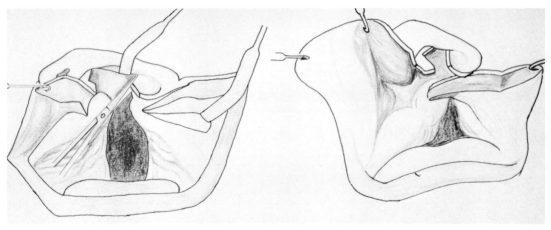

Figure 31-3 Use of skin hooks for rotation of medial lip element.

dermining is performed next to free the or-bicularis oris up to the alar base on the non-cleft side (Fig. 31–2). With skin hooks, the medial lip element is then rotated downward so that the levels of the cupid's bow peaks (points 1 and 3) are equal (Fig. 31–3).

Lateral Lip Elements.   Full thickness in-cisions connect points 9, 10 and 11. Wide supraperiosteal undermining of the lateral lip elements is extremely important in order to free the soft tissue from the maxilla (Figs. 31–2 and 31–3).

Anatomic Rebuilding of the Alar Wing. The alar base on the cleft side and its cu-taneous base (point 12) should be properly elevated from the muscle and the inferior meatus in the following manner: At the mu-cocutaneous border of the nasal floor (begin-ning at the anterior border of the choana) on the cleft side and from the inferior meatus (beginning at the inferior conchae), the sur-geon makes an incision that ends at point 12 and should join with the incision from 12 to 13, forming a right (90-degree) angle. With scissors a blunt dissection is made, and the muscle from the dermal portion of the alar base is elevated. A small incision should be made with the scissors in front of the inferior conchae; it should form a right (90-degree) angle with the incision made before, in order to obtain a free alar wing that will be easy to handle.

SUTURING

The alar base on the cleft side (point 12) is brought medially (to point 6) with a horizon-

tal mattress suture, which should transfix the nasoseptum and is tied in the normal nostril. By this procedure a muscular portion is freed which enables the operator to manage the nose and lips surgically as separate entities (Fig. 31–4).

The quadrangular flap, represented by points 10, 11, 12 and 13, is sutured into the back cut incision with a catgut simple stitch. At this point, it will be noted that the medial rotation flap (points 3, 4 and 7) fits easily into the lateral defect, and a few loose catgut simple sutures in the muscle layer allow tension-free skin closure with 6-0 nylon su-tures (Fig. 31–5).

In the photographic sequence of Figure 31–6 the principal steps of the surgical proce-dure are presented.

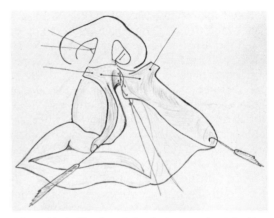

Figure 31-4 Fixation of the alar base on the cleft side.

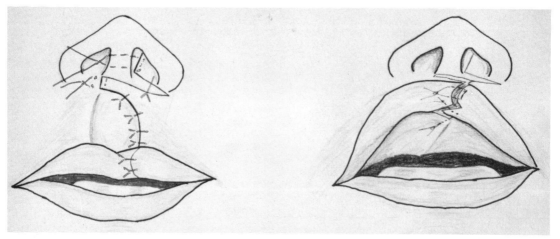

Figure 31–5 Suturing of quadrangular flap and medial rotation flap, allowing tension-free skin closure.

RESULTS

This procedure has been performed on 167 patients with unilateral cleft lip at the Instituto Estomatologico in Antigua, Guatemala, and on 43 patients at Stanford University. Figures 31–7 to 31–10 show the results obtained with our variation of the rotation-advancement technique.

DISCUSSION

The Millard rotation-advancement operation is one of the most excellent and widely used types of repair for unilateral cleft lip. Two problems have occurred, however, when using this technique for wide clefts:

1. Shortness of vertical lip length.
2. Inadequate length from nasal floor to vermilion or shortness of lateral vermilion.[11]

In 1964 Millard advocated a sharp turning down of the rotation incision in the form of a "back cut," which he emphasized could overcome the problem of vertical shortness.[8, 9] In addition, he suggested extension of the upper horizontal incision around the alar base on the cleft side. This would enable the use of more cheek tissue in wide clefts and additional rotation of the alar base, resulting in improved alar symmetry. Poole noted a sharp increase in vertical length when the incision was carried past the ala but felt that, nonetheless, adequate vertical length was difficult to obtain with the rotation-advancement technique when the lateral lip was short in both horizontal and vertical dimensions.[4]

According to Bernstein, the most common problem resulting from the Millard repair is the contraction of the vertical scar in patients with wide clefts. He stated that tension causes foreshortening in the region of the vertical scar, and he therefore introduces a small triangular flap at the bottom of the philtrum in order to obtain extra lip length.[1]

Williams pointed out that the distance from the nasal floor to the commissure and the vertical length of the lip are both decreased in the rotation-advancement technique. He felt this might indicate that this operative technique shortens the entire involved side, particularly in cases of wide clefts.[16]

In order to make the advancement flap long enough in wide clefts, the vermilion of the lateral or cleft side must often be sacrificed. This results in a thin lateral lip segment on the cleft side. To correct this, Millard proposed the vestibular extension of the lateral flap for use in wide clefts. This eliminated the redundant tissue blocking the airway and allowed for reduction of tightness in the closure. He also noted that insufficient length from the nasal floor to the commissure was less of a problem since he began carrying the horizontal incision past the alar base.

The modification presented in this chapter is an attempt to overcome the two major shortcomings of the standard rotation-advancement technique when applied to wide unilateral cleft lips. First, the square-ended vestibular flap provides a substantial length of tissue in one of the two areas in which tension is greatest in the Millard repair. The flap is relatively large, is easily sutured into position, and fits well into the rotation gap

(Text continued on page 1846)

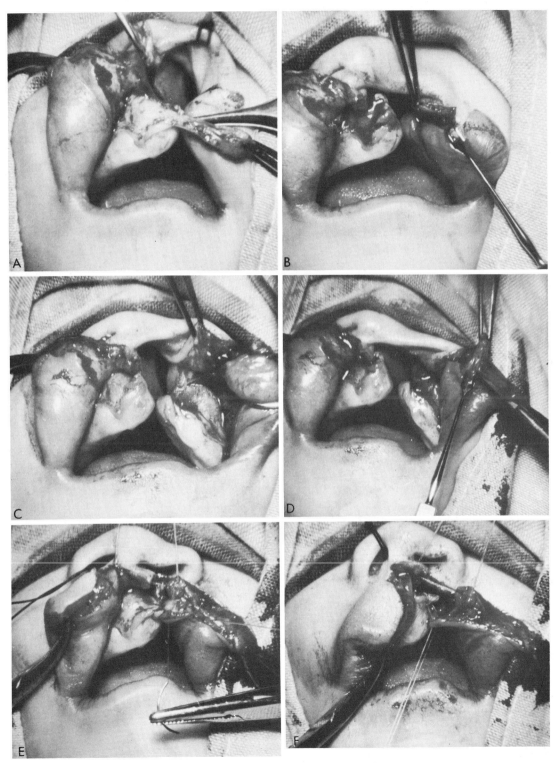

Figure 31–6 Major steps in surgical procedure.

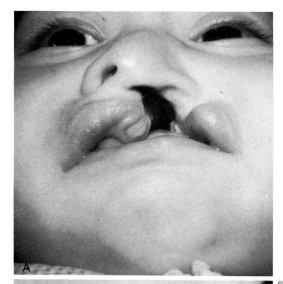

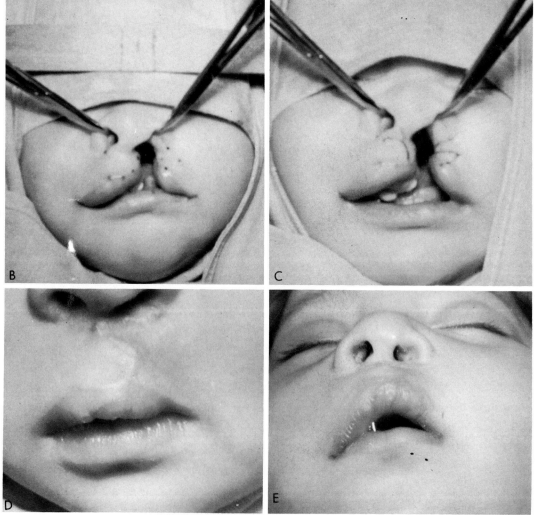

Figure 31–7 *A*, Preoperative appearance. *B*, Showing marking. *C*, Design of incisions. *D* and *E*, One-month postoperative appearance.

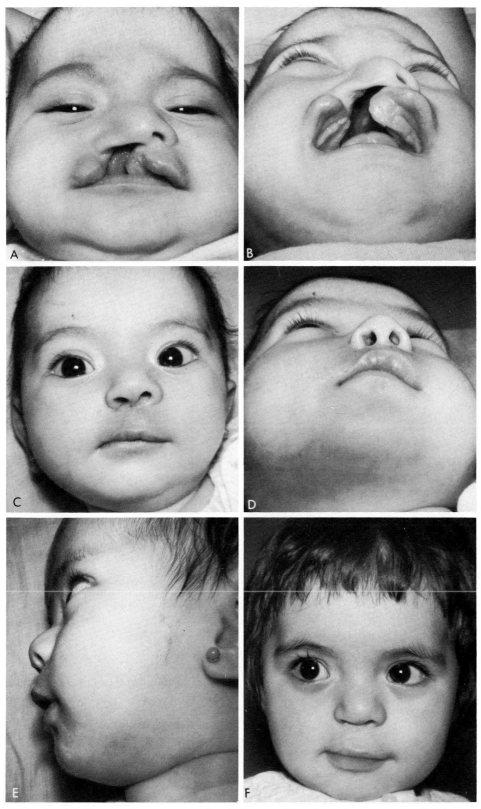

Figure 31–8 *A* and *B*, Preoperative appearance. *C* to *E*, Two-month postoperative appearance. *F*, Nine-month postoperative appearance.

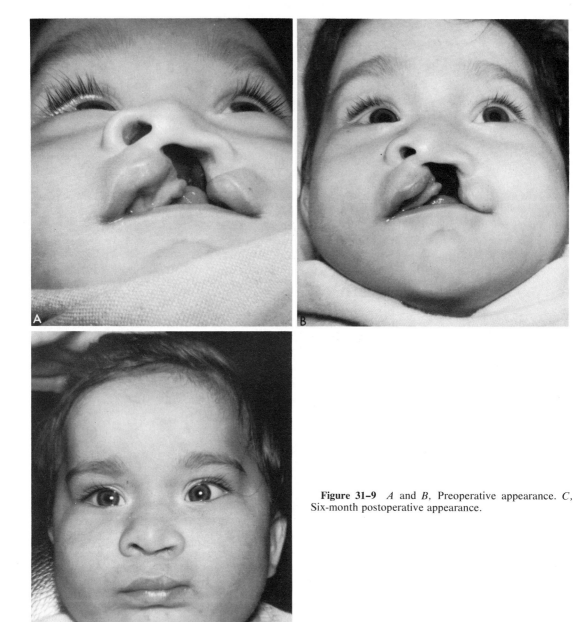

Figure 31–9 *A* and *B*, Preoperative appearance. *C*, Six-month postoperative appearance.

created by the back cut. Necrosis of the tip of the advancement flap has not been a problem with this technique. Furthermore, the triangular excision allows for relaxation of tension in the vertical suture line and provides for increased vertical lip height and advancement flap length without the necessity of sacrificing lateral lip vermilion. Thus, the horizontal length and thickness of the lateral lip segment are not encroached upon. It is important to stress at this point that the incision of the lateral lip element must not be extended lateral to point 9, if the cupid's bow peak–to–commissure distance is to be equal bilaterally.

This method can be a "modify as you go" technique similar to that mentioned by Millard in his writings; that is, the markings on the lateral side (points 9, 10 and 11) can be made after the medial elements are cut. The rotation flap of the medial side can be grasped with a skin hook and laid over the lateral lip elements; the lateral elements are marked

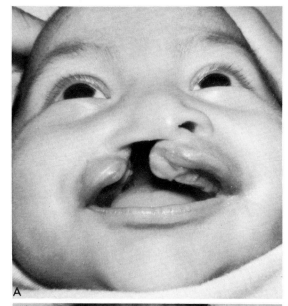

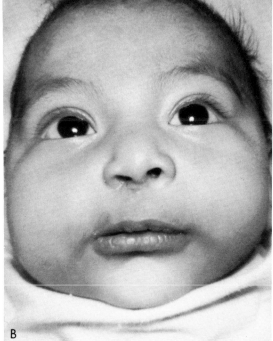

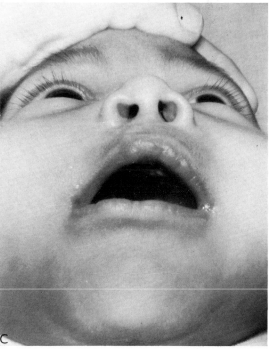

Figure 31–10 *A*, Preoperative appearance. *B* and *C*, One-month postoperative appearance.

where the rotation flap overlaps, so that it fits in precisely. A back cut can also be made in the lateral lip element so that additional length can be obtained if it is needed at this time.

Hence, this modification of the rotation-advancement technique evolved out of the surgeon's dissatisfaction with the latter when faced with the problem of repairing a wide unilateral cleft lip. It should be mentioned that this dissatisfaction was not based on purely theoretical grounds, *i.e.,* that one should discard a minimal amount of tissue. Rather, lateral mucosa sacrificed to gain lip length may result in a cupid's bow–to–commissure distance on the cleft side that is shorter than that on the noncleft side. The major advantage of this technique is that it supplies adequate length on the lateral side without sacrificing lateral lip vermilion. To accomplish this, a small wedge-shaped excision (points 9, 10 and 11) is of course necessary, and although this may seem to violate a cardinal rule ("discard no tissue"), the results have been gratifying and, in our opinion, worthy of trial by other surgeons.

REFERENCES

1. Bernstein, L.: Modified operation for wide unilateral cleft lips. Arch. Otolaryngol., *91:*11–18, 1970.
2. Blair, V. P., and Brown, J. B.: Mirault operation for single harelip. Surg. Gynecol. Obstet., *51:*81–91, 1930.
3. Brauer, R. O.: A comparison of the Tennison and Le Mesurier lip repairs. Plast. Reconstr. Surg., *23:*249–259, 1959.
4. Clifford, R. H., and Poole, R., Jr.: The analysis of the anatomy and geometry of the unilateral cleft lip. Plast. Reconstr. Surg., *24:*311–320, 1959.
5. Davies, D.: The repair of the unilateral cleft lip. Br. J. Plast. Surg., *18:*254–264, 1965.
6. Le Mesurier, A. B.: The treatment of complete unilateral harelips. Surg. Gynecol. Obstet., *95:*17–27, 1952.
7. Le Mesurier, A. B.: A method of cutting and suturing the lip in treatment of complete unilateral clefts. Plast. Reconstr. Surg., *4:*1–12, 1949.
8. Millard, D. R.: Extensions of the rotation-advancement principle for wide unilateral cleft lips. Plast. Reconstr. Surg., *42:*535–544, 1968.
9. Millard, D. R.: Refinements in rotation-advancement cleft lip technique. Plast. Reconstr. Surg., *33:*26–38, 1964.
10. Millard, D. R.: A radical rotation in single harelip. Am. J. Surg., *95:*318–322, 1958.
11. Poole, R. M.: The configurations of the unilateral cleft lip, with reference to the rotation advancement repair. Plast. Reconstr. Surg., *37:*558–565, 1966.
12. Randall, P.: A triangular flap operation for the primary repair of unilateral clefts of the lip. Plast. Reconstr. Surg., *23:*331–347, 1959.
13. Steffenson, W. H.: Further experience with the rectangular flap operation for cleft lip repair. Plast. Reconstr. Surg., *11:*49–55, 1953.
14. Steffenson, W. H.: A method for repair of the unilateral cleft lip. Plast. Reconstr. Surg., *4:*144–152, 1949.
15. Tennison, C. W.: The repair of the unilateral cleft lip by the stencil method. Plast. Reconstr. Surg., *9:*115–120, 1952.
16. Williams, H. B.: A method of assessing cleft lip repairs: Comparison of Le Mesurier and Millard techniques. Plast. Reconstr. Surg., *41:*103–107, 1968.

CHAPTER 32

SURGICAL REPAIR OF THE CLEFT PALATE

HERBERT J. BLOOM, D.D.S.

OBJECTIVES OF CLEFT PALATE SURGERY

The primary purpose of cleft palate repair (palatorrhaphy) is to create a mechanism capable of producing normal speech and deglutition. Secondary objectives include decreasing the potential chances for development of middle ear disease and consequent hearing loss, insuring normal growth patterns of the bones of the midface and providing an environment for the normal development and eruption of the teeth.

Although acceptable speech is not exclusively dependent upon the availability of the required structures, without the physical capacity to achieve the minimal needs for velopharyngeal valving, good speech is beyond the patient's ability, regardless of the level of intelligence, adequacy of hearing or degree of training. Unless the surgical procedure contemplated has reasonable likelihood of producing an effective valve at the junction of the soft palate and pharyngeal walls, its undertaking may be open to challenge, if the patient's best interests are considered. Under certain circumstances the patient may fare better with a functioning prosthetic obturator than with a nonfunctioning surgically repaired palate.

TIMING THE PALATE SURGERY

The optimum time for palatal repair is as controversial as that for lip surgery. The appropriate time for surgery is dependent not only on the age of the patient, but also on the aspect of the palate to be closed first.

In accordance with the respective philosophy of the doctor or the treatment center consulted, the palate may be operated upon when the patient is between 1 and 6 years of age, with few advising surgery at earlier or later ages. Also, there are surgeons who choose to follow one of three sequences: (*a*) closing the entire palate in one stage, (*b*) closing the alveolar and hard-palate clefts as a first stage, or (*c*) closing the soft palate early, with subsequent closure of the anterior palate.

Valid support is given to each sequence, but regardless of individual preferences, there has been strict adherence to the axiom that better speech is obtained when the components for velopharyngeal valving are available at the time speech patterns are developing. Once the pattern of abnormal speech has been established, acceptable speech through surgery and other therapy is difficult to achieve. This alone would suggest the necessity for a closed palate with a pliable functioning velum before the child is 2 years old, and consensus favors performing initial palatal surgery on the child when he is between 18 and 24 months old.

SURGICAL TECHNIQUE

The variation characteristic of lip clefts also occurs in palatal clefts. Palatal defects may be wide or narrow, bilateral or unilateral, complete or incomplete, and may have addi-

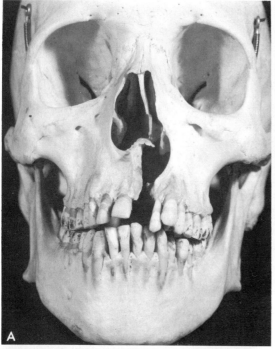

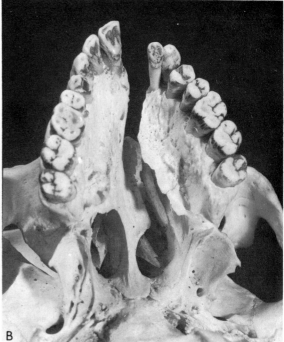

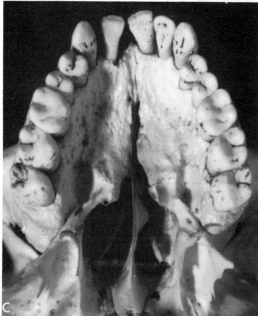

Figure 32-1 *A* and *B*, Front skeletal and palatal views of a left complete cleft palate. *C*, Incomplete midline cleft of the bony palate.

tional classifying factors. Procedures for closure must, therefore, be adjusted to allow for defect contingencies, and innumerable clinicians have, through the years, introduced modifications of established techniques that, in their respective opinions, achieve the all-important goal: velopharyngeal competence with minimal subsequent maxillary deformity.

In 1861 Von Langenbeck introduced a technique that for more than a century has remained the basis for all cleft palate surgery. Frequently referred to as the Von Langenbeck operation, it involves elevating and displacing the palatal mucoperiosteum toward the midline to secure closure without tension. Von Langenbeck added to his surgical design a device reported by Dieffenbach 40 years earlier, the use of relaxing incisions on the

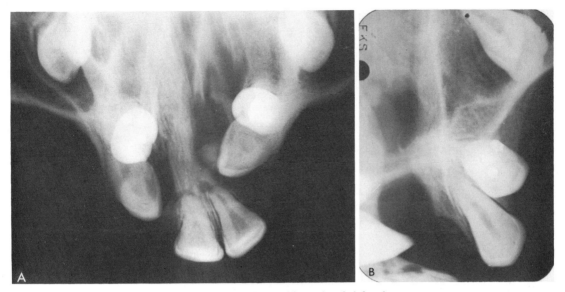

Figure 32-2 Occlusal radiographs of cleft palate.

medial side of the alveolar process. The incisions, made posteriorly around the maxillary tuberosity, are extended along the lateral walls of the soft palate. The Von Langenbeck technique is the sine qua non in cleft palate surgery.

The patient's preoperative status must be compatible with standards of safety in anesthesia and quality in tissue repair. The patient is placed at the extreme end of the operating table, and his neck is carefully hyperextended. His head is allowed to fall back slightly, and an oblong sandbag is placed beneath him at the upper level of his shoulders. Care must be exercised to avoid subluxation of the cervical vertebrae during cervical hyperextension or surgical manipulation.

General anesthesia is administered through an orally placed endotracheal tube. A Dingman or similar type of mouth gag is placed in position with an appropriately sized tongue blade, the endotracheal tube being held by the blade in position against the tongue. Caution must be taken to prevent compression of the tube between blade and tongue, and the blade, being of sufficient length to depress the entire tongue free of the soft palate, must not touch the posterior wall of the pharynx. The surgeon must have unobstructed vision of all palatal and oropharyngeal structures.

The patient receives an intravenous infusion of 5 per cent dextrose in water, which supplies nutritional and fluid needs during surgery and in the immediately postoperative recovery period. Equally important, a venous avenue is assured in the event that medication is required during and after the operation. The sites of the contemplated incisions are infiltrated with a solution (0.5 per cent lidocaine) containing epinephrine (1 : 100,000). This significantly aids in decreasing blood loss, and at the same time the infiltration produces a turgidity which facilitates incision and dissection.

Temporary traction sutures are placed on the medial side of the tip of each half of the uvula. With the soft palate under tension, and using a No. 11 scalpel blade, the surgeon pares the margins of the cleft at right angles to the surface. Excision of tissue should be minimal, sufficient only to expose the full thickness of the palatal tissue from oral to nasal mucosa (Fig. 32-3).

The lateral relaxing incision is made with a No. 15 scalpel blade, through the mucoperiosteum to the bone, at a position on the alveolar process midway between the major palatal vessels and gingival margin. This incision extends posteriorly from the location of the first premolar tooth around the maxillary tuberosity and along the line of the pterygomandibular raphe, terminating at the end of the palatal closure (Fig. 32-4).

A curved periosteal elevator is inserted into the lateral relaxing incision; the mucoperiosteum is elevated from the surface of the palatal shelf along the entire length of the incision. The neurovascular bundle exiting from the greater palatine foramen is identified; it can be stretched by blunt dissection of the mucoperiosteal flaps, but it must be left intact (Fig. 32–5).

Elevator or closed curved Metzenbaum scissors are inserted into the incision extending to the velum. By dissection within planes lateral to the pterygoid hamulus and pharyngeal wall, the musculature of the palate is mobilized. When the width of the cleft suggests the probability of closure under tension, the palatal aponeurotic attachment may be detached from the posterior edge of the palatal shelf, and the hamular process may be fractured by direct pressure at its base. The void created deep in the relaxing incision is firmly packed to control bleeding, while the identical procedure is being carried out on the opposite side.

Finally, the nasal mucosa is transected and detached from the nasal side of the palatal shelves by the use of a small right-angle knife (Fig. 32–6). Where the vomer is unilaterally

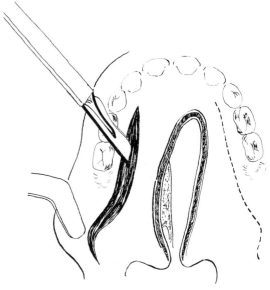

Figure 32–4 The lateral relaxing incision is made through the entire thickness of the mucoperiosteum to the bone. Care is taken to include the blood supply within the flap to be mobilized.

attached, a vomer flap may be reflected to form the nasal floor (Fig. 32–7).

To close the entire palate, 0000 or 5-0 chromic catgut may be used, although surgeons vary in their choice of suture mate-

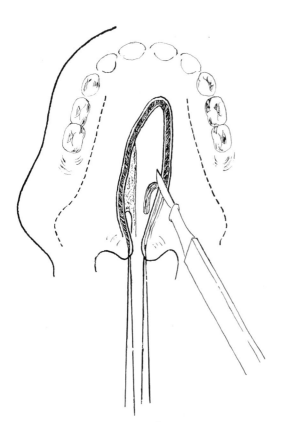

Figure 32–3 Temporary traction sutures placed at the top of the uvula allow for precise paring of the margins of the cleft.

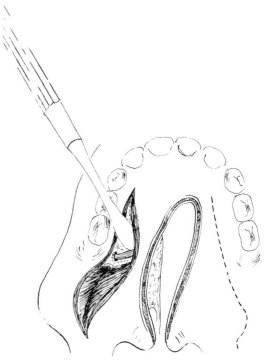

Figure 32–5 A periosteal elevator mobilizes the mucoperiosteal flap. The neurovascular bundle may be stretched, but it remains intact.

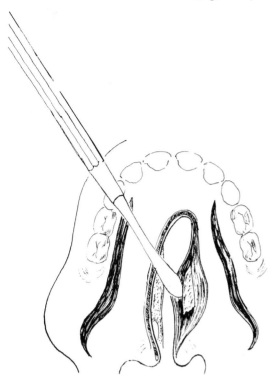

Figure 32–6 The nasal mucosa is transected and detached from the nasal side of the palatal shelves.

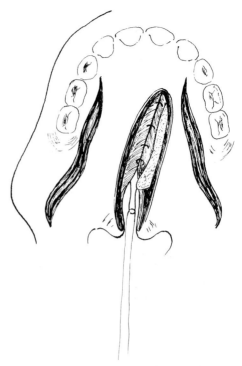

Figure 32–8 The nasal mucosa is approximated with interrupted sutures; knots are tied on the nasal side.

rial. Currently, 0000 chromic catgut for deep tissues, including nasal mucosa, and 0000 black silk for oral mucosa are preferred by most surgeons. For closure of all layers, 0000 or 5-0 Mersilene is gaining in popularity.

With interrupted sutures tied on the nasal side, the nasal mucosa is approximated in a single layer (Fig. 32–8); the muscle is sutured in layers, and the oral surface is closed with interrupted vertical mattress sutures to evert the wound edges (Fig. 32–9). Closure of all layers without tension is imperative. The de-

fects caused by the lateral relaxing incisions may be closed by two or three interrupted sutures, if this is possible without creating lateral tension.

Not all clefts of the palate can or should be closed in one stage. When the deformity is such that closure can only be accomplished

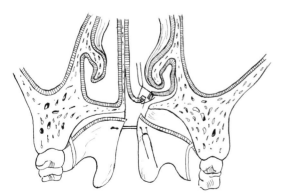

Figure 32–7 A vomer flap may be detached and sutured to the opposite nasal mucosal flap to form the nasal floor. The cleft is closed in two layers over the bony palate.

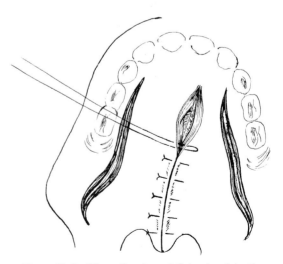

Figure 32–9 The soft palate cleft is closed in three layers: nasal, muscular and oral. The oral surface is closed with vertical mattress sutures to create slight eversion of the wound margins.

with the wound under tension, or when closure requires extensive undermining and displacement of tissue, a two-stage procedure is preferred. Surgical trauma conducive to formation of scar tissue leads to surgical catastrophe: a short inert palate and restricted development of the bony components of the midface.

Closure of the anterior or posterior aspect of the palate allows for some physiologic molding without inhibition of growth. The second stage of the operation often can be performed at a later date with only minimal need for undermining and shifting of tissue. Those surgeons who follow the practice of hard-palate closure as the first stage do so with the belief that the initial operation creates improved alveolar arch contour, and spontaneously progressive decrease in the width of the soft-palate cleft. The second stage of the operation, usually from 3 to 6 months later, is attended by little surgical trauma, with a resultant soft palate that more closely approximates the normal structure.

The rationale for primary closure of the soft palate is that this procedure provides the mechanical requirements for velopharyngeal valving at the age when it is most needed. The mucoperiosteum is left undisturbed at the time of operation, since there is evidence that the undermining and shifting of mucoperiosteal tissue of the palatal shelves may have an inhibitory effect on development of the central part of the face. In any event, one cannot overemphasize the importance of retaining anatomic components in a close-to-normal functioning relationship, by means of atraumatic surgical techniques and minimal distortion of tissue segments, to achieve the objectives of cleft palate surgery.

PROCEDURES SECONDARY TO CLEFT PALATE SURGERY

Procedures that follow initial cleft palate surgery are almost invariably limited to attempts to correct hypernasal speech by improving velopharyngeal competence. Fistulas that develop in the hard palate are annoying to the patient because they often are attended by poor oral hygiene and the escape of fluid and air into the nose. The speech deficit caused by a hard-palate fistula, however, is usually a manifestation of poor articulation

and is typically less severe than that resulting from an incompetent soft palate.

Most of the larger postoperative fistulas of the hard palate are best closed by prosthetic obturators. The dense, immobile, relatively avascular tissue surrounding these fistulas is not compatible with shifting of flaps or normal healing, and the reparative undertaking is not without a substantial risk of tissue breakdown. Descriptions of designs of a variety of advancement, pedicle and turnover flaps for repair of openings in the hard palate and the alveolus have been reported in detail in the literature.

Normal speech is made possible by rapidly successive elevations of the soft palate against the posterior pharyngeal wall, and with the additional action of the lateral pharyngeal musculature, this palatopharyngeal neuromuscular system creates a valve that seals off the nasal from the oral cavity during the emission of most sounds. The severity of speech hypernasality is a reflection of the volume of air that escapes nasally as a result of the incompetence of the system. Hypernasality is the chief complaint in more than one third of the patients who have undergone initial cleft palate surgery.

Techniques to lengthen the soft palate and enhance velopharyngeal valving have been utilized both as initial and as secondary operations. The V–Y and W–V palatal retropositioning procedures, developed by Ganzer and later modified by Veau, Wardill, Kilner and others, are performed during initial surgery. The use of a flap from the posterior wall of the pharynx to the velum as a secondary procedure was tried by Passavaut in the midnineteenth century. Since then there have been many innovations in an effort to decrease the quality of hypernasality in the speech of postoperative cleft palate patients. Stark employs the pharyngeal flap as part of the initial staphylorrhaphy; Blocksma inserts Silastic in the posterior pharyngeal wall to gain its forward displacement; Hynes's operation produces a shelf on the posterior pharyngeal wall; Moore and Sullivan developed what is referred to as "bilateral palatopharyngeous flaps"; and other ingenious clinicians have introduced surgical devices to control this most prevalent cause of failure of palatal surgery.

Palatal retropositioning at the time of the initial surgery, especially without a combined

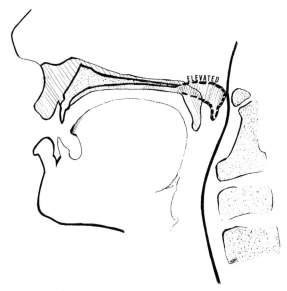

Figure 32–10 Upward and backward movement of the velum during normal speech.

pharyngeal flap, rarely accomplishes its intended purpose. The surgical maneuvers result in additional scarring, and controlled investigation has led to the opinion that anticipated additional length of the palate cannot be attained solely by this method. Likewise, the theoretical advantages of the complex palatopharyngeoplasties are yet to be confirmed.

Currently, the most widely used operation for correction of hypernasality, with unequivocal benefits, is the inferiorly or superiorly based posterior pharyngeal wall flap. The trend is toward use of the latter, but the inferiorly based flap does offer a few advantages: relative technical ease, its position at the site of maximal lateral movement of the pharyngeal wall and the fact that its attachment does not necessitate opening the previously repaired soft palate.

The superiorly based pharyngeal flap has one highly important advantage: its base is located at the position of contact of the velum with the pharyngeal wall during normal speech, approximately at the atlas (Fig. 32–10). This position enhances the possibilities for normal physiologic action—upward and backward movement of the velum—and thus the pharyngeal flap may be able to assume a dynamic function, rather than simple mechanical obturation. The sparsity of scientific data related to accurate preoperative and postoperative evaluations makes the selection of this second procedure an arbitrary judg-

ment, but many formerly inferiorly based flaps are now being transposed to a superiorly based position to improve the quality of speech.

SURGICAL TECHNIQUE TO CORRECT VELOPHARYNGEAL INCOMPETENCE (SUPERIORLY BASED PHARYNGEAL FLAP)

The position of the patient on the operating table is the same as that for initial closure of the cleft palate. Anesthesia is maintained through an orally placed endotracheal tube held firmly against the tongue by a Dingman mouth gag. The tongue blade depresses the entire length of the tongue to provide unrestricted vision and access to the entire oropharyngeal wall. Dilute epinephrine (0.5 per cent lidocaine with epinephrine, 1:100,000) is injected into the soft palate and pharynx. As the needle is passed through the superior constrictor muscle and the solution is deposited within the buccopharyngeal fascial plane, the pharyngeal musculature pouches forward, facilitating its elevation from the retropharyngeal space. Transient arrhythmias occasionally may accompany injections at this site.

Traction sutures are placed on each side of the tip of the uvula, and with a No. 15 scalpel blade, the surgeon divides the soft palate ver-

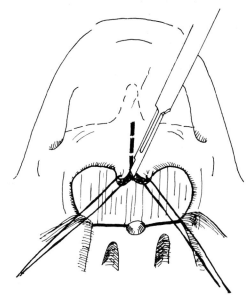

Figure 32–11 With the velum under tension, a midline incision divides the soft palate to just short of the posterior border of the hard palate.

tically forward from the tip of the uvula to a level just short of the posterior border of the hard palate (Fig. 32–11). The upper extent of the pharyngeal wall is now accessible, allowing for placement of the base of the flap near the level of the atlas promontory.

Two parallel incisions can now be made through the superior constrictor muscle and the overlying mucosa down to the buccopharyngeal fascia. Both incisions should be as high and as far apart as possible, care being taken to avoid impingement upon the orifices of the eustachian tube. The incisions are joined at their lower extent to form a rounded V, allowing for adaptation of the tip of the flap to the anterior pole of the created palatal defect (Fig. 32–12).

The flap is separated from the underlying fascia by blunt dissection through each incision with curved scissors and a palate elevator. The lower end of the flap is detached, and with a traction suture inserted at its tip, the entire flap is raised to its superiorly placed base. The lateral margins of the donor site are now approximated with interrupted 000 chromic catgut sutures. By inclusion of the buccopharyngeal fascia in these sutures,

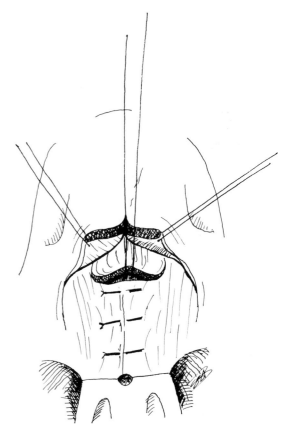

Figure 32–13 The mucosal-muscular flap is detached; the lateral margins of the donor site are approximated to the underlying fascia.

the dead space is obliterated, thereby reducing the possibility of the formation of a retropharyngeal hematoma (Fig. 32–13).

With the flap inverted and carried to the forward extent of the palatal incision, the nasal mucosa of the palate is sutured to the pharyngeal mucosa of the flap. The interrupted 0000 chromic catgut sutures are tied on the nasal side. A horizontal mattress suture, with the knot tied over the oral mucosa, secures the tip of the flap to its anterior position in the soft palate (Fig. 32–14).

Closure of the oral surface over the cut pharyngeal wall flap is accomplished by advancing each side of the soft palate toward the midline. To facilitate this advancement of tissue, the oral surface of the soft palate can be slightly undermined, by tiny splitting incisions of the cut palatal margins, before the flap is sutured into position. Vertical sutures (0000 black silk or Mersilene), which include the muscle of the flap, close the oral mucosal surface along the midline (Figs. 32–15 and 32–16).

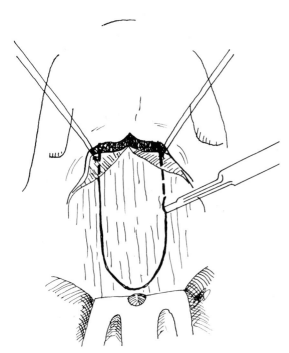

Figure 32–12 The divided palate offers visual access to the upper recess of the pharynx. Parallel incisions outline the pharyngeal flap, with the base placed superiorly and the lower extent of the incisions joined by a rounded V.

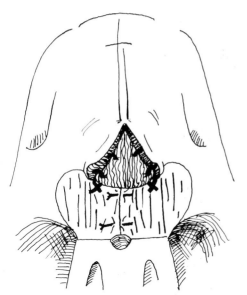

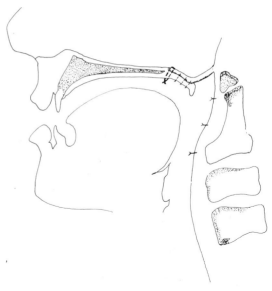

Figure 32–14   The flap is inverted into the created palatal defect. The tip is attached under the peak of the defect by a mattress suture tied on the oral side; sutures tied on the nasal side approximate the flap mucosa to palatal nasal mucosa.

Figure 32–16   Sagittal section of the positioned superiorly based pharyngeal flap.

POSTOPERATIVE CARE OF THE CLEFT PALATE PATIENT

Food intake during the first 48 hours after palate surgery is limited to clear liquids. Thereafter, the patient is maintained on a full liquid diet during the first week and on semiliquids through the fourteenth postoperative day. Arm restraints may be used when (and as long as) they are necessary to keep the pa-

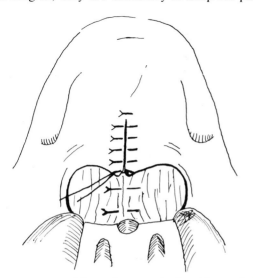

Figure 32–15   The oral mucosa is closed by vertical mattress sutures that include the underlying musculature of the pharyngeal flap.

tient's fingers and also foreign objects from the mouth during healing.

Elevation of temperature occurring on the first day, which may persist through the third day, is considered within the limits of physiologic response to the surgery. Persistence of elevated temperature, or an abrupt rise after the second or third day, is considered an indication of a complication, most frequently infection. As a prophylactic measure, many clinicians advocate routine use of antibiotics, but there is no conclusive evidence of their effectiveness when used in this manner.

Throughout the first 24 to 48 hours, humidity supplied through a cold-steam tent may prevent dehydration of the respiratory tract and preclude pulmonary complications. Steroids and antihistamines also have been administered during the early postoperative period, but with doubtful benefit. Drug therapy should be initiated in accordance only with specific indications.

Most patients who have undergone cleft palate repair are discharged from the hospital between the fifth and seventh postoperative days. Strict supervisory instructions to parents should include avoidance of mechanical objects, such as spoons, about the patient's face that are likely to disrupt the healing process; discouraging the patient from blowing and sucking actions; and preparation of food in a blender or otherwise thinning it so that it flows easily from a cup. Physical activity must be carefully controlled, and all precautions should be taken to prevent exposure to infection.

Patients who have undergone pharyngeal-flap surgery require additional postoperative supervision, particularly during the first two days after surgery. Hemorrhage and respiratory embarrassment are threats that demand vigilant monitoring, and vital signs are recorded as a strictly routine regimen. On occasion, edema at the eustachian orifice causes obstruction with concomitant mild otitis. This condition usually is transitory, subsiding spontaneously as the pharyngeal edema resolves.

REHABILITATION OF THE PATIENT WITH A CONGENITAL OROFACIAL CLEFT

Notwithstanding heroic efforts by surgeons and commensurate technical progress, the congenital orofacial cleft profoundly affects the individual, in whom nature, in its complex process of facial and jaw development, has produced a devastating result. Despite carefully planned and executed therapeutic programs, few of these patients completely escape all the potential hazards consistent with the deformity: facial disfigurement, deficient oral tissue, defective speech, disturbances in dentition and upper respiratory tract and ear disease. It is highly unfortunate that a normal intelligence neither masks the physical deformity nor prevents the consequently traumatized personality.

Modern rehabilitation of the cleft lip or cleft palate patient focuses on the patient's functional needs, handicaps, and physical and sociopsychologic problems. The goal is to have the patient achieve self-dependence and self-respect; it cannot be attained by, nor is it the sole responsibility of, the surgeon. A team of specialists, working for the welfare of the total child, is the basis for a broadening of knowledge beyond that which each individual brings into the setting and is the most effective means of achieving total rehabilitation of the patient. Depending upon the age and problems of the patient, the rehabilitation team may include any combination or all of the following specialists: the oral surgeon, speech pathologist, prosthodontist, orthodontist, otolaryngologist, pedodontist, plastic surgeon, pediatrician, psychologist, psychiatrist or social service worker. The most effec-

tive treatment of the patient may be achieved by coordinating the skills of these individuals in a medical center where examination and evaluation of the patient can be made by the team as a unit. This method affords the opportunity for discussion between members of different specialties and formulation of an adequate sequential rehabilitative program.

Total rehabilitation of the patient necessitates that each specialist interest himself in the specialties of the other members of the team, so that sharp individuality and exact professional identity are blended functionally within the total group personality. The unified team of specialists examines the patient, and treats the total patient. The surgeon, despite his remarkable contributions toward the physical cure of deformities, provides only the initial step toward the cure of birth deficiencies.

REFERENCES

1. Barsky, A. J.: Pierre Franco, father of cleft lip surgery: His life and times. Br. J. Plast. Surg., 17:335, 1964.
2. Bill, A. H., Moore, A. W., and Coe, H. E.: The time of choice for repair of cleft palate in relation to the type of surgical repair and its effect on bony growth of the face. Plast. Reconstr. Surg., 18:469, 1956.
3. Blocksma, R.: Correction of velopharyngeal insufficiency by Silastic pharyngeal implant. Plast. Reconstr. Surg., 31:286, 1963.
4. Bloom, H. J.: Sinai cleft palate habilitation center. Bull. Sinai Hosp. (Detroit), 5:8, 1957.
5. Boo-Chai, K.: An ancient Chinese text on a cleft lip. Plast. Reconstr. Surg., 38:89, 1966.
6. Brauer, R. O.: Observations and measurements of nonoperative setback of premaxilla in double cleft patients. Plast. Reconstr. Surg., 35:148, 1965.
7. Brown, J. B., and McDowell, F.: Surgical repair of cleft lips. Arch. Surg., 56:750, 1948.
8. Bunke, H. L., Page, P., Price, B., Blazine, C., and Fraser, F.: The evaluation of management of velopharyngeal insufficiency. Cleft Palate J., 4:171, 1966.
9. Calman, J. S.: Movement of the soft palate. Br. J. Plast. Surg., 5:286, 1953.
10. Castiglioni, A.: A History of Medicine. 2nd ed. New York, Alfred A. Knopf, Inc., 1958.
11. Dingman, R. O., and Bloomer, H. H.: Clinical observations on the use of the pharyngeal flap in the habilitation of cleft palate patients. Cleft Palate Bull., 11:6, 1961.
12. Dingman, R. O., and Grabb, W. C.: A new mouth gag. Plast. Reconstr. Surg., 31:563, 1963.
13. Dorrance, G. M.: The Operative Story of Cleft Palate. Philadelphia, W. B. Saunders Co., 1933.
14. Georgiade, N. C.: Anterior palatal alveolar closure

by means of interpolated flaps. Plast. Reconstr. Surg., *39:*162, 1967.

15. Guerrero-Santos, J., Garay, J., and Altamirano, J. T.: The use of lingual flaps in repair of fistulae of the hard palate. Plast. Reconstr. Surg., *38:*123, 1966.

16. Hynes, W.: Pharyngoplasty by muscle transplantation. Br. J. Plast. Surg., *3:*128, 1956.

17. Ivy, R. H., and Curtis, L.: Procedures in cleft palate surgery: Experiences with the Veau and Dorrance technic. Ann. Surg., *100:*502, 1934.

18. Kahn, S., and Winston, J.: Surgical approaches to the bilateral cleft lip problem. Br. J. Plast. Surg., *13:*13, 1960.

19. Kilner, T. P.: The management of the patient with cleft lip and/or palate. Am. J. Surg., *93:*204, 1958.

20. Le Mesurier, A. B.: A method of cutting and suturing the lip in the treatment of complete unilateral clefts. Plast. Reconstr. Surg., *4:*1, 1949.

21. McNeil, C. K.: Orthopedic principles in the treatment of lip and palate clefts. *In* Holtz, R. (Ed.): Early Treatment of Cleft Lip and Palate. Berne, Huber, 1964.

22. Millard, D. R., Jr.: Refinements in rotation-advancement cleft lip technique. Plast. Reconstr. Surg., *33:*26, 1964.

23. Millard, D. R., Jr.: Complete unilateral clefts of the lip. Plast. Reconstr. Surg., *25:*595, 1960.

24. Millard, D. R., Jr.: A radical rotation in single harelip. Am. J. Surg., *95:*318, 1958.

25. Mladick, R., Pickrell, K., and Gingrass, R.: Blood volume determinations in cleft lip-palate surgery. Plast. Reconstr. Surg., *39:*71, 1967.

26. Morley, M. E.: Cleft Palate and Speech. 6th ed. Edinburgh, Livingstone, 1966.

27. Morris, H. L., and Spriestersbach, D. C.: Pharyngeal flap as a speech mechanism. Plast. Reconstr. Surg., *39:*66, 1967.

28. Obregon, G., and Smith, J. K.: The posterior pharyngeal flap palatoplasty. Arch. Otolaryngol., *69:*174, 1959.

29. Ousley, J. Q., Lawson, L. I., Miller, W. R., and Blackfield, H. M.: Experience with the high attached pharyngeal flap. Plast. Reconstr. Surg., *38:*232, 1966.

30. Pierson, A. L.: Early operations for hare-lip. Boston Med. Surg. J., *47:*134, 1852.

31. Randall, P.: A lip adhesion operation in cleft lip surgery. Plast. Reconstr. Surg., *35:*371, 1965.

32. Randall, P.: A triangular flap operation for the primary repair of unilateral clefts of the lip. Plast. Reconstr. Surg., *23:*331, 1959.

33. Reid, D. A. C.: Fistulas in the hard palate following cleft palate surgery. Br. J. Plast. Surg., *15:*377, 1962.

34. Rogers, B. O.: Palate surgery prior to von Graefe's pioneering staphylorrhaphy 1816: An historical review of the early causes of surgical indifference in repairing the cleft palate. Plast. Reconstr. Surg., *39:*1, 1967.

35. Skoog, T.: A design for the repair of unilateral cleft lips. Am. J. Surg., *95:*223, 1958.

36. Slaughter, W. B., and Pruzansky, S.: The rationale for velar closure as a primary procedure in the repair of cleft palate defects. Plast. Reconstr. Surg., *13:*341, 1954.

37. Stark, R. B., and DeHaan, C. R.: The addition of a pharyngeal flap to primary palatoplasty. Plast. Reconstr. Surg., *26:*378, 1960.

38. Steffensen, W. H.: Collective review: Palate lengthening operations. Plast. Reconstr. Surg., *10:*380, 1952.

39. Stevens, A. H.: Staphylorrhaphe, or palate suture, successfully performed. North Am. Med. Surg. J., *3:*233, 1827.

40. Sullivan, D.: Bilateral pharyngoplasty as an aid to velopharyngeal closure. Plast. Reconstr. Surg., *27:*31, 1961.

41. Tennison, C. W.: The repair of unilateral cleft lip by the stencil method. Plast. Reconstr. Surg., *9:*115, 1952.

42. Whalen, J. S., and Conn, A. W.: Improved technics in anesthetic management for repair of cleft lips and palates. Anesth. Analg. (Cleveland), *46:*355, 1967.

INDEX

In this index *italic* page numbers indicate illustrations,
and (t) indicates a table; "vs." is used to
mean "differential diagnosis from."

Allergy(ies) (*Continued*)
   antibiotic, 417
   emergencies in, 417, 1545, 1546
   food, swelling from, vs. dentoalveolar infection, 514
   history taking and, 423
   penicillin and, 412
Allogeneic homograft, definition of, 1512. See also
   Graft(s), homogenous, allogeneic.
Allograft, definition of, 1512
Alloplast, in cystic cavities, 563
Alveolalgia, 1627–1630, 1634
   and pain, 1683
   curettage in, 1629
   drugs in, 1628
   etiology of, 1628
   in history taking, 423
   mouthwash in, 1628
   patient's physical status and, 1629
   saliva and, 1629
   trauma in, 1628
   treatment of, 1630
   vs. myofascial pain syndrome, 1684
Alveolar cyst, median, 518
Alveolar neurovascular bundle, inferior. See
   Mandibular alveolar canal.
Alveolar process. See *Ridge(s), alveolar.*
Alveolar ridge. See *Ridge(s), alveolar.*
Alveolectomy, atypical facial neuralgia following,
      1708
   definition of, 179
   following radiation therapy, 110
   for dentures, 180
   in radiation treatment, 1813
   mucoperiosteal flaps for, *179*
   objectives of, 182
   of edentulous jaws, tray set-up for, *433*
   partial, 180–182. See also *Alveoplasty.*
   prophylaxis for, 416
   radical, preradiation, 106, *107,* 1813
   tray set-up for, *30*
   with odontectomy, *180, 181*
      tray set-up for, *432*
Alveolitis. See *Alveolalgia.*
Alveolotomy, definition of, 181
Alveolus, cancer of, incidence of, 1811
   healing, carcinoma of, 1675–1677, *1676*
   maxillary sinus herniation through, *825,* 1606, *1606*
Alveoplasty, 54, 55, 179
   definition of, 100, 179
Ameloblastic adenoid tumor. See *Adenoameloblastoma.*
Ameloblastic fibroma. See *Fibroma, ameloblastic.*
Ameloblastic fibro-odontoma, *781*
Ameloblastic hemangioma, 735
Ameloblastic neurinoma, classification of, 735
Ameloblastic odontoma. See *Odontoma(s), ameloblastic.*
Ameloblastic odontosarcoma, classification of, 735
Ameloblastic sarcoma. See *Sarcoma(s), ameloblastic.*
Ameloblastoma(s), 735–752, *736–753*
   arising from cysts, 626
   classification of, 735
   cysts vs., 635
   development from tooth follicle, 273
   etiology of, 735
   from dentigerous cyst, 735, 736
   marsupialization and, 555
   simple, classification of, 735

Ameloblastoma(s) (*Continued*)
   terminology of, 635
   treatment of, *737, 739*
American Association of Oral and Plastic Surgeons, 7
American Board of Oral Surgery, 8
American College of Dentists, Committee on Hospital
      Dental Service, 9, 10
   Committee on Oral Surgery, 10
American College of Surgeons, 11
American Dental Association, Council on Dental
      Education, 8–10
American Society of Anesthesiologists (A.S.A.),
      assessment of physical status (P.S.), 419
American Society of Exodontia, 7
American Society of Oral Surgeons, 8
American Society of Oral Surgery and Exodontia, 8
Ammonia, and chemical leukoplakia, *907*
Amnesia, in head injury, 1034
Ampicillin, 412
Amputation neuroma. See *Neuroma, amputation.*
Analgesia, local. See *Anesthesia, local.*
Analysis, archial, 1435, *1436*
   cephalometric, in dentofacial orthopedics, 1435
Anatomic space. See *Space(s), anatomic.*
Anatomy, facial, *1596, 1597*
   radiographic, of facial bones and jaws, 1015–
      1030.
      See also *Radiograph(s).*
   landmarks in, 1434, 1435
Anemia, acute cerebral, 1540
   and bald tongue, *900*
   and impaction, 255
   oral surgery and, 18
   symptoms of, 18
Anesthesia(s), administration of, and ecchymosis,
      1556
   alcohol injections for, in alveolalgia, 1630
   endotracheal, complications in, *1552–1554*
      for neck surgery, 1782
   facial, nerve trauma and, 1664
   for buccal surgery, 1751
   for lip surgery, 1741, 1743, 1746, 1748
   for tongue surgery, 1759, 1762
   general, and dislocation of mandible, 1644
   history taking and, 423
   hypoxia during, 978, 980
   in children, 405, 406, 409
   in cleft palate surgery, 1851
   in fracture management, 1063, 1066, 1068, 1069
   in geriatric patient, 979, 980
   in hemophiliacs, *1572,* 1575–1577
   in segmental surgery, 1387
   local, administration of, *1556, 1582*
      and lip biting, *909*
   premedication for, 22–24, 24(t)
      in children, 405, 406
      in geriatric patients, 979
   selection of, 22–24
      during pregnancy, 21
Anesthetist, and anesthetic choice, 421
   in operating room routine, 429
Aneurysmal bone cyst(s), 654, *655*
   differential diagnosis of, 654
   treatment of, 654
   vs. odontogenic cysts, 635
Aneurysmal giant cell tumor. See *Aneurysmal
   bone cyst.*